Aminoff's Electrodiagnosis in Clinical Neurology

Commissioning Editor: Lotta Kryhl
Editorial Assistant: Emma Cole
Project Manager: Nancy Arnott/Maggie Johnson
Design: Stewart Larking
Illustration Manager: Gillian Richards
Illustrator: Jennifer Rose
Marketing Manager (USA/UK): Helena Mutak/Gaynor Jones

Aminoff's Electrodiagnosis in Clinical Neurology

SIXTH EDITION

Michael J. Aminoff, M.D., D.Sc., F.R.C.P
Distinguished Professor
Department of Neurology
School of Medicine
University of California, San Francisco
San Francisco, California, USA

With 49 Contributing Authors

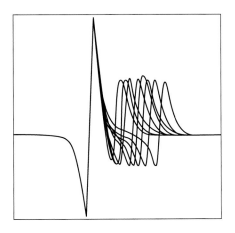

ELSEVIER
SAUNDERS

Chapter 1: "The Emergence of Electrophysiology as an Aid to Neurology" by Mary A. B. Brazier is in the Public Domain.

Chapter 20: "Electrophysiologic Evaluation of Movement Disorders" by Mark Hallett is in the Public Domain.

First edition 1980
Second edition 1986
Third edition 1992
Fourth edition 1999
Fifth edition 2005

Notices

Knowledge and best practice in this field are constantly changing. As new research and experience broaden our understanding, changes in research methods, professional practices, or medical treatment may become necessary.

Practitioners and researchers must always rely on their own experience and knowledge in evaluating and using any information, methods, compounds, or experiments described herein. In using such information or methods they should be mindful of their own safety and the safety of others, including parties for whom they have a professional responsibility.

With respect to any drug or pharmaceutical products identified, readers are advised to check the most current information provided (i) on procedures featured or (ii) by the manufacturer of each product to be administered, to verify the recommended dose or formula, the method and duration of administration, and contraindications. It is the responsibility of practitioners, relying on their own experience and knowledge of their patients, to make diagnoses, to determine dosages and the best treatment for each individual patient, and to take all appropriate safety precautions.

To the fullest extent of the law, neither the Publisher nor the authors, contributors, or editors assume any liability for any injury and/or damage to persons or property as a matter of products liability, negligence or otherwise, or from any use or operation of any methods, products, instructions, or ideas contained in the material herein.

Saunders

British Library Cataloguing in Publication Data

Electrodiagnosis in clinical neurology. – 6th ed.

1. Electrodiagnosis. 2. Nervous system–Diseases–Diagnosis.

616.8'07547-dc22

ISBN-13: 9781455703081
eBook ISBN: 9781455726769

Printed in China

Last digit is the print number: 9 8 7 6 5 4 3 2

To my wife, Jan

Contributors

VIVIEN C. ABAD, M.D., M.B.A
Sleep Disorders Center
Palo Alto Foundation
Palo Alto, California, USA
Chapter 33: Polysomnographic Evaluation of Sleep Disorders

DAVID C. ADAMS, M.D.
Associate Professor
Department of Anesthesiology
University of Vermont College of Medicine
Burlington, Vermont, USA
*Chapter 30: Intraoperative Monitoring by Evoked Potential
Techniques*

JAMES W. ALBERS, M.D., Ph.D.
Emeritus Professor
Department of Neurology
University of Michigan Medical School
Ann Arbor, Michigan, USA
*Chapter 36: Electrophysiologic Techniques in the Evaluation
of Patients with Suspected Neurotoxic Disorders*

MICHAEL J. AMINOFF, M.D., D.Sc.
Distinguished Professor
Department of Neurology
School of Medicine
University of California, San Francisco
San Francisco, California, USA
*Chapter 3: Electroencephalography: General Principles
and Clinical Applications*
Chapter 11: Clinical Electromyography
Chapter 21: Evaluation of the Autonomic Nervous System
Chapter 26: Somatosensory Evoked Potentials
*Chapter 27: Somatosensory Evoked Potentials in Infants
and Children*
*Chapter 36: Electrophysiologic Techniques in the Evaluation of
Patients with Suspected Neurotoxic Disorders*

EILEEN E. BIRCH, Ph.D.
Director, Pediatric Eye Research Laboratory
Retina Foundation of the Southwest;
Adjunct Professor
Department of Ophthalmology
University of Texas Southwestern Medical Center
Dallas, Texas, USA
Chapter 23: Visual Evoked Potentials in Infants and Children

THOMAS P. BLECK, M.D.
Professor
Department of Neurological Sciences
Rush Medical College
Chicago, Illinois, USA
*Chapter 35: Electrophysiologic Evaluation of Brain Death:
A Critical Appraisal*

CHARLES F. BOLTON, M.D.
Adjunct Professor
Department of Medicine
Queen's University
Kingston, Ontario, Canada
*Chapter 34: Electrophysiologic Evaluation of Patients
in the Intensive Care Unit*

MARY A.B. BRAZIER, Ph.D. (deceased)
Professor, Departments of Anatomy and Physiology
David Geffen School of Medicine at UCLA
Los Angeles, California, USA
*Chapter 1: The Emergence of Electrophysiology as an Aid
to Neurology*

JEFFREY W. BRITTON, M.D.
Associate Professor
Department of Neurology
Mayo Clinic College of Medicine
Rochester Minnesota, USA
Chapter 5: Electroencephalographic Artifacts and Benign Variants

MARK B. BROMBERG, M.D., Ph.D.
Professor
Department of Neurology
School of Medicine
University of Utah
Salt Lake City, Utah, USA
Chapter 12: Quantitative Electromyography

DAVID BURKE, M.D., D.Sc.
Bushell Professor of Neurology
Royal Prince Alfred Hospital;
Associate Dean [Research]
Sydney Medical School
University of Sydney
Sydney, New South Wales, Australia
Chapter 14: Microneurography and its Potential Clinical
Applications

JOHN A. CADWELL, B.S.E.E, M.D.
Director of Engineering
Cadwell Laboratories, Inc.
Kennewick, Washington, USA
Chapter 2: Electrophysiologic Equipment and Electrical Safety

MICHAEL S. CARTWRIGHT, M.D.
Assistant Professor
Department of Neurology
Wake Forest University School of Medicine
Winston-Salem, North Carolina, USA
Chapter 16: Neuromuscular Ultrasound as a Complement to the
Electrodiagnostic Evaluation

GREGORY D. CASCINO, M.D.
Whitney MacMillan, Jr, Professor of Neurosciences
Department of Neurology
Mayo Clinic College of Medicine
Rochester, Minnesota, USA
Chapter 9: Intraoperative Electroencephalographic Monitoring
During Carotid Endarterectomy and Cardiac Surgery

ROBERT CHEN, M.A., M.B.B.Chir., M.Sc.
Professor
Division of Neurology
Department of Medicine
University of Toronto;
Senior Scientist
Toronto Western Research Institute
Toronto, Ontario, Canada
Chapter 28: Diagnostic and Therapeutic Role of Magnetic
Stimulation in Neurology

PEDRO COUTIN-CHURCHMAN, M.D., Ph.D.
Technical Director
Department of Clinical Neurophysiology
Ronald Reagan UCLA Medical Center
Los Angeles, California, USA
Chapter 8: Topographic Mapping, Frequency Analysis, and Other
Quantitative Techniques in Electroencephalography

JASPER R. DAUBE, M.D.
Professor
Department of Neurology
Mayo Clinic College of Medicine
Rochester, Minnesota, USA
Chapter 13: Nerve Conduction Studies

ANDRÉE DURIEUX-SMITH, Ph.D.
Professor Emeritus
University of Ottawa;
Scientific Director
Institut de Recherche de l'Hôpital Montfort
Ottawa, Ontario, Canada
Chapter 25: Brainstem Auditory Evoked Potentials in Infants
and Children

ANDREW EISEN, M.D.
Professor Emeritus
Division of Neurology
Department of Medicine
University of British Columbia
Vancouver, British Columbia, Canada
Chapter 26: Somatosensory Evoked Potentials

RONALD G. EMERSON, M.D.
Adjunct Professor
Department of Neurology
Columbia University College of Physicians
    and Surgeons
New York, New York, USA
Chapter 30: Intraoperative Monitoring by Evoked Potential
Techniques

JEROME ENGEL, Jr., M.D., Ph.D.
Jonathan Sinay Distinguished Professor of Neurology,
    Neurobiology, and Psychiatry and Biobehavioral
    Sciences
David Geffen School of Medicine at UCLA
Los Angeles, California, USA
Chapter 6: Video-EEG Monitoring for Epilepsy

MORRIS A. FISHER, M.D.
Professor
Department of Neurology
Loyola University Chicago Stritch School of Medicine
Maywood, Illinois, USA
Chapter 18: H-Reflex and F-Response Studies

JOSEPH M. FURMAN, M.D., Ph.D.
Professor
Departments of Otolaryngology, Neurology,
    Bioengineering, and Physical Therapy
University of Pittsburgh School of Medicine
Pittsburgh, Pennsylvania, USA
Chapter 32: Vestibular Laboratory Testing

DOUGLAS S. GOODIN, M.D.
Professor
Department of Neurology
School of Medicine
University of California, San Francisco
San Francisco, California, USA
Chapter 29: Event-Related Potentials

ARI J. GREEN, M.D., M.C.R.
Debbie and Andy Rachleff Distinguished Professor
    of Neurology
Departments of Neurology and Ophthalmology
University of California, San Francisco
San Francisco, California, USA
*Chapter 22: Visual Evoked Potentials, Electroretinography, and
    Other Electrodiagnostic Approaches to the Visual System*

**CHRISTIAN GUILLEMINAULT, M.D., D.M.,
D. Biol.**
Professor
Department of Psychiatry and Behavioral Science
Stanford University School of Medicine
Stanford, California, USA
Chapter 33: Polysomnographic Evaluation of Sleep Disorders

JIN S. HAHN, M.D.
Professor
Department of Neurology and Neurological Sciences
Stanford University School of Medicine
Stanford, California, USA
Chapter 4: Neonatal and Pediatric Electroencephalography

MARK HALLETT, M.D.
Chief, Human Motor Control Section
National Institute of Neurological Disorders and Stroke
National Institutes of Health
Bethesda, Maryland, USA
Chapter 20: Electrophysiologic Evaluation of Movement Disorders

MATTHEW C. KIERNAN, Ph.D., D.Sc.
Professor
Department of Neurology
Prince of Wales Clinical School
University of New South Wales & Neuroscience
    Research Australia
Randwick, Sydney, New South Wales, Australia
Chapter 15: Nerve Excitability: A Clinical Translation

KENNETH D. LAXER, M.D.
Professor Emeritus
Department of Neurology
School of Medicine
University of California, San Francisco;
Director, Sutter Pacific Epilepsy Program
California Pacific Medical Center
San Francisco, California, USA
*Chapter 7: Invasive Clinical Neurophysiology in Epilepsy
    and Movement Disorders*

ALAN D. LEGATT, M.D., Ph.D.
Professor
Department of Neurology
Albert Einstein College of Medicine
Bronx, New York, USA
*Chapter 24: Brainstem Auditory Evoked Potentials: Methodology
    Interpretation, and Clinical Application*

CINDY SHIN YI LIN, Ph.D.
School of Medical Sciences
University of New South Wales
Randwick
Sydney, New South Wales, Australia
Chapter 15: Nerve Excitability: A Clinical Translation

WILLIAM J. MARKS, Jr., M.D.
Professor
Department of Neurology
School of Medicine
University of California, San Francisco
San Francisco, California, USA
*Chapter 7: Invasive Clinical Neurophysiology in Epilepsy
    and Movement Disorders*

MARC R. NUWER, M.D., Ph.D
Professor
Department of Neurology
David Geffen School of Medicine at UCLA
Los Angeles, California, USA
*Chapter 8: Topographic Mapping, Frequency Analysis, and
    Other Digital Techniques in Electroencephalography*

NICOLAE PETRESCU, M.D.
Division of Neurology
Department of Medicine
University of Toronto
Toronto, Ontario, Canada
*Chapter 28: Diagnostic and Therapeutic Role of Magnetic
    Stimulation in Neurology*

TERENCE W. PICTON, M.D., Ph.D., F.R.S.C.
Professor Emeritus
Departments of Medicine and Psychology
University of Toronto
Toronto, Ontario, Canada
*Chapter 25: Brainstem Auditory Evoked Potentials in Infants
    and Children*

SIMON PODNAR, M.D., D.Sc.
Associate Professor
Institute of Clinical Neurophysiology
Division of Neurology
University Medical Center Ljubljana
Ljubljana, Slovenia
*Chapter 31: Electrophysiologic Evaluation of Sacral
    Function*

DEVON I. RUBIN, M.D.
Associate Professor
Department of Neurology
Mayo Clinic College of Medicine
Jacksonville, Florida, USA
Chapter 13: Nerve Conduction Studies

DONALD B. SANDERS, M.D.
Professor
Division of Neurology
Department of Medicine
Duke University School of Medicine
Durham, North Carolina, USA
*Chapter 17: Electrophysiologic Study of Disorders of
    Neuromuscular Transmission*

FRANK W. SHARBROUGH III, M.D.
Professor Emeritus
Department of Neurology
Mayo Clinic College of Medicine
Rochester, Minnesota, USA
*Chapter 9: Intraoperative Electroencephalographic
    Monitoring During Carotid Endarterectomy
    and Cardiac Surgery*

JOHN M. STERN, M.D.
Associate Professor
Department of Neurology
David Geffen School of Medicine at UCLA
Los Angeles, California, USA
Chapter 6: Video-EEG Monitoring for Epilepsy

VIDHYA SUBRAMANIAN, Ph.D.
Postdoctoral Fellow
Pediatric Eye Research Laboratory
Retina Foundation of the Southwest
Dallas, Texas, USA
*Chapter 23: Visual Evoked Potentials in Infants and
    Children*

WILLIAM W. SUTHERLING, M.D.
Director, Neuromagnetism Laboratory
Huntington Medical Research Institutes;
Medical Director
Epilepsy and Brain Mapping Center
Huntington Hospital, Pasadena, California, USA
Chapter 10: Magnetoencephalography

MARGOT J. TAYLOR, Ph.D.
Professor
Departments of Paediatrics and Psychology
Hospital for Sick Children
University of Toronto
Toronto, Ontario, Canada
*Chapter 25: Brainstem Auditory Evoked Potentials in Infants
    and Children*

JOSEP VALLS-SOLÉ, M.D., Ph.D.
Professor
Department of Medicine (Neurology)
University of Barcelona
Barcelona, Spain
*Chapter 19: The Blink Reflex and Other Cranial Nerve
    Reflexes*

RICHARD A. VILLARREAL, B.S.E.
Principal Design Engineer
Cadwell Laboratories, Inc.
Kennewick, Washington, USA
Chapter 2: Electrophysiologic Equipment and Electrical Safety

DAVID B. VODUŠEK, M.D., D.Sc.
Professor
Department of Neurology
Medical School
University of Ljubljana
Ljubljana, Slovenia
Chapter 31: Electrophysiologic Evaluation of Sacral Function

FRANCIS O. WALKER, M.D.
Professor
Department of Neurology
Wake Forest University School of Medicine
Winston-Salem, North Carolina, USA
*Chapter 16: Neuromuscular Ultrasound as a Complement to the
   Electrodiagnostic Evaluation*

FLORIS L. WUYTS, Ph.D.
Professor
Department of Medical Physics
University of Antwerp
Antwerp, Belgium
Chapter 32: Vestibular Laboratory Testing

G. BRYAN YOUNG, M.D.
Professor
Department of Clinical Neurological Sciences
University of Western Ontario
London, Ontario, Canada
*Chapter 34: Electrophysiologic Evaluation of Patients in the
   Intensive Care Unit*

Preface to the Sixth Edition

Electrophysiologic techniques provide an important means of investigating the function of the nervous system in health and disease and of defining the pathophysiologic relevance of the anatomic abnormalities that are often defined so exquisitely by neuroimaging procedures. They also make it possible to distinguish between disorders that clinically may resemble each other, to recognize disorders at a preclinical or subclinical stage, and to monitor disease progression or the functional integrity of different parts of the nervous system during procedures that put them at risk. In addition, the electrophysiologic findings have been incorporated into a number of disease classifications. Both neurologists and clinical neurophysiologists therefore need to keep abreast of advances in the field to ensure that testing is used appropriately, interpreted correctly, and performed optimally, and that regulatory or recommended standards are met. This volume encompasses the latest advances in the field while providing details of the basic principles of the various electrophysiologic techniques in current use for neurologic purposes. The electrophysiologic findings are integrated with the clinical context in which they are obtained to ensure that their significance is appreciated. Common artifacts are described to ensure that they are not misinterpreted.

Over the last 50 years, electrodiagnosis has evolved from an obscure and somewhat erudite field into an established subspecialty (clinical neurophysiology) that is an integral part of clinical neurology, with its own journals, professional societies, national and international conferences, and testing organizations. It would be erroneous, however, to conclude that the specialty, with its established clinical role, is no longer at the forefront of medical advances, having yielded its place to neuroimaging, neuroimmunology, and molecular biology. Indeed, nothing could be further from the truth. New techniques such as nerve excitability studies using threshold tracking, microneurography, neuromuscular ultrasonography, and methods of studying cranial nerve reflexes have increased the scope of the electrodiagnostic examination and provided new insights into disease mechanisms, in some instances at the ionic level, and into treatment strategies. The refinement of evoked-potential techniques to study the function of small fibers in the peripheral nervous system and the development of a more comprehensive approach to the evaluation of the visual system, using multifocal as well as full-field visual evoked potentials, combined with various ancillary techniques, promise to extend the diagnostic scope, utility, and reliability of these electrophysiologic methods of evaluating portions of the nervous system. New surgical treatments for epilepsy and certain movement disorders have not only extended the role of clinical neurophysiologists in guiding operative intervention but have provided them with remarkable opportunities for gaining fresh insights into the operation of the nervous system by electrophysiologic studies. Magnetic stimulation, once a research technique, is developing not only an important diagnostic role but also a place for itself in the therapy of certain neurologic disorders. A number of other electrophysiologic techniques, previously regarded essentially as investigative tools with limited clinical relevance, have now gained importance in the evaluation and management of patients with neurologic disease.

These advances have prompted the production of a new—sixth—edition of this book, thirty-two years after the first edition was published. New chapters have been added, or existing ones expanded, to cover the methods or applications that have developed in recent years. The bibliography in most chapters has been limited to references published in the last 25 years or to classic older publications, but interested readers can refer to previous editions for other older references. More comprehensive bibliographies are provided in chapters dealing with developing topics, for the convenience of readers. The focus continues to be on the clinical application of various techniques for evaluating the nervous system, and methods that have little or no clinical utility are not discussed. The generous acceptance of previous editions has encouraged me to believe that this approach is the correct one and that the book will remain useful for clinicians, clinical neurophysiologists, and trainees in these fields.

I am grateful to all the contributors to this new edition. They were generous with their time, tolerant of my requests, and went to a great deal of trouble either to update their chapters from the last edition or—in the case of new authors—to provide a summary of developments in their own particular field of interest. It was my pleasure and privilege to work with them. Some of the illustrations in the book are taken from previously published sources, as is acknowledged in the text, and I am grateful for permission to reproduce them here. Ms. Charlotta Kryhl, at Elsevier, was of enormous help to me in the preparation of this edition, and I appreciate all her assistance and kindness. I am grateful also to project manager Maggie Johnson and the production team at Elsevier for their efforts in bringing the volume to fruition.

My wife, Jan, supported and encouraged me without complaint as I worked on this book, and it is to her that the volume is again dedicated. Our three children have been a source of great pleasure and pride to us both over the years, and I thank them for the many ways in which they have enriched our lives. This book has grown with them. When the first edition was published in 1980, our daughter was a toddler and neither of our two sons had been born. Alexandra is now a pediatrician undergoing subspecialty training in rheumatology; Jonathan, an attorney, is a federal public defender in Los Angeles; and Anthony is a final-year law student at Harvard. I can but admire their energy, enthusiasm, intellectual curiosity, and professional focus, which I hope will bring them much satisfaction. My own parents, now dead, would have been pleased to see this new edition, for I recall the excitement with which they greeted earlier ones. Finally, as I contemplate the pages of this sixth edition, I recall with warmth and affection those who encouraged my own interest in clinical neurology and neurophysiology when I was training at University College Hospital, the National Hospitals for Nervous Diseases at Queen Square and Maida Vale, and the Middlesex Hospital in London, England. I would like to believe that they—my teachers—would have taken pride in this volume, and I thank them for all that they did for me.

Michael J. Aminoff,
San Francisco, 2011

Preface to the First Edition

Fifty years have passed since Hans Berger's first paper on the human electroencephalogram. Over this time, electroencephalography has evolved into an investigative technique of undoubted practical value, and technologic advances have permitted the development of a number of new electrophysiologic approaches to neurologic diagnosis. These developments have led to certain difficulties for clinicians and neurophysiologists alike. On the one hand, the present-day physician is tempted to avail himself of investigative procedures that he does not entirely understand and that provide him with information which he is often unable to interpret. On the other hand, the neurophysiologist is commonly faced with clinical problems that he fails to appreciate or to which there is no ready solution by the means at his disposal. There is therefore a need for a conveniently sized monograph that provides a general introduction to the role of electrodiagnosis in neurology and is directed at the clinical relevance of the investigative procedures that are now within the province of the electrophysiologist. In preparing the present volume, it has therefore been my aim, and that of the other contributors, to provide in simple terms a comprehensive but concise account of the clinical application of various electrophysiologic methods of investigating the function of the central and peripheral nervous systems. Some of these methods, such as electroencephalography and electromyography, are admirably covered in encyclopedic detail in certain textbooks aimed at specialists or trainees in these fields. The chapters covering these topics in the present volume are in no way intended to take the place of such works; rather, they are directed at those who need to know the principles, uses and limitations of the methods, and who have to relate the information derived from such studies to the clinical context of individual cases. Certain quantitative aspects of these subjects have also been considered, however, because of their potential clinical utility. A number of the other electrophysiologic methods that are covered in this book—such as the various evoked potential techniques—have been developed comparatively recently, and their clinical applications are as yet incompletely defined. In view of the obvious interest shown by increasing numbers of clinicians and neurophysiologists in setting up facilities to undertake such studies for clinical purposes, the technical aspects of some of these subjects have been reviewed in somewhat greater detail, although the emphasis has remained on the practical relevance of the methods. Electrophysiologic techniques that are of more limited clinical utility at the present time, such as recording of the contingent negative variation, have deliberately not been considered.

I am greatly indebted to the contributors to this book, all of whom have taken much time and trouble to survey developments in their own particular fields of interest. I am grateful also to those authors, editors, and publishers who have allowed us to reproduce illustrations previously published elsewhere, and whose permission is acknowledged in the text. The advice and understanding that I received from Ms. Carole Baker and Mr. Bill Schmitt of Churchill Livingstone, the publishers, are greatly appreciated. Finally, it is a pleasure to acknowledge the help, encouragement, and support that my wife, Jan, gave me during all stages of the preparation of this book.

Michael J. Aminoff, M.D.

Contents

Section IV: Evoked Potentials and Related Techniques

Introduction

The Emergence of Electrophysiology as an Aid to Neurology

MARY A. B. BRAZIER

ELECTROTHERAPY

ELECTRODIAGNOSIS

From the time of the ancients to well into the eighteenth century, electricity was regarded as a strange, invisible power. It was differentiated from magnetism in 1600 by Gilbert,[1] but its nature remained a mystery. Gradually the role of electricity in relation to the nervous system was to emerge, first from observation of the effect of applying it to the body, and eventually from the discovery that both muscle and nerve could themselves be sources of this power. The first of these—observation of its application—had had to wait for the technical development of instruments to deliver electricity; the second, for the more delicate instrumentation necessary for detection of the fine currents of nerve. The first technique became the ancestor of electrotherapy; the second became the basis of electrodiagnosis.

ELECTROTHERAPY

The experimenters of the eighteenth century inherited from Robert Boyle,[2,3] who in 1673 and 1675 described electric attraction as "a Material Effluvium, issuing from and returning to, the Electrical Body." This concept, when applied to the nervous system, retained a flavor of galenism's nervous fluids and the vis nervosa of von Haller,[4] and permeates nearly all the writings of the experimenters in this field until vitalism finally gave way to materialism.

Working at first only with frictional machines as a source of electricity, experimenters in the early eighteenth century played with many demonstrations of its strange action at a distance. This was a period when interest in electricity was so keen that it was invoked to explain many natural phenomena, not only of animals but also of plants.

According to Fée (1832),[5] Elizabeth, the daughter of the great Linnaeus, noticed in her father's garden near Uppsala that some of the orange-colored flowers, such as marigolds and firelilies, appeared to give off flashes of light at twilight. (It was Goethe,[6] in 1810, who showed this to be a retinal contrast effect and not an electrical flash.) But those who speculated about animals and man felt that they were on surer ground. Did not the cat's fur crackle when you rubbed it, and had not Theodoric the Visigoth thrown off sparks as he marched?

In the early part of the century it had been discovered empirically that the human body could be charged electrostatically, provided that it was insulated. At first it was thought that a layer of air had to be present between the subject and the ground, for the characteristics of conductors and nonconductors were only beginning to be understood. Stephen Gray,[7] who died in 1736, discovered in 1731 that the distribution of electric charges varies with the insulating or conducting properties of the material employed, and he had reported these findings in a series of letters to the Royal Society. These terms were not used at the time, nor was induction understood (which he had demonstrated and called "Electrical Attraction at a Distance"). He wrote of "Electrick Virtue," and said that his experiments showed that animals "receive Electrick Effluvia." In 1742 his teacher, Desaguliers,[8] a demonstrator for Newton, clarified the distinction between conductors and nonconductors, showing the former to be essentially the "non-electrics" of Gilbert[1] that conveyed electricity away, and the latter to be the "electrics" that could be charged.

In many countries the phenomenon by which the human body could carry a charge was exploited for entertainment. Outstanding examples were the Abbé

The author is deceased

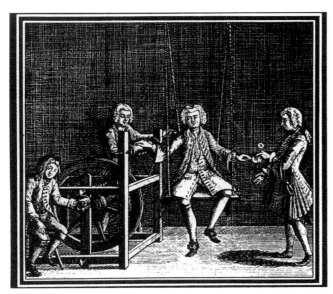

FIGURE 1-1 ▪ Electrification of the human body by frictional electricity. (From Krüger JG: Zuschrift an seine Zuhörer worinnen er ihren seine Gedancken von der Electricität mittheilet. Hemmerde, Halle, 1745.)

Nollet at the Court of Louis XV,[9] Winkler[10] and Hausen at Leipzig,[11] Du Fay in Paris,[12] and Kratzenstein in Halle[13] (Fig. 1-1). Many delightful illustrations survive.

The next step was the discovery that the application of electricity to muscles, even those of the dead, could evoke a contraction. Inevitably, this led to the exploitation of this effect as a therapy despite a complete lack of understanding of its modus operandi. Some attempts were deliberate hoaxes; others—for example, those of the physicians at the center at Montpellier—were the efforts of true believers.

Among these believers was a young physician named Kratzenstein, who was raised in the unlikely atmosphere of the Stahlian school in Halle but was greatly influenced by his teacher, Gottlob Krüger.[14] Krüger, beginning to draw away from the influence of Georg Ernst Stahl (who taught that the soul was the vital force that caused muscles to contract[15]), had experimented widely with the electrification of animals and encouraged his pupil to engage in electrotherapeutic studies. These were first printed in 1744 in the form of letters entitled "Abhandlung von dem Nutzen der Electricität in der Arzenwissenschaft."

Still using frictional electricity, and noting from experiments on himself that electrification of his body caused him to sweat (the "effluvium" of Boyle?), Kratzenstein advanced the hypothesis that this loss of salt-containing fluid could have beneficial medicinal effects. No doubt this proposal stemmed from the age-old concept that bloodletting had therapeutic value.

The cures he claimed consisted of two cases in which there was restoration of movement in contracted fingers.

He also noted the induction of sound sleep, forerunner of that observed in electrosleep. As the news spread around Europe, attempts at cures were made in many centers. These were at first mostly in cases of paralysis. The fact that contraction of a muscle could be obtained at the moment of direct stimulation yet could not be maintained as a cure failed to find correct interpretation, for the role of innervation was not yet understood.

The rare case of success anteceded the understanding of hysterical paralysis and encouraged the establishment of many centers for the treatment of paralytic conditions, among the most famous being the school of Montpellier under the leadership of Boissier de la Croix de Sauvages.[16] In 1749, one of de Sauvages's pupils, Deshais, published a thesis boldly entitled "De Hemiplegia per Electricitatem Curanda,"[17] which showed his thinking to be creeping toward the recognition of the role of the nerve supply, although this was still versed in galenist terms. Deshais wrote, "paralysis is caused by the arrest of nervous fluid destined to circulate in the brain because it meets an insuperable resistance in the nerve fibres. Thus we must increase the pressure of the nervous fluid when hemiplegia resists ordinary remedies." He added that hemiplegia could be cured or, at any rate, improved by electrification (Fig. 1-2).

At this time, electricity and its effects on the human body were a favorite subject for theses. In the collection of unpublished manuscripts (1750–1760) by Jacques de Romas that is preserved in the City Archives of Bordeaux, there is one on electricity that includes observations on the electrification of two paralytic patients. Another example is found in the thesis collection at the University of Montpellier, written in 1750 by Jean Thecla Dufay, who restricts himself to the electrical nature of the nervous fluid and does not discuss therapy.[18] His thesis does, however, give a useful review of the experiments and knowledge of his time. He concludes his account boldly: "Ergo Fluidum nerveum est Fluidum electricum." Montpellier was at that time a center of great interest in electricity, and it was there that Boissier de Sauvages endowed a convent hospital solely for electrical therapy (1740–1760). In 1748, de Sauvages had himself received a prize from the Académie Royale des Sciences at Toulouse for a dissertation on hydrophobia; this was published in 1758. In this paper, in what he termed a "Digression sur l'électricité," he championed the existence of animal electricity and evolved a bizarre hypothesis about nerve and muscle activity in hydrophobia. This went as follows: given that muscular movement is proportional to the force of the nervous fluid, the venom of rabies, on mixing with it, doubles the velocity and also doubles the density of the nervous fluid; hence the nerve force and the resultant

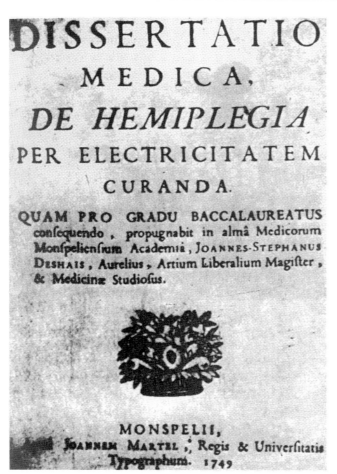

FIGURE 1-2 ■ Title page of the doctoral thesis of J. E. Deshais on the cure of hemiplegia by electricity. (Courtesy of the University of Montpellier.)

muscular movement are eight times stronger than normal. By this tortuous piece of arithmetic, de Sauvages explained the violent muscular spasms in hydrophobia.

Academies were generous with prizes for the medical uses of electricity, which no doubt accounts in part for the plethora of such theses at this time. Another winner was Jean-Paul Marat, who was to meet a violent death in the French Revolution. His essay[19] won the prize of the Paris Academy but drew the rebuke that his criticisms of other workers were too forcefully expressed. Many absurd claims for electrotherapy were made by physicians, and at their doors must be laid the blame for much subsequent quackery. A contemporary critic ridiculed these claims but published only anonymously; however, his gay and witty touch betrayed his identity to Nollet as that of another gentleman of the Church, the Abbé Mangin.[20] Nollet, who had himself gathered acclaim through his use of electrotherapy (though he had also done his part to expose the quacks), scolded Mangin "d'avoir confondu les temps, les lieux, les personnes et les choses."

A more efficient source of electricity was to come to the aid of electrotherapists, although a natural one had, in fact, been used for some years: namely, the shock delivered by the marine torpedo. On being applied to the soles of the feet, this was said to relieve the pain of gout. The rationale for the treatment, however, received no elucidation from the great surgeon, John Hunter,[21] whose exquisite dissections revealed the anatomy of these electric fish, for he thought that "the will of the animal does absolutely controul the electric powers of its body." The reflex nature of the discharge was not established until the serial experiments of Matteucci and Savi[22] in 1844.

By the middle of the eighteenth century, eager electrotherapists were no longer dependent on the frictional machines for producing electricity, for van Musschenbroek, Professor of Physics at Leiden, almost by chance invented a device for storing electricity and discharging it as a shock.[23] This, the ancestor of the condenser, was the Leyden jar.

In 1746, van Musschenbroek, striving to conserve electricity in a conductor and to delay the loss of its charge in air, attempted to use charged water as the conductor, insulating it from air in a nonconducting glass jar. However, when he charged the water through a wire leading from a frictional electrical machine, he found the electricity dissipated as quickly as ever. An assistant who was holding the jar containing charged water accidentally touched the inserted wire with his other hand and got a frightening shock. With one hand he had formed one "plate," the charged water being the other "plate," and the glass jar the intervening dielectric. A condenser was born. Experimental electricity had reached the stage when such a development was due, for a similar discovery was made by the Dean of the Cathedral of Kamin in Pomerania, whose followers gave the jar his name, "Kleiste Flasche."

One of the many to espouse this new electrifying technique was the Abbé Bertholon,[24,25] who traveled widely in Europe, bringing back reports of strange cures that others could not replicate. He was not alone in the variety of claims he made, for this form of "therapy" had spread widely through Europe. So diverse were the diseases for which cures were being claimed that academies in several countries offered prizes, including the Académie at Lyons. It offered a prize in 1777 for the answer to the questions, "Quelles sont les maladies qui dépendent de la plus ou moins de grande quantité de fluide électrique dans le corps humain, et quels sont les moyens de remédier aux unes et aux autres?" This was a spur to many, including Bertholon, who, in his two volumes on the electricity of the human body in health and disease, claimed to examine his cases as to whether electrification was the only ameliorator of the patient's condition or was an additive to other therapies. A great believer in a "latent electricity" within the body, he held that it was manipulation of this inherent electricity that formed the basis of the cures he claimed. This concept was a rewording of "animal spirits," and in no way did he foresee the intrinsic electricity of nerve and muscle found (but little understood) by Galvani.[26,27]

We owe the next step in the invention of sources of electricity to the controversy that developed with Volta over the explanation of Galvani's results[28]; the voltaic pile, which soon replaced the Leyden jar in the hands of those espousing electrotherapy, was the ancestor of the batteries of today. By the turn of the century, books were beginning to appear on the history of medical electricity (e.g., by Vivenzio[29] in 1784 and Sue[30] in 1802).

The early ventures in applying electricity to patients with various diseases were gradually sorted out and achieved a rational basis, thanks to the development of knowledge of basic neurophysiology with its elucidation of the relationship of nerve to muscle, of spinal cord to nerve, and of brain to all. However, one method, for which therapeutic claims were made, has still not reached the first stage of scientific rationale. This is electroconvulsive shock.

Many early experimenters (e.g., Fontana[31] in 1760 and Caldani[32] in 1784) noted the convulsions of their frogs when electricity was applied to their brains, although Galvani attempted this without success. ("Si enim conductores non dissectae spinale medullae, aut nervis, ut consuevimus, sed vel cerebro-contractiones vel nullae, vel admodum exiguae sunt.") In the first decade of the nineteenth century, his nephew, Aldini, was to experiment with electroshock in humans.[33] Impressed by the muscular contractions he obtained on stimulating animals and cadavers, he stood close to the guillotine to receive heads of criminals in as fresh a condition as possible. He found that passing a current either through the ear and mouth or through the exposed brain and mouth evoked facial grimaces. The fresher the head, the more remarkable the grimace. He then proceeded to apply electrical stimulation from a voltaic pile to the living. His theory was that the contractions were excited by "le développement d'un fluide dans la machine animale," and this he held to be conveyed by the nerves to the muscles. We recognize here the explanation popularized by Bertholon.[24]

One set of these early experiments on humans reaches into the twentieth century, for Aldini applied his galvanism to the mentally ill (Fig. 1-3). Having experimented on himself with electrodes in both ears or in one ear and his mouth, or on forehead and nose, he experienced a strong reaction ("une forte action"), followed by

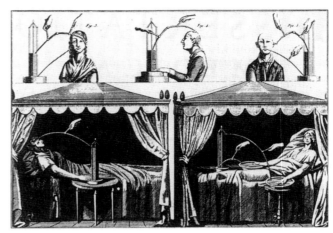

FIGURE 1-3 ■ Aldini's experiments with electroshock "therapy" in humans. Above, mental patients with the electrodes in various positions connecting to voltaic piles for stimulation. Below, two recently dead patients connected directly, or by saline baths, to voltaic piles. (From Aldini G: Essai Théorique et Expérimental sur le Galvanisme. Fournier, Paris, 1804.)

prolonged insomnia lasting several days. He found the experience very disagreeable but thought the changes it produced in the brain might be salutary in the psychoses ("la folie"). Passing the current between the ears produced violent convulsions and pain, but he claimed good results in patients suffering from melancholia.

Aldini had no instrument to tell him the amount of current passed (he recorded only the number of copper and zinc discs in the voltaic pile). In the twentieth-century adaptation of this technique, we are also not told by the originator what current flowed between electrodes placed bilaterally on the frontoparietal regions, only the voltage (although it is current, and not voltage, that stimulates). "I decided to start cautiously with a low-intensity current of 80 volts for 1.5 seconds ... The electrodes were applied again and a 110-volt discharge was applied for 1.5 seconds."[34] We are not surprised to be told of the resultant convulsion, apnea, and cyanosis.

This report related the results of the first experiments made by Cerletti in 1932, but even now, many years later, no rationale has been found for the salutary effects claimed by the users, and one is reminded again of Aldini's concept of a rearrangement of functions in the brain such as take place from a hit on the head: "Une chute, un coup violent porté sur la tête, ont souvent produit des altérations très sensibles dans les facultés intellectuelles."

In the years following Aldini's application of electricity to humans, a revival of electrotherapy resulted from the work of Duchenne,[35,36] who stimulated paralyzed muscles, at first through punctures of the skin but later percutaneously. Although considerable controversy arose from his work, he had, in fact, a greater understanding of electric currents than his predecessors, and by careful exploration he found the motor points for the muscles he was stimulating. From his work grew some understanding of the anatomy underlying the induced contractions of muscles, and in 1868 he published a small book on muscular paralysis, in which he illustrated the muscle fiber abnormalities he found by light microscopy.[37] It may be said that it was Duchenne who built the bridge between electrotherapy and electrodiagnosis, leaving his name to Duchenne dystrophy.

A less controversial ancestor of modern electrical techniques (the cardiac stimulator) is found in a report given to the Accademia di Torino[38] in 1803, in which the hearts of three decapitated felons were found to retain excitability long after the voluntary muscles ceased to respond to galvanic stimulation. The reporters were Vassalli, Giulio, and Rossi.

Before the end of the nineteenth century, stimulation of the heart by alternating currents was being used in France for resuscitation by Prévost and Batelli, and it developed into a standard procedure in the twentieth century.[39]

ELECTRODIAGNOSIS

The several forms of electrodiagnosis used in neurology have much shorter histories than electrotherapy, for they have their basis in fundamental neurophysiology rather than in quasiquackery. They include electroencephalography, electromyography, cerebral and spinal potentials evoked by sensory stimulation (EPs), the recording of the action potentials of nerve, the electroretinogram, and the contingent negative variation (CNV). Of these, the CNV, up to this time, has proved of more interest to the psychologist than to the neurologist.

In the period under review, only electroencephalography, electromyography, the action potential of nerve, and the evoked cortical potential have a history. This history, which they largely share, essentially stems from the discoveries of Galvani.

The epoch-making researches of Galvani have been described so many times that they are well known to all who work in electrophysiology. Best known is his *Commentarius*,[26] in which he first made public his claims for intrinsic animal electricity, but this was only the culmination of years of experimentation about which he has left copious notes, now in the Archives of the University of Bologna.

These laboratory notes, written in the vernacular and plentifully illustrated by his own sketches (often including himself), begin in 1780 (Fig. 1-4). Retaining still the analogy of an electric fluid, Galvani declared his goal in the title of his notes: "Dell'azione del fluido elettrico applicato a nervi in varie maniere."

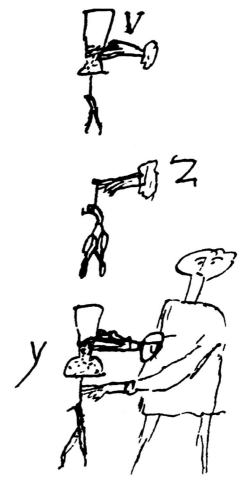

FIGURE 1-4 ▪ Galvani's sketch of himself experimenting on a frog nerve–muscle preparation that he likened to a Leyden jar. (From notes made December 10, 1781, preserved in the Archives of the University of Bologna.)

The three chief observations that stand out from the many experiments that Galvani included in 1791 in his published *Commentarius* were (1) that a frog's nerve preparation, although at a distance from a sparking electrostatic machine, would twitch when touched by an observer; (2) that the atmospheric electricity of a thunderstorm could be used to stimulate frogs' legs if a long wire was stretched across the roof (the principle of the lightning conductor); and (3) that frogs' legs twitched when hung by hooks from the railing of his house, even in the absence of a thunderstorm. Galvani interpreted this as evidence that the muscle contraction was caused by electricity originating in the animal tissues themselves.

It was this last experiment (Fig. 1-5) that raised the most controversy. It was eventually attacked by Volta and explained as merely the current that flows between dissimilar metals.[28] In fact, despite the title of Volta's famous letter, two dissimilar metals are not enough to

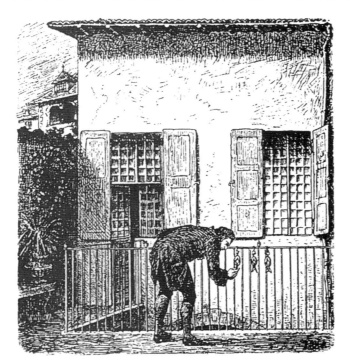

FIGURE 1-5 ▪ Drawing that Du Bois-Reymond had made by an artist from his own original sketch. It shows Galvani hanging frogs' legs on the railings of his house in the Strada San Felice in Bologna. (From Reden von Emil Du Bois-Reymond, vol 2. Veit, Leipzig, 1887.)

cause a current to flow; they need to be separated by an electrolyte. In Galvani's case, the metals were the brass of the hooks and the iron of the railings, with the frog providing the electrolyte. Volta's insistence on the metallic origin of all of the electricity in all Galvani's experiments on frogs caused him, and more especially his eager but less prudent nephew, Aldini,[40] to press on to experiments omitting the dissimilar metals. Finally, in 1794, an experiment was evolved and published anonymously (but quite certainly the work of Galvani), in which no external source of electricity was present.[41] A twitch was demonstrated in a frog's nerve–muscle preparation when the cut end of another nerve was placed on the muscle. In this case, the source of the electricity was what we now recognize as the current of injury from the cut nerve, or as it came to be called, the demarcation potential (Fig. 1-6).

It seems strange, in the light of history, that this challenge based on bimetallic electricity was the one to throw the greatest doubt on Galvani's claim of intrinsic animal electricity. He had himself, in 1786, made intensive tests of touching the frog (on a metal hook) with a second metal (e.g., gold, silver, tin, and lead), and his notes, recorded on September 20 of that year, make it clear that he was fully familiar with this metallic source. In fact,

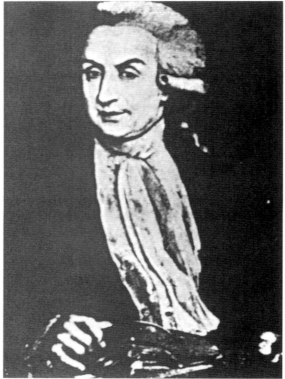

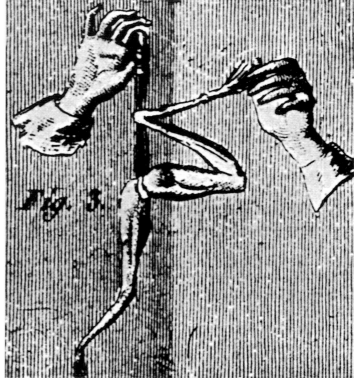

FIGURE 1-6 ▪ Left, a portrait of Galvani from the oil painting in the library of the University of Bologna. (Courtesy of the late Dr. Giulio Pupilli.) Right, an illustration of his experiment on muscle contraction in the absence of all metals. (From Aldini G: Essai Théorique et Expérimental sur le Galvanisme. 2 Vols. Fournier, Paris, 1804.)

he described experiments with dissimilar metals in his *Commentarius* but failed to interpret them correctly.

Alexander von Humboldt is the first great name in support of Galvani, for he recognized that both protagonists had made discoveries of real phenomena and that Volta's brilliant development of the current flow between dissimilar metals did not preclude the existence of animal electricity.[42] Humboldt exposed the erroneous parts, not only of Galvani's and Volta's interpretations, but also of the writers who had rushed in so precipitously to take up arms for one or the other protagonist; Pfaff,[43] Fowler,[44] Valli,[45] and Schmück[46] each received his rebuke.

The next step, once the skeptics had been persuaded that nerve–muscle preparations could emit electricity, was to establish that this phenomenon was not dependent on injury. The clear proof of demarcation currents we owe to Matteucci,[22,47] Professor of Physics in Pisa, who established in 1842 (publishing his findings in 1843 and 1844) that a current flowed from an injured point in a muscle to its uncut surface. By this time, thanks to their invention by Oersted in 1820 in Copenhagen,[48] galvanometers had come to the aid of the electrophysiologist, and Matteucci could determine not only the presence of a current but also its direction. Matteucci became convinced (but did not prove) that in an uninjured limb a current normally flowed from the tendon to the belly, and this he called the "muscle current," but he doubted the electricity of nerve.

The main center of research on this problem moved from Italy to Berlin, where Hermann[49] and Du Bois-Reymond,[50,51] with their superior instrumentation, were able to differentiate currents of injury from normal electric potentials recorded from the surface of a muscle on contraction. With Du Bois-Reymond's demonstration of this in humans, electromyography was born (Fig. 1-7).

But the kind of electricity that Galvani was searching for was the "fluido elettrico," what we now call transmission (i.e., the transmission of the nerve impulse that exerts control of muscle movement by the nervous system). In this concept Galvani was unquestionably correct, although it was another 50 years before the electrical nature of the nerve impulse was indubitably demonstrated by Du Bois-Reymond. Improving on Oersted's invention of passing a current through a single coil of wire to deflect the needle, Du Bois-Reymond increased the number of coils to 2,500 and thereby provided himself with an induction coil sufficiently sensitive to detect the change in potential when an impulse passed down a nerve trunk. This he detected as a "negative variation" in the demarcation potential that his predecessors had described. It was what we now know as the action potential of nerve and is the basis of electroneurography. When, in 1850, von Helmholtz designed an instrument for

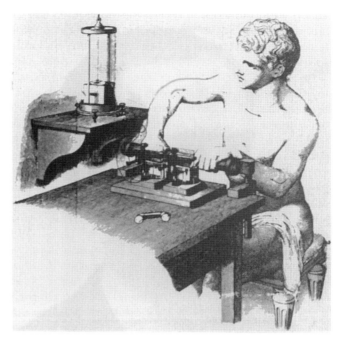

FIGURE 1-7 ■ Du Bois-Reymond's experiment on muscle currents in humans. (The subject plunged two fingers into cups of saline.) On contraction of the right arm muscles, a difference of potential developed that, through wires to the solenoid, produced a deflection of the needle. (From Du Bois-Reymond E: Untersuchungen über thierische Electricität, 2 vols. Reimer, Berlin, 1848, 1849.)

measuring the conduction velocity of nerve, he opened the way for the modern neurologist's detection of demyelinating diseases.[52]

Du Bois-Reymond did not underestimate the importance of his discovery. He wrote:

> If I do not greatly deceive myself, I have succeeded in realizing in full actuality (albeit under a slightly different aspect) the hundred years' dream of physicists and physiologists to wit, the identification of the nervous principle with electricity.

His discovery did indeed have importance, an importance that led even beyond his dreams of biologic electricity. Within 25 years of the publication of his massive book *Untersuchungen über thierische Electricität*, the idea occurred to a young lecturer at Liverpool, in the north of England, that as nerve impulses flowed in and out of the brain, their passage might be detectable. In 1874, he obtained a grant from the British Medical Association (BMA) and within a year reported his findings to a meeting of the BMA on August 25, 1875. His name was Richard Caton[53–57] (Fig. 1-8).

Caton had already experimented on the peripheral nerve–muscle currents, but he began to search for their cerebral counterparts; he not only detected them but also noticed that when both of his electrodes lay on the cortical surface there was a continuous waxing and waning

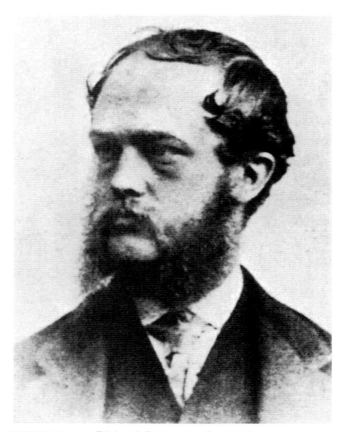

FIGURE 1-8 ■ Richard Caton, the first to discover the electroencephalogram and to detect the evoked potential change on visual stimulation and realize its application to cortical localization. (From a photograph taken in his thirties when he was working in electrophysiology: a generous gift to the author from his daughter.)

of potential. This oscillation of the baseline was present in the unstimulated animal, and Caton proved it to be unrelated to respiratory or cardiac rhythms. He also proved these fluctuations to be biologic in origin by showing them to be vulnerable to anoxia and to anesthesia and to be abolished by the death of the animal. Caton had discovered the electroencephalogram (EEG).

The report of Caton's demonstration that the BMA published contained (in part) these statements[53]:

Feeble currents of varying direction pass through the multiplier when the electrodes are placed on two points of the external surface, or one electrode on the grey matter, and one on the surface of the skull. . . . When any part of the grey matter is in a state of functional activity, its electric current usually exhibits negative variation. . . . Impressions through the senses were found to influence the currents of certain areas . . .

Caton had found not only the EEG but also the cerebral potential change evoked by sensory stimulation. In these potential swings superimposed on the baseline oscillations, Caton immediately recognized a meaning for studies of cortical localization, a discovery basic

to the use of evoked potentials in today's clinical neurology.

Caton's great contribution, in addition to discovering the EEG, was in providing experimentalists for the first time with a method for mapping the localization of sensory areas in the cortex, supplanting the crude ablation techniques that had until then been the only approach, other than Gall and Spurzheim's[58] claims for bumps on the skull. This was an era of intense interest in cortical localization owing to the prominence of David Ferrier's mapping of the motor cortex from 1873 to 1874,[59] and in his subsequent work it was this aspect of his discoveries that Caton pursued.

In 1875, electronic amplifiers were unthought of and cameras had not yet come into the laboratory. To gain acceptance of his discovery, Caton had to demonstrate the "brain waves" of his animals by optical magnification of the movements of the meniscus in his Thompson's galvanometer.

He went on to expand his experiments, reporting them more fully in 1877 in a Supplement to the *British Medical Journal*[55] and again at the Ninth International Medical Congress in Washington, D.C., in 1887.[56] At this meeting, he reported experiments on 45 animals (cats, rabbits, and monkeys) and described his operating technique, electrodes, and instrumentation.

Among these many experiments is one of special interest to electroencephalographers; he found the flicker response of the EEG, a phenomenon found again in humans by Adrian and Matthews[60] in 1934. Caton wrote:

I tried the effect of intervals of light and darkness on seven rabbits and four monkeys, placing electrodes on the region (13) stimulation of which causes movement of the eyes . . . In those five experiments in which I was successful the relation between the intervals of light and darkness and the movements of the galvanometer needle was quite beyond question . . .

Strangely enough, despite the prominent groups before whom Caton gave his demonstrations and the popular medical journal in which he reported them, his work received no attention among English-speaking physiologists.

In Poland, 15 years later, a young assistant in the physiology department of the University of Jagiellonski in Crakow, Adolf Beck,[61-63] not knowing of Caton's work, was searching initially for the same phenomenon: namely, for electrical signs in the brain of impulses reaching it from the sense organs (Fig. 1-9). Like Caton before him, he succeeded, and he also found the brain wave. His animals were dogs and rabbits, and because he lacked a camera, he published the protocols of all his experiments in the Polish language for a doctoral thesis.[61] In order to reach a greater audience, he sent a short account to the most widely read journal in Germany, the *Centralblatt für Physiologie*.[62] A spate of claims for priority for finding sensorily evoked potentials

By the end of the century, the electrical activity of the brain had reached the textbooks,[67] and cameras were beginning to reach the laboratory scientist. In 1913 and 1914 came the first photographs of EEGs from Pravdich-Neminsky in Russia[68] and from Beck's old professor, Cybulski, in Poland.[69] It was Neminsky who gave us the first photograph of an evoked potential recorded at the cortex of a dog on stimulation of the sciatic nerve (Fig. 1-10). He also demonstrated that the EEG could be recorded from the intact skull. From Cybulski came the first photograph of experimentally induced epilepsy (Fig. 1-11), although such a result had been reported previously in 1912 in Russia by Kaufmann,[70] who lacked a camera. Kaufmann had read the works of Caton and Beck and the other claimants, and, in fact, had written a review of them. From this study, he argued that an epileptic attack must surely be accompanied by abnormal discharges and, on provoking one in his animals, he found both the tonic and clonic phases.

Although successful with light as the stimulus, Caton had been disappointed by his failure to record cortical potential swings evoked by sounds, for he was searching for the auditory cortex. "Search was made," he wrote, "to discover an area related to perceptions of sound. The electrodes were placed on various parts of the brain, and loud sounds were made close to the rabbit's ears by means of a bell, etc. No results were obtained."[55] Beck, independently, had searched for a cortical area that

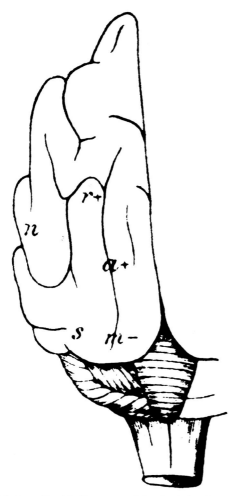

FIGURE 1-9 ■ Beck's diagram of the dog's brain on which he marked the positions of electrodes that gave him a response to light (m−, a+) and a faint response to sound (n, s). (From Beck A: Doctoral Thesis. Polska Akademija Umiejetnosci Series 2:187, 1891.)

followed the German publication of Beck's findings. The first came in 1890 from Fleischl von Marxow,[64] professor of physiology (and teacher of Freud) in Vienna; his claim was based on a letter he had sealed in 1883. Other claims came from Gotch and Horsley[65] and from Danilevsky.[66]

It is noticeable that it was the electrical response of the brain to sensory stimulation that drew the most interest, for this was a finding that lay directly in the mainstream of current thinking about cortical localization of function.*

The completely novel idea of a continuously fluctuating electric potential intrinsic to the "resting" brain, although confirmed by every worker, was of interest at that time only to its two independent discoverers, Caton and Beck.

*For a fuller account of this early work on the EEG and the use of the evoked cortical potential, see Brazier MAB: A History of the Electrical Activity of the Brain. Pitman, London, 1961.

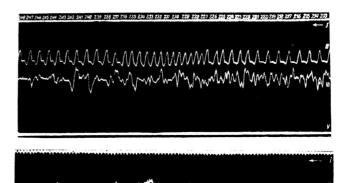

FIGURE 1-10 ■ The first photograph to be published of electroencephalograms (EEGs) and of an evoked potential. The upper record shows (in trace III) the brain potentials of a curarized dog with the pulsations of an artery in the brain recorded above them. In the lower record, the sciatic nerve is being stimulated from time to time, and the decrease in activity noted by Neminsky (and by Beck before him) can be seen. The record reads from right to left, line I being a time-marker in fifths of a second, line III the EEG, and line V the signal for stimulation at each break. (From Pravdich-Neminsky VV: Ein Versuch der Registrierung der elektrischen Gehirnerscheinungen. Zentralbl Physiol 27:951, 1913.)

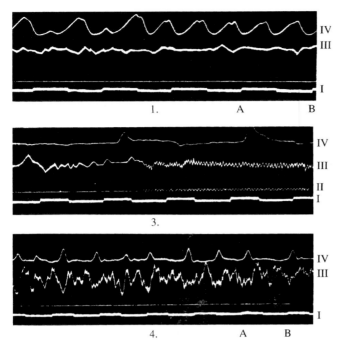

FIGURE 1-11 ■ The first published record of the electroencephalogram (EEG) in experimental epilepsy induced by cortical stimulation in a dog. The record reads from right to left, the uppermost trace IV being the heart, III the cortex, II the stimulus (which leaks onto the EEG), and I the time line. The lower strip is continuous with the upper one. A–B = 1 second. (From Cybulski N, Jelehska-Macieszyna: Action currents of the cerebral cortex (in Polish). Bull Internat Acad Sci Crac B:776, 1914.)

responded electrically to sound but was rarely successful. He did, however, discover the desynchronization of the ongoing oscillatory activity on sensory stimulation, which is what we now call "alpha blocking of the EEG."

At the turn of the century, this question of the localization of the auditory cortex was taken up by a student of the famous Bechterev in St. Petersburg. Larionov by name, he started to attempt localization by extirpation experiments but, on learning of Caton's success with visual stimuli, changed to a search for the evoked potential.[71,72] He was fortunate in having far more sensitive instrumentation than that of his predecessors (a Wiedermann–d'Arsonval galvanometer), and with this he was able to map out, in cats, the topographic centers on the temporal cortex of response to the pitch of different tuning forks (Fig. 1-12).

In America and in Western Europe, there was no sign of interest in these many revelations of the electrical activity of the brain despite their obvious meaning for cortical localization. In Germany, however, there was a psychiatrist who had read all the publications and who hoped to find in the electrical activity of the brain the source of "psychic energy." This was Hans Berger at

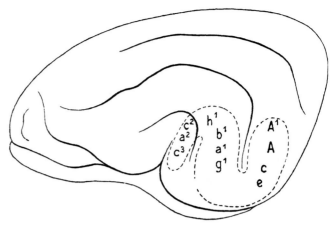

FIGURE 1-12 ■ Schema for localizations of tones in the dog's cortex. (From Larionov VE: Über die musikalischen Centren des Gehirns. Pflüg Arch ges Physiol 76:608, 1899.)

the University of Jena. He worked in secrecy and did not publish until 1929,[73] but he kept copious notebooks and diaries, from which we know that he began experiments in 1902, rapidly confirmed Caton's discovery of the EEG in animals, but failed to find the potential changes evoked by sensory stimulation. He made further attempts in 1907 and again in 1910, by which time he had a more sensitive galvanometer, but again he failed. This was a great disappointment to him, for he eagerly wanted to relate such to psychic functions. Berger's failure to find these changes in his animal experiments lacks an explanation, for Caton's findings had by that time been confirmed by many workers in four different countries, all of whose works were read by Berger.[61-63,66,68–72,74,75] In none of Berger's publications,[73,76–78] which began in 1929 (Fig. 1-13) and continued with rapidity to 1938, do we find him claiming the discovery of the EEG for himself; the claim he made, and justly, was that he was the first to demonstrate that, in having electrical activity in the brain, humans were no different from other vertebrates, and it was he who named the spontaneous ongoing activity "Das Elektrenkephalogram."

Being of an abnormally reclusive nature, he kept his first success (the recording from a patient with a skull defect) a secret for 5 years, although he jotted down in his notebook that this gave him the opportunity to apply Caton's observations to humans and the hope that "we may learn the physical basis of consciousness."

Disappointed as he was in his search for a physiologic basis for psychic phenomena, on which he had published a monograph[76] in 1921 and one on telepathy[78] in 1940, he had, as the world knows, launched the EEG as a clinical neurologic test—a test now employed in every neurologic institution in the world.

Über das Elektrenkephalogramm des Menschen.

Von

Professor Dr. **Hans Berger**, Jena.

(Mit 17 Textabbildungen.)

(Eingegangen am 22. April 1929.)

Wie *Garten* [1], wohl einer der besten Kenner der Elektrophysiologie, mit Recht hervorgehoben hat, wird man kaum fehlgehen, wenn man jeder lebenden Zelle tierischer und pflanzlicher Natur die Fähigkeit zuschreibt, elektrische Ströme hervorzubringen. Man bezeichnet solche Ströme als bioelektrische Ströme, weil sie die normalen Lebenserscheinungen der Zelle begleiten. Sie sind wohl zu unterscheiden von den durch Verletzungen künstlich hervorgerufenen Strömen, die man als Demarkations-, Alterati oder Längsquerschnittsströme bezeichnet hat. Es war von vornherein zu erwarten, daß auch im Zentralnervensystem, das doch eine gewaltige Zellanhäufung darstellt, bioelektrische Erscheinungen nachweisbar seien, und in der Tat ist dieser Nachweis schon verhältnismäßig früh erbracht worden.

Caton [2] hat bereits 1874 Versuche an Kaninchen- und Affenhirnen veröffentlicht, bei denen unpolarisierbare Elektroden entweder an der Oberfläche beider Hemisphären oder die eine Elektrode an der Hirnrinde, die andere an der Schädeloberfläche angelegt worden waren. Die Ströme wurden zu einem empfindlichen Galvanometer abgeleitet. Es fanden sich deutliche Stromschwankungen, die namentlich beim Erwachen aus dem Schlaf und beim Eintritt des Todes sich verstärkten, nach dem Tode schwächer wurden und dann vollständig schwanden. Schon *Caton* konnte nachweisen, daß starke Stromschwankungen bei Belichtung des Auges sich an der Hirnrinde einstellten, und er sprach bereits die Vermutung aus, daß unter Umständen diese Rindenströme zur Lokalisation innerhalb der Hirnrinde verwendet werden könnten.

Fleischl von Marxow [3] hat im Jahre 1883 zuerst beobachtet, daß bei verschiedenen Tieren bei Ableitung von zwei symmetrisch gelegenen

---
[1] *Garten:* Die Produktion von Elektrizität. *Wintersteins* Handbuch der vergleichenden Physiologie 3. Bd., 2. Hälfte, S. 105.
[2] *Caton:* Brit. med. J. 2, 278 (1875). Ref. Zbl. Physiol. 4, Nr 25 (1890). Nach *Bechterew:* Die Energie des lebenden Organismus. S. 102. Wiesbaden 1902.
[3] *Fleischl von Marxow:* Gesammelte Abhandlungen S. 410. Leipzig: J. A. Barth 1893 und Zbl. Physiol. 4 (1890).

Archiv für Psychiatrie. Bd. 87. 35

FIGURE 1-13 ■ The opening page of the first publication reporting the electroencephalogram of humans. Note the acknowledgment to Caton. (From Berger H: Über das Elektrenkephalogram des Menschen. Arch Psychiatr Nervenkr 87:527, 1929.)

REFERENCES

1. Gilbert W: De Magnete, Magneticisque Corporibus et de Magno Magnete Tellure. Peter Short, London, 1600
2. Boyle R: Essays of the Strange Subtility, Determinate Nature, Great Efficacy of Effluviums, to which are Annext New Experiments to Make Fire and Flame Ponderable Together with a Discovery of the Perviousness of Glass. Pitt, London, 1673
3. Boyle R: Experiments and Notes about the Mechanical Origine or Production of Electricity. London, 1675
4. von Haller A: Elementa Physiologiae Corporis Humani. 8 Vols, Bousquet, Lausanne, 1757
5. Fée A: Vie de Linné. In: Mémoires de la Société Royale des Sciences de Lille, 1832
6. Goethe JW: Farbenlehre. Tübingen, 1810
7. Gray S: A letter to Cromwell Mortimer, M.D., Secretary of the Royal Society containing several experiments concerning electricity. Phil Trans, 37–38:18 and 405, 1731
8. Desaguliers JT: A Dissertation Concerning Electricity. Innys and Longman, London, 1742
9. Nollet JA: Recherches sur les Causes Particulières des Phénomènes Électriques. Guérin, Paris, 1749
10. Winkler JH: Gedanken von den Eigenschaften Wirkungen und Ursachen der Electricität. Breitkopf, Leipzig, 1744
11. Hausen CA: Novi Profectus in Historia Electricitatis. Schwann, Leipzig, 1743
12. Du Fay C: Quatrième mémoire sur l'électricité. p. 457. In: Mémoires de l'Académie Royale des Sciences. Paris, 1735
13. Kratzenstein JH: Abhandlung von dem Nutzen der Electricität in der Arznenwissenschaft. Hemmerde, Halle, 1744
14. Krüger JG: Zuschrift an seine Zuhörer worinnen er ihren seine Gedancken von der Electricität mittheilet. Hemmerde, Halle, 1745
15. Stahl GE: Theoria Medica Vera. Halle, 1708
16. Boissier de la Croix de Sauvages F: Dissertation sur la nature et cause de la rage. In: Pièces qui ont Remporté le Prix de l'Académie Royale des Sciences, Inscriptions, et Belles Lettres de Toulouse depuis l'Année 1747 jusqu'à 1750. Forest, Toulouse, 1758
17. Deshais JE: De Hemiplegia per Electricitatem Curanda. Martel, Montpellier, 1749
18. Dufay JTF: An Fluidum Nerveum sit Fluidam Electricum? Martel, Montpellier, 1750
19. Marat JP: Mémoire sur l'Électricité Médicale. Meguignon, Paris, 1784
20. Mangin, L'Abbé de : Histoire Générale et Particulière de l'Électricité ou ce qu'en Ont Dit de Curieux et d'Amusant Quelques Physiciens de l'Europe. 3 Vols. Rollin, Paris, 1752
21. Hunter J: Anatomical observations on the torpedo. Phil Trans, 63:481, 1773
22. Matteucci C: Traité des Phénomènes Électro-physiologiques des Animaux. Suivi d'Études Anatomiques sur le Système Nerveux et sur l'Organe Électrique de la Torpille par Paul Savi. Fortin & Masson, Paris, 1844
23. van Musschenbroek P: Quoted in JA Nollet. In: Mémoires de l'Académie des Sciences. Paris, 1746
24. Bertholon N: De l'Électricité du Corps Humain dans l'État de Santé et de Maladie. 2 Vols. Croulbois, Paris, 1780
25. Bertholon N: De l'Électricité des Végétaux. Didot, Paris, 1783
26. Galvani L: De viribus electricitatis in motu musculare commentarius. De Bononiensi Scientiarum et Artium Instituto atque Academia Commentarii, 7:363, 1791
27. Galvani L: Memorie ed Esperimenti Inediti di Luigi Galvani. Capelli, Bologna, 1937
28. Volta AGA: Letter to Sir Joseph Banks, March 20, 1800 on electricity excited by the mere contact of conducting substances of different kinds. Phil Trans, 90:403, 1800
29. Vivenzio G: Istoria dell'Elettricità Medica. Naples, 1784
30. Sue P: Histoire du Galvanisme. 4 Vols. Bernard, Paris, 1802
31. Fontana FGF: Letter to Urbain Tosetti. p. 159. In: von Haller A (ed): Mémoires sur les Parties Sensibles et Irritables du Corps Animal. 3rd Ed. D'Arnay, Lausanne, 1760
32. Caldani L: Institutiones Physiologicae et Pathologicae. Luchtmans, Leiden, 1784
33. Aldini G: Essai Théorique et Expérimental sur le Galvanisme. 2 Vols. Fournier, Paris, 1804

34. Cerletti U: Electroshock therapy. J Clin Exp Psychopathol, 15:191, 1954

35. Duchenne GBA: De l'Électrisation Localisée, et de son Application à la Pathologie et à la Thérapeutique. Ballière, Paris, 1855

36. Duchenne GBA: Physiologie des Mouvements Démontrée à l'Aide de l'Expérimentation Électrique et de l'Observation Clinique et Applicable à l'Étude des Paralysies et des Déformations. Ballière, Paris, 1867

37. Duchenne GBA: De la Paralysie Musculaire, Pseudohypertrophique ou Paralysie Myo-sclérosique. Asselin, Paris, 1868

38. Comitato di Torino : Classe di Scienza esatta dell'Accademia di Torino. Thermidor Année, 10:27, 1803

39. Prévost JL, Batelli F: La mort par les courants électriques alternatifs à bas voltage. J Physiol Pathol Gén, 1:399, 1899

40. Aldini G: De Animali Electricitate Dissertationes Duae. Lucheron, Bologna, 1794

41. Galvani L: Dell'Uso e dell'Attività dell'Arco Conduttore nelle Contrazioni dei Muscoli. University of Bologna, 1794

42. von Humboldt FA: Versuche über die gereizte Muskel und Nervenfaser. 2 Vols. Decker, Posen & Rottman, Berlin, 1797

43. Pfaff CH: Abhandlung über die sogennante thierische Electrizität. Gren's Journal der Physik, 8:196, 1798

44. Fowler R: Experiments and Observations Relative to the Influence Lately Discovered by M. Galvani, and Commonly Called Animal Electricity. Duncan, Edinburgh, 1793

45. Valli E: Experiments in Animal Electricity. Johnson, London, 1793

46. Schmück EJ: Beiträge zur neuern Kenntniss der thierische Elektricität. Mannheim, 1792

47. Matteucci C: Mémoire sur l'existence du courant électrique musculaire dans les animaux vivants ou récemment tués. Ann Chim, 7:425, 1843

48. Oersted C: Experimenta circa Effectum Conflictis Electrici in Acum Magneticum. J Chem Phys, 29:275, 1820

49. Hermann L: Über sogennanten secondärelectromotorische Erscheinungen an Muskeln und Nerve. Arch Physiol, 33:103, 1884

50. Du Bois-Reymond E: Untersuchungen über thierische Electricität. 2 Vols. Reimer, Berlin, 1848

51. Du Bois-Reymond E: Gesammelte Abhandlungen zur Allgemeinen Muskel- und Nerve-physik. Veit, Leipzig, 1877

52. von Helmholtz H: Messungen über den zeitlichen Verlauf der Zuchung animalischer Muskeln und die Fortpflanzungsgeschwindigkeit der Reizung in den Nerven. Arch Anat Physiol, 276, 1850

53. Caton R: The electric currents of the brain. Br Med J, 2:278, 1875

54. Caton R: On the electric relations of muscle and nerve. Liverpool Med Chir J, 1875

55. Caton R: Interim report on investigation of the electric currents of the brain. Br Med J Suppl, 1:62, 1877

56. Caton R: Researches on electrical phenomena of cerebral grey matter. Ninth International Medical Congress, Trans Cong, 3:246, 1887

57. Caton R: Die Ströme des Centralnervensystems. Centralbl Physiol, 4:758, 1891

58. Gall FJ, Spurzheim JC: Anatomie et Physiologie du Système Nerveux en Général et du Cerveau en Particulier, avec des Observations Intellectuelles et Morales de l'Homme et des Animaux, par Configuration de leur Têtes. Schoell, Paris, 1810

59. Ferrier D: The localisation of function in the brain. Proc R Soc Lond, 22:229, 1873

60. Adrian ED, Matthews BHC: The Berger rhythm: potential changes from the occipital lobes in man. Brain, 57:355, 1934

61. Beck A: The determination of localization in the brain and spinal cord by means of electrical phenomena (in Polish). Rozprawy Wydzialu Matematycvno-przyrodniczych Polska Akademia, series II, 1:186, 1890

62. Beck A: Die Ströme der Nervencentren. Centralbl Physiol, 4:572, 1890

63. Beck A, Cybulski N: Further research on the electrical phenomena of the cerebral cortex in monkeys and dogs (in Polish). Rozprawy Wydzialu Matematycvno-przyrodniczych Polska Akademia, 32:369, 1891

64. Fleischl von Marxow E: Mitteilung betreffend die Physiologie der Hirnrinde. Centralbl Physiol, 4:538, 1890

65. Gotch F, Horsley VAH: Über den Gebrauch der Elektricität für die Lokalisierung der Erregungsscheinungen im Centralnervensystem. Centralbl Physiol, 4:649, 1891

66. Danilevsky VY: Zu Frage über die elektromotorische Vorgänge im Gehirn als Ausdruck seines Tätigkeitzustandes. Centralbl Physiol, 5:1, 1891

67. Schäfer EA: Textbook of Physiology. Pentland, London, 1898

68. Pravdich-Neminsky VV: Ein Versuch der Registrierung der elektrischen Gehirnerscheinungen. Zentralbl Physiol, 27:951, 1913

69. Cybulski N, Jelénska-Macieszyna : Action currents of the cerebral cortex (in Polish). Bull Internat Acad Sci Crac, B:776, 1914

70. Kaufmann PY: Electrical phenomena in cerebral cortex (in Russian). Obzory Psikhiatrii Nevrologii i Eksperimental'noi Psikhologii, 7–8:403, 1912

71. Larionov VE: Galvanometric determination of cortical currents in the area of the tonal centres under stimulation of peripheral acoustic organs (in Russian). Nevrologicheskii Vestnik, 7:44, 1899

72. Larionov VE: Über die musikalischen Centren des Gehirns. Pflüg Arch ges Physiol, 76:608, 1899

73. Berger H: Über des Elektrenkephalogram des Menschen. Arch Psychiatr Nervenkr, 87:527, 1929

74. Verigo BF: Action currents of the brain and medulla (in Russian). Vestnik Klinicheskoi i sudebnoi Psikhiatrii i Nevropathologii, 7:1889

75. Verigo BF: Action currents of the frog's brain. Report of the 3rd Congress of Russian physiologists and biologists, St. Petersburg (in Russian). Vrach, 10:45, 1889

76. Berger H: Psychophysiologie in 12 Vorlesungen. Fischer, Jena, 1921

77. Berger H: Das Elektrenkephalogram des Menschen. Acta Nova Leopoldina, 6:173, 1938

78. Berger H: Psyche. Fischer, Jena, 1940

Electrophysiologic Equipment and Electrical Safety

JOHN A. CADWELL and RICHARD A. VILLARREAL

The development and refinement of instrumentation has been a great asset in the diagnosis of neurologic diseases. With advances in instrumentation, however, physiologists are in danger of making more technologically advanced misinterpretations than previously, so it is important to have an understanding of the basic functions and limitations of modern instrumentation. This chapter will enhance the practitioner's ability to understand how the instrumentation and its limitations may influence the interpretation of signals recorded during routine electrophysiologic studies.

MAJOR COMPONENTS OF AN ELECTRODIAGNOSTIC INSTRUMENT

The major components of an electrodiagnostic instrument are shown in Figure 2-1.

Electrodes

The electrode is the interface between the patient and the instrumentation. The proper application and use of electrodes is one of the most fundamental requirements for

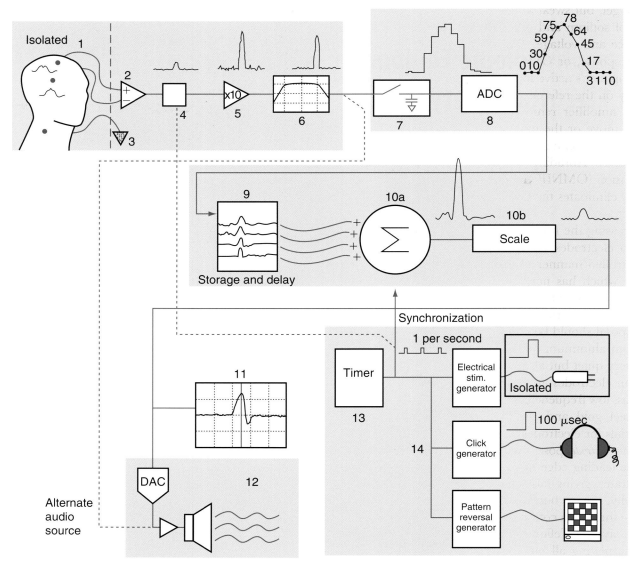

FIGURE 2-1 ■ Major components of an electrodiagnostic instrument. 1, Electrodes pick up electrical signals. 2, Differential input of amplifier removes noise sources common to both active and reference inputs but passes signals that are different at the two inputs. 3, Isolated ground serves as a reference to differential inputs to improve isolation mode rejection ratio. 4, Synchronous switch prevents stimulus artifact from propagating through amplifier. 5, Gain stage of amplifier increases signal to a convenient amplitude for further processing. 6, Filters separate excess noise from signal. 7, Sampling (sample and hold) circuit captures and freezes the signal at frequent intervals. 8, Digitizer converts the continuously variable analog signal to a number proportional to its amplitude. 9, Storage provided for the digital values needed for one sweep. 10, Averager (10a) adds the sweeps together and scales (10b) the results. 11, Data are displayed (along with graticule, cursors, and numerical readouts of certain values). 12, A speaker provides auditory representation of the signal. 13, Timing circuitry (manual or automatic) generates the start-of-sweep, start-of-stimulus, and amplifier switch control signals. 14, Stimulus generator produces electrical shock, auditory, or visual stimulus as appropriate. ADC, analog-to-digital converter; DAC, digital-to-analog converter.

obtaining good signals, but it is often neglected. Electrode characteristics can affect the response. Electrodes can be classified into at least two different types: (1) surface and (2) needle.

Surface electrodes applied with conductive gel form a battery. The voltage of the battery (usually less than 600 mV)

depends primarily on the type of electrode material and secondarily on how good a contact is achieved at the microscopic level. The electrode metals are usually not homogeneous and consist of numerous microscopic or sometimes visible grains. Each grain produces a slightly different battery voltage. The electrolyte is assumed to be the gel, but sweat and serum change the concentrations of sodium and other ions, thus affecting the impedance and voltage. (This is the basis of the galvanic skin response, or GSR.) Most of the battery effect on the amplifier's active input is canceled by an equivalent battery on the reference input. Direct current blocking in the amplifier removes any imbalance. If the electrodes move or the patient sweats, however, the small changes in potential can easily be larger than the signals of interest. Abrading the skin with a ground quartz suspension (OMNIPREP) or puncturing the skin completely eliminates the GSR and much of the movement artifact.

Increasing the homogeneity of the material results in quieter electrodes. Silver electrodes can be corroded in a controlled manner to form a uniform silver chloride finish, which has noise and impedance characteristics better than those of the bare metal. If a silver electrode is abraded, its performance is reduced, and rechloriding or disposal should be considered. Aluminum electrodes form an aluminum oxide layer, which is very uniform and very quiet but also has a very high resistance. Aluminum electrodes are almost purely capacitive and do not pass low frequencies effectively. Tin, platinum, stainless steel, gold, and carbon are also used as fairly stable materials for electrodes.[1]

Needle electrodes pose other problems. Microscopic burrs on the leading edge of the needle damage muscle as it penetrates, giving false evidence of injury in electromyography. These burrs can be detected by passing the needle through a cotton gauze. Monopolar needles have a thin layer of Teflon (polytetrafluoroethylene) or parylene insulating all but the tip. If the insulation cracks or abrades, or if there is a break in the insulation, the needle will be noisy and should be discarded. Materials, manufacturing problems, and damage during transport and handling can also result in increased noise, even in the absence of visible defects. Additional information on the care and testing of needles and electrodes is found elsewhere.[2]

Electrode materials should not be mixed. The battery potentials created by two different materials will not cancel, and if direct-current (DC) blocking does not occur at the first stage of the amplifier, a large offset will be present. This offset may saturate the amplifier or decrease the headroom for saturation, so that clipping of the waveform occurs. The offset may contribute to unacceptable shock artifact. It may also change the operating point of the amplifier, which will degrade noise and performance. Fortunately, most modern amplifiers are designed to tolerate electrode offset.

Amplifier

The amplifier increases the amplitude of the desired response while it rejects unwanted noise. The first and most crucial stage of the amplifier consists of a differential input. A differential input amplifies the difference in potential presented at its two inputs (active and reference), while rejecting any signal common to both of these inputs. *Reference* is often used to mean a neutral input, but this only refers to a location on the body that has very little signal compared with the site of the active electrode. Both *active* and *reference* inputs are equally effective at generating potentials, and there is no *neutral* input on a differential amplifier.

An amplifier's ability to reject common signals is known as its common mode rejection ratio (CMRR). The higher the CMRR, the better the rejection. Another important parameter of the amplifier input is the input impedance. Input impedance has resistive, capacitive, and inductive components. An input impedance of 10 Mohm or higher is desirable because a low input impedance attenuates the signal slightly and degrades the active-to-reference signal matching necessary for high CMRR. The higher-frequency components of a response are affected more by the input capacitance than by the input resistance. Input inductance is usually negligible. Another amplifier differential input characteristic of concern is input voltage noise and input current noise generated by the input circuitry itself. Input noise is added to the response signal.

Gain and Sensitivity

Amplifier *gain* describes how much the input signal is increased in voltage. The units are volts per volt, and gains of 10 to 10,000 are common. *Display sensitivity* describes the visible waveform and is expressed as volts per division or volts per centimeter. Smaller numerical values represent increased sensitivity; thus, 1 mV/cm is more sensitive than 10 mV/cm. A graphic display shows a vertical deflection proportional to the voltage, and changing the gain alters the size of the display. A computer displays the digital representation of the analog signals, which maintains the concept of sensitivity at any convenient gain setting for which the amplifier is designed. In most newer systems, the amplifier gain either is fixed or has a few discrete steps, and the display system is changed digitally.

Analog Filters

The stages following the differential input amplify and filter the response signal. Low-cut (low-frequency cutoff) and high-cut (high-frequency cutoff) filters are used to

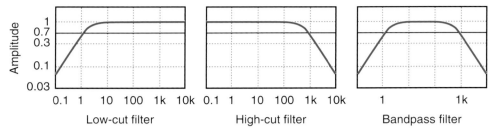

FIGURE 2-2 ■ Relationship of amplitude to frequency for single-pole filters at 1 Hz and 1 kHz.

narrow the frequency range of the incoming signal (Fig. 2-2), and thus eliminate that portion of the noise outside the bandpass of the response signal. (Signal processing textbooks generally refer to highpass, lowpass, and bandpass filters for mathematical reasons. A bandpass from 10 to 1,000 Hz has a 10-Hz highpass and a 1,000-Hz lowpass. The designations *low-cut* and *high-cut* sidestep this confusing terminology and are used in this chapter.) The signal will also be affected if it has frequency components outside the bandpass; the filters are therefore adjustable to keep most of the signal and reject most of the noise. A component of the noise will always overlap the signal and cannot be reduced without distorting the signal (Fig. 2-3).

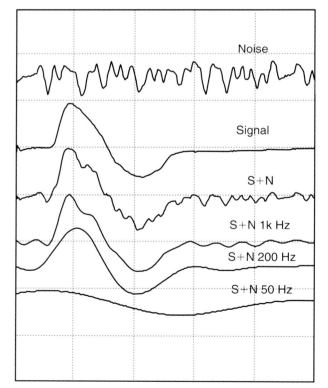

FIGURE 2-3 ■ A signal (S) with peak energy at 150 Hz and noise (N) with peak energy at 1 kHz are added and then high-cut filtered at 1,000, 200, and 50 Hz. Optimal signal-to-noise ratio is achieved at 200 Hz.

Notch filters provide precise band-reject capability and are tuned for 50- or 60-Hz operation. The "Q" (quality) of a filter is a mathematical measure of its resonance. High-Q filters respond to a narrow but precise range of frequencies. They are used for 50- and 60-Hz notches because signals that are only a few Hertz above or below the notch frequency are passed transparently. Low-Q filters respond to a wide range of frequencies and are used for bandpass applications. Comb filters function like multiple-notch filters, which are tuned to successive harmonics of the mains frequency (Fig. 2-4). Combs remove these harmonics, which make the "buzzing" sound commonly heard from 50- or 60-Hz interference.

The cutoff frequency of a filter is the frequency at which the output power is half of the input power (–6 dB) or the output voltage is 0.707 times the input voltage (–3 dB). Except for brickwall filters, the output power increases or decreases smoothly with frequency, as shown in Figure 2-2. Changes in frequency are measured in octaves (doubling or halving of the frequency) or decades (increases or decreases tenfold). The simplest filters have a single pole and will roll off, or attenuate, the signal by 6 dB for every doubling of the frequency (6 dB per octave or 10 dB per decade), but they will also cause attenuation and phase shift well away from the –3 dB point, as shown in Table 2-1. (The word *pole* is an engineering term used in describing transfer functions; one pole represents a single resistance-capacitance [RC] filter.)

TABLE 2-1 ■ Effect of a 1,000-Hz Single-Pole High-Cut Filter			
Input (Hz)	Amplitude	Percent Decrease	dB Decrease
100	0.99	1	0.04
500	0.89	11	1
1,000	0.707	29	3
2,000	0.44	56	7
10,000	0.10	90	20
100,000	0.01	99	40

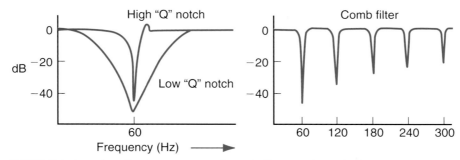

FIGURE 2-4 ■ Amplitude responses of notch filters and comb filter.

To separate noise and signal more effectively, steeper filters are used. Two-pole and four-pole filters are common. Each additional pole adds 6 dB per octave (10 dB per decade) attenuation. These filters are usually more than cascaded one-pole filters, having feedback and feedforward paths. Varying the amount of feedback and feedforward varies the overshoot, phase, rolloff characteristics, and amplitude ringing. Special cases of filters have specific designations, but all are part of a continuum consisting of just a few distinct topologies (Fig. 2-5). Thus, the Butterworth has the flattest passband at the expense of poor rolloff; the Bessel has constant phase delay for all frequencies; the Chebyshev has maximal transition steepness at the expense of passband ripple; the elliptic filter has infinite rolloff with rebound in the stopband; the notch is a special elliptic filter that rebounds back to 0 dB; and a brickwall filter has infinite slope without rebound at the expense of maximum "ringing." (For analog circuits, anything over 100 dB per decade is a brickwall.) Further discussion of analog filters is provided elsewhere.[3]

Analog-to-Digital Conversion

Analog-to-digital conversion requires a circuit to "freeze" the signal for a few microseconds, the sample and hold (S/H), and a circuit to convert the amplitude of the "frozen" signal to a digital value, the analog-to-digital converter (ADC). Sometimes these circuits are implemented in one device, and so they will be referred to collectively as the ADC. The ADC is specified by its conversion rate and its resolution (number of bits).

Digital Circuitry

The digital section consists of three major parts: processor, memory, and averager. The processor is the "brain" of the instrument; it coordinates all data flow and interface functions. Processors are classified by the number of bits processed in parallel and by the processing speed.

Memory is used for processor instruction storage and for digitized signal storage. The amount of memory is expressed in bytes. The averager adds and scales synchronized signal responses to improve the signal-to-noise ratio and may be implemented by the processor.

ADVANTAGES OF DIGITAL CIRCUITRY

Operations on digital signals are precise. Adding two analog signals gives a result with a percentage error, and the errors are cumulative. Two digital signals added together will always give precisely the same result. The chip or the components that add two analog signals will shift or drift with time, temperature, humidity, power supply voltage, and other factors. They may require calibration or compensation, and sometimes they cannot be made to work at all. The chip that adds two digital signals always gives exactly the same answer and is insensitive to its environment. Digital systems eliminate analog drift with time and temperature, and eliminate some of the need to recalibrate. Analog component values vary, but digital coefficients are absolute. A capacitor with ±0.1 percent tolerance in a filter is an exotic part, but a 16-bit digital system has 0.001 percent accuracy, is easy and inexpensive to build, and never changes with time or temperature. Every digital unit is also exactly like every other unit, so fabrication and characterization are simplified. Digital systems can perform functions that are not practical and sometimes not possible with analog systems. Almost all analysis is easier to perform digitally. Processor performance has increased tenfold with each of the last two editions of this book, and the price and power requirements have fallen. There are now few problems or solutions that are not easier, less expensive, and more reliable to solve or implement digitally.

DIGITAL FILTERS

In most electrodiagnostic instruments, analog filters are used sparingly and have been replaced by digital filters. Digital filters can duplicate analog filters, but they can

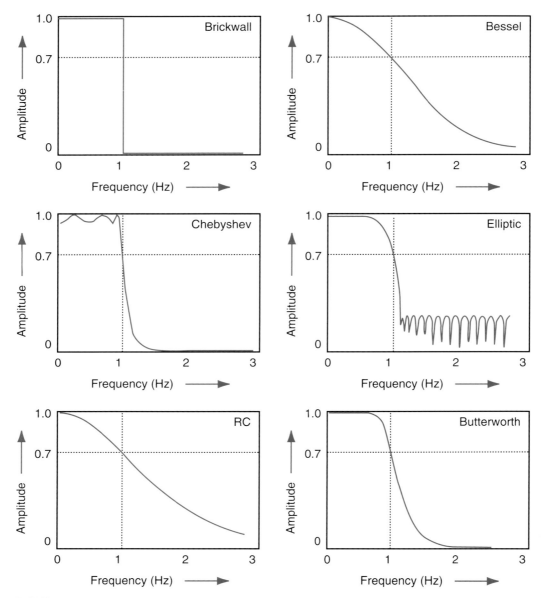

FIGURE 2-5 ■ The relationship of amplitude to frequency for six different filter types. RC, resistance-capacitance.

also create classes of filters not readily implemented from analog components. If implemented correctly, multipole digital filters can be superior to the analog equivalent. Multipole analog filters require components that are subject to temperature and aging variations; these act to "detune" the filter.

Two major types of digital filters are the infinite impulse response (IIR) and the finite impulse response (FIR) filters. In an IIR filter (Fig. 2-6), a portion of the output data is fed back to the input. If the output does not feed back, the filter is nonrecursive and is classified as an FIR filter. The feedback term in an IIR represents the contribution of previous data points to the output. Because only a few terms are needed (two terms for each two poles), efficient filters

are realizable. IIRs act much like analog filters. The *infinite* means that, like an RC network, the output approaches its final value asymptotically.

FIRs (Fig. 2-7) compute each output from weighted portions of a limited number of past, present, and future input data points. Each point used in the computation is called a filter tap, and each tap requires a multiply-and-accumulate operation. If the FIR is symmetric (i.e., uses the same number of taps and matching coefficients into the future as into the past), then there is zero phase shift. Evoked potentials can be smoothed without changing their latency. (Three-point smoothing algorithms are FIRs.) Obviously, the future is never known in the real world, even for the upcoming few milliseconds.

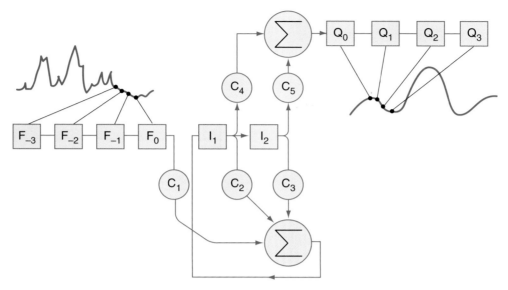

FIGURE 2-6 ▪ A two-pole (biquad) infinite impulse response filter uses five coefficients that determine the filter frequency and type, and requires only two intermediate terms.

An FIR filter avoids this problem by delaying the output for half the number of taps and moving the time reference by the same amount. In a real-time system, all frequencies are delayed by the same amount and only the relative phases have zero shift. This trick has a small price. Steep-skirted filters are accompanied by ringing whenever an edge or impulse occurs; this is called *Gibbs' phenomenon*. Because zero has been shifted out in time, half of the ringing occurs before the impulse and can sometimes be seen

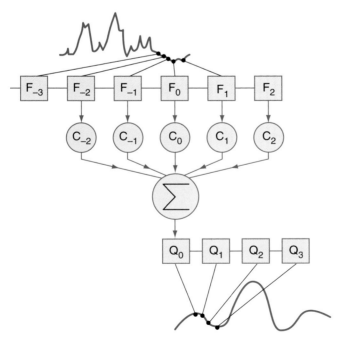

FIGURE 2-7 ▪ A five-tap finite impulse response filter. Computation of Q_0 is delayed until F_{-2} is loaded. If coefficient C_2 equals C_{-2}, and C_1 equals C_{-1}, phase shift is eliminated.

before the stimulus. The additional peaks created by Gibbs' phenomenon are artifact, as is their occurrence before the stimulus. Such peaks have been interpreted and presented as new responses previously hidden by the noise or as anticipatory potentials.[4]

Digital filter characteristics, including cutoff frequency and the number of poles, are determined by their coefficients. Adjustable frequencies do not require more resistors, capacitors, and analog switches; they only require changing a set of numbers in the processor and adding computational power. High-cut, low-cut, and notch filters for multiple channels are typically implemented with a single processor.

Fast Fourier transforms (FFT) are a class of algorithms that turn time data into frequency-phase data and vice versa. They are especially convenient for looking at a signal's frequency characteristics and for implementing brickwall or other arbitrary filters. Fast refers to algorithms implementing the Fourier transform by eliminating redundant calculations to speed up computation. A brickwall filter is implemented by performing the FFT, zeroing out all unwanted frequency terms, and then performing an inverse FFT. Brickwall filters show maximum Gibbs' phenomenon but are maximally effective at reducing noise outside the passband.

Display

A response can be presented visually and audibly. Historically, electromyographic instruments (EMG) used analog oscilloscope displays, where the response signal vertically deflects an electron beam as it sweeps horizontally across the face of a phosphor-coated tube. All modern systems use digital displays, which create pictures by illuminating individual pixels (dots) on a screen to create a picture. Digital displays have inherent persistence supplied by video memory instead of by long-persistence phosphors. Other advantages that oscilloscopes once had can be simulated with clever programming, and the ability to combine waveforms and graphical and textual information on one display has eliminated oscilloscope technology.

Auditory presentation of the response is useful not only in helping to classify a response but also in detecting and identifying noise. Types of interference from power lines, fluorescent lights, cathode ray tube (CRT) displays, biologic artifact such as EMG activity, electrode artifact, and sterilizing ovens are easily identified by their characteristic sounds.

Stimulators

ELECTRICAL STIMULATORS

Stimulation occurs when the voltage across the nerve membrane is decreased enough to initiate depolarization. The nerve has sodium ion pumps that normally maintain a resting potential, and the stimulating current must overwhelm the pumping capability. To do this requires a fairly constant charge per stimulus. The charge is the area under the curve of an amplitude–duration plot, and accounts for intensity, pulse width, and wave shape. The most common wave shape is a square wave because it is easy to generate. Other wave shapes will not change the charge requirements, although wild claims have been made to the contrary. If the charge is introduced very slowly with the use of a low-amplitude, long-duration pulse, the nerve is able to compensate partially for the stimulus and requires more total charge for depolarization. The strength–duration curve shows this relationship, which varies for different tissues.

Several caveats and exceptions are well known. If the nerve is initially hyperpolarized and then depolarized, the total charge required can be reduced. A biphasic stimulus can also be used to achieve zero net charge transfer, which may eliminate electrolysis and possible tissue injury in direct nerve stimulation. In polysynaptic systems (the brain), both inhibition and potentiation are observed with paired pulses, depending on the interstimulus intervals.

Constant, as in constant current, means that the output remains at the specified, adjustable level. Constant-current stimulators have high output impedance and allow the output voltage to change to maintain the desired current. Constant-voltage stimulators have low output impedance and allow the output current to vary to maintain the desired voltage. Other stimulators have finite output

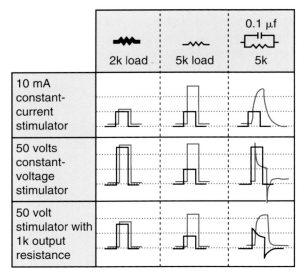

FIGURE 2-8 ■ Current and voltage outputs of three stimulator types and three loads. Body impedance is similar to load 3, with both resistive and capacitive components. One vertical division represents 10 mA (black line) and 20 volts (lighter line, offset slightly above and to the right).

impedance and allow both voltage and current to change as the load impedance changes (Fig. 2-8).

Constant current has the theoretical advantage that the product of duration and current determines the stimulator's effectiveness. Some authors claim that constant current is less painful, but this is both subjective and sensitive to technique and methodology. Constant-current stimulators will deliver the same current as electrode gel dries out, an advantage for those who do not or cannot check electrodes.

Constant-voltage stimulators will deliver a stimulus to the nerve, even if a small amount of gel or body fluid is shorting the leads. It will charge the body capacitance quickly and then deliver full current, and so it is a more powerful stimulator.

Electrical stimulators produce large voltages that can introduce artifact into the waveform. Some of the artifact occurs if the amplifier saturates and has a long recovery time. In 1980 the authors began turning the amplifiers off during the stimulus to reduce amplifier recovery time. Clamping the stimulator output immediately after the stimulus or putting out a biphasic wave to remove the charge stored by the body, or both, is also useful. If the stimulus is completely isolated, very little current should be common to both stimulator and amplifier. Complete isolation is difficult to obtain; instead, the upgoing voltage on one stimulator electrode and the downgoing voltage on the other are designed to have equal capacitive coupling back to ground to cancel out amplifier-stimulator leakage currents.

AUDITORY STIMULATORS

The brainstem auditory evoked potential (BAEP) is generated by acoustic signals between 4 and 8 kHz. A 100-μsec square-wave click has most of its energy in this band. The click is amplitude-controlled between 0 and 130 dB, a range of over 3,000,000 : 1. Careful attention to noise and inadvertent feedthrough is needed for this dynamic range. Headphones capable of faithfully reproducing the electric pulse generate an auditory click. Both magnetic transducers and piezoelectric transducers are used. The magnetic transducers mounted on a headband generate a small electrically coupled artifact at the beginning of the sweep. Piezoelectric transducers are usually placed about a foot away from the ear on a hollow acoustic coupling tube, using spongy inserts to hold the tube in the ear canal and to suppress ambient noise. Because the click takes about 1 msec to traverse the tube, all components of the response are separated from the artifact by 1 msec.

VISUAL STIMULATORS

Visual stimulators for eliciting evoked potentials depend on the rapidly changing contrast along the edges of checks to produce a response. Raster scan, plasma and liquid-crystal display (LCD) TV monitors and light-emitting diode (LED) checkerboards are used. The LED checkerboard generators can reverse the on-off pattern almost instantly. The raster scanned displays take from 0 to 16.7 msec to change patterns, related to the time it takes for the beam to sweep the display. This stimulus lag shows up as a smearing and an 8-msec latency shift of the responses compared with the LED responses, Other display technologies have delays that vary by manufacturer and user setup, and require calibration and normal values for the stimulator used. Check size, contrast, intensity, and the subject's visual acuity also affect the response, as discussed in Chapter 22.

MAGNETIC STIMULATORS

Magnetic stimulators generate a 1- to 2-Tesla magnetic field in 50 to 100 μsec, which induces a voltage in peripheral nerves or cerebral cortex sufficient to achieve depolarization. The principle is the same as that for a transformer, in which a changing magnetic field induces a voltage around it. The stimulator is the primary of the transformer, and the cortex is the single-turn secondary. The body is almost perfectly transparent to the magnetic field, and so currents can be induced below the skin with minimal or no pain. Magnetic stimulators allow measurement of motor evoked potentials, which are discussed in Chapter 28.

Software

The algorithms used to control the instrument are known as the *software*. The resources allocated to write the software exceed the effort to design the modern electrodiagnostic instrument. To partition the design effort, most systems have multiple processors, each of which controls a portion of the system. The various stimulators and the amplifier may each have a dedicated processor and associated software or firmware. The software may reside in various formats in an instrument. Software that is programmed into nonvolatile memory is called *firmware*. Software resides on hard disk or CD-ROM and is loaded into system memory during initialization. The design and reliability of the software have a large influence on the utility of an instrument.

As EMG instruments, and especially the reports and data they generate, become less stand-alone and more integrated into electronic records and connected computer systems, software design becomes more demanding. The user interface becomes more critical; it must appear simple and intuitive when, in fact, increased effort is needed to make it more intuitive. The underlying software components have to be cleanly partitioned so that maintenance and testing of the hardware, acquisition, and user interface can be verified. Awareness of and adherence to software standards allow other systems to access, utilize, and display the results, and may allow collaboration in ways that proprietary solutions preclude.

FACTORS THAT REDUCE SIGNAL FIDELITY

Noise

Physiologic signals are mixed with noise. Low-level signals of all sorts are plagued with noise, and it is noise that limits the resolution and precision of the signal measurement. Noise usually refers to *white noise*, but several other types of noise, with multiple sources and varied solutions, are worth considering. Advances in technology have also introduced new noise sources.

WHITE NOISE

Random noise or white noise sounds like a harsh "shhhhhh." It is generated by processes that are statistical in nature, and has uniform energy in all frequency bands (energy per band = constant). A 10 k-ohm resistor at room temperature generates about 0.3 μV of white noise across its leads just lying on a bench. This thermal noise, generated by agitated electrons, places an absolute lower limit on amplifier quietness unless the system is cooled to absolute zero or unless the input impedance is reduced to zero. Passing a current through the resistor creates additional pink noise (energy per band = 1/frequency), which has a more musical "shhhhh" sound. Because cooling (of patients) is not practical, skin preparation and conductive gel are required to decrease impedance, and high-impedance amplifiers are necessary for decreasing current flow. The preamplifier has additional noise determined by engineering choices, and generally cannot be improved easily. The electroencephalogram (EEG) is nearly random noise (in evoked potential studies), as is weak background EMG activity; these are usually the dominant sources of white noise.

IMPULSE NOISE

Impulse noise sounds like a "pop," "crack," or "click" and includes transistor "popcorn" noise, static discharge, EMG artifact, artifact from metal dental fillings touching intermittently, and electrode movement. *Impulse noise*, as used here, is present for a short time in only one epoch, unlike random noise, which is present uniformly throughout each epoch.

MAINS NOISE

Mains 50- or 60-Hz interference (assumed 60 Hz in this discussion) produces a continuous audible buzz if harmonics are present, but it is inaudible or barely audible otherwise. It is induced by magnetic induction and by capacitive coupling. Harmonics are present when iron-core transformers, dimmers, and fluorescent lights are nearby. The energy is all at 60 Hz, 120 Hz, 180 Hz, and so forth, and is usually biggest in the odd harmonics (e.g., 180 Hz, 300 Hz); the energy in high-order harmonics drops rapidly.

IN-BAND NOISE SOURCE

Cellular telephones, high-efficiency fluorescent lights, switching power supplies for laptops, and blood pressure cuffs with digital readouts are examples of the profusion of noise sources. Regulatory mandates to control such sources are growing in response to the awareness of their adverse effect on sensitive measurements. Most of these emit electrical noise in the 1,000- to 100,000-Hz range, which either steps on the signal of interest or is poorly rejected by the amplifier. Awareness and avoidance are essential.

SYNCHRONOUS NOISE

Synchronous noise is time-locked with stimulation and averaging. It can be generated by numerous sources:

1. The instrument processor generating the stimulus executes the same instruction sequence and may radiate a characteristic burst of energy.
2. The timer used to generate the stimulus rate may radiate electrical noise.
3. Electrical stimulator recovery may have an abrupt turnoff after many milliseconds.
4. The power supply may be modulated by the slightly increased power demands during stimulation.
5. Headphones with a low-frequency resonance may ring down for several milliseconds.
6. The patient may blink or track the target used to elicit visual evoked potentials (VEPs), thereby introducing electroretinogram (ERG) signals.

SIGNAL-TO-NOISE RATIO (SNR)

The relative size of the signal to the noise determines how well the signal can be visualized or even detected. The evoked potential signal present in any one epoch is 1 to 100 times smaller than the background noise. The electrodiagnostic equipment must obtain an SNR that is better than 3 : 1 for reproducible testing. Figure 2-9 is a graphic presentation of SNR values.

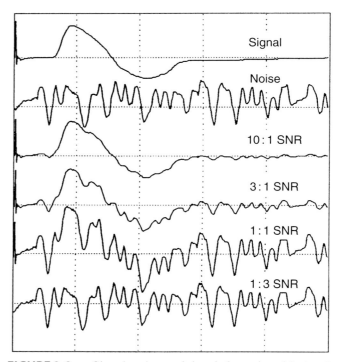

FIGURE 2-9 ■ Signal, noise, and signal plus noise with signal-to-noise ratios of 1:3, 1:1, 3:1, and 10:1.

SNR is expressed as an integer ratio or in dB:

$$\mathrm{SNR} = \frac{\mathrm{signal}}{\mathrm{noise}}$$

or

$$\mathrm{SNR_{dB}} = 20 \ \log \left(\frac{\mathrm{signal}}{\mathrm{noise}}\right)$$

Decibel notation is convenient because both large ratios (e.g., $100{,}000{:}1 = 100$ dB) and small ratios (e.g., $0.25{:}1 = -12$ dB) are easily represented, and because gain calculations use addition instead of multiplication (e.g., the product of a gain of 5 and a gain of 15 is a gain of 75, which is the same as 14 dB + 23.5 dB = 37.5 dB). The slope of analog filters is constant when plotted on a log-log scale, and the slope is then numerically the rolloff in dB per decade. Decibels are a relative scale given in logarithmic values. The reference (denominator of the ratio) must be specified for the decibel notation to be useful. For filters and amplifiers or attenuators, the reference is the input voltage. For SNR, the reference is the noise voltage. The audiometric reference uses an absolute pressure value of 0.0002 dyne/cm^2 to define 0 dB SPL (sound pressure level).

Most noise in electrodiagnostic instruments originates at the amplifier input and is measured at the output. Noise measurements are specified "referred to the input" by taking the noise on the display and dividing by the gain to get an equivalent noise at the amplifier jacks. Amplifier noise is measured with the inputs shorted (there will be additional noise with a patient connected) and is usually specified in μV RMS. The average or root-mean-square (RMS) noise relates to the heating capability of the signal. It has convenient mathematical properties and can be measured with an RMS voltmeter, but the heating capability is not intuitive on inspection. White noise has a gaussian distribution, and so a few large spikes will appear above a surface of more average spikes. Peak-to-peak noise voltage is seen directly on the display. To estimate peak-to-peak noise, exclude the largest single excursion in each direction to eliminate the right-sided tail of the gaussian curve (Fig. 2-10). To convert from peak-to-peak to RMS, multiply by 0.14 for white noise and by 0.35 for sine waves.

Amplifier noise should be measured periodically or when problems are suspected. Static discharge (even without visible or sensible sparks) can damage sensitive input transistors, which have no input protection, decreasing the input impedance and adding enormous

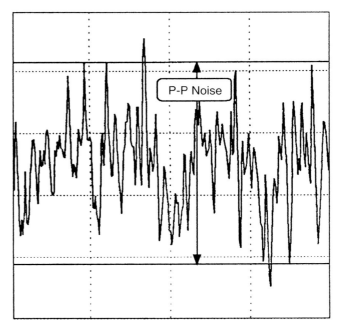

FIGURE 2-10 ▪ Peak-to-peak noise measurement uses the typical largest peaks found by excluding the single largest upgoing and downgoing peak.

amounts of noise. The measurement is performed by running an average with inputs shorted. Set gains to 10 μV per division (settings vary by system, but use the same settings each time and save a copy of the results for future reference); filters 10 to 3 k; scale × 100; average count to 1,000 trials; and measure the peak-to-peak voltage. Channels with more than twice as much noise as the others are suspect.

Filters

Fidelity means that the observed signal is the same as the originating signal. Fidelity requires that the bandwidth of the system be adequately wide, that amplitude is scaled linearly, and that phase relationships of the component sine waves are preserved. Filters can reduce fidelity, but in most cases fidelity has less value than good SNR. Moreover, the originating signal cannot be determined precisely unless excellent SNRs are obtainable. It is important to understand the results of intended or incidental distortion. Signals that are smoother have fewer high-frequency components and distort less (e.g., VEPs). Square waves and signals with fast rising and falling edges have the largest high-frequency components and distort more easily (e.g., potentials recorded by the needle EMG).

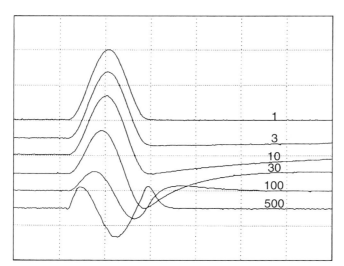

FIGURE 2-11 ■ A frequency limited impulse is low-cut filtered at six different frequencies, showing undershoot and later an overshoot. The gain of the bottom waveform has been increased tenfold.

Increasing the low-cut filters stabilizes the baseline, but it also removes low-frequency signals and adds a phase to the trailing edge of the signal (Fig. 2-11). Two-pole and higher-order low-cuts can add an additional small trailing phase. Digital low-cut filters can add a phase to the leading edge of the signal.

Decreasing the high-cut filter frequency reduces white noise and results in smoother waves. Single-pole high-cuts round the edges of fast signals but do not add overshoot. Most filters of two or more poles cause overshoot and undershoot, creating what appears to be an additional phase (Fig. 2-12). Digital high-cut filters can do worse, adding lightly damped ripple both preceding and following the edges (Fig. 2-13). Digital high-cuts can be made to act exactly like analog filters, but the steeper skirts available digitally allow better noise control, especially for evoked potential studies.

Filters are a special source of synchronous noise. Steeply skirted filters and notch filters are resonant circuits that feed forward a signal equal in amplitude but opposite in phase to the noise presumed present. If the skirts or notch are in the signal passband, the resonance will create ringing artifact (Fig. 2-14). Large shock artifact, motor nerve conduction responses, and the expected responses of evoked potentials all can cause this ringing. Digital filters, as explained before, can cause ringing that precedes the response. VEPs and the compound muscle action potential have peak energy centered at about 60 Hz and are grossly distorted by 50- or 60-Hz notch filters. All filters tend to smear sharp pulses and can obscure the signal.

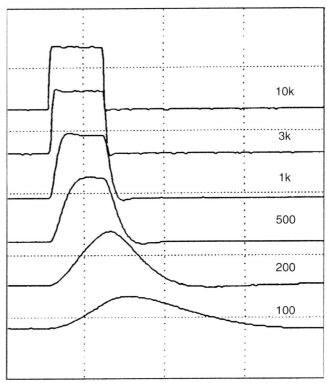

FIGURE 2-12 ■ A square-wave input is high-cut filtered at six different frequencies, showing increasing rounding of the leading and trailing edges.

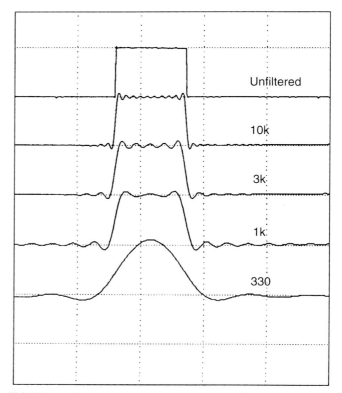

FIGURE 2-13 ■ A 3-msec square wave is filtered at four different frequencies by a brickwall zero phase-shift digital filter. The amplitude of the overshoot is constant for all four settings.

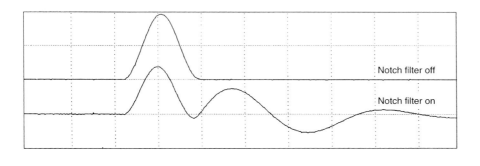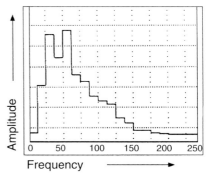

FIGURE 2-14 ▪ An 8-msec frequency limited impulse has peak energy between 25 and 60 Hz, as shown by its frequency analysis. When the 60-Hz notch is turned on, the impulse is grossly distorted.

Saturation

Saturation is inherent in all systems when the output signal nears the power supply voltage. The incremental gain is then near zero, and further input causes no change in the output. If the amplifier gain is turned up, large noise-spikes will be clipped sooner, reducing the noise contribution. However, sometimes allowing the amplifier or filters to block can generate long, exponentially decaying artifact after the overvoltage as the amplifier comes back to life. Large power-supply currents and voltage changes can also couple into other circuits. By designing a voltage clamp, instead of waiting for saturation to occur, large-amplitude noise can be removed with immediate recovery after the spike. Clamping can be implemented with analog or digital circuits.

Aliasing

Analog signals are continuous in time and amplitude. They are digitized by taking samples at intervals and recording a numerical value for each sample. Sampling is usually done at regular intervals. Events occurring between samples are lost. If the sampling rate is too slow for a rapidly changing event that covers multiple data points, the event is grossly distorted and reappears at a different frequency: this is called aliasing. Aliasing appears on television when wagon wheels that are moving rapidly forward appear to be moving slowly backward. Limiting the frequency range of the signal limits the allowable complexity of an event. Sampling the frequency-limited event at twice the maximum signal frequency (known as the Nyquist sampling rate) just barely captures the event without aliasing. If a blip does occur between samples, it must have high-frequency components and the assumption about the maximum signal frequency is untrue (Fig. 2-15). White noise and other noise often have high frequencies. After sampling, noise frequency components above the half-Nyquist rate will reappear below the half-Nyquist rate and will be added back in as increased noise at a lower frequency. If averaging is used, the new noise will average out as described earlier, although the noise can still be excessive. In EEG, EMG, and nerve conduction studies that do not use averaging, the high-frequency noise appears as increased signal noise. Mains interference has continuous sinusoidal components that alias as new sinusoidal components at a lower frequency, possibly in the delta, theta, alpha, or beta bands of the EEG signal, causing confusion or misinterpretation. EMG artifact is several times worse in an EEG record without adequate antialiasing.

To avoid aliasing, either the higher frequencies must be removed with analog filters prior to sampling or the sampling rate must be increased. Practical systems use sampling rates well above the Nyquist rate, usually 3 to 10 times higher than needed (i.e., 6 to 20 times the

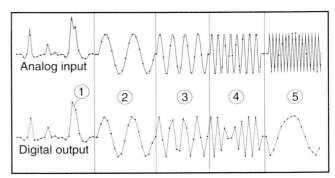

FIGURE 2-15 ▪ Effect of sampling on various signals. In Section 1, the pointer shows that the output is missing one serration present on the input electromyographic signal. Section 2 is adequately sampled (9 times the signal frequency). Section 3 is marginally sampled (4×). Section 4 is inadequately sampled (2×). Section 5 is aliased, and the output frequency is less than the input frequency.

highest signal frequency). The higher sampling rate eases analog antialiasing filter requirements, and it makes waveform reconstruction possible with the use of a straight-line segment to connect the samples.

Quantization

Each analog sample is converted to a number by the ADC. The precision of that number determines how accurately it represents the original analog value. Whatever precision is chosen, the leftover is rounded up or down and the difference is called the quantizing error. The bit length of a word can be picked by choosing an acceptable quantizing error. One decimal place of precision equals 3.3 digital bits. If 1 percent accuracy is needed, the product of 2 decimal places and 3.3 (i.e., 6.6 or 7 bits) is used. Accuracy of 0.1 percent requires 10 bits, and so on. Nonlinearity, nonmonotonicity, and other ADC errors further decrease the digitizing accuracy.

As in the decimal system, where the rightmost digit is the least significant digit, the rightmost bit is the least significant bit (lsb) in the binary system. The term *lsb* as a percentage of full-scale error is used to describe the noise characteristics of the system. The quantization error is, by definition, one-half lsb for an ideal ADC. For example, an 8-bit ADC has 0.4 percent resolution (i.e., 1 part in 256), and the largest quantizing error would be ± 0.2 percent. Quantization error is a problem if the data are too "grainy" for the application because such error is a noise source. Quantization is also a problem when a small difference between two large digitized values is computed. This may occur internally as an intermediate step in a computation for digital filters, FFTs, and other algorithms. If quantization error is minimal and the data are sampled at an adequate rate, the analog and digital representations of the signal are equally valid. Further information is available elsewhere.[4]

Instrument Malfunction

CALIBRATION

Modern electrodiagnostic instruments typically do not have any user-adjustable calibration controls. If the instrument requires some sort of calibration, the calibration is performed internally, usually at power-up. The operator's manual should be consulted for any user-initiated calibration requirements.

Most electrophysiologic systems have built-in signal generators that help to verify basic operation. More advanced systems have software-controllable signal generators and amplifier settings to allow automatic verification of all gain,

filter, and montage setups. Other verification functions may include self-test of random access memory (RAM), read-only memory (ROM), and communication links. Overall system performance becomes more difficult to ascertain as the amount of data manipulation increases. System verification must be performed on a regular basis. Such verification requires that prerecorded input data are processed correctly and that all gains and filter settings are correct.

BAD ELECTRODES

Broken and damaged electrodes are one of the most common causes of poor responses. Electrodes are subject to repeated twisting, bending, and pulling, as well as to chemical attack from solvents and conductive gels. Broken or intermittent contact of the electrode wire can cause anything from loss of signal to increased noise. Intermittent contact caused by a wire broken inside the insulation is difficult to detect. Using pre-gelled disposable electrodes after the expiration date may result in excessive impedance. Using disposable electrodes or replacing electrodes on a regular basis will help to prevent electrode problems.

DAMAGED ACOUSTIC TRANSDUCERS

It is difficult to tell whether the audible click of an auditory stimulator has the needed 4 to 8 kHz components. A good telephone connection, for example, has no frequencies above 2,700 Hz, and the loss of higher frequencies is hardly detectable. Headphones that are used at high stimulus intensities will degrade rapidly, producing subsequent BAEPs of poor quality.

SIGNAL-ENHANCING TECHNIQUES

Common Mode Rejection Ratio

Signals of interest may be as small as 0.1 μV, and the ambient noise at 60 Hz may be a full volt (−120 dB SNR) or more. Averaging will add only 30 dB to the SNR, so a lot of help is needed to obtain a good response. The amplifier is responsible for most of the noise control. The 60-Hz noise is common to both active and reference inputs, and is called a common mode voltage (CMV). By subtracting reference from active, the CMV will disappear. Any "signal" common to both active and reference inputs will also disappear (Fig. 2-16). The efficacy of the differential amplifier at rejecting common mode signals is the common mode rejection ratio (CMRR) and is typically between 10,000:1 and 100,000:1 (80 to 100 dB).

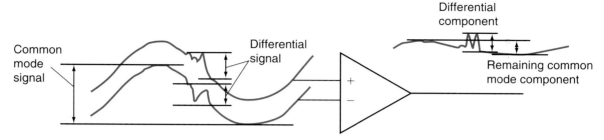

FIGURE 2-16 ▪ A differential amplifier with a common mode rejection ratio of 10:1 will reduce the output 60-Hz signal by the same ratio. Any difference between active and reference inputs is amplified.

The high CMRR of an amplifier is produced by subtracting two extremely similar signals. Any signal mismatch between active and reference inputs causes a difference-error that decreases CMRR. One such mismatch results from unequal electrode impedance. Because the amplifier has finite input impedance, any mismatch in patient electrode impedance will produce different voltages at each input. In 1970, a typical 1-Mohm impedance amplifier required electrode matching within 1 k ohm to achieve 60 dB of CMRR. Modern (FET and MOSFET) amplifiers have typical inputs of 5 picofarad capacitance in parallel with 10^9 to 10^{12} ohms resistance, which gives about 5×10^8 ohms impedance at 60 Hz. The new CMRR computation, assuming 10 k ohms electrode impedance mismatch, is 100 dB. Thus, impedance mismatch is a smaller factor in determining actual CMRR for the modern instrument.

CMRR drops rapidly with increasing frequency and will not effectively remove 15-kHz TV noise, AM radio stations, or similar signals. (Radio frequency filters and appropriate high-cut filters are used instead.) CMRR is usually specified with inputs shorted and at a frequency of 50 or 60 Hz.

An amplifier CMRR above 100 dB does not necessarily improve the rejection of 50- or 60-Hz interference. This is because of the presence of induced currents flowing in the body. Microamp currents are induced by the body's capacitance to noise sources and to earth. The current flowing through the body results in a differential voltage between two spatially separated electrodes that the amplifier will not reject.

Grounding

PATIENT GROUNDING

By tying the body to earth ground, the 50- or 60-Hz mains interference can be reduced by 10 to 100 times. Earth ground is not a reference for each of the differential amplifiers; rather, it is used to drain off the excess common mode voltage. The voltage induced on the body is capacitively coupled. It is induced by coupling between the exposed area of the body; the dielectric of free space; and the area of wire, lamp, or whatever equipment has large noise voltages. Ground forms a low (1 to 100 k ohm) impedance shunt for these signals. Tying the body to earth is a potential safety hazard to the patient and is *not* recommended as a means of reducing common mode interference. Modern equipment connects the patient to an isolated ground, instead of to earth ground, to eliminate the potential safety hazard when earth ground is utilized.

INSTRUMENT GROUNDING

The chassis of the electrophysiologic instrument is connected to earth ground by a ground wire in the power cord. If the electrical outlet ground lead is not connected, if the building has a poor connection to earth ground, or if the ground line is broken along its path from instrument to earth, a high-impedance connection results. Instrument noise will be excessive and noise generated by other devices will be carried back to the instrument and will couple into the pickup electrodes. A dedicated ground wire from the power receptacle to earth is an optimal solution. Figure 2-17 shows the building ground, equipment ground, and potential leakage pathways of concern to the neurophysiologist.

Isolation

Another method of reducing the effect of common mode voltage (which complements high CMRR and balanced electrode impedances) is to float the amplifier from ground and connect it solely to the patient. High isolation is now mandated for safety reasons. The amplifier circuitry will electrically ride the common mode voltage on the body. This is comparable to a fishing bobber in the ocean, which rises and falls with the waves. The measurement used to describe the rejection of common mode

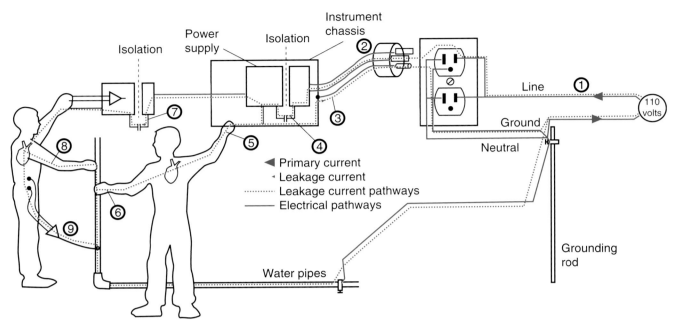

FIGURE 2-17 ■ Grounding techniques and leakage current pathways. Leakage current is generated by the mains voltage (1) applied across the inherent capacitance of the line cord and power supply (4). If the ground lead is intact, the leakage current returns to ground by that route (3). If the ground is faulty, current can flow through the operator if one hand (5) contacts the instrument and another touches a sink, radiator, or other grounded equipment (6). The amplifier is secondarily isolated but still has a certain unavoidable capacitance across the isolation. A smaller leakage current (7) can flow through this capacitance and through the patient to earth ground (8) or through other attached equipment (9), especially if the other equipment is nonisolated. If line and neutral at the outlet or power cord are reversed (2), the leakage usually increases but must still be within agency specifications. Transcardiac current and possible fibrillation dictate the maximum leakage currents allowed.

noise is the isolation mode rejection ratio (**IMRR**) and is typically above 100 dB. Isolation requires coupling the power, the signals, and the control lines across a very low capacitance barrier. Transformers, optocouplers, and capacitive couplers using frequency modulation, pulse width modulation, or linear modulation techniques are typically used. Isolation also increases patient safety because fault currents cannot flow through the amplifier and the patient.

An IMRR of 120 dB means that a 1-volt signal should be reduced to 1 μV. Measured values would probably be 10 or more times higher. The ground electrode impedance forms a voltage divider with the amplifier's capacitive coupling to earth ground, so the amplifier does not exactly float with the common mode voltage. (The fishing bobber sinks a little.) Also, small currents that flow through the body generate voltage drops (the product of current and resistance). The resulting voltage is a differential signal, not a common mode signal, and is amplified instead of rejected (Fig. 2-18). Induced currents from magnetic fields also produce differential signals. As a result, a specified **IMRR** above 100 dB

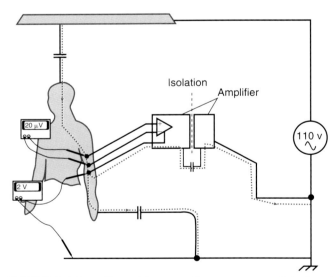

FIGURE 2-18 ■ Capacitive coupling causes small induced currents to flow through the body. The current creates a voltage drop between the electrodes, which is a differential signal. Increased isolation mode rejection ratio and common mode rejection ratio have no effect on this residual 60-Hz interference.

produces little or no improvement in rejecting 60-Hz noise. CMRR and IMRR have the same units and the same effect, but describe different processes.

Interference Reduction

Interference from external noise sources couples to the patient and electrode wires by magnetic induction and capacitive coupling. The best remedy for the interference problem is to remove the noise source or to move the instrument to a different location. Some of the more common noise waveforms are shown in Figure 2-19.

If the source of noise cannot be removed, other measures can be taken to minimize the interference. Twisting active and reference electrode wires together minimizes the loop area. The larger the loop area, the more interference is "caught." Shielding the electrode wires with a continuous metal foil will also reduce external pickup. The shield must be tied to the amplifier's ground to be effective. Placing amplifiers on the electrodes optimally reduces loop area and can sometimes improve noise performance.

Interference reduction is especially difficult during intraoperative monitoring (IOM) because of the proximity of noise-generating devices and the use of long electrode wires. In some cases, techniques such as twisting and conventional shielding may not eliminate the noise. The authors have developed a shielding method effective in the operating room that utilizes a ferrous metal shield material.[5]

Nonlinear Filtering

Nonlinear filters can improve SNR by selectively attenuating data that are likely to be noise. Slew-rate limiting eliminates large fast transients. The slew-rate is how fast the output signal is allowed to change, and is expressed in volts per second. For small signals, slew-rate limiting has no effect. For large signals (which are mostly noise), it limits the output excursion, decreasing the amount of signal passed. Sometimes a small signal is riding on a large signal. Slew-rate limiting flattens the leading and trailing edges of the noise, creating triangles on the screen. A small signal on the side of the triangle is squashed and lost, and so the averaged value will be smaller. High slew-rates are not especially useful, and low slew-rates distort the signal excessively. For evoked potential studies, 20 to 50 μV per msec is reasonable.

Averaging

Averaging is the most useful technique for improving the SNR. Averaging is performed by adding successive traces and dividing the result by the number (n) of samples. If the noise is unrelated to the signal, the SNR will be improved in proportion to the square root of the number of trials ($\sqrt{n}$), independent of the noise spectrum (Table 2-2). The buried signal is often assumed to have the same size and shape on each sweep. This assumption is good for monosynaptic or oligosynaptic responses and becomes less valid for polysynaptic cortical potentials,

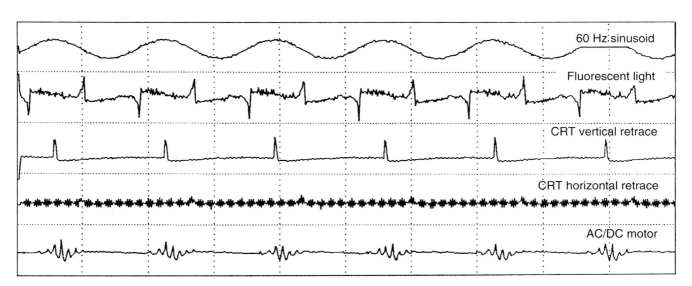

FIGURE 2-19 ▪ Electrical artifact arising from five types of sources is shown. Sinusoidal 60-Hz activity is generated by incandescent bulbs, heaters, and ungrounded equipment. Fluorescent lights and some electrical motors generate characteristic artifact at exact 16.6-msec intervals. The cathode ray tube (CRT) vertical retrace may be close to 50 or 60 Hz or may range from 40 to 75 Hz. The CRT horizontal retrace is aliased, appearing as shown, but may have other envelopes.

TABLE 2-2 ■ Effects of Averaging with 10-mV Root-Mean-Square Noise Present in the Signal

Number of Averages	Noise (μV)	Time to Average at 3 Hz
1	10	NA
10	3	3 sec
1,000	0.3	5 min
10,000	0.1	1 hr

whose average is the average of numerous different responses.

Each trace is added to the preceding traces, and the result is divided by the total number. The signal value increases with the number of trials because the response in each trace is assumed to be in-phase and, when normalized by "n," remains constant. The noise component is variable in phase and amplitude; each point is independent of the preceding points. Large positive values tend to cancel with large negative values, medium with medium, small with small. The total increases by the square root of the number of trials but, when normalized by "n," tends to zero at the rate of $1/\sqrt{n}$.

$$\left(\frac{\sqrt{n}}{n} = \frac{1}{\sqrt{n}} \right)$$

REJECT

Impulse noise can be considered a single event that is unrelated to the stimulus. Because the event is not present, except in one sweep, it averages out faster than random noise and tends to zero at the rate of $1/n$. However, most impulses are huge compared with the signal, and so even $1/n$ is not good enough. A better solution is to delete sweeps that have large artifacts. A voltage-sensitive trigger detects these large-amplitude impulses and inhibits the averager for that sweep. The stimulus artifact can also trigger the reject circuitry, and so rejects are implemented to ignore the stimulus artifact. By selecting the reject level and delay appropriately, the troublesome impulses are effectively controlled. Electrocautery can generate huge artifacts that affect multiple sweeps, and another version of artifact rejection is to stop the averager for a short period after any rejected signal.

STIMULUS RATE

The choice of stimulus rate affects the averaging process. Mains interference is neither random nor unrelated to a fixed stimulus rate. The 60-Hz artifact can be made random (relative to the stimulus) by using a random stimulus rate.

In evoked potential studies, a stimulus rate that is an exact submultiple of 60 Hz (e.g., 2.00 or 3.00 Hz) becomes synchronous with mains noise, and the 60-Hz noise is averaged in instead of out. For nerve conduction studies, only a single unaveraged sweep is desired, but several sequential stimuli are applied until the desired response is obtained. Having an exact submultiple then makes the 60-Hz activity in the baseline appear to stand still, and small responses are easier to identify. EMG that is made synchronous with the 60-Hz noise is easier to look at for the same reason. Common EMG sweep speeds for EMG are 100 msec and 200 msec, and both are exactly synchronous at 50 or 60 Hz.

When averaging is performed for a specified number of sweeps, there are stimulus rates whose 60-Hz average is null, and other rates where the mains noise is additive. Selecting the exact stimulus rate within a fraction of a percent will optimize the noise reduction. Reduction is generally better than $1/\sqrt{n}$, and changes in noise can be striking with small changes in stimulus rate. Variations in stimulus rate, variations in the actual mains frequency, any rejected waveforms, and variations in noise level from sweep to sweep may prevent the complete elimination of the mains as a noise source.

If the stimulus can be made to fire randomly between desired limits (e.g., 2.5 to 3.5), the mains noise will be uncorrelated and will reduce at about $1/\sqrt{n}$. Random stimulus rates are very effective at reducing noise in an averaged response when the noise is caused by multiple uncorrelated sources.

Synchronous noise cannot be averaged out. Placing the electrodes and ground in saline or water and averaging may reveal noise sources creating nonphysiologic responses. Solutions include eliminating the noise source (if possible), making it asynchronous by adding jitter to the source, or subtracting the noise from the signal. Of these, the last solution works well only if the average of the noise is repeatable. The extracted noise reference will inevitably have additional white noise, which will then add back into the signal when the synchronous noise is subtracted. Subtracting such noise templates may create new and more interesting problems.

SAFETY

A patient connected to an electrodiagnostic instrument is potentially at risk for excessive electric current if special precautions are not taken. Normally the skin's high impedance (100 k ohms) offers some protection from electric shock; however, electrodes applied to abraded skin with conductive gel can lower the impedance to below

1,000 ohms. There are two major sources of shock hazard: (1) leakage current and (2) dielectric breakdown. Leakage current may potentially flow from the instrument itself or from another source connected to the patient. In the operating room, a patient connected to a variety of other monitoring and life-support instruments could conduct leakage current if any of the instruments fails. Dielectric breakdown (an electric arc through or around the insulation) usually requires thousands of volts. Two sources are large transients on the mains (e.g., from a lightning strike) and intentional cardiac defibrillation. The primary safety concerns are unintentional cardiac arrest or fibrillation and burns.

Regulatory agencies have created standards for safety. Medical equipment has its own safety standards, and they give substantial assurance that inadvertent injury to the patient or operator, especially because of electrical leakage, is unlikely, even with improper grounding or multi-instrument configurations. Most countries have a national agency or agencies that specify or create the safety standards as dictated by national law. States and municipalities may also have special requirements, as may hospital accreditation bodies. Even individual hospitals may have their own safety requirements. Fortunately, most agencies have harmonized their requirements to conform to the International Electrotechnical Commission (IEC) standards. IEC601 is the standard applied to medical equipment. The IEC601 standard is a substantial collection of requirements for medical equipment, including electrical and mechanical safety, electromagnetic radiation, electromagnetic susceptibility, software design, and equipment accuracy. The standard also stipulates specific requirements for EMG/evoked potential and EEG equipment.

Electrical and Mechanical Safety

The maximum allowable leakage current varies with the type of medical instrument. The maximum leakage current for patient-connected parts is chosen to give a safety margin by a factor of 10, assuming that a conductive line from ground to the sinoatrial node has been inserted. The IEC601 standard has three different values based on three different classifications: (1) type B (nonisolated); (2) type BF (isolated); and (3) type CF (ultra-isolated for direct cardiac contact). Loss of earth ground to the instrument is considered a possible fault condition, and the safety standards limit the leakage current that could possibly flow from the instrument through the operator or patient to earth ground.

The safety standards also deal with a variety of other possible hazards, including flammability of the instrument, maximal temperatures, mechanical stability and strength, and warning labels. The protection of the patient from inadvertent stimuli during power-up and power-down and from an instrument malfunction is also considered. The standards require that exposed metal be connected to earth ground via the power cord to prevent inadvertent coupling from electrical sources inside the system (e.g., a broken wire) to the patient or operator.

Electromagnetic Interference and Susceptibility

The proliferation of electrical devices leads to an increase in the possibility that the electromagnetic radiation produced by these devices may interfere with electrodiagnostic studies. The potential for interference depends on factors such as the distance from the interference source; carrier frequency, modulation frequency, and strength of the electromagnetic radiation; electrode wire orientation; electrode impedance; and the design of the amplifier input circuitry. The majority of electrical devices are regulated to produce low electromagnetic radiation in certain frequency bands. However, some devices (e.g., electrosurgical units and portable communication devices) are allowed to radiate significant radio frequency energy.

Because electrodiagnostic instruments are used increasingly as monitors in the operating room, the ability of the instrument to continue to operate correctly after being subjected to severe conditions becomes important. The amplifier or stimulator inputs should survive static discharges of 8,000 to 12,000 volts. A static discharge to any part of the instrument should not cause the instrument to malfunction. Electromagnetic radiation must not couple to the instrument's internal circuitry and cause disruption or cause the system to display a signal that is indistinguishable from physiologic data. A large transient on the input power must also not cause any disruption.

Misuse of Equipment

Despite all the safety standards, instrumentation safety and the interpretation of results can still be compromised by operator misuse. During stimulation, electrical stimulators must generate large currents to depolarize the nerves. Normally, the current is confined to a small volume close to the electrodes. However, attaching stimulator leads across the chest or between contralateral sites across the chest (e.g., to both median nerves) creates a pathway that includes the heart. This is often done inadvertently, as shown in Figure 2-20.

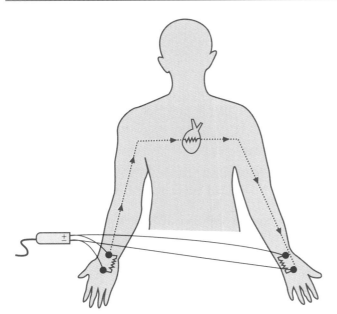

FIGURE 2-20 ■ Use of one stimulator for both median nerves allows transcardiac current to flow.

Electrical stimulators can cause burns if the power dissipation, as determined by the pulse width, current, and repetition rate, is too great or is applied for too long. Other hazards include possible chemical injury from metal ion transport similar to iontophoresis, which is used to carry beneficial drugs across the skin. Overabraded skin may develop scar tissue. Connecting two electrical stimulators in parallel by jumpering them together may not work because the outputs of stimulators are commonly clamped to decrease shock artifact. The clamped stimulator will then short the active stimulator,

and no current will flow in the patient. The screen display will appear normal if a constant-current stimulator is used. Auditory stimulators can also cause hearing damage if high stimulus intensities are employed for extended durations. The equipment operator's manual is an important source for learning of the limitations and safe use of the instrument.

CONCLUDING COMMENTS

Accurate and reliable electrophysiologic recordings require an understanding of the principles and pitfalls of the technology used. A knowledge of the characteristics of the equipment allows the user to eliminate or avoid problems and to obtain technically superior results. Equipment will change and technology advances, but principles remain the same.

REFERENCES

1. Geddes LA, Baker LE: Principles of Applied Biomedical Instrumentation. 3rd Ed. John Wiley & Sons, New York, 1989
2. Reiner S, Rogoff JB: Instrumentation. p. 498. In Johnson EW (ed): Practical Electromyography. 2nd Ed. Williams & Wilkins, Baltimore, 1988
3. Horowitz P, Hill W: The Art of Electronics. 2nd Ed. Cambridge University Press, New York, 1989
4. Sheingold DH (ed): Analog-Digital Conversion Handbook. Prentice-Hall, Englewood Cliffs, NJ, 1986
5. Villarreal RA: System and Devices for Reducing Signal Interference in Patient Monitoring Systems. US Patent No. 6,870,109

Electroencephalography and Magnetoencephalography

Electroencephalography: General Principles and Clinical Applications

MICHAEL J. AMINOFF

The electroencephalogram (EEG) represents the electrical activity of the brain as recorded from electrodes placed on the scalp. Many clinical neurologists and neurosurgeons do not fully appreciate the potential value or the limitations of electroencephalography, and this lack of information is reflected in the manner in which they use this technique in clinical practice. On the one hand, patients are often referred indiscriminately for study with little, if any, information provided about their clinical background. On the other hand, patients for whom electroencephalography might be expected to provide clinically useful information are not investigated by this means at all.

Electroencephalography is most useful in the investigation and management of patients with epilepsy. The presence of "epileptiform" activity (p. 49) in the EEG of a patient with suspected epilepsy does not establish the diagnosis beyond doubt because similar activity may occasionally be found in patients who have never had a seizure. It is, however, one more factor that must be taken into account when patients are evaluated clinically. In patients with behavioral or other disturbances that could be epileptic in nature, but about which there is some uncertainty, the presence of such activity increases considerably the likelihood that the attacks are indeed epileptic. In patients with an established seizure disorder, the EEG findings may help to classify the disorder, identify a focal or lateralized epileptogenic source, indicate the most appropriate medication that should be prescribed, provide a guide to prognosis, and follow the course of the disorder.

Electroencephalography also provides a noninvasive means of localizing structural abnormalities, such as brain tumors. Localization is generally by an indirect means, however, depending on the production of abnormalities by viable brain in the area of the lesion. Moreover, it is sometimes disappointingly inaccurate, and the findings themselves provide no reliable indication of the type of underlying pathology. In this context, it is hardly surprising that advances in neuroimaging techniques for the detection of structural abnormalities in the brain—in particular, by the development of computed tomography (CT) scanning and magnetic resonance imaging (MRI)—have led to a reduction in this use of electroencephalography as a screening procedure. Nevertheless, the EEG reflects the function of the brain and is therefore a complement, rather than an inconsequential alternative, to these newer procedures.

The third major use of electroencephalography is in the investigation of patients with certain neurologic disorders that produce characteristic EEG abnormalities which, although nonspecific, help to suggest, establish, or support the diagnosis. These abnormalities are exemplified well by the repetitive slow-wave complexes sometimes seen in herpes simplex encephalitis, which should suggest this diagnosis if the complexes are found in patients with an acute cerebral illness. The electrical findings are best regarded as one more physical sign, however, and as such should be evaluated in conjunction with the other clinical and laboratory data. A further use of electroencephalography—one that may increase in importance with the development of quantitative techniques for assessing the data that are obtained—is in the screening or monitoring of patients with metabolic disorders, because it provides an objective measure of the improvement or deterioration that may precede any change in the clinical state of the patient.

Electroencephalography is also an important means of evaluating patients with a change in mental status or an altered level of consciousness. Continuous EEG monitoring provides dynamic information that allows for the early detection of functional changes and may thereby improve clinical outcome. This is especially useful when the clinical examination is limited or in patients at particular risk of deterioration, as after head injury or subarachnoid hemorrhage. Technical advances have made long-term monitoring practical, but review of the raw EEG traces remains important in ensuring the validity of any conclusions.[1] Finally, the EEG is used for studying natural sleep and its disorders, and as help in the determination of brain death. Further comment on these aspects is deferred to Chapters 33 and 35, and the clinical utility of the EEG in the investigation of infants and children is considered separately in Chapter 4.

The EEG is now recorded with simultaneous functional MRI (fMRI) in various research contexts. The approach was originally developed to improve the localization of the generators of certain EEG abnormalities in epilepsy by mapping their hemodynamic correlates, but has developed into a sophisticated investigative tool.[2]

In describing the EEG findings in various seizure disorders, the revised terminology for the organization of seizures and epilepsies proposed by the International League Against Epilepsy has been adopted,[3] but the older terms are retained in parentheses for the convenience of readers.

PRACTICAL CONSIDERATIONS

Recording Arrangements

The EEG is recorded from metal electrodes placed on the scalp. The electrodes are coated with a conductive paste, then applied to the scalp and held in place by adhesives, suction, or pressure from caps or headbands.

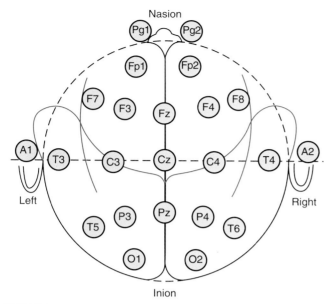

FIGURE 3-1 ■ The International 10–20 system of electrode placement. A, earlobe; C, central; F, frontal; Fp, frontal polar; P, parietal; Pg, nasopharyngeal; T, temporal; O, occipital. Right-sided placements are indicated by even numbers, left-sided placements by odd numbers, and midline placements by z.

Alternatively, needle electrodes can be inserted directly into the scalp. The placement of recording electrodes is generally based on the international 10–20 system, in which the placement of electrodes is determined by measurements from four standard positions on the head: the nasion, inion, and right and left preauricular points (Fig. 3-1). When this system is used, most electrodes are about 5 to 7 cm from the adjacent electrodes, in an adult. If closer spacing is required (e.g., to define the site of an epileptogenic focus), electrodes can be placed in intermediate positions. The potential differences between electrodes are amplified and then recorded on continuously moving paper by a number of pen-writers or displayed on an oscilloscope screen. Relatively inexpensive digital systems are now widely available commercially, and these have many advantages over the older analog systems. They permit reconstruction of the EEG with any desired derivation or format and also permit data manipulation for added analysis. They also facilitate access to any desired portion of the record and obviate storage problems. Further discussion of such systems is provided in Chapter 8.

Electrodes are connected with amplifiers in predetermined patterns, or montages, to permit the electrical activity of various areas to be recorded in sequence. The recording arrangements can be varied, or the EEG can be reconstructed after digital recording, so that the potential difference is measured either between pairs of scalp electrodes (bipolar derivation) or between individual electrodes and a common reference point. In the latter arrangement, the reference point can be either a relatively inactive site on the scalp or elsewhere (e.g., the vertex or the linked ears) or a point connected to all the electrodes in use so that it reflects the average of the potentials at these electrodes. Each technique has its own advantages and drawbacks, but for routine purposes at least two of these methods for deriving the EEG are used. Montages are generally selected so that recordings are made from rows of equidistant electrodes running from the front to the back of the head or transversely across it. In most North American laboratories, traces from the left side of the head are displayed above those from the right, and those from anterior regions are displayed above those from more posterior areas.

The more detailed technical and practical aspects of EEG recording are beyond the scope of this chapter. There is, however, one general point that must be made clear. As already indicated, the potential difference between pairs of electrodes—or between an electrode and its reference point—is amplified before being displayed on moving paper or an oscilloscope screen. The input leads of the individual amplifiers are designated as black (input terminal 1, or G1) and white (input terminal 2, or G2). They are arranged so that when the electrode connected with the black lead is relatively more negative than that connected with the white one, an upward deflection of the trace occurs. The relationship between the two inputs, then, determines the direction in which the trace is deflected, not the absolute value of any discharge that is recorded. With bipolar derivations, the conventional American recording arrangement is for the most anterior electrode of each pair to be connected with the black lead when recording from the front to the back of the head, and for the left-hand electrode of any pair to be connected with the black lead when recording across the head. With the reference derivations, each of the active scalp electrodes is connected to the black lead of an amplifier, and all the white leads are connected with the common reference point.

Interpretation of specific events in the EEG derived with a common reference point may be confounded if the reference electrode itself lies within the active field, whereas a voltage peak involving two adjacent electrodes to the same extent may not be detected in the bipolar derivation because no potential difference will be recorded between these electrodes. Both the bipolar derivation and the use of a common reference permit abnormalities to be localized, but the former method is less satisfactory for localizing widespread changes or for demonstrating areas in which activity is suppressed. With linked bipolar derivations, the source of localized EEG abnormalities is determined by locating the common electrode at which the deflections of the traces show a reversal of phase or polarity when recordings are made simultaneously from at least two rows of electrodes at right angles to each other (i.e., from rows of electrodes in the anteroposterior and transverse axes of the head). Changes in amplitude may be misleading in bipolar recordings. For example, a greater amplitude in one channel does not necessarily reflect the origin of a particular discharge but signifies only that a larger potential difference exists between the two electrodes connected to that amplifier; a lower amplitude may reflect inactivity or equal activity at the two electrode sites. By contrast, with common reference derivations, localization of abnormalities is accomplished primarily on the basis of amplitude.

Various *special electrodes* have been devised for recording the activity of inaccessible regions of the brain, because electrodes placed on the scalp may not detect such activity. A nasopharyngeal electrode, consisting of a flexible, insulated rod or wire with a small silver electrode at its tip, can be inserted into the nostril and advanced until the terminal electrode is in contact with the mucosa of the posterior nasopharynx. This permits recording of electrical activity from the anteromedial surface of the temporal lobe. Insertion of these electrodes is generally undertaken by technologists without the application of any local anesthetic, and not all patients tolerate the procedure. Furthermore, recordings from them may be contaminated by pulse, muscle, and respiratory movement artifact, and only rarely do they reveal abnormalities that are not seen with the usual scalp electrodes. Sphenoidal electrodes can record activity from the anteroinferior portion of the temporal lobe. These electrodes are less likely to lead to artifacts than are nasopharyngeal electrodes, but their application is more difficult. The electrode consists of a sterile needle or fine wire that is insulated, except at its tip, and a physician inserts it percutaneously under local anesthesia so that it lies adjacent to the sphenoid bone, a little in front of the foramen ovale. Other accessory electrodes that are commonly used in the electrophysiologic evaluation of patients with focal seizures and impaired consciousness (previously called complex partial seizures) are surface sphenoidal electrodes, minisphenoidal electrodes, and anterior temporal electrodes. There is no consensus of opinion regarding the relative merits of these different electrodes.

The *EEG examination* usually is undertaken in a quiet, relaxed environment, with the patient seated or lying comfortably with the eyes closed. Recordings initially are made for up to about 5 minutes from each of several different standard montages, for a total of about 30 minutes. Depending on the findings, the examination can then be continued by recording with less conventional montages. During the recording of activity from each montage, the patient should be asked to lie with the eyes open for about 20 seconds before closing them again, so that the responsiveness of the background activity can be assessed.

When this routine part of the examination has been completed, recording continues while activation procedures are undertaken in an attempt to provoke abnormalities.

Activation Procedures

Hyperventilation for 3 or 4 minutes is a generally well-tolerated method of provoking or accentuating EEG abnormalities, but it should not be performed in patients who have recently had a stroke, transient ischemic attack, or subarachnoid hemorrhage, or in those with moyamoya disease, significant cardiac or respiratory disease, hyperviscosity states, or sickle cell disease or trait. The patient is asked to take deep breaths at a normal respiratory rate until instructed to stop. The resultant fall in arterial PCO_2 leads to cerebral vasoconstriction and thus to mild cerebral anoxia. This anoxic state is held by many to bring out the EEG abnormalities, although cogent criticisms of this view exist and the precise mechanism involved remains unclear.[4] Certain quantitative techniques have been suggested in an endeavor to establish a more uniform procedure, but these methods are not in routine use. The EEG is recorded during the period of hyperventilation and for the following 2 minutes, with the use of a montage that encompasses the area where it is suspected, based on clinical or other grounds, that abnormalities may be found; or, in the absence of any localizing clues, an area that covers as much of the scalp as possible. The eyes are generally kept closed during the procedure, apart from a brief period at its conclusion to evaluate the responsiveness of any induced activity. Hyperventilation usually causes more prominent EEG changes in children than in adults. There is considerable variation, however, in the response of individual subjects, and this variation makes it difficult to define the limits of normality. It may also produce or enhance various bioelectric artifacts.

Recording during *sleep* or after a 24-hour period of *sleep deprivation* may also provoke EEG abnormalities that might otherwise be missed, and this technique is similarly harmless. This approach has been used most widely in the investigation of patients with suspected epilepsy.

Abnormalities may also be elicited with an electronic stroboscope to cause rhythmic *photic stimulation* while the EEG is recorded with the use of a bipolar recording arrangement that covers particularly the occipital and parietal regions of the scalp. The flash stimulus is best monitored on one channel either with a photocell or directly from the stimulator. Abnormalities are more likely to be elicited when the patient is awake for the procedure. At any given flash rate, the EEG is recorded with the patient's eyes open for about 5 seconds and then while the eyes are closed for a further 5 seconds. Flash rates of up to 30 Hz are generally used, but an even wider range of frequencies is employed in some laboratories. The manner by which abnormalities are produced is unknown.

Various *auditory stimuli* may also precipitate EEG abnormalities in patients with epilepsy, but they are not used routinely in the EEG laboratory, except in the evaluation of comatose patients (p. 79). Other stimuli that may induce paroxysmal EEG abnormalities include tactile stimuli and reading.

A number of different pharmacologic activating procedures have been described. These procedures are not in general use, however, and may carry some risk to the patient; thus, they are not discussed in this chapter.

Artifacts

A variety of *artifacts* may arise from the electrodes, recording equipment, and recording environment. Examples are the so-called electrode "pop" resulting from a sudden change in impedance (seen as an abrupt vertical deflection of the traces derived from a particular electrode, superimposed on the EEG tracing, as shown in Fig. 3-2); distorted waveforms resulting from inappropriate sensitivity of the display; excessive "noise" from the amplifiers; and environmental artifacts generated by currents from external devices, electrostatic potentials (as from persons moving around the patient), and intravenous infusions (generating sharp transients coinciding with drops of the infusion, possibly caused by electrostatic charges). Bioelectric artifacts are noncerebral potentials that arise from the patient and include ocular, cardiac, swallowing, glossokinetic, muscle, and movement artifacts.

With reference derivations, artifacts may be introduced because of the location of the reference electrode or because the reference electrode is within the cerebral field under study. No single site is ideal as a reference point. The ear or mastoid placements are commonly used but may be contaminated by muscle, electrocardiogram

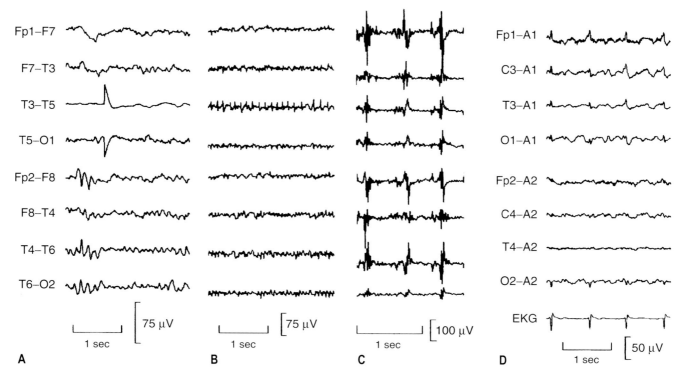

FIGURE 3-2 ▪ **A**, Electrode artifact arising at the T5 electrode. **B**, Electromyographic artifact in the left temporal region. **C**, Chewing artifact. **D**, Electrocardiographic artifact.

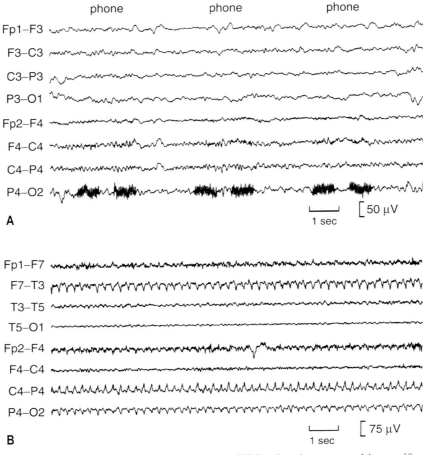

FIGURE 3-3 ▪ **A**, Electroencephalogram (EEG) showing a repetitive artifact that coincided with the ringing of the telephone ("phone"). **B**, EEG showing a rhythmic discharge with an unusual field, which related to continuous venous-to-venous hemodialysis. When hemodialysis was briefly stopped, the rhythmic activity ceased.

(ECG), or temporal spike discharges. The vertex, which is also widely used, is very active during sleep and is sometimes contaminated by vertical eye movements during wakefulness.

In general, artifacts are recognized because of their temporal relationship to extracerebral monitors such as the ECG, because of their unusual appearance, or because the electrical field of the event is hard to interpret in a biologically plausible manner (Fig. 3-3). They are discussed in detail in Chapter 5, but brief comment concerning them is also made here.

BIOELECTRIC ARTIFACTS

Eye-movement artifacts are generated by the corneoretinal potential, which is in the order of 100 mV and has been likened to a dipole with the positive pole at the cornea and the negative pole at the retina. Eye movement leads to a positive potential recorded by the electrodes closest to the cornea. Thus, with upward movement of the eyes (such as occurs during a blink), a positive potential is recorded at the frontopolar (supraorbital) electrodes relative to more posteriorly placed electrodes, and thus a downward deflection occurs at these electrodes. Such eye movement is easily distinguished from frontal slow EEG activity by recording from an infraorbital electrode referenced to the mastoid process; the former leads to activity that is out of phase between the supra- and infraorbital electrodes, whereas frontal EEG activity is in phase. Similarly, horizontal eye movements lead to a positivity at the frontotemporal electrode on the side to which the eyes are moved and a corresponding negativity on the opposite side (Fig. 3-4). Nystagmus or eyelid flutter, for example, produces a rhythmic discharge in the frontal electrodes (see Fig. 3-4). Oblique eye movements and asymmetric eye movements may be confusing, but are usually easily distinguished by experienced electroencephalographers.

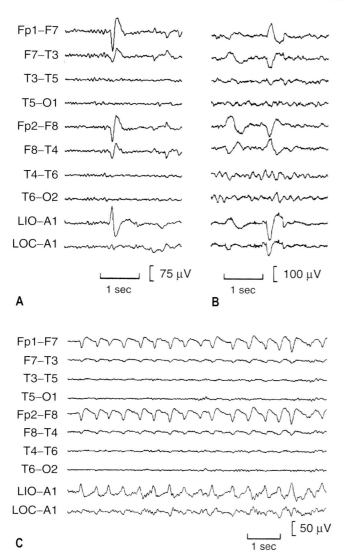

FIGURE 3-4 ■ Eye movements. **A**, Eye closure. **B**, Lateral eye movement. **C**, Eyelid flutter. LIO, left infraorbital; LOC, left outer canthus.

Cardiac artifacts are related to the ECG or ballistocardiogram and are especially conspicuous when monitoring for electrocerebral inactivity in brain-death suspects or in referential recordings involving the ears (see Fig. 3-2). The ECG can be monitored by electrodes placed on the chest and recorded on a separate channel, thereby facilitating recognition of such artifacts in the scalp recording, which may otherwise be misinterpreted as sharp waves or spike discharges. Conspicuous ECG artifact may obscure underlying low-voltage electrocerebral activity, a point of concern when comatose patients are being examined for possible brain death. Pulse artifact may occur at any site but typically is localized to a single electrode and appears as a recurrent slow wave that sometimes has a saw-toothed appearance and is time-locked to the ECG.

It occurs when an electrode is placed over or close to an artery, and movement of the electrode will eliminate it. Pacemaker artifacts consist of spike discharges that precede the ECG.

Muscle artifact is composed of brief-duration spike discharges that are too rapid to be cerebral in origin. Chewing artifacts are electromyographic (EMG) artifacts produced by the temporalis muscles (see Fig. 3-2). Sucking artifact (in infants) is characterized by bitemporal sharp activity that may be difficult to identify without careful observation of the baby. Lateral rectus spikes are recorded from the anterior temporal electrodes and relate to horizontal eye movements; they are out of phase on the two sides of the head. Attempting to relax or quieten the patient should reduce muscle artifact. In most instances, high-frequency filters should not be used for this purpose, except as a last resort, because they simply alter the appearance of the artifact (sometimes so that it looks more like EEG fast activity) and also influence the background EEG.

Movement produces artifact in addition to muscle activity. Any movements may produce such artifacts, and these will vary in appearance depending on the nature and site of the movement. Movements arising at a consistent site may be monitored by a pair of electrodes and recorded on a separate channel. Hiccups produce a brief generalized movement artifact that may have a pseudoperiodic quality; this is not confined to the EEG but is seen also in, for example, the ECG channel. Glossokinetic artifact relates to the difference in potential between the tip of the tongue and its base; tongue movements generate slow waves that are recorded over one or both temporal regions (Fig. 3-5). When suspected, tongue movements may be monitored by a submental electrode.

Sweat artifact is common and is characterized by high-amplitude potentials of very low frequency. Low-frequency filters can attenuate these slow waves.

INSTRUMENTAL ARTIFACTS

Background 60-Hz noise in a restricted number of channels is often related to mismatched electrical impedance of electrode pairs or to the poor application of electrodes so that slight movement alters transiently the impedance of an individual electrode. A 60-Hz interference signal normally is common to the pair of electrodes connected to an amplifier; the differential amplifier essentially discards this common signal. If the electrical impedance of one of the electrodes is altered, however, the current flowing across that electrode–skin interface will be altered, thereby leading to voltage differences between one electrode and the other of the pair. The differential amplifier will magnify these differences so that the 60-Hz

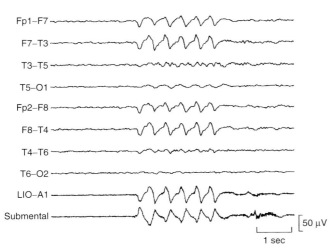

FIGURE 3-5 ■ EEG showing rhythmic slow waves in the temporal regions relating to glossokinetic artifact. It can be seen that the cerebral activity is in phase with activity recorded infraorbitally (indicating that it is not eye movement artifact) and out of phase with activity recorded submentally.

artifact then becomes obtrusive. In addition, other artifacts related to movement arise at that electrode and are limited to the channel with which the faulty electrode is connected, causing "mirror-image" phase reversals when these channels are part of a linked bipolar montage. Widespread 60-Hz artifact is of concern because it may indicate a safety problem warranting attention as discussed in Chapter 2, where the various artifacts that arise in digital equipment also are considered.

EEG Interpretation

Evaluation of the EEG for clinical purposes involves definition of the frequency, amplitude, and distribution of the electrical activity that is present, and of its response to external stimulation such as eye-opening. The degree of synchrony and symmetry over the two sides of the head is noted. The presence of any focal activity is determined and its nature characterized. The findings must be interpreted in relation to the patient's age and level of arousal. For descriptive purposes, EEG activity is usually characterized on the basis of frequency.

ACTIVITY RECORDED IN THE EEG

The mechanisms responsible for the presence of widespread rhythmic activity in the brain are not known. Some means of generating rhythmic activity must be involved, as also must some method of synchronizing the activity of different cerebral regions. Experiments on animals have produced considerable evidence to suggest that the rhythmic activity normally recorded from the

scalp has a cortical origin, being derived from the graded postsynaptic potentials of cortical neurons. It is the pyramidal neurons—cells that are vertically oriented with regard to the cortex, have a large apical dendrite extending toward the surface, and are located in cortical layers III, V, and VI—that are important in this respect. The origin of the scalp-recorded EEG primarily from postsynaptic potentials, rather than action potentials, is in keeping with the former's longer duration and synchronous occurrence over a large area of cell membrane. Potentials arising from neuronal activity in subcortical structures or from horizontally oriented cortical cells contribute little, if anything, to the normal scalp-recorded EEG. The factors that determine whether a cortical potential is recorded over the scalp include its voltage, the extent to which the generator cells are discharging synchronously, the area of cortex involved, and the site of cortical involvement with respect to the sulcal convolutions. Potentials arising in the sulcal depths are less likely to be recorded over the scalp by conventional EEG than are those arising at the surface. Spatial summation of cortical activity is important in producing the voltage fields that are recorded as the scalp EEG because of the attenuating properties of the skull and other interposed tissues.[5]

The cortical activity has a regular rhythmicity that seems to depend on the functional integrity of subcortical mechanisms. It has been accepted generally that the thalamus serves as the pacemaker of certain of the cortical rhythms that are recorded during electroencephalography, but intracortical circuitries may also be involved significantly.[6] The precise details are beyond the scope of this chapter. The physiologic basis of the abnormal rhythms that are encountered at electroencephalography is defined even less clearly. It has become apparent, however, that a cortical area of 10 to 20 cm^2 is often required to generate an interictal spike or ictal rhythm recognizable at the scalp.[7] It also remains unclear whether it is possible to record at the scalp the EEG from sources deeper than the most superficial cortex,[8,9] but source area is clearly important in this regard.

The EEG is a two-dimensional representation of three-dimensional activity that fails to provide sufficient information to allow for the unique localization of the neuronal generators of an intracranial current source (the "inverse problem").

Alpha Activity

ALPHA RHYTHM

Alpha rhythm may have a frequency of between 8 and 13 Hz, but in most adults it is between 9 and 11 Hz. This rhythm is found most typically over the posterior portions of the head during wakefulness, but it may also be present in the central or temporal regions. Alpha rhythm is seen best when the patient is resting with the eyes closed. Immediately after eye closure, its frequency may be increased transiently (the "squeak" phenomenon). The alpha rhythm is not strictly monorhythmic but varies over a range of about 1 Hz, even under stable conditions. It is usually sinusoidal in configuration, may wax and wane spontaneously in amplitude, and sometimes has a spiky appearance; a spindle configuration denotes a *beating* phenomenon that results from the presence of two (or more) dominant frequencies.

The alpha rhythm is attenuated or abolished by visual attention (Fig. 3-6) and affected transiently by other sensory stimuli and by other mental alerting activities (e.g., mental arithmetic) or by anxiety. The term *paradoxical alpha rhythm* refers to the appearance of alpha rhythm on eye-opening in drowsy subjects; this represents an alerting response. Alpha activity is well formed and prominent in many normal subjects but is relatively inconspicuous or absent in about 10 percent of instances. Its precise frequency is usually of little diagnostic significance unless information is available about its frequency on earlier occasions. In children, the dominant, posterior responsive rhythm reaches about 8 Hz by the age of 3 years and reaches 10 Hz by approximately 10 years of age. Slowing occurs with advancing age; as a consequence of certain medication (e.g., anticonvulsant drugs); and in patients with clouding of consciousness, metabolic disorders, or virtually any type of cerebral pathology. The alpha activity may increase in frequency in children as they mature and in older subjects who are thyrotoxic. A slight asymmetry is often present between the two hemispheres with regard to the amplitude of alpha activity and the degree to which it extends anteriorly. In particular, alpha rhythm may normally be up to 50 percent greater in amplitude over the right hemisphere, possibly because this is the nondominant hemisphere or because of variation in skull thickness. A more marked asymmetry of its amplitude may have lateralizing significance but is difficult to interpret unless other EEG abnormalities are present, because either depression or enhancement may occur on the side of a hemispheric lesion. Similarly, a persistent difference in alpha frequency of more than 1 to 2 Hz between the two hemispheres is generally regarded as abnormal. The side with the slower rhythm is more likely to be the abnormal one, but it is usually difficult to be certain unless other abnormalities are also found.

Unilaterally attenuated or absent responsiveness of the alpha rhythm sometimes occurs with lesions of the parietal or temporal lobe (Bancaud phenomenon).[10] Asymmetric attenuation of the alpha rhythm during mental alerting procedures with the eyes closed may also be helpful for lateralizing any impairment of cerebral function.[10]

Some normal adults have an alpha rhythm that is more conspicuous centrally or temporally than posteriorly, or has a widespread distribution. Care must be taken not to misinterpret such findings as evidence of abnormality. The so-called slow alpha variant resembles normal alpha rhythm in distribution and reactivity but has a frequency of about 4 to 5 Hz, which approximates one-half that of any alpha rhythm in the same record. This variant is of no pathologic significance.

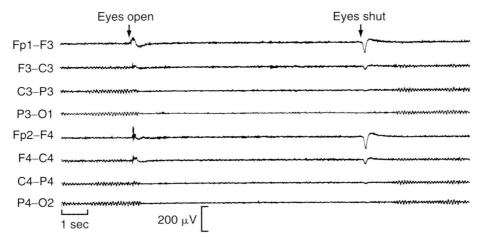

FIGURE 3-6 ■ Normal 9- to 10-Hz alpha rhythm recorded in the electroencephalogram of a 64-year-old man. The posterior distribution and responsiveness to eye-opening of the rhythm can be seen.

OTHER RHYTHMS OF ALPHA FREQUENCY

Not all activity having a frequency of 8 to 13 Hz is necessarily an alpha rhythm. Alpha-frequency activity that is widespread in distribution and unresponsive to external stimulation is found in some comatose patients (p. 79). Temporal alpha activity is sometimes found in elderly subjects and may be asynchronous, episodic, and persistent during drowsiness. Runs of activity in the alpha range of frequencies are occasionally found frontally in children immediately after arousal from sleep (frontal arousal rhythm) and are not of pathologic significance.

Mu rhythm has a frequency that usually is in the alpha range, is seen intermittently over the central region of one or both hemispheres, is unaffected by eye-opening, and is blocked unilaterally or bilaterally by movement or the thought of movement (Fig. 3-7). It is also blocked by sensory stimulation. Bilateral mu rhythm is often asynchronous and may exhibit amplitude asymmetries between the two hemispheres. The negative portions of the waves are sharpened, and the positive portions are generally rounded. Mu rhythm is often associated with a centrally located beta rhythm that is also attenuated by contralateral movement. In most instances, mu rhythm has no diagnostic significance. It is found in about 20 percent of young adults. When recorded over a skull defect, it may be mistaken for a potential epileptogenic abnormality.

Beta Activity

Any rhythmic activity that has a frequency greater than 13 Hz is referred to as beta activity. Activity of this sort is present anteriorly in the EEG of normal adults. Beta activity, responsive to eye-opening, is sometimes found over the posterior portions of the hemispheres and is then best regarded as a *fast variant of the alpha rhythm*. Beta activity that fails to respond to eye-opening is a common finding and usually has a generalized distribution, but in some instances it is located centrally and is attenuated by tactile stimulation or contralateral movements. It usually has an amplitude of less than about 30 μV. The amount of such activity varies considerably among normal subjects. Activity having a frequency between 18 and 25 Hz is usually more conspicuous during drowsiness, light sleep, and rapid eye movement (REM) sleep than during wakefulness. It may also be augmented by cognitive tasks. Beta activity may be induced by a number of different drugs, particularly barbiturates and the benzodiazepine compounds, but also neuroleptics, antihistaminics, D-amphetamine, methylphenidate, and cocaine.[11] Drug-induced fast activity is typically diffuse and symmetric over the two hemispheres. Focal or lateralized spontaneous beta activity, or asymmetric drug-induced fast activity, raises the possibility of localized cerebral pathology. In such circumstances, however, it must be borne in mind that the amplitude of beta activity may be increased either ipsilateral or contralateral to a lesion involving one cerebral hemisphere; and that an amplitude asymmetry is common in normal subjects, with beta activity being up to 30 percent lower on one side than the other. Beta activity is increased in amplitude over the area of a skull defect owing to the greater proximity of the recording electrodes to the surface of the brain and the low-impedance pathway. It is reduced in amplitude over a subdural collection of fluid or localized swelling or edema of the scalp, and transiently in either a localized or lateralized manner after a focal seizure.

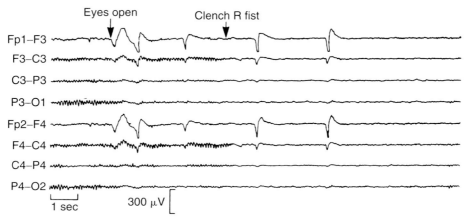

FIGURE 3-7 ■ Bilateral mu rhythm recorded in the electroencephalogram of a 26-year-old woman with no neurologic disorder. The effect on the rhythm of clenching the right fist can be seen.

Generalized *paroxysmal fast activity* is a rare finding, occurring in less than 1 percent of EEG recordings; it may be mistaken for muscle artifact, drug effect, or sleep spindles, depending on the circumstances. In one study of 20 patients with such activity, all had seizure disorders, usually with seizures of more than one type, and most were cognitively impaired.[12] The paroxysmal EEG disturbance occurred almost always during sleep, often with associated clinical seizures that were commonly of the tonic variety.[12]

Theta Activity

Activity with a frequency between 4 and 7 Hz is referred to as theta activity. Theta and slower activity is usually very conspicuous in children but becomes less prominent as they mature. Some theta activity is often found in young adults, particularly over the temporal regions and during hyperventilation, but in older subjects theta activity with amplitude greater than about 30 μV is seen less commonly, except during drowsiness. Focal or lateralized theta activity may be indicative of localized cerebral pathology. More diffusely distributed theta activity is a common finding in patients with a variety of neurologic disorders, but it also may be caused by nothing more than a change in the patient's state of arousal.

Rhythmic trains of *midline theta activity*, occurring especially at the vertex and having an arciform, sinusoidal, or spiky configuration, have been described as a nonspecific finding in patients with many different disorders. Such activity may be persistent or intermittent; may be present during wakefulness or drowsiness; and shows variable reactivity to eye-opening, movement, alerting, and tactile stimulation.[10] It is not present during sleep. Its origin is uncertain.

Delta Activity

Activity that is slower than 4 Hz is designated delta activity. Activity of this sort is the predominant one in infants and is a normal finding during the deep stages of sleep in older subjects. When present in the EEG of awake adults, delta activity is an abnormal finding.

Delta activity, responsive to eye opening, is commonly seen posteriorly (intermixed with alpha activity) in children and sometimes in young adults; it is then designated *posterior slow waves of youth*. The spontaneous occurrence interictally of posterior, rhythmic slow waves is well described in patients with absence seizures. The slow activity has a frequency of about 3 Hz, is present during wakefulness, is responsive to eye-opening, and may be enhanced by hyperventilation. The symmetric or asymmetric occurrence of rhythmic delta activity over the posterior regions of the head after eye closure is rare. Such activity usually lasts for no more than 2 or 3 seconds and is a nonspecific finding that has been described in a number of different neurologic disorders.[10]

POLYMORPHIC DELTA ACTIVITY

Polymorphic delta activity is continuous, irregular, slow activity that varies considerably in duration and amplitude with time; it persists during sleep, and shows little variation with change in the physiologic state of the patient (Fig. 3-8). It has been related to deafferentation of the involved area of the cortex and to metabolic factors. Such activity may be found postictally and in patients with metabolic disorders. It is commonly seen, with a localized distribution, over destructive cerebral lesions involving subcortical white matter (Fig. 3-9), but it generally is not found with lesions restricted to the cerebral

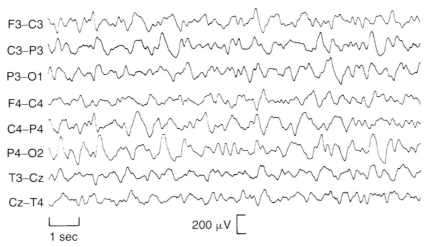

FIGURE 3-8 ■ Electroencephalogram of a 19-year-old patient with encephalitis, showing a background of diffuse, irregular theta and delta activity.

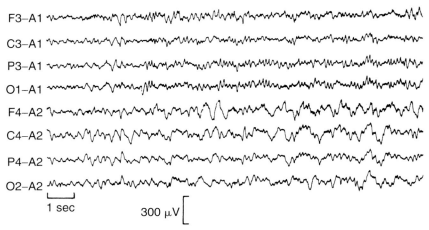

FIGURE 3-9 ▪ Electroencephalogram of a 52-year-old man who had a right parietal glioma. Note the polymorphic slow-wave focus in the right central region and the diffusely slowed background.

cortex itself. It may be found either unilaterally or bilaterally in patients with thalamic tumors or lesions of the midbrain reticular formation, but its distribution in such circumstances is somewhat variable. Thus, although diffuse irregular slow activity is found over one hemisphere in some cases, in others it has a more restricted distribution.

The EEG finding of focal polymorphic delta activity correlates with the presence of focal abnormalities on neuroimaging, but nonfocal abnormalities (e.g., diffuse atrophy or cerebral edema) are sometimes found. The maximal delta focus may not always overlie the structural abnormality, even though it is in the same hemisphere. The amplitude, frequency, and distribution of focal slow waves do not relate to lesion size or to mass effect. In some patients with focal polymorphic slow-wave activity, no abnormalities whatsoever are present on CT scans; such patients usually have seizure disorders, cerebral trauma, or cerebral ischemia.

Diffuse polymorphic delta activity occurs in patients with white matter encephalopathies and following acute or extensive lesions of the upper brainstem.

INTERMITTENT RHYTHMIC DELTA ACTIVITY

Intermittent rhythmic delta activity is paroxysmal, has a relatively constant frequency, and is usually synchronous over the two hemispheres. It is often more prominent occipitally in children or frontally in adults (Fig. 3-10), may be enhanced by hyperventilation or drowsiness, and usually is attenuated by attention. Its origin is unclear, but it probably relates to dysfunction of subcortical centers influencing the activity of cortical neurons. Its significance is considered on page 51.

Breach Rhythm

Breach rhythm is a mu-like rhythm found in patients with skull defects after surgical operations. It has a frequency of between 6 and 11 Hz, usually with faster components, and the waves often have spike-like negative phases. The rhythm recorded parasagittally is often responsive to fist-clenching and other stimuli, whereas that recorded more laterally (at the T3 or T4 electrode) is generally unresponsive to any stimuli. The presence of a breach rhythm has no predictive value for the development of seizures or the recurrence of the intracranial pathology that necessitated the original surgery.

Lambda Waves

Lambda waves are electropositive sharp waves that may occur in the occipital region in normal subjects who are looking at and scanning something (e.g., reading) in a well-illuminated field, particularly if their attention and interest are aroused. Morphologically similar activity is sometimes seen during non-REM sleep. The nature of these potentials is unclear, and they have no known diagnostic significance at present. They are sometimes asymmetric over the two hemispheres but can be distinguished from sharp transients of pathologic significance by their response to eye closure or reduction in the level of background illumination.

Triphasic Waves

Triphasic waves typically consist of a major positive potential preceded and followed by smaller negative waves. They are found most characteristically in metabolic

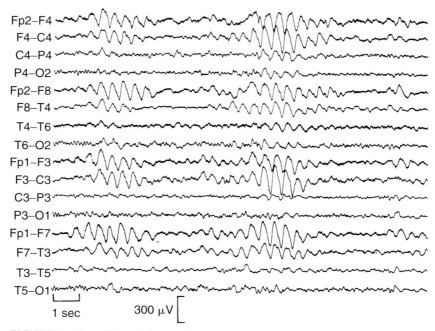

FIGURE 3-10 ▪ Frontal intermittent rhythmic delta activity recorded in the electroencephalogram of a 14-year-old boy with obstructive hydrocephalus.

encephalopathies, when they usually are generalized, bilaterally synchronous, and frontally predominant. They are sometimes reactive to external (painful) stimulation. Triphasic waves were originally thought to be specific for hepatic encephalopathy, but in fact are found in a variety of metabolic encephalopathies and suggest a poor prognosis for survival.[13] They have also been described in hypothermia,[14] myxedema coma,[15] neuroleptic malignant syndrome,[16] and a variety of other neurologic disorders, including dementia.[13] Triphasic waves may occur in patients receiving pentobarbital, especially as the drug is being tapered after treatment of status epilepticus,[17] during which time they should not be mistaken for epileptiform activity. Similarly, they have been noted in patients with primary generalized epilepsy at a time when they had a postictal depression in level of consciousness.[18] The periodic complexes found in certain conditions (p. 52), especially Creutzfeldt–Jakob disease, may take the form of triphasic waves.

Spike Discharges

One of the major uses of electroencephalography is in the investigation of patients with suspected epilepsy. In this regard, the presence in the EEG of interictal spike discharges or sharp waves is often held to be suggestive of an epileptic disturbance. *Epileptiform activity* is defined as abnormal paroxysmal activity consisting, at least in part, of spikes or sharp waves resembling those found in many patients with epilepsy. It is not synonymous with an *electrographic seizure*, which typically consists of rhythmic repetitive activity having a relatively abrupt onset and termination, a characteristic evolution, and lasting at least several seconds. A spike is defined arbitrarily as a potential having a sharp outline and a duration of 20 to 70 msec, whereas a sharp wave has a duration of between 70 and 200 msec. The distinction between epileptiform and nonepileptiform sharp transients usually is made intuitively but bearing in mind certain guidelines. *Epileptiform sharp transients* are usually asymmetric in appearance, are commonly followed by a slow wave, have a duration that differs from that of the ongoing background activity, may be biphasic or triphasic, and often occur on a background containing irregular slow elements (Fig. 3-11). These criteria distinguish between epileptiform activity and background activity that is sharp and variable in amplitude (e.g., a spiky alpha rhythm).

Pathologic spike discharges have different clinical implications depending on their characteristics and location. Focal epileptiform spike discharges arise from a localized cerebral region. The likelihood of spikes arising from a particular area depends on the age of the patient, type of underlying lesion, and epileptogenicity of the involved region. Slowly progressive lesions are more likely to be associated with such activity than are rapidly progressive ones, and the frontal and temporal lobes are more epileptogenic than the parietal and occipital lobes. The benign epileptiform discharges that occur in drowsy subjects (p. 54) have a different significance from that of

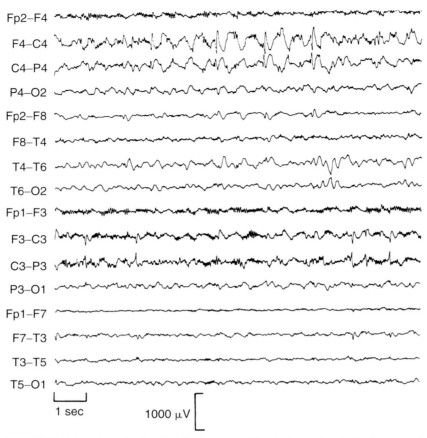

FIGURE 3-11 ■ Interictal spike discharges arising independently in the central region of either hemisphere in a patient with seizures since infancy.

the anterior or mesial temporal spike discharges found interictally in patients with focal (partial) seizures with impaired consciousness (complex partial seizures). Similarly, 3-Hz, 6-Hz, and 1- to 2-Hz spike-wave discharges differ in their clinical and prognostic relevance. Moreover, the significance of frankly epileptiform discharges depends on the clinical circumstances in which they are found.

Epileptiform spike discharges arising focally in the temporal region are associated most commonly with focal (partial) seizures accompanied by an impairment of consciousness and are activated during drowsiness or sleep. Intermittent delta activity may also be present. Frontal epileptiform spike discharges have been associated with seizures of different types, including focal seizures with impaired external awareness and focal motor seizures, posturing, and drop attacks.[19] Occipital discharges of very short duration may occur in congenitally blind children without seizures. In general, occipital spikes tend to be benign, although they sometimes are related to structural abnormalities or occipital seizures, especially in older persons. One form of benign epilepsy of childhood is associated with spike-wave discharges that occur in one or both occipital regions after eye closure.[20]

Focal epileptiform spike discharges relate to paroxysmal depolarizing shifts occurring synchronously (as a result of disinhibition and excitation) in a population of neurons. Such shifts consist of a 20- to 30-mV depolarization of the cell membrane for up to about 100 msec, with a superimposed train of action potentials and followed by an afterhyperpolarization that may last for approximately 2 seconds. The slow wave that is recorded from the scalp after many epileptiform spikes ("spike-wave discharge") has been attributed to this afterhyperpolarization. Inhibitory activity is also triggered in the surrounding cortex as well as contralaterally, and this activity may be responsible for the focal slow activity that often occurs intermittently in association with an active spike focus.

Generalized spike-wave discharges are discussed in detail in the next section.

Paroxysmal Activity

Paroxysmal activity has an abrupt onset and termination, and it can be distinguished clearly from the background activity by its frequency and amplitude. It may occur as a normal phenomenon during hyperventilation in young adults and in response to arousal or sensory stimuli during sleep. The epileptiform transients just described are one example of paroxysmal activity. Abnormal paroxysmal activity that consists, at least in part, of epileptiform sharp transients (*epileptiform activity*) has a high correlation with the occurrence of epileptic seizures. It does not necessarily represent seizure (ictal) activity, however, and scalp-recorded electrographic seizures may not contain any epileptiform activity.

SPIKE-WAVE ACTIVITY

Generalized, bilaterally symmetric and bisynchronous 2.5- to 3-Hz *spike-wave activity* is the expected finding in patients with primary or idiopathic generalized epilepsy; it is enhanced by hyperventilation or hypoglycemia. More is known about the fundamental mechanisms underlying the absence seizures that occur in primary generalized epilepsy than about other types of generalized seizure. Gloor and Fariello related the generalized spike-wave activity associated with absence seizures to abnormal oscillatory discharges between cortical and thalamic neurons.[21,22] This oscillation involves the regular alternation of brief periods of neuronal excitation (associated with a markedly increased firing probability) during the spike phase with longer periods of neuronal silence during the slow-wave phase. Large populations of cortical and thalamic neurons are affected in near-synchrony, and the brainstem reticular formation also participates.

Generalized 2.5- to 3-Hz spike-wave activity may also be found in secondary generalized epilepsy (i.e., in patients with generalized seizures secondary to known pathology), but it is then superimposed on a diffusely abnormal background and is often accompanied by other EEG abnormalities. In the secondary generalized epilepsies, however, slow (p. 62) or atypical (p. 63) spike-wave activity is found more commonly. Generalized, bisynchronous spike-wave activity rarely may arise from a unilateral cortical focus, particularly on the medial surface of the hemisphere; this phenomenon is referred to as *secondary bilateral synchrony*. In such circumstances, the paroxysmal activity usually has a faster or slower frequency than that in primary generalized epilepsy, and the form and relationship of the spike to the wave component of the complex are less regular. Further, a consistent asymmetry of amplitude and waveform may exist between the hemispheres, the activity being either more or less conspicuous on the affected side. Recognition of the cortical origin of such activity is facilitated when isolated focal discharges arise from one side, particularly if they consistently precede the bursts of bilaterally synchronous activity; otherwise, recognition can be difficult unless the paroxysmal discharges have a focal or lateralized onset.

The mechanisms generating secondary bilateral synchrony of spike-wave discharges are not fully established but may involve either the propagation of discharges from one hemisphere to the other along the forebrain commissures or the activation by a cortical focus of diencephalic or other midline structures, which then elicit a synchronous discharge from both hemispheres. Studies have shown diminished but persistent bisynchronous epileptiform discharges after corpus callosotomy in patients with seizure disorders, suggesting that both mechanisms may be important.

It should be noted that bilaterally synchronous spike-wave activity may also be seen in rare instances in patients with structural subtentorial or midline lesions, as well as in unselected nonepileptic patients and in the clinically unaffected siblings of patients with primary generalized epilepsy.

Generalized paroxysmal EEG disturbances, consisting of either slow activity, spike-wave activity, or sharp transients, occur in patients with a diffuse encephalopathic process involving predominantly the cortical and subcortical gray matter, but not when the white matter alone is involved. If both gray and white matter are affected, generalized paroxysmal activity occurs on a background of continuous polymorphic slow activity. Bilaterally synchronous spike-wave activity is seen in diffuse gray matter encephalopathies and is usually more slow and irregular than that in patients with primary epilepsy.

INTERMITTENT RHYTHMIC DELTA ACTIVITY

Intermittent rhythmic delta activity (see Fig. 3-10) with a frontal predominance (often designated FIRDA) in adults and an occipital emphasis in children was referred to on page 48. It may result from a destructive lesion or from pressure and concomitant distortion affecting midline subcortical structures, in particular the diencephalon and rostral midbrain; it also occurs with deep frontal lesions. However, such activity is nonspecific and of no particular diagnostic significance. There is no means of clearly distinguishing the EEG pattern in deep midline lesions from that in diffuse cortical or subcortical encephalopathies or in metabolic encephalopathies. In most patients with FIRDA a diffuse encephalopathic process is present rather than a lesion limited to deep midline structures. FIRDA is occasionally present in otherwise healthy subjects during hyperventilation.[23]

BURST-SUPPRESSION PATTERN

The so-called *burst-suppression pattern* is characterized by bursts of high-voltage, mixed-frequency activity separated by intervals of marked quiescence or apparent inactivity that may last for no more than a few seconds or as long as several minutes. It occurs with a generalized distribution during the deeper stages of anesthesia; in patients who are comatose following overdosage with central nervous system (CNS) depressant drugs; and in any severe diffuse encephalopathy, such as that following anoxia (Fig. 3-12). The bursts may be asymmetric or bisynchronous. The prognostic significance of a burst-suppression pattern depends on the circumstances in which it is found. When it follows cerebral anoxia, it is associated with a poor outcome. Spontaneous eye-opening, nystagmoid movements, pupillary changes, facial movements,[24] myoclonus,[25] and limb movements have occasionally been associated with the EEG bursts,[25] and these sometimes mimic volitional activity.[24] In other instances, movements occur exclusively between EEG bursts.[26] Experimental studies in animals indicate that approximately 95 percent of cortical neurons become hyperpolarized and then electrically silent during periods of EEG suppression; this results from increased inhibition at cortical synapses, which also leads to functional disconnection of the cortex from its thalamic input.[27]

PERIODIC COMPLEXES

Repetitive paroxysmal slow- or sharp-wave discharges, or both, may occur with a regular periodicity in a number of conditions. Such *periodic complexes* are seen most conspicuously and with a generalized distribution in subacute sclerosing panencephalitis and Creutzfeldt–Jakob disease, and are sometimes found in patients with liver failure. Periodic complexes that exhibit, to a greater or lesser extent, a regular rhythmicity in their occurrence may also be found in patients with certain lipidoses, progressive myoclonus epilepsy, drug toxicity, anoxic encephalopathy, head injury, subdural hematoma, occasionally after tonic-clonic seizures, and in rare instances in other circumstances. Their diagnostic value therefore depends on the clinical circumstances in which they are found.

PERIODIC LATERALIZED EPILEPTIFORM DISCHARGES

Repetitive epileptiform discharges sometimes occur periodically as a lateralized phenomenon (designated *periodic lateralized epileptiform discharges*, or PLEDs), although they are often reflected to some extent over the homologous region of the opposite hemisphere as well. Their amplitude has ranged between 50 and 300 μV, and their periodicity between 0.3 and 4 seconds in different series.[28] Structural cortical or subcortical lesions often—but not

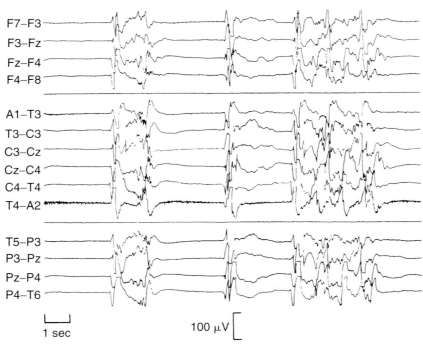

FIGURE 3-12 ■ Burst-suppression pattern recorded in the electroencephalogram of a 70-year-old man after a cardiac arrest from which he was resuscitated.

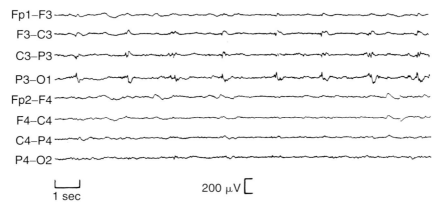

FIGURE 3-13 ▪ Periodic lateralized epileptiform discharges over the left hemisphere in the electroencephalogram of a 78-year-old woman with a recent stroke.

always—underlie the occurrence of these discharges.[29] They typically are seen in patients with hemispheric lesions caused, most commonly, by cerebral infarction (Fig. 3-13), hemorrhage, or tumors. In patients with acute hemispheric stroke, PLEDs are more likely when there are associated metabolic derangements, especially hyperglycemia and fever.[30] Patients with herpes simplex encephalitis may have PLEDs, especially in the first 2 weeks of the illness, but their absence in no way excludes the diagnosis. Other infections occasionally associated with PLEDs include neurosyphilis, cysticercosis, bacterial meningitis, mononucleosis encephalitis, and early Creutzfeldt–Jakob disease. PLEDs may also be found in patients with chronic seizure disorders or long-standing static lesions (e.g., old infarcts), sometimes as a persistent phenomenon but more often for a brief period, especially when seizures or toxic metabolic disturbances have occurred recently. They or more generalized periodic epileptiform discharges are found occasionally with metabolic disorders that more typically produce diffuse EEG disturbances (e.g., anoxia, hepatic encephalopathy, and abnormal blood levels of glucose or calcium), and PLEDs also have been reported with head injury, lupus cerebritis,[31] subdural hematoma, cerebral abscess or other cystic lesions, and sickle cell disease. In many cases, no specific cause can be found.

In one series, acute stroke, tumor, and CNS infection were the most common causes of PLEDs, accounting for 26, 12, and 12 percent of cases, respectively. Acute hemorrhage and traumatic brain injury combined were responsible for another 12 percent. Other, previously unreported, causes included posterior reversible encephalopathy syndrome, familial hemiplegic migraine, and cerebral amyloidosis. In 9 cases, chronic PLEDs were related to underlying cortical dysplasia or severe remote cerebral injury, all with an accompanying partial seizure disorder. Alcohol withdrawal was sometimes a precipitant,

and in a few cases was seemingly the sole cause. Seizure activity occurred in 85 percent of patients. The overall mortality rate was 27 percent.[32]

During the acute stage of illness, patients with PLEDs are usually obtunded and commonly have seizures (especially focal seizures) and a focal neurologic deficit. The PLEDs themselves are usually an interictal pattern, being replaced or obscured by other activity as a seizure develops. They may also occur ictally, however, particularly in patients with partial seizures, status epilepticus, or epilepsia partialis continua.[33] The intense hypermetabolism and increased blood flow revealed by positron emission tomography (PET) and single-photon emission computed tomography (SPECT) scans provide some support for the belief that this EEG pattern is sometimes ictal in nature.[34] Moreover, patients have been described with recurrent or prolonged confusional episodes during which PLEDs were present in the EEG; with clinical improvement, the EEG normalized.[35]

PLEDs typically occur every 1 to 2 seconds; vary in morphology in different patients; and usually (but not always) disappear over the course of a few days or weeks, to be replaced by a focal or lateralized polymorphic slow-wave disturbance or by isolated spike discharges. The underlying disease determines the prognosis of patients with PLEDs. The absence of clinical seizures when PLEDs are detected is also associated with a poor prognosis for survival.[36]

The pathophysiologic basis of PLEDs is not understood. Some have considered PLEDs to be equivalent to the terminal phase of status epilepticus; others have reported their association with rhythmic discharges that have a stereotyped distribution, frequency, configuration, and amplitude for individual patients, and that may be obscured by the development of frank electrographic seizure discharges.[37]

PLEDs may occur independently over both hemispheres; they are then designated BiPLEDs. The complexes over the two hemispheres differ in their morphology and repetition rate. BiPLEDs are caused most commonly by anoxic encephalopathy, multiple vascular lesions, and CNS infection with either herpes simplex or other agents, but they may also be found in patients with chronic seizure disorders or with recent onset of seizures. BiPLEDs are usually found in comatose patients and are associated with a much higher mortality than are PLEDs.[32]

Low-Voltage Records

A number of normal subjects have generally low-voltage EEGs, consisting of an irregular mixture of activity with a frequency ranging between 2 and 30 Hz and an amplitude of less than 20 μV. A little alpha activity may, however, be present at rest or during hyperventilation, and it is sometimes possible to enhance the amplitude of background rhythms by simple or pharmacologic activating procedures. This low-voltage EEG pattern may occur on a hereditary basis. Similar low-voltage records are occasionally encountered in patients with Huntington disease or myxedema, but they are of no diagnostic value. Such records should be distinguished from those consisting primarily of low-voltage delta activity.

Other EEG Patterns

Over the years, special pathologic significance has been attributed (without adequate justification) to a number of EEG patterns that are now known to occur as a normal phenomenon in some healthy subjects, particularly during drowsiness or sleep. They do not predict the occurrence of seizures. These patterns are therefore of dubious clinical relevance, but—although recent studies[38] suggest that their prevalence is relatively low—they merit brief comment to prevent their misinterpretation and thus to avoid misdiagnosis and unnecessary investigations. Further details are provided in Chapter 5.

14- AND 6-HZ POSITIVE SPIKES

During drowsiness and light sleep, especially in adolescents, runs of either 14- or 6-Hz positive spikes, or both, may occur, superimposed on slower waves; generally they last for less than about 1 second. They are found especially in the posterior temporal or parietal regions on one or both sides and are best seen as surface-positive waveforms on referential recordings. They are of no pathologic relevance, although bursts

of such activity have been described in comatose patients with Reye syndrome and in adults with hepatic or renal disease.

SMALL SHARP SPIKES OR BENIGN EPILEPTIFORM TRANSIENTS OF SLEEP

Small sharp spikes or benign epileptiform transients of sleep are found during drowsiness or light sleep in as many as one-quarter of normal adults. Generally, they consist of monophasic or biphasic spikes; they are sometimes followed by a slow wave but are unaccompanied by sharp waves or rhythmic focal slowing of the background. They usually occur independently over the two hemispheres with sporadic shifting localization, but are best seen in the anteromesial temporal regions. Their appearance varies in different patients. They are distinguished from transients of pathologic significance by their bilateral occurrence, failure to occur in trains, and disappearance as the depth of sleep increases, and by the absence of abnormal background activity. Although commonly less than 50 μV, they are sometimes larger, so that size is not a reliable distinguishing feature. Such discharges are best regarded as normal and are of no diagnostic help in the evaluation of patients with suspected epilepsy.

6-HZ SPIKE-WAVE ACTIVITY

Brief bursts of 6-Hz spike-wave activity, usually lasting for less than 1 second, may occasionally be seen in normal adolescents or young adults, especially during drowsiness, and are sometimes referred to as phantom spike-waves. They disappear during deeper levels of sleep, unlike pathologically significant spike-wave discharges. In some instances, the discharges are bilaterally symmetric and synchronous, but in others they are asymmetric. The spike is usually small compared with the slow wave and may be hard to recognize; when the spike is large, the discharges are more likely to be of pathologic significance. Discharges that are frontally predominant are also more likely to be associated with epilepsy than are discharges that are accentuated occipitally.

WICKET SPIKES

A wicket spike pattern usually is found in adults, most commonly in drowsiness or light sleep but also during wakefulness. It may consist of intermittent trains of sharp activity resembling a mu rhythm, or of sporadic single spikes that are surface-negative and essentially monophasic. Its frequency is usually between 6 and 12 Hz.

Wicket spikes are generally best seen over the temporal regions, either bilaterally or independently over the two sides, and sometimes have a shifting lateralized emphasis. The spikes are not associated with a subsequent slow wave or with any background abnormality. Wicket spikes have no diagnostic significance and, in particular, do not correlate with any particular symptom complex, including epilepsy. When these spikes occur singly, however, they may be mistaken for interictal temporal spike discharges.

RHYTHMIC TEMPORAL THETA BURSTS OF DROWSINESS (PSYCHOMOTOR VARIANT)

During drowsiness or light sleep, especially in young adults, bursts of rhythmic sharpened theta waves with a notched appearance sometimes occur, predominantly in the midtemporal regions either unilaterally or bilaterally (Fig. 3-14). If bilateral, they may occur synchronously or independently, with a shifting emphasis from one side to the other. Individual bursts commonly last for at least 10 seconds. Unlike electrographic seizure discharges, the bursts of activity do not show an evolution in frequency, amplitude, or configuration. They are of no pathologic significance.

RHYTHMIC THETA DISCHARGES

In patients older than about 40 years, bursts of rhythmic sharpened theta activity at about 5 to 7 Hz may occur, often with an abrupt onset and termination. In contrast to seizures, they typically show no evolution of their frequency, distribution, or configuration, and they are not followed by focal or diffuse slow activity. These subclinical rhythmic electrographic discharges in adults (known by the acronym SREDA) usually are distributed bilaterally and diffusely, but occasionally are focal or lateralized. When diffuse, the discharges are often most conspicuous over the parietal and posterior temporal regions. They can occur at rest, during hyperventilation, or with drowsiness. The bursts may last up to 1 or 2 minutes, or even longer, and may be mistaken for a subclinical seizure. Digital analysis has revealed that the bursts are maximal in the parietal or parietocentrotemporal region and that they consist of a complex mixture of rapidly shifting frequencies that show little spatial or temporal correlation.[39] Such discharges are probably of no diagnostic relevance and do not correlate with epilepsy or any specific clinical complaints.

Unusual variants of SREDA include predominantly delta frequencies, notched waveforms, or discharges having a frontal or more focal distribution; bursts that are more prolonged in duration; and discharges that occur during sleep.[40]

EEG Changes with Aging

A number of EEG changes occur with senescence, but the extent to which they occur varies widely in different subjects. It is widely believed that the mean alpha frequency slows in elderly subjects compared with young adults, but whether such slowing occurs in completely healthy and cognitively intact elderly subjects is unclear; if it does, it is to a minimal degree.[41] In subjects older

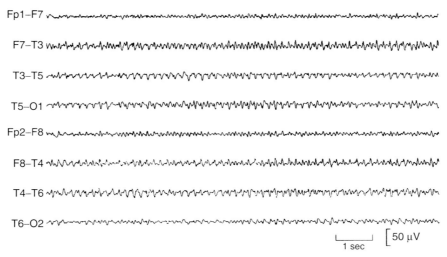

FIGURE 3-14 ■ Rhythmic sharpened theta activity seen bilaterally during drowsiness in the electroencephalogram of a 16-year-old boy. Bursts of such activity are a normal variant (sometimes called psychomotor variant) without pathologic significance.

than 50 years, alpha-like activity is sometimes seen in one or both temporal regions and may be more conspicuous than the occipital alpha rhythm.[41]

The effect of aging on beta activity is less clear, and review of the published accounts is confounded by differences in the methods of analysis and recording circumstances, differences in the types of patients studied, and a failure to consider medical and drug histories and the state of intellectual function. No consistent effects on beta rhythms have been found in elderly subjects, although various alterations have been described by different authors.

Diffuse theta and delta activity is significantly increased in elderly persons and is clearly related to intellectual deterioration and life expectancy. Polymorphic or rhythmic focal slow activity, encountered fairly commonly in the elderly, usually is localized to the left anterior temporal region. Such slow activity may be enhanced or brought out during drowsiness or hyperventilation. It is of little pathologic significance, showing no obvious correlation with life expectancy, neurologic disease, or intellectual changes.[42] It should not be regarded as abnormal if it occurs infrequently in bursts on an otherwise normal background; however, the bounds of normality are unclear.

EEG sleep patterns also change with age, with a reduction in total sleep time and especially in the duration of stage 3 and 4 sleep.

EEG RESPONSES TO SIMPLE ACTIVATING PROCEDURES

Hyperventilation

The response to hyperventilation (p. 40) varies considerably in different subjects and is enhanced by hypoglycemia. Typically, there is a buildup of diffuse slow activity, first in the theta- and then in the delta-frequency ranges, with the activity settling in the 30 to 60 seconds after the conclusion of overbreathing. As indicated earlier, these changes are often attributed to a fall in arterial PCO_2, which leads to cerebral vasoconstriction and thus to reduced cerebral blood flow; however, other mechanisms also have been suggested.[4] The EEG response depends very much on the age of the subject. In normal children or in young adults it may be quite striking, with continuous or paroxysmal rhythmic, high-voltage delta activity coming to dominate the EEG record. By contrast, many elderly persons show little or no response. This lack of response has been attributed to an inability of these persons to alter their arterial PCO_2 and has been related to

reduced cerebrovascular reactivity. Persistence of any response for an excessive period after hyperventilation has ceased generally is regarded as abnormal, as is an asymmetric response. However, individual variability in the response to hyperventilation can make it difficult to evaluate the findings provoked by the maneuver.

In some patients, hyperventilation leads to the reproduction of symptoms. The occurrence of symptoms should be noted by the technologist so that electroclinical correlations can be made.

Spike-wave discharges can be provoked in patients with generalized epilepsy, especially in patients with absence seizures. Focal abnormalities may be enhanced in patients with partial epilepsy. Delta rhythm notched by faster activity (beta activity or muscle artifact) is an occasional nonspecific finding that may simulate spike-wave discharges; however, it should not be taken as evidence of epilepsy. Review of the background activity usually permits the nature of this activity to be recognized. Hyperventilation is widely believed to be a safe and useful method for activating seizures or provoking interictal epileptiform activity,[43,44] although some have questioned its utility.[45] In patients with cerebrovascular disease, irregular theta and delta activity appears earlier and more conspicuously on the affected side than on the other, and in some instances repetitive paroxysmal discharges may be seen in a restricted distribution. In patients with tumors, hyperventilation may enhance the abnormalities seen on the resting record or provoke changes that are otherwise not apparent.

Photic Stimulation

In response to photic stimulation (p. 40), it is usual to observe the so-called driving response over the posterior regions of the head. This response consists of rhythmic activity that is time-locked to the stimulus and has a frequency identical or harmonically related to that of the flickering light. Not all normal subjects exhibit a driving response, and many show it at only some stimulus frequencies. Moreover, a mild amplitude asymmetry is sometimes seen in normal subjects. Even when the amplitude difference between the two hemispheres is greater than 50 percent, an underlying structural lesion is unlikely unless other EEG abnormalities are present (e.g., a gross amplitude asymmetry of the alpha rhythm or the presence of focal slow waves or sharp transients). Focal hemispheric lesions may lead to an ipsilateral reduction in amplitude or, less commonly, to enhanced responses. An asymmetry in the development of a driving response is more likely to be associated with focal slowing and other EEG abnormalities and with the presence of a structural lesion.

Enhanced responses—bilateral high-amplitude spikes—may occur posteriorly at low flash rates (less than 5 Hz) in patients with diffuse encephalopathies such as Creutzfeldt–Jakob disease or progressive myoclonic epilepsy.[4]

Paroxysmal activity is sometimes found during photic stimulation, even when the EEG is otherwise normal. Polyspike discharges following each flash of light may be seen, particularly during stimulation while the eyes are closed. The discharges are muscular in origin; are most conspicuous frontally; stop when stimulation is discontinued; and may occur without clinical accompaniments, although in other cases a fluttering of the eyelids is seen. Activity of this sort is generally referred to as a *photomyogenic (or photomyoclonic) response* and is regarded as a normal response to high-intensity light stimulation, being not uncommon in healthy persons. It must be distinguished from a photoparoxysmal response (Fig. 3-15).

A *photoparoxysmal response* occurs in some (less than 5 percent) epileptic patients, particularly in those with generalized (myoclonic, tonic-clonic, or absence) seizures. Juvenile myoclonic epilepsy is closely associated with photosensitivity. Approximately 70 to 90 percent of subjects with a generalized response to photic stimulation have epilepsy.[4] An abnormal response occurs occasionally in patients with diverse CNS and metabolic disorders. Early reports of photoparoxysmal responses in alcohol and drug withdrawal syndromes were not

supported by the study of Fisch and colleagues, who studied 49 subjects during acute alcohol withdrawal without finding a single instance of such a response.[46] It may also occur on a familial basis or spontaneously in subjects without neurologic or metabolic disorders, and it is rare for such subjects to go on to develop epilepsy.

A photoparoxysmal response consists of bursts of slow-wave and spike or polyspike activity that has a discharge frequency unrelated to that of the flashing light and may outlast the stimulus. The activity is cerebral in origin and is usually generalized, bilaterally symmetric, and bisynchronous, although it may have a frontocentral emphasis. It is sometimes associated with clinical phenomena such as speech arrest, transient absence, or deviation of the eyes or head: if photic stimulation is continued, a generalized tonic-clonic seizure may result. There is no difference in the incidence of seizures in patients with photoparoxysmal responses that outlast or are limited to the time of stimulation or stop spontaneously.[47] Photoparoxysmal activity sometimes occurs with a more restricted distribution in the occipital region, particularly in patients with an epileptogenic lesion in that area; such activity may be unilateral or bilateral.

Natural Sleep

The electrophysiologic changes that occur during sleep are discussed in Chapter 33; only brief mention of them is made here. As the patient becomes drowsy (stage 1), the alpha rhythm becomes attenuated and the EEG is

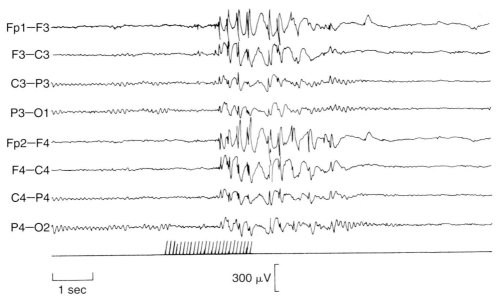

FIGURE 3-15 ■ Photoparoxysmal response recorded in a patient with epilepsy. The lowest trace records the light flashes, which were occurring at 12 Hz.

characterized mainly by theta and beta rhythms. During light sleep (stage 2), theta activity becomes more conspicuous, and single or repetitive vertex sharp transients occur spontaneously or in response to sensory stimuli. Bursts of high-voltage biphasic slow waves (K-complexes) also occur spontaneously or with arousal, and are often associated with bursts of diffuse 12- to 14-Hz activity (sleep spindles). The spindles are usually most prominent in the central regions and may occur independently of the K-complexes, which have been related to outward dendritic currents in the middle and upper cortical layers and held to represent an isolated cortical "down-state."[48] Positive occipital sharp transients (POSTs) may also occur spontaneously, either singly or (more commonly) repetitively in runs during this stage of sleep; they are bilaterally synchronous, but may be markedly asymmetric (Fig. 3-16).[49] As sleep deepens, the EEG slows further until up to 50 to 60 percent (stage 3) or more (stage 4) of the record consists of irregular delta activity at 2 Hz or less; vertex sharp waves and spindles may also be found in stage 3 sleep. Stage 3 and 4 sleep generally is referred to as slow-wave sleep. During REM sleep, the heart and respiratory rates become irregular, irregular eye movements occur, and the EEG comes to resemble that of stage 1 sleep.

A new staging system for sleep has been described by the American Association of Sleep Medicine (AASM) and designates three stages of non-REM sleep (N1, N2, N3) and one stage of REM sleep (R). N1 is equivalent to stage 1 non-REM sleep, N2 to stage 2 non-REM sleep, N3 to stages 3 and 4 non-REM sleep, and R to stage REM sleep.[50] Further details of this staging system are provided in Chapter 33.

Focal cerebral lesions may lead to abnormalities of normal sleep activity, most often causing a voltage asymmetry of vertex sharp waves or sleep spindles. In some instances, such activity may be absent unilaterally. In rare instances, sleep spindles may show a frequency asymmetry, being slower on one side (usually that of the lesion) than the other.[51]

The EEG is sometimes recorded during sleep or following a period of sleep deprivation in the hope of activating abnormalities, especially when patients with suspected epilepsy are being evaluated. The incidence of epileptiform discharges is increased when the EEG is recorded during sleep as well as wakefulness, and the additional yield is greatest when patients are being investigated for suspected focal seizures involving an impairment of consciousness (complex partial seizures). However, both the extent of this additional yield and the manner in which sleep recordings are best obtained in patients with suspected epilepsy are controversial. In particular, there is disagreement as to whether activation is best achieved with natural or drug-induced sleep. Nevertheless, in all patients with a suspected seizure disorder, the EEG probably should be recorded during both wakefulness and natural sleep because this may be helpful and involves no additional cost or risk.

Slow or atypical spike-wave discharges are usually (but not always) more conspicuous during sleep. Focal spike

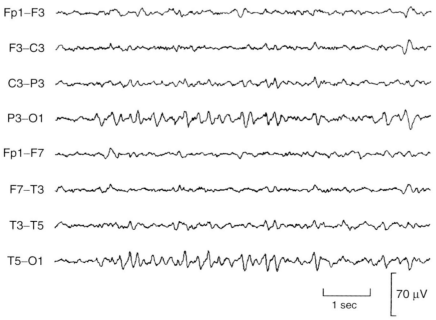

FIGURE 3-16 ■ Runs of positive occipital sharp transients recorded during drowsiness in a subject with a normal electroencephalogram.

discharges can be enhanced or precipitated during any stage of non-REM sleep; but most interictal epileptiform discharges, whether focal or generalized, are usually seen less commonly during REM sleep. Classic 3-Hz spike-wave activity is seen more often but is less well organized during non-REM sleep than during wakefulness, whereas it occurs less frequently during REM sleep but is similar in form, rhythmicity, and regularity to its appearance in the waking record.

Thus, recording during sleep can be useful, especially in patients with suspected focal seizures when the EEG recorded during wakefulness does not show focal or lateralized epileptiform activity. However, the interpretation of EEGs obtained in such circumstances can be complicated by difficulty in determining whether particular findings represent the normal electrical accompaniments of sleep or are of pathologic significance.

Sleep Deprivation

Sleep deprivation is a harmless activating procedure, especially in patients with epilepsy, and is therefore undertaken in many laboratories. It is more likely than sedated sleep to elicit useful information (precipitation or enhancement of epileptiform discharges, presence of a new independent focus, or new type of epileptiform discharge) and activates epileptiform discharges independent of the activating effects of sleep.[52]

EEG FINDINGS IN PATIENTS WITH NEUROLOGIC DISORDERS

Epilepsy

Although the EEG is recorded from a very restricted portion of the brain and for only a limited time, it is an invaluable adjunct to the management of patients with epilepsy. The recording of electrocerebral activity during one of the patient's clinical attacks may be particularly helpful in determining whether the attacks are indeed epileptic in nature and whether they have a focal or lateralized origin. Because attacks usually occur unpredictably, however, the chances of a recording actually being in progress during an attack are not particularly good unless prolonged recordings are made or attacks are deliberately provoked. Moreover, even if an attack can be recorded, the EEG may be so obscured by muscle and movement artifact that little useful information can be gained from it.

The interictal EEG is also abnormal in many epileptic patients and may exhibit features that help to establish the diagnosis. In this connection, the presence of paroxysmal activity consisting of spike, polyspike, or sharp-wave discharges, either alone or in association with slow waves, is of prime importance. Such epileptiform activity may be focal, multifocal, or diffuse and may appear unilaterally or bilaterally; if bilateral, it may be synchronous or asynchronous and symmetric or asymmetric. When multiple foci are present, one of them may be the primary one, generating a mirror focus in the homologous region of the contralateral hemisphere, although the development of such mirror foci in humans is not well documented. Alternatively, a single deep focus may discharge to homologous regions of the cortex so that the EEG reveals either a focus that shifts from side to side or bilaterally synchronous discharges. In many patients with multiple foci, however, the foci are distinct from each other, with discharges arising from them asynchronously. Such patients often have extensive bilateral cerebral lesions and many experience clinical seizures of more than one type.

Epileptiform activity is found in between 2 and 4 percent of subjects who have never experienced a seizure. Accordingly, the presence of epileptiform activity, in itself, does not establish the diagnosis of epilepsy. Among patients with epilepsy, the initial EEG contains epileptiform activity in about 50 to 55 percent of cases. Because the incidence of epilepsy in the general population is only 0.5 percent, however, epileptiform activity is actually more likely to be encountered in EEGs from nonepileptics than in those from epileptics if recordings are made from an unselected group of subjects. By contrast, among patients with episodic behavioral or cerebral disturbances that could well be epileptic in nature, the presence of epileptiform activity in the EEG markedly increases the likelihood that epilepsy is the correct diagnosis.[53] The presence of epileptiform activity can therefore be very helpful in establishing the diagnosis of epilepsy beyond reasonable doubt, depending on the clinical context in which the EEG is obtained.[53] The absence of such activity cannot be taken to exclude this diagnosis.

Several factors (e.g., the age of the patient and the type and frequency of seizures) bear on the presence or absence of epileptiform activity in the EEG of patients with undoubted epilepsy on clinical grounds. Some of these factors should influence the manner in which the EEG is obtained. First, epileptiform activity is more likely to be found if repeated records are obtained. Second, the diagnostic yield is increased by the routine use of activation procedures (e.g., hyperventilation, photic stimulation, sleep, and sleep deprivation for 24 hours; see pp. 56–59) to precipitate epileptiform discharges. Third, the timing of the examination may influence the yield. Epileptiform activity is found more commonly if the EEG is recorded soon after (particularly within 24 hours of) a clinical seizure.[54,55] If seizure frequency is influenced by external or situational factors (e.g., the menstrual period), the EEG should be scheduled with these factors in mind. In patients with one of the reflex epilepsies, it may be possible to reproduce the provocative stimulus while the EEG is recorded.

King and associates examined the possibility of diagnosing specific epilepsy syndromes by clinical evaluation, EEG, and MRI in 300 patients who presented with a first unexplained seizure.[54] They were able to diagnose a generalized or focal epilepsy syndrome on clinical grounds in 141 (47 percent of) patients, and subsequent analysis showed that only 3 of these diagnoses were incorrect. When the EEG data were also utilized, an epilepsy syndrome was diagnosed in 232 patients (77 percent). Neuroimaging revealed 38 epileptogenic lesions; there were no lesions in patients with generalized epilepsy confirmed by EEG. The EEG recorded within the first 24 hours was more useful in detecting epileptiform abnormalities than a later EEG (51 percent vs. 34 percent). This study emphasizes the utility of the EEG in evaluating patients with a single seizure for determining the precise diagnosis, and thereby the prognosis and need for treatment.

In reviewing the EEG findings in patients with seizure disorders, attention has been confined to the more common types of seizures encountered in clinical practice.

PRIMARY (IDIOPATHIC) GENERALIZED EPILEPSY

The background activity of the interictal record is usually relatively normal, although some posterior slow (theta and delta) activity may be present in patients with absence (petit mal) seizures. Generalized, bilaterally symmetric, and bisynchronous paroxysmal epileptiform activity often is seen, especially during activation procedures such as hyperventilation or photic stimulation.

Absence (Petit Mal) Seizures

In patients with absence seizures, epileptiform activity consists of well-organized 2.5- to 3-Hz spike-wave discharges (Fig. 3-17) that may be seen both interictally (especially during hyperventilation, which increases the discharges in about 75 percent of patients, or with hypoglycemia) and ictally. The presence of observed clinical accompaniments depends on the duration of the discharges and the manner in which the patient's clinical status is evaluated. With sufficiently sensitive techniques, it may well be found that this type of epileptiform activity is generally associated with behavioral disturbances (i.e., is usually an ictal phenomenon). For example, auditory reaction time is commonly delayed during the first 2 seconds of a generalized spike-wave discharge, even when there is no clinically obvious impairment of external awareness. The characteristics of the spike-wave complexes are best defined in referential derivations.

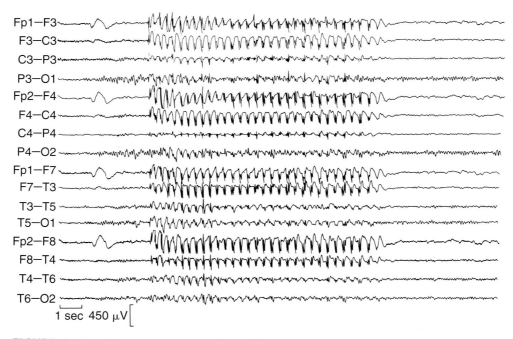

FIGURE 3-17 ■ Paroxysmal, generalized, bilaterally synchronous and symmetric 2.5- to 3-Hz spike-wave activity recorded interictally in the electroencephalogram of a patient with absence (petit mal) seizures.

They are often maximal in amplitude in the frontocentral regions, and careful analysis has shown that the spike has several components; it is not a simple, monophasic phenomenon. The frequency of the complexes is often a little faster than 3 Hz at onset and tends to slow to about 2 Hz before terminating. Sleep may influence the morphology of the complexes (p. 59). In some instances, the discharges cease with eye-opening or in response to alerting. There may be inconstantly lateralized amplitude asymmetries or inconsistent asynchronous onsets over the two hemispheres when the recordings on different occasions are compared, but such findings are of no clinical help. The background between the generalized bursts of activity occasionally contains isolated spike discharges that may be focal (usually, frontal) in distribution; this finding is also without special significance. Similarly, high-voltage intermittent rhythmic delta activity may be found occipitally, especially in children during the first decade of life. EEG findings that are repeatedly normal in a child with clinical attacks resembling absence seizures suggest that a diagnosis of primary generalized epilepsy is incorrect.

Absence epilepsy of childhood onset usually presents before the age of 12 years and commonly remits in late adolescence. By contrast, juvenile absence epilepsy presents in the second decade and is associated with less frequent absences but a greater likelihood that seizures will continue into adulthood and that generalized tonic-clonic convulsions will occur. Further details of these disorders are provided in Chapter 4. The absences that occur in juvenile myoclonic epilepsy are associated with spike- or polyspike-wave activity that has a frequency of 2.5 to 4 Hz (with a range of 2 to 7 Hz) and that is enhanced by hyperventilation; there is much intra- and interdischarge variation, and discharges may be interrupted for brief periods.

When absence attacks continue to occur in adults, they are often difficult to recognize because of their short duration.[56,57] Such patients usually also have generalized tonic-clonic seizures. Michelucci and colleagues found in adults that the interictal EEG background is normal but may be interrupted by generalized bursts of spike-wave or polyspike-wave discharges and, occasionally, by independent focal spikes; runs of polyspikes sometimes occur during non-REM sleep.[56] Ictally, 3-Hz spike-wave discharges are characteristic, sometimes preceded by polyspikes with or without intermixed spike-wave or polyspike-wave discharges. Similar findings have been reported by others.[57]

Myoclonic Seizures

Bursts of generalized spike-wave or polyspike-wave activity are found both ictally and interictally, often with a frequency of 3 to 5 Hz and an anterior emphasis; they may be enhanced especially by photic stimulation or sleep. In juvenile myoclonic epilepsy, discussed in detail in Chapter 4, the interictal EEG usually has a normal background; however, this is interrupted by bursts of generalized, frontally predominant polyspikes or of polyspike-wave or spike-wave discharges having a variable frequency that is often between 3 and 5 Hz but may be higher. Photic stimulation provokes or enhances such abnormalities in 25 to 30 percent of cases, and hyperventilation also activates the epileptiform abnormalities. Focal or lateralizing features or shifting asymmetries are sometimes found. Ictally, the myoclonic seizures are associated with anteriorly dominant polyspike or polyspike-wave bursts followed by rhythmic delta activity. Absence seizures in this syndrome are accompanied by irregular spike-wave or polyspike-wave discharges of variable frequency.

Tonic-Clonic (Grand Mal) Seizures

Generalized, bilaterally synchronous spike discharges, or bursts of spike-wave or polyspike-wave activity, or both, may be seen interictally (Fig. 3-18), the latter sometimes being identical to that found in absence attacks. The earliest change during a tonic-clonic convulsion is often the appearance of generalized, low-voltage fast activity. This activity then becomes slower, more conspicuous, and more extensive in distribution and, depending on the recording technique, may take the form of multiple spike or repetitive sharp-wave discharges that have a frequency of about 10 Hz and are seen during the tonic phase of the attack. In other instances, seizure activity may be initiated by a flattening (desynchronization) of electrocerebral activity or by paroxysmal activity, such as that which occurs in the interictal period. In any event, as the seizure continues into the clonic phase, a buildup of slow waves occurs and the EEG comes to be characterized by slow activity with associated spike or polyspike discharges. Following the attack, the EEG may revert to its preictal state, although there is usually a transient attenuation of electrocerebral activity, followed by the appearance of irregular polymorphic slow activity that may persist for several hours or even longer. In a few cases, the postictal EEG is characterized by periodic complexes.

SECONDARY (SYMPTOMATIC) GENERALIZED EPILEPSY

In patients with secondary generalized epilepsy (i.e., with generalized seizures relating to known pathology, such as Lennox–Gastaut syndrome), the background activity of the interictal EEG is usually abnormal, containing an excess of diffuse theta or delta activity that is poorly

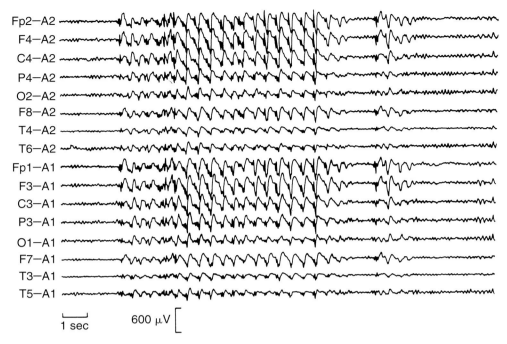

FIGURE 3-18 ■ Paroxysmal, generalized, bilaterally synchronous spike-wave and polyspike-wave discharges seen interictally in the electroencephalogram of a 62-year-old woman with tonic-clonic seizures caused by primary generalized epilepsy.

responsive to eye-opening and may show a focal or lateralized emphasis. Single or independent multiple spike discharges also may be found. However, interictal paroxysmal activity characteristically consists of *slow spike-wave* or polyspike-wave discharges that are usually less well organized than in the primary generalized epilepsies, with a frequency that varies between 1.5 and 2.5 Hz (Fig. 3-19). This activity exhibits a characteristic variability in frequency, amplitude, morphology, and distribution on different occasions, even during the same examination. In some instances it is generalized and exhibits bilateral symmetry and synchrony; in others it is markedly asymmetric, showing a clear emphasis over one hemisphere or even over a discrete portion of that hemisphere. Hyperventilation and flicker stimulation are generally less effective as activating agents than in the primary generalized epilepsies, but non-REM sleep can increase the frequency of the paroxysmal discharges.

Such paroxysmal activity may also occur as an ictal phenomenon accompanying absence and myoclonic attacks. The most common EEG changes associated with tonic seizures are relative or total desynchronization (flattening), with sudden disappearance of any ongoing spike-wave activity, or the development of rhythmic activity (usually at about 10 Hz, or faster) that usually increases in amplitude, has a generalized distribution, and is followed by irregular slow waves (Fig. 3-20). In some instances, an initial desynchronization of the traces is followed by this pattern of generalized rhythmic fast activity. The ictal EEG features of tonic-clonic seizures

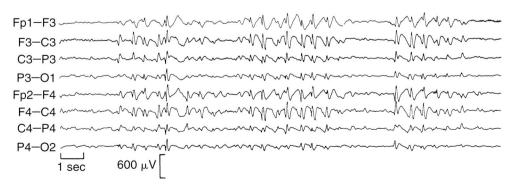

FIGURE 3-19 ■ Interictal 2-Hz spike-wave activity in the electroencephalogram of 17-year-old boy with Lennox–Gastaut syndrome.

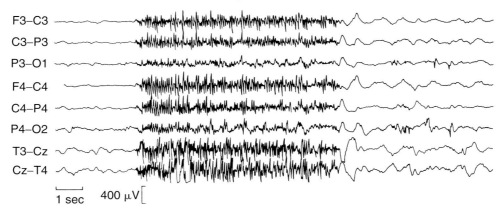

F3–C3

C3–P3

P3–O1

F4–C4

C4–P4

P4–O2

T3–Cz

Cz–T4

1 sec   400 μV

FIGURE 3-20 ■ Tonic seizure recorded in the electroencephalogram of an 11-year-old girl with Lennox–Gastaut syndrome.

are as described for patients with primary generalized epilepsy. *Atonic (astatic) seizures* are associated with polyspike-wave discharges, an attenuation of the background, or a brief burst of generalized fast activity or spikes.

Generalized *atypical spike-wave discharges* have a more irregular appearance than that of 3-Hz or slow spike-wave activity, and range in frequency between 2 and 5 Hz. They occur ictally or interictally, may be activated by sleep and sometimes by photic stimulation, and have been associated with various types of generalized seizures.

In patients with myoclonus epilepsy the background is diffusely slowed, and bursts of spikes, polyspikes or sharp waves, or spike-wave discharges are seen either unilaterally or bilaterally. Flicker stimulation may lead to bursts of spike- or polyspike-wave activity. The spike activity is sometimes time-locked to the myoclonic jerking that the patient exhibits.

EPILEPSIES PRODUCING FOCAL (PARTIAL) SEIZURES

Several varieties of so-called benign focal (partial) epilepsy have been described in children. These include benign epilepsy with centrotemporal (rolandic) spikes; occipital, or frontal, epilepsy; benign partial epilepsy of adolescence; and benign epilepsy associated with multiple spike foci. They are considered in Chapter 4.

The interictal EEG findings may vary considerably at different times in patients with focal (partial) epilepsy, especially in those with impairment of consciousness or awareness (commonly described as complex symptomatology). The interictal record (see Fig. 3-11) may exhibit intermittent focal sharp waves or spikes, continuous or paroxysmal focal slow-wave activity, localized paroxysmal spike-wave discharges, or any combination of these features. There is some correlation between the site of epileptiform discharges and the clinical manifestations of seizure phenomena. For example, among patients with

epilepsy, focal seizures with impaired external awareness (complex partial seizures) are more likely in those with interictal anterior temporal spike discharges, visual hallucinations are more common in those with occipital spikes, and hemifacial seizures occur more often in those with centrotemporal (rolandic) spikes.

In patients with temporal lobe abnormalities, spike discharges may be confined to one hemisphere, may be found either independently or synchronously over both hemispheres, or may occur in the homologous region of both hemispheres with a consistent temporal relationship between the spikes. In the latter case it is presumed that the discharge originates from one side and spreads to the other via commissural connections (e.g., the corpus callosum) to produce a so-called mirror focus that eventually becomes independent of the original focus, although the evidence to support this concept is incomplete in humans.

Focal epileptiform discharges may be restricted to the vertex electrodes, in which case they can be hard to distinguish from the normal vertex sharp activity seen during sleep. The occurrence of such discharges during wakefulness, the presence of associated focal slowing, or a tendency for the discharges to lateralize to one side of the midline would suggest that they are abnormal, as also would fields of distribution that differ from those of normal vertex sharp waves.

Bilaterally synchronous spike-wave activity is an occasional finding in patients with focal (partial) seizures. Unless this activity is markedly asymmetric, has a focal onset, or is preceded by focal or lateralized discharges, it can be difficult to distinguish from the similar activity seen in patients with primary generalized epilepsy.

Interictal abnormalities may be provoked by such harmless activation procedures as hyperventilation, sleep, or sleep deprivation (pp. 56–59), but flicker stimulation is not helpful in most patients with partial epilepsy. When these abnormalities arise in the anterior temporal region

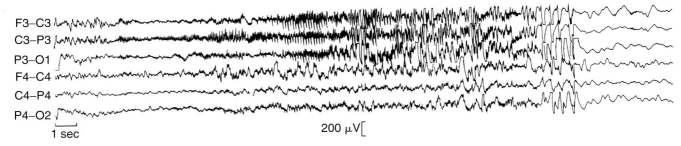

FIGURE 3-21 ■ Focal seizure recorded in the electroencephalogram of a 12-year-old girl. The seizure commences with rhythmic left-sided fast activity that increases in amplitude and becomes intermixed with slower elements, with some spread to the contralateral hemisphere. Slow waves with some associated spike discharges occur in the later part of the seizure. This activity is followed by lower-voltage, diffuse slow activity with a left-sided emphasis. Clinically, the seizure was characterized by clonic jerking of the side of the face and the limbs on the right side, followed by unresponsiveness as slow activity became conspicuous in the later part of the trace.

they may be recorded only from nasopharyngeal, sphenoidal, or other accessory electrodes. The site of focal interictal abnormalities does not necessarily correspond to the region in which seizures usually originate, however, and this must be kept in mind when patients are being evaluated (see Chapter 6). Moreover, the possibility of an underlying structural abnormality (e.g., a tumor) must be remembered in patients with focal seizures. The presence of a focal polymorphic slow-wave disturbance may reflect such a lesion, and the significance of this finding should be indicated clearly to referring physicians. A repeat examination after an appropriate interval will help to exclude the common alternative possibility that the abnormality is postictal in nature. The presence of independent bilateral spike discharges makes a unilateral structural lesion unlikely.

In some patients with focal seizures, and especially those with elementary symptomatology, the scalp-recorded EEG shows no change during the ictal event. More commonly, however, the EEG shows localized

discharges (Figs. 3-21 and 3-22) or more diffuse changes during the ictal period. In some patients, the ictal EEG shows a transient initial desynchronization, which is either localized or diffuse and is followed by synchronous fast activity; in others, the initial flattening of the traces does not occur. In still other cases, rhythmic activity of variable frequency, with or without associated sharp transients, is seen during a seizure. The ictal discharge often is succeeded by a transient flattening of the traces and then by slow activity that may have a localized distribution. If focal slow activity is present, the EEG examination may have to be repeated after several days to distinguish postictal slowing from that caused by a structural lesion.

For practical purposes, temporal lobe epilepsy is divided into medial and neocortical (lateral) temporal lobe epilepsy, and different ictal EEG patterns have been reported, depending on the site at which seizures arise. In seizures arising medially, lateralized rhythmic activity is typically maximal over the ipsilateral temporal lobe,

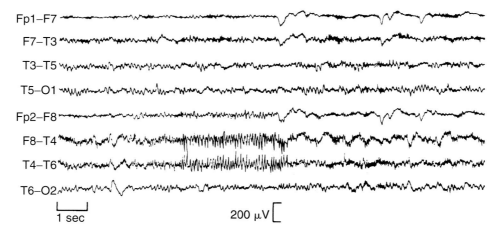

FIGURE 3-22 ■ Electroencephalogram of a 13-year-old boy with frequent attacks of "dimming out." A burst of repetitive spikes is seen to occur in the right temporal region; during this time he experienced an attack.

whereas for seizures arising laterally such ictal activity often has a hemispheric distribution and a lower maximal or irregular frequency.[58,59] In some (13 percent) patients with medial temporal lobe epilepsy, the electrographic seizure recorded over the scalp is contralateral to the side of seizure origin, as determined by depth recordings and curative surgery; lateralized postictal slowing, however, is a reliable lateralizing finding.[60]

When a focal seizure becomes generalized as a secondary phenomenon, patients usually go on to experience a tonic-clonic convulsion. Focal EEG abnormalities then are replaced by the more diffuse changes occurring during such seizures.

ANTICONVULSANT DRUGS, SEIZURE CONTROL, AND THE EEG

The EEG findings are influenced by antiseizure medication. An analysis of 23 controlled trials with therapeutic drug monitoring and serial EEG observations was made by Schmidt.[61] Suppression of "paroxysmal" discharges correlated well with an increase in the plasma concentrations of diazepam, phenobarbital, or phenytoin, either alone or in combination with phenobarbital or primidone. A more limited correlation was reported for carbamazepine and in patients with focal discharges receiving sodium valproate. Epileptiform discharges sometimes became more profuse with carbamazepine despite clinical improvement. An increase in beta activity correlated with increased plasma concentrations of clonazepam, phenytoin, and phenobarbital. Background slowing occurred with high plasma concentrations of diazepam or phenytoin, either alone or in combination with phenobarbital or primidone. Slowing of background activity usually was associated with clinical evidence of toxicity to carbamazepine, phenytoin, phenobarbital, or primidone.

The effects of newer anticonvulsant agents on the EEG are less clear. Lamotrigine reduces the frequency and duration of electrographic seizures and diminishes interictal epileptiform discharges without affecting background activity.[62] Ictal and interictal EEG abnormalities are reduced or unaffected by vigabatrin independently of seizure control, which is improved by the drug in most patients, and the EEG background may be slowed.[63]

The extent to which the suppression of interictal epileptiform discharges reflects the degree of seizure control is variable. In patients with clinical absences associated with generalized 3-Hz spike-wave activity, a good correlation usually exists between seizure control by pharmacologic agents and the amount of interictal epileptiform activity, but the relationship is otherwise more complex. Intravenous phenytoin and benzodiazepines acutely suppress both clinical seizures and interictal epileptiform activity, but in other contexts any correlation of the clinical and EEG effects of anticonvulsant drugs is hard to define. In one recent study, no clear association was found to exist between the presence or frequency of interictal epileptiform discharges and seizure frequency or antiepileptic drug use in patients with focal-onset seizures.[64]

Antiepileptic drug treatment, particularly with carbamazepine or phenytoin, may lead to a paradoxical increase in seizure frequency, sometimes with the appearance of new seizure types or even absence or myoclonic status epilepticus, and a deterioration of the EEG in patients with primary generalized epilepsy.[65] Other drugs that may worsen seizures in this context include lamotrigine, vigabatrin, and gabapentin.

STATUS EPILEPTICUS

Tonic-Clonic (Convulsive) Status

The EEG findings during the seizures may consist of diffuse repetitive spikes, sharp waves, or spike-wave complexes. Alternatively, the findings may resemble those seen during a single seizure, except that the electrographic seizures occur repetitively and there is usually no transient postictal attenuation of the EEG. If seizures have a focal onset, the EEG may show focal spikes, which then spread diffusely. The interictal background is usually, but not always, abnormal, with an excess of irregular, asynchronous, diffuse slow activity, often with intermixed spikes and spike-wave complexes. The main value of recording the EEG during convulsive status epilepticus is to determine whether seizures are continuing when any motor manifestations are subtle because of associated brain damage, the duration of the epileptic state, or pharmacologic neuromuscular blockade. The EEG is also useful in monitoring treatment that involves induction of anesthesia, being important as a means of ensuring that adequate doses are given, and helps in determining whether involuntary motor activity that emerges when medication is being withdrawn relates to recurrence of seizures or is nonepileptic in nature.

Patients in postanoxic status epilepticus typically have a poor prognosis for useful recovery and, in consequence, their seizures generally are not treated aggressively. However, patients having preserved brainstem reactions, somatosensory evoked potentials, and EEG reactivity may do well if their status epilepticus is treated vigorously.[66]

Nonconvulsive and Focal Status Epilepticus

This is suggested clinically by the occurrence of a fluctuating abnormal mental status with confusion, reduced responsiveness, lethargy, somnolence, automatisms, inappropriate behavior, or some combination of these and other symptoms. In patients without a history of prior seizures the epileptic basis of symptoms often is not recognized initially, and a primary psychiatric disorder is suspected until an EEG is obtained. EEG monitoring has shown that nonconvulsive status epilepticus occurs more commonly than previously appreciated in the neurologic intensive care unit, and that it is also a common sequela to convulsive status epilepticus but generally will not be recognized in the absence of an EEG.[67–70] Nonconvulsive status epilepticus has been subdivided into generalized (absence) status and focal status with impairments of consciousness or awareness (complex partial status). These may resemble each other clinically, but their EEG features are quite distinct. The EEG is therefore important in establishing the diagnosis, distinguishing between the different types of nonconvulsive status, and monitoring the response to treatment. In absence status, which may occur in either children or adults, the EEG shows diffuse, bilaterally synchronous, continuous or discontinuous spike-wave and polyspike-wave discharges occurring at about 2 or 3 Hz. Less commonly, irregular arrhythmic spike-wave or polyspike-wave complexes may occur on a diffusely slowed background. By contrast, in focal status epilepticus with impaired consciousness (complex partial status), the EEG generally shows focal or lateralized electrographic seizures, although they sometimes are more generalized. Thus, paroxysmal activity (e.g., repetitive spikes, spike-wave discharges, slow waves, or beta rhythm) may be found unilaterally, bilaterally, or on alternating sides.

In patients with focal status epilepticus, the EEG findings may show intermittent electrographic seizures, merging EEG seizures, continuous ictal discharges, or periodic epileptiform discharges (either PLEDs or BiPLEDs). When PLEDs occur in this context, they may be the initial rather than a terminal ictal pattern.[33] Outcome is related more to age and etiology than to specific ictal EEG patterns.[33]

Myoclonic Status Epilepticus

The most common cause of this disorder is anoxic encephalopathy. The EEG may show generalized periodic or pseudoperiodic complexes (usually consisting of spikes or sharp waves), often with an attenuated background between the complexes or a burst-suppression pattern.[25,71] In some patients, no epileptiform activity is seen.[71]

Recent reports suggest that the use of inappropriate antiepileptic medication in patients with idiopathic generalized epilepsy may result in absence or myoclonic status, often with atypical features.[65] Myoclonic status epilepticus also may occur in patients with juvenile myoclonic epilepsy as a result of drug withdrawal and responds to benzodiazepines.[72]

Status Epilepticus and Sleep

In rare instances, an EEG appearance suggesting status epilepticus may occur during sleep. Such an EEG consists of almost continuous, generalized spike-wave activity that is present primarily during non-REM sleep, which may make it impossible to recognize the normal sleep architecture.

Epilepsia Partialis Continua

This may be regarded as a type of focal status epilepticus and is characterized clinically by rhythmic clonic movements of a group of muscles (Fig. 3-23). In some cases the EEG is normal. Epileptiform abnormalities may have been obscured, however, by the background rhythms or by muscle or movement artifact; alternatively, these abnormalities may not have been detected because they arose from infolded regions of the cortex and were therefore not picked up by the recording scalp electrodes. Focal EEG abnormalities, which sometimes are enhanced by hyperventilation, are present in some patients and consist of abnormal slow waves, sharp transients, or both. It is sometimes possible to identify a relationship between the EEG and muscle activity when the frequency of the jerking is slow. The background activity is frequently slowed or asymmetric, and in occasional instances shows PLEDs.

LONG-TERM EEG MONITORING FOR EPILEPSY

Long-term EEG recordings are generally performed to distinguish between attacks that are epileptic or psychogenic in nature, to determine the frequency of seizure activity, and to localize an epileptogenic source. Monitoring procedures are considered in detail in Chapter 6.

VALUE OF THE EEG IN THE MANAGEMENT OF PATIENTS WITH EPILEPSY

In addition to the aforementioned help that the EEG findings provide in supporting a clinical diagnosis of epilepsy, in permitting a precise epilepsy syndrome to be identified, and in excluding an underlying structural cause of the seizures, the findings are useful in a number of other ways with regard to the management of patients with epilepsy. They are an important aid to the clinician who is attempting to classify the seizure disorder of individual patients and may therefore influence the choice of anticonvulsant drugs that are prescribed. For example,

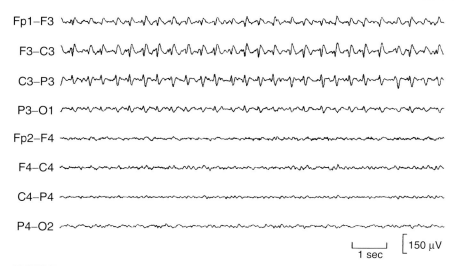

FIGURE 3-23 ■ Electroencephalogram of 46-year-old woman with epilepsia partialis continua. Sharp waves can be seen arising from the left central region and were accompanied by repetitive jerking of the right arm. The seizures were found to result from neurosarcoidosis.

unless the EEG findings are taken into account, it may be difficult to distinguish between certain types of partial seizures, absence seizures, and the so-called atypical absences that occur in patients with Lennox–Gastaut syndrome. The EEG may enable a focal or lateralized epileptogenic source to be identified, even when it is not apparent on clinical grounds. This identification may be of prime importance when the etiology or surgical treatment of the disorder is under consideration. Further comment on this aspect is made in Chapters 6 and 7.

The EEG is particularly helpful in the diagnosis of absence and focal status epilepticus with altered consciousness; indeed, it is often the only means that permits these diagnoses to be made with any confidence. In tonic-clonic (grand mal) status epilepticus, EEG monitoring is invaluable for monitoring the level of induced anesthesia and for determining whether seizure activity is continuing, as discussed earlier.

The EEG can provide a limited guide to the prognosis of patients with epilepsy. Thus, an EEG that is normal and remains so following the standard activation procedures, discussed earlier, generally implies a more favorable prognosis than otherwise, although this prognosis is not always supported by the outcome in individual cases. In patients with absence attacks, 1- to 2-Hz spike-wave discharges suggest a poorer prognosis than bilaterally symmetric and bisynchronous 3-Hz spike-wave activity. The presence of abnormal background activity also implies a poor prognosis. The EEG findings have, however, proved to be disappointingly unreliable as a means of determining the prognosis for the subsequent development of seizures in children experiencing their first febrile convulsion or in patients with head injuries.

Emphasis is sometimes placed on the EEG findings when the feasibility of withdrawing anticonvulsant drugs is under consideration after epileptic patients have been free from seizures for some years. However, the EEG provides no more than a guide to the outlook in such circumstances, and patients certainly can have further attacks after withdrawal of medication despite a normal EEG or, conversely, can remain seizure-free despite a continuing EEG disturbance. The difficulty in obtaining reliable, definitive data concerning the utility of the EEG in this circumstance was underscored in the meta-analysis of Berg and Shinnar.[73] In patients with partial epilepsy, a more recent study suggests that the risk of relapse after drug withdrawal is not predicted by the findings in EEGs recorded before the beginning of drug withdrawal; by contrast, the changes that occur in the EEG recorded during drug withdrawal or in the 3 years thereafter do have prognostic value.[74] Therefore, decisions concerning withdrawal of medication must be based on clinical grounds, with the context of individual cases, as well as the EEG findings, taken into account.

Syncope

Loss of consciousness may occur because of diffuse cerebral hypoxia or ischemia. The clinical features of a syncopal event may be similar to those of a seizure. Conspicuous motor activity, for example, may accompany loss of consciousness in patients with syncope due to malignant cardiac arrhythmias, as well as with certain seizures. Thus, the possibility of syncopal episodes must be borne in mind when a patient presents with the late onset of an apparent seizure disorder. Recent studies show that neurocardiogenic syncope continues to be misdiagnosed as epilepsy,[75] and that such patients are often over-investigated and inappropriately treated, risking a fatal outcome.

During a syncopal episode, the EEG generally is said to show a diffusely slowed background initially and then high-voltage delta activity, usually after an interval of about 10 seconds or so, and followed sometimes by transient electrocerebral silence if the hypoperfusion persists. Recovery occurs in the reverse order. In fact, the EEG changes are more variable; in some instances there is no attenuation of electrocerebral activity, whereas in other instances electrocerebral quiescence develops with little or no preceding change in the frequency of background rhythms.[76,77] The precise temporal relationship of the EEG changes to the loss of consciousness is also variable,[76] depending in part on the cause of the syncope.[78]

Infections

EEG changes are generally more marked in patients with encephalitis than in patients with uncomplicated meningitis. In most of the acute meningitides and viral encephalitides, the EEG is characterized by diffuse rhythmic or arrhythmic slow activity, although focal abnormalities sometimes are found as well. The degree of slowing reflects, at least in part, the severity and extent of disease, the level of consciousness, and any metabolic and systemic changes. These EEG findings are not really helpful for diagnostic purposes, although they may be useful in following the course of the disorder, especially if the clinical features are relatively inconspicuous. Persistence or progression of the EEG abnormalities suggests advancing disease, complications, or residual brain damage, but clinical improvement and EEG improvement do not necessarily follow the same time course. The presence of focal abnormalities raises the possibility that an abscess is developing, although localized electrical abnormalities also may arise for other reasons (e.g., secondary vascular changes or scarring). Residual neurologic deficits, or complications such as a seizure disorder, may develop even if the EEG returns to normal after the acute phase of the illness.

In the chronic meningitides, the EEG may show little change, although in other instances it may show diffuse slowing. Similarly, the findings in aseptic meningitis generally are normal or consist of mild diffuse slow activity,

usually in the theta-frequency range. Such findings are sometimes helpful in following the course of the disorder.

The findings in patients with the encephalopathy associated with infection by human immunodeficiency virus (HIV) are discussed on page 75.

An encephalopathy may occur in patients with systemic sepsis but no evidence of intracranial infection or other identifiable cause for its occurrence; it is probably multifactorial in etiology. The EEG is more sensitive than clinical evaluation for detecting such sepsis-associated encephalopathy. It becomes increasingly slowed, may show triphasic waves, and—in some cases—exhibits a burst-suppression pattern or becomes increasingly suppressed.[79] Recovery may occur, however, even when a burst-suppression pattern is present.[79]

HERPES SIMPLEX ENCEPHALITIS

The EEG findings in herpes simplex encephalitis are sometimes characteristic, especially if serial recordings are made. Initially, diffuse slow activity is found, often with a lateralized or focal emphasis, especially over the temporal lobe on the affected side. Subsequently, stereotyped repetitive sharp- or slow-wave complexes, with a duration of up to about 1 second, may come to be superimposed on the slow background, usually developing between the 2nd and 15th days of the illness but occasionally not arising until even later (Fig. 3-24). These complexes may be found over one or both hemispheres, particularly in the temporal regions, and occur with a regular repetition rate, the interval between successive complexes usually being between 1 and 4 seconds in different patients. When the complexes are bilateral, they may occur synchronously or independently on the two sides. Such bilateral involvement generally implies a more serious outlook than otherwise. The occurrence of focal electrographic seizure activity may obliterate the periodic activity temporarily on the involved side. In time, the amplitude of the repetitive complexes becomes less conspicuous until they can no longer be recognized, the EEG showing instead a focal slow-wave disturbance; attenuation of activity over the affected region; or, in cases that have a fatal outcome, a progressive reduction in frequency and amplitude of background activity.

These changes, when found during the course of an acute cerebral illness, may have considerable diagnostic value in suggesting the possibility of herpes simplex encephalitis. Periodic complexes are not, however, an invariable finding in herpes simplex encephalitis, and their absence does not exclude the possibility of this disorder. Moreover, similar activity may occur in rare cases of infectious mononucleosis encephalitis.

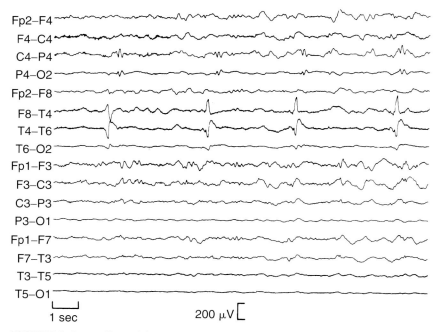

FIGURE 3-24 ▪ Repetitive complexes seen in the right temporal region of a child with herpes simplex encephalitis.

SUBACUTE SCLEROSING PANENCEPHALITIS

Recurrent slow-wave complexes, sometimes with associated sharp transients, occur with a regular periodicity in this disease, which is now rarely encountered in the developed world (Fig. 3-25). The complexes usually last for

up to 3 seconds, but their form may show considerable variation in different patients or in the same patients at different times, as may the interval (usually 4 to 14 seconds) between successive complexes. In most instances, they have a generalized distribution and occur simultaneously

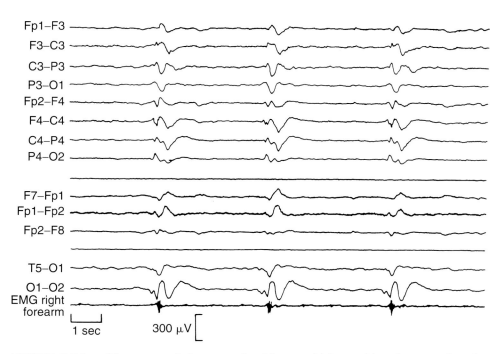

FIGURE 3-25 ▪ Electroencephalogram of a 16-year-old boy with subacute sclerosing panencephalitis of 8 months' duration. Generalized slow-wave complexes are seen to occur approximately every 4 seconds and last for up to 1 second. Each complex is accompanied by a brief electromyographic discharge from the right forearm extensor muscles.

over the two hemispheres, but in the early stages of the illness they are sometimes more conspicuous over one side. Sleep may have a variable influence on the complexes; in some patients it has no effect, but in others the complexes are either brought out, enhanced, or lost during sleep. Occasionally, they seem to disappear for a time but this is unusual, except in the terminal stages of the illness. When myoclonic jerking is a clinical feature of the patient's illness, the jerks are usually time-related to the periodic complexes, occurring just before or just after them. Although the background EEG activity is sometimes relatively normal, it generally is characterized by a reduction or loss of alpha rhythm and the presence of diffuse slow activity. Randomly occurring spikes or sharp waves may be found, especially in the frontal regions, as may bilaterally synchronous spike-wave activity or rhythmic frontal delta activity. Transient, relative quiescence of the background following a complex is an occasional finding.

Periodic complexes similar in form and repetition rate to those just described also may occur in patients with phencyclidine (PCP) intoxication.

CREUTZFELDT–JAKOB DISEASE

In Creutzfeldt–Jakob disease, the EEG is also characterized by periodic complexes occurring on a diffusely abnormal, slowed background (Fig. 3-26). The complexes differ from those occurring in subacute sclerosing panencephalitis. They consist of brief waves (generally less than 0.5 second in duration) of variable (often triphasic) form and sharpened outline; these waves recur with an interval of 0.5 to 2 seconds between successive complexes and may show a temporal relationship to the myoclonic jerking that patients commonly exhibit. This periodic activity is usually present diffusely and is then bilaterally synchronous, but it may have a more restricted focal

or lateralized distribution in the early stages of the disorder. Such a restricted distribution correlates with clinical cerebral dysfunction and with the findings on MRI.[80] Asymmetries occasionally persist, even at advanced stages. In the Heidenhain variant of the disease, periodic complexes may remain confined to the occipital regions and initially may be unilateral.

The typical periodic discharges may not be found in the early and terminal stages of the disease. When the disease is sufficiently advanced that it is strongly suspected on clinical grounds or has been confirmed pathologically, typical EEG abnormalities have been reported in more than 90 percent of patients.[81]

The periodic discharges are not present in certain familial forms of Creutzfeldt–Jakob disease[82] or in the new-variant disease, in which the EEG is often abnormal in a nonspecific manner.[83,84] They are also absent in Gerstmann–Straussler–Scheinker syndrome.

Both the clinical features of a rapidly progressive encephalopathy and the EEG appearance of periodic complexes suggesting Creutzfeldt–Jakob disease have been reported in patients with lithium or baclofen toxicity, indicating the need to take a careful drug history in such circumstances.[85,86] Bismuth subsalicylate toxicity may lead to a prolonged encephalopathy that is mistaken for Creutzfeldt–Jakob disease, but the EEG usually is diffusely slowed, without more characteristic features.[87]

ABSCESS

In patients with acute supratentorial cerebral abscess, the EEG is characterized by low-frequency, high-amplitude, polymorphic focal slow activity such as that shown in Figure 3-9. PLEDs have been reported over the involved hemisphere in occasional cases. The EEG changes are often much more dramatic than those encountered with

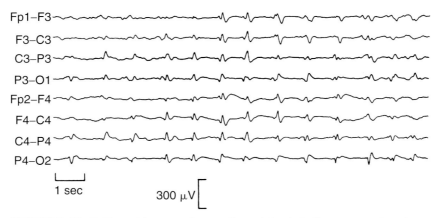

FIGURE 3-26 ▪ Repetitive complexes, often triphasic in form, occurring about once every second on a rather featureless background in the electroencephalogram of a 66-year-old patient with Creutzfeldt–Jakob disease.

other focal cerebral lesions. Depending on the degree to which consciousness is depressed, however, focal changes are sometimes obscured by a more generalized slow-wave disturbance or by frontal intermittent rhythmic delta activity.

Infratentorial abscesses generally produce less marked EEG abnormalities characterized by intermittent rhythmic delta rhythms or diffuse slow activity.

The EEG changes produced by chronic supratentorial abscesses may be indistinguishable from those produced by focal lesions such as tumors (p. 73).

Vascular Lesions

In considering the changes that occur in patients with vascular lesions of the nervous system, it must be borne in mind that the EEG findings fail to provide a reliable means of distinguishing such lesions from other types of structural pathology (e.g., cerebral tumors). Similarly, the EEG findings do not provide a way of distinguishing the underlying pathologic basis of the vascular disturbance, and this drawback limits the utility of the technique. It may, however, become an increasingly important means for the continuous monitoring of patients at special risk for certain vascular complications.

In patients with cerebral ischemia caused by occlusive disease of major vessels, the normal background activity often is depressed in the affected portion of the hemisphere, and a slow-wave (theta or delta) disturbance may be found, sometimes associated with sharp transients or PLEDs. Changes are usually most conspicuous in the ipsilateral midtemporal and centroparietal regions in patients who have involvement of the middle cerebral or internal carotid artery, in the frontal region when the

anterior cerebral artery is affected, and in the occipital region when the posterior cerebral artery is occluded. The topographic extent of these changes varies in individual patients, however, depending on factors such as the site of occlusion, rapidity of its development, and adequacy of the collateral circulation. The EEG may revert to normal with time despite a persisting clinical deficit, but sharp transients become more conspicuous in some cases. In patients with ischemia restricted to the internal capsule, the EEG usually is normal or shows only minor changes. Similarly, discrete subcortical vascular lesions (e.g., lacunar infarcts) generally do not alter the EEG. In patients with vertebrobasilar ischemia, the EEG is often normal, although it may show minor equivocal changes. In some cases of infarction of the lower brainstem (Fig. 3-27), however, widespread, poorly reactive alpha-frequency activity is found. With involvement of more rostral brainstem regions and of the diencephalon, the EEG is characterized by predominant slow activity, which often is organized into discrete, bilaterally synchronous runs without constant lateralization.

Following acute nonhemorrhagic stroke, the EEG may show focal abnormalities (e.g., a polymorphic slow-wave disturbance) at a time when CT scans are normal. Thus, in this context, the EEG may reflect dysfunction not yet apparent morphologically. Such changes may be helpful in distinguishing between a hemispheric and brainstem lesion. They also have been used to distinguish between a cortical and a lacunar infarct when such distinction is clinically difficult, although studies indicate that lateralized minor abnormalities are more common than is generally appreciated after lacunar infarction.[88]

In patients with mild atherosclerotic cerebrovascular disease, hyperventilation may induce focal or lateralized

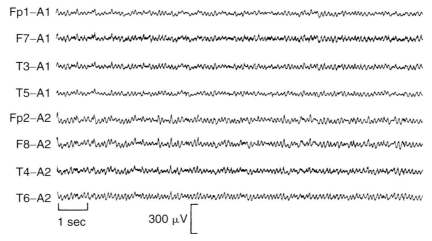

FIGURE 3-27 ■ Generalized, rhythmic 9- to 10-Hz activity, unresponsive to sensory stimuli, in the electroencephalogram of a 68-year-old woman following cardiopulmonary arrest.

EEG abnormalities that are not apparent otherwise. Carotid compression sometimes is used to provoke EEG changes caused by inadequacies of the collateral circulation. This maneuver is not always innocuous, however, and may give misleading information (e.g., positive responses in patients without vascular disease or a lack of response in patients with well-established disease).

In patients with intracerebral hematomas, the extent of the EEG changes depends on the site and size of the hematoma and on the rapidity of its development. Background activity is depressed over part or all of the affected side, and focal polymorphic delta activity is seen. Especially in the elderly, this slow activity is sometimes localized preferentially to the temporal region, regardless of the site of the lesion. Sharp transients are seen more commonly than in patients with nonhemorrhagic vascular lesions, especially in the temporal region, and intermittent bilateral rhythmic delta activity also may be found, especially where secondary displacement of brainstem structures has occurred. EEG changes are often inconspicuous in patients with hemorrhage into the lower brainstem, but widespread, poorly reactive alpha-like activity may be noted. Cerebellar hemorrhage is associated with little, if any, change unless tonsillar herniation complicates the clinical picture, in which case diffuse slowing results.

The EEG findings in patients with cerebral venous or venous sinus thrombosis are similar to, but often more extensive than, those in patients with occlusive arterial disease. When the superior sagittal sinus is involved, the changes are usually bilateral, often variable, and commonly asymmetric.

It is unclear whether the EEG has any role in indicating the prognosis following stroke, and no definite conclusions can be reached on the basis of the few published studies on this point. The EEG has been used to monitor patients undergoing carotid endarterectomy, and this is discussed further in Chapter 9.

A reversible posterior leukoencephalopathy has been related to hypertensive encephalopathy. It is associated with characteristic abnormalities on neuroimaging that suggest subcortical edema without infarction.[89] Occipital lobe seizures may occur,[90] and variable EEG abnormalities may be encountered. The diagnosis, however, is based on the clinical and neuroimaging abnormalities.

SUBARACHNOID HEMORRHAGE

Although the EEG may be normal following subarachnoid hemorrhage, diffuse slowing is a common finding, especially in patients with clouding of consciousness. Focal abnormalities also may be observed and can be related to the presence of a local hematoma; to the source of hemorrhage, especially when it is an angioma; or to secondary ischemia by arterial spasm. Continuous EEG monitoring in the intensive care unit is being used increasingly to detect focal changes caused by vasospasm while they are still subclinical or at least at a time when the vasospasm may still be reversible.[91]

SUBDURAL HEMATOMA

The background activity sometimes is reduced in amplitude or virtually abolished over the affected hemisphere in patients with a chronic subdural hematoma (Fig. 3-28). In other instances, however, a focal ipsilateral slow-wave disturbance is the most conspicuous abnormality, and little suppression of background rhythms is found. In either

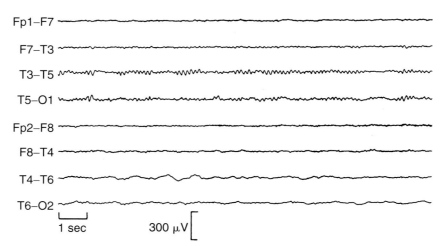

FIGURE 3-28 ▪ Focal slowing in the right posterior quadrant and suppression of normal background rhythms over this side in the electroencephalogram of a patient with a suspected right subdural hematoma.

case, generalized changes (e.g., frontal intermittent rhythmic delta activity) may be present as well, and repetitive periodic complexes have been described in rare instances.

Because the EEG is sometimes normal in patients with a chronic subdural hematoma, the possibility of such a lesion cannot be excluded just because the electrophysiologic findings are unremarkable. Indeed, even when abnormalities are found, it can sometimes be difficult, if not impossible, to localize the lesion with any certainty owing to the interplay of the various changes described earlier. Moreover, the EEG findings do not reliably distinguish a chronic subdural hematoma from other space-occupying lesions. In all instances, therefore, detailed neuroradiologic assessment is necessary if cases are to be managed correctly.

INTRACRANIAL ANEURYSMS AND ARTERIOVENOUS MALFORMATIONS

The findings in subarachnoid hemorrhage have been described already. Focal slow activity is an occasional finding in patients with aneurysms that have not bled, but in uncomplicated cases there is often little to find in the EEG. Following subarachnoid hemorrhage, focal or lateralized abnormalities are sometimes present and may be a guide to the site of bleeding. Focal slow activity or epileptiform discharges may be found in the EEG of patients with intracranial arteriovenous malformations.

STURGE–WEBER SYNDROME

Together with depression of normal background activity and the responses to hyperventilation and photic stimulation over the affected hemisphere, irregular slow activity and sharp transients are often seen. The reduction in background activity is not necessarily related to the presence and degree of intracranial calcification. Abnormalities sometimes have a more generalized distribution that can be confusing, but in such circumstances they are commonly more conspicuous over the involved side.

Headache

Electroencephalography has little relevance to the diagnosis of migraine. In uncomplicated cases, the EEG is usually normal, or shows only minor nonspecific changes between and during migrainous attacks. Focal or unilateral slow-wave disturbances are common, however, particularly in patients developing lateralized aura or neurologic deficits in association with their attacks. Such localized abnormalities usually settle rapidly once the clinical disturbance has resolved, unless infarction has

occurred or there is an underlying structural abnormality. Paroxysmal epileptiform activity sometimes is found, but the proportion of cases with such a disturbance varies greatly in different series. It is unclear whether the association of migraine with such paroxysmal activity is genetic or related to cerebral ischemic damage. The EEG disturbance, in itself, is insufficient evidence to permit the headaches to be regarded as the manifestation of an epileptic disorder.

There is always some concern that an underlying structural lesion may have been missed in patients with chronic headache syndromes that fail to respond to medical treatment. Although the EEG has been used by some as a screening procedure for patients requiring further investigation, the EEG is less sensitive than cranial CT scanning or MRI and—given the implications of delay in the diagnosis of an intracranial mass lesion—it is hard to justify its use in place of imaging studies when these modalities are readily available and intracranial pathology is suspected clinically.[92]

There is little, if any, evidence that the EEG has a useful role in the routine evaluation of patients presenting with headache, and it is not helpful for predicting prognosis or in selecting therapy.[92]

Tumors

Tumors may affect the EEG by causing compression, displacement, or destruction of nervous tissue; by interfering with local blood supply; or by leading to obstructive hydrocephalus. Considerable variation exists in the presence, nature, and extent of abnormalities in different subjects, depending, at least in part, on the tumor's size and rate of growth and on the age of the patient. An abnormal record is more likely to be found in patients with a supratentorial tumor than an infratentorial one, and in patients with a rapidly expanding tumor rather than a slowly growing lesion. Superficial supratentorial lesions generally produce more localized EEG changes than do deep hemispheric lesions; the latter may lead to abnormalities over the entire side involved or to even more diffuse changes. EEG abnormalities are more common with rostral than with caudal infratentorial lesions. In general, abnormalities are more conspicuous with tumors in children than adults. Even if the EEG is abnormal, however, the changes may be generalized rather than focal. Thus, they would not be particularly helpful in the diagnosis or localization of the underlying neoplasm, although they would provide information about the extent of cerebral dysfunction produced by it.

Diffuse abnormalities are common in all patients with cerebral tumors when the level of consciousness is depressed; therefore, in this context, these abnormalities are particularly probable in patients with infratentorial lesions. In addition to diffuse slowing, intermittent bilateral rhythmic delta activity may be seen with a frontal emphasis in adults, or more posteriorly in children. In these circumstances, localization of the tumor by EEG is often less feasible than at an earlier period in the natural history, although a gross asymmetry of such activity between the two hemispheres raises the possibility of a lateralized hemispheric lesion. Earlier records sometimes permit more definite localization, but they may show only subtle changes, which are easily missed.

Depression of electrical activity over a discrete region of the brain is a reliable local sign of an underlying cerebral lesion, but this sign may be masked by volume conduction of activity from adjacent areas. The presence of a focal polymorphic slow-wave disturbance (Fig. 3-29) is also important, although such an abnormality has less localizing significance when it is found over the temporal lobe. Focal ictal or interictal sharp activity is of some, but lesser, localizing value unless it is associated with an underlying focal slow-wave disturbance. However, epileptiform activity may precede the appearance of more reliable focal EEG abnormalities by several months or even longer. It usually occurs at the margins of the lesion and is more likely with slowly growing tumors than with rapidly expanding ones, and more likely with hemispheric tumors than with brainstem lesions. Some correlation exists between the presence of epileptiform activity in patients with brain tumors and the development of seizures, but in general this correlation is not close enough to be of prognostic relevance. Many patients with such EEG discharges do not have seizures; conversely, many patients with seizures from brain tumors do not have spikes and sharp waves in their EEGs.

Epileptiform discharges may occur bilaterally, without obvious focality, in patients with parasagittal or mesial hemispheric lesions, but then are often asymmetric in distribution over the two sides or confined to the vertex. A number of other abnormalities have been described in patients with discrete cerebral lesions, including an asymmetry of drug-induced fast activity, a local increase in beta activity, and the presence of a mu rhythm; but these findings are of much less significance and can lead to difficulty in determining which of the two sides is the abnormal one.

In assessing the findings in patients with suspected brain tumors, the main value of the EEG is in indicating which patients require more detailed investigation, especially when facilities for CT scanning or MRI are not readily available. Its value even in this regard is limited, however, because a normal or equivocal EEG does not exclude the possibility of a tumor. Deep-seated supratentorial tumors may produce no abnormalities whatsoever at an early stage, and the EEG is likely to be normal in patients with pituitary tumors unless the lesion has extended beyond the pituitary fossa or has caused hormonal changes. Furthermore, there are no abnormalities that will allow the differentiation of neoplastic lesions from other localized structural disorders, such as an infarct. The EEG can provide no information about the nature of the tumor in individual cases; the findings in patients with tumors of different histologic types or in different locations are therefore not discussed in this chapter.

Although its place as a noninvasive screening procedure has been taken over largely by CT scanning or MRI in the developed countries, the EEG still has an

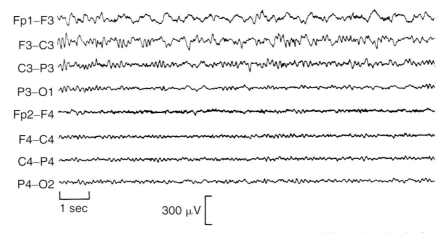

FIGURE 3-29 ■ Polymorphic slow-wave activity in the left frontal region in the electroencephalogram of a 62-year-old man with a glioma.

important complementary role in the evaluation of patients with known or suspected brain tumors. In particular, the EEG is helpful in the evaluation of episodic symptoms that might either be epileptic in nature or have some other basis, and it provides information about the extent of cerebral dysfunction.

Tuberous Sclerosis

There are no pathognomonic EEG features of tuberous sclerosis, but epileptiform activity or changes suggestive of space-occupying lesions may be found. The EEG is often normal in mild cases, but in others focal slow- or sharp-wave disturbances are seen. In more advanced cases, a hypsarrhythmic pattern may be seen during infancy, whereas in older patients the record may contain generalized spike-wave activity or independent multifocal spike discharges. Thus, focal or generalized changes may be found in this disorder.

Pseudotumor Cerebri

In pseudotumor cerebri, or benign intracranial hypertension, the EEG is often normal, but abnormalities, consisting of a diffusely slowed background and bursts of activity in the alpha-, theta-, or delta-frequency ranges, sometimes are found.

Dementia

The EEG changes in most patients with dementia are nonspecific and do not discriminate between the different types of dementing processes. In early cases, the findings may be normal. As the dementia advances, however, the amount and frequency of the alpha rhythm decline, and irregular theta and slower activity appears, sometimes with a focal or unilateral emphasis, and especially in the temporal region. In patients with Alzheimer disease, the alpha rhythm often is lost at a relatively early stage compared with patients with other disorders that cause dementia. As a general rule, abnormalities occur earlier and are much more conspicuous in Alzheimer disease than in frontotemporal dementia. In the latter disorder, the EEG is often normal[93]; even if diffuse slow-wave activity is present, the alpha rhythm commonly is preserved.

In some cases, the cause of dementia may be suggested by the EEG findings. Both Creutzfeldt–Jakob disease and subacute sclerosing panencephalitis are associated commonly with characteristic EEG changes, as described earlier. When a focal structural lesion (e.g., a tumor or chronic subdural hematoma) is responsible for the intellectual decline, there may be localized depression of electrocerebral activity or a focal polymorphic slow-wave disturbance, sometimes with relative preservation of the alpha rhythm. In multi-infarct dementia, significant asymmetries in background activity often occur over the two hemispheres, and focal slow-wave disturbances are common. The findings in patients with parkinsonism, Huntington disease, hepatolenticular degeneration, and Steele–Richardson–Olszewski syndrome are discussed on page 81 but are of no help in distinguishing the intellectual decline occurring in those disorders from other diseases associated with dementia.

In patients with the dementia sometimes associated with HIV infection, the EEG may be normal or diffusely slowed. Focal slow-wave disturbances in these patients raise the possibility of neoplastic involvement or opportunistic infection.

Considerable overlap exists between the EEG findings in patients with dementia of the Alzheimer type and mentally normal elderly subjects; thus, the EEG cannot be used to indicate reliably whether an elderly patient has dementia. Indeed, the diagnostic or prognostic utility—if any—of either routine or quantitative EEG in the evaluation of patients with cognitive impairment is unclear.[94] However, the presence of diffuse slow-wave activity supports the diagnosis of dementia rather than pseudodementia (depression). Again, the EEG findings cannot be used to distinguish with any confidence between an acute and a chronic disturbance of cognitive function, although in the former circumstance abnormalities are more likely to reverse with time. However, a markedly abnormal EEG in patients with clinically mild cognitive disturbances should suggest an acute process, such as a toxic or metabolic encephalopathy.

Metabolic Disorders

The EEG has been used to detect and monitor cerebral dysfunction in patients with a variety of metabolic disorders, and changes may certainly precede any alteration in clinical status. The EEG findings may also be helpful in suggesting that nonspecific symptoms have an organic basis. Diffuse (rather than focal) changes characteristically occur in metabolic encephalopathies unless there is a pre-existing or concomitant structural lesion. Typically, desynchronization and slowing of the alpha rhythm occur, with subsequent appearance of theta, and then of delta, activity. These slower rhythms initially may be episodic or paroxysmal and are enhanced by hyperventilation. Triphasic waves (p. 48), which consist of a major positive potential preceded and followed by smaller negative waves, may also be found and usually are generalized, bilaterally synchronous, and frontally predominant. They are sometimes reactive to external (painful) stimulation. Although triphasic waves were thought originally to be specific for hepatic encephalopathy, they are found in a variety of metabolic encephalopathies and may suggest a poor prognosis for survival.[13]

Diffuse slowing of the EEG has been described in hyperglycemia or hypoglycemia, Addison disease, hypopituitarism, pulmonary failure, and hyperparathyroidism. In hypoparathyroidism, similar changes are found in advanced cases, but spikes, sharp waves, and slow spike-wave discharges also may be seen. A low-voltage record in which the alpha activity classically is preserved but slowed characterizes myxedema, and there may be some intermixed theta or slower elements. These changes may pass unrecognized, however, unless premorbid records are available for comparison. In hyperthyroidism, the alpha rhythm is usually diminished in amount but increased in frequency, beta activity is often conspicuous, and scattered theta elements may be present. The findings in Cushing disease and pheochromocytoma are usually unremarkable.

Water intoxication or hyponatremia may cause diffuse slowing of the EEG, and bursts of rhythmic delta activity are also commonly present. Hypernatremia and abnormalities of serum potassium concentration usually have little effect on the EEG.

HEPATIC ENCEPHALOPATHY

The EEG shows progressive changes in patients with advancing hepatic encephalopathy, and in general a good correlation exists between the clinical and electrical findings. In early stages the alpha rhythm slows, gradually being replaced by theta and delta activity, but in some instances it may coexist with this slow activity. As the disorder progresses, triphasic complexes usually (but not invariably) occur symmetrically and synchronously over the two hemispheres, with a frontal emphasis (Fig. 3-30). With further clinical deterioration, the EEG in patients with hepatic encephalopathy comes to consist of continuous triphasic and slow-wave activity, which shows a marked anterior emphasis and may be interrupted by periods of relative quiescence. The amplitude of the slow-wave activity gradually decreases as death approaches.

After orthotopic liver transplantation, epileptiform activity may be encountered in the EEG, especially in those who ultimately fail to survive.[95] Other EEG abnormalities in liver transplantation recipients include diffuse slowing,

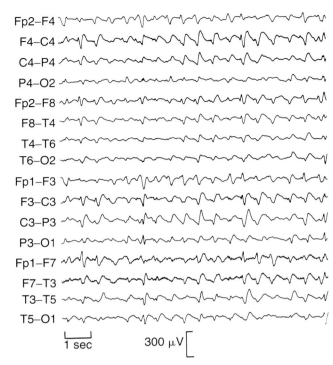

FIGURE 3-30 ■ Triphasic and slow-wave activity in the electroencephalogram of a 79-year-old woman with hepatic encephalopathy.

local or generalized suppression of electrocerebral activity, the presence of triphasic waves, electrographic seizures that may be subclinical, and PLEDs.[95] Focal or generalized abnormalities may be related to cerebrovascular complications or to infective processes to which patients are prone because of their immunosuppressed status. Generalized abnormalities may also be related to other metabolic disturbances, central pontine myelinolysis, and medication effects.

RENAL INSUFFICIENCY

In patients with renal insufficiency, the EEG may be normal initially but the background eventually slows; theta and delta activity develops in increasing amounts and is sometimes paroxysmal; and, ultimately, the record is dominated by irregular slow activity that does not respond to external stimuli. Triphasic complexes are an occasional finding but usually are not as well formed as those in hepatic encephalopathy. Spike and sharp-wave discharges may also be seen in some patients, as may photoparoxysmal responses.

During hemodialysis, the EEG findings are often dramatic, even in patients who previously had a relatively normal record, consisting of bursts of generalized, high-voltage rhythmic delta activity occurring on either

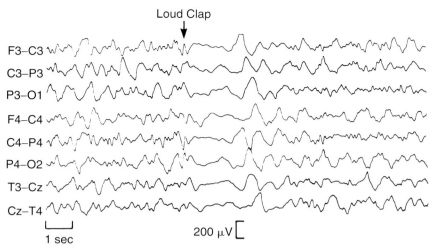

FIGURE 3-31 ▪ Electroencephalogram of a comatose child showing attenuation of the diffuse background slow activity in response to a sudden loud noise.

a relatively normal or a generally slowed background. In patients developing the progressive encephalopathy that sometimes occurs during chronic hemodialysis, the EEG contains diffuse slow-wave activity interrupted by bilaterally synchronous complexes of slow, sharp, triphasic, and spike waves.

ANOXIC ENCEPHALOPATHY

The EEG changes occurring during acute pancerebral hypoperfusion or hypoxia were discussed earlier in the section on syncope (p. 67). If cerebral hypoxia or anoxia is prolonged, it leads to an encephalopathy that may be irreversible. Diffuse slowing of variable degree is found in the EEG of some comatose patients, and short runs of fast activity also may be present. The responsiveness of the background to external stimulation (Fig. 3-31) provides important prognostic information in such circumstances (p. 79). In patients with more severe brain damage, the EEG may show continuous or intermittent epileptiform discharges, diffuse unresponsive alpha-frequency activity (p. 79), a burst-suppression pattern (see Fig. 3-12 and p. 52), or electrocerebral inactivity. Generalized periodic epileptiform complexes and BiPLEDs suggest a poor prognosis for survival.[96] A detailed discussion of the EEG findings in brain death and neocortical death is provided in Chapter 35.

Effects of Drugs and Alcohol on the EEG

Various medications may affect the EEG depending on timing, dose, and metabolic factors, and on whether there are pre-existing or iatrogenic systemic disorders. Drug effects are usually symmetrical and typically occur diffusely. A lateralized asymmetry may relate to

suppression over one hemisphere (reflecting localized pathology) or enhancement on the other (as with a breach rhythm).[97]

Excessive fast activity is a common consequence of medications such as barbiturates or benzodiazepines, and may be accompanied by some slowing (theta) of the background. Other causes of increased fast activity include tricyclic antidepressants, amphetamines, cocaine or its withdrawal,[98] and drug or alcohol withdrawal states. Diffuse slowing of the background EEG may occur with anticonvulsant toxicity, as well as with use of tricyclic agents and clozapine.[99] Narcotic drugs may lead to a reduction of alpha frequency and duration and, with chronic administration, to slowing of the record. Lithium causes slowing of the alpha rhythm and paroxysmal slow-wave activity that may have a focal or lateralized emphasis. Periodic complexes resembling those occurring in Creutzfeldt–Jakob disease have been described with lithium[85] or baclofen toxicity.[86]

Bursts of epileptiform activity (spike or spike-wave discharges) occurring spontaneously or during photic stimulation may relate to use of clozapine,[100] lithium, neuroleptics, selective serotonin reuptake inhibitors, or tricyclic antidepressants. Acute withdrawal from barbiturates or benzodiazepines after chronic usage also may be responsible, and a reduction of antiepileptic medications may enhance epileptiform discharges.

Triphasic waves occur on a diffusely slowed background in patients intoxicated with several medications, as also with any metabolic encephalopathy. They are well described in the hyperammonemic encephalopathy associated with valproic acid, but also have been reported with baclofen, levodopa, lithium, pentobarbital and in the serotonin syndrome. Various coma patterns have been reported with drug intoxications, including spindle coma, alpha-pattern coma, burst-suppression, and electrocerebral inactivity. Recovery occurs as the causal drug is eliminated.

Alcohol causes mild slowing during chronic intoxication. Paroxysmal activity occasionally is found during alcohol withdrawal, following which the EEG reverts to normal unless there is any coexisting pathology. Photomyogenic or photoparoxysmal responses may occur, but these responses were encountered rarely in one study of 49 subjects during acute alcohol withdrawal.[46] In most patients with alcohol-withdrawal seizures, the EEG is either normal or mildly slowed; epileptiform discharges are uncommon. Focal abnormalities suggest the possibility of a structural lesion or may be the postictal sequelae of partial seizures.

Multiple Sclerosis

Patients with multiple sclerosis commonly have abnormal EEGs. Focal or generalized activity in the theta and delta ranges may be found, as may diffuse or localized spike discharges. Focal changes are often evanescent and probably are related to foci of acute demyelination. The findings are of no help in the diagnosis of the disorder, however, and usually bear little relationship to the clinical signs.

Trauma

Electroencephalography generally is undertaken to provide some guide as to the nature and severity of head injuries, the prognosis for recovery, and the likelihood of developing post-traumatic seizures. In addition, it often is requested when patients with post-traumatic syndromes are being evaluated at a later stage, in the hope that it will provide an indication of whether nonspecific symptoms have an organic etiology; however, its use in this regard has no rational basis.

No specific EEG abnormalities develop after head injury. In evaluating the findings at electroencephalography, one must bear in mind that abnormalities may have existed before the injury and that the significance of any findings will depend, in part, on the time at which the study was undertaken in relation to the trauma. This is important because the correlation between clinical and electrophysiologic findings is often poor when the EEG is recorded 3 or more months after the injury was sustained.

The presence of a localized abnormality is often of particular concern because it may point to the existence of an intracerebral, subdural, or extradural hematoma.

Unfortunately, there is no reliable way of distinguishing electroencephalographically between surgically remediable intracranial lesions, such as a subdural hematoma, and pathology that does not necessitate operative treatment. In such circumstances, the judicious use of imaging procedures clearly facilitates the rational management of individual patients.

The EEG findings in individual cases depend, in greater part, on the patient's level of consciousness. The abnormalities that may be seen in comatose subjects are discussed separately, and there is further comment on this aspect in Chapter 35. Other abnormalities that may be found following head trauma include local or generalized depression of normal activity; slowing of the alpha rhythm; focal or diffuse slow-wave disturbances, especially in the temporal region in adults; and spike or paroxysmal discharges. These changes may develop progressively with time, if serial recordings are undertaken. Focal abnormalities may be related directly to local injury but also may occur as a sequela to complications of cerebral trauma, such as ischemia or edema. They may be obscured initially by more generalized changes in the EEG, becoming conspicuous only as the latter diminish. Before pathologic implications can be attributed to a localized depression of electrocerebral activity, however, extracerebral factors (e.g., subcutaneous edema or hemorrhage) must be excluded by careful scrutiny of the patient. Localized or lateralized paroxysmal discharges are sometimes the sole evidence of a structural abnormality, such as a hematoma, and indicate the need for further neuroradiologic investigations.

The EEG findings do not improve the accuracy of predicting which patients are likely to go on to develop post-traumatic epilepsy. Patients with EEG abnormalities may remain free from seizures, whereas those who go on to develop post-traumatic epilepsy may have one or more normal records in the 3 months following injury.

Continuous EEG monitoring in the intensive care unit of patients with traumatic brain injury helps to detect seizures that might be clinically inapparent and to guide early prognostication. Vespa and colleagues found, in a study of 94 patients monitored during the initial 14 days after injury, that 22 percent had seizures; more than half of these were nonconvulsive and were diagnosed solely on the basis of the EEG.[69] In another study, monitoring during the first 3 days after injury, with particular attention to the percentage of alpha variability, was found to be sensitive and specific in this regard, improving prognostic ability independently of traditional clinical indicators of outcome.[101] Such findings suggest an important role for EEG monitoring of patients after severe head injury.

Coma

Altered states of consciousness may result from many causes, and it is therefore not surprising that the EEG findings in comatose patients are variable. A few general points require emphasis. First, although the EEG changes are never specific to any particular disorder, they may direct attention to diagnostic possibilities that otherwise might be overlooked. Second, in evaluating patients with depressed levels of consciousness, it is particularly important, both for prognostic purposes and for following the course of the disorder, that serial records are obtained so that the direction of any change can be determined. Automated "trending" of the EEG may be particularly helpful in the context of the intensive care unit. Finally, any spontaneous variation in the EEG and the responses evoked by external stimuli must be considered when the comatose patient is being evaluated or followed electrophysiologically (see Fig. 3-31). A change in electrocerebral activity can be expected to occur following stimulation of a patient with a mildly depressed level of consciousness; this reactivity becomes inconstant, delayed, or lost as the depth of coma increases. More specifically, stimulation during light coma results in an attenuation of the background rhythms or, especially as coma deepens, a paradoxical arousal response in which slow-wave activity briefly becomes more profuse and conspicuous. With further progression, repeated stimulation may be needed to produce any EEG change, and finally the EEG becomes unresponsive.

When consciousness is impaired, the EEG becomes slowed, the degree of slowing often (but not always) corresponding to the extent to which consciousness is depressed. The slow-wave activity may be episodic or continuous and, in the former instance, often shows a frontal emphasis and bilateral synchronicity. As the depth of coma increases, the EEG becomes unresponsive to afferent stimuli, and its amplitude diminishes until eventually it becomes flat and featureless, sometimes preceded by a burst-suppression pattern. Such a record should not be taken to indicate that irreversible brain death has occurred; similar changes may be found in severe hypothermia or in coma caused by intoxication with CNS depressant drugs (see Chapter 35). Records characterized by rhythmic generalized fast activity intermixed with slower rhythms are found in patients who have taken excessive quantities of certain drugs, particularly benzodiazepines or barbiturates. In any severe diffuse encephalopathy, the EEG may show a burst-suppression pattern; its prognostic significance varies with the cause (p. 52).

In some comatose patients, the EEG resembles that found during normal wakefulness, in that it consists predominantly of activity in the alpha-frequency range (see Fig. 3-27). Such activity is distributed more widely than normal alpha rhythm, however, and, unlike the latter, is often unresponsive to sensory stimuli. This alpha-pattern coma has been reported particularly in patients with brainstem strokes or following hypoxia caused by cardiopulmonary arrest and with drug intoxication.[102] It also has been described after trauma and in association with encephalitis, Reye syndrome, thalamic tumor, or hyperglycemia with hyperosmolality.[103] Certain differences can be seen in the EEG, depending on whether hypoxia or a brainstem lesion is responsible. In particular, the alpha-frequency activity is often maximal posteriorly and may retain some reactivity to sensory stimulation (e.g., passive eye-opening or pain) with brainstem pathology, whereas it is generalized or more prominent anteriorly and usually unreactive in hypoxic coma. The designation theta-pattern coma is used when widespread, persistent, unreactive theta-frequency activity is present in the EEG of a comatose patient. It has the same significance as alpha-pattern coma. Indeed, in some recordings, the two patterns coexist (alpha-theta coma).[103] Alpha-pattern coma usually has been associated with a poor prognosis for survival, although recovery sometimes occurs. In fact, prognosis appears to depend more on the cause of the coma than on the presence of the alpha pattern in itself.[102] Kaplan and co-workers found that EEG reactivity in alpha-pattern coma predicted survival, in that most patients with reactivity recovered consciousness, whereas most without such reactivity died.[102] Others have noted that alpha- or theta-pattern coma, or alpha-theta coma, is a transient clinical phenomenon that usually changes to a more definitive pattern by 5 days after coma onset. EEG reactivity then implies a more favorable prognosis, and a burst-suppression pattern implies a gloomy outcome.[103]

The term *spindle coma* is used when the EEG shows activity resembling sleep spindles in patients who are comatose. Such spindles are, however, much more diffuse in distribution than normal sleep spindles. It has been postulated that they relate to functional derangement of the midbrain reticular formation. There is no relationship between the occurrence of spindle activity and clinical deficit, depth or cause of coma, or outcome. EEG reactivity seems predictive of outcome, however, as does the cause of the coma.[104] In general, patients with brainstem or cerebral infarction have the poorest outcome, and those with cerebral hypoxia or a cardiopulmonary arrest also have a high likelihood of death or of remaining in a persistent vegetative state.[104]

The EEG may be diagnostically helpful in the evaluation of comatose patients. Sometimes electrographic seizure activity is found; in some instances, this may have been unsuspected clinically, as when nonconvulsive status epilepticus is found in obtunded patients in the intensive care unit or in those recovering from convulsive status epilepticus. In other instances, localized changes in frequency and amplitude suggest the presence of a structural supratentorial lesion. Repetitive complexes are seen in the EEGs of some comatose patients. The character and distribution of the complexes, the degree to which they exhibit a regular periodicity, and the interval between successive complexes may be helpful in suggesting the cause of the coma if the clinical circumstances surrounding the case are obscure. The clinical significance of PLEDs and BiPLEDs is discussed on page 52; either of these two patterns may be found in obtunded or comatose patients. In general, PLEDs occur most commonly with acute hemispheric lesions (e.g., infarcts or tumors), but occasionally occur with more diffuse disturbances (e.g., hypoxia). In contrast, the most common cause of BiPLEDs is diffuse pathologic involvement of the brain (e.g., anoxic encephalopathy or CNS infections), and this EEG pattern generally is associated with a higher mortality rate than when the epileptiform discharges are restricted to one side. The findings in subacute sclerosing panencephalitis, Creutzfeldt–Jakob disease, herpes simplex encephalitis, and hepatic encephalopathy have been described earlier. Periodic complexes may be found in a number of other disorders, including postanoxic coma.

Despite the different EEG changes that may occur in comatose patients, the limited information that can be gleaned from some of these changes, and the advent of more sophisticated investigative techniques, the EEG remains useful for prognostic purposes. In one study, for example, it was found that the outcome of postanoxic coma could be predicted most accurately by combining the results of the Glasgow Coma Scale at 48 hours with the findings obtained by recording somatosensory evoked potentials (see Chapter 26) and, if these data were inconclusive, with the EEG.[105] In another study involving a systematic review of the literature, the prognostic value of early neurologic and neurophysiologic findings in anoxic-ischemic coma was examined. The recording of somatosensory evoked potentials was found again to be the most useful method to predict poor outcome, but the EEG was also helpful, with an isoelectric or burst-suppression pattern having a specificity of 100 percent in five of six relevant studies.[106] Young has reviewed the topic and found that a single EEG indicates no possibility of recovery of consciousness with 100 percent

specificity when there is complete generalized suppression (less than 10 μV) after the first day following a cardiac arrest.[107] Less marked suppression, a burst-suppression pattern, periodic complexes, and an alpha-theta pattern usually but not invariably indicate a grim outlook. Generalized periodic epileptiform complexes and BiPLEDs after an anoxic insult also are associated with a poor prognosis for survival and suggest that aggressive treatment is not warranted.[96]

Continuous EEG (CEEG) monitoring of comatose patients in the intensive care unit is an important approach to monitoring cerebral function. It seems especially valuable in monitoring for the occurrence—and guiding treatment—of seizures or cerebral ischemia, in prognostication, and in adjusting levels of sedation for pharmacologically paralyzed patients.[108] It may well improve outcomes and shorten the duration of stay in hospital or the intensive care unit, but this remains to be demonstrated. A number of technical issues need to be resolved, however, before CEEG monitoring comes into widespread use.

Persistent Vegetative State

The EEG findings in the persistent vegetative state are too variable to be of any clinical utility. The EEG may be relatively normal or show continuous or intermittent generalized slowing, background suppression, generalized periodic patterns, PLEDS, or triphasic waves. The findings show no relation to etiology and may vary with time in the same patient.[109]

De-Efferented State (Locked-In Syndrome)

Patients with locked-in syndrome may be regarded mistakenly as comatose. Although alert, these patients are mute and quadriplegic, and have a supranuclear paralysis of facial and bulbar muscles either from the pathologic involvement of major portions of the basis pontis with relative sparing of the tegmentum, or owing to bilateral midbrain lesions. The EEG is usually normal or shows minor nonspecific abnormalities, with preserved reactivity to pain, sound, and flicker stimulation. Prolonged polygraphic recording may show preserved sleep architecture or, in some instances, no REM stage and variable disorganization of non-REM sleep.

Miscellaneous Disorders

The EEG abnormalities in a number of disorders are of little diagnostic help and are considered here only briefly.

Spinocerebellar Degeneration

In spinocerebellar degeneration, the EEG is usually normal, but focal or generalized slowing sometimes occurs. In patients with an associated seizure disorder, epileptiform activity also may be found.

Parkinson Disease

Mild nonspecific changes, consisting usually of background slowing that may or may not be lateralized, are found occasionally in patients with Parkinson disease, but in most patients the EEG is normal.

Paroxysmal Choreoathetosis

Epileptiform activity is not a feature of the EEG obtained in patients with paroxysmal choreoathetosis. Records usually are normal or show only an excess of generalized slow activity.

Huntington Disease

Patients with Huntington disease characteristically have a low-voltage, featureless record in which the predominant background activity is sometimes in the beta range. Irregular slow activity, however, may be present in some cases, whereas in others the record is normal. Paroxysmal disturbances occasionally are found. The EEG findings have no value in determining which of the apparently unaffected offspring of patients with this inherited disorder will develop the disease.

Sydenham Chorea

EEG abnormalities are common but nonspecific in Sydenham chorea, consisting usually of diffuse slow activity in the theta- or delta-frequency ranges. Focal or lateralized slow-wave disturbances also may be found, and epileptiform discharges are seen occasionally. Improvement occurs with time but does not necessarily parallel the time course of clinical changes.

Hepatolenticular Degeneration

The EEG is normal in most patients with hepatolenticular degeneration, but in others either generalized or paroxysmal slowing is found, sometimes together with spike discharges or sharp waves. In uncomplicated cases, the presence of EEG abnormalities shows no clear correlation with the clinical or biochemical state, and patients with predominantly hepatic or neural involvement show similar changes. Abnormalities are found most often when there are complications of the disease; these improve with clinical improvement.

Progressive Supranuclear Palsy

The EEG is often normal but sometimes shows nonspecific changes such as an excess of theta activity, minor lateralizing asymmetries, or frontal intermittent rhythmic delta activity. There are no characteristic EEG features of the disorder.

Transient Global Amnesia

Most EEGs recorded during or shortly after an episode of transient global amnesia are completely normal.

Psychiatric Disorders

Although a vast literature has accumulated on the EEG findings in patients with psychiatric disorders, there is little evidence that the EEG is of any use in the diagnosis and management of such patients, apart from when it suggests the possibility of an organic disturbance.

REFERENCES

1. Kurtz P, Hanafy KA, Claassen J: Continuous EEG monitoring: is it ready for prime time? Curr Opin Crit Care, 15:99, 2009
2. Rosenkranz K, Lemieux L: Present and future of simultaneous EEG-fMRI. MAGMA, 23:309, 2010
3. Berg AT, Berkovic SF, Brodie MJ et al: Revised terminology and concepts for organization of seizures and epilepsies: report of the ILAE Commission on Classification and Terminology, 2005–2009. Epilepsia, 51:676, 2010
4. Mendez OE, Brenner RP: Increasing the yield of EEG. J Clin Neurophysiol, 23:282, 2006
5. Olejniczak P: Neurophysiologic basis of EEG. J Clin Neurophysiol, 23:186, 2006
6. Buzsaki G, Traub RD, Pedley TA: The cellular basis of EEG activity. p. 1. In Ebersole JS, Pedley TA (eds) Current Practice of Clinical Electroencephalography. 3rd Ed. Lippincott Williams & Wilkins, Philadelphia, 2003
7. Tao JX, Baldwin M, Hawes-Ebersole S et al: Cortical substrates of scalp EEG epileptiform discharges. J Clin Neurophysiol, 24:96, 2007
8. Ebersole JS: Cortical generators and EEG voltage fields. p. 12. In Ebersole JS, Pedley TA (eds): Current Practice of Clinical Electroencephalography. 3rd Ed. Lippincott Williams & Wilkins, Philadelphia, 2003
9. Alarcon G, Guy CN, Binnie CD et al: Intracerebral propagation of interictal activity in partial epilepsy: implications

for source localisation. J Neurol Neurosurg Psychiatry, 57:435, 1994

10. Westmoreland BF, Klass DW: Unusual EEG patterns. J Clin Neurophysiol, 7:209, 1990

11. Kojelka JW, Pedley TA: Beta and mu rhythms. J Clin Neurophysiol, 7:191, 1990

12. Brenner RP, Atkinson R: Generalized paroxysmal fast activity: electroencephalographic and clinical features. Ann Neurol, 11:386, 1982

13. Bahamon-Dussan JE, Celesia GG, Grigg-Damberger MM: Prognostic significance of EEG triphasic waves in patients with altered state of consciousness. J Clin Neurophysiol, 6:313, 1989

14. Reutens DC, Dunne JW, Gubbay SS: Triphasic waves in accidental hypothermia. Electroencephalogr Clin Neurophysiol, 76:370, 1990

15. River Y, Zelig O: Triphasic waves in myxedema coma. Clin Electroencephalogr, 24:146, 1993

16. Blatt I, Brenner RP: Triphasic waves in a psychiatric population: a retrospective study. J Clin Neurophysiol, 13:324, 1996

17. Lancman ME, Marks S, Mahmood K et al: Atypical triphasic waves associated with the use of pentobarbital. Electroencephalogr Clin Neurophysiol, 102:175, 1997

18. Ogunyemi A: Triphasic waves during post-ictal stupor. Can J Neurol Sci, 23:208, 1996

19. Westmoreland BF: Epileptiform electroencephalographic patterns. Mayo Clin Proc, 71:501, 1996

20. Andermann F, Zifkin B: The benign occipital epilepsies of childhood: an overview of the idiopathic syndromes and of the relationship to migraine. Epilepsia, 39: Suppl 4. S9, 1998

21. Gloor P, Fariello RG: Generalized epilepsy: some of its cellular mechanisms differ from those of focal epilepsy. Trends Neurosci, 11:63, 1988

22. Gloor P: Epilepsy: relationship between electrophysiology and intracellular mechanisms involving second messengers and gene expression. Can J Neurol Sci, 16:8, 1989

23. Accolla EA, Kaplan PW, Maeder-Ingvar M: Clinical correlates of frontal intermittent rhythmic delta activity (FIRDA). Clin Neurophysiol, 122:27, 2011

24. Reeves AL, Westmoreland BF, Klass DW: Clinical accompaniments of the burst-suppression EEG pattern. J Clin Neurophysiol, 14:150, 1997

25. Jumao-as A, Brenner RP: Myoclonic status epilepticus: a clinical and electroencephalographic study. Neurology, 40:1199, 1990

26. Pourmand R: Burst-suppression pattern with unusual correlates. Clin Electroencephalogr, 25:160, 1994

27. Steriade M, Amzica F, Contreras D: Cortical and thalamic cellular correlates of electroencephalographic burst-suppression. Electroencephalogr Clin Neurophysiol, 90:1, 1994

28. Pohlmann-Eden B, Hoch DB, Cochius JI et al: Periodic lateralized epileptiform discharges: a critical review. J Clin Neurophysiol, 13:519, 1996

29. Kalamangalam GP, Diehl B, Burgess RC: Neuroimaging and neurophysiology of periodic lateralized epileptiform discharges: observations and hypotheses. Epilepsia, 48: 1396, 2007

30. Neufeld MY, Vishnevskaya S, Treves TA et al: Periodic lateralized epileptiform discharges (PLEDs) following stroke are associated with metabolic abnormalities. Electroencephalogr Clin Neurophysiol, 102:295, 1997

31. Lim KS, Cheong KL, Tan CT: Periodic lateralized epileptiform discharges in neuropsychiatric lupus: association with cerebritis in magnetic resonance imaging and resolution after intravenous immunoglobulin. Lupus, 19:748, 2010

32. Fitzpatrick W, Lowry N: PLEDs: clinical correlates. Can J Neurol Sci, 34:443, 2007

33. Garzon E, Fernandes RM, Sakamoto AC: Serial EEG during human status epilepticus: evidence for PLED as an ictal pattern. Neurology, 57:1175, 2001

34. Hughes JR: Periodic lateralized epileptiform discharges: do they represent an ictal pattern requiring treatment? Epilepsy Behav, 18:162, 2010

35. Terzano MG, Parrino L, Mazzucchi A et al: Confusional states with periodic lateralized epileptiform discharges (PLEDs): a peculiar epileptic syndrome in the elderly. Epilepsia, 27:446, 1986

36. Orta DS, Chiappa KH, Quiroz AZ et al: Prognostic implications of periodic epileptiform discharges. Arch Neurol, 66:985, 2009

37. Reiher J, Rivest J, Grand'Maison F et al: Periodic lateralized epileptiform discharges with transitional rhythmic discharges: association with seizures. Electroencephalogr Clin Neurophysiol, 78:12, 1991

38. Santoshkumar B, Chong JJ, Blume WT et al: Prevalence of benign epileptiform variants. Clin Neurophysiol, 120:856, 2009

39. O'Brien TJ, Sharbrough FW, Westmoreland BF et al: Subclinical rhythmic electrographic discharges of adults (SREDA) revisited: a study using digital EEG analysis. J Clin Neurophysiol, 15:493, 1998

40. Westmoreland BF, Klass DW: Unusual variants of subclinical rhythmic electrographic discharge of adults (SREDA). Electroencephalogr Clin Neurophysiol, 102:1, 1997

41. Klass DW, Brenner RP: Electroencephalography of the elderly. J Clin Neurophysiol, 12:116, 1995

42. Oken BS, Kaye JA: Electrophysiologic function in the healthy, extreme old. Neurology, 42:519, 1992

43. Guaranha MS, Garzon E, Buchpiguel CA et al: Hyperventilation revisited: physiological effects and efficacy on focal seizure activation in the era of video-EEG monitoring. Epilepsia, 46:69, 2005

44. Drury I: Activation of seizures by hyperventilation. p. 575. In Luders HO, Noachtar S (eds): Epileptic Seizures: Pathophysiology and Clinical Semiology. Churchill Livingstone, Philadelphia, 2000

45. Holmes MD, Dewaraja AS, Vanhatalo S: Does hyperventilation elicit epileptic seizures? Epilepsia, 45:618, 2004

46. Fisch BJ, Hauser WA, Brust JCM et al: The EEG response to diffuse and patterned photic stimulation during acute untreated alcohol withdrawal. Neurology, 39:434, 1989

47. So EL, Ruggles KH, Ahmann PA et al: Prognosis of photo-paroxysmal response in nonepileptic patients. Neurology, 43:1719, 1993

48. Cash SS, Halgren E, Dehghani N et al: The human K-complex represents an isolated cortical down-state. Science, 324:1084, 2009

49. Rey V, Aybek S, Maeder-Ingvar M et al: Positive occipital sharp transients of sleep (POSTS): a reappraisal. Clin Neurophysiol, 120:472, 2009

50. AASM Manual for the Scoring of Sleep and Associated Events: Rules, Terminology and Technical Specification. American Academy of Sleep Medicine, Darien, IL, 2007

51. Reeves AL, Klass DW: Frequency asymmetry of sleep spindles associated with focal pathology. Electroencephalogr Clin Neurophysiol, 106:84, 1998

52. Fountain NB, Kim JS, Lee SI: Sleep deprivation activates epileptiform discharges independent of the activating effects of sleep. J Clin Neurophysiol, 15:69, 1998

53. Goodin DS, Aminoff MJ: Does the interictal EEG have a role in the diagnosis of epilepsy? Lancet, 1:837, 1984

54. King MA, Newton MR, Jackson GD et al: Epileptology of the first-seizure presentation: a clinical, electroencephalographic, and magnetic resonance imaging study of 300 consecutive patients. Lancet, 352:1007, 1998

55. Gotman J, Koffler DJ: Interictal spiking increases after seizures but does not after decrease in medication. Electroencephalogr Clin Neurophysiol, 72:7, 1989

56. Michelucci R, Rubboli G, Passarelli D et al: Electroclinical features of idiopathic generalised epilepsy with persisting absences in adult life. J Neurol Neurosurg Psychiatry, 61:471, 1996

57. Panayiotopoulos CP, Chroni E, Daskalopoulos C et al: Typical absence seizures in adults: clinical, EEG, video-EEG findings and diagnostic/syndromic considerations. J Neurol Neurosurg Psychiatry, 55:1002, 1992

58. Foldvary N, Lee N, Thwaites G et al: Clinical and electrographic manifestations of lesional neocortical temporal lobe epilepsy. Neurology, 49:757, 1997

59. Ebersole JS, Pacia SV: Localization of temporal lobe foci by ictal EEG patterns. Epilepsia, 37:386, 1996

60. Williamson PD, French JA, Thadani VM et al: Characteristics of medial temporal lobe epilepsy: II. Interictal and ictal scalp electroencephalography, neuropsychological testing, neuroimaging, surgical results, and pathology. Ann Neurol, 34:781, 1993

61. Schmidt D: The influence of antiepileptic drugs on the electroencephalogram: a review of controlled clinical studies. p. 453. In Buser PA, Cobb WA, Okuma T (eds): Kyoto Symposia. (Electroencephalogr Clin Neurophysiol Suppl 36). Elsevier, Amsterdam, 1982

62. Marciani MG, Spanedda F, Bassetti MA et al: Effect of lamotrigine on EEG paroxysmal abnormalities and background activity: a computerized analysis. Br J Clin Pharmacol, 42:621, 1996

63. Marciani MG, Stanzione P, Maschio M et al: EEG changes induced by vigabatrin monotherapy in focal epilepsy. Acta Neurol Scand, 95:115, 1997

64. Selvitelli MF, Walker LM, Schomer DL et al: The relationship of interictal epileptiform discharges to clinical epilepsy severity: a study of routine electroencephalograms and review of the literature. J Clin Neurophysiol, 27:87, 2010

65. Thomas P, Valton L, Genton P: Absence and myoclonic status epilepticus precipitated by antiepileptic drugs in idiopathic generalized epilepsy. Brain, 129:1281, 2006

66. Rossetti AO, Oddo M, Liaudet L et al: Predictors of awakening from postanoxic status epilepticus after therapeutic hypothermia. Neurology, 72:744, 2009

67. DeLorenzo RJ, Waterhouse EJ, Towne AR et al: Persistent nonconvulsive status epilepticus after the control of convulsive status epilepticus. Epilepsia, 39:833, 1998

68. Towne AR, Waterhouse EJ, Boggs JG et al: Prevalence of nonconvulsive status epilepticus in comatose patients. Neurology, 54:340, 2000

69. Vespa PM, Nuwer MR, Nenov V et al: Increased incidence and impact of nonconvulsive and convulsive seizures after traumatic brain injury as detected by continuous electroencephalographic monitoring. J Neurosurg, 91:750, 1999

70. Young GB, Jordan KG, Doig GS: An assessment of non-convulsive seizures in the intensive care unit using continuous EEG monitoring: an investigation of variables associated with mortality. Neurology, 47:83, 1996

71. Celesia GG, Grigg MM, Ross E: Generalized status myoclonicus in acute anoxic and toxic-metabolic encephalopathies. Arch Neurol, 45:781, 1988

72. Larch J, Unterberger I, Bauer G et al: Myoclonic status epilepticus in juvenile myoclonic epilepsy. Epileptic Disord, 11:309, 2009

73. Berg AT, Shinnar S: Relapse following discontinuation of antiepileptic drugs: a meta-analysis. Neurology, 44:601, 1994

74. Tinuper P, Avoni P, Riva R et al: The prognostic value of the electroencephalogram in antiepileptic drug withdrawal in partial epilepsies. Neurology, 47:76, 1996

75. Josephson CB, Rahey S, Sadler RM: Neurocardiogenic syncope: frequency and consequences of its misdiagnosis as epilepsy. Can J Neurol Sci, 34:221, 2007

76. Aminoff MJ, Scheinman MM Griffin JC et al: Electrocerebral accompaniments of syncope associated with malignant ventricular arrhythmias. Ann Intern Med, 108:791, 1988

77. Clute HL, Levy WJ: Electroencephalographic changes during brief cardiac arrest in humans. Anesthesiology, 73:821, 1990

78. Brenner RP: Electroencephalography in syncope. J Clin Neurophysiol, 14:197, 1997

79. Young GB, Bolton CF, Archibald YM et al: The electroencephalogram in sepsis-associated encephalopathy. J Clin Neurophysiol, 9:145, 1992

80. Cambier DM, Kantarci K, Worrell GA et al: Lateralized and focal clinical, EEG, and FLAIR MRI abnormalities in Creutzfeldt–Jakob disease. Clin Neurophysiol, 114:1729, 2003

81. Bortone E, Bettoni L, Giorgi C et al: Reliability of EEG in the diagnosis of Creutzfeldt–Jakob disease. Electroencephalogr Clin Neurophysiol, 90:323, 1994

82. Tietjen GE, Drury I: Familial Creutzfeldt–Jakob disease without periodic EEG activity. Ann Neurol, 28:585, 1990

83. Zeidler M, Stewart GE, Barraclough CR et al: New variant Creutzfeldt–Jakob disease: neurological features and diagnostic tests. Lancet, 350:903, 1997

84. Will RG, Zeidler M, Stewart GE et al: Diagnosis of new variant Creutzfeldt–Jakob disease. Ann Neurol, 47:575, 2000

85. Smith SJM, Kocen RS: A Creutzfeldt–Jakob like syndrome due to lithium toxicity. J Neurol Neurosurg Psychiatry, 51:120, 1988

86. Hormes JT, Benarroch EE, Rodriguez M et al: Periodic sharp waves in baclofen-induced encephalopathy. Arch Neurol, 45:814, 1988

87. Gordon MF, Abrams RI, Rubin DB et al: Bismuth subsalicylate toxicity as a cause of prolonged encephalopathy with myoclonus. Mov Disord, 10:220, 1995

88. Petty GW, Labar DR, Fisch BJ et al: Electroencephalography in lacunar infarction. J Neurol Sci, 134:47, 1995

89. Hinchey J, Chaves C, Appignani B et al: A reversible posterior leukoencephalopathy syndrome. N Engl J Med, 334:494, 1996

90. Bakshi R, Bates VE, Mechtler LL et al: Occipital lobe seizures as the major clinical manifestation of reversible posterior leukoencephalopathy syndrome: magnetic resonance imaging findings. Epilepsia, 39:1381, 1998

91. Vespa PM, Nuwer M, Juhasz C et al: Early detection of vasospasm after acute subarachnoid hemorrhage using continuous EEG ICU monitoring. Electroencephalogr Clin Neurophysiol, 103:607, 1997

92. Gronseth GS, Greenberg MK: The utility of the electroencephalogram in the evaluation of patients presenting with headache: a review of the literature. Neurology, 45:1263, 1995

93. Pasquier F, Petit H: Frontotemporal dementia: its rediscovery. Eur Neurol, 38:1, 1997

94. Jelic V, Kowalski J: Evidence-based evaluation of diagnostic accuracy of resting EEG in dementia and mild cognitive impairment. Clin EEG Neurosci, 40:129, 2009

95. Steg R, Wszolek ZK: Electroencephalographic abnormalities in liver transplant recipients: practical considerations and review. J Clin Neurophysiol, 13:60, 1996

96. San-Juan OD, Chiappa KH, Costello DJ et al: Periodic epileptiform discharges in hypoxic encephalopathy: BiPLEDs and GPEDs as a poor prognosis for survival. Seizure, 18:365, 2009

97. Blume WT: Drug effects on EEG. J Clin Neurophysiol, 23:306, 2006

98. Herning RI, Guo X, Better WE et al: Neurophysiological signs of cocaine dependence: increased electroencephalogram beta during withdrawal. Biol Psychiatry, 41:1087, 1997

99. Freudenreich O, Weiner RD, McEvoy JP: Clozapine-induced electroencephalogram changes as a function of clozapine serum levels. Biol Psychiatry, 42:132, 1997

100. Malow BA, Reese KB, Sato S et al: Spectrum of EEG abnormalities during clozapine treatment. Electroencephalogr Clin Neurophysiol, 91:205, 1994

101. Vespa PM, Boscardin WJ, Hovda DA et al: Early and persistent impaired percent alpha variability on continuous electroencephalography monitoring as predictive of poor outcome after traumatic brain injury. J Neurosurg, 97:84, 2002

102. Kaplan PW, Genoud D, Ho TW et al: Etiology, neurologic correlations, and prognosis in alpha coma. Clin Neurophysiol, 110:205, 1999

103. Young GB, Blume WT, Campbell VM et al: Alpha, theta and alpha-theta coma: a clinical outcome study utilizing serial recordings. Electroencephalogr Clin Neurophysiol, 91:93, 1994

104. Kaplan PW, Genoud D, Ho TW et al: Clinical correlates and prognosis in early spindle coma. Clin Neurophysiol, 111:584, 2000

105. Bassetti C, Bomio F, Mathis J et al: Early prognosis in coma after cardiac arrest: a prospective clinical, electrophysiological, and biochemical study of 60 patients. J Neurol Neurosurg Psychiatry, 61:610, 1996

106. Zandbergen EG, de Haan RJ, Stoutenbeek CP et al: Systematic review of early prediction of poor outcome in anoxic-ischaemic coma. Lancet, 352:1808, 1998

107. Young GB: The EEG in coma. J Clin Neurophysiol, 17:473, 2000

108. Young GB: Continuous EEG monitoring in the ICU: challenges and opportunities. Can J Neurol Sci, 36 Suppl 2: S89, 2009

109. Kulkarni VP, Lin K, Benbadis SR: EEG findings in the persistent vegetative state. J Clin Neurophysiol, 24:433, 2007

Neonatal and Pediatric Electroencephalography

JIN S. HAHN

The electroencephalogram (EEG) is an important tool in the evaluation of an infant or child with symptoms referable to the central nervous system (CNS). EEGs are used to assess seizure disorders, monitor the progression of a disease, and determine the prognosis for recovery or the development of long-term sequelae. Many EEGs are obtained to "rule out neurologic disorder" or simply to verify a diagnosis that has been well established clinically without much thought from the clinician as to the potential value or yield of such a test. However, the EEG may be overinterpreted by an electroencephalographer with little pediatric experience or training. The clinician, faced with a report of an abnormal EEG, may then feel obliged to undertake additional diagnostic tests, such as magnetic resonance imaging (MRI), or even to advise unnecessary therapy.

This chapter is an overview of pediatric EEG with particular emphasis on newborns and young infants. It illustrates the value of the EEG in the era of neuroimaging, and provides a source of references for those interested in a particular topic. Not all facets of pediatric EEG are reviewed. Rather, the normal patterns seen during infancy and childhood are discussed in detail, with emphasis on those that are often misinterpreted or "over-read." Most EEG abnormalities are nonspecific and, in the absence of a clinical history, are of little diagnostic value, except to indicate the possibility of a pathologic process involving the CNS. Therefore, neurologic disorders that are often associated with specific and, in some cases, pathognomonic EEG patterns are emphasized.

NEWBORN INFANTS

The EEG is an important adjunct to the neurologic evaluation of the sick newborn infant. It provides an excellent, noninvasive method of assessing at-risk newborns and formulating a prognosis for long-term neurologic outcome. EEGs are commonly utilized in the United States for the evaluation of premature and full-term infants. Improvements in the obstetric management of high-risk pregnancies and major advances in neonatal medicine have decreased the mortality and lessened the morbidity of small premature infants. Although neonatal mortality has declined since the advent of neonatal intensive care units (NICUs), morbidity statistics have been changed less dramatically. The neurologic assessment of critically ill newborns is an important aspect of their initial care because preservation of cerebral function is the goal of the intensive supportive care. The major long-term sequelae of surviving newborn infants are neurologic in nature: cerebral palsy, intellectual disability, and other more subtle motor and cognitive deficits.

The major areas in which the EEG can provide unique information in the assessment of newborn full-term and preterm infants are:

1. Diagnosis and treatment of seizures.
2. Evaluation of infants with compromised cerebral function caused by primary neurologic disorders (e.g., hypoxic-ischemic encephalopathy and cerebral infarction) and those with significant systemic disease (e.g., severe respiratory distress syndrome or sepsis) who are at risk for secondary encephalopathies.
3. Estimation of the conceptional age (CA), which is defined as the estimated gestational age (EGA) plus the legal age. The EGA is the age in weeks of the infant at birth calculated from the date of the mother's last menstrual period or by ultrasound study or a standardized physical examination. Legal age is that of the infant since birth.
4. Identification of specific neurologic entities (e.g., intraventricular hemorrhage, periventricular leukomalacia, congenital brain malformations, viral encephalitis, and metabolic encephalopathies).
5. Determination of prognosis and long-term neurologic outcome.

The EEG is also used in neonatal research concerned with the study of infant behavior and the assessment of physiologic functions that are dependent on the sleep state. For example, studies of neonatal apnea have demonstrated marked differences in the quantity and quality of apneas in active and quiet sleep.[1]

The neurologic disorders of newborn infants are often unique to this period of life. Asphyxia is a common cause of neurologic compromise in the newborn and leads to hypoxic-ischemic encephalopathy. Placental dysfunction, particularly infection, can cause periventricular leukomalacia in premature infants. Metabolic encephalopathies (e.g., hypoglycemia) may cause transient EEG abnormalities, yet permanently impair cerebral function. Transient and more benign metabolic abnormalities (e.g., hypocalcemia) cause seizures but are becoming less common with improvements in neonatal intensive care. Meningitis, traumatic lesions (including subarachnoid hemorrhage), congenital malformations of the CNS, drug withdrawal, and inherited disorders of CNS metabolism (e.g., amino or organic acidurias) constitute the bulk of the remaining neurologic syndromes of relevance to the electroencephalographer.

Technical Considerations

Many technical aspects of EEG recording are unique to the newborn infant. It is beyond the scope of this chapter to detail the nuances of EEG recording in the newborn nursery, which is reviewed elsewhere.[2,3] Table 4.1 is a summary of some major technical areas in which EEG recording in neonates differs from that in older children and adults. This recording method is used for preterm and full-term infants until approximately 1 to 2 months after term. The American Clinical Neurophysiology Society (formerly the American Electroencephalographic Society) has published guidelines for the recording of EEGs in infants.[4]

The technologist should have additional training in a laboratory that is already recording from neonates, should become familiar with nursery procedures, and should develop a good rapport with the nursery staff. The technologist should annotate normal and abnormal body and facial movements of newborn infants. In conjunction with the respirogram, electro-oculogram, and EEG, the infant's movements provide the necessary data to determine the behavioral or sleep state. An EEG lacking such clinical observations and polygraphic (non-EEG) variables is extremely difficult, if not impossible, to interpret unless it is grossly abnormal. The use of digital EEG and simultaneous video recordings of the newborn is helpful for detecting movements and artifacts, but does not obviate the need for good annotation and physiologic monitors.

Normal EEG

There is extensive literature on the normal cerebral electrical activity of the premature and full-term newborn.[3,5] Only a summary of the salient characteristics of the normal EEG at each conceptional age is given here.

CNS MATURATION AND ONTOGENIC SCHEDULING

Spontaneous electrocerebral activity in premature newborn infants evolves more rapidly than at any other time during human life. A close and consistent relationship exists between the changes in the EEG and the maturational changes of the nervous system. To understand and interpret neonatal EEGs, it is important to recognize the

TABLE 4-1 ■ EEG Recording in the Neonatal Period

Recording Techniques	Comments

Electrodes and placement
  Paste or collodion attachment
  Minimum of 9 scalp electrodes applied in premature infants and entire 10–20 array in term infants
  Fp1 and Fp2 placements replaced by Fp3 and Fp4 (halfway between 10–20 placements Fp and F)
  At least 16-channel recording is preferred
	Electrodes and placement
	  Needle electrodes are never used; collodion may not be allowed in some nurseries
	  Small head limits electrodes to frontal, central, occipital, midtemporal, and Cz in premature infants
	  Frontal sharp waves, delta, and other activity are of higher amplitude in prefrontal than frontopolar region
	  Many polygraphic parameters must be measured; all brain areas can be monitored with one montage

Polygraphic (non-EEG) variables recorded routinely—respiration (thoracic, with or without nasal thermistor); extraocular movements (primarily in infants older than 34 weeks CA); and electrocardiogram	These variables are essential in the determination of the behavior state (awake, active sleep, or quiet sleep) and the recognition of artifacts
Single montage used for entire recording, particularly with 16-channel recording	Generalized changes in background activity and state-related changes are more important than exact localization of focal abnormalities
Screen display of 15 to 20 sec for entire record. Long time constant—between 0.25 and 0.60 sec	It is easier to recognize interhemispheric synchrony and slow background activity
Frequent annotations by the technologist of baby's body movement and, in small premature infants, eye movement	Important information for the determination of behavioral state and possible artifact
Technologist attempts to record active and quiet sleep, particularly in older premature and term infants. Duration of record may exceed 60 min	Presence or absence of well-developed sleep states is important for interpretation; some pathologic patterns are seen primarily in quiet sleep
Accurate notation of EGA, CA, recent drug administration, recent changes in blood gases	Interpretation is dependent on knowledge of CA of infant. The EEG is very sensitive to abrupt changes in blood gases and certain medications

rapid maturational changes that take place in the brain during the last trimester. Such development takes place in an extrauterine environment in the premature infant. There is a rapid enlargement of the brain, with the weight increasing fourfold from 28 weeks to 40 weeks CA. Its appearance changes from a relatively primitive-looking structure before 24 weeks when the surfaces of the cerebral hemispheres are smooth, to 28 weeks when the major sulci make their appearance. The sulci and gyri continue to develop, until ultimately the complex brain of the full-term infant is achieved. Rapid maturational changes are also apparent in the neurochemical milieu; in interneuronal connectivity, with the development of dendritic trees and synaptogenesis; and in the myelination of axons.

Despite the apparent simplicity of the anatomy of the premature infant's brain, its repertoire of function is rather extensive. The premature infant of 28 weeks CA is capable of complex, spontaneous motor activity, vigorous crying, and response to stimuli. Behavioral states are also relatively well developed at 28 weeks CA.

In parallel with the developmental maturation of the brain, there is maturation of the bioelectric cerebral activity. According to the rule of ontogenic scheduling, the bioelectric maturation of cerebral activity of the healthy infant occurs in a predictable, time-linked manner. This maturational process is dependent primarily on the age of the brain (i.e., CA), and is independent of the number of weeks of extrauterine life. Therefore, the EEG of a premature infant born at 30 weeks EGA whose legal age is 10 weeks (CA 40 weeks) is similar to that of a 38-week EGA infant who is 2 weeks old. Some minor differences exist in the EEGs of premature infants who mature to term and those of full-term newborns, but these differences appear to be of little clinical significance. Consequently, an accurate estimate of the CA is essential for the correct interpretation of neonatal EEGs.

The EEG patterns of the newborn infant are dependent not only on the CA, but also on the behavioral states of the infant during the recording. Distinct EEG patterns of active (rapid eye movement or REM) and quiet (non-REM) sleep can be identified easily in normal infants by 35 weeks CA and in many infants as early as 27 to 28 weeks CA (Fig. 4-1). It is important to record both sleep states whenever possible, as abnormalities may be found only in one sleep state.

BEHAVIORAL STATES

The full-term newborn has easily recognizable waking and sleeping behavioral states that are very similar to those of older children and adults. These states are generally classified as waking, active sleep (REM sleep), quiet sleep (non-REM sleep), and indeterminate or transitional sleep (a sleeping state that cannot be classified definitely as either active or quiet sleep). Active sleep is the most common sleep-onset state in newborn infants and remains so for the first 2 to 4 months of post-term life[6]; it constitutes approximately 50 percent of the sleeping time in term infants

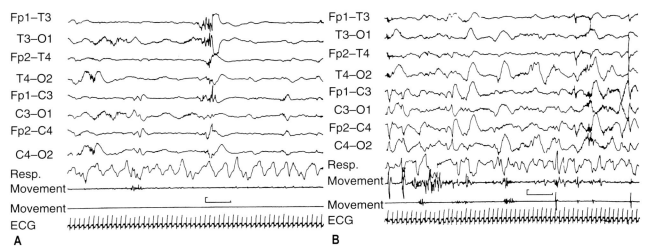

FIGURE 4-1 ■ **A**, Recording of quiet sleep of a healthy premature infant (29 weeks conceptional age). Discontinuous background is associated with infrequent limb movements. Note the burst of high-amplitude theta in the left frontotemporal region. Resp, abdominal respiration. Upper movement channel, movement monitor located under the baby's body. Lower movement channel, surface electromyogram on the right leg. Calibration: 50 μV; 2 seconds. **B**, Active sleep recorded in the same infant. Continuous background is associated with frequent body and limb movements. Bilateral brushes in the central regions are present in the right half of the tracing. Respirations are slightly less regular than in *A*. Calibration: 50 μV; 2 seconds.

and a slightly higher proportion in premature infants. The duration of active sleep at onset is usually 10 to 20 minutes but may exceed 40 minutes in some newborns.

A normal infant is considered awake if the eyes are open. Behavior may vary from quiet wakefulness to crying with vigorous motor activity. Transient eye closures may accompany crying and also occur during quiet wakefulness. If the eyes remain closed for an extended period of time (usually for more than 1 minute), the infant is considered asleep.

Active sleep in infants older than 29 weeks CA is characterized by eye closure, bursts of rapid horizontal and vertical eye movements, irregular respirations, and frequent limb and body movements ranging from brief twitches of a limb to gross movements of one limb or the entire body, grimacing, smiling, frowning, and bursts of sucking.

Quiet sleep in infants older than 29 weeks CA is characterized by the infant lying quietly with eyes closed, regular respiration, and the absence of rapid eye movements. There is a paucity of body and limb movements, although occasional gross body movements, characterized by brief stiffening of the trunk and limbs, may occur and sometimes are associated with brief clonic jerks of the lower extremities.

DISTINCTIVE PATTERNS IN NEONATAL EEGS

Certain distinct EEG patterns are common in the newborn, especially in the premature infant. These specific patterns serve as useful findings for determining the CA of the infant's nervous system. Figure 4-2 depicts some of these waveforms.

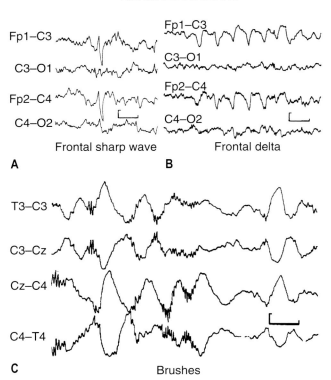

FIGURE 4-2 ■ **A**, Bilateral frontal sharp waves (*encoches frontales*) in a healthy full-term infant. **B**, Frontal rhythmic delta activity (anterior slow dysrhythmia) in a healthy preterm infant. **C**, Central delta brushes in a healthy premature infant (35 weeks conceptional age). Calibration: 50 μV; 1 second.

Theta Bursts (Sawtooth Waves)

Occipital theta bursts consist of rhythmic, medium- to high-amplitude, 4- to 7-Hz activity located in the occipital regions. These occipital theta bursts are present as a physiologic pattern in very premature infants (maximal between 24 and 26 weeks CA) and disappear by 32 weeks CA.[7,8] This pattern serves as a useful hallmark in determining CA.

Temporal theta burst activity is seen commonly in the EEGs of slightly older premature infants. This activity appears at approximately 26 weeks CA, with the maximal incidence between 27 and 31 weeks, and is seen rarely beyond 35 weeks.[9] The bursts consist of sharply contoured, high-amplitude (50 to 150 μV, occasionally 200 to 300 μV), 4- to 6-Hz activity; they are maximal in the temporal areas, but often become diffuse and, commonly, bilateral and synchronous (see Fig. 4-1).

These regular theta rhythms originate in the occipital regions in very premature infants and with increasing CA migrate toward temporal regions.[8] The gradient of occipitotemporal maturation of this pattern appears to coincide with the timing of gyral development in these regions.

Delta Brushes

Delta brushes are a hallmark of prematurity and are most abundant between 32 and 35 weeks CA (see Fig. 4-2). They consist of short bursts of 8- to 20-Hz rhythmic activity, often with spindle morphology, superimposed on high-amplitude slow waves (0.8 to 1.5 Hz). The amplitude of the fast activity may range from 10 to 100 μV (usually 20 to 50 μV), and that of the slow waves from 25 to 200 μV. Typically, delta brushes occur asynchronously in the homologous areas of the two hemispheres. Delta brushes predominate in the central (rolandic) region in very young premature infants (younger than 32 weeks CA), and extend to the occipital and temporal regions in older premature infants. Brushes are more abundant in active sleep in younger infants (up to 32 weeks CA) and in quiet sleep in infants older than 33 weeks CA. Delta brushes peak in abundance between 31 and 33 weeks CA, and decrease in number with increasing CA. In full-term infants, they are infrequent during quiet sleep and virtually absent in active sleep.

Frontal Sharp Transients (*Encoches Frontales*)

Frontal sharp transients are biphasic sharp waves (initially a negative deflection, followed by a wider positive deflection); they are of maximal amplitude in the prefrontal regions (Fp3, Fp4) and occur primarily during sleep, particularly during the transition from active to quiet sleep. The typical amplitude is 50 to 150 μV and

the duration of the initial surface-negative component is 200 msec. They usually appear bilaterally and synchronously, although they may be asymmetric in amplitude. Sometimes they appear unilaterally, shifting from one side to the other during the record. Typical frontal sharp transients appear at 35 weeks CA and persist until several weeks after term (see Fig. 4-2).

Rhythmic Frontal Delta Activity (Anterior Slow Dysrhythmia)

Rhythmic frontal delta activity consists of bursts and short runs of 1.5- to 4-Hz, 50- to 200-μV delta activity that is often monomorphic and of maximal amplitude in the frontal regions (see Fig. 4-2). Like frontal sharp transients, rhythmic frontal delta activity is most prominent during transitional sleep. This activity appears at approximately 37 weeks CA and lasts until approximately 6 weeks after term. Rhythmic frontal delta activity is often intermixed with frontal sharp transients. This activity should be distinguished from prolonged runs of monorhythmic bifrontal delta activity that persists in all sleep states, which is an abnormal finding.

Tracé Discontinu

In very young premature infants, the electrical activity of the brain is interrupted by long periods of quiescence. This pattern, called *tracé discontinu*, may be present in all states of sleep in very premature infants and persists to some degree in infants of 34 to 36 weeks CA. During periods of quiescence, the EEG is very low in amplitude (less than 30 μV) and may even be flat at standard amplification. The active periods increase in duration as the CA increases (Fig. 4-3). They are composed of bursts containing monomorphic delta, theta, and faster activity, delta brushes, and temporal theta bursts. The mean duration of interburst intervals in the healthy premature infant decreases with increasing gestational age; the mean interval at 27 to 29 weeks CA is approximately 6 seconds, and at 30 to 34 weeks is approximately 4 to 5 seconds. The maximum interburst intervals should not exceed approximately 30 seconds at any age beyond 27 weeks CA (Fig. 4-4).[1,10] In healthy, very preterm infants, the maximum interburst interval duration can be much longer: 126 seconds at 21 to 22 weeks CA, 87 seconds at 23 to 24 weeks CA, and 44 seconds at 25 to 26 weeks CA.[11]

Tracé Alternant

As the CA increases, the periods of relative electrocerebral inactivity become shorter in duration, and the interburst intervals display generalized amplitude attenuation

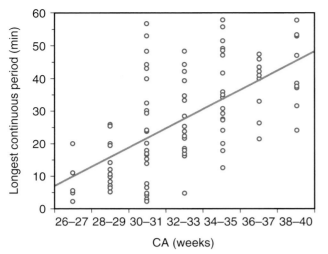

FIGURE 4-3 ▪ Longest continuous period of cerebral activity at various conceptional ages (CAs). The regression line was determined by the least-squares method. (From Hahn JS, Monyer H, Tharp BR: Interburst interval measurements in the EEG of premature infants with normal neurologic outcome. Electroencephalogr Clin Neurophysiol, 73:410, 1989, with permission.)

rather than quiescence. This pattern, called *tracé alternant*, is the discontinuous pattern that characterizes the quiet sleep of the full-term newborn (Fig. 4-5). *Tracé alternant* consists of 3- to 6-second bursts of high-amplitude delta

and theta activity (1 to 6 Hz, 50 to 100 μV) admixed with lower-amplitude beta and theta activity, which occur at intervals of 3 to 6 seconds. The bursts may also contain scattered isolated sharp transients. The interburst intervals contain diffuse moderate-amplitude (25 to 50 μV), mixed-frequency (usually 4- to 12-Hz) activity, similar to that occurring during wakefulness and active sleep following quiet sleep.

A gradual transition from *tracé discontinu* to *tracé alternant* occurs as the premature infant approaches term, although even in the healthy full-term infant, occasional short, very-low-amplitude interburst intervals are seen. *Tracé discontinu*, therefore, differs from *tracé alternant* primarily on the basis of the amplitude of the activity during the interburst interval.

Interhemispheric Synchrony

Interhemispheric synchrony is defined as the relatively simultaneous appearance in both hemispheres of bursts of cerebral activity during discontinuous portions of the record. In the very young premature infant (younger than 29 weeks CA) the EEG activity during *tracé discontinu* is hypersynchronous, with the degree of synchrony approaching 90 to 100 percent. The degree

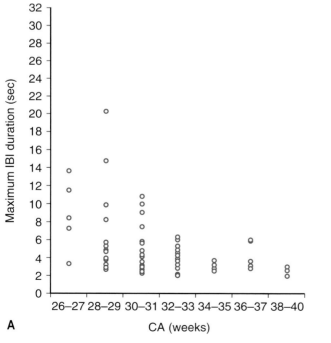

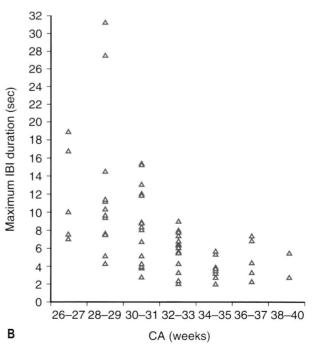

FIGURE 4-4 ▪ The maximum interburst interval (IBI) versus conceptional age (CA). **A**, For type 1 IBIs (intervals of at least 2 seconds containing no cerebral activity greater than 15 μV in any channel). **B**, For type 2 IBIs (similar to type 1 IBIs, except for a transient lasting less than 2 sec in one or two electrodes or continuous cerebral activity greater than 15 μV in one electrode). (Modified from Hahn JS, Monyer H, Tharp BR: Interburst interval measurements in the EEG of premature infants with normal neurologic outcome. Electroencephalogr Clin Neurophysiol, 73:410, 1989, with permission.)

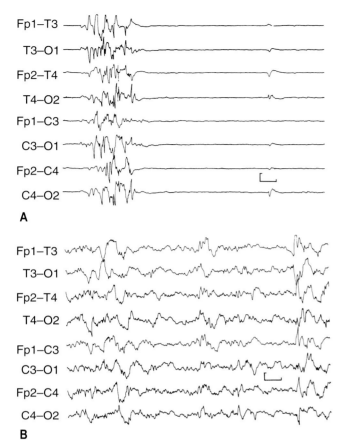

FIGURE 4-5 ■ **A**, Burst-suppression (paroxysmal) pattern during quiet state in a stuporous, full-term infant with severe hypoxic-ischemic encephalopathy. **B**, *Tracé alternant* pattern in quiet sleep of a healthy full-term infant. Calibration: 50 µV; 1 second.

of interhemispheric synchrony decreases to 60 to 80 percent for the next 4 to 5 weeks (30 to 35 weeks CA) and gradually approaches 100 percent as the infant reaches term.

AGE-SPECIFIC BACKGROUND PATTERNS

Normal Patterns at 23 to 26 Weeks CA

The EEG in very preterm infant is consistently discontinuous (*tracé discontinu*), although some variability in the organization of discontinuous patterns can be observed. In some phases bursts can be longer and intervals shorter, whereas at other times the discontinuity is more marked.[8] In a study of five subjects in this age group, the maximum interburst interval duration ranged between 20 and 62 seconds and the minimum burst length was 1 to 2 seconds.[8] Another study found that the maximum interburst interval duration was 87 seconds at 23 to 24 weeks CA and 44 seconds at 25 to 26 weeks CA.[11] Occipital theta bursts are

prominent (maximal at 25 weeks CA). Temporal theta bursts can be seen, but are less common than in older preterm infants. Some delta brushes are observable, but the incidence is generally low (between 9 and 21 percent of bursts).

Normal Patterns at 27 to 29 Weeks CA

The EEG at 27 to 29 weeks CA is characterized by a discontinuous background, *tracé discontinu*, that consists of mixed-frequency activity, primarily in the delta range. Bursts contain runs of high-amplitude, very slow, rhythmic occipital delta activity; and somewhat lower-amplitude, more arrhythmic central and temporal delta activity.[10] The maximum interburst intervals are generally less than 30 seconds.[10]

Beginning as early as 27 weeks CA, there may be behavioral and EEG differentiation of active and quiet sleep states.[10] During active sleep, REMs are observed with burst of slow waves admixed with theta activity. During quiet sleep, REMs are absent and the background becomes more discontinuous.

High-amplitude temporal theta bursts (see Fig. 4-1) become prominent during this period. Isolated frontopolar slow waves with superimposed faster activity (so-called "delta crests") are also common in this age group. Delta brushes are present primarily in the central (rolandic) and occipital regions.[10]

Normal Patterns at 30 to 32 Weeks CA

Two distinct types of background predominate at 30 to 32 weeks CA. A discontinuous background (*tracé discontinu*) composed of an admixture of occipital delta (1 to 2 Hz, 25 to 100 µV) and centrotemporal delta-, theta-, and alpha-range activity occurs when the child is in quiet sleep. More continuous background occurs with eye movements and more active body movements, consistent with active sleep. Synchrony during *tracé discontinu* reaches a nadir during this period (approximately 60 to 75 percent).

Delta brushes are very abundant at this age; they are located in the occipital, central, and temporal regions with a higher incidence during the continuous portions of the record (active sleep). There are fewer temporal theta bursts than at earlier ages, and the delta crests and occipital theta bursts are less common.

Normal Patterns at 33 to 35 Weeks CA

Sleep states at 33 to 35 weeks CA are becoming more clearly defined. Discontinuous activity (*tracé discontinu*) is associated with quiet sleep. During wakefulness and active sleep, continuous background slow activity (primarily 1 to 2 Hz, 25 to 100 μV) that is maximal in the temporal, central, and occipital regions is more abundant. In general, an increasing amount of lower-amplitude theta and faster activity is also present in all states. Synchrony approaches 80 percent at 35 weeks CA.

Delta brushes are still abundant but fewer than at an earlier age, and they are more frequent during quiet sleep. Typical frontal sharp transients (encoches frontales) appear at 34 to 35 weeks CA. Temporal theta activity should be much less common.[9]

Normal Patterns at 36 to 38 Weeks CA

Three different EEG patterns predominate at 36 to 38 weeks CA. (1) Continuous, diffuse, low-amplitude, 4- to 6-Hz activity (usually less than 50 μV) characterizes quiet wakefulness (activité moyenne). This activity is often admixed with 50- to 100-μV delta (2- to 4-Hz) activity and is the predominant rhythm of sleep-onset active sleep.[3] Delta brushes are rare in active sleep. (2) A discontinuous pattern (tracé alternant) with bursts of mixed-frequency slow activity and occasional delta brushes, separated by low- to medium-amplitude background, typifies quiet sleep. During this period, there is a transition from tracé discontinu to tracé alternant. The tracé alternant pattern persists until 4 to 8 weeks after term. (3) The active sleep that follows quiet sleep is characterized by low- to moderate-amplitude theta activity with occasional delta waves at lower amplitude than that occurring during sleep-onset active sleep.[3] Synchrony approximates 90 percent during the discontinuous portions of the EEG.

Delta brushes are less abundant during quiet sleep and are virtually absent during active sleep. Frontal sharp transients and rhythmic frontal delta activity are prominent, particularly during the transition from active sleep to quiet sleep.

Normal Patterns at 38 to 42 Weeks CA (Full-Term Newborn)

Sleep and waking cycles are well established at 38 to 42 weeks CA. Four distinctive patterns occur during sleep. (1) Low- to medium-amplitude theta activity with superimposed delta activity (2 to 4 Hz, less than 100 μV), the latter appearing as continuous activity or in short runs or bursts, characterizes active sleep, particularly at sleep onset. (2) Diffuse continuous delta activity (0.5 to 2 Hz, 25 to 100 μV) is found at the beginning and end of quiet sleep periods and occasionally is found during long portions of such sleep (slow-wave quiet sleep).

(3) Tracé alternant is characteristic of well-established quiet sleep. (4) Activité moyenne is a continuous low-amplitude activity (25 to 50 μV) at 1 to 10 Hz (predominantly 4 to 7 Hz) that characterizes wakefulness and active sleep, particularly following a period of quiet sleep. Interhemispheric synchrony during tracé alternant approaches 100 percent, but transient asynchrony may occur at its onset.

Delta brushes are rare in the EEGs of term infants; they occur primarily during quiet sleep. Frontal sharp transients and rhythmic frontal delta activity are abundant, particularly during the transitional period between active sleep and quiet sleep. The amplitude of the background activity is relatively symmetric over the two hemispheres, although transient asymmetries are common, particularly in the temporal regions. Rhythmic theta-alpha bursts, which consist of bursts or short runs (1 to 3 seconds) of sharply contoured, primarily surface-negative, rhythmic theta- and alpha-range activity, are common in the central and midline frontocentral areas, particularly during quiet sleep. Scattered isolated sharp waves are common in the temporal regions and are less common in the central and midline regions. These sharp transients usually are incorporated within the bursts of the tracé alternant.

Figure 4-6 summarizes the various EEG patterns that are seen in the neonatal EEG and how these patterns change as the premature infant matures to term. By knowing which maturational patterns become prominent at a particular CA, an estimation of the CA can be determined.

PITFALLS IN NEONATAL EEG INTERPRETATION

Inexperienced electroencephalographers often mistakenly characterize the frontal sharp transients and rhythmic frontal delta activity of the older premature infant and the temporal theta bursts of the very premature infant as "epileptiform" or "paroxysmal." The abundant brushes in the EEGs of younger premature infants may also give the background a "spiky" or "paroxysmal" appearance, especially when a compressed screen display (20 seconds) is used. Multifocal sharp waves are also noted, particularly in the temporal and central regions of healthy infants.

The various discontinuous background patterns of healthy premature infants must be distinguished from the abnormal paroxysmal patterns discussed in the next section. Transient interhemispheric amplitude asymmetries are common in all age groups, as is asynchrony of the bursts during the discontinuous portions of the tracings in

FIGURE 4-6 ▪ A summary depicting the various maturational patterns seen in the electroencephalogram of preterm and term infants as a function of the conceptional age (CA). These patterns include the number of temporal theta bursts and delta brushes, the durations of interburst intervals and bursts, and the degree of interhemispheric synchrony.

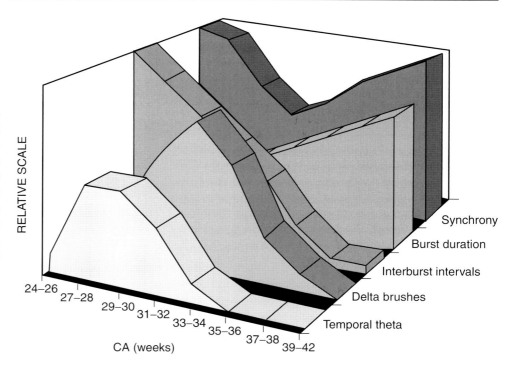

premature infants (approximately 31 to 35 weeks CA). There may be significant asymmetries in the onset of the *tracé alternant* pattern in normal infants, with *tracé alternant* appearing in one hemisphere 1 to 5 minutes before it emerges in the other.[1]

Abnormal EEG

It is beyond the scope of this chapter to discuss all the deviations from normal that are encountered in the EEGs of newborn infants. Rather, emphasis is placed on the patterns most commonly seen, those associated with certain specific neurologic disorders, and those that appear to be of prognostic value.

ABNORMAL BACKGROUND PATTERNS

Only the most common EEG abnormalities that occur in the neonatal EEG are discussed in this section. Additional discussions of the prognostic value of the EEG in full-term newborns can be found elsewhere.[3,12] One of the more common causes of a severely abnormal EEG background is hypoxic-ischemic encephalopathy. An EEG performed early can be valuable in predicting the severity of the encephalopathy and prognosis.[13] The following section discusses the various abnormal EEG patterns and their prognostic significance (Table 4-2).

Before interpreting the EEG, it is important to consider any acute changes in metabolic status, administration of neuroactive medications, or changes in respiratory status

TABLE 4-2 ▪ Prognostic Significance of Neonatal Background EEG Patterns

EEG Background Patterns	Percentage with Favorable Outcome
Isoelectric	0–5
Burst-suppression	0–15
Low-voltage undifferentiated	15–30
Excessively discontinuous	40–50
Diffuse slow activity	15–20
Gross asynchrony	10–20

Favorable outcome includes those with normal and mildly abnormal outcomes. See text on the importance of the timing of the EEG with respect to prognosis. (Data from Tharp BR, Cukier F, Monod M: The prognostic value of the electroencephalogram in premature infants. Electroencephalogr Clin Neurophysiol, 51:219, 1981; Takeuchi T, Watanabe K: The EEG evolution and neurological prognosis of perinatal hypoxia neonates. Brain Dev, 11:115, 1989; and Ortibus EL, Sum JM, Hahn JS: Predictive value of EEG for outcome and epilepsy following neonatal seizures. Electroencephalogr Clin Neurophysiol, 98:175, 1996.)

(e.g., oxygenation or pH) that may affect the background EEG acutely. For example, the EEG may become transiently abnormal and even isoelectric during acute hypoxemia. Many drugs used in nurseries (e.g., intravenous diazepam, lorazepam, midazolam, and opioids) may cause an acute but reversible depression of the EEG. The synthetic opioid, sufentanil, increases the discontinuity of the background in premature infants.[14] Intravenous morphine infusions may cause excessive discontinuity, sharp waves, and even burst-suppression patterns.[15] Therefore if these drugs are being administered at the time of the EEG, the record should be interpreted with caution and another record should be obtained after their discontinuance.

Electrocerebral Inactivity (Isoelectric)

Electrocerebral inactivity implies that there is no discernible cerebral electrical activity, even at high sensitivities. Such an EEG pattern is seen in various clinical settings, most commonly following severe asphyxia, circulatory collapse, and massive intracerebral hemorrhage. It can also be seen in bacterial meningitis, encephalitis, severe malformations of the brain (e.g., hydranencephaly or massive hydrocephalus), and inborn errors of metabolism. The same technical requirements for recording isoelectric records in adults are applied to infants. High sensitivities (equal to or exceeding 2 μV/mm), long time constants (0.1 seconds or more, or low-frequency filter of 1 Hz), and long interelectrode distances should be used. The technologist should also perform various auditory and nociceptive stimulations to confirm lack of reactivity.

In the absence of drug intoxication, acute hypoxemia, hypothermia, and postictal state, this EEG pattern carries a grave prognosis in neonates; however, it does not necessarily indicate "brain death." The vast majority of neonates with inactive EEGs either die in the neonatal period or survive with severe neurologic deficits. The neuropathology of the brains of neonates with inactive EEGs reveals widespread encephalomalacia and ischemic neuronal necrosis involving the cerebral cortex, corpus striatum, thalamus, midbrain, pons, and medulla.

In newborns, the return of EEG activity may be seen after an isoelectric EEG recorded in the first 24 hours of life or immediately after an acute hypoxic-ischemic event. If recovery occurs, the isoelectric EEG usually is followed by other abnormal patterns (particularly, diffusely slow backgrounds), but occasionally a flat EEG persists for many months following the acute neurologic insult.

Inactive EEG and Brain Death

There are no universally agreed criteria for brain death determination in newborn infants. The Task Force for the Determination of Brain Death in Children established the criteria for determining brain death in children, but did not provide guidelines for diagnosing brain death in infants under the age of 7 days.[16] For infants between the ages of 7 days and 2 months, the Task Force recommended that two physical examinations and EEGs separated by 48 hours be performed routinely.

During the first week after birth, an isoelectric EEG is not a reliable test for determining brain death. However, some believe that brain death can be diagnosed in the full-term newborn, even when less than 7 days of age.[17] If the initial EEG in the newborn shows electrocerebral inactivity in the absence of barbiturates, hypothermia, or cerebral malformations (e.g., hydranencephaly or hydrocephalus), and if the findings on neurologic examination remain unchanged after 24 hours, electrocerebral inactivity is confirmatory of brain death. Based on available data, the risk of misdiagnosis appears exceedingly low. Most neurologists believe that the EEG is a useful adjunct to the determination of brain death if it is performed by an experienced technologist using the standards of the American Clinical Neurophysiology Society (formerly the American Electroencephalographic Society[18]) and is interpreted by an experienced electroencephalographer.

Burst-Suppression (Paroxysmal) Pattern

The burst-suppression pattern (see Fig. 4-5, *A*) is characterized by an isoelectric background interrupted by nonperiodic bursts of abnormal activity: delta and theta activities with admixed spikes, beta activity, or both; less commonly, bursts or short runs of diffuse or focal alpha or theta activity that is occasionally rhythmic. The bursts, which are usually highly synchronous between hemispheres, contain no age-appropriate activity. In the most severe form, this pattern is invariant and minimally altered by stimuli, and persists throughout waking and sleeping states. This abnormal pattern must be differentiated from the normal discontinuous patterns seen in the quiet sleep of premature infants.

Burst-suppression patterns are seen following a variety of severe brain insults (e.g., asphyxia, severe metabolic disorders, CNS infections, and cerebral malformation). A burst-suppression pattern can be induced pharmacologically with high doses of barbiturates and other neuroactive medications. In the absence of significant concentrations of neuroactive medications, a burst-suppression pattern usually is associated with a very poor prognosis (85 to 100 percent unfavorable prognosis, depending on the study). Infants who have a burst-suppression pattern that changes with stimulation have a somewhat better prognosis.[19] A burst-suppression pattern in the first 24 hours of life that is replaced rapidly by a less severely abnormal EEG is followed occasionally by a normal neurologic outcome.[19]

Variants of Burst-Suppression Pattern

In a small group of full-term newborns with neonatal hypoxic-ischemic encephalopathy, Sinclair and co-workers compared different types of burst-suppression patterns with outcome.[20] Burst-suppression pattern was defined as a background with bursts lasting 1 to 10 seconds alternating with periods of marked background attenuation (amplitude consistently less than 5 μV). A modified burst-suppression pattern was defined as a burst-suppression pattern that was not constantly discontinuous throughout the recording, had periods of attenuation that contained activity higher than 5 µV, or both. Those newborns with a burst-suppression pattern had poor outcome: death in 6 of 15, severe disability in 4, and normal outcome in 2 of 9 survivors. The outcome in those with a modified burst-suppression pattern was more favorable: neonatal death in 1 of 8, severe disabilities in 1, and normal outcome in 3 of 7 survivors.[20] The EEGs were performed within the first week of life, but the timing of the EEG in regard to the timing of the insult was not provided. The study did not assess whether the burst-suppression pattern could be modified with stimulation.

Instead of rigidly distinguishing between burst-suppression and other constantly discontinuous patterns based on the amplitude of activity during the suppressions, Biagioni and colleagues examined EEG parameters of discontinuity and correlated these scores with the outcome.[21] In 32 full-term infants with hypoxic-ischemic encephalopathy who had an EEG with a constantly discontinuous pattern, they noted the minimum burst duration (activity greater than 45 µV), maximum interburst interval duration (interburst interval was defined as a period of activity less than 45 µV), and mean interburst interval amplitude. The best indicators predictive of a normal outcome were maximum interburst interval duration shorter than 10 seconds, mean interburst interval amplitude greater than 25 µV, and minimum burst duration longer than 2 seconds.[21] The maximum interburst interval duration correlated with the severity of the hypoxic-ischemic encephalopathy. It was also lengthened significantly (more than double) in children who received phenobarbital. The timing of the EEG was also an important factor in determining prognosis; of the nine subjects who had a constantly discontinuous EEG after the eighth day from birth none had a normal outcome. All of the 32 EEGs in this study would be compatible with the definition of modified burst-suppression pattern, as defined by Sinclair and colleagues,[20] because there were no records with interburst interval amplitudes less than 5 µV.

Menache and co-workers also examined several EEG parameters of discontinuity in 43 term or near-term infants who had a variety of neurologic disorders.[22] They included EEGs with constantly or transiently discontinuous patterns. Only 7 had a burst-suppression pattern as defined above. A predominant interburst interval duration (defined as the duration of more than 50 percent of all interburst intervals with amplitudes less than 25 µV) of longer than 30 seconds correlated with the occurrence of both unfavorable neurologic outcome and subsequent epilepsy.[22] Infants with this finding had 100 percent probability of severe neurologic disabilities or death

(all had hypoxic-ischemic encephalopathy) and an 86 percent chance of developing subsequent epilepsy.

Excessively Discontinuous Background

The background EEG is normally discontinuous in very premature infants, with periods of total absence of cerebral activity lasting many seconds. With the maturation of the brain, the duration of these flat periods, or interburst intervals, decreases as the preterm infant approaches term.[1,5,11] Conversely, the duration of the longest period of continuous EEG increases with CA (see Figs. 4-3 and 4.4).[11,23] In healthy, very preterm infants the maximum interburst interval duration in one study was 126 seconds at 21 to 22 weeks CA, 87 seconds at 23 to 24 weeks CA, and 44 seconds at 25 to 26 weeks CA.[11]

There are some differences among studies regarding the duration of normal interburst intervals, owing in part to the various criteria used to define them. Nevertheless, a conservative statement is that the maximum duration of interburst intervals should not exceed 60 seconds at 24 to 27 weeks CA, 30 seconds at 28 to 29 weeks CA, and 20 seconds at 30 to 31 weeks.[5] In full-term infants the maximum interburst interval should not exceed 6 seconds.[12] Excessively long interburst intervals are indicative of encephalopathy at all CAs, and generally have unfavorable prognostic implications.[12]

Unlike the burst-suppression pattern, there is some reactivity to tactile stimulation and often preservation of sleep-state transitions in an EEG with an excessively discontinuous background. Furthermore, in the premature infant, periods of EEG activity separated by excessively long interburst intervals may contain many of the normal transients that are abundant at this age (e.g., delta brushes and temporal theta bursts), whereas the bursts within the burst-suppression pattern of term infants are composed of abnormal EEG activity.

Low-Voltage Undifferentiated Pattern

A low-voltage pattern is usually defined as activity between 5 and 15 µV during all states.[24] Faster frequencies tend to be depressed or obliterated. Differentiation of sleep state in low-voltage records may be difficult, although some amplitude differences may exist between sleep states, with amplitudes being slightly higher in quiet sleep than in active sleep.

Low-voltage records are seen in a variety of severe CNS disorders, including hypoxic-ischemic encephalopathy; toxic-metabolic disturbances; congenital hydrocephalus; and severe intracranial hemorrhage, including large subdural hematomas. The prognostic value of the low-voltage EEGs depends strongly on the timing of recording after a presumptive brain injury. The pattern is ominous, especially when it persists beyond the first week after the insult; there is high probability of neurologic sequelae or death.[25] Therefore, EEGs obtained shortly after an acute event should be interpreted with caution, and a follow-up study should be performed.

Several caveats about the interpretation of low-voltage EEGs are required. It is important that the recording is long enough to include periods of quiet sleep (which are generally higher in amplitude than active sleep). Neuro-depressive medications and surfactant treatment may depress EEG amplitude. Severe scalp edema, subgaleal hematomas, subdural hematomas, and extra-axial fluid collections may also attenuate the EEG amplitude artifactually.

Low-Voltage Background with Theta Rhythms

The low-voltage background with theta rhythms is a variant of the low-voltage pattern. Continuous low-voltage background (5 to 25 μV) is accompanied by low-voltage (5 to 15 μV) theta activity that occurs in bursts of varying lengths or sometimes continuously. The theta activity may be diffuse but is more often focal or multifocal. The EEG shows no reactivity to stimulation and, usually, no discernible sleep states. This pattern is usually seen in neonates with hypoxic-ischemic encephalopathy and is highly associated with unfavorable outcomes.[3]

Diffuse Slow Activity

The pattern of diffuse slow activity, also called the mono-morphic medium-voltage pattern, consists of widespread amorphous delta activity that persists throughout the recording and is not altered significantly by sensory stimuli (Fig. 4-7). The faster patterns in the theta and beta range, which are normally abundant in the EEGs of term infants, are absent. The background is devoid of the normal patterns seen in the premature infant, such as delta brushes, temporal theta bursts, and occipital theta bursts. This pattern may emerge during the recovery phase after hypoxic-ischemic encephalopathy, replacing more severe patterns such as electrocerebral inactivity, low-voltage undifferentiated pattern, or burst-suppression. When a pattern of diffuse slow activity persists beyond 1 month in full-term neonates after hypoxic-ischemic encephalopathy, the prognosis appears to be poor, with two-thirds of the subjects having neurologic sequelae.[25]

This type of abnormal background must be distinguished from the high-amplitude, slow-wave pattern that

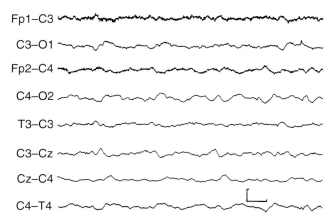

FIGURE 4-7 ■ Diffusely slow background with absence of normal patterns for the conceptional age (CA). Premature infant (34 weeks CA) with hypoxic encephalopathy, severe respiratory distress syndrome, and bloody cerebrospinal fluid. The infant died at 6 days of age, and autopsy revealed subarachnoid hemorrhage, cerebral edema, and widespread anoxic encephalopathy. Calibration: 50 μV; 1 second.

occurs during a portion of the normal quiet sleep of preterm and term infants, and that gradually replaces the *tracé alternant* pattern during the first 4 to 6 weeks after term. This pattern should also be distinguished from frontal rhythmic delta activity (anterior slow dysrhythmia), which is a normal pattern seen in transitional sleep that appears at 37 weeks CA and persists for several weeks after term.

Grossly Asynchronous Records

The degree of interhemispheric synchrony is dependent on the CA. A record is considered to be grossly asynchronous if, during the discontinuous state, all background rhythms are persistently asynchronous between the hemispheres (estimated less than 25 percent synchrony for infants older than 30 weeks CA). The majority of records with gross interhemispheric asynchrony have paroxysmal backgrounds (Fig. 4-8). Records with markedly asynchronous burst-suppression patterns are often seen in infants with severe hypoxic-ischemic encephalopathy, congenital malformations (e.g., agenesis of corpus callosum or Aicardi syndrome), and periventricular leukomalacia. A grossly asynchronous pattern usually is associated with an unfavorable outcome.

Amplitude Asymmetry Pattern

A persistent amplitude asymmetry in the background activity between the hemispheres (Fig. 4-9) that exceeds 50 percent and is present in all states is thought to be significant. This pattern commonly correlates with lateralized

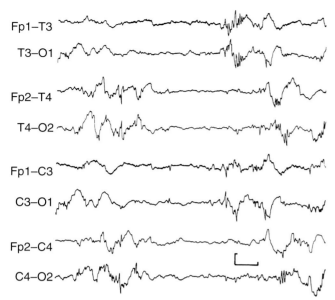

FIGURE 4-8 ■ Excessive interhemispheric asynchrony. Premature infant with hypoxic encephalopathy and severe bronchopulmonary dysplasia (estimated gestational age 28 weeks; legal age 11 weeks). The child exhibited severe developmental delay and seizures by the age of 16 months. Calibration: 50 µV; 1 second.

structural pathologies (e.g., intraparenchymal hemorrhages, strokes, or congenital malformations). It is important to exclude the presence of asymmetric scalp edema or cephalohematomas and technical pitfalls (e.g., electrode "salt bridges" or asymmetric electrode placement).

Transient amplitude asymmetries have nonspecific prognostic significance. Transient unilateral attenuation of background EEG activity, usually lasting about 1 minute, may occur rarely during slow-wave quiet sleep in normal newborns. These episodes usually occur within minutes of the time the infant first enters slow-wave quiet sleep and are accompanied by normal background activity. Transient asymmetries also may occur after subclinical electrographic seizures.

Focal Abnormalities

Focal abnormalities usually consist of localized amplitude attenuation of background activity, with or without spikes (see Fig. 4-9). Again, it is important to exclude electrode placement errors, salt-bridge formation, localized scalp edema, and cephalohematoma, any of which can cause localized attenuation of amplitudes. Less commonly seen is focal high-amplitude slowing, often accompanied by spikes and sharp waves; it is seen more commonly in older premature and term infants. This pattern may correlate with focal cerebral lesions (e.g., hemorrhage, cerebral infarction, and periventricular

leukomalacia). However, the sensitivity and specificity of the EEG for diagnosing focal cerebral abnormalities seem to be poor.

Disturbance of Sleep States

Sleep-state differentiation should be readily apparent after 34 weeks CA. EEGs that lack distinct sleep states despite a long period of recording (1 hour) usually occur in infants with encephalopathies from a variety of causes. The background is usually persistently low in amplitude or is excessively discontinuous. It is important to ensure that this lack of change in sleep state is not caused by excessive environmental stimulation in the NICU, hypothermia, toxic factors, or administration of neuroactive medications. If these causes can be eliminated, an EEG that contains no recognizable states generally is associated with a poor prognosis. If the EEG is performed within the first 24 hours, it should be repeated after several days.

Several types of abnormalities of sleep states can be encountered in an EEG. They include the lack of well-developed active and quiet sleep; poor correlation (concordance) between the behaviors characterizing a particular state and the EEG; excessive transient or "indeterminate" sleep; excessive lability of sleep states; and deviations from the normal percentages of specific behavioral states. Much variability exists in the interpretation of these patterns, and few normative data are

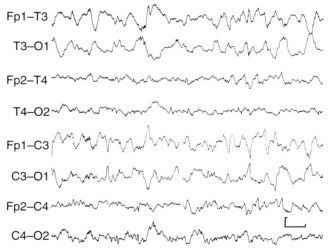

FIGURE 4-9 ■ Attenuation of the amplitude of the background activity over the right hemisphere, maximal in the right temporal region, in a full-term 3-day-old child who had occasional seizures but was alert and without abnormality on neurologic examination. Neuroimaging studies showed localized hemorrhage in the right temporal lobe and an arteriovenous malformation. Calibration: 50 µV: 1 second.

available. These patterns occur in babies with mild hypoxic or metabolic encephalopathies or subarachnoid hemorrhage, or following complicated pregnancies or deliveries. As the abnormal clinical state resolves, the EEG rapidly returns to normal. These abnormalities are etiologically nonspecific and apparently have little predictive value.

Other Nonspecific Background Disturbances

Many abnormalities are of little prognostic value in isolation but often accompany the severe abnormalities just discussed. These disturbances include excessive amounts of anterior slow dysrhythmia; increased incidence of *encoches frontales* (frontal sharp transients); excessive amounts of fast background rhythms, particularly beta activity; and a transiently dysmature background. These abnormalities are etiologically nonspecific and have little predictive value.

DYSMATURE PATTERNS

EEGs are considered dysmature if they contain patterns that are at least 2 weeks immature for the CA. EEG patterns that have been used as benchmarks for determining maturity include the degree of interhemispheric synchrony, number of delta brushes during active and quiet sleep, number of temporal theta bursts, and duration and morphology of the interburst intervals during discontinuous sleep. Normative scales for these patterns have been developed by several investigators[1,9,26]; however, the determination of dysmaturity usually is performed subjectively. The determination of dysmaturity is made more easily when the infant's CA is near term. Dysmature patterns that resolve on serial EEGs (transient dysmaturity) are not significant with respect to outcome; however, persistently dysmature patterns on serial EEGs may indicate a poor prognosis (e.g., neurologic sequelae or early death).[27–29]

A variety of exogenous and endogenous factors may disturb the maturational schedule of the EEG. Seizures may produce a temporary dysmaturity or regression. When dysmaturity results from seizures, it does not consistently correlate with a poor outcome. Dysmature EEG patterns may be caused by prolonged physiologic disturbances, such as chronic lung disease or patent ductus arteriosus, that cause an arrest or delay in brain maturation.[28] Dysmature EEG patterns are often observed in infants with severe bronchopulmonary dysplasia[27] and cystic periventricular leukomalacia.[29]

Biagioni and co-workers obtained EEGs within the first 2 weeks in 63 preterm infants (28 to 34 weeks

EGA) and scored the degree of dysmaturity using precise maturational criteria.[30] They found that a normal EEG was associated with a favorable prognosis (in 25 of 26 infants), but a highly dysmature EEG was not necessarily associated with a poor prognosis (only 2 of 9 infants had severe neurologic sequelae). The fact that some infants had a normal evolution despite very dysmature EEGs may reflect transient effects on the EEG of metabolic or circulatory disturbance early in the course of the preterm infant.

VALUE OF SERIAL EEGS IN NEWBORN INFANTS

Serial EEG recordings beginning shortly after birth are useful to assess the timing and mode of brain injuries and also may assist in elucidating their pathogenesis in preterm infants.[31] Serial EEGs may help to distinguish between acute and chronic pathologic processes. The former are characterized by EEG findings of acute depression (e.g., increased discontinuity, decreased faster frequencies, and low amplitudes); the latter may consist of dysmature and disorganized EEG patterns. The timing of brain insults may be assessed by considering the stage of EEG abnormalities in relation to the time of birth. For example, serial EEGs in preterm infants may be useful for determining the timing of injury. Hayakawa and colleagues performed serial EEGs and categorized background EEG abnormalities into acute- or chronic-stage abnormalities in infants with cystic periventricular leukomalacia.[32] The timing of injury was judged to be postnatal if the EEG was normal during the early neonatal course but afterward developed acute-stage followed by chronic-stage abnormalities. Insults just before or around birth would result in acute-stage abnormalities during the early neonatal period, whereas antenatal insults would result in chronic-stage abnormalities during this period. In infants whose initial EEG displayed chronic-stage abnormalities, the mean age of cystic degeneration on ultrasonography was 4 days earlier than those with acute-stage abnormalities, presumably because the injury occurred several days before birth.[32]

Serial EEGs in Preterm Infants

The recording of serial EEGs is an important aspect of the evaluation of premature infants. The EEG should be obtained at the time of acute neurologic insult and repeated 1 to 2 weeks later, particularly if the initial EEG is normal or only moderately abnormal. In premature infants, abnormal outcomes have been associated with patterns including isoelectric EEG; positive rolandic sharp waves; a burst-suppression pattern that is distinct from the *tracé discontinu* seen in normal, early premature infants (see Fig. 4-1); excessive interhemispheric asynchrony (see Fig. 4-8); persistent and significant (greater than 50 percent) interhemispheric amplitude asymmetries; and an excessively slow background of variable amplitude (10 to 100 μV) that is unresponsive to stimulation and devoid of normal rhythms such as delta brushes (see Fig. 4-7). Other less severe EEG abnormalities, such as mild asymmetries and asynchrony for the conceptional age, transient excessively discontinuous backgrounds, and alterations in the amount of background faster rhythms, do not seem to have prognostic value. The worsening of background pattern on serial recordings is associated with higher probability of neurologic sequelae.[1]

Tharp and colleagues prospectively studied all premature infants (birth weight less than 1,200 g) admitted to an NICU and reported that neurologic sequelae occurred in all infants whose neonatal EEGs were markedly abnormal and in the majority of those with two or more moderately abnormal tracings (recorded at weekly intervals).[33] The EEG was more sensitive than the neurologic examination in predicting poor outcome (72 percent vs. 39 percent), whereas both were equally effective in predicting normal outcome. The EEG also proved more sensitive than cranial computed tomography (CT) and ultrasonography in establishing the severity of the encephalopathy. The combination of EEG and ultrasonography may be particularly useful in detecting brain injury in preterm infants. In a recent study, EEG abnormalities (within 72 hours) in conjunction with abnormal ultrasonography detected periventricular leukomalacia with a sensitivity of 94 percent and a specificity of 64 percent.[34]

Maruyama and colleagues evaluated acute EEG background abnormalities in 295 preterm infants (EGA 27 to 32 weeks) on the basis of continuity, frequency spectrum, and amplitude, and graded them on a five-point scale.[35] The EEGs were performed within the first week of life. The maximal grade of the acute background abnormalities correlated with the subsequent development of cerebral palsy (mostly because of periventricular leukomalacia) and its severity, but the presence of significant acute background abnormalities also had a high false-positive rate.

Serial EEGs in Term Infants

Serial EEGs have also been utilized in the assessment of full-term newborns. Takeuchi and Watanabe assessed 173 high-risk, full-term infants with hypoxic-ischemic encephalopathy (defined as an episode of fetal distress or an Apgar score of 5 or less at 1 or 5 minutes after delivery).[36]

The severity of the depression of EEG background activity and its persistence correlated with the neurologic outcome. Infants with normal EEGs and with only minimal or mild background depression that disappeared during the first few days of life had good outcomes. By contrast, neurologic sequelae occurred in infants with a major depression of the background at any time (burst-suppression, or nearly isoelectric background); with moderate depression (abnormal *tracé alternant*, a discontinuous background, or a very-low-voltage irregular pattern) lasting longer than 4 days; or with mild depression present after 9 days. Similarly, in a study of nine term infants with hypoxic-ischemic encephalopathy, Pressler and colleagues found that an early EEG was an excellent prognostic indicator for a favorable outcome if normal within the first 8 hours after birth.[37] The outcome was unfavorable if major background abnormalities persisted beyond 8 to 12 hours. However, an inactive or very depressed EEG within the first 8 hours correlated with a good outcome if the EEG activity recovered within 12 hours.

Zeinstra and colleagues confirmed that serial EEGs are better than a single study performed early. They performed two EEGs, the first 12 to 36 hours after birth and the second at 7 to 9 days in 36 term infants with acute neonatal asphyxia.[38] Several infants with a burst-suppression pattern on the initial EEG showed a significant improvement on the second EEG, and had a favorable outcome. If the first EEG was normal or mildly abnormal, the second EEG did not add substantially to the prognostic value.

ABNORMAL EEG TRANSIENTS

Spikes and sharp waves are seen commonly in neonatal EEGs and must be interpreted conservatively. In older infants and children, interictal spikes and sharp waves are signatures of an epileptogenic disturbance. In term and premature newborns, however, such sharp or fast transients may be seen in asymptomatic newborns with a normal outcome.[39] Even when seen in "excessive" amounts, they tend to be relatively nonspecific and do not necessarily imply an epileptogenic abnormality. Unless they are repetitive, periodic, or confined to specific regions, pathologic significance should be assigned with caution. This section focuses on some EEG transients that may have a pathologic significance. The relationship between sharp transients and neonatal seizures is discussed later.

Positive Rolandic Sharp Waves

Positive rolandic sharp waves are moderate- to high-amplitude (50 to 200 μV), surface-positive transients lasting 100 to 250 msec (Fig. 4-10). The morphology is

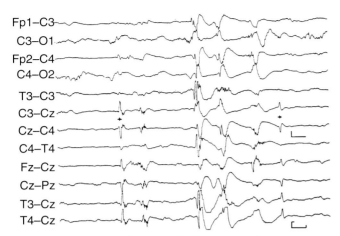

FIGURE 4-10 ■ Positive rolandic sharp waves in a premature infant with intraventricular hemorrhage on computed tomographic scan. +, positive sharp waves at Cz. Calibration: 50 μV; 1 second.

variable: simple, notched, or with superimposed fast rhythms.[3] They may occur in the central regions (C3, C4), either unilaterally or bilaterally, or in the central vertex (Cz) region. Positive rolandic sharp waves correlate with deep white matter lesions, particularly periventricular leukomalacia.[40,41] They may be an early marker of white matter injury, often preceding the ultrasonographic detection of cystic changes.[41] They may be associated with intraventricular hemorrhage, if there is a component of white matter injury. Positive rolandic sharp waves usually are associated with an unfavorable outcome. However, infants with these sharp waves often have other EEG background abnormalities that may confound determination of their prognostic significance. In studies of premature infants, the occurrence of positive rolandic sharp waves with a frequency exceeding 2 per minute was highly associated with motor disabilities or early mortality.[3,40]

In late premature infants (CA exceeding 34 weeks), low-amplitude positive rolandic sharp waves that are sometimes difficult to distinguish from the background may be present. They occur in short bursts lasting 3 to 7 seconds, with a repetition rate of 1 to 4 Hz.[3] This type of positive rolandic sharp waves has unclear prognostic significance.

Temporal Sharp Transients

Abnormal temporal sharp transients must be distinguished from normal, usually sharply contoured theta bursts of activity that are seen in the temporal areas during the discontinuous (*tracé discontinu*) background in normal premature infants (26 to 32 weeks CA), with highest incidence between 29 and 31 weeks CA. These temporal theta bursts or "sawtooth" waves are normal patterns and are not associated with seizures.

Positive Temporal Sharp Waves

Positive temporal sharp waves have a morphology and polarity similar to those of positive rolandic sharp waves but occur over the midtemporal regions (T3 and T4). In a study of premature infants (31 to 32 weeks CA) they were seen in approximately half of asymptomatic infants and in three-quarters of children with various disorders (asphyxia, metabolic disorders, and cystic periventricular leukomalacia).[42] Their incidence was higher in the asphyxia group when compared with the asymptomatic group, but not in the other disorders. In the asymptomatic group, their frequency tended to decrease rapidly on subsequent EEGs, whereas they persisted in the pathologic groups. Scher and colleagues found that positive temporal sharp waves were present in a population of healthy, asymptomatic infants, with the peak at 33 to 36 weeks CA.[43] They were uncommon in term infants but persisted in premature infants who had matured to term. These authors postulated that the persistence of these sharp waves in the latter group may represent an electrographic pattern of dysmaturity.[43] Others have found a correlation with hypoxic-ischemic insult in the newborn period. Full-term infants who have positive temporal sharp waves appear to have a high incidence of focal or diffuse structural lesions on neuroimaging studies and a high incidence (80 percent) of other EEG background abnormalities.[44] From this study, the prognostic implication of positive temporal sharp waves is unclear. There is no consistent association with neonatal seizures.

Excessive Frontal Sharp Transients

Frontal sharp transients are physiologic patterns seen in infants between 35 and 45 weeks CA. These sharp waves are seen more abundantly in mild encephalopathies and are absent in severe encephalopathies. Nunes and colleagues found increased density and asynchrony of frontal sharp transients in symptomatic hypoglycemic neonates compared with normal controls.[45] However, it is not clear whether hypoglycemia was responsible because serum glucose concentrations were not recorded around the time of the EEG and the infants had encephalopathies of various etiologies, including asphyxia, hydrocephalus, and sepsis.

Periodic Discharges

Focal periodic discharges and periodic lateralized epileptiform discharges (PLEDs) are pathologic patterns that occur in various encephalopathic conditions, but do not necessarily imply ictal events. The distinction between

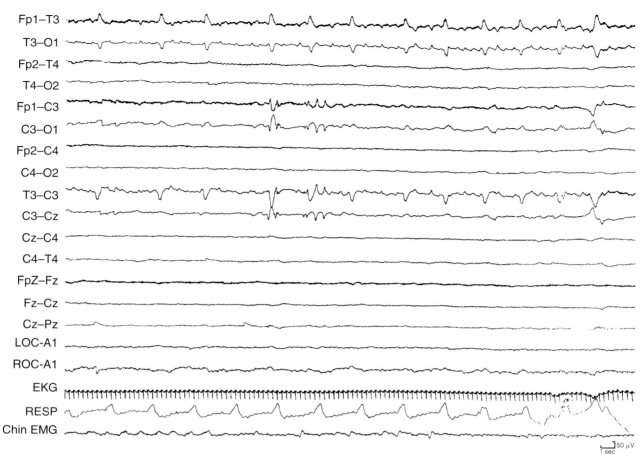

FIGURE 4-11 ■ Periodic sharp discharges located in the left hemisphere (maximal in the left temporal region) in an infant of 33 weeks estimated gestational age with bacterial meningitis and multicystic abscesses, resulting in seizures. Calibration: 50 µV; 1 second

these two patterns is sometimes difficult to define but may relate to their duration and persistence. *Focal periodic discharges* consist of broad-based, often biphasic discharges that may occur focally or independently at various locations (Fig. 4-11). They may last from a few seconds to several minutes and sometimes become faster in frequency. The usual lack of evolution in the morphology, frequency, or field of the discharge differentiates them from electrographic seizures. However, focal periodic discharges sometimes may represent a "slow" ictal pattern, often associated with focal clonic seizures.

Focal periodic discharges may occur in a variety of CNS disorders, such as cerebrovascular insults (strokes), hypotension, bacterial meningitis, viral encephalitis, and brain malformation, and in the course of metabolic disorders. Scher and Beggarly studied 34 infants with focal periodic discharges in EEGs recorded in the neonatal period.[46] Cerebral infarction was the most common underlying pathology. Most (75 percent) of these infants had an unfavorable prognosis (death or neurodevelopmental sequelae).

Focal periodic discharges may occur in neonates without clinical seizures. However, they sometimes follow a high-frequency EEG discharge (with focal clinical seizures occurring during the high-frequency discharge). In preterm infants, focal periodic discharges are associated less commonly with electrographic seizures and a demonstrable cerebral lesion.

PLEDs are defined as stereotyped, repetitive, paroxysmal complexes occurring with a regular periodicity (between 1 and 10 seconds). The morphology may be variable: slow waves, sharp waves, or spikes that are bi-, tri-, or polyphasic, lasting 200 to 400 msec.[3] Duration is at least 10 minutes. They often last much longer. PLEDs exhibit no evolution in morphology, frequency, or field, and they are not associated with ictal manifestations. PLEDs have been seen in patients with focal pathology (e.g., cerebral infarcts) or more diffuse encephalopathies (e.g., perinatal asphyxia).

In infants with severe encephalitis, the periodic discharges may be multifocal and often are located in the temporal, frontal, and central regions. The periodic slow waves or sharp slow waves have a periodicity of 1 to

4 seconds and persist throughout the tracing, interrupted only by focal seizures.

Focal periodic discharges and PLEDs may represent a continuum of a similar pathophysiologic process, appearing in brain-injured infants who sometimes exhibit clinically detectable seizures and who usually display other EEG background abnormalities and disorganized states. The prognosis appears poor for either pattern, although it may depend more on the underlying etiology.

Rhythmic Theta-Alpha Activity

The EEG of preterm and term infants sometimes shows excessive amounts of rhythmic theta- or alpha-frequency activity. In a study of term infants (37 weeks CA or older) by Hrachovy and O'Donnell, such patterns were found in a variety of conditions, including congenital heart diseases, congenital brain abnormalities, and hypoxemia, as well as in infants receiving neuroactive medications.[47] They concluded that this pattern was diagnostically nonspecific and may be seen occasionally in infants without overt CNS disease.

Rhythmic theta-alpha bursts, which consist of bursts or short runs (1 to 3 seconds) of sharply contoured, primarily surface-negative, rhythmic theta- and alpha-range activity, are common in the central and frontocentral midline areas, particularly during quiet sleep (Fig. 4-12).[48] These are called *wickets* or *rhythmic sharp theta burst* by some authors. Such bursts occur in healthy infants, although some authors believe that they are often seen in infants who have suffered various CNS insults, particularly when clearly defined sharp waves or spikes are intermixed with these bursts. However, in a study of newborns with electrographic seizures, the presence of this activity seemed to have a favorable prognostic value.[49]

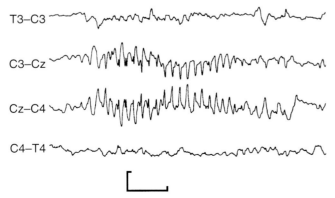

FIGURE 4-12 ■ Rhythmic theta-alpha burst at the vertex (Cz) region. Calibration: 50 μV; 1 second. (Modified from Ortibus EL, Sum JM, Hahn JS: Predictive value of EEG for outcome and epilepsy following neonatal seizures. Electroencephalogr Clin Neurophysiol, 98:175, 1996, with permission.)

Biagioni and associates investigated the significance of rhythmic theta-alpha bursts and other "abnormal" EEG transients in preterm and full-term neonates.[50] They scored the EEGs based on the abundance of isolated sharp transients (surface positive or negative), rhythmic sharp theta bursts, rhythmic delta activities, and rhythmic low-amplitude alpha discharges. The overall incidence of abnormal transients was low, with 21 percent of the EEGs having frequent abnormal transients. In the EEGs of full-term newborns or preterm infants reaching term, the score correlated with the outcome. During the preterm age, the EEG score did not correlate significantly with the outcome. Surprisingly, the authors considered these transients to be abnormal at any CA and attributed the lack of correlation with outcome in premature infants to the fact that the immature brains have a limited ability to generate them. However, based on their study, it is not clear whether patterns such as rhythmic theta-alpha bursts represent clearly abnormal activity because such transients do not correlate consistently with outcome.

NEONATAL SEIZURES

Neonatal seizures are a common problem in the newborn nursery; they can occur in infants at any CA and have diverse etiologies. The vast majority of neonatal seizures today are due to hypoxic-ischemic brain injury and intracranial hemorrhage. The clinical spectrum of neonatal seizures is quite different from that of older children. Generalized tonic-clonic seizures are exceedingly rare in the newborn, especially in the premature infant. The most common seizure types are focal or multifocal clonic, tonic, and myoclonic phenomena, and motor automatisms, such as oral-buccal-lingual movements, and progression movements (e.g., pedaling, stepping, and rotatory arm movements).[51,52]

The EEG is of particular diagnostic value in those infants whose seizures are subclinical, subtle, or easily confused with nonepileptic motor behavior. Studies using video-EEG monitoring of infants with CNS dysfunction have shown that several types of abnormal paroxysmal motor activity previously considered to be seizures are not associated with ictal EEG patterns.[51,52] Included are generalized tonic posturing, motor automatisms, and some myoclonic jerks. The investigators contend that these behaviors may be elaborated by "brainstem release" or other nonepileptic mechanisms. Therefore, EEG monitoring is crucial in determining the epileptic nature of all but the most obvious "seizure-like" behavior (e.g., clonic and migrating clonic activity and tonic eye deviation). The EEG can also be useful in the evaluation of jittery babies and of infants who have abnormal motor activity that is confused easily with seizures.

Electrographic seizures and status epilepticus often occur without recognizable clinical accompaniments, particularly in depressed newborns. Possible reasons include the use of pharmacologic paralyzing agents (for management of neonates on mechanical ventilators), the administration of anticonvulsants that decouple the clinical behavior and the EEG, and the inability of some immature neonatal cortex to generate the clinical expression of epileptic activity. In other cases, subclinical electrographic seizures occur in infants who are obtunded or comatose and who have suffered a significant hypoxic-ischemic insult; the seizures usually are associated with long-term neurologic sequelae. EEGs are essential in monitoring CNS function in such babies and in determining the effectiveness of anticonvulsant therapy.

Ictal EEG

The criteria of an electrographic seizure in neonates are the subject of debate.[52,53] The electrographic patterns of neonatal seizures are highly variable, with complex and varied morphology and frequencies (Fig. 4-13). Most groups operationally define electrographic seizures as clear ictal events characterized by the appearance of sudden, repetitive, evolving stereotyped waveforms that have a definite beginning, middle, and end, and last a minimum of 10 seconds.[49,52] During a seizure, there is a progressive buildup of rhythmic activity at almost any frequency or repetitive sharp waves and spikes. Neonatal seizures are usually electrographically focal and have variable spread over the ipsilateral and often the contralateral hemispheres. Two or more focal seizures may appear concomitantly in the same hemisphere (Fig. 4-14) or, more commonly, appear in both hemispheres and progress independently at different frequencies. Multifocal seizures are common in severe encephalopathies. Multifocal ictal activity is more often associated with neurologic sequelae than unifocal seizure discharges, particularly if there are two or more independent foci.[54,55] Status epilepticus, defined as total seizure duration lasting more than 30 minutes or seizures occupying more than 50 percent of the EEG, is also highly associated with severe neurologic sequelae or death.[49,56]

The electroclinical correlation is rather poor, with a limited number of ictal EEG patterns accompanying a variety of clinical manifestations. Certain types of EEG patterns are reported to be associated commonly with certain clinical seizures (e.g., rhythmic alpha-frequency activity with apneic seizures, and rhythmic delta waves with tonic seizures), but the relationships

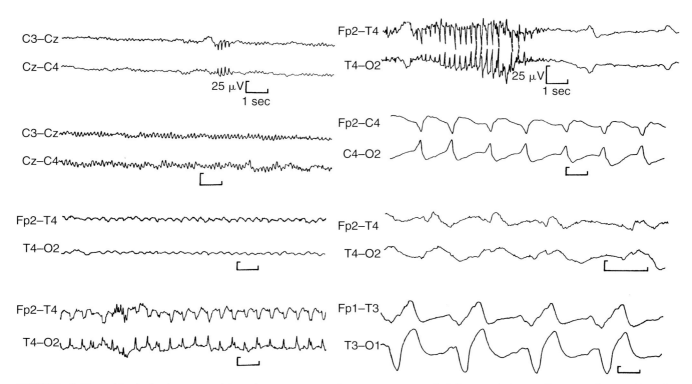

FIGURE 4-13 ■ Typical electrographic seizure patterns in premature and full-term infants. Except where otherwise indicated, calibration: 50 μV; 1 second.

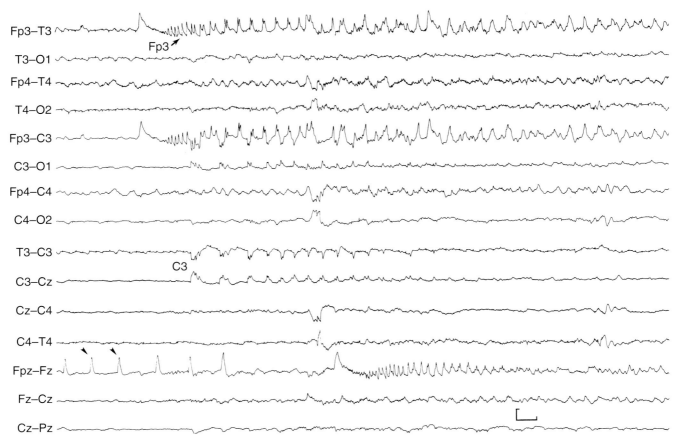

FIGURE 4-14 ■ Multifocal electrographic seizures in a 1-day-old infant (estimated gestational age 38 weeks; birth weight 3,100 g) with severe respiratory distress syndrome and hypoxemia. Independent ictal discharges are seen in the left frontal (Fp3) and central (C3) regions. In the midline frontopolar region, there are focal periodic discharges (arrowheads), followed by a brief seizure discharge. Calibration: 25 μV, 1 second.

are rather tenuous. In benign familial neonatal convulsions, there appears to be a characteristic pattern of electroclinical seizures; the seizures begin with a diffuse flattening of the background, accompanied by apnea and tonic motor activity, and are followed by rhythmic theta or delta activity that evolves into bilateral spike and sharp-wave discharges during bilateral clonic activity.[57,58] Others have found that the seizures in benign familial neonatal convulsions are focal in onset with secondary generalization.[59,60]

Figure 4-15 illustrates some of the artifacts that may be confused with seizure discharges.

Interictal EEG

Interictal background patterns are extremely variable and can range from normal background activity to isoelectric records. The interictal background reflects the severity of the underlying encephalopathy responsible for the seizures. The background activity may be worsened transiently by altered cerebral metabolism and perfusion associated with a seizure, by intravenously administered anticonvulsant drugs, or by systemic postictal changes. Therefore, the final interpretation of the EEG should be made on the basis of the entire record, particularly the preictal background. If a seizure occurs in the early portions of the EEG, a prolonged recording session may be necessary to allow sufficient recovery from the postictal state before judgment of the interictal background is made. Regardless of the presence of electrographic seizures, the interictal EEG patterns (which reflect the severity of the underlying encephalopathy) can be most helpful in the prediction of neurologic sequelae.[49,61] Severely abnormal background patterns are highly associated with early neonatal mortality or severe neurologic outcome.[49,54,55] In one study the presence of an isoelectric pattern was always associated with unfavorable outcome, whereas a burst-suppression or a low-voltage undifferentiated pattern was associated with 70 to 80 percent unfavorable outcome.[49] Serial EEGs in neonates with seizures may have better prognostic value than a single EEG.[62]

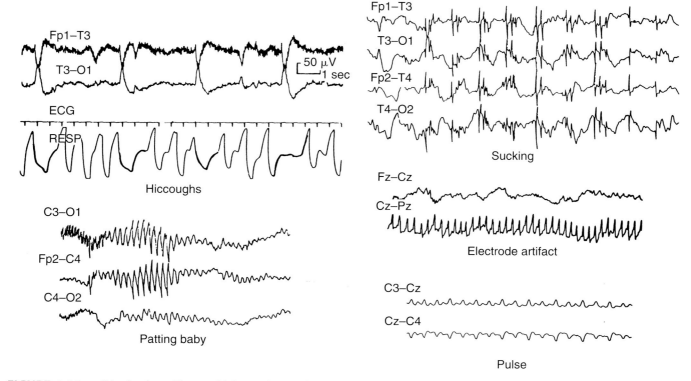

FIGURE 4-15 ■ Rhythmic artifacts, which can be confused with ictal patterns. Calibration: 50 μV; 1 second.

Spikes, Sharp Waves, and Seizures

In older infants and children, interictal spikes and sharp waves are signatures of an epileptogenic disturbance. In the neonate, however, such sharp transients are relatively nonspecific and do not necessarily imply an epileptogenic abnormality. Most consider sharp transients occurring over the frontal, rolandic, and temporal areas to be abnormal if they are excessively frequent for the CA, appear in short runs, or are consistently unilateral or polyphasic. They are particularly abnormal if they occur during the attenuated phase of *tracé alternant* or persist during the more continuous pattern of REM sleep or wakefulness. Multifocal sharp waves are also considered to be abnormal, although they do not show a statistically significant association with neonates having seizures.

In newborns, sharp waves occur in a variety of pathologic situations (e.g., infarcts, hemorrhages, and leukomalacia). In our experience, sporadic isolated negative or biphasic spikes and sharp waves occurring in an otherwise normal record should be interpreted conservatively. A record may be interpreted as abnormal solely on the basis of an excessive numbers of spikes or repetitive focal spikes or sharp waves, but its value as a predictor of long-term neurologic outcome remains uncertain unless other abnormalities exist.

Whether spikes and sharp waves represent interictal epileptiform discharges in a neonatal EEG is still debated.

Clancy quantified the number and location of sharp transients (central and temporal only) in infants with electrographically proven seizures and found more focal and multifocal sharp transients than in a control population.[63] The sharp transients also tended to occur in bursts (runs) in the group with seizures. However, there was a significant overlap in the frequency of such discharges between the two populations, and there was no comparison group of encephalopathic infants without seizures.

In a study of 81 neonates with EEG-proven seizures, the abundance of negative temporal sharp waves in the interictal EEG was correlated significantly with the development of postneonatal seizures.[49] Furthermore, a direct relation existed between the severity of the postneonatal seizure disorder and the number of temporal sharp waves. However, until further studies are completed in neonatal seizures with a control group, spikes and sharp waves in a neonatal EEG cannot be construed to indicate an "epileptogenic" disturbance. The diagnosis of neonatal seizures must be made in the clinical context, ideally with the recording of ictal discharges. Nevertheless, the authors believe that the presence of frequent (three or more per minute) negative temporal sharp waves is abnormal, and in their population was highly correlated with an unfavorable outcome and frequent postneonatal seizures.[49]

In the same study, the presence of rhythmic theta-alpha bursts in both the ictal and the interictal EEGs strongly correlated with a favorable outcome and a decreased likelihood of developing postneonatal seizures.[49] The authors believe that these patterns are a normal phenomenon of healthy newborns and may be a predictor of favorable outcome. They are depressed in neonates with severe encephalopathies who are destined to develop postneonatal seizures and neurologic sequelae.

Brief Rhythmic Discharges

Although isolated sharp waves in neonates do not seem to correlate with an epileptic process, brief rhythmic discharges may have a stronger correlation. The EEG ictal pattern of neonatal seizures has been defined arbitrarily as one that lasts at least 10 seconds. However, brief rhythmic discharges (less than 10 seconds) may at times have an epileptic correlation.[53] The significance of such discharges was investigated in a study of 340 neonates (30 to 40 weeks CA).[64] Rhythmic discharges were defined as runs of repetitive, rhythmic, monomorphic, stereotyped, sinusoidal, or sharply contoured waveforms occurring within a frequency of 0.5 to 20 Hz. The cohort was subdivided into three groups: (1) 67 with brief rhythmic discharges with maximal duration less than 10 seconds; (2) 63 with long rhythmic discharges (exceeding 10 seconds); and (3) 210 without rhythmic discharges. In 40 percent of the subjects with rhythmic discharges accompanied by a clinical seizure, the electrographic discharge lasted less than 10 seconds. The authors hypothesized that brief rhythmic discharges occurring without clinical accompaniments may represent brief epileptic seizures or an interictal pattern. The incidence of postneonatal epilepsy was similar in all three groups. The presence of brief rhythmic discharges was associated with periventricular leukomalacia, and long rhythmic discharges with hypoxic-ischemic encephalopathy. The presence of any rhythmic discharges (brief or long) correlated with an abnormal neurodevelopmental outcome. Therefore, the presence of brief rhythmic discharges in the neonatal EEG (unaccompanied by longer seizures) may be correlated with either an underlying epileptogenic process or an interictal pattern.

NEONATAL NEUROLOGIC DISORDERS WITH CHARACTERISTIC EEG PATTERNS

Most of the neurologic syndromes encountered in neonates are associated with nonspecific EEG abnormalities. The EEG changes are usually generalized and reflect the severity of the cerebral insult. A burst-suppression pattern, for example, can be caused by severe meningitis,

hypoxic-ischemic encephalopathy, or subarachnoid hemorrhage. Usually the EEG pattern, in itself, does not suggest the etiology of the neurologic problem. A few specific neurologic disorders, however, may be associated with characteristic EEG abnormalities that suggest certain etiologic considerations to the clinician.

In *holoprosencephaly* there are characteristic EEG abnormalities attributable to the distinct neuroanatomic features. When a large fluid-filled dorsal cyst is present, the EEG is low in amplitude or isoelectric over the affected region. The EEG recorded from scalp regions overlying the abnormal telencephalon is often grossly abnormal and manifests a variety of bizarre patterns. These include multifocal asynchronous spikes and polyspikes, and prolonged runs of rhythmic alpha, theta, or delta activity that may represent ictal activity (Fig. 4-16). Fast beta activity may also occur and probably represents subclinical seizures. In patients with semilobar holoprosencephaly, the background often shows excessive hypersynchronous theta activity in all states and hypersynchronous beta activity during sleep.[65] This hypersynchronous activity correlates with the severity of the thalamic and hemispheric abnormalities in the various types of holoprosencephaly.

The EEG in *lissencephaly* (agyria-pachygyria) is said to show a characteristic EEG pattern of "major fast dysrhythmia," characterized by rapid, very-high-amplitude, alpha-beta activity during wakefulness and 14-Hz spindles during sleep in infants.[66] High-amplitude (often greater than 300 μV), rhythmic 5- to 11-Hz activity and conspicuous beta activity predominate as the child grows.

Another rare anomaly, *Aicardi syndrome*, is associated with rather typical EEG abnormalities. This syndrome occurs in girls and is characterized by the association of infantile spasms appearing during the first few months of life and multiple congenital anomalies. The major CNS anomalies consist of agenesis of the corpus callosum, cortical heterotopias, porencephalic cysts, and ocular lesions. The characteristic EEG feature is a burst-suppression pattern that is completely asynchronous between the two hemispheres. Hypsarrhythmia may also develop in patients with Aicardi syndrome, and is quite asynchronous and discontinuous. A patient may have hypsarrhythmia in one hemisphere and a completely independent burst-suppression pattern in the other.

Inborn errors of metabolism of the newborn are associated with a variety of nonspecific EEG abnormalities. One of these disorders may be suspected when a grossly abnormal EEG background develops in a previously normal infant who deteriorates after the initiation of feedings. The absence of a history of intrauterine distress, neonatal hypoxia, signs of infection, or extracerebral anomalies would suggest that another etiology is responsible for

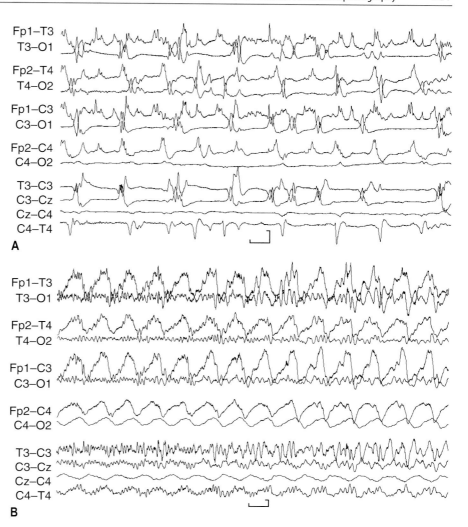

FIGURE 4-16 ■ Electroencephalogram (EEG) of a 3-hour-old male infant (estimated gestational age 34 weeks) with alobar holoprosencephaly, macrocephaly, and frequent myoclonic/clonic seizures. **A**, Background shows multifocal sharp waves, pseudoperiodic sharp waves, and absence of normal background rhythms and interhemispheric asynchrony. The amplitude in posterior head regions is attenuated due to a large dorsal cyst. Calibration: 100 μV; 1 second. **B**, During clinical seizures, the EEG discharges consist of high-amplitude synchronous 1-Hz rhythmic activity anteriorly, with superimposed diffuse rhythmic 7-Hz activity. Calibration 200 μV; 1 second.

the marked disturbance of cerebral electrical activity. In the neonatal form of *maple syrup urine disease*, a characteristic pattern is seen in the first few weeks of life.[67] Runs and bursts of 5- to 7-Hz, primarily monophasic negative (mu-like or comb-like) activity in the central and midline central regions are present during all states, with the most abundant bursts occurring in non-REM sleep (Fig. 4-17). This pattern gradually disappears after the institution of dietary therapy. Similar patterns have been noted in propionic acidemia. Positive rolandic sharp waves may be seen in certain inborn errors of metabolism (e.g., propionic acidemia) that are associated with white matter lesions.

Herpes Simplex Encephalitis

Herpes simplex encephalitis is one of the common fatal viral encephalitides in the neonatal period. The neonatal form is most often caused by the type 2 herpes simplex

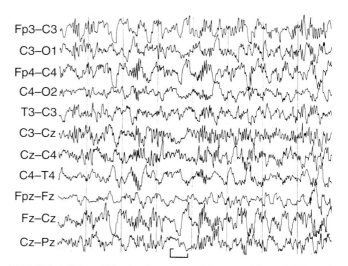

FIGURE 4-17 ■ Rhythmic runs and bursts of 5- to 8-Hz, primarily monophasic, negative (mu-like) activity in the central and central parasagittal regions during sleep in a 3-week-old, full-term infant with the neonatal form of maple syrup urine disease. Calibration: 50 μV; 1 second.

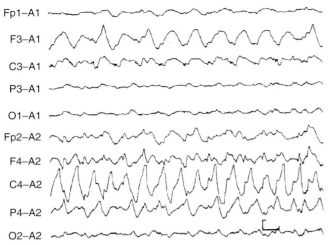

FIGURE 4-18 ■ Herpes simplex encephalitis in a full-term infant. Moderate-amplitude periodic sharp waves in the right central region and independent delta activity in the left frontal region, which persisted throughout the entire recording. The child died at 3 months of age with severe cortical atrophy. Calibration: 25 µV; 1 second.

virus, which the newborn acquires during delivery from maternal genital lesions. Herpes simplex encephalitis in older children and adults is most often caused by type 1 herpes simplex virus and is often associated with characteristic periodic EEG patterns that typically appear in the temporal regions. In the newborn the encephalitis involves the brain more diffusely and is often preceded by characteristic skin lesions. The EEG in severe, disseminated herpes encephalitis may show multifocal periodic or pseudoperiodic discharges with an interval of 1 to 4 seconds in the temporal regions, as well as the frontal and central regions (Fig. 4-18). This pattern is usually invariant throughout the tracing but may be intermixed at times with focal seizures. Since the introduction of acyclovir therapy, this severe electrographic pattern has become uncommon, and more nonspecific EEG abnormalities are usually recorded.[68]

Other EEG Analysis Techniques

In recent years, automated techniques for analyzing neonatal EEGs have been utilized.[69] These include two-channel EEGs, spectral edge frequency, and amplitude-integrated EEG. Recently amplitude-integrated EEG has been used to monitor neonates with hypoxic-ischemic encephalopathy and assess various encephalopathies in premature infants.[70] This method uses signal processing for rectifying and integrating the EEG amplitudes with a compressed time scale.[71] It has been used as a bedside measure of the EEG background and found to be useful for

identifying infants with more severe encephalopathy and worse outcomes,[72] particularly when combined with the neurologic examination.[73] The technique relies on a limited number of channels, usually single bipolar derivation from the parietal regions. In a comparative study of amplitude-integrated EEG and standard neonatal EEG, the former was very good at detecting severely abnormal patterns (e.g., a burst-suppression pattern, low-voltage undifferentiated pattern, and inactivity).[74] The ability to detect seizures was fairly good (sensitivity 80 percent, specificity 100 percent), although brief seizure discharges could be missed.

Spectral edge frequency has been used in studying preterm infants who are at risk for cerebral white matter injury. Those with white matter injury had a marked decrease in the spectral edge frequency, representing loss of faster background frequencies.[75] This method, which tracks frequencies without regard to amplitude, may be more suitable for premature infants.

These methods have several limitations. Because they utilize a limited array of electrodes, focal transients and ictal discharges distant from the electrodes may be missed. The interpretation of various patterns (e.g., seizures and sharp waves) requires experience, as well as frequent correlation with routine EEGs. Management decisions about hypoxic-ischemic encephalopathy or treatment of neonatal seizures should not be made solely on the basis of these methods. Newer monitoring devices allow simultaneous monitoring of real-time waveforms and compressed data, which allows better correlation by the clinical neurophysiologist.

OLDER INFANTS AND CHILDREN

Normal Patterns During the First 2 Years

The brain grows rapidly during the first 2 years of life, and significant maturational changes also occur in the cerebral electrical patterns, although they are less dramatic than those encountered during the neonatal period. A brief summary of the more important maturational features is given here, and several normal patterns are discussed. More comprehensive reviews are provided elsewhere.[76]

THE EEG DURING WAKEFULNESS

The predominant occipital rhythm, destined to become the alpha rhythm at 24 to 36 months of age, appears in normal infants at 3 to 6 months of age. This activity has a frequency of 3.5 to 4.5 Hz with maximal amplitude (50 to 100 µV) in the midline occipital region (Oz), particularly in younger infants, and appears when the child's eyes are gently and passively closed. The occipital rhythm often reaches 5 Hz by 5 months (50 to 100 µV) and 6 to 7 Hz by 12 months (50 to 75 µV).[6] A central theta rhythm (4 to 6 Hz), which is usually 1 to 2 Hz faster than the occipital rhythm, is present at 3 months of age; it gradually increases in frequency and reaches 8 to 9 Hz at 2 to 3 years of age. This activity does not attenuate with eye-opening and may represent the precursor of the mu rhythm. In addition, rhythmic theta activity may appear over the parieto-occipital and temporal regions during periods of crying. Runs of 4-Hz activity (50 to 200 µV) are also present in the temporal regions of many normal infants.

Lambda activity may occur in healthy babies as early as the first few months of life (Fig. 4-19). These infants usually have a prominent driving response at the slower rates of photic stimulation. In some healthy children, high-amplitude (often reaching 100 to 200 µV), biphasic slow transients that are sharply contoured may be seen in the posterior head regions following eye-blinks. These transients are present between 6 months and 10 years of age, with the peak incidence between 2 and 3 years. Both lambda activity and blink-related transients may be high in amplitude and occur asymmetrically; they should not be confused with epileptiform discharges.

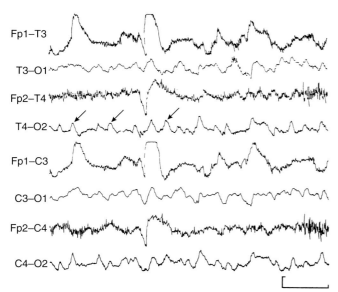

FIGURE 4-19 ■ Lambda activity (arrows) in a healthy full-term infant, 2 months old. There was respiratory distress during the neonatal period. The child's eyes were open and scanning the room during the electroencephalographic examination. High-amplitude evoked responses to low-frequency photic stimulation were present later in the record. Calibration: 50 µV; 1 second.

THE EEG DURING DROWSINESS

Drowsiness produces many interpretative problems for most electroencephalographers. The EEG patterns of drowsiness are often seen paradoxically when the child appears awake with eyes open. These patterns are noted particularly after arousal from a long period of sleep, when sedating drugs are administered, or following a prolonged period of vigorous crying. Most healthy full-term infants have definite EEG changes during drowsiness; these usually are characterized by an increase in the amplitude and a slowing of the frequency of the background rhythms. The EEG patterns of drowsiness are sometimes difficult to identify during the first few months of life, however, perhaps because they are admixed with sleep activity. At 4 to 6 months of age a distinctive pattern of *hypnagogic hypersynchrony* emerges during drowsiness. This pattern consists of runs of high-amplitude (100 to 200 µV), rhythmic 3- to 5-Hz activity lasting seconds to many minutes that appear in the parieto-occipital and temporal regions during the first year of life. During the second year, the drowsy state is often ushered in by a gradual decrease in the amplitude of the background activity and a slowing of the predominant waking occipital rhythm. In older infants and children, monorhythmic theta activity appears over the anterior scalp derivations, particularly in the frontocentral or central regions, and is encountered most commonly between the ages of 3 months and 2 years.[76]

Hypnagogic hypersynchrony often appears as bursts of high-amplitude, 4- to 5-Hz activity in the central and frontal regions. Spikes and sharp waves are often admixed with the slow waves, resulting in an "epileptiform" appearance (Fig. 4-20). This pseudoepileptiform pattern has been described in approximately 8 percent of normal children aged 1 to 16 years,[76] and was reported in a high percentage of children with a history of febrile seizures. Such activity is considered normal if it occurs only in drowsiness; if it disappears when typical sleep complexes, such as vertex waves and spindles, appear; and when the spikes or sharp waves have a random temporal relationship to the theta waves (compared with epileptogenic spike-wave activity, in which there is a more fixed temporal relationship between the spikes and the waves).

THE EEG DURING SLEEP

Active sleep (a precursor to REM sleep), characterizes sleep onset in newborns. Between 2 and 3 months of age, quiet sleep (possibly a precursor to non-REM sleep) replaces active sleep as the initial stage of sleep in the EEG laboratory setting. REM sleep is often recorded

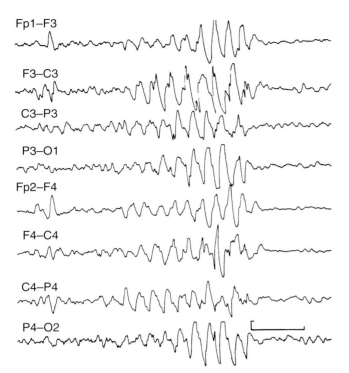

FIGURE 4-20 ■ Hypnagogic hypersynchrony during drowsiness in a healthy 3-year-old girl. Time constant: 0.035 seconds. Calibration: 50 µV; 1 second.

during the first year of life, but it is seen rarely thereafter in routine clinical EEGs. The low- to moderate-amplitude, mixed-frequency, slow background is usually easily distinguishable from non-REM sleep. Rhythmic, sharp 3- to 6-Hz activity occurring in bursts, or runs, may be seen in the posterior head regions. These sharp waves are confined to the midline occipital electrode (Oz) until 4 months of age, after which they can be recorded from more widespread areas posteriorly. This activity is often associated temporally with rapid eye movements. It should be considered an entirely normal pattern.

Rapid maturational changes occur in the EEG during the first 3 months after term. The *tracé alternant* pattern gradually disappears (between 3 and 9 weeks) and is replaced by diffuse slow-wave quiet sleep. Frontal sharp waves and delta brushes also disappear. The onset of sleep shifts from active to quiet sleep with a decrease in the percentage of time spent in active sleep.

The 12- to 14-Hz *sleep spindles* over the central regions that characterize stage 2 and 3 sleep in older children and adults can be seen in the non-REM sleep of some infants between 4 and 9 weeks post-term and are well established throughout non-REM sleep in most infants by 12 weeks post-term.[6] Initially, sleep spindles may be slower (10 to 12 Hz). Approximately 86 percent of spindles are 12 to 14 Hz by 6 months of age.[77] Spindles are usually present symmetrically over the central

regions but are often asynchronous during the first year. The percentage of asynchronous spindles is 36 percent at 1.5 months and falls to 25 percent thereafter.[77] This asynchrony may persist until 2 years of age and is often seen in older children during the early stages of non-REM sleep.

In the first year of life, spindles have a monophasic and often a mu or "comb-like" morphology (a spiky negative component and a rounded positive component), and may exceed 10 seconds in duration. The longest spindles appear at 3 to 4 months of age (up to 21 seconds).[6] As the child enters the second year of life, the duration of sleep spindles decreases, the interval between spindles increases, and their incidence declines. The incidence during non-REM sleep remains low until 4 to 5 years of age, when there may be a moderate increase. This apparent decrease in incidence is explained partially by the tendency for spindles to occur in deeper stages of sleep than those during the first year. Therefore, the absence of sleep spindles in infants between 5 and 12 months of age is unusual and considered abnormal, whereas in older infants in very light stages of sleep, spindles tend to be sparse or absent. Hypothyroid infants have a markedly reduced number of spindles.

In some normal infants, sleep spindles may be more abundant over one hemisphere during the entire tracing. Only major and persistent amplitude asymmetries or the absence of spindles during quiet sleep in the second half of the first year should be considered abnormal. Asymmetry of the background activity will probably accompany the spindle asymmetry in infants with cerebral pathology.

Slower spindles (10 to 12 Hz) can also occur in older children, are usually more frontal in location than the 12- to 14-Hz spindles, and tend to wane after 13 years of age.[6]

Vertex sharp waves usually can be identified during non-REM sleep after 3 to 4 months of life.[76] Their voltage field is more diffuse in infants than adults, and they often blend into the background activity, making identification difficult. In newborns during the first month of life, repetitive sharp waves confined to the midline central region (Cz) may represent precursors of vertex waves. Vertex waves consist primarily of monophasic (negative) or biphasic (negative–positive) sharp waves during the first 2 years of life. They are higher in amplitude and sharper in children than in adults. In older children, vertex activity may occur in bursts and runs of repetitive, high-amplitude sharp waves, which are often admixed with sleep spindles. Such high-amplitude, short-duration, and repetitive vertex waves should not be classified as epileptiform. Vertex waves are usually symmetric and synchronous, but transient amplitude asymmetries may occur, and often a series of vertex waves will appear unilaterally for several seconds over one hemisphere. In the author's experience, typical *K-complexes* do not appear until 2 to 3 years of age. These are high-amplitude, biphasic slow waves (surface-positive transient followed by a slower, surface-negative component) that occur spontaneously over the vertex region, occasionally as a response to sound or other environmental stimuli during sleep.

The background activity during sleep consists of an admixture of delta and theta rhythms, with the former appearing at highest amplitude in the occipital regions and the latter appearing frontally at lower amplitudes. From about 3 months to 10 years, during stage 2 sleep, a frequency–amplitude gradient is present which consists of a progressive decrement in voltage from occipital to frontal areas, with an accompanying decrease in slow frequencies in the same posterior to anterior direction. The pattern was poorly developed or absent in a group of infants and children with a variety of acute and chronic illnesses.[78] In children, particularly 1 to 2 years of age, the transition from light to deep stages of sleep may be associated with the appearance of bilateral, moderate- to high-amplitude biphasic slow transients (cone waves) over the occipital regions.[76]

Post-arousal hypersynchrony (hypnapompic hypersynchrony) occurs during transition from sleep to arousal, and consists of runs or bursts of diffuse bisynchronous 75- to 350-μV, 3- to 4.5-Hz activity, maximal over the central, frontal, or frontocentral regions.[6] This pattern is seen as early as 3 to 4 months, peaks between 1 and 3 years, and disappears by 4 years of age.

Normal Patterns after the First 2 Years

THE EEG DURING WAKEFULNESS

The normal EEG patterns of childhood and adolescence are described in several published reviews,[6] and are summarized briefly here.

The dominant posterior rhythm (i.e., the *alpha rhythm* that attenuates with eye-opening) remains in the 4- to 7-Hz range between 12 and 30 months. By 3 years of age it reaches 8 Hz in most normal children.[6,76] Over the next several years, the frequency of the alpha rhythm increases slowly; most of children reach the adult alpha frequency of 9 to 11 Hz by 8 years of age. Compared with adults, children show higher amplitude of the occipital rhythm.

Posterior slow activity in the delta and theta range is common in children of all ages during wakefulness. There are no definite guidelines as to what constitutes excessive posterior slowing; each electroencephalographer must develop his or her own normative range. A conservative approach is suggested. Many EEGs are over-read because of an exaggerated concern about slightly excessive theta activity during wakefulness. In many instances, the slowing is caused by drowsiness. For this reason, technologists should stimulate all cooperative children for at least a portion of the record by engaging the patient in conversation, and should attempt to record the EEG before sleep. "Excessive slowing" is very common after arousal from sleep. The child should be given several minutes to awaken fully before the EEG can be considered to represent a truly waking state.

Occipital slow waves (slow-fused transients, posterior slow waves of youth) consist of single, high-amplitude delta waves that are admixed with the ongoing rhythm.[76] The alpha activity immediately preceding the slow transient often has a higher amplitude than that of preceding alpha waves and, in conjunction with the slow wave, creates a sharp and slow-wave complex that may be misinterpreted as an epileptiform discharge. The maximal incidence is between the ages of 8 and 14 years.

Episodic runs or bursts of moderate-amplitude, rhythmic 2.5- to 4.5-Hz activity in the temporo-occipital regions is common in children (25 percent) and reaches maximal expression at 5 to 7 years of age.[6] This activity may have a sharp morphology, particularly when it is admixed with the alpha activity, and usually appears in short runs or bursts.

Bursts and runs of occipital delta are commonly seen in children with nonconvulsive generalized (petit mal) epilepsy. The delta activity in epileptic children usually occurs in high-amplitude bursts and is often admixed with spikes, forming a typical 3-Hz spike-wave complex. A unique posterior delta rhythm provoked by eye closure may be seen occasionally in normal children between 6 and 16 years (*phi rhythm*).[79] This rhythm consists of rhythmic high-amplitude (100 to 250 μV) slow waves of 3 to 4 Hz, lasting for 1 to 5 seconds after eye closure. The phi rhythm is not associated with epilepsy, and it often lacks the sinusoidal morphology and accentuation with hyperventilation that are characteristic of the pathologic occipital delta patterns. The phi rhythm occurs only after eye closure, usually after a period of concentrated visual attention, and lasts less than 3 seconds.[79]

A *mu rhythm* is seen occasionally in young children; the incidence increases progressively with age. Runs of rhythmic 7- to 11-Hz activity with either a sinusoidal or comb-like appearance are present in central derivations in relaxed wakefulness. Monophasic, sharply contoured mu often occurs unilaterally in the central regions, where it may be misinterpreted as an abnormal pattern. Mu activity persists with eye-opening and blocks with tactile stimulation or movements of the contralateral limb.

Hyperventilation usually produces a buildup of high-amplitude mixed delta and theta activity in normal children at all ages. This response most commonly consists of an increase in the pre-existing posterior slow activity (e.g., posterior slow waves of youth), or a buildup of posteriorly dominant or diffuse slow-wave activity. In children younger than 7 years, the slow-wave buildup is maximal posteriorly. After 7 or 8 years, it is maximal over the anterior head regions. A buildup with hyperventilation is abnormal only if persistent focal slow waves or epileptiform potentials appear, if generalized spike-wave activity is activated, or if the buildup is markedly asymmetric. If the buildup is asymmetric, the hemisphere with the lower amplitudes is the one that is often more involved pathologically. A generalized buildup of delta activity, even if it has a paroxysmal appearance, should be considered normal unless definite spikes are admixed with the slow waves. The admixture of high-amplitude alpha waves and a prominent buildup of occipital delta waves often leads to the appearance of sharp and slow-wave complexes that can be misinterpreted easily as epileptiform activity. Some children may overbreathe so vigorously that they transiently lose contact with the environment and fail to respond to the technologist's commands. This behavior, which may resemble an absence seizure, is accompanied by diffuse high-amplitude delta activity without spikes. North and colleagues described 18 children with this unusual response, which they called "pseudoseizures caused by hyperventilation."[80]

Intermittent photic stimulation is performed routinely in most EEG laboratories. The main value of this technique is to provoke epileptiform activity (photoparoxysmal response). Photoparoxysmal responses may be provoked in normal children and have been reported in 7 to 9 percent of the normal population.[81] A photoparoxysmal response is characterized by: (1) bursts of high-amplitude slow activity, often with admixed spikes, or (2) bitemporo-occipital sharp and slow-wave or spike and slow-wave activity. Photoparoxysmal response appears to be a genetically determined trait, which occurs more often in the siblings of epileptic children with the response than in a control population.[81] Photic stimulation is not performed routinely on newborns and young infants; however, even premature infants may manifest photic driving responses at flash frequencies of 2 to 10 Hz.

Occipital spikes may be provoked in a very small number of nonepileptic children in the absence of a photoparoxysmal response by using a photostimulator with a fine grid pattern.[82] These spikes, which are confined to the occipitoparietal regions, gradually increase in amplitude as the stimulus is continued. They occur in a wide variety of nonepileptic disorders and are of doubtful pathologic significance.

Familial and twin studies have shown the individual characteristics of the EEG are determined largely genetically. A low-amplitude background, for example, is known to have an autosomal-dominant mode of inheritance, and the gene has been localized to the distal part of chromosome 20q.[83] Doose and colleagues have reported that alpha activity extending into the frontal regions is more common in the parents of children with primary generalized epilepsy (18 percent) than in those parents whose children have focal epilepsy (8 percent) or in control subjects (9 percent).[84] The authors concluded that their study "reveals a clear correlation between the type of EEG background activity in parents and the EEG characteristics in their children."

THE EEG DURING DROWSINESS AND SLEEP

Drowsiness and sleep present as many interpretative problems in older children as they do in those 2 years of age or younger. High-amplitude paroxysmal hypnagogic hypersynchrony, maximally expressed between 3 and 5 years of age, is still encountered in the EEGs of children as old as 12 years (see Fig. 4-20). Drowsiness in children usually is characterized by a gradual disappearance of the alpha rhythm, an increase in the amount of fronto-central beta activity, and the appearance of rhythmic posterior 2.5- to 6-Hz activity. Artifacts from slow horizontal eye movements may be noted in the lateral frontal leads. More slow rhythms are noted anteriorly in children older than 10 to 12 years.

During light sleep, runs of high-amplitude, repetitive, sharp vertex waves are common and frequently are admixed with central sleep spindles, leading to complexes often classified as epileptiform. Sleep spindles may appear to have a spiky appearance when recorded with bipolar montages (Fig. 4-21). A referential montage reveals the benign morphology of this paroxysmal sleep activity.

Postarousal hypersynchrony (hypnapompic hypersynchrony) in children reaches 4 to 5 Hz and may persist until 4 years of age.

EEG Patterns of Dubious Significance

Certain EEG patterns that present difficulties in interpretation are reviewed here. These patterns often have an epileptiform appearance, although their relationship to pathologic processes has not been established clearly.

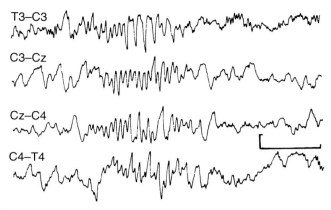

FIGURE 4-21 ■ Sleep spindle (sigma) and vertex waves in a healthy 3-year-old girl (the same child as in Fig. 4-20). Calibration: 50 μV; 1 second.

Positive spike bursts of 14 and 6 Hz are recorded commonly in the EEGs of adolescents during drowsiness and sleep, and are considered a benign pattern by most electroencephalographers.[85] They consist of brief (0.5- to 1-second) rhythmic arciform discharges that are maximal in the posterior temporal regions. The 14-Hz activity is most prevalent and may often appear without the 6- to 7-Hz activity. They may be seen in children as young as 3 to 4 years of age, but peak at 13 to 14 years of age.[86] Similar positive spikes have been reported in various encephalopathies, including hepatic coma and Reye syndrome.[1]

Rhythmic temporal theta bursts of drowsiness (psychomotor variant discharges) consist of 5- to 7-Hz sharply contoured activity that is often flat or notched in appearance. This pattern is most prevalent in young adults, but can also be seen in adolescents. Originally, this pattern was considered to be abnormal and was associated with vegetative states, psychiatric disorders, and temporal lobe epilepsy; however, this pattern has been found subsequently in a variety of benign conditions and is now regarded as a nonspecific finding. It has no significance with regard to epilepsy.

Benign sporadic sleep spikes (also known as sharp transients of sleep or small sharp spikes) are seen commonly in the normal population, particularly if nasopharyngeal electrodes are used. These sleep-activated spikes are usually low in amplitude (less than 50 μV), brief in duration (less than 50 msec), and have a simple waveform with a mono- or biphasic spike that has a rapidly ascending limb and steep descending limb. They are best seen in anterior to midtemporal derivation during non-REM sleep.[85] They are present in 10 percent of individuals between 10 and 20 years of age, and are rare in children younger than 10 years of age. They can be seen in up to a quarter of normal adults.

Abnormal EEGs

The EEG can be helpful in evaluating children with a variety of proven or suspected neurologic disorders. In most instances, the EEG is used to verify the organic nature of a particular neurologic disturbance, confirm a clinical suspicion as to the location of a particular lesion, follow the progression of a disease and the response to therapy, investigate the possibility that episodic behavioral or motor phenomena are epileptic in nature, or provide data that will help the clinician classify a seizure disorder and develop rational therapy. This section discusses some of the EEG patterns seen in children after the age of 1 month that are relatively specific for certain diseases, contribute significantly to the therapy of the patient, assist in reaching a diagnosis, or are of prognostic value.

Epilepsy

The EEG is important in the evaluation of children with episodic disorders and in defining childhood epileptic syndromes; however, the episodic nature of the problem results in a significant number of nondiagnostic EEGs. To increase the yield of abnormal records, the clinician should be familiar with the factors that may promote the appearance of epileptiform activity. These factors include obtaining adequate recordings during wakefulness and sleep at a time of day when the child is more likely to be having seizures; activating procedures, such as hyperventilation, photic stimulation, and sleep deprivation (in older children); and the recording of an EEG in close proximity to a seizure, particularly if a previous EEG was normal or nonspecifically abnormal. Occasionally, antiepileptic drugs should be discontinued, particularly if the diagnosis of epilepsy is uncertain or if the patient is being evaluated for the surgical resection of a focal epileptogenic area. During and immediately after antiepileptic drug withdrawal, bursts of generalized spike-wave activity may appear transiently in the EEGs of patients with focal epileptogenic lesions, as well as in nonepileptic patients who are withdrawing from short-acting barbiturate drugs. Studies in adult patients with partial seizures have not found significant EEG changes in the period of drug withdrawal and have suggested that the increase in seizure frequency and the appearance of new epileptiform patterns represents the unmasking of pre-existing foci.[87]

The type of epileptiform activity in an individual child with a single seizure type may change over serial records. Camfield and colleagues reported 159 children with epilepsy who had at least two EEGs (excluding those with absences, akinetic-atonic and myoclonic seizures).[88] A 40 to 70 percent *discordance* for the type of abnormality was found on the second EEG. For example, of the 42 children with major focal abnormalities on the first EEG, 7 had only generalized spike-wave activity on the second. A total of 7 of the 17 with only generalized abnormalities on the initial recording showed only focal abnormalities on the second EEG.

Lombroso followed 58 neurologically and cognitively normal patients with idiopathic generalized epilepsy for 9 to 20 years.[89] Ultimately, 56 percent developed focal EEG features, particularly in the temporal or frontal regions. For example, focal EEG spikes and slowing emerged over time in 60 percent of the children with idiopathic generalized nonconvulsive (absence) seizures only.

These reports emphasize that caution should be used when trying to establish the child's seizure type from the EEG alone. Certainly, generalized 3-Hz spike-wave activity with a clinical absence is diagnostic of generalized absence epilepsy. If the same EEG or subsequent recordings contain focal spikes or slowing, the clinical diagnosis should not necessarily be changed to localization-related epilepsy.

It should also be emphasized that epileptiform activity, including focal and generalized discharges, may persist in children whose seizures have stopped and who are no longer in need of chronic anticonvulsant drugs. In the long-term study of Shinnar and colleagues, epileptiform abnormalities were not associated with an increased risk of seizure recurrence in children withdrawn from medication after a mean seizure-free interval of 2.9 years.[90]

Video-EEG monitoring, reliable ambulatory EEG monitoring, and telemetry have expanded our ability to investigate episodic disorders of behavior. These techniques are providing electroclinical correlative data that were previously unavailable. Further discussion of this aspect is provided in Chapters 6 and 7.

The EEGs of patients with various types of epileptic syndromes, defined according to the International Classification of Epilepsies and Epileptic Syndromes,[91] are detailed in Chapter 3. The International League Against Epilepsy has recently published the Revised Terminology and Concepts for Organization of Seizures and Epilepsies.[92] Certain additional aspects that relate particularly to children are discussed here.

Childhood Absence Epilepsy

Childhood absence (petit mal) epilepsy often begins between 4 and 6 years of age, but on rare occasions, under the age of 1 year. In patients with childhood absence epilepsy, epileptiform activity consists of well-organized, generalized 3-Hz spike-wave discharges that may be seen ictally (during the absence seizures) and interictally (particularly during drowsiness and sleep). A detailed electroclinical study found the average seizure duration was 9.4 seconds (range 1 to 44 seconds).[93] In the population under study, about one-quarter of the absence seizures (with clinical signs including arrest of activity, eyelid movement, eye-opening, altered awareness, and automatisms) lasted less than 4 seconds.

The morphology of the 3-Hz spike-wave discharge is modified by sleep. The bursts during non-REM sleep are shorter in duration and more irregular in morphology, with generalized polyspike and polyspike-wave discharges replacing the typical 3-Hz spike-wave bursts. This polyspike activity does not appear to predict the concurrence or future appearance of generalized convulsions.

Bilateral posterior delta activity (occipital intermittent rhythmic delta) is seen commonly in this disorder and often has a notched appearance.[93] Purely focal epileptiform discharges may be seen in addition to the generalized spike-wave discharges in approximately 15 percent of patients.[93,94] The EEG is only rarely normal in children with untreated childhood absence epilepsy. Repeatedly normal EEGs in a child with episodes of impaired external awareness are therefore more consistent with a focal seizure disorder or nonepileptic phenomena.

The EEG is of limited value in formulating a long-term prognosis for a child with childhood absence epilepsy. Some studies have suggested a favorable long-term prognosis for remission in the setting of a normal IQ, absence of hyperventilation-induced spike-waves, male sex, and normal neurologic findings. Other studies have not found a prognostic value of the EEG in predicting duration of absence or ultimate remission.[95,96] The remission rate without antiepileptic medication is approximately 80 percent.[96] The presence of polyspike-wave activity does not seem to predict the development of generalized tonic-clonic seizures[94]; rather, a family history of generalized tonic-clonic seizures and age of onset at 8 years or older are more predictive of future generalized tonic-clonic seizures.

Other Epileptic Syndromes with Absence Seizures

Absence seizures are seen in four childhood epilepsy syndromes: (1) childhood absence epilepsy; (2) juvenile absence epilepsy; (3) epilepsy with myoclonic absences; and (4) juvenile myoclonic epilepsy. Childhood absence epilepsy often begins between 4 and 6 years of age, whereas the absence seizures in the other syndromes occur later in the first decade or in the teenage years.

Panayiotopoulos and colleagues analyzed the clinical and electrographic features of 20 patients with absence syndromes.[97] They found that in childhood absence epilepsy there was often a cessation of hyperventilation with an absence seizure because of a more profound loss of consciousness. They also found that the ictal discharge in juvenile absence epilepsy was longer than in childhood absence epilepsy or juvenile myoclonic epilepsy. Janz has pointed out that the paroxysmal discharges in the childhood form of absence epilepsy occur more commonly at 2.5 to 3.5 Hz, whereas in other forms that begin later in childhood or adolescence, the frequency is faster.[98] He also noted that a photoparoxysmal response is equally common among male and female patients with the childhood form of absence epilepsy, but is significantly more common in females with other syndromes, particularly those with juvenile myoclonic epilepsy. Seizure frequency is much higher in childhood absence epilepsy, as are complex absences, including those with retropulsive movements.

In juvenile myoclonic epilepsy, the characteristic EEG pattern consists of generalized bursts of spike-wave activity, polyphasic spike-wave activity (often accompanied by a myoclonic jerk), fragmentation of the discharges, and multiple spike complexes with a compressed capital W appearance.[99] The repetition rate of the individual spike-wave complexes is usually 3 to 5 Hz, occasionally up to 10 Hz. In some individuals the epileptiform activity is attenuated or eliminated on eye-opening. In juvenile myoclonic epilepsy the epileptiform discharges contain more polyspikes and are more likely to be disorganized (fragmented) than those in childhood or juvenile absence epilepsy.[100] Approximately 25 percent of patients have photoparoxysmal responses and hyperventilation commonly activates the epileptiform activity. The EEG may occasionally be normal, particularly in individuals receiving antiepileptic medication.

Focal and asymmetric EEGs and clinical features can be observed in juvenile myoclonic epilepsy. Aliberti and colleagues found focal slow waves, spikes and sharp waves, and focal onset of the generalized discharge in 37 percent of 22 patients with this disorder.[101] They also noted that transient discontinuation of the discharges, called "fragmentation," is characteristic, as are multiple spikes preceding the slow waves resulting in a compressed W shape. Clinical and EEG asymmetries often delay the diagnosis because of the concern that the patient has partial seizures.[102] In Lombroso's long-term follow-up study of patients with idiopathic generalized epilepsy, focal abnormalities ultimately appeared in 56 percent; they were particularly common in individuals with both absence and generalized tonic-clonic seizures, and were least common in patients with juvenile myoclonic epilepsy (11 percent).[89]

The myoclonic jerks are temporally related to the generalized spike- or polyspike-wave discharges. These rapid shock-like contractions may involve either the proximal or distal muscles of the limbs, the face, and occasionally the trunk. There may be a transient post-myoclonic inhibition of the involved musculature leading to a loss of tone, and in occasional patients, to a flapping movement. This inhibition is coincident with the aftergoing slow wave of the generalized paroxysm.[103]

An understanding of these syndromes allows prognostic statements about the duration of the epilepsy and the risk for the appearance of other seizure types. For example, the outcome in patients with juvenile absence epilepsy is less favorable than in children with childhood absence epilepsy, with less than half achieving remission, particularly if they have experienced a generalized tonic-clonic seizure.[104] In many cases, however, the patient does not fit easily into one of the classic syndromes, and absence epilepsy may be a "biologic continuum."

Epilepsies Associated with Encephalopathies

Three major and characteristic electroclinical syndromes occur in children with static or progressive encephalopathies: (1) hypsarrhythmia; (2) Lennox–Gastaut syndrome; and (3) the pattern of multiple independent focal spikes. These syndromes are characterized primarily on the basis of specific EEG abnormalities and are associated with a heterogeneous group of diseases. They are the electrographic expression of a diffuse encephalopathy. Any neurologic disorder that is associated with a diffuse involvement of the neocortex may manifest one or all of these EEG patterns.

Hypsarrhythmia is the electrophysiologic expression of an encephalopathy that occurs primarily in the first year of life and is caused by any diffuse insult to the developing brain. The EEG is characterized by a diffusely abnormal background composed of high-amplitude (generally greater than 200 μV) delta activity admixed with multifocal spikes and sharp waves. The typical pattern is best expressed in non-REM sleep. The syndrome is expressed clinically by infantile spasms, delay of developmental milestones, and a very poor prognosis for ultimate intellectual development. During the spasms the ictal event is represented by three different EEG patterns: positive-vertex slow waves; spindle-like beta activity; and diffuse flattening (electrodecremental activity).[105,106]

Infantile spasms can be the sequelae of a specific severe neonatal insult such as hypoxic-ischemic encephalopathy and viral encephalitis (symptomatic infantile spasms), or they may be caused by a genetic disorder such as tuberous sclerosis complex. In approximately 10 to 15 percent of infants, no etiology is discovered (cryptogenic infantile spasms) despite examinations, neuroimaging studies, and metabolic and genetic testing. Neurodevelopmental outcome is more favorable in the cryptogenic group.

It has been recommended that the word *infantile* be discarded because spasms can occur at any age. *Epileptic spasms* is the preferred term to designate a specific seizure involving the axial musculature that tends to occur in clusters.[92] In older children (e.g., those with the Lennox–Gastaut syndrome), typical infantile spasms may gradually evolve into more prolonged tonic seizures and yet maintain the typical electrodecremental ictal EEG pattern.

Infants in the symptomatic group are often neurologically abnormal in the neonatal period and have abnormal EEGs. In many cases, however, the EEG and the neurologic examination normalize during the first few months of life. Subsequently, minor abnormalities such as focal sharp waves gradually appear in the EEG and evolve into a pattern of full-blown hypsarrhythmia. Partial seizures may evolve into infantile spasms.

Approximately 25 percent of children with hypsarrhythmia do not have infantile spasms, but rather have other types of seizures. These children tend to have a poorer prognosis than those with spasms, because of more serious underlying etiologies.

Children with the clinical syndrome of infantile spasms may have EEG abnormalities other than typical hypsarrhythmia. Modified or atypical hypsarrhythmia is any pattern that differs from the classic pattern, and includes disorganized patterns with preserved interhemispheric synchronization, patterns with little or no spike and sharp-wave activity, unilateral hypsarrhythmia, and those with focal abnormalities.[107] The presence of modified features may depend on the stage or treatment of infantile spasms, but seems to have little prognostic significance.[107]

Asymmetric spasms involve only one side of the body or are more intense on one side than the other,[108] and are usually associated with an asymmetric hypsarrhythmia pattern and regional pathology. Ictal patterns that accompany asymmetric spasms include focal spikes and sharp waves and unilateral or asynchronous paroxysmal fast activity in the hemisphere contralateral to the asymmetric spasms.[108]

Focal abnormalities and asymmetric hypsarrhythmia have assumed a more important role with the advent of surgical treatment of infantile spasms.[108,109] A subgroup of children with refractory spasms and focal seizures has been identified whose EEGs or seizure symptomatology suggest focal cortical pathology and who appear to be benefited by resection of the involved cortex. The major abnormalities identified pathologically include cystic-gliotic encephalomalacia and a variety of dysgenic or dysplastic lesions. These focal lesions may not be seen on early conventional MRI studies and may be found only by positron emission tomography or single photon emission computerized tomography.[110,111]

The EEG is of little value in formulating a prognosis for ultimate intellectual development. There is a tendency for full recovery in those infants whose initial EEGs are less severely abnormal, and in those with typical, symmetric hypsarrhythmia. Two-thirds of these infants with cryptogenic infantile spasms may have a favorable neurodevelopmental outcome.[112] The prognosis is clearly worse in those with symptomatic spasms (e.g., patients with tuberous sclerosis, with static encephalopathies from perinatal events, or with known metabolic or chromosomal syndromes).

The *Lennox–Gastaut syndrome* includes a heterogeneous group of static and progressive encephalopathies that are grouped together on the basis of the presence of slow (2- to 2.5-Hz or less) spike-wave discharges on the EEG. The clinical spectrum that accompanies this particular EEG pattern includes cognitive disturbances; high incidence of abnormalities on neurologic examination; and frequent occurrence of tonic, akinetic, atypical absence, and generalized tonic-clonic seizures, which are characteristically refractory to antiepileptic drugs.[113] The EEG pattern is recorded commonly during the first two decades of life, but seizure onset is most frequent between 6 months and 3 years of age. Occasional patients have had the onset of seizures in the teenage years. The interictal EEG may also show slowing of the background activity, focal or multifocal spikes and sharp waves, and diffuse polyspike-wave activity. The EEG abnormalities are enhanced during sleep. During sleep, bursts of activity at approximately 10 Hz ("recruiting rhythm") may be associated with subtle tonic seizures. The pathology underlying the syndrome varies widely, ranging from encephalopathies dating to the prenatal or neonatal period to progressive neurodegenerative diseases. Approximately one-third of patients have a prior history of infantile spasms and hypsarrhythmia. In a study of 15 children with drop attacks ("epileptic fall") Ikeno and colleagues described 7 with seizures characterized by flexor spasms resembling infantile spasms with the typical slow-wave and electrodecremental ictal pattern.[114] All had spasms in infancy.

A striking pattern of non-REM sleep–activated, nearly continuous spike-wave activity can be seen in several syndromes, including Landau–Kleffner syndrome, the syndrome of continuous spike-waves during slow-wave sleep, and so-called atypical benign partial epilepsy of childhood.[115,116]

The pattern of *multiple independent focal spikes* is seen often in children with a prior history of hypsarrhythmia or the Lennox–Gastaut syndrome. This pattern is defined as "epileptiform discharges (spikes, sharp waves, or both) which, on any single recording, arise from at least three noncontiguous electrode positions with at least one focus in each hemisphere."[117] This EEG pattern is seen most often in patients during the first two decades of life. Among children with this EEG pattern, most (84 percent) have seizures, usually of more than one type, but most commonly of the generalized tonic-clonic variety. Many patients have cognitive disabilities, particularly if seizures started before the age of 2 years, and many have abnormal neurologic examinations. Multifocal spikes on a *normal* EEG background can sometimes be seen in children with benign partial epilepsies who are neurologically and cognitively normal. The normal neurodevelopmental history and the benign form of their epilepsy differentiate these patients from those with the multifocal spike pattern.

Early-Onset Epilepsies Associated with Encephalopathies

Early myoclonic encephalopathy is characterized by erratic, fragmentary myoclonic jerks that begin in the first month of life. These jerks are replaced by partial seizures; massive myoclonus; infantile spasms; and infrequently, tonic seizures. The EEG shows a characteristic burst-suppression pattern; bursts are composed of spikes, sharp waves, and slow activity lasting 5 to 6 seconds and alternating with 4- to12-second periods of attenuation.[118] The burst-suppression pattern often evolves into hypsarrhythmia or multifocal spikes and sharp waves. Etiology often is not determined, although some cases are familial in nature. Known etiologies include inborn errors of metabolism (particularly nonketotic hyperglycinemia), pyridoxine dependency, and brain malformations such as hydranencephaly. The infants have marked developmental delay, abnormal tone, and microcephaly.

Ohtahara syndrome (early infantile epileptic encephalopathy with suppression-burst) is characterized by frequent tonic spasms with onset in the neonatal period or early infancy and a burst-suppression pattern.[119] The burst-suppression pattern is composed of bursts lasting 1 to 3 seconds and the nearly flat suppression phase lasts 2 to 5 seconds (Fig. 4-22). The *tonic* spasms are associated with the bursts or with an abrupt attenuation of cerebral activity (desynchronization). Focal seizures are seen in one-third of the infants, but myoclonic seizures are rare. The seizure types may evolve from tonic spasms to infantile spasms with hypsarrhythmia (West syndrome), Lennox–Gastaut syndrome, or both. The infants have severe encephalopathy. Etiology is varied but often related to structural abnormalities, including cerebral dysgenesis, porencephaly, hemimegalencephaly, Aicardi syndrome, and diffuse or focal cortical dysplasias. Less commonly, metabolic disorders are associated with Ohtahara syndrome.

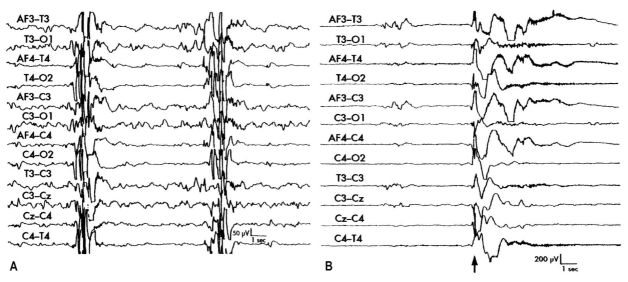

FIGURE 4-22 ▪ A 2-week-old term infant with Ohtahara syndrome. Since birth the infant had experienced tonic seizures every few minutes. **A**, Electroencephalogram (EEG) shows a burst-suppression pattern, with bursts composed of spikes and sharp waves admixed with slow waves. **B**, EEG during a brief tonic seizure shows a high-amplitude sharp wave (arrow) followed by a complex slow wave and low-amplitude fast activity, much of the latter representing artifact. (Modified from Tharp BR: Neonatal seizures and syndromes, Epilepsia 43:2, Suppl. 3, 2002, with permission.)

Ohtahara syndrome and early myoclonic encephalopathy have overlapping etiologies and EEG patterns, which may lead to confusion in their nosology. The initial seizure types in the two syndromes are quite different. The burst-suppression pattern in early myoclonic encephalopathy may be seen only during sleep, whereas it is observed in waking and sleeping states in Ohtahara syndrome.

Focal Seizures

Focal (partial) seizures are very common in infants and children. Many occur in normal children and have a benign prognosis. Although it is reasonably easy in older children and adults to distinguish focal and generalized seizures clinically, it may be quite problematic in younger children, particularly infants. The 1981 International Classification of Epileptic Seizures was developed primarily for use in adults and is difficult to use in children, particularly those under 2 years of age. This has led to proposals for a new classification specifically for infants (Table 4-3).[120,121]

It is difficult to classify seizures in infants because the clinical manifestations are quite different from those of older children and adults. In a video-EEG study,[121] two skilled epileptologists were asked to determine whether seizures were focal or generalized in a group of children under 26 months of age. There was very poor agreement between the observers when they viewed *only* video recordings of ictal events. The inter-rater agreement on seizure onset when they used only the EEG was better for generalized-onset seizures (0.79) than for focal seizures (0.54). These and other authors[120] found that it was virtually impossible to determine the level of consciousness or awareness in a seizing infant, thus making it impossible to classify focal seizures as simple or complex. Seizures in infants may be so subtle that even a skilled observer is unable to determine if they are focal or generalized. Many tonic motor events may be bilateral in a focal seizure, whereas asymmetric tonic posturing may be associated with a generalized ictal EEG discharge. Well-developed complex automatisms are much less common than in older children, whereas simple oral-buccal movement (e.g., sucking) is more common. Focal dystonic posturing, a helpful lateralizing feature of focal seizures in older children and adults, is seen less commonly in infants and has less lateralizing value. Versive movements, particularly of the eyes, have little lateralizing value.

The EEG may be a helpful adjunct in determining the etiology of focal seizures. If the background activity is normal, and the child is neurologically and cognitively normal, it is probable that the seizures will fall into one of the benign syndromes. In these disorders, the frequency of the epileptiform activity may be very high and is often enhanced by sleep. The morphology of the abnormal activity is also rather distinctive, particularly in benign rolandic epilepsy and childhood occipital epilepsies.

Benign Childhood Epilepsy with Centrotemporal Spikes (Benign Rolandic Epilepsy)

Benign rolandic epilepsy is one of the most common focal epilepsy syndromes of childhood. It is characterized clinically by the occurrence of seizures in an otherwise normal child between the ages of 5 and 12 years. The seizures are typically focal (usually hemifacial, often associated with somatosensory symptoms) when they occur during waking hours and tend to generalize during sleep.

TABLE 4-3 ■ Proposed Classification of Seizures in Infants	
Seizure Type	Seizure Semiology
Astatic (atonic)	Sudden loss of tone involving one or more muscle groups or entire body
Behavioral	Sudden change of behavior (usually an arrest or marked reduction of motor activity—hypomotor seizure); automatisms usually simple and consist primarily of oral-buccal movements
Clonic	Clonic jerking of one or more limbs, or generalized and occasionally involving face and/or eyelids only; may alternate from side to side or be asynchronous between each half-body (resembling a generalized motor seizure)
Tonic	Symmetric or asymmetric tonic posturing, occasionally asymmetric tonic neck-like posturing, sometimes with eye and head version; may be followed by clonic phase
Infantile spasm/myoclonic epileptic spasm	In older children, it may be difficult to distinguish a spasm from true myoclonus or a short tonic seizure
Versive	May involve the eyes only or eyes and head; may be associated with behavioral changes or tonic involvement of limb(s)
Unclassified seizures	Seizures that cannot be categorized in the above classification

Adapted from Acharya JN, Wyllie E, Luders HO et al: Seizure symptomatology in infants with localization-related epilepsy. Neurology, 48:189, 1997; and Nordli DR, Brazil CW, Scheuer ML et al: Recognition and classification of seizures in infants. Epilepsia, 38:553, 1997, with permission.

Ictal EEG patterns of rolandic seizures consist of slow waves intermixed with spikes from the hemisphere contralateral to the symptoms.[116]

The interictal EEG features biphasic, high-amplitude (100 to 300 µV) sharp waves in the centrotemporal (rolandic) regions and a normal background activity. The epileptiform discharges are often bilateral and asynchronous, and may increase markedly in frequency during sleep. A characteristic EEG feature of the spike in this syndrome is the "horizontal dipole:" a surface negative spike in the central region and simultaneous positive spike in the frontal region.[122,123] The central negative spikes can be of maximum amplitude anywhere along the central sulcus. They have been divided into "high central foci" and "low central foci," both foci occurring with equal frequency. Gregory and Wong found that children without the dipole discharges were more likely to have more frequent seizures, developmental delay, school difficulties, and an abnormal neurologic examination compared with a group having rolandic discharges with a horizontal dipole.[122]

A more detailed EEG analysis found that a topographic pattern of non-stationary fields represented by a "double" spike-wave complex was highly correlated with seizure occurrence[124]; by contrast, children without seizures were more likely to have a topographic pattern of stationary potential fields (i.e., a single spike-wave complex). The complex spike consisted of a sequence of dipoles with a small initial spike that was negative in the frontal region and positive in the centrotemporal regions, followed by a more obvious higher-amplitude spike that was negative centrotemporally and, when present, positive frontally. There were no significant morphologic (as differentiated from topographic) differences of the spike that provided a clue to its "epileptogenicity" or to the presence or absence of an organic lesion.[125] Other authors, by contrast, were able to distinguish children with uncontrolled benign focal epilepsy from those with focal spikes and other syndromic categories (e.g., symptomatic, cryptogenic, and Landau–Kleffner) on the basis of spike morphology using a single morphologic index, the composite spike parameter, which was derived from the amplitude, duration, and sharpness of the spike.[126]

Magnetoencephalographic analysis of rolandic discharges has shown that the prominent negative sharp wave appears as a tangential dipole in the rolandic region, with the positive pole situated anteriorly, and presumably is generated through a mechanism similar to that for the middle-latency components of the somatosensory evoked responses from stimulation of the lower lip.[123]

The EEGs of a significant percentage of children with benign rolandic epilepsy also contain generalized spike-wave discharges typical of an idiopathic generalized epilepsy (approximately 10 to 15 percent); bilateral or shifting foci (34 percent); multiple independent foci (9.8 percent); and, occasionally, a photoparoxysmal response to intermittent photic stimulation.[116,127,128]

Long-term follow-up studies reveal that most children with benign rolandic epilepsy become seizure-free in their midteens. Rarely is any focal pathology demonstrable on neuroimaging studies if the seizure symptomatology and EEG are characteristic. An autosomal-dominant gene with age-dependent penetrance is presumably responsible for the EEG trait. Focal centrotemporal spikes are therefore quite common in siblings of children with this syndrome and can also occur sporadically in normal children (3.7 percent of 1,057 normal children studied by Okubo and colleagues[129]).

Although benign rolandic epilepsy has an excellent prognosis with regard to seizure remission, behavior problems and cognitive dysfunctions may sometimes develop in its course. Comprehensive neuropsychologic studies have shown that children with rolandic epilepsy have a high incidence of learning disabilities, developmental language disorders, and attention deficits.[130] Children with significant learning or behavioral problems were more likely to have long spike-wave clusters, generalized 3–4 Hz spike-wave discharges, asynchronous bilateral spike-wave foci, and focal slow waves.[131] Rarely, rolandic epilepsy may evolve to a more severe syndrome with linguistic, behavioral and neuropsychological deficits, such as Landau–Kleffner syndrome, atypical focal epilepsy of childhood, or epilepsy with continuous spike wave during sleep.[116]

Panayiotopoulos Syndrome

Panayiotopoulos syndrome (early-onset benign childhood occipital epilepsy) is a common childhood-related electroclinical syndrome with onset between 3 and 7 years and seizures that have a pronounced autonomic component. The seizures are characterized by prominent ictal vomiting, as well as pallor, urinary incontinence, hypersalivation, and cyanosis. These autonomic symptoms are often followed by tonic eye and head deviation, progressive alteration of consciousness, and hemifacial convulsive movements. The seizures may end with hemiconvulsions or generalized tonic-clonic seizures. Prolonged focal seizures may develop into status epilepticus. Seizures in this syndrome are predominantly nocturnal and infrequent (with half of the children having only one or two seizures). The epilepsy course is shorter, and in most children the seizures subside within 1 to 2 years.[132] The ictal EEG shows discharges consisting mainly of unilateral rhythmic slow activity, usually intermixed with fast rhythms and small spikes.[116] The onset is in the occipital or posterior region. Interictally, the EEG reveals multifocal, high-amplitude spikes or sharp waves that may appear in any area, but predominate in the occipital regions. The spikes often appear in clone-like repetition.

Idiopathic Childhood Occipital Epilepsy of Gastaut

Idiopathic childhood occipital epilepsy of Gastaut is a relatively rare form of occipital epilepsy. The onset of seizures occurs in slightly older children (usually 7 to 10 years of age). Seizures are characterized by initial visual symptoms (e.g., simple or complex visual hallucinations, blindness, or both). The visual symptoms may be followed by a tonic deviation of the eyes, vomiting, and hemiclonic or generalized tonic-clonic seizures. Frequently, the seizures are followed by headaches that have a migrainous quality. Seizures are diurnal and, if left untreated, are more likely to be multiple in a day or week.

The EEG demonstrates bilateral paroxysms of high-amplitude, rhythmic spikes or sharp waves in the occipital regions. These epileptiform discharges attenuate with eye-opening and are activated by the elimination of central vision and fixation (fixation-off sensitivity). Ictal EEG shows seizure onset in the occipital region, consisting of fast rhythms or spikes, or both. During the blindness phase, pseudoperiodic slow waves are seen.[116] As the seizure progresses, spikes spread to the centrotemporal regions.

The outcome in idiopathic childhood occipital epilepsy of Gastaut is not as well defined as that in Panayiotopoulos syndrome, but seems less favorable. Seizures respond usually to carbamazepine. However, only approximately half of the patients may achieve a remission off antiepileptic drugs.[133]

Occipital spikes may also occur in various brain disorders with or without seizures, in symptomatic occipital epilepsy, and in children with visual impairment that is either congenital or acquired.[134] Spikes associated with visual impairment initially have short durations, but as the child grows they increase in duration and amplitude, and become associated with a slow wave. They disappear by the teenage years or in young adulthood.

Febrile Seizures

The EEG is of little value in the evaluation of children with typical (simple) febrile seizures. The majority of children with febrile seizures have normal EEGs during the following week,[135] although some may show nonspecific disturbances such as excessive posterior slowing. Epileptiform activity rarely occurs in the immediate postseizure period. Another etiology must be considered if focal spikes or generalized epileptiform discharges are present. A review study revealed that focal slowing is the predominant EEG abnormality seen acutely in children with febrile status epilepticus, occurring in about one-third of cases.[136] The relationship between the focal slowing and epilepsy is uncertain.

The EEG does not appear to be of value in predicting which child will have future febrile seizures or develop epilepsy. Risk factors for epilepsy after febrile seizures are clinical: family history of nonfebrile seizures, pre-existing neurologic abnormality such as cerebral palsy, and a complex febrile seizure (greater than 15 minutes' duration, more than one seizure in 24 hours, focal features).

Acquired Epileptic Aphasia (Landau–Kleffner Syndrome)

Acquired epileptic aphasia, a disorder first described by Landau and Kleffner, is characterized by the appearance of a progressive aphasia in a previously healthy child. The degree of aphasia roughly appears to parallel the EEG abnormalities. Seizures commonly occur after the onset of the aphasia but are treated easily with antiepileptic medication. Standard antiepileptic treatment usually has no effect on the aphasia, which may improve over years but infrequently disappears completely. The etiology is unknown.

The EEG is characterized by slow spike-wave discharges that are of higher amplitude over the temporal regions and spread diffusely through both hemispheres, giving the appearance of a generalized discharge. A striking EEG abnormality often occurs during sleep, also called "continuous spikes and waves during slow sleep" or "electrical status epilepticus during slow-wave sleep."[115] This latter syndrome can occur independently of the Landau–Kleffner syndrome and is often associated with progressive cognitive and behavioral deterioration.[137–139] With neurophysiologic techniques, including invasive electrical recording and evoked potential studies, as well as radiologic procedures including positron emission tomography, the focal epileptiform disturbance can be localized to the language cortex in one temporal lobe, with evidence of spread to homologous regions of the contralateral hemisphere.

INFECTIOUS DISEASES

The EEG abnormalities in children with CNS infections are usually nonspecific. Localized slowing or epileptiform activity may indicate focal pathology (e.g., abscesses or subdural empyemas), and a unilateral attenuation of the background activity may suggest a subdural effusion. As a rule, however, the EEG has not been of particular value in the detection of subdural effusions and has been replaced by CT scans or MRI. Certain infections may cause characteristic periodic or pseudoperiodic patterns, such as herpes simplex encephalitis (with short intervals of 1 to 4 seconds) and subacute sclerosing panencephalitis (with long intervals of 4 to 14 seconds). More details on the EEG findings in CNS infections are available in Chapter 3.

GENETIC SYNDROMES WITH CHARACTERISTIC EEG PATTERNS

Angelman Syndrome

Angelman syndrome is characterized by severe intellectual disability, inappropriate laughter, jerky movements, ataxic gait, severe speech impairment, and epilepsy. It is usually caused by a de novo deletion of maternally inherited chromosome 15 in the 15q11–q13 critical region. A small percentage show mutations of the *UBE3A* gene. The EEG often has many of the features of the Lennox–Gastaut syndrome, as well as other unique abnormalities that may suggest the diagnosis. The typical EEG findings in young children consist of: (1) high-amplitude persistent rhythmic 4- to 6-Hz theta waves; (2) runs of high-amplitude, usually anterior, delta waves (2 to 3 Hz), often admixed with spikes; and (3) spikes mixed with high-amplitude 3- to 4-Hz components posteriorly that are facilitated or seen only with eye closure.[140] A notched-delta pattern (a variant of the anterior delta pattern) may be somewhat specific for Angelman syndrome.[141] The epileptiform activity is often quite striking and at times may be associated with jerky motor behavior that resembles facial or upper-limb myoclonus.[142] After 4 years of age, the typical pattern is replaced by focal epileptiform activity. Occasionally, girls with Angelman syndrome clinically resemble those with Rett syndrome. The strikingly different EEG findings in these two disorders, particularly during the second year of life, are helpful in arriving at the proper diagnosis.[143]

Rett Syndrome

Rett syndrome, a progressive encephalopathy in girls, is characterized by severe intellectual disability with autistic features, stereotyped hand-wringing movements, episodic hyperventilation, seizures, and acquired microcephaly. The diagnosis is made by well-established clinical criteria. Approximately 80 percent of females with classic Rett syndrome have a mutation in the *MECP2* gene (chromosomal locus Xq28). The EEG may also be helpful in confirming the diagnosis, particularly in the later stages of the disorder.

The EEG is usually normal or nonspecifically abnormal during stage I and early stage II of the disease.[144] Epileptiform activity (consisting primarily of spikes and sharp waves in the centrotemporal region) and slowing of the background appear in stage II (Fig. 4-23). The spikes may be repetitive, enhanced by sleep, and occasionally triggered by tactile stimulation.[144] In stage III (the postregression stage, characterized by increasing seizures, intellectual disability, gait difficulties, and pyramidal signs), the EEG background continues to deteriorate and multifocal spikes and slow spike-wave discharges resembling those of Lennox–Gastaut syndrome are common. The epileptiform activity often wanes during stage IV, which is associated with severe motor and intellectual handicaps, the necessity for the patient to use a wheelchair, and a gradual decline in the frequency of the seizures. During stages III and IV, monorhythmic slow (theta) activity frequently is recorded in the central or frontocentral region.[144] Less frequently, generalized periodic 1-Hz spikes (which resemble those occurring in Creutzfeldt–Jakob disease) are seen.

Other syndromes that may resemble Rett syndrome, particularly during the early years of life, include autism, biotin-dependency disorders, and Angelman syndrome.[143]

MECP2 Duplication Syndrome

MECP2 duplication syndrome is an X-linked neurodevelopmental syndrome affecting males, characterized by intellectual disability, autistic features, treatment-resistant epilepsy, and infantile hypotonia progressing to lower-limb spasticity.[145] The duplication in the Xq28 region is usually submicroscopic, but is detectable by comparative genomic hybridization. Multiple seizure types may occur, but absences, myoclonic, and myoclonic-astatic seizures often occur together. The EEG shows slowing of the dominant posterior rhythm, paroxysmal rhythmic theta activity posteriorly, and multifocal or generalized spike or spike-wave discharges.[145,146]

CDKL5 Mutation Syndrome

Mutations in the X-linked gene *CDKL5* have been found in several girls with X-linked infantile spasm syndrome, girls with atypical Rett syndrome, and boys with severe early-onset encephalopathy and intractable epilepsy.

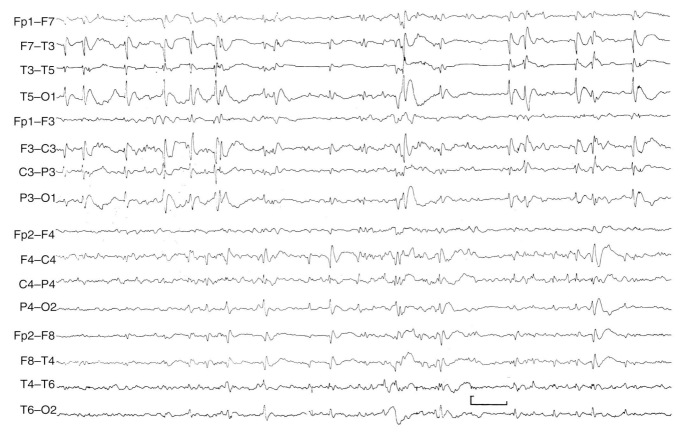

FIGURE 4-23 ■ Centrotemporal spikes during sleep in a 6-year-old girl with stage III Rett syndrome. The spikes are repetitive and predominate in the left hemisphere. Calibration: 50 μV; 1 second.

The common features are early-onset seizures, intellectual disability, and, very often, features suggestive of Rett syndrome. The epilepsy tends to be polymorphic, with myoclonic, tonic, and partial seizures or spasms. The EEG pattern changes with age and is characterized by focal, multifocal, and diffuse pseudoperiodic epileptiform (spikes and polyspikes) discharges.[147,148]

PROGRESSIVE NEUROLOGIC SYNDROMES

The EEG abnormalities accompanying most of the progressive neurologic syndromes of childhood are nonspecific and consist of variably slowed background activity and focal or generalized epileptiform discharges. In the early phases of the diffuse encephalopathies, a distinction sometimes can be made between a primary gray or white matter disorder on the basis of the EEG pattern. Continuous nonparoxysmal, polymorphic delta activity is associated more commonly with leukoencephalopathies, whereas multifocal cortical or generalized epileptiform activity in association with bilateral, paroxysmal slow activity is more consistent with neuronal disease, including

cortical and subcortical gray matter. As the disease progresses, this distinction becomes less prominent. Several neurodegenerative disorders have EEG abnormalities that are sufficiently characteristic to warrant discussion (Table 4-4).

Neuronal Ceroid Lipofuscinosis

Neuronal ceroid lipofuscinosis is a group of inherited, progressive, lysosomal-storage disorders characterized by progressive intellectual and motor deterioration, visual loss, seizures, and early death. Among the many clinical and pathologic subgroups in this disease, three have been reported with peculiar EEG abnormalities (see Table 4-4).

Infantile neuronal ceroid lipofuscinosis (Santavuori–Haltia type) has onset in the first two years of life, and is characterized clinically by a regression of developmental milestones followed by myoclonus. Serial EEGs in this form reveal a progressive diminution in amplitude, culminating in isoelectricity.[149] The rapid development of an isoelectric EEG in conjunction with gradual loss of

TABLE 4-4 ■ EEG Patterns and Associated Disorders	
EEG Pattern	**Disorder**
Comb-like rhythm	Maple syrup urine disease
	Propionic acidemia
Fast central spikes	Tay–Sachs disease
Rhythmic vertex positive spikes	Sialidosis (type I)
Vanishing EEG	Infantile neuronal ceroid lipofuscinosis
High-amplitude 16- to 24-Hz activity	Infantile neuroaxonal dystrophy
Diminished spikes during sleep	Progressive myoclonic epilepsy
Giant somatosensory evoked potentials	Progressive myoclonic epilepsy
Marked photosensitivity	Progressive myoclonic epilepsy and neuronal ceroid lipofuscinosis, particularly late infantile type
Burst-suppression	Neonatal citrullinemia
	Nonketotic hyperglycinemia
	Propionic acidemia
	Leigh disease
	D-Glyceric acidemia
	Molybdenum cofactor deficiency
	Menkes syndrome
	Holocarboxylase synthetase deficiency
	Neonatal adrenoleukodystrophy
Hypsarrhythmia	Zellweger syndrome
	Neonatal adrenoleukodystrophy
	Neuroaxonal dystrophy
	Nonketotic hyperglycinemia
	Phenylketonuria
	Carbohydrate-deficient glycoprotein syndrome (type III)

Adapted from Nordli DR, De Vivo DC: Classification of infantile seizures: implications for identification and treatment of inborn errors of metabolism. J Child Neurol, 17:Suppl 3, 3S3–3S8, 2002 with permission.

the electroretinogram (ERG) and visual evoked potentials (VEPs) is unique to this form of neuronal ceroid lipofuscinosis.

In the classic late-infantile form (Jansky–Bielschowsky type), the EEG shows pseudoperiodic epileptiform discharges and a characteristic high-amplitude response to photic stimulation.[150] A high-amplitude VEP and low-amplitude or absent ERG are noted. This disease begins at 2 to 4 years of age, usually with seizures.

In juvenile neuronal ceroid lipofuscinosis (Spielmeyer–Vogt–Sjögren type), progressive visual loss begins at 4 to 7 years of age. The EEGs contain distinctive runs of high-amplitude spike-wave complexes. The ERG disappears at an early stage of the illness and the VEP gradually becomes of low amplitude.

Mitochondrial Encephalopathy

An increasing number of progressive and often familial neurologic syndromes have been associated with an abnormality of mitochondrial metabolism, including a variety of defects in respiratory chain and phosphorylation system enzymes. Two common phenotypes are myoclonic epilepsy and ragged-red fibers (MERRF); and mitochondrial encephalomyopathy, lactic acidosis, and stroke-like episodes (MELAS). Other disorders now considered to fall into this category include the Ramsay Hunt syndrome and other progressive myoclonic epilepsy syndromes, Alpers disease, Leigh disease, and some of the "system degenerations."

So and colleagues described the electrophysiologic features of 13 patients with MERRF syndrome.[151] These included generalized, bilaterally synchronous, atypical spike-wave discharges; multiple spike-wave bursts; and focal, often occipital, spikes with a slowed background. Only three patients had a photoparoxysmal response.

Alpers disease (infantile hepatocerebral syndrome) is characterized by a progressive encephalopathy with intractable seizures and liver disease leading to cirrhosis.[152] Mutation on *POLG1* gene encoding the catalytic subunit of mitochondrial DNA polymerase has been reported in this condition.[153] The EEG shows, in addition to diffuse background abnormalities, unusual, high-amplitude (200 to 1,000 μV) slow activity (1 Hz or less), with superimposed lower-amplitude polyspikes that are often asymmetric and are more prominent over the posterior head regions, where the most significant neuronal loss is found at autopsy.[154]

Infantile Neuroaxonal Dystrophy

Infantile neuroaxonal dystrophy is a progressive neurodegenerative disorder of infancy with brain iron accumulation, characterized pathologically by accumulations of large eosinophilic axonal swellings or spheroids. Mutations in the *PLA2G6* gene have been identified in this syndrome. A characteristic EEG pattern has been described consisting of high-amplitude, unreactive 16- to 22-Hz rhythms and an absence of responses to a variety of sensory stimuli.[155]

BRAIN DEATH

The Task Force for the Determination of Brain Death in Children has set forth the criteria for determining brain death in children.[16] The Task Force recommended that EEGs be obtained routinely in children between the ages of 7 days and 1 year, but not in older children if an irreversible cause exists. Most neurologists believe that the EEG is a useful adjunct to the determination of brain death if it is performed by an experienced technologist and interpreted by an experienced electroencephalographer, as is discussed in Chapter 35. The criteria for irreversible brain death are not established clearly in infants less than 1 week of age.

ACKNOWLEDGMENT

The author thanks Dr. Barry Tharp, who was the co-author of this chapter in earlier editions of this book.

REFERENCES

1. Hahn JS, Tharp BR: Neonatal and pediatric electroencephalography. p. 85. In Aminoff MJ (ed): Electrodiagnosis in Clinical Neurology. 5th Ed. Elsevier, Philadelphia, 2004

2. Clancy RR, Bergqvist AG, Dlugos DJ: Neonatal electroencephalography. p. 161. In Ebersole JS, Pedley TA (eds): Current Practice of Clinical Electroencephalography. 3rd Ed. Lippincott William & Wilkins, Philadelphia, 2003

3. Andre M, Lamblin MD, d'Allest AM et al: Electroencephalography in premature and full-term infants. Developmental features and glossary. Neurophysiol Clin, 40:59, 2010

4. American Electroencephalographic Society: Guideline 2: Minimum technical standards for pediatric electroencephalography. J Clin Neurophysiol, 23:92, 2006

5. Vecchierini MF, Andre M, d'Allest AM: Normal EEG of premature infants born between 24 and 30 weeks gestational age: terminology, definitions and maturation aspects. Neurophysiol Clin, 37:311, 2007

6. Grigg-Damberger M, Gozal D, Marcus CL et al: The visual scoring of sleep and arousal in infants and children. J Clin Sleep Med, 3:201, 2007

7. Hughes JR, Miller JK, Fino JJ et al: The sharp theta rhythm on the occipital areas of prematures (STOP): a newly described waveform. Clin Electroencephalogr, 21:77, 1990

8. Biagioni E, Frisone MF, Laroche S et al: Occipital sawtooth: a physiological EEG pattern in very premature infants. Clin Neurophysiol, 111:2145, 2000

9. Biagioni E, Bartalena L, Boldrini A et al: Background EEG activity in preterm infants: correlation of outcome with selected maturational features. Electroencephalogr Clin Neurophysiol, 91:154, 1994

10. Selton D, Andre M, Hascoet JM: Normal EEG in very premature infants: reference criteria. Clin Neurophysiol, 111:2116, 2000

11. Hayakawa M, Okumura A, Hayakawa F et al: Background electroencephalographic (EEG) activities of very preterm infants born at less than 27 weeks gestation: a study on the degree of continuity. Arch Dis Child Fetal Neonatal Ed, 84:F163, 2001

12. Holmes GL, Lombroso CT: Prognostic value of background patterns in the neonatal EEG. J Clin Neurophysiol, 10:323, 1993

13. Van Lieshout HBM, Jacobs JWFM, Rotteveel JJ et al: The prognostic value of the EEG in asphyxiated newborns. Acta Neurol Scand, 91:203, 1995

14. Nguyen The Tich S, Vecchierini MF, Debillon T et al: Effects of sufentanil on electroencephalogram in very and extremely preterm neonates. Pediatrics, 111:123, 2003

15. Young GB, da Silva OP: Effects of morphine on the electroencephalograms of neonates: a prospective, observational study. Clin Neurophysiol, 111:1955, 2000

16. Task Force for the Determination of Brain Death in Children: Guidelines for the determination of brain death in children. Ann Neurol, 21:616, 1987

17. Ashwal S: Brain death in the newborn. Current perspectives. Clin Perinatol, 24:859, 1997

18. American Electroencephalographic Society: Guideline 3: Minimum technical standards for EEG recording in suspected cerebral death. J Clin Neurophysiol, 23:97, 2006

19. Douglass LM, Wu JY, Rosman NP et al: Burst suppression electroencephalogram pattern in the newborn: predicting the outcome. J Child Neurol, 17:403, 2002

20. Sinclair DB, Campbell M, Byrne P et al: EEG and long-term outcome of term infants with neonatal hypoxic-ischemic encephalopathy. Clin Neurophysiol, 110:655, 1999

21. Biagioni E, Bartalena L, Boldrini A et al: Constantly discontinuous EEG patterns in full-term neonates with hypoxic-ischaemic encephalopathy. Clin Neurophysiol, 110:1510, 1999

22. Menache CC, Bourgeois BF, Volpe JJ: Prognostic value of neonatal discontinuous EEG. Pediatr Neurol, 27:93, 2002

23. Hahn JS, Monyer H, Tharp BR: Interburst interval measurements in the EEG of premature infants with normal neurological outcome. Electroencephalogr Clin Neurophysiol, 73:410, 1989

24. Holmes G, Rowe J, Hafford J et al: Prognostic value of the electroencephalogram in neonatal asphyxia. Electroencephalogr Clin Neurophysiol, 53:60, 1982

25. Mariani E, Scelsa B, Pogliani L et al: Prognostic value of electroencephalograms in asphyxiated newborns treated with hypothermia. Pediatr Neurol, 39:317, 2008

26. Nunes ML, Da Costa JC, Moura-Ribeiro MV: Polysomnographic quantification of bioelectrical maturation in preterm and fullterm newborns at matched conceptional ages. Electroencephalogr Clin Neurophysiol, 102:186, 1997

27. Hahn JS, Tharp BR: The dysmature EEG in infants with bronchopulmonary dysplasia and its prognostic implications. Electroencephalogr Clin Neurophysiol, 76:106, 1990

28. Hayakawa F, Okumura A, Kato T et al: Dysmature EEG pattern in EEGs of preterm infants with cognitive impairment: maturation arrest caused by prolonged mild CNS depression. Brain Dev, 19:122, 1997

29. Biagioni E, Bartalena L, Boldrini A et al: Electroencephalography in infants with periventricular leukomalacia: prognostic features at preterm and term age. J Child Neurol, 15:1, 2000

30. Biagioni E, Bartalena L, Biver P et al: Electroencephalographic dysmaturity in preterm infants: a prognostic tool in the early postnatal period. Neuropediatrics, 27:311, 1996

31. Watanabe K, Hayakawa F, Okumura A: Neonatal EEG: a powerful tool in the assessment of brain damage in preterm infants. Brain Dev, 21:361, 1999

32. Hayakawa F, Okumura A, Kato T et al: Determination of timing of brain injury in preterm infants with periventricular leukomalacia with serial neonatal electroencephalography. Pediatrics, 104:1077, 1999

33. Tharp BR, Scher MS, Clancy RR: Serial EEGs in normal and abnormal infants with birth weights less than 1200 grams: a prospective study with long term follow-up. Neuropediatrics, 20:64, 1989

34. Kubota T, Okumura A, Hayakawa F et al: Combination of neonatal electroencephalography and ultrasonography: sensitive means of early diagnosis of periventricular leukomalacia. Brain Dev, 24:698, 2002

35. Maruyama K, Okumura A, Hayakawa F et al: Prognostic value of EEG depression in preterm infants for later development of cerebral palsy. Neuropediatrics, 33:133, 2002

36. Takeuchi T, Watanabe K: The EEG evolution and neurological prognosis of perinatal hypoxia neonates. Brain Dev, 11:115, 1989

37. Pressler RM, Boylan GB, Morton M et al: Early serial EEG in hypoxic ischaemic encephalopathy. Clin Neurophysiol, 112:31, 2001

38. Zeinstra E, Fock JM, Begeer JH et al: The prognostic value of serial EEG recordings following acute neonatal asphyxia in full-term infants. Eur J Paediatr Neurol, 5:155, 2001

39. Scher MS, Bova JM, Dokianakis SG et al: Physiological significance of sharp wave transients on EEG recordings of healthy pre-term and full-term neonates. Electroencephalogr Clin Neurophysiol, 90:179, 1994

40. Marret S, Parain D, Ménard J et al: Prognostic value of neonatal electroencephalography in premature newborns less than 33 weeks of gestational age. Electroencephalogr Clin Neurophysiol, 102:178, 1997

41. Baud O, d'Allest AM, Lacaze-Masmonteil T et al: The early diagnosis of periventricular leukomalacia in premature infants with positive rolandic sharp waves on serial electroencephalography. J Pediatr, 132:813, 1998

42. Vecchierini-Blineau MF, Nogues B, Louvet S et al: Positive temporal sharp waves in electroencephalograms of the premature newborn. Neurophysiol Clin, 26:350, 1996

43. Scher MS, Bova JM, Dokianakis SG et al: Positive temporal sharp waves on EEG recordings of healthy neonates: a benign pattern of dysmaturity in pre-term infants at postconceptional term ages. Electroencephalogr Clin Neurophysiol, 90:173, 1994

44. Chung HJ, Clancy RR: Significance of positive temporal sharp waves in the neonatal electroencephalogram. Electroencephalogr Clin Neurophysiol, 79:256, 1991

45. Nunes ML, Penela MM, da Costa JC: Differences in the dynamics of frontal sharp transients in normal and hypoglycemic newborns. Clin Neurophysiol, 111:305, 2000

46. Scher MS, Beggarly M: Clinical significance of focal periodic discharges in neonates. J Child Neurol, 4:175, 1989

47. Hrachovy RA, O'Donnell DM: The significance of excessive rhythmic alpha and/or theta frequency activity in the EEG of the neonate. Clin Neurophysiol, 110:438, 1999

48. Zaret BS, Guterman B, Weig S: Circumscribed midline EEG activity in neurologically normal neonates. Clin Electroencephalogr, 22:13, 1991

49. Ortibus EL, Sum JM, Hahn JS: Predictive value of EEG for outcome and epilepsy following neonatal seizures. Electroencephalogr Clin Neurophysiol, 98:175, 1996

50. Biagioni E, Boldrini A, Bottone U et al: Prognostic value of abnormal EEG transients in preterm and full-term neonates. Electroencephalogr Clin Neurophysiol, 99:1, 1996

51. Mizrahi EM, Kellaway P: Diagnosis and management of neonatal seizures. Lippincott-Raven, Philadelphia, 1998

52. Scher MS: Controversies regarding neonatal seizure recognition. Epileptic Disord, 4:139, 2002

53. Shewmon DA: What is a neonatal seizure? Problems in definition and quantification for investigative and clinical purposes. J Clin Neurophysiol, 7:315, 1990

54. Bye AME, Cunningham CA, Chee KY et al: Outcome of neonates with electrographically identified seizures, or at risk of seizures. Pediatr Neurol, 16:225, 1997

55. Pisani F, Copioli C, Di Gioia C et al: Neonatal seizures: relation of ictal video-electroencephalography (EEG) findings with neurodevelopmental outcome. J Child Neurol, 23:394, 2008

56. Pisani F, Cerminara C, Fusco C et al: Neonatal status epilepticus vs recurrent neonatal seizures: clinical findings and outcome. Neurology, 69:2177, 2007

57. Hirsch E, Velez A, Sellal F et al: Electroclinical signs of benign neonatal familial convulsions. Ann Neurol, 34:835, 1993

58. Ronnen GM, Rosales TO, Connolly M et al: Seizure characteristics in chromosome 20 benign familial neonatal convulsions. Neurology, 43:1993

59. Aso K, Watanabe K: Benign familial neonatal convulsions: generalized epilepsy? Pediatr Neurol, 8:226, 1992

60. Bye AME: Neonate with benign familial neonatal convulsions: recorded generalized and focal seizures. Pediatr Neurol, 10:164, 1994

61. Legido A, Clancy RR, Berman PH: Neurologic outcome after electroencephalographically proven neonatal seizures. Pediatrics, 88:583, 1991

62. Khan RL, Nunes ML, Garcias da Silva LF et al: Predictive value of sequential electroencephalogram (EEG) in neonates with seizures and its relation to neurological outcome. J Child Neurol, 23:144, 2008

63. Clancy RR: Interictal sharp EEG transients in neonatal seizures. J Child Neurol, 4:30, 1989

64. Oliveira AJ, Nunes ML, Haertel LM et al: Duration of rhythmic EEG patterns in neonates: new evidence for clinical and prognostic significance of brief rhythmic discharges. Clin Neurophysiol, 111:1646, 2000

65. Hahn JS, Delgado MR, Clegg NJ et al: Electroencephalography in holoprosencephaly: findings in children without epilepsy. Clin Neurophysiol, 114:1908, 2003

66. Mori K, Hashimoto T, Tayama M et al: Serial EEG and sleep polygraphic studies on lissencephaly (agyria-pachygyria). Brain Dev, 16:365, 1994

67. Tharp BR: Unique EEG pattern (comb-like rhythm) in neonatal maple syrup urine disease. Pediatr Neurol, 8:65, 1992

68. Toth C, Harder S, Yager J: Neonatal herpes encephalitis: a case series and review of clinical presentation. Can J Neurol Sci, 30:36, 2003

69. de Vries LS, Toet MC: Amplitude integrated electroencephalography in the full-term newborn. Clin Perinatol, 33:619, 2006

70. Hellstrom-Westas L: Continuous electroencephalography monitoring of the preterm infant. Clin Perinatol, 33:633, 2006

71. Rosen I: The physiological basis for continuous electroencephalogram monitoring in the neonate. Clin Perinatol, 33:593, 2006

72. Toet MC, Hellstrom-Westas L, Groenendaal F et al: Amplitude integrated EEG 3 and 6 hours after birth in full term neonates with hypoxic-ischaemic encephalopathy. Arch Dis Child Fetal Neonatal Ed, 81:F19, 1999

73. Shalak LF, Laptook AR, Velaphi SC et al: Amplitude-integrated electroencephalography coupled with an early neurologic examination enhances prediction of term infants at risk for persistent encephalopathy. Pediatrics, 111:351, 2003

74. Toet MC, van der Meij W, de Vries LS et al: Comparison between simultaneously recorded amplitude integrated electroencephalogram (cerebral function monitor) and standard electroencephalogram in neonates. Pediatrics, 109:772, 2002

75. Inder TE, Buckland L, Williams CE et al: Lowered electroencephalographic spectral edge frequency predicts the presence of cerebral white matter injury in premature infants. Pediatrics, 111:27, 2003

76. Kellaway P: An orderly approach to visual analysis: elements of the normal EEG and their characteristics in children and adults. p. 100. In Ebersole JS, Pedley TA (eds): Current Practice of Clinical Electroencephalography. 3rd Ed. Lippincott Williams & Wilkins, Philadelphia, 2003

77. Louis J, Zhang JX, Revol M et al: Ontogenesis of nocturnal organization of sleep spindles: a longitudinal study during the first 6 months of life. Electroencephalogr Clin Neurophysiol, 83:289, 1992

78. Aucelio CN, Niedermeyer E, Melo AN: The frequency–amplitude gradient in the sleep EEG of children and its diagnostic significance. Arq Neuropsiquiatr, 65:206, 2007

79. Silbert PL, Radhakrishnan K, Johnson J et al: The significance of the phi rhythm. Electroencephalogr Clin Neurophysiol, 95:71, 1995

80. North K, Ouvrier R, Nugent M: Pseudoseizures caused by hyperventilation resembling absence epilepsy. J Child Neurol, 5:288, 1990

81. Doose H, Waltz S: Photosensitivity—genetics and clinical significance. Neuropediatrics, 24:249, 1993

82. Harding GF, Fylan F: Two visual mechanisms of photosensitivity. Epilepsia, 40:1446, 1999

83. Steinlein O, Anokhin A, Yping M et al: Localization of a gene for the human low-voltage EEG on 20q and genetic heterogeneity. Genomics, 12:69, 1992

84. Doose H, Castiglione E, Waltz S: Parental generalized EEG alpha activity predisposes to spike wave discharges in offspring. Hum Genet, 96:695, 1995

85. Tatum WOT, Husain AM, Benbadis SR et al: Normal adult EEG and patterns of uncertain significance. J Clin Neurophysiol, 23:194, 2006

86. Mizrahi EM: Avoiding the pitfalls of EEG interpretation in childhood epilepsy. Epilepsia, 37 Suppl 1:S41, 1996

87. Marks DA, Katz A, Scheyer R et al: Clinical and electrographic effects of acute anticonvulsant withdrawal in epileptic patients. Neurology, 41:508, 1991

88. Camfield P, Gordon K, Camfield C et al: EEG results are rarely the same if repeated within six months in childhood epilepsy. Can J Neurol Sci, 22:297, 1995

89. Lombroso C: Consistent EEG focalities detected in subjects with primary generalized epilepsies monitored for two decades. Epilepsia, 38:797, 1997

90. Shinnar S, Berg AT, Moshé SL et al: Discontinuing antiepileptic drugs in children with epilepsy: a prospective study. Ann Neurol, 35:534, 1994

91. Commission on Classification and Terminology of the International League Against Epilepsy: Proposal for revised classification of epilepsies and epileptic syndromes. Epilepsia, 30:389, 1989

92. Berg AT, Berkovic SF, Brodie MJ et al: Revised terminology and concepts for organization of seizures and epilepsies: report of the ILAE Commission on Classification and Terminology, 2005–2009. Epilepsia, 51:676, 2010

93. Sadleir LG, Farrell K, Smith S et al: Electroclinical features of absence seizures in childhood absence epilepsy. Neurology, 67:413, 2006

94. Vierck E, Cauley R, Kugler SL et al: Polyspike and waves do not predict generalized tonic-clonic seizures in childhood absence epilepsy. J Child Neurol, 25:475, 2010

95. Bouma PA, Westendorp RG, Van Dijk JG et al: The outcome of absence epilepsy: a meta-analysis. Neurology, 47:802, 1996

96. Callenbach PM, Bouma PA, Geerts AT et al: Long-term outcome of childhood absence epilepsy: Dutch Study of Epilepsy in Childhood. Epilepsy Res, 83:249, 2009

97. Panayiotopoulos CP, Obeid T, Waheed G: Differentiation of typical absence seizures in epileptic syndromes. Brain, 112:1039, 1989

98. Janz D: The idiopathic generalized epilepsies of adolescence with childhood and juvenile age of onset. Epilepsia, 38:4, 1997

99. Panayiotopoulos CP, Obeid T, Tahan AR: Juvenile myoclonic epilepsy: a 5-year prospective study. Epilepsia, 35:285, 1994

100. Sadleir LG, Scheffer IE, Smith S et al: EEG features of absence seizures in idiopathic generalized epilepsy: impact of syndrome, age, and state. Epilepsia, 50:1572, 2009

101. Aliberti V, Grünewald RA, Panayiotopoulos CP et al: Focal electroencephalographic abnormalities in juvenile myoclonic epilepsy. Epilepsia, 35:297, 1994

102. Lancman ME, Asconapé JJ, Penry JK: Clinical and EEG asymmetries in juvenile myoclonic epilepsy. Epilepsia, 35:302, 1994

103. Oguni H, Mukahira K, Oguni M et al: Video-polygraphic analysis of myoclonic seizures in juvenile myoclonic epilepsy. Epilepsia, 35:307, 1994

104. Tovia E, Goldberg-Stern H, Shahar E et al: Outcome of children with juvenile absence epilepsy. J Child Neurol, 21:766, 2006

105. Fusco L, Vigevano F: Ictal clinical electroencephalographic findings of spasms in West syndrome. Epilepsia, 34:671, 1993

106. Pellock JM, Hrachovy R, Shinnar S et al: Infantile spasms: a U.S. consensus report. Epilepsia, 51:2175, 2010

107. Lux AL, Osborne JP: A proposal for case definitions and outcome measures in studies of infantile spasms and West syndrome: consensus statement of the West Delphi group. Epilepsia, 45:1416, 2004

108. Gaily EK, Shewmon DA, Chugani HT et al: Asymmetric and asynchronous infantile spasms. Epilepsia, 36:873, 1995

109. Vinters HV, DeRosa MJ, Farrell MA: Neuropathological study of resected tissue from patients with infantile spasms. Epilepsia, 34:772, 1993

110. Miyazaki M, Hashimoto T, Fujii E et al: Infantile spasms: Localized cerebral lesions on SPECT. Epilepsia, 35:988, 1994

111. Chugani HT, Conti JR: Etiologic classification of infantile spasms in 140 cases: role of positron emission tomography. J Child Neurol, 11:44, 1996

112. Dulac O, Plouin P, Jambaque I: Predicting favorable outcome in idiopathic West syndrome. Epilepsia, 34:747, 1993

113. Arzimanoglou A, French J, Blume WT et al: Lennox–Gastaut syndrome: a consensus approach on diagnosis, assessment, management, and trial methodology. Lancet Neurol, 8:82, 2009

114. Ikeno T, Shigematsu H, Miyakoshi M et al: An analytic study of epileptic falls. Epilepsia, 26:612, 1995

115. Nickels K, Wirrell E: Electrical status epilepticus in sleep. Semin Pediatr Neurol, 15:50, 2008

116. Panayiotopoulos CP, Michael M, Sanders S et al: Benign childhood focal epilepsies: assessment of established and newly recognized syndromes. Brain, 131:2264, 2008

117. Yamatogi Y, Ohtahara S: Severe epilepsy with multiple independent spike foci. J Clin Neurophysiol, 20:442, 2003

118. Lombroso CT: Early myoclonic encephalopathy, early infantile epileptic encephalopathy, and benign and severe infantile myoclonic epilepsies: a critical review and personal contributions. J Clin Neurophysiol, 7:380, 1990

119. Yamatogi Y, Ohtahara S: Early-infantile epileptic encephalopathy with suppression-bursts, Ohtahara syndrome; its overview referring to our 16 cases. Brain Dev, 24:13, 2002

120. Acharya JN, Wyllie E, Lüders HO et al: Seizure symptomatology in infants with localization-related epilepsy. Neurology, 48:189, 1997

121. Nordli DR, Bazil CW, Scheuer ML et al: Recognition and classification of seizures in infants. Epilepsia, 38:553, 1997

122. Gregory DL, Wong PK: Clinical relevance of a dipole field in rolandic spikes. Epilepsia, 33:36, 1992

123. Minami T, Gondo K, Yamamoto T et al: Magnetoencephalographic analysis of rolandic discharges in benign childhood epilepsy. Ann Neurol, 39:326, 1996

124. Van der Meij W, Van Huffelen AC, Wienecke GH et al: Sequential EEG mapping may differentiate "epileptic" from "non-epileptic" rolandic spikes. Electroencephalogr Clin Neurophysiol, 82:408, 1992

125. Van der Meij W, Wieneke GH, Van Huffelen AC et al: Identical morphology of the rolandic spike-and-wave complex in different clinical entities. Epilepsia, 34:540, 1993

126. Frost JD, Hrachovy RA, Glaze DG: Spike morphology in childhood focal epilepsy: relationship to syndromic classification. Epilepsia, 33:531, 1992

127. Gelisse P, Genton P, Bureau M et al: Are there generalised spike waves and typical absences in benign rolandic epilepsy? Brain Dev, 21:390, 1999

128. Beydoun A, Garofalo EA, Drury I: Generalized spike-waves, multiple loci, and clinical course in children with EEG features of benign epilepsy of childhood with centro-temporal spikes. Epilepsia, 33:1091, 1992

129. Okubo Y, Matsuura M, Asai T et al: Epileptiform EEG discharges in healthy children: prevalence, emotional and behavioral correlates, and genetic influences. Epilepsia, 35:832, 1994

130. Doose H, Neubauer B, Carlsson G: Children with benign focal sharp waves in the EEG—developmental disorders and epilepsy. Neuropediatrics, 27:227, 1996

131. Massa R, de Saint-Martin A, Carcangiu R et al: EEG criteria predictive of complicated evolution in idiopathic rolandic epilepsy. Neurology, 57:1071, 2001

132. Ferrie CD, Beaumanoir A, Guerrini R et al: Early-onset benign occipital seizure susceptibility syndrome. Epilepsia, 38:285, 1997

133. Caraballo RH, Cersosimo RO, Fejerman N: Childhood occipital epilepsy of Gastaut: a study of 33 patients. Epilepsia, 49:288, 2008

134. Biagioni E, Cioni G, Cowan F et al: Visual function and EEG reactivity in infants with perinatal brain lesions at 1 year. Dev Med Child Neurol, 44:171, 2002

135. Maytal J, Steele R, Eviatar L et al: The value of early post-ictal EEG in children with complex febrile seizures. Epilepsia, 41:219, 2000

136. Nordli DR, Moshe SL, Shinnar S: The role of EEG in febrile status epilepticus (FSE). Brain Dev, 32:37, 2010

137. Tassinari CA, Bureau M, Dravet C et al: Epilepsy with continous spikes and waves during slow sleep—otherwise described as ESES (epilepsy with electrical status epilepticus during slow sleep). p. 245. In Roger J, Bureau M, Dravet C et al (eds): Epileptic syndromes in infancy, childhood and adolescence. 2nd Ed. John Libbey, London, 1992

138. Perez ER, Davidoff V, Despland P et al: Mental and behavioral deterioration of children with epilepsy and CSWS: acquired epileptic frontal syndrome. Dev Med Child Neurol, 35:661, 1993

139. Morrell F, Whisler WW, Smith MC et al: Landau–Kleffner syndrome. Treatment with subpial intracortical transection. Brain, 118:1529, 1995

140. Buoni S, Grosso S, Pucci L et al: Diagnosis of Angelman syndrome: clinical and EEG criteria. Brain Dev, 21:296, 1999

141. Korff CM, Kelley KR, Nordli DR, Jr: Notched delta, phenotype, and Angelman syndrome. J Clin Neurophysiol, 22:238, 2005

142. Guerrini R, DeLorey T, Bonanni P et al: Cortical myoclonus in Angelman syndrome. Ann Neurol, 40:39, 1996

143. Laan LA, Brouwer OF, Begeer CH et al: The diagnostic value of the EEG in Angelman and Rett syndrome at a

young age. Electroencephalogr Clin Neurophysiol, 106: 404, 1998

144. Glaze DG: Neurophysiology of Rett syndrome. J Child Neurol, 20:740, 2005

145. Ramocki MB, Tavyev YJ, Peters SU: The MECP2 duplication syndrome. Am J Med Genet A, 152A:1079, 2010

146. Echenne B, Roubertie A, Lugtenberg D et al: Neurologic aspects of MECP2 gene duplication in male patients. Pediatr Neurol, 41:187, 2009

147. Elia M, Falco M, Ferri R et al: CDKL5 mutations in boys with severe encephalopathy and early-onset intractable epilepsy. Neurology, 71:997, 2008

148. Pintaudi M, Baglietto MG, Gaggero R et al: Clinical and electroencephalographic features in patients with CDKL5 mutations: two new Italian cases and review of the literature. Epilepsy Behav, 12:326, 2008

149. Vanhanen SL, Sainio K, Lappi M et al: EEG and evoked potentials in infantile neuronal ceroid-lipofuscinosis. Dev Med Child Neurol, 39:456, 1997

150. Veneselli E, Biancheri R, Buoni S et al: Clinical and EEG findings in 18 cases of late infantile neuronal ceroid lipofuscinosis. Brain Dev, 23:306, 2001

151. So N, Berkovic S, Andermann F et al: Myoclonus epilepsy and ragged-red fibers (MERRF) 2. Electrophysiological studies and comparisons with other progressive myoclonus epilepsies. Brain, 112:1261, 1989

152. Harding BN: Progressive neuronal degeneration of childhood with liver disease (Alpers–Huttenlocher syndrome): a personal review. J Child Neurol, 5:273, 1990

153. Ferrari G, Lamantea E, Donati A et al: Infantile hepatocerebral syndromes associated with mutations in the mitochondrial DNA polymerase-gamma A. Brain, 128:723, 2005

154. Wolf NI, Rahman S, Schmitt B et al: Status epilepticus in children with Alpers' disease caused by POLG1 mutations: EEG and MRI features. Epilepsia, 50:1596, 2009

155. Kurian MA, Morgan NV, MacPherson L et al: Phenotypic spectrum of neurodegeneration associated with mutations in the PLA2G6 gene (PLAN). Neurology, 70:1623, 2008

Electroencephalographic Artifacts and Benign Variants

JEFFREY W. BRITTON

The electroencephalogram (EEG) is a valuable tool in neurologic diagnosis. However, its value depends on the correct identification of abnormalities so that benign variants and artifacts are not mistaken for pathologic findings.[1-5] The characteristic features of benign variants and artifacts are discussed in the present chapter. Reference to some of these artifacts was also made in Chapter 3.

BENIGN EEG VARIANTS

Benign variants are EEG waveforms that bear a resemblance to epileptogenic abnormalities.[1,2,6] Many benign variants initially were thought to be pathologic but careful clinical correlation showed an unreliable association with neurologic disease and verified their presence in normal populations. The erroneous designation of these waveforms as epileptogenic may lead to clinical and socioeconomic consequences for patients. Their presence is best considered a nonspecific finding that is not predictive of an epileptic disorder or other neurologic disease. However, just as patients with epilepsy and other diseases of the central nervous system (CNS) can have a normal EEG, the presence of a benign variant should not be misinterpreted as excluding such diagnoses.

Benign variants are not rare; the prevalence in one EEG laboratory was determined to be 18.3 percent.[7] Benign variants are often confused with epileptogenic EEG abnormalities, given their rhythmic and occasionally spike-like morphologic characteristics. Examples of the most common rhythmic and spike-like benign variants are summarized in Table 5-1 and in Figures 5-1, 5-2, and 5-3. In general, benign EEG variants are most prominent in drowsiness and resolve with wakefulness and deeper levels of sleep. Although there are exceptions, as discussed below, this feature can help in distinguishing them from epileptogenic abnormalities.

Rhythmic Benign Variants

WICKET WAVES

Wicket waves are sharply contoured, arciform or "mu"-shaped waveforms which most commonly are localized to the midtemporal regions. Wicket waves are

TABLE 5-1 ■ Benign EEG Variants Categorized by Morphologic Characteristics
RHYTHMIC WAVEFORMS
Wicket waves
Rhythmic temporal theta of drowsiness
Slow alpha variant
Subacute rhythmic electrographic discharges of adults
Midline rhythmic theta
Breach rhythm
SPIKE-LIKE WAVEFORMS
Small sharp spikes
14- and 6-Hz positive spikes
6-Hz (phantom) spike-wave

characteristically present during drowsiness and resolve with wakefulness and deeper levels of sleep. However, they have also been described in rapid eye movement (REM) sleep.[8] The importance of identifying wicket waves is to avoid incorrectly labeling them as temporal sharp waves.[9] The prevalence of wicket waves in an analysis of findings listed in EEG reports ranges from 0.03 to 1.0 percent.[10,11] Others have estimated the prevalence to be higher, perhaps reflecting differences in the documentation practices of different laboratories with respect to the rate at which benign waveforms are specified in reports.[6,12]

Wicket waves may predominate in one temporal region, but are often bilateral. They typically appear in clusters lasting for 1 to 2 seconds, occurring at theta frequency. Wicket-wave clusters often exhibit a "crescendo–decrescendo" onset and offset, which aids in their identification. They may be sharply contoured and characteristically show phase reversal on bipolar montages over the midtemporal region, giving rise to a "vampire" or "piranha teeth" appearance (see Fig. 5-1). Occasionally, isolated wicket spikes may be present and can be difficult to differentiate from temporal sharp waves. In such cases, resemblance of the isolated wicket spike to waveforms found in more typical wicket-wave clusters in the same patient, and the lack of a succeeding slow wave, help distinguish them from epileptogenic temporal sharp waves.

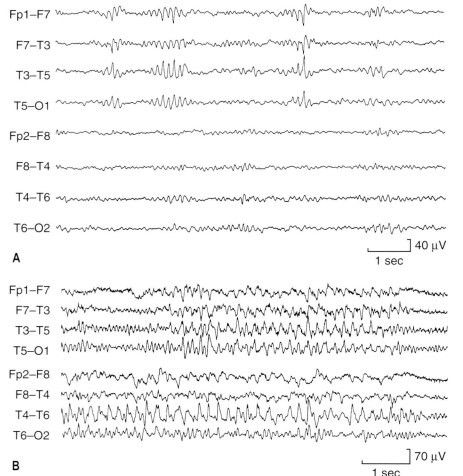

FIGURE 5-1 ■ Rhythmic benign electroencephalographic variants. **A**, Wicket waves. These waves characteristically are sharply contoured but, unlike epileptiform discharges, are not associated with after-coming slow waves. The typical midtemporal localization and crescendo–decrescendo morphology are shown in this patient. (Modified from Klass DW, Westmoreland BF: Electroencephalography: general principles and adult electroencephalograms. In Daube JR (ed): Clinical Neurophysiology. FA Davis, New York, 1996.) **B**, Rhythmic temporal theta of drowsiness. Discharges may be sharply contoured or may have a notched appearance. The frequency of the discharge does not evolve over its duration, unlike seizure discharges.

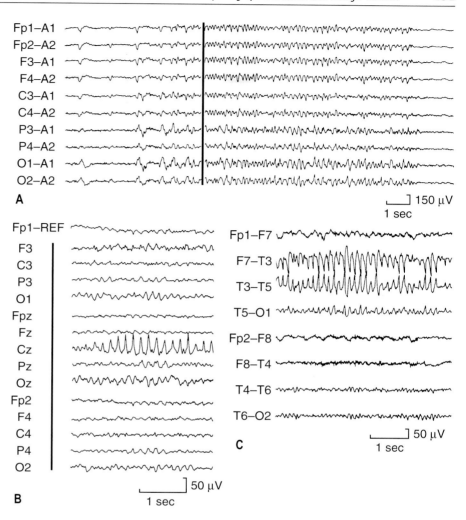

FIGURE 5-2 ■ Rhythmic benign electroencephalographic variants (continued). **A,** Subclinical rhythmic epileptiform discharge of adults. Discharges often show evolution to higher frequencies as they continue, as shown. The waveforms are often maximal over the parietal or posterior temporal region. **B,** Midline theta rhythm. The discharge, which is maximal over the vertex, shows minimal change in frequency over time, unlike seizure activity. **C,** Breach rhythm in a patient with previous left temporal lobectomy. The electroencephalogram shows a significant increase in amplitude over a previous craniotomy. Breach rhythms may show sharply contoured waveforms, which can be misinterpreted as epileptogenic activity.

RHYTHMIC TEMPORAL THETA OF DROWSINESS

Rhythmic temporal theta of drowsiness (RTTD), also known as rhythmic midtemporal discharges and the "psychomotor variant", consists of rhythmic theta discharges localized to the midtemporal region. Bursts of RTTD range from a few seconds to a few minutes in duration.[6] They may be unilateral, bilateral independent, or bisynchronous. RTTD characteristically resolves during deeper levels of sleep and upon arousal. Magnetoencephalography suggests the generators of RTTD may be localized to the posterior inferior temporal region.[13]

RTTD has characteristic morphologic features (see Fig. 5-1).[4,14] The individual waveforms may be sharply contoured and sometimes show a "notched" appearance. RTTD discharges typically stand out prominently on the EEG, which may result in their being mistaken for paroxysmal epileptogenic activity. Features that allow distinction from seizure discharges include resolution upon arousal, absence of clinical disturbance during the discharge, the notched waveform morphology when present, and lack of evolution of the discharge to other frequencies or spread to other regions.[15] These attributes contrast with electrographic seizures, which tend to show evolution from one frequency to another and propagation to other brain regions.[16]

SLOW ALPHA VARIANT

Slow alpha variant consists of theta activity present over the posterior head regions, with a frequency typically measuring 50 percent of the alpha rhythm.[6] The slow alpha variant is thought to represent a frequency subharmonic of the alpha rhythm. Slow alpha variant waveforms may be notched in appearance, similar to RTTD. Failure to recognize slow alpha variant may lead to a misdiagnosis of a posterior cerebral dysrhythmia.

SUBACUTE RHYTHMIC EPILEPTIFORM DISCHARGES OF ADULTS

Subacute rhythmic epileptiform discharges of adults (SREDA) are rhythmic EEG discharges of moderate to high amplitude that produce an abrupt change on the

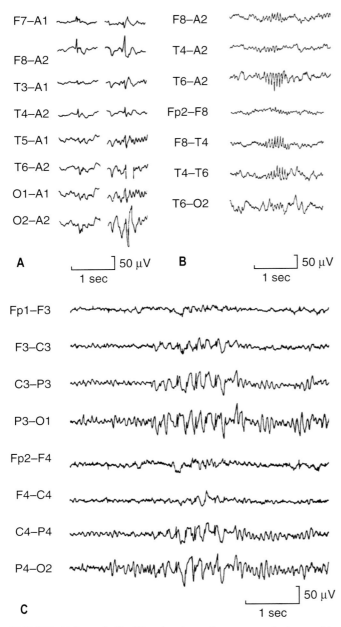

FIGURE 5-3 ■ Spike-like benign electroencephalographic variants. **A,** Small sharp spike (left side of image) contrasted with an anterior temporal sharp wave (right side of image). Note the low amplitude and steep descending slope of the biphasic small sharp spike in the F8–A2 derivation, as well as the low-amplitude after-coming slow wave. **B,** Discharges of 14- and 6-Hz positive spikes (ctenoids). Maximal amplitude is often seen over the posterior and temporal regions. Note surface positivity at T6–A2. **C,** "Phantom" 6-Hz spike-wave discharges, posterior variant.

EEG that may be mistaken for electrographic seizure activity.[6,17] Clinical testing during SREDA, however, shows no evidence of neurologic impairment during the discharge, and clinical follow-up does not suggest an association with epilepsy.[18] Although SREDA is less common than the other benign variants discussed in this chapter,[10] it is important to recognize it as distinct from epileptogenic activity.

SREDA typically consists of a mixture of frequencies, with theta activity predominating.[15] The bursts last from 20 seconds to a few minutes.[17] It is characteristically widespread in distribution, but is often maximal in amplitude over the parietal and posterior temporal regions.[15,19] The discharges are usually bisynchronous, but unilateral SREDA has been described. In contrast to other benign variants, SREDA can be seen during wakefulness, and it can also be seen in REM sleep.[20] While it often begins with the abrupt onset of diffuse, sharply contoured activity of mixed, but predominantly theta, frequency,[15] it may also begin with a single bisynchronous sharp complex followed by semirhythmic sharp activity, which eventually merges into a sustained discharge.[21] The onset of a SREDA discharge is depicted in Figure 5-2. Clinical testing during the discharge by a technologist or clinician helps to confirm the benign nature of this variant rhythm.

MIDLINE RHYTHMIC THETA

Midline rhythmic theta was originally described as a potentially epileptogenic abnormality correlating with the diagnosis of temporal lobe epilepsy. It was determined subsequently to be a nonspecific finding, occurring in patients without a clear diagnosis of epilepsy.[6,11,22] As its name suggests, this benign variant consists of moderate-amplitude theta activity present over the central midline vertex region (see Fig. 5-2). The waveform morphology can be rounded, arciform, mu-shaped, or sinusoidal in appearance. Although this discharge is an unreliable indicator of seizures, parasagittal lesions can give rise to rhythmic slowing in this same region and should be considered when this waveform is encountered on the EEG.

BREACH RHYTHM

"Breach rhythm" refers to the EEG alterations involving derivations from electrodes placed over the region of a skull defect. In a breach rhythm, the EEG characteristically shows an increase in background amplitude and an increased representation of lower-frequency waveforms in the affected area.[23] The waveforms in a breach rhythm also appear sharply contoured, which may cause confusion with epileptogenic sharp waves.[6] Figure 5-2 shows a breach rhythm in a patient who had undergone temporal lobectomy previously; the increased amplitude, slow-wave changes, and sharp contour of the electrocerebral activity in the left temporal derivations are evident. The EEG interpreter should be cautious not to overcall the epileptogenicity of sharply contoured waveforms in patients with a breach rhythm, as doing so may overestimate their seizure potential.

Spike-like Benign Variants

SMALL SHARP SPIKES

Small sharp spikes, also known as benign sporadic sleep spikes and benign epileptiform transients of sleep, are monophasic or biphasic spikes localized to the temporal regions. On ipsilateral ear-reference recordings, the field may involve the bifrontal regions. The waveforms sometimes show a downward deflection on ear-referential montages due to surface negativity at the ear reference, giving a "stalactite" or "icicle" appearance. They may be unilateral or bilateral, and are typically present in drowsiness and light sleep, resolving upon arousal and during deeper levels of sleep. Their reported prevalence ranges from 2.5 to 24 percent.[7,24] Although some investigators have reported small sharp spikes to be more prevalent in patients with focal epilepsy than in nonepilepsy populations,[24,25] the general consensus is that they are nonspecific and not uncommon in the nonepileptic population.[26,27]

The morphologic features of small sharp spikes are well described.[26] They are typically low-amplitude waveforms (less than 50 μV) of short duration (less than 50 msec), with a monophasic or biphasic morphology. Biphasic waveforms typically show a steep descending slope (see Fig. 5-3). In contrast to epileptogenic temporal spike-wave discharges, the slow waves associated with small sharp spikes (if present at all) are much lower in amplitude and brief (less than 100 msec duration).

14- AND 6-HZ POSITIVE SPIKES (CTENOIDS)

Discharges of 14- and 6-Hz positive spikes, previously referred to as "ctenoids", consist of arciform discharges featuring surface-positive spikes which are usually maximal in amplitude over the temporal and posterior head regions (see Figure 5-3). They are best seen in montages utilizing long interelectrode distances. The discharges typically last for 1 to 2 seconds and are most often bilateral in distribution. This EEG finding at one time was thought to correlate with juvenile delinquency, as well as a number of other neurologic conditions including migraine and attention deficit–hyperactivity disorder.[28,29] However, no clinical condition has been found to be associated specifically with 14- and 6-Hz activity, and they can be found in the normal population.[30] Discharges of

14- and 6-Hz positive spikes are most common in adolescents and young adults, and have a reported prevalence ranging from 0.5 to 5.7 percent.[7,10,28]

6-HZ ("PHANTOM") SPIKE-WAVE ACTIVITY

"Phantom" or 6-Hz spike-wave activity consists of 1- to 2-second clusters of moderate-amplitude theta activity having a frequency ranging from 5 to 7 Hz. These complexes characteristically are associated with a low-amplitude spike, referred to as a "phantom" spike.[31] Occasionally, the spike cannot be seen at all, resulting in a rhythmic theta discharge over the posterior or anterior head regions. As is typical for benign EEG variants, 6-Hz spike-wave complexes are characteristically present in drowsiness and resolve in deeper levels of sleep and upon arousal. Their prevalence in the EEG laboratory has been reported to be 2.5 percent.[7]

There are two forms of 6-Hz spike-wave activity, known as the anterior and posterior variants.[32] The posterior variant is known by the acronym FOLD (female, occipital, low amplitude, and drowsiness), and the anterior variant has been referred to as WHAM (wake, high amplitude, anterior, and male). Over the years, it has become less clear that there is a significant gender difference between the two forms. However, the distinction between anterior and posterior variants still has some clinical merit, as the anterior variant may be seen in patients with idiopathic generalized epilepsy on antiepileptic medication, in whom generalized spike-wave activity may emerge upon medication withdrawal. An example of the posterior variant of 6-Hz spike-wave activity is shown in Figure 5-3.

ARTIFACTS

Artifacts are unavoidable in EEG practice. The potential sources of EEG artifact are almost innumerable and change with the times.[3,33] For example, in the era before air conditioning, sweat artifact was ubiquitous in hot seasons but it is very uncommon now; conversely, laptop computer artifact did not exist in previous generations but is not rare now, particularly in the setting of epilepsy monitoring units. Artifacts may resemble cortical activity and in some cases can obscure the EEG, thereby posing many challenges for the electroencephalographer. Artifacts can mimic rhythmic or sporadic delta activity, sharp waves, spikes, and electrographic seizures. Failure to recognize artifacts may lead to false-positive reports, which may contribute to errors in clinical management. Artifacts can be categorized as physiologic, technical, and environmental, based

TABLE 5-2 ▪ Sources of EEG Artifact Categorized by Type

PHYSIOLOGIC SOURCES

Eyes (eye blinks, flutter, slow eye movements, nystagmus, electroretinogram)

Cardiorespiratory (electrocardiogram, ballistocardiogram, pulse, pacemaker, resuscitation, respirations)

Muscle (frontalis and temporalis myogenic activity, nuchal rhythmic muscle artifact, myokymia, hemifacial spasm, palatal myoclonus)

Sweat (sweat artifact, psychogalvanic response)

Tongue (glossokinetic)

EQUIPMENT AND TECHNICAL SOURCES

Electrode-associated (high impedance, interchanged electrodes, salt-bridging)

Acquisition settings (filter selection, sensitivity)

Plug, jack box, amplifier, equipment switches

ENVIRONMENTAL SOURCES

60-Hz sources

Oscillating devices (ventilators, percussion beds, sequential compression devices, intravenous pumps)

Personal electronic equipment (cell phones, laptop computers)

Patient care (patting, rocking, chest physiotherapy, cardiorespiratory resuscitation)

on their source. Some of the more common and interesting artifacts encountered in clinical EEG are summarized in Table 5-2. Recognition and prevention of EEG artifacts rely on the experience and diligence of both the EEG technologist and the interpreter. Video recording may facilitate their detection and identification of their source, particularly in patients undergoing prolonged EEG telemetry.

Physiologic Sources and Artifact Types

EYE-MOVEMENT ARTIFACTS

The eye has dipole properties that can affect the EEG. The polarity of the eye is such that the cornea is surface positive and retina is negative.[34,35] Accordingly, eye movements can cause significant changes in the EEG, particularly in those regions most closely situated to them. Some artifacts related to the eye are shown in Figure 3-4 and Figure 5-4. During an eye blink, the cornea deviates upward, leading to an *eye blink artifact*, which is identified readily as a brief high-amplitude deflection of positive polarity over the frontopolar regions. Eye blink artifacts are typically symmetric, except in patients with significant unilateral ocular pathology or eye enucleation, and in those with restricted movement of one eye (see Fig. 5-4).

Downward eye movements, such as in downbeat nystagmus (see Fig. 5-4), result in eye movement artifact with the opposite polarity of eye blinks, due to movement of

the negatively charged retina towards the frontopolar electrodes. Downbeat nystagmus artifact may be mistaken for a periodic frontal dysrhythmia if an ocular source is not considered.

Slow roving horizontal eye movements appear as 0.2 to 1.0 Hz *slow eye movement* artifacts on the EEG. Their presence is a defining characteristic of drowsiness. Slow eye movement artifacts are highest in amplitude over the left (F7) and right (F8) frontotemporal regions. A characteristic feature is that the polarity at F7 and F8 is out of phase at any given point in time, at least in patients with conjugate eye movements. For example, when the eyes move to the left, a surface positive waveform is present at F7 due to movement of the left cornea into its field, and at the same time F8 shows a surface negative waveform as the retina moves nearer to it.

Eye flutter consists of characteristic 3- to 6-Hz oscillations which primarily involve the frontopolar region. Eye flutter can be distinguished from a frontal dysrhythmia by its restriction to the most anterior derivations.

Saccadic eye movements or jerk nystagmus give rise to rhythmic delta waveforms over the frontotemporal regions. When accompanied by *lateral rectus spikes*, these artifacts may resemble spike-wave activity. Jerk nystagmus can be distinguished from cerebral delta or spike-wave activity by its characteristic morphology, which consists of a steep initial slope followed by a more gradual return to baseline, giving rise to a "shark-fin" or "sail-shaped" morphology. In horizontal nystagmus, the left and right frontotemporal waveforms are out of phase.

Electroretinogram (*ERG*) artifact may be observed during photic stimulation because of activation of retinal potentials. It consists of low-amplitude sharply contoured waveforms localized to the frontal regions that are time-locked to the flash frequency of the strobe (see Fig. 5-4). Confirmation can be achieved by covering one eye during stimulation, which results in attenuation of the artifact on that side, followed by its return when the eye is uncovered.

MYOGENIC AND TREMOR ARTIFACTS

Myogenic artifact is typically most prominent over the temporal and frontal derivations due to the proximity of those electrodes to the temporalis and frontalis muscles. *Chewing artifact* (see Fig. 3-2) can obscure the temporal channels, rendering the temporal regions unreadable. Temporal myogenic activity can be alleviated by instructing the patient to open the mouth slightly (Fig. 5-5). Myogenic artifact is typically decreased during drowsiness and usually resolves in slow-wave and REM

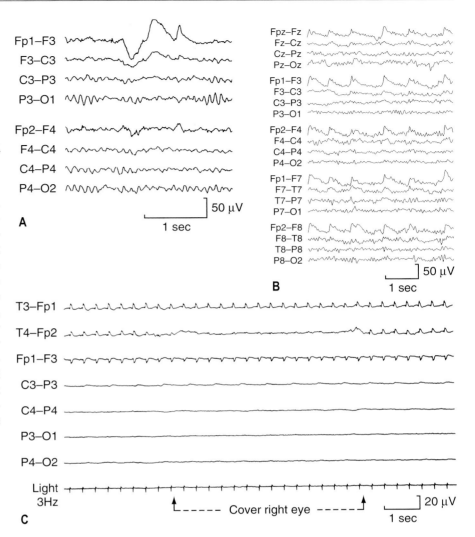

FIGURE 5-4 ▪ Eye-related artifacts. **A,** Asymmetric eye blink in a patient with right eye enucleation. (By permission of Mayo Foundation for Medical Education and Research. All rights reserved.) **B,** Downbeat nystagmus in a patient with a degenerative cerebellar disorder. Recording shows upgoing waveforms in frontopolar derivations, due to upward movement of the negatively charged retina. The waveforms also show an initial steep slope followed by slower descent, typical of the fast and slow phases of jerk nystagmus. (The F7/8 electrode placements are over the anterolateral frontal/anterior inferior temporal regions, and the T7/8 placements are over the inferior midtemporal regions.) **C.** Electroretinogram artifact over frontopolar regions, verified by attenuation at Fp2 upon shielding the right eye from the photic stimulus.

sleep. *Rhythmic nuchal myogenic* artifact may occur in patients with head and neck tremors and in the presence of nuchal muscle tension (see Fig. 5-5). In the latter situation, propping the head forward with a pillow may resolve it.

Finally, certain movement disorders affecting muscles of the scalp, jaw, or upper facial regions may give rise to alterations on the EEG. *Myokymia* is characterized by periodic bursts of low-amplitude high-frequency discharges, each burst lasting approximately 200 to 400 msec and recurring at 1- to 5-second intervals in affected regions (Fig. 5-6). *Hemifacial spasm* typically gives rise to prolonged high-frequency bursts involving electrode derivations overlying the affected regions, which last for the duration of the clinical spasm. Finally, *palatal myoclonus* may give rise to low-amplitude 2-Hz periodic 100- to 200-msec bursts on the EEG, which are thought to stem from detection of myogenic potentials arising from the pharyngeal muscles involved with the palatal

contractions. Artifact from palatal myoclonus is best seen on ear referential recordings, but they are not always detectable on the scalp EEG due to their low amplitude and distance from the recording electrodes (see Fig. 5-6).

CARDIOVASCULAR ARTIFACTS

Electrocardiographic (ECG) monitoring during the EEG facilitates identification of *ECG artifact*. ECG artifact tends to be most prominent on ear-referential recordings. Cardiac conduction abnormalities such as bundle branch block may produce rhythmic, sharply contoured, longer-duration artifacts that can be confused with periodic sharp complexes. Correlation with the ECG monitor allows clarification of the cardiac nature of the discharges in such cases (Fig. 5-7; see also Fig. 3-2).

Pulse artifact (see Fig. 5-7) consists of focal delta-frequency activity typically involving a high-impedance

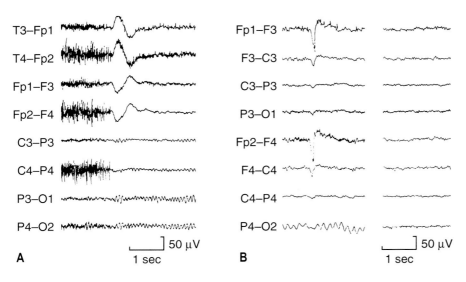

FIGURE 5-5 ■ Myogenic and tremor artifacts. **A**, Myogenic artifact from frontalis and temporalis muscles (left side of figure). This was attenuated by instructing the patient to open his jaw (right side of figure after eye blink). **B**, Tremulous myogenic artifact in P4–O2 secondary to tension in nuchal muscles (left side of figure). This was alleviated by propping the patient's head up with a pillow during the recording (right side of figure).

electrode situated over a scalp arteriole. Pulse artifact typically involves a single electrode distribution. Its nature can be confirmed by correlation of the waveform frequency with the heart rate on the ECG. The etiology can be established further by manual compression of the causative arteriole, which should suppress the artifact temporarily. Refilling the affected electrode to improve impedance, or moving the affected electrode to a nearby location, may be necessary to resolve the artifact. Failure to recognize pulse artifact may result in misdiagnosis of focal delta activity.

Other cardiac-related artifacts include *pacemaker*, *ballistocardiographic*, and *resuscitation artifacts*. Pacemaker activity may give rise to spike-like waveforms on the EEG. Ballistocardiographic artifact results from rhythmic body movement secondary to cardiac pulsations in high cardiac-output states. Finally, during cardiopulmonary resuscitation, artifact may be present due to chest compressions and may mimic periodic lateralized epileptiform discharges (PLEDs) or electrographic seizure activity.[36]

RESPIRATORY ARTIFACTS

Respiratory artifact typically consists of intermittent slow-wave activity correlating with the respiratory rate. It may present as delta-frequency waveforms occurring at 3- to 5-second intervals concordant with respiratory effort. This may be particularly prominent in patients on ventilator support.

SWEAT-ASSOCIATED ARTIFACTS

Excessive sweat may affect the EEG. *Sweat artifact* consists of very-low-frequency long-duration oscillations of the baseline. Sweat artifact typically involves more than one electrode region. The waveform duration generally ranges from 3 to 6 seconds. Observation of sweating by the technologist helps to identify the etiology.

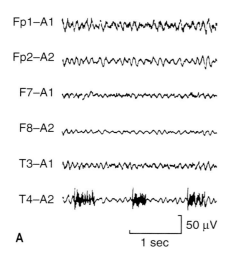

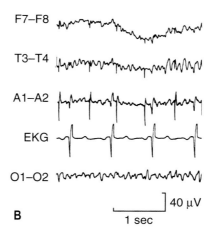

FIGURE 5-6 ■ Myogenic artifact in association with specific movement disorders. **A**, Myogenic artifact in a patient with myokymia, manifested by periodic bursts of intermittent high-frequency discharges maximal over the right temporalis region in this case. **B**, Intermittent low-amplitude spike discharges at 2 Hz in a patient with palatal myoclonus, demonstrated best in the A1–A2 derivation.

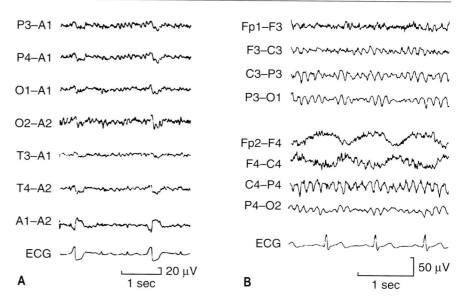

FIGURE 5-7 ■ Cardiovascular artifacts. **A**, Electrocardiographic artifact in a patient with a bundle branch block, resembling periodic sharp complexes. **B**, Pulse artifact mimicking focal delta activity over the right frontal region. Correlation of waveform frequency with the electrocardiogram (ECG) and limitation of the distribution of the waveform to a single electrode facilitates identification. (By permission of Mayo Foundation for Medical Education and Research. All rights reserved.)

Smooth muscle fibers associated with eccrine sweat gland secretion sometimes give rise to 1- to 2-second, bi- or triphasic potentials over the frontal regions. These discharges have been referred to as the *psychogalvanic* or *sympathetic skin response*.[37] The psychogalvanic response can be elicited by startle and noise, suggesting an association with adrenergic activity. It is uncommon, but when present can be confused with frontal delta activity.

GLOSSOKINETIC POTENTIALS

Glossokinetic potentials present as rhythmic 3- to 5-Hz activity that is diffuse but maximal over the anterior head regions. They are illustrated in Figure 3-5. Glossokinetic potentials may resemble frontal intermittent rhythmic delta activity (FIRDA), but their benign nature can be confirmed by demonstrating their correlation with tongue movement. This is achieved by having the patient repeat certain words involving lingual activity, such as "lilt," "Tom Thumb," or "la la la." Glossokinetic potentials result from the presence of dipole properties in the tongue, with the tip showing surface negativity and the base positivity. Glossokinetic potentials stem from direct-current potential changes occurring when the tongue tip moves into the vicinity of the anterior electrodes.[38]

Technical and Equipment-Related Artifacts

Technical and equipment artifacts are those EEG alterations that result from factors related to the EEG recording system. These artifacts can arise from a disturbance anywhere along the pathway between the patient and the EEG acquisition system. Potential sources of technical and equipment artifact include disturbances involving the electrodes, wires, electrode inserts, jack box, amplifier, and acquisition unit.

ELECTRODE ARTIFACTS

Most electrode artifacts occur when there is relatively high impedance between the recording electrode and skin. High electrode impedance may result in artifactual findings ranging from isolated electrode "pops" and focal continuous slow-wave activity to rhythmic pseudo-discharges mimicking seizures (Fig. 5-8). Rhythmic electrode artifact can be distinguished from an electrographic seizure by recognizing that the activity arises from one electrode derivation, with sparing of neighboring channels. In contrast, most electrographic seizure discharges involve more than one electrode region at onset and spread to neighboring cortical areas during propagation. Some exceptions to this are worth noting; neonatal seizures may be limited to a single electrode distribution.

Excessive electrode paste between two electrodes contributing to the same derivation may cause the EEG in that channel to be isoelectric This results from a "salt bridge" artifact due to equalization of the surface potentials at each electrode because of the increased conductance between them due to the excess electrode paste (Fig. 5-9).[39]

ELECTRODE PLUG, JACK BOX, FILTERING, AND AMPLIFIER CONNECTION ERRORS

Plugging an electrode into the incorrect insert on the jack box will give rise to an erroneous recording. This can be prevented by testing all electrodes at the beginning of the recording. If the error is not identified and corrected, the resulting EEG will show an unusual configuration compared to that expected because of misrepresentation of

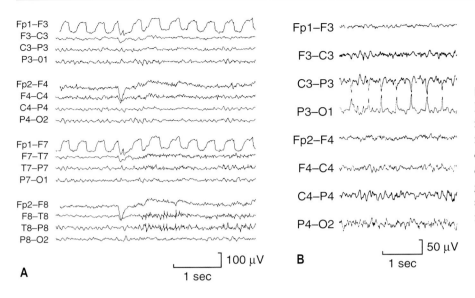

FIGURE 5-8 ■ Electrode artifacts. **A,** Electrode artifact at Fp1 resembling left frontal delta activity. This was later corrected by refilling the Fp1 electrode with electrode paste (not shown). **B,** Repetitive electrode artifact at P3 resembling electrographic seizure. Isolation of discharge to a single electrode helps to distinguish this from electrographic seizure activity.

the electrode location on the EEG (see Fig. 5-9). Recognition of these artifacts is challenging and requires significant experience with the normal appearance of the EEG.

Occasionally, electrostatic artifact due to switches on the EEG equipment may lead to a *switch artifact*. An example of switch artifact due to turning on a strobe light to test photic stimulation is shown in Figure 5-10. This is less common in the era of digital EEG.

Use of low- and high-frequency filters may obscure pathologic findings and make benign waveforms appear abnormal. For example, a low-frequency (high-pass) filter setting of 5 Hz may smooth out motion artifact but

can also interfere with detection of slow-wave abnormalities. Similarly, use of high-frequency (low-pass) filters may "round off" high-frequency myogenic potentials, converting a muscle twitch into a waveform resembling a spike or sharp wave.

In low-voltage recordings, such as in brain death, it is essential to confirm that all connections are intact and that the sensitivity and filter settings are appropriate so as to avoid the erroneous diagnosis of electrocerebral inactivity. An example of "pseudo-electrocerebral silence" corrected by replugging the jack box into the amplifier is shown in Figure 5-10.

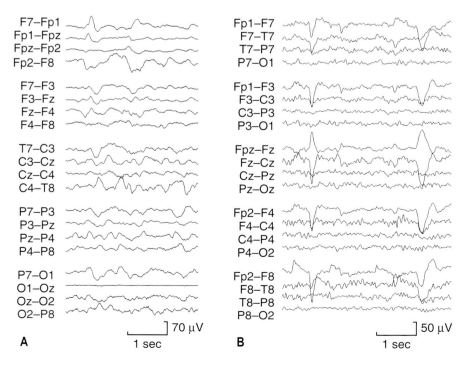

FIGURE 5-9 ■ Electrode artifacts (continued). **A,** Salt bridge artifact. Continuity of conduction paste between O1 and Oz results in an isoelectric recording at O1–Oz derivation. **B,** Artifact due to incorrect electrode insertion. In this case, Fz was plugged into the Fpz insert and vice versa, giving rise to erroneous eye-blink localization to Fz instead of Fpz.

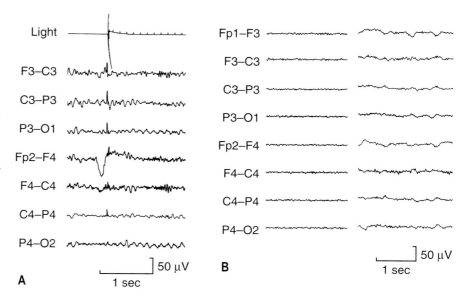

FIGURE 5-10 ■ Electroencephalographic artifacts due to equipment. **A**, Artifactual spike resulting from switching on a strobe light. **B**, Electroencephalogram (EEG) initially showing pseudo-electrocerebral silence in a critically ill patient (left half of figure). After correction of the inadequate jack box connection, the EEG shows that cerebral activity is present.

Environmental Artifacts

Electrical activity in the immediate vicinity of the recording may produce disturbances in the EEG. Given the high amplification needed for EEG acquisition, unwanted detection of alternate current from the facility's electrical infrastructure or other devices in the immediate environment, such as in the intensive care unit (ICU) setting, may affect the recording adversely.[40]

60-Hz Artifact

Alternating current in the recording facility may give rise to characteristic low-amplitude 60-Hz artifact that can obscure the EEG. Proper grounding helps mitigate this to some extent. It also should be recalled that the electrode wires may serve inadvertently as an antenna for environmental 60-Hz activity, which can be resolved by moving the wires. The 60-Hz artifact is often diffuse, but it may sometimes also be focal, involving electrodes with relatively high impedance. Refilling affected electrodes may help eliminate it in these cases (Fig. 5-11). The 60-Hz notch filter should be used sparingly, at least during acquisition, so as to not attenuate high-frequency cerebral waveforms.

Artifact from Personal Electronic Equipment

Use of a personal laptop computer during the EEG, which occurs commonly in the setting of the epilepsy monitoring unit, can give rise to a high-frequency artifact which may obscure the EEG (see Fig. 5-11). Cell phones also may introduce artifact, particularly when being charged in close proximity to the patient. A repetitive artifact that coincides with the ringing of a telephone is shown in Figure 3-3.

Intravenous Drip Artifact

Intravenous drips occasionally cause periodic brief electrostatic potentials on the EEG. This is seen particularly in high-sensitivity recordings such as in the ICU setting.

Patting and Percussion Artifact

Chest percussion during respiratory therapy and patting of the back, such as when consoling a small child or infant, may give rise to rhythmic "*patting*" artifact (Fig. 5-12). In the absence of direct observation via video monitoring, such artifacts may be confused with seizure activity.

Artifact from Oscillating Medical Devices

Periodic or oscillating devices in the immediate vicinity of the patient, such as intermittent compression devices, ventilators, and perfusion beds, may give rise to corresponding changes on the EEG. Careful observation by the technologist is required to identify the source in such cases. Rhythmic activity caused by a percussion bed is shown in Figure 5-12.

CONCLUDING COMMENTS

Identification of benign variants and artifacts is an important aspect of EEG interpretation. Benign variants may resemble potentially epileptogenic abnormalities, leading to misdiagnosis. Similarly, artifacts can be

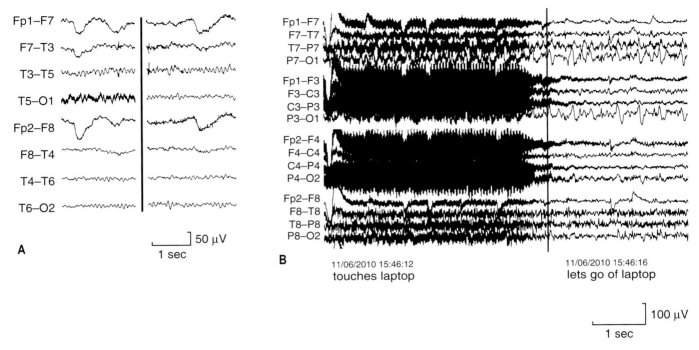

FIGURE 5-11 ▪ Environmental electroencephalographic artifacts. **A**, High impedance at O1 leading to 60-Hz artifact (shown in left half of figure at T5–O1), corrected by refilling the electrode with conductive paste. **B**, Laptop artifact in epilepsy monitoring unit recording. The artifact was present when the computer was touched while it was charging, and resolved after release of the computer.

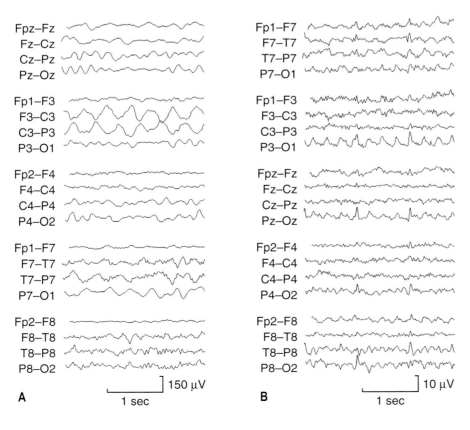

FIGURE 5-12 ▪ Environmental electroencephalographic (EEG) artifacts (continued). **A**, "Patting" artifact. Rhythmic delta activity identified over C3 and P7, correlating with the nurse patting the infant while the left side of the head rested against the nurse's chest. **B**, Percussion bed artifact. Diffuse rhythmic EEG alteration (best seen at P3–O1) in an intensive care unit patient correlating with use of a percussion bed.

mistaken for pathologic abnormalities. Correct identification requires astute observation, experience, and skill on the part of both the technologist and the EEG interpreter. Supplementation of the EEG recording with video can help clarify the source of artifact in some cases, and is particularly important in the ICU setting. Artifacts and benign variants should be considered possible explanations if an EEG interpretation conflicts with the clinical presentation. In such cases, repeating the EEG for the purposes of confirmation may be justifiable when such discrepancies cannot be resolved otherwise.

REFERENCES

1. Westmoreland BF: Benign electroencephalography variants and patterns of uncertain significance. p. 235. In Ebersole JS, Pedley TA (eds): Current Practice of Clinical Electroencephalography. Lippincott Williams & Wilkins, Philadelphia, 2003

2. Westmoreland BF: Electroencephalography: adult normal and benign variants. p. 119. In Daube JR, Rubin DI (eds): Clinical Neurophysiology. Oxford University Press, New York, 2009

3. Goldensohn ES, Legatt AD, Koszer S et al: Artifacts: patient generated and externally generated. p. 392. In Goldensohn's EEG interpretation: Problems of Overreading and Underreading. Wiley-Blackwell, Armonk, NY, 1999

4. Goldensohn ES, Legatt AD, Koszer S et al: Normal activity that resembles abnormal activity. p. 396. In Goldensohn's EEG interpretation: Problems of Overreading and Underreading. Wiley-Blackwell, Armonk, NY, 1999

5. Benbadis SR, Tatum WO: Overinterpretation of EEGs and misdiagnosis of epilepsy. J Clin Neurophysiol, 20:42, 2003

6. Westmoreland BF, Klass DW: Unusual EEG patterns. J Clin Neurophysiol, 7:209, 1990

7. Radhakrishnan K, Santoshkumar B, Venugopal A: Prevalence of benign epileptiform variants observed in an EEG laboratory from South India. Clin Neurophysiol, 110:280, 1999

8. Gélisse P, Kuate C, Coubes P et al: Wicket spikes during rapid eye movement sleep. J Clin Neurophysiol, 20:345, 2003

9. Krauss GL, Abdallah A, Lesser R et al: Clinical and EEG features of patients with EEG wicket rhythms misdiagnosed with epilepsy. Neurology, 64:1879, 2005

10. Santoshkumar B, Chong JJR, Blume WT et al: Prevalence of benign epileptiform variants. Clin Neurophysiol, 120:856, 2009

11. Mushtaq R, Van Cott AC: Benign EEG variants. Am J Electroneurodiagnostic Technol, 45:88, 2005

12. Westmoreland BF: Epileptiform electroencephalographic patterns. Mayo Clin Proc, 71:501, 1996

13. Lin YY, Wu ZA, Hsieh JC et al: Magnetoencephalographic study of rhythmic mid-temporal discharges in non-epileptic and epileptic patients. Seizure, 12:220, 2003

14. Klass DW, Westmoreland BF: Nonepileptogenic epileptiform electroencephalographic activity. Ann Neurol, 18:627, 1985

15. O'Brien TJ, Sharbrough FW, Westmoreland BF et al: Subclinical rhythmic electrographic discharges of adults (SREDA) revisited: a study using digital EEG analysis. J Clin Neurophysiol, 15:493, 1998

16. Foldvary N, Klem G, Hammel J et al: The localizing value of ictal EEG in focal epilepsy. Neurology, 57:2022, 2001

17. Westmoreland BF, Klass DW: A distinctive rhythmic EEG discharge of adults. Electroencephalogr Clin Neurophysiol, 51:186, 1981

18. Begum T, Ikeda A, Takahashi J et al: Clinical outcome of patients with SREDA (subclinical rhythmic EEG discharge of adults). Intern Med, 45:141, 2006

19. Zumsteg D, Andrade DM, Del Campo JM et al: Parietal lobe source localization and sensitivity to hyperventilation in a patient with subclinical rhythmic electrographic discharges of adults (SREDA). Clin Neurophysiol, 117:2257, 2006

20. Fleming WE, Avidan A, Malow BA: Subclinical rhythmic electrographic discharge of adults (SREDA) in REM sleep. Sleep Med, 5:77, 2004

21. Westmoreland BF, Klass DW: Unusual variants of subclinical rhythmic electrographic discharge of adults (SREDA). Electroencephalogr Clin Neurophysiol, 102:1, 1997

22. Westmoreland BF, Klass DW: Midline theta rhythm. Arch Neurol, 43:139, 1986

23. Cobb WA, Guiloff RJ, Cast J: Breach rhythm: the EEG related to skull defects. Electroencephalogr Clin Neurophysiol, 47:251, 1979

24. Saito F, Fukushima Y, Kubota S: Small sharp spikes: possible relationship to epilepsy. Clin Electroencephalogr, 18:114, 1987

25. Hughes JR, Gruener G: Small sharp spikes revisited: further data on this controversial pattern. Clin Electroencephalogr, 15:208, 1984

26. White JC, Langston JW, Pedley TA: Benign epileptiform transients of sleep. Clarification of the small sharp spike controversy. Neurology, 27:1061, 1977

27. Gutrecht JA: Clinical implications of benign epileptiform transients of sleep. Electroencephalogr Clin Neurophysiol, 72:486, 1989

28. Wang PJ, Tseng CL, Lin LH et al: Analysis and clinical correlates of the 14 and 6 Hz positive electroencephalographic spikes in Chinese children. Chung-Hua Min Kuo Hsiao Erh Ko i Hsueh Hui Tsa Chih, 32:272, 1991

29. Boutros N, Fristad M, Abdollohian A: The fourteen and six positive spikes and attention-deficit hyperactivity disorder. Biol Psychiatry, 44:298, 1998

30. Jabbari B, Russo MB, Russo ML: Electroencephalogram of asymptomatic adult subjects. Clin Neurophysiol, 111:102, 2000

31. Thomas JE, Klass DW: Six-per-second spike and wave complex: the wave and spike phantom. Neurology, 18:587, 1968

32. Hughes JR: Two forms of the 6/second spike and wave complex. Electroencephalogr Clin Neurophysiol, 48:535, 1980

33. Ebersole JS, Bridgers SL, Silva CG: Differentiation of epileptiform abnormalities from normal transients and artifacts on ambulatory cassette EEG. Am J Electroneurodiagnostic Technol, 23:113, 1983

34. Iwasaki M, Kellinghaus C, Alexopoulos AV et al: Effects of eyelid closure, blinks, and eye movements on the electroencephalogram. Clin Neurophysiol, 116:878, 2005

35. Lins OG, Picton TW, Berg P et al: Ocular artifacts in EEG and event-related potentials. I: Scalp topography. Brain Topogr, 6:51, 1993

36. Schauble B, Klass DW, Westmoreland BW: Resuscitation artifacts during electroencephalography. Am J Electroneurodiagnostic Technol, 42:16, 2002

37. Gutrecht JA: Sympathetic skin response. J Clin Neurophysiol, 11:519, 1994

38. Klass DW, Bickford RG: Glossokinetic potentials appearing in the electroencephalogram. Electroencephalogr Clin Neurophysiol, 12:239, 1960

39. Tenke CE, Kayser J: A convenient method for detecting electrolyte bridges in multichannel electroencephalogram and event-related potential recordings. Clin Neurophysiol, 112:545, 2001

40. White DM, Van Cott AC: EEG artifacts in the intensive care unit setting. Am J Electroneurodiagnostic Technol, 50:8, 2010

Video-EEG Monitoring for Epilepsy

JOHN M. STERN and JEROME ENGEL, Jr

Video-EEG monitoring (VEM) includes a variety of techniques used simultaneously to record electrical and behavioral characteristics of paroxysmal disturbances in cerebral function over extended periods.[1,2] It has been called "long-term monitoring" in the past; however, the increasing availability of the recording technology has resulted in it being used in a larger variety of clinical circumstances and for a greater range for durations. Clinically valuable results may require recording durations shorter than an hour or longer than a month. Overall, VEM is useful for investigating events that are difficult to record during routine electroencephalography (EEG) or involve key behavioral changes that are to be assessed in the context of the ongoing EEG. It is employed for four purposes: (1) to distinguish between epileptic seizures and other intermittent behaviors; (2) to characterize the electroclinical features of habitual ictal events in order to diagnose seizure type and, when possible, a specific epileptic syndrome; (3) to determine the frequency and temporal pattern of ictal events to identify precipitating factors and assess the effectiveness of therapeutic interventions; and (4) to localize the site of seizure origin in patients with medication-resistant seizures as part of the evaluation for surgical treatment.[3-6]

VEM is designed for the diagnosis of intermittent abnormalities that include behavioral change. Clinical situations wherein behavior is unchanging, but neurologic monitoring is needed, such as for a critically ill patient with neurologic disease, typically do not require video recording. Continuous EEG monitoring alone often is sufficient. However, if the critically ill patient is manifesting episodic behaviors of unknown neurologic significance, then simultaneously recording video and EEG provides insight into the underlying cause for the episodes. Simultaneous recording allows a direct comparison of behavior and electrocerebral activity. As such, VEM's usefulness includes recording for prolonged periods to capture an infrequent and unpredictable behavioral change, as well as recording for brief periods when the behavior is predictable or frequent. For brief recordings, an outpatient setting may be possible.[1,2]

VEM became readily available for long-term monitoring and as a clinical diagnostic tool in the 1960s as a result of two independent technologic developments. First, the use of stereotactically implanted chronic depth electrodes provided a means of easily recording ictal EEG discharges during complex partial and secondarily generalized epileptic seizures without contamination by muscle artifact.[7,8] Second, EEG telemetry was devised by scientists working with the National Aeronautics and Space Administration (NASA) in order to record electrophysiologic changes occurring in animals (and later, humans) put into earth's orbit. Combining telemetry technology with depth electrodes chronically implanted into brains of epileptic patients allowed artifact-free ictal EEGs to be recorded during spontaneous seizures occurring unpredictably over prolonged periods. Since then, many advances in VEM have occurred, and a variety of approaches are currently available. No specific approach is generally accepted for standard use; rather, each of the various technologies and methods has relative strengths and weaknesses that allow specific equipment and configurations to be chosen, depending on the needs and limitations of individual clinical facilities.

The American Clinical Neurophysiology Society and the International Federation of Clinical Neurophysiology have issued "Guidelines for Long-Term Monitoring for Epilepsy,"[1,2] which reviews available technologies and methods, and makes recommendations concerning indications for their use. The technology for VEM continues to advance. Nevertheless, the suggestions for a standard terminology for the most common subcategories of VEM, shown in Table 6-1, are still appropriate.

This chapter is concerned with the indications for VEM, the available monitoring equipment and methods of procedure, the interpretation of data, and recommendations for specific diagnostic purposes. The equipment and procedures discussed here are appropriate for VEM of adults and children; more details on adaptations necessary for application to infants and neonates can be found elsewhere.[9,10]

INDICATIONS

VEM can be expensive and labor-intensive, but it is cost-effective in many circumstances. Its use should be limited to diagnostic problems that cannot be resolved easily in the routine EEG laboratory.

Differential Diagnosis

VEM is often used as the ultimate test in the differential diagnosis between epilepsy and other disorders associated with intermittent or paroxysmal disturbances that resemble epileptic seizures.[11] A definitive diagnosis is made easily when habitual events are shown to consist of clinical behaviors characteristic of epilepsy and are associated with well-defined ictal EEG discharges, or when other etiologies can be clearly demonstrated (e.g., cardiac arrhythmias or sleep disturbances). Often, however, the events in question occur without obvious EEG or other electrophysiologic changes. In this case, a diagnosis usually is reached with reasonable confidence based on features of the ictal behavior in association with other clinical and laboratory information.

Focal seizures without amnesia or alteration of consciousness (traditionally called simple partial seizures) usually have no EEG correlates that can be recorded with extracranial electrodes.[12] Consequently, seizures without impaired consciousness are diagnosed most often by characteristic behavioral features and, at times, elevated serum prolactin levels,[13] rather than by the occurrence of ictal EEG discharges. Myoclonic jerks may also have no EEG correlates but usually can be diagnosed on the basis of characteristic motor signs.[14] Many other nonepileptic disorders can be recognized readily by clinical examination during the habitual event, by review of video recordings, or both. In most of these situations, however, the results of VEM merely confirm the clinical impression derived from historical and other information, and are not diagnostic in themselves.

The most difficult, and most important, differential diagnosis for which VEM is used is the distinction between epileptic seizures and psychogenic nonepileptic seizures. Because, by definition, psychogenic nonepileptic seizures have no abnormal EEG correlates, this diagnosis is usually one of exclusion. Certain features may distinguish them from epileptic seizures. These include: gradual

---

TABLE 6-1 ■ Terminology for Subcategories of Long-Term Monitoring for Epilepsy

Long-term EEG monitoring: scalp/sphenoidal electrodes; direct cable, no video

Long-term intracranial EEG monitoring: depth, subdural, epidural, or foramen ovale electrodes; direct cable, no video

Long-term EEG recording with video monitoring: scalp/sphenoidal electrodes; direct cable, video

Long-term intracranial EEG recording with video monitoring: depth, subdural, epidural, or foramen ovale electrodes; direct cable, video

Long-term EEG telemetry: scalp/sphenoidal electrodes, cable or radio telemetry, no video

Long-term intracranial EEG telemetry: depth, subdural, epidural, or foramen ovale electrodes; cable or radio telemetry, no video

Long-term EEG telemetry with video monitoring: scalp/sphenoidal electrodes, cable or radio telemetry, video

Long-term intracranial EEG telemetry with video monitoring: depth, subdural, epidural, or foramen ovale electrodes; cable or radio telemetry, video

EEG ambulatory recording: scalp/sphenoidal electrodes, ambulatory recording

onset, eye closure, waxing and waning motor activity, uncoordinated nonsynchronous thrashing or undulation of the limbs, quivering, pelvic thrusting, side-to-side head movements, opisthotonic posturing, weeping, screaming and talking throughout the ictal episode, prolongation for many minutes or even hours, abrupt termination without postictal confusion, evidence of some recall during the ictal event, and features that are not stereotyped but differ from one episode to another.[11,15,16] Any of these symptoms, however, can be epileptic phenomena, and differential diagnosis between nonepileptic psychogenic seizures and complex partial seizures is particularly difficult.[17] Furthermore, nonepileptic psychogenic seizures may be associated with autonomic changes (e.g., pupillary dilatation, depressed corneal reflexes, Babinski responses, cardiorespiratory changes, and urinary and fecal incontinence) as well as self-injury induced by falling or biting the lips and tongue.[11,16,18] Consequently, a definitive diagnosis cannot be made solely on the basis of ictal clinical features observed during VEM; other positive evidence (e.g., secondary gain) is necessary.

A conclusion that an ictal event captured by VEM is nonepileptic and psychogenic does not, in itself, rule out the existence of an epileptic condition, because some patients with epilepsy also have nonepileptic psychogenic seizures.[11,16] When the two phenomena coexist, it should be possible to obtain a history of more than one seizure type and to use VEM to record examples of each type to determine which are nonepileptic and which are epileptic. Based on this information, the patient and family can be instructed to record these events separately to determine the effects of antiepileptic and psychiatric interventions on each independently.

Nonepileptic psychogenic seizures, which are involuntary and as disabling as epileptic events, need to be distinguished from malingering, which is voluntary simulation, and from factitious disorder, which is self-induction of epileptic attacks for the purpose of gaining patient status.[19] This differential diagnosis sometimes can be accomplished by data obtained during VEM, but usually it depends on historical information.

Characterization and Classification

Patients with known epileptic seizures that do not respond to antiepileptic medication may be undergoing treatment for the wrong type of epilepsy. In this situation, VEM can provide crucial information that characterizes the epileptic events so that the physician can make a seizure diagnosis and, when possible, a diagnosis of a specific epilepsy syndrome.[5] Seizure type usually determines

the most appropriate antiepileptic drugs and whether a patient might be a candidate for surgical intervention. A specific epilepsy syndrome is often associated with a known prognosis, which is helpful information for the patient and physician.[20]

VEM is particularly useful for distinguishing focal from generalized seizures on the basis of characteristic ictal EEG features. It is important to distinguish the different epileptic causes of brief loss of consciousness, which can be a typical absence seizure, an atypical absence seizure, or a focal seizure characterized by impaired consciousness only. It may be impossible to distinguish between atypical absences resulting from bilateral or diffuse brain damage and focal seizures originating primarily from frontal lobe lesions with secondary bilateral synchrony.[21]

VEM is also useful for determining the degree of alteration of consciousness during focal seizures, particularly when trained personnel are available to examine the patient during the ictal event. Although this information usually has no direct therapeutic relevance, because all focal seizures are treated with the same medications, a definitive diagnosis can at times have medicolegal implications (e.g., a patient without alteration of consciousness might be allowed to drive), and it is important for counseling patients regarding activities of daily living. Documentation of the degree of disability during and after the seizure can be important in the decision about whether surgical treatment is warranted. More detailed tests (e.g., reaction time tasks) during ictal events can be used to identify subtle disturbances of function for the same purposes.

Determination of Frequency and Temporal Pattern of Seizures

When patients are known to have epileptic seizures of a specific type, but it is unclear how often these seizures are occurring, VEM can be used to determine the frequency of ictal events. Patients with seizures that involve relatively brief lapses of consciousness may not be aware of each ictal event; therefore they depend on observers to know whether therapeutic interventions have resulted in benefit. In these situations, VEM is a more accurate way of documenting seizure frequency before and after treatment. Unexplained deterioration in mental function can be caused by unrecognized brief daytime seizures or more severe nocturnal events. Knowledge about the occurrence and frequency of such ictal events is important for medicolegal reasons, for counseling patients regarding the activities of daily living, and for deciding whether surgical intervention is warranted.

VEM can reveal when seizures are most likely to occur. At times, this information is useful for identifying specific precipitating factors that might be avoided.[21] Combining VEM with serum drug level assessments can help to determine whether seizures occur because serum levels are subtherapeutic at specific times of the day, and it can aid in suggesting more effective drug dosing schedules.[22]

Localization of the Epileptogenic Region

The most common use of VEM is for localization of a discrete epileptogenic region in patients with drug-resistant epilepsy who are candidates for surgical therapy. Consideration for surgical therapy is essentially the only situation in which detailed information about localization is of clinical value. This localization includes not only identification of an area that can be removed when localized resection is contemplated, but also demonstration that no such well-defined epileptogenic region exists in patients who are candidates for nonlocalized therapeutic surgical procedures such as hemispherectomy and corpus callosum section.[6]

VEM is capable of revealing clinical signs and symptoms of habitual ictal events that have localizing value (see Appendix 6-1); however, these clinical behaviors may result from propagation to distant cortical areas and can never be considered definitive evidence of an epileptogenic region.[23] Consequently, identification of the area to be surgically resected usually requires clear demonstration of the site of electrographic ictal onset. Reliable localization of an epileptogenic region can often be determined with scalp EEG recordings, in association with a variety of other confirmatory tests; but at times VEM with intracerebral, epidural, or subdural recordings is necessary.[6,24,25] A variety of electrode types are used for this purpose, including depth, strip, grid, and foramen ovale electrodes. The performance of intracranial VEM requires specialized technical and clinical expertise to place electrodes, to guarantee patient safety in the recording unit, and to interpret the EEG data obtained.

In large part as a result of technical advances in VEM, approximately twice as many patients underwent surgical treatment for medically refractory epilepsy in 1991 as did so in 1985.[26] For some surgical procedures (e.g., standard anterior temporal lobectomy), 70 to 90 percent of patients with medically refractory focal seizures with dyscognitive features can expect to become seizure-free, whereas almost all of the remainder experience worthwhile improvement.[27–29] The results of VEM techniques are also used increasingly to guide extratemporal cortical resections with beneficial results,[25,28] and patients with secondary generalized epilepsies who would not have been considered surgical candidates only a few years ago are now benefiting from large multilobar resections and, to a much lesser extent, corpus callosum sections.[30,31]

TECHNICAL CONSIDERATIONS

Equipment, methods of procedure, and typical system configurations used for VEM are considered in this section, which is adapted, with permission, from guidelines published elsewhere.[1,2,32]

Equipment for EEG Recording

ELECTRODES

Disk electrodes are used for scalp EEG recordings; needles and electrode caps are not recommended. Electrodes should have a hole in the top to permit periodic re-gelling, and should be applied with collodion and gauze.

Sphenoidal electrodes sometimes are used to record from the mesial or anterior aspects of the temporal lobe in the region of the foramen ovale, but they are used rarely now because true temporal electrodes (T1/T2) usually suffice.[21,33,34] They are constructed of fine, flexible, braided stainless steel wire, insulated except at the tip, and are inserted through a needle guide, as illustrated in Figure 6-1. Sphenoidal electrodes may be left in place from days to several weeks. Nasoethmoidal, supraoptic, and auditory canal electrodes have also been used but are difficult to place; nasopharyngeal electrodes cannot lateralize and their use is discouraged.[21] Some investigators prefer to use a variety of basal electrodes (e.g., sphenoidal plus T1/T2, and other placements on the face and ear) to define the fields of basal epileptiform transients better.[35]

Recordings from the surface of the brain are performed with strip electrodes or grid electrodes, which can be placed epidurally or subdurally. Strip electrodes are inserted through burr holes, whereas grid electrodes require a craniotomy for placement.[25] Electrode strips consist of a row of stainless steel or magnetic resonance imaging (MRI)–compatible platinum disks embedded in Silastic, or a bundle of fine wires with recording contacts at the tips. Electrode grids consist of 4 to 64 small platinum or stainless steel disks arranged in two to eight rows and embedded in soft Silastic. The disks in strip and grid electrodes typically are spaced so that there is 1 cm from disk center to disk center. Strip and grid electrodes are

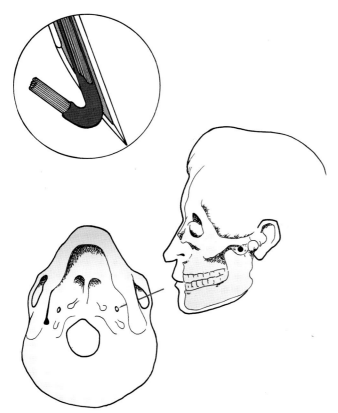

FIGURE 6-1 ■ The placement of sphenoidal electrodes. The needle is inserted approximately 2.5 cm anterior to the tragus immediately under the zygomatic bone (black dot on lateral view). The tip of the electrode should lie close to the foramen ovale (basilar view). Inset shows how multistranded Teflon-coated wire protrudes from the tip of the insertion needle and is bent backward on the Teflon coating to prevent breakage of wire strands. Inner lip of the needle can also be beveled to ensure further against breakage of the sphenoidal wire. (From Engel J, Jr: Seizures and Epilepsy. FA Davis, Philadelphia, 1989, with permission.)

preferred in patients with focal seizures whose epileptogenic region is likely to be in the lateral neocortex. Strips are easier to insert than grids and can be used bilaterally. Grids usually are used only unilaterally because bilateral craniotomy is rarely justified, but their extensive coverage allows not only accurate topographic mapping of interictal and ictal epileptic events but also detailed functional mapping of normal essential cortex.[36]

A variety of rigid and flexible depth electrodes are used for intracerebral recording.[25] Most are multicontact and are constructed of either stainless steel or metals compatible with MRI, such as platinum and nickel-chromium alloy. They are inserted stereotactically by several techniques that enter the skull from the side, back, or top of the head.[25] Depth electrodes are best suited for recording from structures deep within the

brain (e.g., the hippocampus and amygdala), orbital frontal cortex, and cortex in the interhemispheric fissure (e.g., supplementary motor area and anterior cingulate). Consequently, depth electrode evaluations usually are preferred in patients with focal seizures of limbic origin.[25] Depth electrodes also are useful when the evaluation requires bilateral coverage or coverage over a large region, although electrode strips also may be used in these situations, depending on the experience and preference of the surgeon.

Intermediately invasive electrodes are used at some centers. Foramen ovale electrodes are constructed of flexible stainless steel or MRI-compatible metals and contain one to four recording contacts.[24] They are placed in the ambient cistern through a needle inserted into the foramen ovale and record from hippocampal gyrus in a manner similar to the most mesial contacts of subtemporally inserted strip or grid electrodes. Although foramen ovale electrodes cannot record directly from hippocampus and amygdala, as do depth electrodes, and do not record as broad a field as strip and grid electrodes, they do have a definite advantage over sphenoidal and other extracranial basal electrodes. Epidural peg electrodes are inserted through twist drill holes in the skull; they can record from selected areas of the lateral cortical surface as an alternative to strip or grid electrodes.[24]

Foramen ovale electrodes may be used in association with grid electrodes for more comprehensive recordings of mesial temporal structures, including those on the contralateral side. Also, strip electrodes and epidural pegs may be used contralateral to grid electrodes as sentinel electrodes to identify the occurrence of distant ictal discharge, even though the spatial distribution of these epileptic events cannot be mapped. Similarly, strip or epidural peg electrodes can be used in association with depth electrodes to provide additional information about ictal discharges at the cortical surface.

AMPLIFIERS

Amplifiers used for VEM should have the following performance specifications: low-frequency response of at least 0.5 Hz; high-frequency response of at least 70 Hz; noise level less than 1 μV RMS; input impedance of at least 1 Mohm; common mode rejection of at least 60 dB; and dynamic range of at least 40 dB.[1,2,32] If a preamplifier is used, preamplification input impedance must be greater than 100 Mohm.[32]

Amplifiers should be able to capture a minimum of 24 channels or, more preferably, 32 or more channels at a minimum of 200 samples per second. The analog-to-digital converter should have a minimum of 12-bit resolution with the ability to discriminate the EEG at 0.5 μV steps or less.[32] To prevent aliasing artifacts, a high-frequency antialiasing filter with a minimum rolloff of 12 dB/octave must be used before digitization.[32] The maximum cutoff frequency for the antialiasing filter is determined by the sampling rate. For example, at a sampling rate of 200 Hz, the amplifier must have an antialiasing high-frequency filter no greater than 70 Hz. For higher sampling equipment, proportionately higher-frequency cutoffs can be used. For recording purposes, the low-frequency filter should be set at 0.16 Hz or less. The use of notch filters for acquisition is discouraged. Because VEM systems allow data to be modified when reviewed, frequency filters and gain of the recording system should be set initially to obtain maximum information rather than clean tracings.

Amplifiers may be mounted on the head, carried on the body, or positioned remote from the patient. The closer the amplifier is to the signal source, the shorter are the electrode leads and the less artifact that results from movement or interference. The amplifier is carried most commonly on the body because of size and weight. In scenarios where the patient has violent or continuous movement, the amplifier may be mounted on the head to minimize artifact. Small, lightweight amplifiers and preamplifiers are commercially available for this purpose. Movement and interference artifact is worst with remote amplifiers, and this arrangement is least satisfactory for recording seizures.

TRANSMISSION

Standard cable used for routine EEG is the simplest and most widely available means of transmission, but it greatly impairs patient mobility and is associated with the greatest amount of artifact. Telemetry refers to a system in which the EEG signal is amplified close to the patient, multiplexed, and then transmitted to a remote recording device, where it is decoded.[1,2] With cable telemetry, the multiplexed signal is transmitted over a lightweight cable that consists of a single wire that is long enough to allow the patient to move around the room. Cable telemetry is inexpensive, is associated with low interference, and is the most common form of EEG telemetry used; however, patient mobility is relatively limited. More mobility is possible with radio or infrared telemetry, in which signals are transmitted without a wire, but the range of these devices is still restricted, and there is increased interference with the EEG signal from outside sources. To overcome this patient restriction, some recently developed systems can store the multiplexed signal

directly onto flash memory within the amplifier/headbox and retransmit it to the system at a later time. This allows the patient to be unhooked from the system for moderate periods and to move about freely without loss of data. Although this does not offer the same degree of freedom as radio telemetry, it has the advantage of allowing patients limited periods in which they are not restricted by cable lengths without subjecting the data to radio frequency interference artifacts.

Ambulatory recording for longer periods is a specific form of VEM in which the patient wears the recording device and no remote transmission is necessary. However, because of limitations of storage, the number of channels are limited, and often these devices are event recorders and do not provide continuous long-term records.

Amplification close to the body and multiplexing of the resultant strong signal accounts for the major advantage of telemetry. The low-voltage signal travels only a short distance and so is less prone to movement artifact and interference from outside sources. Recordings of epileptic seizures, which usually are associated with considerable movement, are therefore relatively artifact-free compared with ictal recordings obtained in a routine EEG laboratory. These advances have made feasible VEM with scalp electrodes. Multiplexers typically combine 16 to 64 channels into a single channel of information, which then is demultiplexed at some later point. If the multiplexed signal is recorded and stored, the recording apparatus must have a higher-frequency response than if the signal is demultiplexed before recording and storage.

RECORDING, STORAGE, RETRIEVAL, AND REVIEW

Many methods of EEG recording and storage are currently available.[1,2,37–39] Current systems use analog-to-digital conversion methods, and the data are stored on a computer hard drive, server, or compact disk (CD)/digital video disk (DVD) media. Digital video allows data to be modified easily on review, and it is amenable to computer reduction and analysis. The storage capacity of the system depends on the sampling rate and the number of channels acquired. For 32 channels of EEG sampled at 200 Hz, a CD can hold approximately 20 hours of continuous data, whereas DVD media can store approximately 90 hours. Higher sampling rates and greater numbers of channels decrease this amount proportionately. A minimum recording capability of 30 GB or 24 hours of VEM is the guideline of the American Clinical Neurophysiology Society (formerly the American Electroencephalographic Society).

Systems that permit selected EEG storage employ a built-in time delay so that the data stored include EEG activity recorded both before and after the device is triggered.[1,2,39] Computer-recognized interictal or ictal events are used to activate the system, so only the events of interest are stored. Because computerized detection programs are not completely accurate, false-positive detections and failure to detect genuine events occur. However, this approach greatly reduces the amount of data that needs to be stored. Storage can also be activated by a pushbutton that the patient or an observer uses to identify ictal events. Such an event-recording approach requires that the patient or an observer be able to recognize when a seizure is occurring, and seizures that occur without warning or subclinically may be missed. A portable system is now available that allows computerized detection of ictal and interictal events for use with an ambulatory recorder.[39,40]

Digital video includes the ability to zoom in on the image after recording and the ease of EEG and video time-locking on review, but detailed zooming requires higher image resolution and therefore larger video files. Thus there is a trade-off between the quality of the image and the amount of video that can be stored. To overcome the difficulty with storage, most systems offer the ability to edit and delete unwanted video online before permanent storage, keeping only the clinically necessary video segments.

The most common method for review is to display both the EEG and the video on a high-resolution monitor. This has several advantages, including the ability to reformat the EEG montage, filter settings, and gain. In addition, the digital video image can be time-locked to the EEG via a cursor to correlate clinical behavior easily with the EEG. In order to display the EEG waveform accurately, the display must have certain minimal characteristics. The display should have a minimum scaling ability for each channel such that 1 second of EEG occupies approximately 30 mm, with a resolution of 120 data points per second.[32] Vertical scaling depends on the number of channels displayed, but a minimum of four pixels per vertical millimeter is required for accurate reproduction of the waveforms.[32] The system should also offer the ability to mark the EEG digitally for technologist comments, pushbutton events, and automatic detections.

The major advance in this area of VEM is the capability to record digitally onto disk or flash memory so that the continuous attention of an EEG technologist is not necessary. This has made 24-hour monitoring less expensive. The added refinements of computer-detected and patient-triggered selective identification and/or storage have reduced the amount of data that need to be reviewed. Techniques for rapid review of EEGs have also facilitated data analysis, particularly for ambulatory

recording, in which the addition of an audio channel has enhanced recognition of meaningful events.[37] The development of digital recording systems makes it possible to reproduce data on a high-resolution computer monitor in any montage, gain, or filter setting desired.[37,39] Movable time markers, spike maps, and other programs for analysis permit facilitated interpretation, and networking between workstations at multiple locations is feasible.

Equipment for Monitoring Clinical Behavior

Methods of monitoring behavior include self-reporting, observer-reporting, video and/or audio recording, and detailed monitoring of specific physical or cognitive functions.[1,2,37,38] Self-reporting requires the patient to make notes in a daily diary or log, indicating the occurrence of the specific events in question. This self-reporting can be accompanied by the use of a pushbutton that marks the occurrence of an event on the EEG tracing. Self-reporting is the common method of recording clinical behavior during ambulatory monitoring. Observer-reporting uses the same methods but someone else, such as a parent, maintains a log and activates the event marker. For inpatient VEM, specially trained nurses or technologists can be made available to examine the patient during a seizure in order to elucidate the clinical behavior and to elicit mental and neurologic deficits. A useful approach to the clinical examination during spontaneous epileptic seizures is shown in Table 6-2. Video and/or audio recording ideally is used in association with self- and observer-reporting, and is the usual practice for inpatient VEM. This approach

---

TABLE 6-2 ■ Clinical Examination During Epileptic Seizures

A. ICTAL PHASE

1. Mental status
   a. Determine responsivity to commands, orientation, language function
   b. Present a nonsense phrase for later recall, to determine amnesia
2. Motor
   a. Note site of initiation and pattern of motor symptoms, clonic and/or postural
   b. Note focal or lateralizing motor deficits during spontaneous movements and, if possible, provoke movements to confirm deficits
3. Sensory
   In special situations it might be useful to demonstrate a general analgesia to pinprick or to document a specific sensory deficit, such as ictal blindness

B. POSTICTAL PHASE

1. Observe spontaeous abnormal behaviour (e.g., automatisms, combativeness, or unresponsiveness); determine time course of resolution
2. Examine for specific focal or lateralizing neurologic deficits, including cognitive deficits
3. Test for recall of nonsense phrase given in A-1b, to determine amnesia for ictal event
4. Elicit description, if possible, of aura, behavioral seizure, and postictal symptoms

From Engel J, Jr: Seizures and Epilepsy. FA Davis, Philadelphia, 1989, with permission.

requires one or more video cameras (which are continuously focused on the patient) and a mechanism for synchronizing the video-recorded behavior with simultaneously recorded EEG activity. In selected situations it may also be helpful to use polygraphic instrumentation, continuous reaction time monitoring, or other automated techniques to identify specific physiologic or cognitive disturbances during ictal events. These data usually are recorded along with EEG activity.

A variety of black-and-white and color video cameras are available for use in VEM, including low light–level cameras and infrared cameras that can record in darkened rooms. A common approach is to use two cameras, providing a split-screen image with one camera focused on the entire body and the other on a close-up of the face. Lens irises are available that automatically adjust to changing light conditions. Remote zoom and pan-and-tilt devices allow monitoring personnel to maintain the patient in the desired place on the video screen. For large units with several monitoring beds, a full-time monitoring technologist can be employed for this purpose. For smaller units, nurses or EEG technologists can watch the monitor and make adjustments when they have a chance; however, information may be lost. An alternative approach is to allow the patient's family to maintain the appropriate adjustments of the video equipment.

Four approaches to auto tracking are currently available for video monitoring of patients who are moving around a large room. One depends on a radio frequency transmitter worn by the patient. Another uses a coded pulse of infrared light emitted from the camera, which is reflected off a strip worn by the patient and picked up by a detector on the camera. For the third, multiple cameras surround the room and the recording device determines which camera is recording from the patient by use of a computer that senses contrast. The fourth technique uses image processing to track specific defined features of the patient.

With modern systems, EEG and behavior are synchronized automatically when the data are stored digitally, and simultaneous display of EEG and behavior on the video image occurs with the reformatting technique. Clinical events are marked digitally on the EEG record at the appropriate point in time, and then re-reviewed by reading the EEG with the clinical notes. It is also possible to review the video time-locked to the EEG, simultaneously displayed on a high-resolution computer monitor. In this way, discrete periods of EEG and behavior can be correlated with each other.

Unidirectional and omnidirectional audio microphones can be used during VEM. Ideally, the microphone should eliminate unwanted extraneous noise but record the patient and observers who are describing ictal events. The most bothersome extraneous noise on VEM units is the television in the patient's room. Consequently, it can be useful to wire the pushbutton that the patient uses to signal the occurrence of an event so that it also automatically turns off the television set.

Methods of Procedure

ELECTRODES

Disk and sphenoidal electrodes should be checked periodically for breakage. Re-gelling of disk electrodes should be performed as necessary to maintain balanced, low impedance. Scalp irritation usually can be avoided if the patient uses a strong antidandruff shampoo before the electrodes are applied. Impedance is measured at the beginning, periodically during, and with ambulatory EEG at the end of recording. Impedance should be maintained at less than 5,000 ohms.

Malfunction of intracranial electrodes cannot be corrected after they are inserted; however, problems with the special connectors can be resolved, and these must be inspected periodically. Impedance measurements of intracranial electrodes can be performed safely with currents in the range of 10 nA. For patients with intracranial electrodes, the guidelines for indwelling devices should be followed (in the United States, UL type A patient).

RECORDING SYSTEM

The integrity of the entire recording system from electrode to storage medium should be checked before beginning VEM, and periodically during the monitoring. This is done most easily by observing the ongoing EEG and by having the patient generate physiologic artifacts. In addition, most systems have automatic impedance checks, can identify loose or bad electrode-to-amplifier connections, and have self-diagnostics to ensure proper recording parameters. The technician should also periodically review the record files to ensure that they are being stored properly. All instruments should also be calibrated as suggested by the manufacturer. More specific calibration systems are recommended for ambulatory EEG recorders.

RECORDING TECHNIQUES

Although a minimum of 24 channels is recommended for VEM, 32 or more are used routinely and are particularly necessary when basal electrodes are employed.[1,2,32] Thirty-two channels are standard for scalp and sphenoidal VEM to localize epileptogenic regions for surgery;

96 or more channels are being used increasingly with intracranial electrodes. Ambulatory recordings with 24 channels are now also possible, with selective storage triggered by computerized spike and seizure detection and with an event marker operated by the patient or an observer.[40,41]

With most recording systems it is possible to record extracranially using a common reference, and then to review the data in any desired montage. The most useful montage for extracranial recordings with basal electrodes (e.g., sphenoidal, earlobe, or T1/T2) employs standard lateral temporal bipolar chains in association with independent bipolar chains involving the basal electrode sites (Table 6-3). Normal variants, such as small sharp spikes and 14- and 6-Hz positive spikes, are distinguished more easily from epileptic transients in this manner. Inclusion of C3/C4 electrodes on the basal electrode chain is useful when cancellation occurs between basal electrodes and T3 or T4. Montages used with intracranial electrodes vary greatly depending on the electrodes used and the cerebral areas of suspected involvement.

VEM System Configurations

Table 6-4 lists the common basic system configurations recommended by the American Clinical Neurophysiology Society[2] and the International Federation of Clinical Neurophysiology.[1] Although newer systems all use digitally acquired EEG and video, older systems are still available and in use for VEM, particularly in developing countries. Their configurations are summarized in this section.

Monitoring with paper printout only is appropriate for documentation, characterization, and quantification of clinical and subclinical ictal events and interictal EEG features over a period of hours, as is assessment of the relationship of these EEG events to behavior, performance tasks, naturally occurring events or cycles, or therapeutic intervention. It is not appropriate for evaluations that require the patient to move freely or when continuous monitoring is necessary for days. This form of long-term monitoring is relatively labor-intensive and becomes progressively more cumbersome with duration. At least 16 channels of EEG data and synchronized video monitoring are required for presurgical localization of epileptogenic regions with this and all subsequently described configurations. Because of the limitations of this method, it is no longer considered the standard of care.

TABLE 6-3 ■ Basal Electrode Montages for VEM

BASAL ELECTRODE (PG) MONTAGES INDEPENDENT FROM LATERAL TEMPORAL DERIVATIONS

16-Channel	12-Channel		
Fp1–F7	Fp1–F7		
F7–T3	F7–T3		
T3–T5	T3–T5		
T5–01	T5–01		
Fp2–F8	Fp2–F8		
F8–T4	F8–T4		
T4–T6	T4–T6		
T6-02	T6-02		
C3–T3	T3–PG1	or	C3–PG1
T3–PG1	PG1–PG2		PG1–PG2
PG1–Nz	PG2–T4		PG2–C4
Nz–PG2	ECG		ECG
PG2–T4			
T4–C4			
C4–Cz			
ECG			

BASAL ELECTRODE (PG) MONTAGE NOT INDEPENDENT FROM LATERAL TEMPORAL DERIVATIONS

Fp1–F7	Fp2–F8
F7–PG1	F8–PG2
PG1–T3	PG2–T4
T3–T5	T4–T6
T5–01	T6–02

From Engel J, Jr, Burchfiel J, Ebersole J et al: Long-term monitoring for epilepsy: report of an IFCN committee. Electroencephalogr Clin Neurophysiol, 87:437, 1993, with permission.

TABLE 6-4 ■ Commonly Used VEM System Configurations

MONITORING WITH PAPER PRINTOUT ONLY

 EEG transmission: "hard wire" (standard cable) or telemetry (cable or radio)
 EEG recording/storage: continuous paper printout
 EEG review/analysis: complete manual review
 Behavior monitoring: self, observer, and video

MONITORING WITH CONTINUOUS STORAGE

 EEG transmission: cable or radio telemetry
 EEG recording/storage: analog or video tape, digital media (hard disk, server, CD/DVD)
 EEG review/analysis: selective review of clinical ictal events, random sampling review for subclinical ictal and interictal events
 Behavior monitoring: self, observer, and video

COMPUTER-ASSISTED SELECTIVE MONITORING

 EEG transmission: cable or radio telemetry
 EEG recording/storage: digital tape/disk, computer-assisted selective storage
 EEG review/analysis: selective review of clinical and computer-recognized ictal and interictal events on high-resolution monitor
 Behavior monitoring: self, observer, and video

AMBULATORY CASSETTE–SELECTIVE EVENT RECORDING/EPOCH SAMPLING

 EEG transmission: ambulatory flash memory or hard disk (16- or 24-channel)
 EEG recording/storage: flash memory, hard disk, or digital media (CD/DVD); event recording/epoch sampling (periodic or after trigger)
 EEG review/analysis: epoch review
 Behavior monitoring: self, observer

Monitoring with continuous storage is appropriate for the same purposes as monitoring with paper printout only, but for days and weeks rather than for hours. It is not appropriate for the quantitative analysis of subclinical ictal or interictal features or for evaluations benefiting from complete freedom of movement. Radio telemetry provides more mobility than does cable telemetry; however, video monitoring becomes difficult or impossible when this degree of mobility is required.

Computer-assisted selective monitoring is most appropriate for the same purposes as the previous two configurations, but it also records subclinical as well as clinical ictal EEG events. It is not appropriate for evaluations benefiting from complete freedom of movement. Computerized recognition programs generate false-negative and false-positive errors, so important data may be missed with this technique.

Continuous storage recording with computer-assisted event detection is preferred; it is used at most epilepsy centers. This technique reduces the amount of data that needs to be reviewed while maintaining the continuous data if a more detailed review is desired. Typically, the data are reviewed, and the technologist saves selected segments.

Sixteen- and 24-channel ambulatory monitoring is most appropriate for documentation and quantification of ictal (clinical and subclinical) and interictal EEG features and assessment of their relationship to reported behavior, naturally occurring events or cycles, or therapeutic intervention, when the data are most likely to be obtained outside the hospital or laboratory environment. With the addition of computerized spike and seizure detection, it is also appropriate for detailed characterization of EEG features for classification of seizure types and presurgical evaluation.[42] This configuration, as well as the other ambulatory configurations, can be used in an inpatient setting and is particularly useful when mobility is of benefit. The absence of EEG changes during a reported ictal event does not rule out an epileptic condition.

INTERPRETATION OF RESULTS

Artifacts

EEG data obtained using VEM techniques are likely to contain unusual artifacts that are uncommon, or never encountered, in the standard EEG laboratory (Fig. 6-2). These are often peculiar to the systems in use, and the electroencephalographer working on a VEM unit must become familiar with their appearance.

Scalp and sphenoidal electrodes show the usual biologic artifacts seen with standard EEG, but, in addition,

chewing, talking, and teeth-brushing can produce electromyographic (EMG), glossokinetic, and reflex extraocular movement potentials that are more difficult to identify. Intracranial electrode recordings are usually free from biologic artifacts, except for pulsation and respiration.

Altered electrode–scalp contact and intermittent lead-wire disconnection caused by body movement are the most common sources of mechanical artifacts during VEM. Artifacts induced by movement of a direct-connection standard cable are avoided when telemetry systems are used. Rhythmic mechanical artifacts produced by rubbing or scratching the scalp, or movements of the head or extremity (particularly when associated with accompanying biologic artifacts), can be mistaken for ictal discharges. Interference from nearby electrical equipment, including computers and video players plugged into power transformers, electrostatic potentials from movements of persons with dry clothing, or telephone ringing can also produce bothersome EEG transients. Mechanical artifacts caused by body movement and electrical interference are usually much fewer with intracranial than with extracranial recording.

Electrodes, wires, amplifiers, receivers, switches, reformatters, tape recorders, oscillographs, or any other part of the VEM system can potentially cause artifact. Electrode pops, faulty switches or connectors, and contact between dissimilar metals are common causes of spurious transients, whereas chipped silver–silver chloride coating, instability of the electrode–scalp interface, and electrode wire movement are the most common causes of rhythmic slow waves.

As with routine EEG, diagnosis of an epileptic ictal EEG event is made by recognition of well-formed spike-wave or other characteristic patterns with a believable field and typical ictal progression, followed by postictal slowing and appropriate interictal abnormalities in other portions of the record. Confounding artifacts caused by biologic and mechanical disturbances can usually be identified when simultaneous video-recorded behavior is available. For ambulatory EEG monitoring, when video is not available, it is standard procedure to have the patient and technologist produce common biologic and mechanical artifacts at the beginning or at the end of the recording, where they can be used as a reference for confusing transients on that tape. Conservative interpretation of unusual or equivocal EEG events is recommended.

Epileptic Activity

Interictal spike-wave discharges are identified on VEM, as on standard EEG, using artifact-free segments of the recording for analysis. Interictal spike-wave discharges

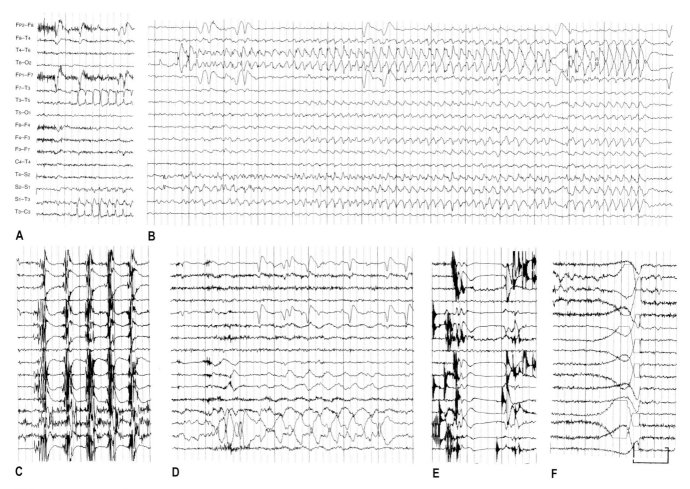

FIGURE 6-2 ■ Artifacts commonly encountered during electroencephalographic telemetry recordings. **A**, Tapping on T3 produces an artifact in S1 as well because the sphenoidal wire is curled under the head-dressing. This gives the false impression of a field; however, careful inspection reveals a double phase reversal. **B**, Scratching over the right posterior head region demonstrates how this apparent field effect can result in rhythms that resemble an ictal discharge. Again, the double phase-reversal provides the clue that this is not a cerebral event but a mechanical artifact. **C**, Rhythmic muscle activity is often seen during chewing. **D**, Many patients will rock their head wrapping back and forth in order to relieve itching and discomfort, producing regular or irregular slow-wave artifacts that have a wide distribution but display multiple phase-reversals. **E**, Intermittent sudden loss of signal usually indicates a poor connection. When the artifact is generalized, but some signal remains, as shown here, the most likely site of disconnection is the montage card, where the end of the card remains connected. **F**, Current telemetry systems are so good that movement artifact other than direct mechanical interference rarely distorts the signal. However, movement artifact, as shown here, can occur as the only consequence of a disconnected ground lead. Calibrations: 1 second and 100 µV.

recorded from depth electrodes are commonly much more widespread than those seen during extracranial recording, and they do not correlate as well with the location of the epileptogenic region.[43,44]

Ictal discharges recorded from depth electrodes can originate focally, from one or two electrode sites, or regionally, from several electrodes simultaneously. Focal onsets are believed to be more localizing, particularly when mesial temporal structures are involved, because regional onsets may represent propagation from a distant epileptogenic area that is not detected by available recording electrodes. Ictal onsets that originate simultaneously from both sides of the brain, or simultaneously from multiple intracranial and extracranial electrodes, are generally not useful for identifying an epileptogenic region.[43,44] Examples of focal and regional ictal onsets recorded with depth electrodes are shown in Figure 6-3.

Two distinctive types of intracranially recorded focal ictal onset-patterns are recognized. One consists of low-voltage fast activity that builds up over several seconds and resembles a localized version of the recruiting

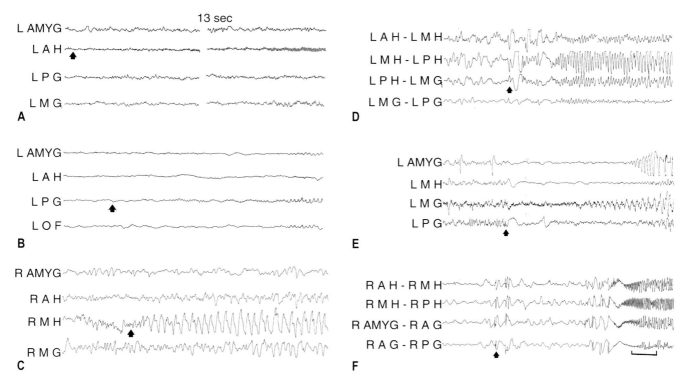

FIGURE 6-3 ▪ Segments of depth electrode electroencephalographic telemetry. Ictal onsets from six patients are shown. These tracings represent examples of progressively decreasing localizing value. **A**, Very-low-voltage fast activity seen initially only as thickening of the trace (arrow) isolated to the left anterior hippocampal pes (LAH); this continues for 17 seconds before it is barely seen at other areas. **B**, Low-voltage fast activity of much lower frequency than that seen in part A begins (arrow) at the left posterior hippocampal gyrus (LPG) and appears in all depth leads on the left after 5 seconds. **C**, Sharp activity of 4 to 5 Hz begins in the right middle hippocampal pes (RMH) (arrow) and 1 second later is reflected slightly in all depth electrodes on the right. **D**, Sharp activity begins with phase reversal in the left posterior hippocampal pes (LPH) (arrow) and remains most prominent there, although it is reflected in all the other depth electrodes. **E**, Ictal rhythmic activity first appears in the left middle hippocampal gyrus (LMG) and later spreads to other depth electrodes; this is preceded by a regional suppression (arrow) involving all left temporal depth electrodes. **F**, Ictal discharges begin with irregular, regionally synchronous spike, polyspike, and slow-wave bursts followed by a buildup of low-voltage fast activity, which is also synchronous in both hippocampal pes and gyrus. Calibration: 1 second. For each sample, channels not shown recorded from homologous contralateral depth sites, extratemporal, skull, and sphenoidal derivations. (From Engel J, Jr, Crandall PH, Rausch R: The partial epilepsies. p. 1349. In Rosenberg RN [ed]: The Clinical Neurosciences. Vol 2. Churchill Livingstone, New York, 1983, with permission.)

rhythm of generalized tonic-clonic convulsions (Fig. 6-4, *A*). A variation of this pattern is suppression of ongoing EEG activity. The second type, typical of hippocampal onset, consists of localized high-amplitude spike or spike-wave discharges, which may resemble interictal spike-waves and can occur at various frequencies (Fig. 6-4, *B* and Fig. 6-5). Some may begin very slowly and increase in frequency as the seizure progresses, whereas others may begin with relatively rapid 3- or 4-Hz discharges. These latter patterns are more often subclinical or associated with auras, and commonly evolve into the low-voltage fast discharges that then propagate and give rise to focal seizures (Fig. 6-4, *B*).[45] Ictal EEG events that have no clinical correlate are seen most often when computerized seizure detection is used; these electrographic seizures are helpful in identifying the epileptogenic region and may also have prognostic significance.[46]

Ictal discharges, as seen with intracranial electrodes, may not be reflected in the scalp or sphenoidal EEG.[12] Particularly with mesial temporal ictal patterns, the initial discharge in the depth will continue for tens of seconds before propagating contralaterally, and only at that time do ictal EEG rhythms appear in the sphenoidal and, later, scalp derivations. On most (85 to 90 percent) occasions, the ictal onset will appear first in the sphenoidal electrode on the side of seizure origin, even though activity in the depth of the brain is usually bilateral at that time.[47] The early sphenoidal ictal pattern consists most often of characteristic 5- to 7-Hz rhythmic activity, which may occur at the outset or may begin after a more

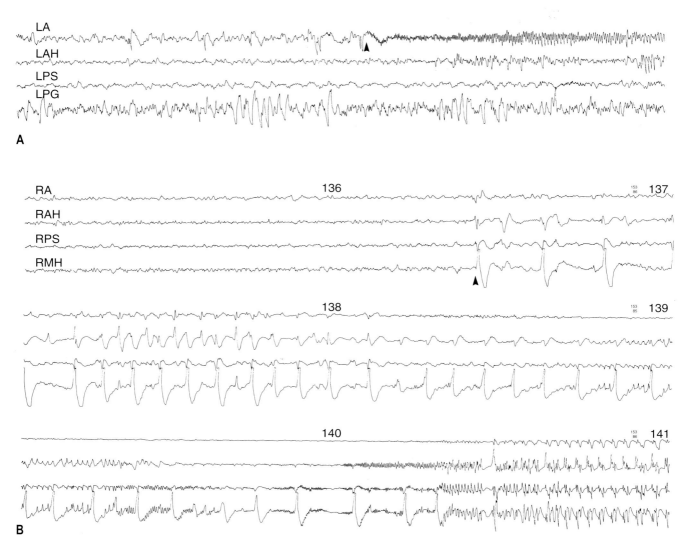

FIGURE 6-4 ■ Segments of telemetry recordings from two patients showing stereoelectroencephalographic activity at selected depth electrode bipolar tips during the onset of complex partial seizures. **A**, The classic depth electrode–recorded ictal onset consisting of a buildup of low-voltage fast discharge, here beginning in a single channel (arrow). **B**, Three continuous segments show a more common ictal onset-pattern, beginning with rhythmic high-amplitude sharp and slow transients (arrow), eventually giving way to a low-voltage fast discharge, which then evolves into higher-amplitude repetitive spikes or spike-waves. L, left; R, right; A, amygdala; AH, anterior hippocampus; MH, mid-hippocampus; PG, posterior hippocampal gyrus; PS, presubiculum. Calibration: 1 second. (From Engel J, Jr: Brain metabolism and pathophysiology of human epilepsy. p. 1. In Dichter MA [ed]: Mechanisms of Epileptogenesis: The Transition to Seizure. Plenum, New York, 1988, with permission.)

diffuse initial ictal EEG change. A delayed focal sphenoidal onset, defined as one in which the characteristic 5- to 7-Hz rhythmic activity develops within 30 seconds after any initial ictal EEG change that is not predominantly contralateral, has been found to be as accurate as an initial focal pattern in localizing the epileptogenic region (Fig. 6-6).[47] The ictal discharge is known to persist for long periods in one mesial temporal structure before propagating to the scalp EEG, and so the temporal relationship of the sphenoidal-recorded ictal onset and behavioral ictal signs

or symptoms was not considered to be important in this classification.

Ictal onsets recorded from both intracranial and extracranial electrodes can be extremely subtle and difficult to recognize. At times, they appear only as a change in the frequency of ongoing activity that is restricted to a few channels and is not consistent with a state change (see Fig. 6-3, *A* and *B*). Usually, the new activity is more rhythmic than the ongoing baseline tracing and may contain faster frequencies that are not seen in the

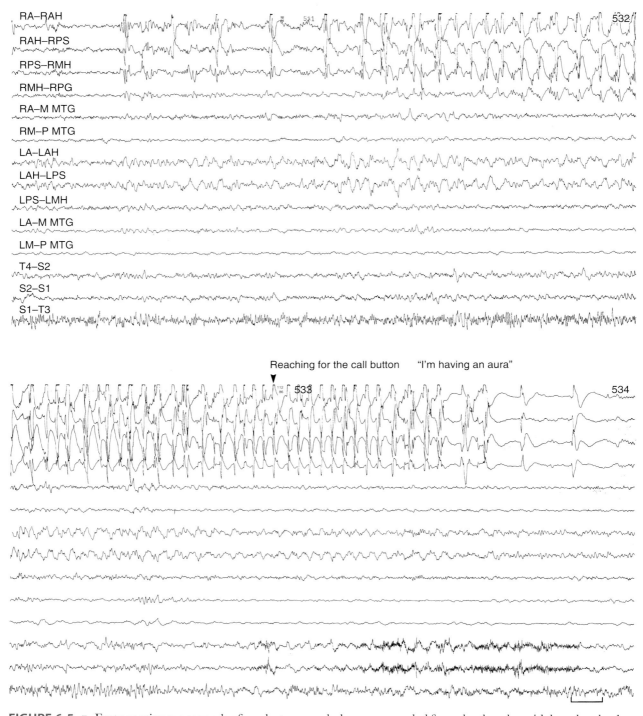

FIGURE 6-5 ▪ Forty continuous seconds of an electroencephalogram recorded from depth, sphenoidal, and scalp electrodes during a simple partial seizure involving the right temporal lobe. The ictal event begins in the left portion of the upper panel as an increase in interictal spike discharges that are maximal at the right anterior hippocampal electrode (RAH). After 8 to 9 seconds, these spikes become regular, eventually developing into a 3-Hz spike-wave pattern involving all derivations from the right mesial temporal lobe before ending abruptly in the right portion of the lower panel. Note that no low-voltage fast ictal activity is seen, either initially or at any part of the ictal episode. Videotape analysis indicated that the patient reached for the call button at the arrow, at which point regular rhythmic slow activity is also seen in the left anterior hippocampus (LAH) and the right sphenoidal (S2) electrode. The patient then indicated that she was having an aura, which consisted of a sensation of fear in her stomach. Calibration: 1 second. RA, right amygdala; RAH, right anterior hippocampal pes; RPS, right presubiculum; RMH, right middle hippocampal pes; RPG, right posterior hippocampal gyrus; RA-M MTG, right anterior-to-middle middle temporal gyrus; RM-P MTG, right middle-to-posterior middle temporal gyrus; LA, left amygdala; LAH, left anterior hippocampal pes; LPS, left presubiculum; LMH, left middle hippocampal pes; LA-M MTG, left anterior-to-middle middle temporal gyrus; LM-P MTG, left middle-to-posterior middle temporal gyrus. (From Engel J, Jr: Brain metabolism and pathophysiology of human epilepsy. p. 1. In Dichter MA [ed]: Mechanisms of Epileptogenesis: The Transition to Seizure. Plenum, New York, 1988, with permission.)

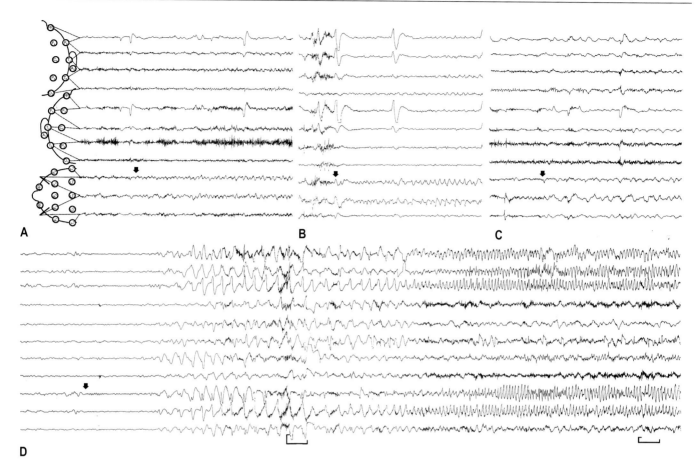

FIGURE 6-6 ■ Examples of electroencephalographic telemetry-recorded ictal onsets from four patients with complex partial seizures. **A,** Low-voltage 6- to 7-Hz rhythmic activity appears at the right sphenoidal electrode (arrow) 5 seconds before it is seen over the right temporal convexity (initial focal onset). **B,** Following a diffuse burst of muscle and eye movement artifact, low-voltage fast activity is recorded by the right sphenoidal electrode (arrow; initial focal onset). This becomes progressively slower, and the amplitude increases; 5 seconds later it is seen diffusely over the right hemisphere. **C,** Irregular, sharply contoured slow waves demonstrate phase reversal at the right sphenoidal electrode (arrow) and are reflected as low-amplitude delta, without phase reversal, over the right hemisphere (of undetermined localizing value). **D,** In this lateralized but not localized ictal onset, voltage suppression and low-voltage fast activity occur over the right frontotemporal area and are best seen at the right sphenoidal electrode (arrow). This precedes by 3 seconds the appearance of diffuse 3-Hz spike-wave discharges, which are also more prominent from the right frontotemporal and sphenoidal derivations. After 10 seconds, this latter activity evolves into high-voltage 7-Hz sharp-waves, which show phase reversal at the right sphenoidal electrode and laterally at the right anterior to midtemporal region (delayed focal onset). Calibrations: 1 second and 100 μV. Note that sensitivity is the same for parts *A*, *B*, and *C*, and the first half of part *D*, but decreased to half in part *D* at the first calibration mark. (From Engel J, Jr, Crandall PH, Rausch R: The partial epilepsies. p. 1349. In Rosenberg RN [ed]: The Clinical Neurosciences. Vol 2. Churchill Livingstone, New York, 1983, with permission.)

interictal recording. Such changes are much more likely to occur with intracranial recordings than with extracranial ones, although they do occasionally appear with scalp and sphenoidal recordings as well. The most common extracranial correlate of this ictal onset-pattern is a cessation of interictal spikes, because interictal and ictal events do not coexist. Consequently, the disappearance of frequent interictal spiking may be the only EEG evidence that a simple partial seizure has occurred, and ongoing interictal spikes often appear to stop several

seconds before a complex partial seizure is recorded from sphenoidal electrodes.

Nonepileptic Abnormal Activity

The presence of continuous focal slowing or focal attenuation of normal fast activity during the interictal state has important localizing value. Such interictal asymmetries recorded with depth electrodes implanted into

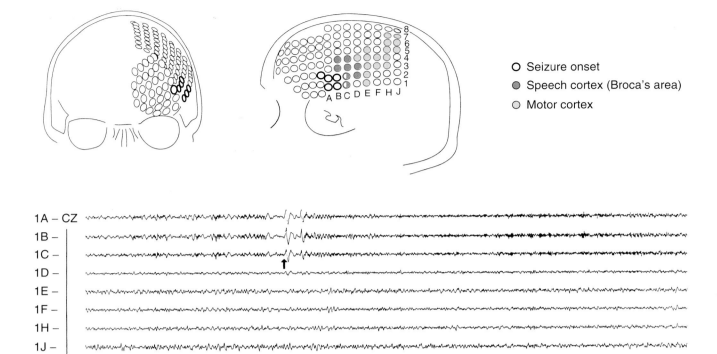

FIGURE 6-7 ■ Extraoperative functional mapping and ictal recording with subdural grid electrodes. Lateral skull radiographic outline shows placement of an anterior and a posterior grid of electrodes over the left lateral convexity. Electrode numbers are shown for the posterior grid, and the electroencephalogram below is derived from the bottom two rows of electrodes. Electrodes are identified where motor and language responses to electrical stimulation were obtained and where a typical seizure originated. This was a simple partial seizure of forced thought and speech arrest followed by a complex partial seizure with ictal vocalization. The electrographic seizure recording shows focal onset of low-amplitude fast activity and sharp waves (arrows) followed by sustained high-amplitude fast activity restricted to electrodes 1A, 1B, 1C, 2A, 2B, and 2C. Note that 1C and 2C are also over Broca's area. Left frontal resection included most of the epileptogenic zone and extended up to Broca's area. Calibrations: 1 second and 100 µV. (Adapted from Sutherling WW, Risinger MW, Crandall PH et al: Focal functional anatomy of dorsolateral frontocentral seizures. Neurology, 40:87, 1990, with permission.)

mesial temporal structures are indicative of hippocampal dysfunction and usually correlate with the presence of hippocampal sclerosis. It is therefore important to make use of VEM to identify nonepileptic abnormalities when the purpose of this evaluation is to localize an epileptogenic region for surgical therapy.

Functional mapping is an essential part of the presurgical evaluation when the epileptogenic region to be removed is adjacent to primary motor, sensory, or language cortical areas that cannot be damaged. Evoked potentials and cortical stimulation can be used to identify these areas extraoperatively, during VEM with subdural grid electrodes.[36] Maps of the epileptogenic region, derived from recording interictal and ictal epileptic abnormalities, can then be combined with the results of functional mapping to determine the boundaries of cortical resection before the patient enters the operating room (Fig. 6-7).

RECOMMENDATIONS

The American Clinical Neurophysiology Society[2] and International Federation of Clinical Neurophysiology[1] have indicated the following minimum standards of VEM practice for specific indications. Also, the American Academy of Neurology has published a practice parameter on epilepsy surgery[28] that impacts on the use of VEM for this purpose. When inpatient VEM is performed, an EEG technologist, monitoring technologist, epilepsy staff nurse, or other qualified personnel must be available to observe the patient, record events, and maintain recording integrity.

Presurgical Evaluation

The most exacting evaluation in VEM is the attempt to localize, by means of extracranial and/or intracranial electrodes, a region of epileptogenic brain tissue that is the site of origin of recurrent seizures and that is amenable to surgical removal. The following are minimum acceptable standards.

EEG TRANSMISSION

Standard cable ("hard wire") or EEG telemetry with at least 16 channels of EEG data is required. Cable telemetry is the most common methodology. Ambulatory EEG is not acceptable for final evaluation but may serve a useful triage function.

EEG RECORDING AND STORAGE

Continuous paper printout with time code is no longer the standard of care. Continuous or computer-assisted selective tape (analog instrumentation, video cassette, or digital) or disk (digital) recording of EEG with a synchronized time code and subsequent selective playback on paper or other high-quality display is recommended.

EEG REVIEW AND ANALYSIS

Detailed visual analysis of all seizures and representative interictal abnormalities from a paper printout or other high-quality display is adequate. Repeat analyses of seizures recorded on tape or disk with variations in playback parameters are preferable. Additional computer analyses of EEG abnormalities (temporal and distribution characteristics) may be beneficial.

BEHAVIOR MONITORING

Continuous video recording synchronized to EEG is recommended. Observer- or self-reported behavior is not sufficient. Time-lapse video recording is discouraged.

Diagnosis of Nonepileptic Seizures

Minimum standards of practice in the differentiation of nonepileptic seizures from epileptic seizures are the same as discussed earlier, although eight channels of EEG data are adequate for identifying most epileptic events. Regardless of the number of channels, however, the absence of clear ictal EEG abnormalities during a behavioral event must be interpreted with reference to the complete clinical evaluation before a diagnosis of nonepileptic seizures can be made.

Classification and Characterization of Epileptic Events

Although four-channel ambulatory EEG is adequate for documentation of certain interictal and ictal electrographic abnormalities, only systems with eight or more channels can provide basic characterization of epileptic EEG events. Classification and characterization of epileptiform EEG features are enhanced by an increased number of EEG channels, and at least 12 (preferably 16 or more) channels of EEG monitoring are needed for detailed analyses. The classification of epileptic seizures usually requires video documentation of the behavioral features, synchronized with EEG data.

Quantification of Electrographic Abnormalities

Four-channel ambulatory EEG is adequate for quantifying the frequency of occurrence of recognizable electrographic interictal or ictal events. In order to differentiate clinical seizures from subclinical ones, however, video monitoring is essential. The identification of the relationship of epileptic events to specific precipitating factors may require video recording or ambulatory capability, depending on features of the provocative stimuli or circumstances.

ACKNOWLEDGMENTS

Dr. Jason Soss contributed to the prior version of this review, which appeared in the last edition of this book. Drs. James Burchfiel, John Ebersole, John Gates, Jean Gotman, Richard Homan, John Ives, Donald King, Jeffrey Lieb, Susumo Sato, and Robert Wilkus participated in the preparation of the "Guidelines for Long-Term Monitoring for Epilepsy," from which large parts of this chapter were adapted. Original research reported by the author was supported in part by Grants NS-02808, NS-15654, and GM-24839 from the National Institutes of Health, and Contract DE-AC03-76-SF00012 from the Department of Energy.

REFERENCES

1. Engel J, Jr, Burchfiel J, Ebersole J et al: Long-term monitoring for epilepsy: report of an IFCN committee. Electroencephalogr Clin Neurophysiol, 87:437, 1993

2. American Clinical Neurophysiology Society: Guideline 12: Guidelines for long-term monitoring for epilepsy. J Clin Neurophysiol, 25:170, 2008

3. Nordli DR: Usefulness of video-EEG monitoring. Epilepsia, 47:Suppl. 1:26, 2006

4. Alving J, Beniczky S: Diagnostic usefulness and duration of the inpatient long-term video-EEG monitoring: findings in patients extensively investigated before the monitoring. Seizure, 18:470, 2009

5. Berg AT, Berkovic SF, Brodie MJ et al: Revised terminology and concepts for organization of seizures and epilepsies: report of the ILAE commission on classification and terminology, 2005–2009. Epilepsia, 51:676, 2010

6. Lüders HO, Comair YG: Epilepsy Surgery. 2nd Ed. Lippincott Williams & Wilkins, Philadelphia, 2001

7. Crandall PH, Walter RD, Rand RW: Clinical applications of studies of stereotactically implanted electrodes in temporal lobe epilepsy. J Neurosurg, 20:827, 1963

8. Talairach J, Bancaud J, Szikla G et al: Approche nouvelle de la neurochirurgie de l'épilepsie: méthodologie stéréotaxique et résultats thérapeutiques. Neurochirurgie, 20:Suppl 1:240, 1974

9. Burgess RC: Neurophysiologic monitoring devices for infants and children. J Clin Neurophysiol, 7:442, 1990

10. Gotman J, Flanagan D, Zhang J et al: Automatic seizure detection in a newborn: methods and initial evaluation. Electroencephalogr Clin Neurophysiol, 103:356, 1997

11. Rowan AJ, Gates JR (eds): Non-epileptic Seizures. 2nd Ed. Butterworth-Heinemann, Boston, 2000

12. Stern JM: Auras and other simple partial seizures. In Sirven J, Stern JM (eds): Atlas of Video-EEG Monitoring. McGraw-Hill, New York, 2011

13. Chen DK, So YT, Fisher RS: Use of serum prolactin in diagnosing epileptic seizures. Neurology, 65:668, 2005

14. Caviness JN, Brown P: Myoclonus: current concepts and recent advances. Lancet Neurol, 3:598, 2004

15. Charcot J-M: Leçons sur les maladies du système nerveux à la Salpêtrière. Recueillies et publiées par Bourneville. Vol 1. Paris, 1886

16. Lesser RP: Psychogenic seizures. Neurology, 46:1499, 1996

17. Krumholz A, Hopp J: Psychogenic (nonepileptic) seizures. Semin Neurol, 26:341, 2006

18. Reuber M, Elger CE: Psychogenic nonepileptic seizures: review and update. Epilepsy Behav, 4:205, 2003

19. American Psychiatric Association: Diagnostic and Statistical Manual of Mental Disorders. (DSM-IV-TR). In 4th Ed. American Psychiatric Association, Washington, DC, 2000

20. Engel J, Jr, Pedley TA (eds): Epilepsy: A Comprehensive Textbook. 2nd Ed. Wolters Kluwer, Philadelphia, 2008

21. Engel J, Jr: Seizures and Epilepsy. FA Davis, Philadelphia, 1989

22. Porter RJ, Penry JK, Lacy JR: Diagnostic and therapeutic re-evaluation of patients with intractable epilepsy. Neurology, 27:1006, 1977

23. Mathern GW, Sperling MR: Presurgical evaluation: general principles and methods. p. 1771. In Engel J, Jr, Pedley TA (eds): Epilepsy: A Comprehensive Textbook. 2nd Ed. Wolters Kluwer, Philadelphia, 2008

24. Wieser HG: Foramen ovale and peg electrodes. p. 1779. In Engel J, Jr, Pedley TA (eds): Epilepsy: A Comprehensive Textbook. 2nd Ed. Wolters Kluwer, Philadelphia, 2008

25. Spencer SS, Sperling MR, Shewmon DA et al: Intracranial electrodes. p. 1791. In Engel J, Jr, Pedley TA (eds): Epilepsy: A Comprehensive Textbook. 2nd Ed. Wolters Kluwer, Philadelphia, 2008

26. Duchowny MS, Harvey AS, Sperling MR et al: Indications and criteria for surgical intervention. p. 1751. In Engel J, Jr, Pedley TA (eds): Epilepsy: A Comprehensive Textbook. 2nd Ed. Wolters Kluwer, Philadelphia, 2008

27. Wiebe S, Blume WT, Girvin JP et al: A randomized, controlled trial of surgery for temporal-lobe epilepsy. N Engl J Med, 345:311, 2001

28. Engel J, Jr, Wiebe S, Fench J et al: Practice parameter: Temporal lobe and localized neocortical resections for epilepsy: report of the quality standards subcommittee of the American Academy of Neurology, in association with the American Epilepsy Society and the American Association of Neurological Surgeons. Neurology, 60:538, 2003

29. Berg AT, Langfitt JT, Vickrey BG et al: Outcome measures. p. 1929. In Engel J, Jr, Pedley TA (eds): Epilepsy: A Comprehensive Textbook. 2nd Ed. Wolters Kluwer, Philadelphia, 2008

30. Chugani HT, Shields WD, Shewmon DA et al: Infantile spasms. I. PET identifies focal cortical dysgenesis in cryptogenic cases for surgical treatment. Ann Neurol, 27:406, 1990

31. Roberts DW: Corpus callosotomy. p. 1907. In Engel J, Jr, Pedley TA (eds): Epilepsy: A Comprehensive Textbook. 2nd Ed. Wolters Kluwer, Philadelphia, 2008

32. Nuwer MR, Comi G, Emerson R et al: IFCN standards for digital recording of clinical EEG. The International Federation of Clinical Neurophysiology. Electroencephalogr Clin Neurophysiol Suppl, 52:11, 1999

33. Sperling MR, Engel J Jr: Electroencephalographic recording from the temporal lobes: a comparison of ear, anterior temporal, and nasopharyngeal electrodes. Ann Neurol, 17:510, 1985

34. Mintzer S, Nicholl JS, Stern JM et al: Relative utility of sphenoidal and temporal surface electrodes for localization of ictal onset in temporal lobe epilepsy. Clin Neurophysiol, 113:911, 2002

35. Lesser RP, Lüders H, Morris HH et al: Commentary: extracranial EEG evaluation. p. 173. In Engel J, Jr, (ed): Surgical Treatment of the Epilepsies. Raven, New York, 1987

36. Jayakar P, Lesser RP: Extraoperative functional mapping. p. 1851. In Engel J, Jr, Pedley TA (eds): Epilepsy: A Comprehensive Textbook. 2nd Ed. Wolters Kluwer, Philadelphia, 2008

37. Legatt AD, Ebersole JS: Options for long-term monitoring. p. 1077. In Engel J, Jr, Pedley TA (eds): Epilepsy: A Comprehensive Textbook. 2nd Ed. Wolters Kluwer, Philadelphia, 2008

38. Bergey GK, Nordli DR: The epilepsy monitoring unit. p. 1085. In Engel J, Jr, Pedley TA (eds): Epilepsy: A Comprehensive Textbook. 2nd Ed. Wolters Kluwer, Philadelphia, 2008

39. LeVan P, Gottman J: Computer-assisted data collection and analysis. p. 1099. In Engel J, Jr, Pedley TA (eds): Epilepsy: A Comprehensive Textbook. 2nd Ed. Wolters Kluwer, Philadelphia, 2008

40. Ives JR, Mainwaring NR, Schomer DL: A solid-state EEG event recorder for ambulatory monitoring of epileptic patients. Epilepsia, 31:661, 1990

41. Gilliam F, Kuzniecky R, Faught E: Ambulatory EEG monitoring. J Clin Neurophysiol, 16:111, 1999

42. Chang BS, Ives JR, Schomer DL et al: Outpatient EEG monitoring in the presurgical evaluation of patients with refractory temporal lobe epilepsy. J Clin Neurophysiol, 19:152, 2002

43. Lieb JP, Engel J, Jr, Gevins A et al: Surface and deep EEG correlates of surgical outcome in temporal lobe epilepsy. Epilepsia, 22:515, 1981

44. Lieb JP, Engel J, Jr, Brown WJ et al: Neuropathological findings following temporal lobectomy related to surface and deep EEG patterns. Epilepsia, 22:539, 1981

45. Velasco AL, Wilson CL, Babb TL et al: Functional and anatomic correlates of two frequently observed temporal lobe seizure-onset patterns. Neural Plast, 7:49, 2000

46. Sperling MR, O'Connor MJ: Auras and subclinical seizures: characteristics and prognostic significance. Ann Neurol, 28:320, 1990

47. Risinger MW, Engel J, Jr, Van Ness PC et al: Ictal localization of temporal lobe seizures with scalp/sphenoidal recordings. Neurology, 39:1288, 1989

APPENDIX

6-1

Behavioral Signs and Symptoms Associated with Electrographic Ictal Discharges Recorded from Specific Cerebral Areas*[†]

SEIZURES ARISING FROM THE TEMPORAL LOBE

Temporal lobe seizures have autonomic signs or symptoms, psychic symptoms, and/or certain sensory symptoms. Seizures of hippocampal-amygdalar (mesiobasal limbic or primary rhinencephalic psychomotor) origin often begin with an indescribable strange sensation, rising epigastric discomfort, or nausea. Other common initial signs and symptoms include fear, panic, and/or marked autonomic phenomena such as borborygmi; belching; pallor; fullness of the face; flushing of the face; arrest of respiration; and pupillary dilatation. Seizures of lateral temporal origin often begin with auditory or visual perceptual hallucinations, illusions, dreamy states, and/or vertiginous symptoms. Language disorders indicate involvement of the language-dominant hemisphere. Gustatory hallucinations may indicate involvement of parietal or rolandic operculum, and olfactory hallucinations may indicate involvement of orbital frontal cortex. Some focal seizures may begin with motor arrest followed by oroalimentary automatisms with amnesia for the ictal event. Common features of this type of seizure include reactive automatisms, duration of more than 1 minute, postictal confusion, and gradual recovery. Secondary generalization occurs occasionally.

---

*Signs and symptoms may be determined by functions of cerebral structures indicated, or their preferential propagation patterns. The information contained in this appendix was adapted in part from deliberations of the Commission on Classification and Terminology of the International League Against Epilepsy, chaired by Dr. J. Roger, and in part from the experiences of Dr. J. Bancaud and his group at the Hôpital Sainte-Anne in Paris. This appendix is reproduced with the permission of Drs. Roger and Bancaud, with the understanding that it often reflects an oversimplification of complicated anatomic interactions that are as yet incompletely identified. Although ictal behavioral signs and symptoms are useful for postulating possible anatomic substrates of epileptogenic dysfunction, such clinical information alone never definitively indicates the site of seizure origin.

[†]From Engel J, Jr: Seizures and Epilepsy. FA Davis, Philadelphia, 1989, with permission.

SEIZURES ARISING FROM THE FRONTAL LOBE

Frontal lobe seizures often have prominent motor manifestations, can include drop attacks, and may be mistaken for psychogenic seizures. Some seizure types commonly are associated with rapid secondary generalization or status epilepticus. Seizures may be brief and frequent, have minimal or no postictal confusion, and can be associated with urinary incontinence. Seizures involving supplementary motor cortex may have postural (including fencing postures) or focal tonic motor signs, vocalization, or speech arrest. Seizures involving cingulate cortex may be associated with changes in mood and affect, vegetative signs, and elaborate motor gestural automatisms at onset. Seizures involving orbital frontal cortex may be associated with olfactory hallucinations and illusions; early motor signs, including gestural automatisms; and autonomic signs and symptoms. Dorsolateral frontal lobe involvement may give rise to simple partial seizures with tonic or, less commonly, clonic signs and versive eye and head movements. The signs and symptoms of seizures involving frontal operculum and prerolandic cortex are described in the following with respect to seizures arising from multilobar regions.

SEIZURES ARISING FROM THE PARIETAL LOBE

Parietal seizures consist of positive somatosensory signs and symptoms, as described for seizures arising from the perirolandic area or an intra-abdominal sensation of sinking, choking, or nausea (particularly with inferior and lateral parietal lobe involvement); rarely, pain (either as a superficial burning dysesthesia or as a vague but severe episodic painful sensation); negative somatosensory symptoms, including numbness, feeling as if a body part were absent, or loss of awareness of part or half of the body (asomatognosia, particularly seen with nondominant hemisphere involvement); severe vertigo or disorientation in space (suggesting inferior parietal lobe involvement); receptive or conductive language disturbances (suggesting dominant parietal lobe involvement); rotary or postural movements; and/or visual symptoms as described for seizures arising from the temporo-parieto-occipital junction.

SEIZURES ARISING FROM THE OCCIPITAL LOBE

Occipital seizures usually, but not exclusively, include visual phenomena. Visual symptoms consist of fleeting visual perceptions, which may be either negative (scotoma, hemianopia, amaurosis) or, more commonly, positive (sparks or flashes, phosphenes), originating in the visual field contralateral to occipital cortical involvement; or visual perceptual illusions or hallucinations described for seizures originating at the temporo-parieto-occipital junction. Motor signs include clonic and/or tonic contraversion (or occasionally ipsiversion) of eyes and head, or eyes only (oculoclonic or oculogyric deviation), palpebral jerks, or forced closure of the eyelids. Nonvisual sensory symptoms include sensations of ocular oscillation, whole-body oscillation, or headache (including migraine). Ictal discharges may spread to produce seizure manifestations of temporal lobe, parietal lobe, or frontal lobe involvement. There is an occasional tendency for seizures to become secondarily generalized.

SEIZURES ARISING FROM MULTILOBAR REGIONS

Some seizure patterns are characteristic of more than one anatomically defined lobe of the brain. Features suggestive of seizures arising from the perirolandic (sensory motor) area can originate in either the precentral (frontal) or the postcentral (parietal) gyrus. Simple partial seizures with motor signs and/or sensory symptoms involve body parts in proportion to their representation on the precentral and postcentral gyrus. Thus involvement of face, tongue, hand, and arm occur most often. Common signs and symptoms, which occasionally may spread in jacksonian manner, include tonic or clonic movements, tingling, a feeling of electricity, a desire to move a body part, a sensation of a part being moved, and/or loss of muscle tone. Lower perirolandic involvement may be associated with speech arrest, vocalization, or dysphasia; movements of the face on the contralateral side; swallowing; tongue sensations of crawling, stiffness, or coldness; and/or facial sensory phenomena, which can occur bilaterally. Movements and sensory symptoms of the contralateral upper extremities occur with involvement of the middle and upper perirolandic area. Sensory symptoms and/or motor signs of the contralateral lower extremity, well-lateralized genital sensations, and/or tonic movements of the ipsilateral foot occur with involvement of the pericentral lobule. Postictal Todd's paralysis and secondary generalization occur commonly with seizures of perirolandic origin.

Features suggestive of seizures arising from the opercular (perisylvian, insular) area can originate in the frontal, parietal, or temporal operculum. Mastication, salivation, swallowing, laryngeal symptoms, epigastric sensations with fear, and/or vegetative phenomena are characteristic of opercular involvement. Focal seizures, particularly with clonic facial movements, are common. Secondary sensory symptoms include numbness, particularly in the hands. Bilateral movement of the upper extremities may be seen.

Features suggestive of seizures arising from the temporo-parieto-occipital junction commonly derive from epileptic discharges involving cortex of more than one lobe. Focal seizures often consist of visual perceptual illusions or formed hallucinations. Visual illusions include a change in size (macropsia or micropsia), a change in distance, an inclination of objects in a given plane of space, distortion of objects, or a sudden change of shape (metamorphopsia, more common with nondominant hemisphere involvement). Formed visual hallucinations may include complex visual perceptions, including colorful scenes in varying complexity; in some cases, the scene is distorted or made smaller, or in rare instances the subject sees his or her own image (autoscopy). Multimodality formed hallucinations may include auditory and occasionally olfactory or gustatory symptoms, and autonomic signs and symptoms appropriate to the visual perceptions. Vertiginous symptoms also arise from this region. Language deficits suggest dominant hemisphere involvement. Complex partial seizures often ensue, presumably owing to mesial temporal spread.

Invasive Clinical Neurophysiology in Epilepsy and Movement Disorders

WILLIAM J. MARKS, Jr, and KENNETH D. LAXER

Invasive recording techniques, in which electrodes are placed on or in the brain to record its activity, are important electrophysiologic tools in the presurgical evaluation and surgical treatment of patients with epilepsy. Similarly, intraoperative microelectrode recordings obtained from deep brain structures are valuable in guiding the surgical treatment of patients with movement disorders, particularly Parkinson disease, essential tremor, and dystonia.

INVASIVE TECHNIQUES IN EPILEPSY

Epilepsy Surgery and Localization of the Epileptogenic Zone

The pioneering work in the 1930s of Penfield and colleagues at the Montreal Neurological Institute established the effectiveness of surgical treatment in controlling seizures in some epileptic patients who do not respond adequately to medical therapy. Despite the wide range of medical treatments for epilepsy currently available, approximately 30 to 35 percent of persons with epilepsy continue to experience seizures.[1] For these patients with medically refractory epilepsy, surgical removal of the epileptogenic brain tissue is often an effective treatment.[1] Surgical resection is predicated on the ability to identify the seizure focus or epileptogenic zone. This area of the brain is responsible for the generation of seizures, and its removal or disconnection results in the cessation of seizures. Techniques for identifying the seizure focus are continually evolving and being refined. Although a number of components typically constitute the contemporary presurgical evaluation of patients with medically refractory epilepsy, ictal electrophysiology remains the "gold standard" in this endeavor. When the scalp-recorded electroencephalogram (EEG) fails to provide adequate electrophysiologic localization of the epileptogenic region, or when it suggests localization that conflicts with the findings from other elements of the preoperative evaluation (e.g., neuroimaging), invasive recordings are necessary to identify clearly the brain region from which seizures arise.

Role and Limitations of Surface EEG in Evaluating Patients with Epilepsy

The ability to record the electrophysiologic activity of the brain with the use of surface electrodes applied to the scalp is rather remarkable when one considers the relatively low amplitude of the signal compared with other biologic signals and with environmental noise, the attenuating effects of tissues intervening between brain and scalp, and the distance between surface electrodes and cerebral generators. Without question, the surface EEG is indispensable in the evaluation of epileptic patients. Its utility includes detection of interictal epileptiform activity, strengthening a suspected diagnosis of epilepsy; identification of focal abnormalities, suggesting a focal structural brain lesion as a possible basis for seizures; and documentation of specific epileptiform patterns associated with particular epilepsy syndromes.

The ictal EEG (i.e., the EEG recorded during a seizure) is especially important in defining the epileptogenic focus in patients with epilepsies producing focal seizures (referred to in past classification schemes as localization-related or partial epilepsy). Long-term recordings of the scalp EEG combined with simultaneous video recordings of clinical behaviors during seizures (video-EEG monitoring) are essential in the evaluation of patients being considered for surgical treatment. For patients to be good candidates for focal resective surgery (e.g., temporal lobectomy or frontal topectomy), their seizures must be localized electrophysiologically to one discrete brain region.

With current EEG technology, electrophysiologic seizure localization can often be accomplished with the scalp-recorded EEG; however, in approximately 30 percent of patients, the surface-recorded ictal EEG is inadequate for this purpose. At times, the surface EEG is simply not helpful in providing information of localizing value, whereas on other occasions it is misleading. For example, the EEG recordings may provide localizing but not lateralizing information, as when simultaneous bitemporal seizure onsets are found (Fig. 7-1). Similarly, the EEG may lateralize the seizure focus to the right or left hemisphere, but may not localize the epileptogenic zone to a particular region. Furthermore, the EEG can be misleading, reflecting activity predominantly in areas to which the seizure has spread and not the area from which it has arisen. To minimize this risk, the EEG findings localizing the seizure focus must begin with or precede the behavioral onset of the seizure as documented by the video recordings.

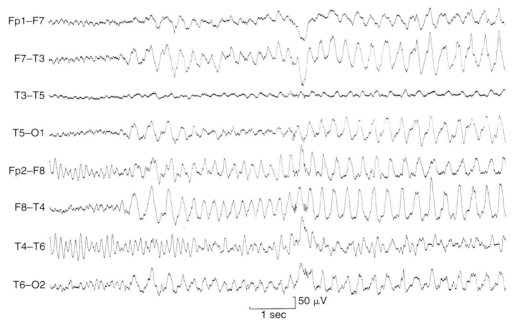

FIGURE 7-1 ■ Example of nonlateralizing ictal electroencephalogram recorded with scalp electrodes. Repetitive, sharply contoured delta-frequency activity at seizure onset is seen simultaneously over both temporal regions.

Role of Invasive Recordings in Evaluating Patients with Epilepsy

In patients with medically refractory epilepsy who are being considered for surgical treatment, invasive recording techniques are used in situations in which the surface EEG (recorded with scalp and sphenoidal electrodes) does not provide adequate localization of the epileptogenic focus or provides discordant localization in relation to other studies. These invasive techniques involve the surgical placement of intracranial electrodes in the subdural or epidural spaces or within the brain parenchyma (Fig. 7-2). No consensus exists among experienced epileptologists concerning the specific indications for one technique rather than another.[2] Regardless of the technique, the rationale is to place recording electrodes close to brain regions thought to be generating seizures in order to identify the epileptogenic region with certainty. In addition to their role in recording the electrical activity of the brain, arrays of electrodes contained on a grid can be located atop the cortical surface and used for mapping studies. These studies use cortical stimulation to identify areas of functional importance that are to be avoided in the surgical resection.

Invasive electrodes, when properly located, provide the obvious advantage of recording seizure activity directly from, or close to, its source. Nevertheless, for practical reasons, the extent of brain area sampled by invasive electrodes is limited, and therefore the ability to survey widespread areas of the brain (accomplished well by the scalp-recorded EEG) is sacrificed to varying degrees in invasive recordings. If invasive electrodes are not near the site of seizure origin, the recordings obtained may be misleading. Thus, the type of electrodes used and the areas in which they are placed in a particular patient are of critical importance. The placement of invasive electrodes is guided by the scalp ictal and interictal EEG, as well as by other studies, such as magnetic resonance imaging (MRI), single photon emission computed tomography (SPECT), and positron emission tomography (PET). Abnormalities identified on high-resolution MRI, especially the features that suggest the structural substrate of the epileptogenic region, provide important information for guiding the placement of invasive electrodes (Fig. 7-3). Other components of the evaluation that may be helpful in directing intracranial electrodes to brain regions likely to yield reliable localizing information include abnormalities identified on neurologic examination, the ictal clinical features (clinical behaviors and signs during the seizure, as discussed in Chapter 6), and abnormalities revealed on functional

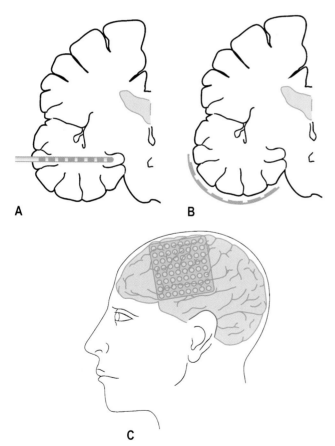

FIGURE 7-2 ■ Various electrodes used for invasive recordings in the evaluation of epilepsy and the representative brain regions from which they record. **A**, Depth electrode implanted with the orthogonal approach to record from the medial and lateral portions of the temporal lobe. **B**, Subdural strip electrode inserted to cover the subtemporal region. **C**, Subdural grid covering the frontoparietal and superior temporal regions.

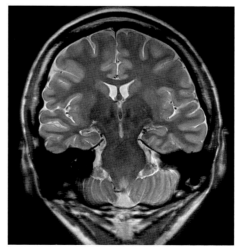

FIGURE 7-3 ■ Coronal T1-weighted magnetic resonance image from a patient with medically refractory temporal lobe epilepsy demonstrating right hippocampal atrophy (left side of image).

imaging studies, including PET, SPECT, and magnetic resonance spectroscopy (MRS). These factors must also be considered when one interprets the recordings provided by invasive electrodes.

Because invasive recording techniques, though generally safe, are associated with potential morbidity, they are reserved for patients who desire operative treatment and in whom surgery is considered appropriate. These approaches are necessary when adequate localizing information cannot be obtained by noninvasive methods. Specific intracranial recording techniques are considered in the following sections.

DEPTH ELECTROENCEPHALOGRAPHY

Definition and Indications

Depth electrodes allow the direct recording of cerebral activity from the brain parenchyma into which they are implanted. The indications for depth electrode recordings are not agreed universally, but the method is particularly well suited to investigating seizures suspected of arising from deep structures such as the hippocampus, amygdala, and medial frontal lobe. Seizures arising from these areas may be difficult to localize with surface recordings because of the closed electric fields and attenuation of the activity by the time it arrives, if at all, at superficial electrode sites. Furthermore, rapid transit of seizures to homologous contralateral regions sometimes precludes the ability to lateralize the area of onset of seizures, even with subdural electrode strips. For example, seizures originating from one hippocampus often spread quickly to the opposite hippocampus,[3] with scalp-sphenoidal or subdural recordings commonly reflecting an apparent synchronous onset of the seizure from both temporal regions. Depth electrodes, because of their unique ability to record seizure activity directly from the hippocampus, are often useful in establishing the hippocampus from which the seizures arise. In addition, the presence of bilateral, independent epileptogenic foci—not always obvious from surface recordings—can often be demonstrated with depth recordings.[4]

Techniques

Rigid and flexible electrodes constructed of a variety of metals and containing a variable number of contacts have been used for chronic depth recordings; the recent availability of electrodes constructed of nonmagnetic materials has allowed postimplantation imaging with MRI to document the anatomic location of the electrodes. Modern placement of depth electrodes utilizing MRI- or computed tomography (CT)-guided stereotactic techniques allows accurate and safe implantation of the electrodes through cranial burr holes with the patient under local or general anesthesia. The trajectory of electrode implantation depends on the location of the suspected epileptogenic focus and on the customary practices at the center where the study is to be undertaken.

Two common depth electrode arrangements are employed to study temporal lobe epilepsy: (1) an orthogonal approach in the horizontal plane, in which three electrodes are implanted on each side through the middle temporal gyrus, with the most distal contacts inserted into the amygdala, anterior hippocampus, and posterior hippocampus; and (2) a longitudinal approach, in which a single electrode is inserted through an occipital burr hole on each side and traverses the long axis of the hippocampus. The orthogonal technique offers the advantage of recording from both the medial and the lateral aspects along the temporal lobe but, compared with the longitudinal approach, requires a greater number of electrodes to do so.

Findings

The interpretation of depth recordings, as with all intracranial recordings, differs from that of surface EEG recordings. First, the electrode is in close proximity to the source of activity, and so the amplitude of the signal is relatively high. Various components of the signal (especially high-frequency activity) are therefore more robust than those recorded with surface electrodes. Second, depth electrodes record activity from a spatially restricted field.

The relevance of background abnormalities recorded by depth electrodes is not clear. Slow-wave disturbances and attenuation of background rhythms may be seen. Such findings do not necessarily correspond to the epileptogenic zone and may represent injury potentials secondary to electrode insertion. In addition, normal background activity is commonly quite sharp in configuration and may assume a rhythmic appearance. Interictal epileptiform abnormalities recorded by depth electrodes are typically of steeper slope, higher amplitude, and briefer duration than those recorded with surface electrodes.[5] The frequency of bitemporal spikes and sharp waves in patients with unilateral temporal lobe epilepsy (defined by ictal depth recordings) is substantially higher in depth recordings than that found in scalp EEG recordings.[6] Ictal patterns recorded at seizure onset with depth electrodes in temporal lobe epilepsy include attenuation of background activity; repetitive, sharp slow waves; rhythmic discharges of beta, alpha, or theta frequency; and irregular slow or sharp waves (Fig. 7-4). In temporal lobe seizures, intraparenchymal recordings

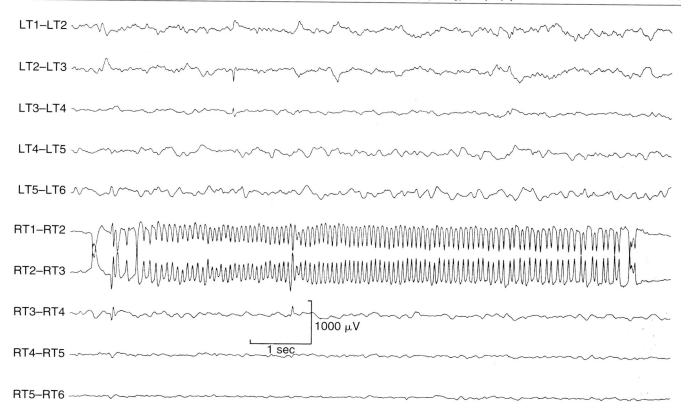

FIGURE 7-4 ▪ Ictal pattern commonly recorded with depth electrodes in medial temporal lobe epilepsy. Rhythmic sharp activity of abrupt onset, phase reversing at RT2 (the contact within the hippocampus) evolves in frequency before slowing and then terminating. Note that the activity remains confined to the right medial temporal region. LT and RT refer to the left and right temporal depth electrodes, respectively, inserted via a posterior approach; each electrode has six contacts, with contact 1 the most anterior and contact 6 the most posterior. Recordings are formatted into a sequential bipolar montage.

commonly demonstrate electrographic onset of the ictus earlier than do subdural recordings. Auras (simple partial seizures), although typically not associated with ictal patterns on scalp recordings, often correlate with electrocerebral changes that are detected by implanted electrodes. Similarly, subclinical seizures are detected more commonly by depth recordings. Focal seizure onsets, in which electrographic changes begin at one or two adjacent contacts of the depth electrode, most commonly are recorded from the hippocampus, but regional onsets may also be seen. Less often, seizures originate in a focal manner from the amygdala. In the absence of a lesion, seizures rarely are seen to arise from the lateral temporal neocortex.

Advantages, Limitations, and Complications

Depth electrode recordings from brain parenchyma provide a sensitive means of recording, with negligible artifact, activity occurring in a limited volume of brain in the vicinity of the electrode. Although the sensitivity and clarity of the signal are heightened with depth recordings, the constricted "field of view" inherent in all intracranial techniques results in the risk that the recorded activity originated from afar and propagated to a brain region sampled by the implanted electrode. Thus interpretation of depth recordings must be performed within the larger context of data provided from other aspects of the evaluation.

Morbidity complicating the use of depth electrodes includes hemorrhage and infection. The risk of hemorrhage is estimated to be less than 2 percent but may result in permanent neurologic sequelae or even death.[7] Most infections respond to antibiotic treatment.

SUBDURAL STRIP ELECTRODE RECORDINGS

Definition and Indications

Subdural strip electrodes consist of a matrix of flexible material in which electrode contacts, arranged in a single row at fixed interelectrode distances (typically 10 mm), are embedded. Each strip is inserted under the dura through a cranial burr hole and directed to overlie the cortical surface of interest. This method is used most commonly to ascertain the *localization* and *lateralization* of an epileptogenic focus in a patient whose surface recordings fail to provide this information. Although subdural electrode recordings have been used in the evaluation of the epileptic brain since the 1930s, the technique gained more routine use in the United States in the early 1980s, when experience indicated that the relatively less invasive subdural approach often supplanted the need for the more invasive depth electrode techniques.

Placement of multiple subdural electrode strips is undertaken typically to survey several cortical regions bilaterally. For example, in patients suspected of having a temporal lobe focus, subdural strips can be inserted through a temporal burr hole and directed laterally and subtemporally on either side to record from neocortical and mediobasal structures, respectively. Additional electrode strips are often placed through a frontal burr hole to record from the dorsolateral or opercular frontal regions; seizures may arise from these areas and spread to temporal regions, with clinical seizure symptomatology and the surface EEG erroneously suggesting temporal lobe onset.

Subdural strip electrodes are also useful in the clarification of whether the epileptogenic region is associated with a lesion evident on MRI when scalp recordings are discordant with the imaging findings. For example, the scalp-recorded EEG tracings depicted in Figure 7-5, *A* are from a patient with medically refractory complex partial seizures whose MRI is shown in Figure 7-5, *B*. These surface recordings suggested that seizures were arising from the left temporal lobe, whereas the MRI revealed a lesion in the right anterior temporal lobe consistent with a cavernous angioma. Because cavernous angiomas are often implicated in an epileptogenic region, the surface EEG localization was questioned and subdural strip electrodes therefore were implanted in both subtemporal regions. Ictal recordings with these electrodes demonstrated that, indeed, the patient's seizures did originate from the area of the lesion (Fig. 7-5, *C*). Resection of the lesion and the immediately adjacent cortex resulted in cessation of the patient's seizures.

The presence of a lesion on MRI does not necessarily imply that it is the site of seizure origination, however, because lesions identified on neuroimaging may be incidental and not related to the epileptogenic region. Further complicating the presurgical evaluation, some patients demonstrate multiple areas of abnormality on imaging (e.g., multiple areas of post-traumatic encephalomalacia, vascular malformations, and areas of cortical malformation); one, some, or none of these areas may be epileptogenic.

Techniques

Strip electrodes are available in a variety of lengths and widths, and with various numbers of contacts and interelectrode spacings. Six-contact strips are often used routinely, although longer or shorter arrays may be employed depending on the locations in which they are to be placed. Strip electrodes are implanted surgically through cranial burr holes, usually with the patient under general anesthesia; multiple strips, directed at different regions, may be inserted through a single burr hole or through multiple burr holes bilaterally. The electrodes typically are placed under fluoroscopic guidance to ensure delivery to the region of interest. Commonly, burr holes are made superior to the zygoma and slightly anterior to the ear for the placement of electrodes in the subtemporal and lateral temporal regions. Strips also can be directed posteriorly to record from the occipital regions, if indicated. Frontal burr holes, located 4 to 6 cm anterior to the coronal suture and slightly lateral to the midline, allow subdural placement of strips along the interhemispheric fissure, to record from medial frontal areas; and across the lateral frontal region, to record from dorsolateral frontal and orbitofrontal regions. With the use of methods similar to those for depth electrodes, the cables from each electrode exit through stab wounds separate from those associated with the burr hole; such an arrangement helps to anchor each strip and reduces cerebrospinal fluid leaks and infection. Skull X-ray, CT, or MRI allows verification of electrode location in relation to the anatomic target.

Both referential and bipolar montages are employed to interpret subdural strip recordings. A scalp electrode can serve as a convenient reference; because of the voltage difference between the scalp and the brain surface, the scalp reference is rarely active but can introduce electromyographic artifact into the recording.

Findings

The interpretation of subdural strip recordings, as with depth electrode recordings, must take into consideration the somewhat restricted sampling of brain activity provided by the technique. Recording from homologous contacts of bilateral strips assists in the assessment of background activity, aids in differentiating localized or lateralized changes in the EEG (or more precisely, the electrocorticogram [ECoG]), and enables a better understanding of seizure propagation patterns.

As with depth recordings, localized disturbances of background rhythms may be seen and do not necessarily correspond to the epileptogenic region. Interictal epileptiform discharges are detected more commonly with subdural than with surface recordings, whereas the frequencies of spikes recorded with subdural and depth recordings are similar.[8] Ictal patterns consist of a distinct alteration of background activity. Similar to depth recordings, electrographic seizure onsets recorded with subdural strips may assume several morphologies, including the abrupt onset of rhythmic spike or sharp-wave activity, low-voltage fast activity, or suppression of background activity (see Fig. 7-5, *C*).

Several series comparing subdural and depth electrode recordings in epilepsy syndromes producing focal seizures (mainly of temporal lobe origin) have been published.[2,3] These reports generally conclude that inferior temporal subdural strip electrodes are somewhat less sensitive than depth electrodes (80 percent compared with 100 percent, respectively) in localizing seizures of medial temporal lobe onset. Importantly, though, the 20 percent of seizures not localized by subdural recordings were not falsely localized; their recordings simply were not localized at all. Thus, a case can be made for subdural recordings as the next phase in evaluating patients with suspected temporal lobe epilepsy where scalp recordings are nonlocalizing. Such recordings are reasonably sensitive, can cover a larger region of brain than depth electrodes, typically are not misleading, and are less invasive and therefore less likely to cause morbidity or mortality compared with depth electrodes. For the minority of patients with temporal lobe epilepsy in whom subdural recordings are also nonlocalizing, depth recordings may then be undertaken. Many epileptologists employ this graduated approach to invasive studies, especially for patients in whom other studies (e.g., MRI or PET) suggest localization.

Subdural recording techniques are valuable in the evaluation of extratemporal lobe epilepsy. Although depth electrodes can be utilized, the large area of cortical surface to be assessed limits their utility. Even in patients with mediofrontal or orbitofrontal epilepsy, subdural electrodes may be superior to depth electrodes in that they cover larger cortical areas, do not need to traverse long distances of brain uninvolved in seizure generation (i.e., white matter), and provide the capacity

to record from a greater cortical volume at each contact. In certain clinical situations, the data provided by subdural and depth electrode recordings are complementary, and their contemporaneous use may be considered.[2]

Advantages, Limitations, and Complications

The technique of recording with multiple subdural strip electrodes offers the advantage of acquiring ictal recordings directly from the cortical surface at many locations in a minimally invasive and relatively safe manner. Compared with depth electrodes, subdural strips are easier to implant as well, because stereotactic procedures are not required. Like other invasive techniques, subdural strip recordings provide a limited sample of cerebral activity. If the electrodes are not placed near the epileptogenic region, recordings may be nonlocalizing or even misleading, detecting propagated activity rather than activity representing the onset of the ictus. As discussed earlier, even when strips are placed subtemporally along the inferior temporal lobe, the subdural recordings may fail to localize hippocampal seizure onsets.

Of all the invasive, extraoperative techniques used for evaluating epilepsy, subdural strip electrodes carry the lowest morbidity rate (less than 1 percent).[9] Infection accounts for the majority of complications and typically is eradicated readily with antibiotics. Other reported complications, which are rare with subdural strips, include unintended extraction of the electrodes by patients in the peri-ictal period (a potential complication of any invasive recording procedure), subdural empyema, and cortical contusion.[3] No mortality has been reported with the technique.

RECORDING AND STIMULATION STUDIES WITH SUBDURAL GRIDS

Definition and Indications

Subdural grids are similar to subdural strips, except that they contain multiple parallel rows of electrode contacts, usually spaced 10 mm apart, embedded in an inert material. Typical arrays are rectangular or square and contain 16 to 64 contacts, although their arrangement can be customized for each patient simply by cutting the grid to conform to the particular need.

The large number of contacts available on subdural grids allows coverage of a relatively widespread cortical area compared with other invasive techniques. Hence subdural grids enable ascertainment of the spatial distribution of epileptiform activity. In addition, grids provide a means of performing chronic extraoperative stimulation studies to identify the localization of various cortical functions in relationship to the epileptogenic zone.

Subdural grids are used to localize the epileptogenic region more precisely when other studies have established lateralization but have failed to define with sufficient certainty the regional localization of the seizure focus. Subdural grids are also employed when previous recordings suggest localization of the epileptogenic zone to a cortical region likely to subserve important neurologic functions. Commonly, grids are used to define the relationship of frontal or parietal

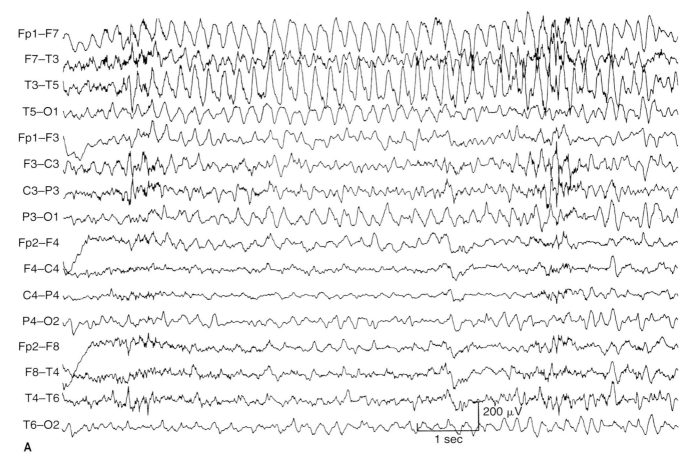

A

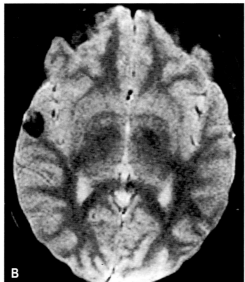

B

FIGURE 7-5 ■ **A**, Scalp-recorded ictal electroencephalogram suggesting onset of seizure from the left temporal region in a patient with medically refractory epilepsy and right temporal lobe lesion. **B**, Axial T2-weighted magnetic resonance image demonstrates the lesion, consistent with a cavernous vascular malformation, in the right temporal lobe (left side of image).

Continued

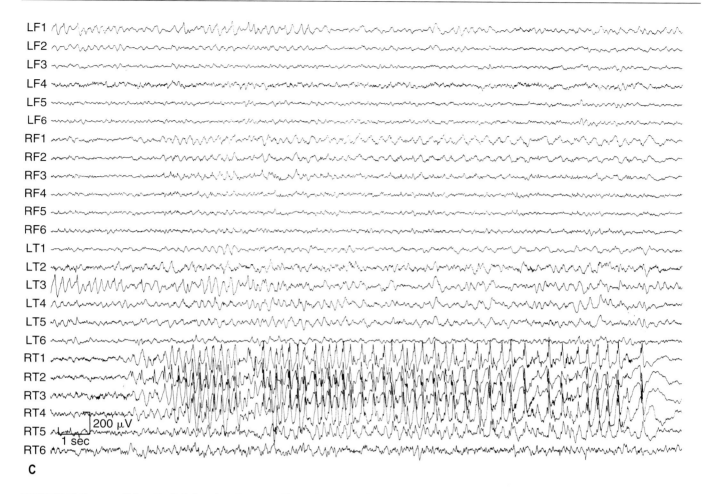

FIGURE 7.5—cont'd **C**, Subdural strip recordings from the left and right frontal (LF, RF) and left and right temporal (LT, RT) regions in the same patient. The ictal recordings demonstrate seizure activity arising from, and remaining confined to, the right temporal region. Repetitive sharp activity is most conspicuous in contacts 2 to 4 of the right temporal electrode in these referential recordings.

epileptogenic foci to motor and sensory areas, or to establish the proximity of frontal or lateral temporal epileptogenic foci to language areas. The ability to identify both epileptogenic cortex and "eloquent" functional cortex is essential in the planning and execution of resective surgery in these regions. Although some functional information can be obtained with the use of intraoperative mapping, the usual lack of ictal recordings in the operating room precludes definite identification of the region from which seizures arise. In addition, from a practical standpoint, young children and some adults do not tolerate intraoperative language mapping, which requires that the patient be awake during the initial portion of the operation. Finally, performing extraoperative recording and stimulation studies over a period of days in an epilepsy monitoring unit allows a more comprehensive evaluation of the epileptogenic region and a more thorough

assessment of language function in a setting where the patient is awake, relaxed, and more cooperative.

Techniques

Subdural electrode grids are placed through a craniotomy, with scalp and bone flaps tailored both to the area of suspected epileptogenicity and to functional areas that the grid is to cover (Fig. 7-6). An osteoplastic bone flap, in which the bone flap is attached to vascularized muscle flaps, reduces the likelihood of osteomyelitis. Typically, the cortical surface is photographed, the grid is inserted to cover the regions of interest, and additional photographs are taken. The intraoperative photographs allow correlation of anatomic landmarks to particular grid contacts, and thus allow the creation of a "map"

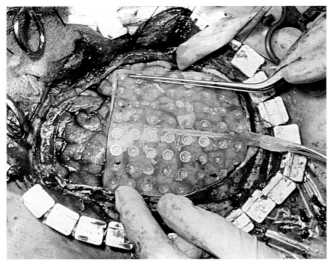

FIGURE 7-6 ■ Intraoperative photograph showing placement of a 64-contact subdural grid following craniotomy.

of the cortical surface that details epileptogenic and functional regions. The grid is sutured to the overlying dura to reduce any tendency to shift. Cerebrospinal fluid leakage is minimized with tunneling and a tight dural closure around the electrode cable. During the course of monitoring with subdural grids, prophylactic antibiotics are administered. For the first 1 to 2 postoperative days, fluid restriction and, sometimes, treatment with steroids are used to reduce the cerebral edema associated with the grid.

Contemporary recording techniques involve the use of computerized equipment to amplify, digitize, analyze, and store data. These techniques are particularly valuable for grid recordings, where the capacity to review data (and to manipulate the manner in which they are presented) from a large number of channels is vital. The recordings are obtained in a monopolar fashion, with the reference being an electrode fastened to the skull at the time of craniotomy, a scalp electrode, or an "inactive" electrode on the grid.

Cortical stimulation studies, in which electrical current is applied to the cortex through the contacts of the grid, provide valuable information concerning cortical function. Such studies typically are performed during the course of monitoring in the epilepsy monitoring unit. Techniques vary from one center to another, but the general approach is to stimulate sequentially, one contact at a time, the cortical surface underlying the grid to identify motor, sensory, language, and other functional areas. This approach has shown a certain amount of variability from subject to subject in the anatomic localization of sensory, motor, and language functions.

Mapping is accomplished by passing current briefly through each contact and observing the patient for motor responses; by inquiring about sensory and other phenomena induced by the stimulation; and by testing the patient's language function with the use of a variety of exercises, including counting and picture-naming. Typical stimulation parameters include bipolar 60-Hz square-wave pulses, of 0.2 to 2.0 msec in duration. The intensity of stimulation is increased progressively until a clinical response is obtained or an afterdischarge (a repetitive discharge evoked by the stimulation) is recorded, usually at 4 to 12 V with constant-voltage stimulation or 2 to 6 mA with constant-current stimulation. The EEG is monitored during stimulation to detect the presence of afterdischarges. Recognition of afterdischarges is important because the propagation of this activity to cortical areas other than those directly beneath the stimulated electrode contact may provide misleading functional information. Additionally, afterdischarges may evolve to become a clinical seizure. Findings from stimulation studies, along with ictal and interictal data, may then be depicted as a map of the cortical surface covered by the grid. This map allows appreciation of the relationship between functionally important areas and epileptogenic areas. Correlation of the map with intraoperative photographs facilitates planning of the surgical resection.

Once a sufficient number of localizing ictal recordings have been obtained and mapping studies are complete, the patient undergoes reopening of the craniotomy under general anesthesia. After the grid position is confirmed, the grid is removed and the resection is undertaken based on the map of epileptogenic and functional areas.

Findings

Interpretation of cortical recordings made with grids is similar to that with strips (previously discussed). One difference is the absence of bilateral information in grid recordings, and this lack can make the assessment of background, interictal, and ictal patterns challenging. As with other invasive recordings, localized background disturbances may be present in the epileptogenic zone. Interictal epileptiform discharges may serve to demarcate regions of potential epileptogenicity or may be geographically distinct from the seizure focus. Ictal recordings, with morphologic features as previously described, provide the primary basis for defining the epileptogenic zone, although no standardized approach to their interpretation exists (Fig. 7-7). Although some authors have found subdural grids rarely to be adequate for seizure localization, others have found the technique generally to be quite useful.[3,10,]

Advantages, Limitations, and Complications

The number and density of contacts contained in a subdural grid allow the localization of epileptogenic and functional cortical regions, and an appreciation of the relationship between the two. The anatomic correlation of these localizations is known precisely because grids are placed under direct visualization. The recordings obtained from grids are restricted to the tops of gyri, however, with little contribution from sulcal cortex. Although generally safe and well tolerated by patients, subdural grids have the highest potential for morbidity (about 4 percent) of any of the invasive techniques because of the requirement for craniotomy and the size of the grid.[11] Infection is the most common complication

but is minimized with meticulous technique, proper maintenance of the craniotomy site and electrode cables, and the use of prophylactic antibiotics. Brain edema can occur but usually responds to fluid restriction and diuresis. Less commonly, subdural hematomas may occur.

EPIDURAL RECORDING TECHNIQUES

Definition, Indications, Techniques, and Findings

Strip or grid electrodes may be placed on top of the dura through burr holes or following craniotomy (rather than in the subdural space) to record activity from the underlying cerebral cortex. Additionally, so-called epidural peg electrodes may be inserted through small skull holes to enable recording in a similar manner, although this technique seems to have fallen out of favor with many epileptologists. The indications for, technical aspects of, and findings with epidural techniques and subdural

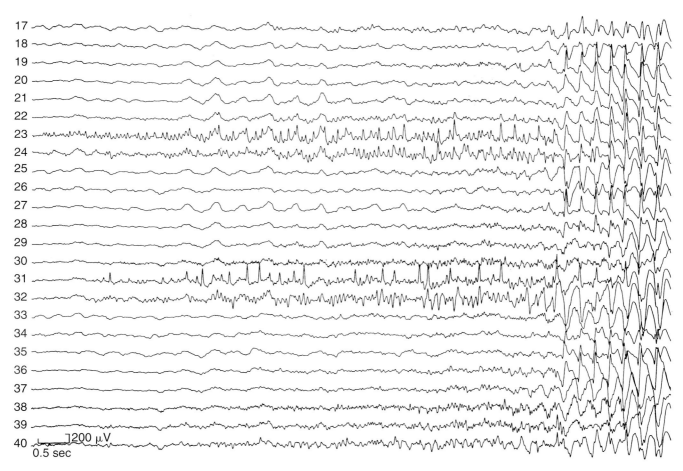

FIGURE 7-7 ■ Ictal recording from an 8-contact × 8-contact subdural grid placed in the right frontal region in a boy with medically refractory epilepsy. Referential recording of selected channels (channels 17 to 40) demonstrates rhythmic sharp beta-frequency activity beginning at electrode 23, followed by rapid spread to adjacent electrodes (24, 31, and 32).

techniques are similar. The epidural approach may be preferable when electrodes must be placed in regions involved in a previous resection, because adhesions may prevent access to the subdural space.

Advantages, Limitations, and Complications

Compared with subdurally placed electrodes, those placed epidurally may be less prone to inciting infection because the intact dura serves as a protective barrier. By the nature of their location, epidural electrodes are easier to place in patients with subdural adhesions from previous surgery. Unlike subdural strips and grids, however, epidural electrode arrays cannot be placed in interhemispheric, basiotemporal, or orbitofrontal regions. Thus, epidural electrodes are reserved mainly for recording from the lateral convexities. Epidural peg electrodes do provide the capacity to obtain relatively extensive coverage of cortex, and these electrodes may be closely spaced to obtain reasonably high-density regional recordings (with the requirement of relatively extensive trephining in such a case). In distinction to subdural electrodes, stimulation studies cannot be undertaken with epidural electrodes unless the exposed dura is denervated before electrode placement to avoid discomfort to the patient during electrical stimulation.

ELECTROCORTICOGRAPHY

Definition and Indications

Electrocorticography (ECoG) consists of the intraoperative recording of electrical activity directly from the exposed cerebral cortex. Developed by Penfield and Jasper in the 1940s, ECoG is used to help delineate the epileptogenic cortical region in more detail than that established by the preoperative, noninvasive evaluation. It is employed, along with electrical stimulation, to identify functional cortical areas, much in the same manner as with grid stimulation studies. Finally, ECoG is performed following the initial resection to assess the completeness of the resection and to identify areas of residual epileptiform activity that may be considered for removal.

The circumstances during which ECoG is employed vary among epileptologists. At some institutions, recordings are made during all cases of epilepsy surgery, and the intraoperative findings are used to tailor the surgical resection to each patient. At other centers, ECoG is used selectively (e.g., only in extratemporal procedures), or it may be performed universally for research purposes but the findings then are not used in determining the

volume of brain tissue to be resected. When resection of central regions is contemplated, motor mapping (in a manner similar to that previously described) may be employed. Such mapping is performed with the patient under general anesthesia but without the use of paralytic agents. Operations undertaken on the language-dominant hemisphere may be performed with the patient under local anesthesia so that intraoperative mapping of language function may be performed, with the findings from this mapping then used to guide the resection. Other centers perform extraoperative language mapping (using subdural grids, as described earlier) for all resections involving the language-dominant hemisphere in which the resection might encroach on cortical areas suspected of being involved in language function. Some surgeons utilize intraoperative language and motor mapping to guide the resection of tumors and other lesions in patients who do not necessarily have epilepsy, with ECoG used primarily to monitor for afterdischarges and to protect the patient from clinical seizures triggered by electrical stimulation.[12]

Techniques

A variety of electrode arrangements may be used in ECoG. Many centers use a crown, attached to the skull, containing a number of electrodes (often 16) that may be directed in various positions atop the cortex following craniotomy. This crown provides a flexible means of covering the exposed cortex of interest while it maximizes the access to and the visibility of the cortex (Fig. 7-8). Electrode strips, such as those used for extraoperative

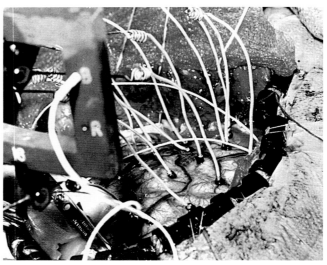

FIGURE 7-8 ■ Intraoperative photograph demonstrating the placement of the crown electrode used for electrocorticography.

subdural recordings, may also be used for intraoperative ECoG, but the fixed interelectrode distances reduce versatility. Particularly for temporal lobe resections, crown or strip electrodes are often supplemented with depth electrodes and individual flexible wire electrodes. In such cases the depth electrodes are inserted typically through the middle temporal gyrus to enable the distal contacts to record from medial structures (the amygdala and hippocampus), providing electrophysiologic information from structures often involved in the epileptogenic process but not readily sampled by means of the cortical surface electrodes. Flexible wire electrodes offer the advantage of insertion beneath the dura, allowing recordings from neocortical subtemporal regions not otherwise accessed. In extratemporal cases, wire electrodes enable recording from the interhemispheric fissure or from other neocortical areas not directly exposed during the craniotomy.

The post of the crown typically is used as the ground, and an electrode clipped to the exposed dura provides the reference. Referential and bipolar montages can be used. Despite the relatively hostile electrical environment of the operating room, high-quality recordings with little artifact can be obtained. Correct selection of filters can limit the interference and amplifier blocking produced during cortical stimulation. The stimulation parameters are similar to those described earlier for grid recordings, although monopolar or bipolar stimulation can be used.

A close working relationship between the epileptologist, the anesthesiologist, and the neurosurgeon is mandatory for obtaining high-quality and useful electrophysiologic data. Although practices vary, many epileptologists find that inducing anesthesia with an opiate (e.g., fentanyl) and maintaining general anesthesia with the opiate and an inhalational agent (e.g., nitrous oxide) provides effective anesthesia and permits acquisition of a satisfactory ECoG. For procedures in which it is desirable for the patient to be awake (e.g., language mapping), local analgesia and sedation with opiates and other agents, including droperidol, are used.[13]

Findings

The activity recorded during ECoG usually is composed of a mixed-frequency background, often with a considerable amount of fast activity; but the frequency, amplitude, and morphology may vary substantially from case to case. The factors influencing the appearance of this activity include the level of consciousness of the patient, the particular anesthetic and sedative agents employed during the operation and their concentrations, the region of the cortex from which the activity is recorded, and the nature of the underlying pathologic disturbance. Halogenated inhalational anesthetic agents (e.g., halothane, enflurane, and isoflurane) invariably increase the amount of fast activity present, and this effect often persists for some time after discontinuation of the drug. A profuse amount of background fast activity obscures the recognition of epileptiform discharges, significantly reducing the usefulness of the recording. In general, ECoG from the central, perirolandic cortex demonstrates predominantly fast activity that can be quite rhythmic and sharp in appearance, mimicking epileptiform activity. Recordings from other regions (e.g., the temporal neocortex) contain predominantly intermediate-frequency activity with less fast activity. When ECoG is undertaken in cases of brain tumors or other structural lesions, suppression and slowing of the activity recorded in the vicinity of the lesion are commonly seen (Fig. 7-9).

In the course of the usual, relatively brief, intraoperative ECoG recording, one rarely records a seizure. Thus, in most cases, identification of interictal epileptiform discharges provides the basis for delineating the epileptogenic zone during epilepsy surgery. Epileptiform discharges recorded by ECoG can assume spike, polyspike, and sharp-wave morphologies and can be of varied amplitude (Figs. 7-10 and 7-11). Many authors maintain that the site of interictal epileptiform discharges is related to the site from which seizures themselves arise and, moreover, that removal of the tissue producing interictal epileptiform abnormalities is important in achieving seizure control.[14] Although some series have found that the absence of epileptiform discharges on postresection ECoG predicts a successful postoperative outcome, and the presence of residual discharges usually is associated with incomplete seizure control following surgery, other reports have concluded that ECoG is of little value in guiding the surgical resection.[3,15]

Pharmacologic activation procedures using intravenous administration of methohexital, etomidate, or other medications may enhance the frequency with which epileptiform discharges are recorded (Fig. 7-12, *A* and *B*), although more significance is placed on the spontaneously appearing discharges than on those that are induced.

Advantages, Limitations, and Complications

Intraoperative ECoG with mapping provides the ability to define epileptogenic and functionally important cortical areas relatively quickly and with more spatial precision than when this information is obtained extraoperatively

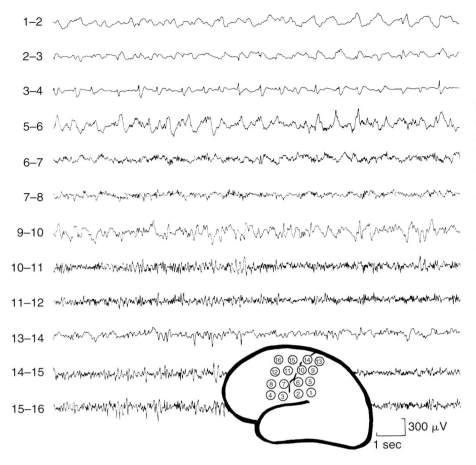

FIGURE 7-9 ■ Intraoperative electrocorticogram from a patient with a left frontoparietal brain tumor. The electrodes were arranged in four rows of four atop the cortical surface, with electrodes 1 to 4 placed along the inferior central region in a posterior-to-anterior fashion and electrodes 5 to 8, 9 to 12, and 13 to 16 placed sequentially more superior. A bipolar montage is depicted and shows irregular slowing and spikes recorded most conspicuously from the inferior frontoparietal region (channels 1 to 3). Note the fast, sharply configured activity present in the bottom half of the recording, which typifies the morphology of activity recorded from the central region.

with the use of implanted, fixed-array electrodes. It allows acquisition of the information, at the time of a single craniotomy, for the resective surgery, and these proximate ECoG findings are then available for the planning of the operation. When intraoperative ECoG provides sufficient information to proceed directly with the resection, it spares the patient the risk (albeit small), discomfort, and cost associated with invasive monitoring.

As previously mentioned, ECoG typically provides only interictal information about the epileptogenic zone, and the relevance of the distribution of interictal discharges to the zone of ictus onset and the requisite tissue that must be resected to abolish seizures is not always clear. At times, the intraoperative recordings contain no epileptiform abnormalities and thus are not helpful. In such cases, when better definition of the epileptogenic region in relation to functional areas is required, a subdural grid usually is placed and extraoperative monitoring carried out before resection.

Performing ECoG prolongs the duration of the operation and the total time during which the patient receives anesthesia. Thus such an operation theoretically carries the risk of increased morbidity compared with an operation of shorter duration, but this concern seems to be of little actual clinical relevance.

MICROELECTRODE RECORDINGS IN THE SURGICAL TREATMENT OF MOVEMENT DISORDERS

Basal ganglia surgery for Parkinson disease and other movement disorders dates back to the 1940s, after it was discovered fortuitously that lesions of the globus pallidus could improve parkinsonian symptoms. Various techniques, including pallidotomy and thalamotomy, gained popularity until the introduction of more effective pharmacologic therapies, particularly levodopa. As the limitations and adverse effects of these medications became clearer, however, surgical options for the treatment of Parkinson disease, essential tremor, dystonia, and other movement disorders provoked renewed interest. The development of deep brain stimulation (DBS) therapy heralded a new era in surgical intervention for movement disorders, and this treatment is now in common use.

Several technologic advances have contributed to the revitalization of surgical therapy for movement disorders. With improvements in modern functional stereotactic neurosurgical techniques and neuroimaging, identification of the neuroanatomic structures of interest and placement of lesions and brain stimulators in these structures has become more precise. Additionally, advances in

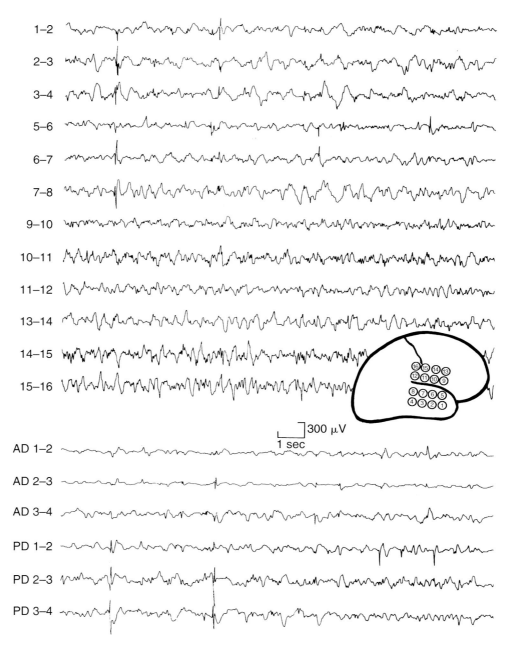

FIGURE 7-10 ■ Intraoperative electrocorticogram from a patient with right temporal lobe epilepsy. The crown electrodes were arranged in four rows of four atop the cortical surface, with electrodes 1 to 4 placed along the middle temporal gyrus, electrodes 5 to 8 placed along the superior temporal gyrus, and electrodes 9 to 12 and 13 to 16 placed sequentially more superior in the suprasylvian region. The top 12 channels of the recording represent a bipolar montage from these electrodes. In addition, four-contact depth electrodes were inserted through the middle temporal gyrus anteriorly and posteriorly to record activity from the amygdala and hippocampus, respectively (AD and PD). Spikes are seen to arise from electrodes 2, 3, 6, 7, PD2, and PD3. In addition, spikes are recorded independently from PD1, the distal contact of the posterior depth electrode.

the understanding of the neurophysiologic underpinnings of Parkinson disease (and, to a lesser extent, other movement disorders) have provided the scientific rationale for a surgical approach to the treatment of these disabling conditions. The advent of DBS therapy provided a nondestructive, adjustable, and reversible treatment with advantages over ablative surgical procedures. Of special interest for the present discussion, neurophysiologic recordings from the basal ganglia and the thalamus have enhanced the precision with which lesions

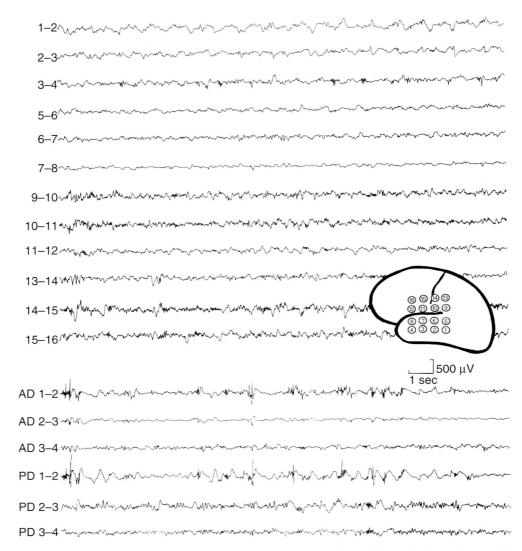

FIGURE 7-11 ■ Intraoperative electrocorticogram from a patient with medically refractory left temporal lobe epilepsy. Recording configuration is similar to that in Figure 7-10. Note isolated epileptiform discharges arising synchronously from the amygdala and hippocampal electrodes (AD1 and PD1).

are made or stimulator leads are placed. The following sections address the use of microelectrode recordings to guide implantation of DBS leads, pallidotomy, and thalamotomy.

Definition and Indications

Microelectrode recordings are obtained with the use of a fine recording electrode, typically having a tip diameter of 15 to 25 μm, through a burr hole or twist-drill hole in the skull with a trajectory toward a stereotactically defined target. The technique enables the recording of extracellular, single-unit neuronal activity. The electrophysiologic properties of the activity so recorded provide an indication of the location of the electrode in relation to the various gray matter nuclei and white matter tracts

encountered along the trajectory. Indeed, the characteristic neurophysiologic signatures of cells within the subthalamic nucleus (STN), globus pallidus internus (GPi), and ventralis intermedius nucleus of the thalamus (Vim) enable identification of the areas targeted in surgical procedures aimed at providing relief from the symptoms of various movement disorders.[16] Furthermore, the motor subterritories within these target nuclei (i.e., the specific regions in which DBS leads are placed or lesions are generated) can be defined because activity in such areas is modulated by active or passive patient movement.

The role of microelectrode recordings in the surgical treatment of movement disorders has not been established fully, yet many clinicians believe that the current limitations of image-based targeting require the addition

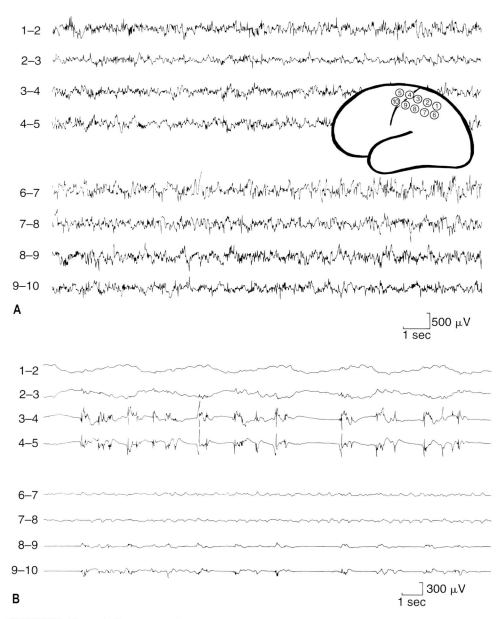

FIGURE 7-12 ■ **A**, Intraoperative electrocorticogram from the left frontoparietal region in a 9-month-old girl with tuberous sclerosis and intractable seizures. The background consists of mixed-frequency activity with a considerable amount of fast activity. No epileptiform discharges are obvious. **B**, Following the administration of methohexital, background activity is suppressed dramatically and frequent spike and polyspike epileptiform discharges emerge, mainly in electrode 4.

of physiologic information to optimize the accuracy of surgical targeting. Current image-guided stereotaxis typically relies upon historical (preoperative) imaging, coupled with fiducial markers provided by a rigid head frame affixed to the patient's head or by frameless markers embedded in the skull. These techniques have inherent in them several factors that diminish the precision of targeting, including mechanical inaccuracies, image distortion (for MRI-based techniques), brain shifts that occur after preoperative images have been obtained,

and variability in the correlation between physiologic function and anatomy.

Whether the employment of microelectrode mapping in surgery for movement disorders results in an improved success rate, greater efficacy, or altered morbidity remains to be settled. One study found that microelectrode recordings significantly altered the ultimate placement of the stimulator lead (by 2 mm or more) relative to the initial site determined by neuroimaging-guided stereotactic techniques in 25 percent of patients.[17]

Techniques

The neurosurgical procedures involved in microelectrode recordings have been well described in the neurosurgical literature and will be outlined here only briefly.[18] The initial target for the microelectrode is determined with the use of CT- or MRI-guided stereotactic techniques. This procedure usually entails attachment of a stereotactic frame to the patient's head, neuroimaging, and calculation of the coordinates for the desired target. Following local analgesia, a small burr hole or twist-drill hole is made in the skull anterior to the coronal suture and lateral to the midsagittal line. The microelectrode, typically constructed of tungsten or platinum-iridium and housed in a protective carrier tube, is inserted under stereotactic guidance and advanced by submillimeter increments with the aid of a microdrive. The neuronal activity is recorded with the use of conventional preamplifiers, AC-DC amplifiers, filters, spike triggers, and processors. In addition to an oscilloscope-type visual monitor, an audio monitor provides an effective means of identifying and differentiating the activity recorded from various structures.

Microelectrode localization of the target (STN for subthalamic DBS, GPi for pallidal DBS or pallidotomy, or Vim for thalamic DBS or thalamotomy) is based on the characteristic patterns of spontaneous neuronal discharges recorded from the various structures, and on the identification of cells whose activity is modulated by limb movement.

Findings

GLOBUS PALLIDUS

DBS of the globus pallidus or pallidotomy for the treatment of Parkinson disease, dystonia, and various other movement disorders relies on identification of the globus pallidus. Once the microelectrode is advanced to the calculated target for the globus pallidus, recordings enable distinction between globus pallidus externus (GPe) and globus pallidus internus (GPi); the latter, and particularly its motor-related region, is the desired location in the globus pallidus in which to implant the stimulator lead or place the lesion. In patients with Parkinson disease, GPe single-cell activity tends to have a lower frequency and a more irregular pattern of firing than does activity recorded from GPi (Fig. 7-13).[18] Two different discharge patterns are characteristic of GPe neurons: (1) a bursting pattern consisting of high-frequency bursts of activity interrupted by pauses; and (2) a low-frequency, irregular pattern.[18-21] Neuronal activity recorded from GPi, by contrast, is distinctly higher in frequency in the

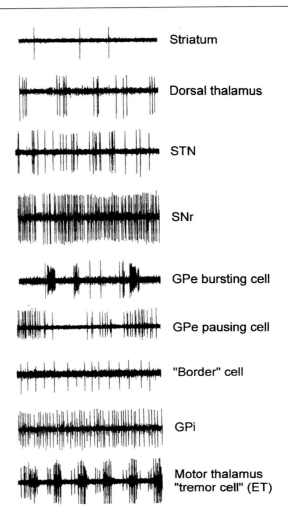

FIGURE 7-13 ▪ Microelectrode recordings of spontaneous neuronal activity from the thalamus and basal ganglia. Each trace represents a 1-second recording in a patient with Parkinson disease (upper eight traces) or essential tremor (bottom trace). STN, subthalamic nucleus; SNr, substantia nigra pars reticulata; GPe, globus pallidus externus; GPi, globus pallidus internus; ET, essential tremor. (From Starr P: Technical considerations in movement disorders surgery. p. 269. In Schulder M, Gandhi CD [eds]: Handbook of Stereotactic and Functional Neurosurgery. Marcel Dekker, New York, 2003, with permission.)

parkinsonian brain; it often assumes a sustained but irregular firing pattern.[18-21] In patients with dystonia, GPi discharge rates tend to be lower.[22] So-called border cells, located in the laminae surrounding GPe and GPi, are identified by their relatively lower frequency and more regular discharge patterns.[17-20] Within both GPe and GPi, cells responsive to active or passive movement, or both, are found.[18-21] Although most of these units respond to contralateral limb movement, some respond in a similar manner with ipsilateral movement. In addition, some cells preferentially respond to one phase of movement more than another (e.g., flexion but not extension, or vice versa).[21]

Identification of the optic tract, located inferior to the inferior margin of GPi, is important so that one can avoid placing the stimulator lead or lesion in this structure and thereby causing visual deficits. Such identification is accomplished by detecting light-evoked action potential discharges at the base of the pallidum.[17-20] Microstimulation, in which 2 to 20 µA of current passed through the microelectrode evokes visual phenomena in the patient's contralateral visual field, is also used for identifying the optic tract.[17-20]

To avoid motor deficits, the internal capsule is identified. As for any white matter region, recordings from this structure are characterized by a relative absence of neuronal action potentials and, occasionally, the presence of axonal spikes. Microstimulation of the internal capsule, resulting in contraction of the tongue, face, or hand, confirms localization.[17-20]

THALAMUS

For the surgical treatment of essential tremor or other forms of tremor, the target for stimulator lead implantation or lesion placement is the Vim. The trajectory of the microelectrode for this procedure usually enters the caudate nucleus first, where recordings demonstrate a slow rate (up to 10 Hz) of spontaneous cellular discharges.[18] As the electrode enters the dorsal thalamus, the recordings are relatively quiescent, except for occasional bursts of activity.[18] On entry of the microelectrode into the ventral aspect of the thalamus, cells responsive to movement may be detected. So-called "tremor cells," cells discharging at the rate of the patient's tremor, may also be encountered (see Fig. 7-13).[18,23] Placement of the surgical lesion or stimulation lead in the area populated by these tremor cells has been shown to correlate with clinical improvement in the patient's tremor.[24] The sensory

thalamus can be identified, and thus avoided, by recording cells responsive to light cutaneous stimuli. Microstimulation, too, enables identification of the sensory thalamus and the internal capsule.[18]

SUBTHALAMIC NUCLEUS

DBS of the STN has emerged as a commonly used procedure to treat the motor symptoms of advanced Parkinson disease when patients experience disabling symptoms despite optimized pharmacologic therapy.[25-28] The STN, a major output nucleus of the basal ganglia, exhibits excessive and abnormally patterned neuronal activity in the parkinsonian brain.[29] Stimulating this structure with high-frequency (greater than 100 Hz) electrical pulses by means of a chronically implanted DBS lead can suppress reversibly the major motor symptoms and signs of Parkinson disease and provide patients with more consistent and higher-quality motor function.[25]

The STN is a small nucleus relative to the other structures targeted in surgery for movement disorders, but its characteristic pattern of neurophysiologic activity enables intraoperative identification with relative ease. With a typical microelectrode trajectory, cells in the caudate nucleus of the striatum and then the dorsal thalamus are recorded en route to the STN. Caudate and thalamic neurons have a relatively low rate of discharge (see Fig. 7-13), and individual units are generally easy to isolate.[18] As the microelectrode is advanced further and the STN is approached, background neuronal activity increases. Upon entering the STN, dense, multi-unit recordings are common; the activity is thus seemingly faster than that observed when single STN units, discharging at rates of 20 to 50 Hz, are isolated.[18]

While recording within the STN, particularly within its dorsal aspect, neurons can be identified that respond to active or passive movement of the patient's contralateral arm or leg (Fig. 7-14).[30] This movement-induced

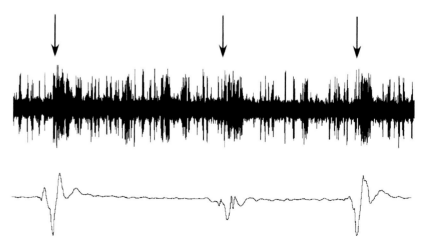

FIGURE 7-14 ▪ Microelectrode recording of movement-related subthalamic nucleus neuronal activity during passive movement of the contralateral upper extremity. The upper trace shows the microelectrode recording and the lower trace shows output of a wrist-mounted accelerometer. Arrows indicate a burst of neuronal activity evoked by limb movement. The trace represents a 4-second recording in a patient with Parkinson disease. (Courtesy of Dr. Philip A. Starr.)

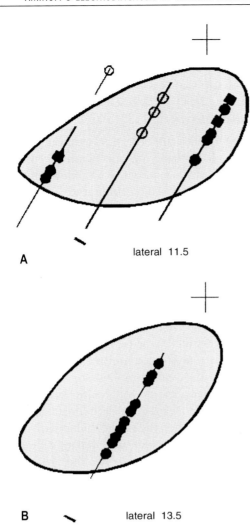

A   lateral 11.5

B   lateral 13.5

FIGURE 7-15 ■ Microelectrode mapping from a case of deep brain stimulation surgery of the subthalamic nucleus, illustrating somatotopy of the motor area. Four microelectrode penetrations were performed in two parasagittal planes. Arm-related cells (filled symbols) are in the anterior, posterior, and lateral aspects of the motor territory, and leg-related cells (open symbols) are in the mediocentral part of the motor territory. Squares represent the most proximal joint (hip, shoulder); circles, the middle joint (knee, elbow); and triangles, the most distal joint (ankle, wrist) for each extremity. A bold line at the end of a microelectrode trajectory indicates the start of substantia nigra pars reticulata. Microelectrode track reconstructions are superimposed on sagittal plane anatomy drawn from a standard brain atlas, with (**A**) 11.5 mm lateral to the midline and (**B**) 13.5 mm lateral to the midline. (From Starr PA, Theodosopoulos PV, Turner R: Surgery of the subthalamic nucleus: use of movement-related neuronal activity for surgical navigation. Neurosurgery, 53:1146, 2003, with permission.)

modulation of activity is perceived most easily as a subtle increase in volume in the audio signal coincident with the movement; this confirms that the electrode is traversing the region of STN subserving motor function—the target for DBS lead implantation. With passage of the microelectrode through the inferior border of STN and into the substantia nigra pars reticulata, the pattern of activity changes abruptly. Higher-frequency activity (50 to 70 Hz), more regular in its pattern and with single units easier to isolate, appears. In clinical practice, mapping with 1 to 3 microelectrode tracks usually allows confident identification of the relevant borders of the STN and its motor subterritory (Fig. 7-15).[31–32] From this information, the desired location of DBS lead implantation can be determined.[17]

Advantages, Limitations, and Complications

Stereotactic neurosurgical procedures for the treatment of Parkinson disease, essential tremor, dystonia, and other movement disorders can diminish the debilitating symptoms of these disorders for many patients. These procedures rely on the precise placement of a stimulator lead or lesion into deep brain structures; thus the exquisite spatial resolution offered by neurophysiologic techniques utilizing microelectrode recording appears to be useful in identifying the target structures of the basal ganglia and thalamus.

REFERENCES

1. Kwan P, Brodie MJ: Early identification of refractory epilepsy. N Engl J Med, 342:314, 2000
2. Arroyo S, Lesser RP, Awad IA, et al: Subdural and epidural grids and strips. p. 377. In Engel J Jr (ed): Surgical Treatment of the Epilepsies. 2nd Ed. Raven, New York, 1993
3. Marks WJ Jr Laxer KD: Invasive clinical neurophysiology in epilepsy and movement disorders. p. 163. In Aminoff MJ (ed): Electrodiagnosis in Clinical Neurology. 5th Ed. Elsevier/Churchill Livingstone, Philadelphia, 2005
4. Sirven JI, Malamut BL, Liporace JD et al: Outcome after temporal lobectomy in bilateral temporal lobe epilepsy. Ann Neurol, 42:873, 1997
5. Ajmone-Marsan C: Chronic intracranial recording and electrocorticography. p. 535. In Daly DD, Pedley TA (eds): Current Practice of Clinical Electroencephalography. Raven, New York, 1990
6. Hirsch LJ, Spencer SS, Williamson MD et al: Comparison of bitemporal and unitemporal epilepsy defined by depth electroencephalography. Ann Neurol, 30:340, 1991

7. Spencer SS, So NK, Engel J Jr et al: Depth electrodes. p. 359. In Engel J Jr (ed): Surgical Treatment of the Epilepsies. 2nd Ed. Raven, New York, 1993

8. Privitera MD, Quinlan JG, Yeh H: Interictal spike detection comparing subdural and depth electrodes during electrocorticography. Electroencephalogr Clin Neurophysiol, 76:379, 1990

9. Wyler AR, Walker G, Somes G: The morbidity of long-term seizure monitoring using subdural strip electrodes. J Neurosurg, 74:734, 1991

10. Masuoka LK, Spencer SS: Seizure localization using subdural grid electrodes. Epilepsia 34 Suppl 6:8, 1993

11. Spencer SS, Lamoureux D: Invasive electroencephalography evaluation for epilepsy surgery. p. 562. In Shorvon SD, Dreifuss F, Fish D et al (eds): The Treatment of Epilepsy. Blackwell Science, Oxford, 1996

12. Berger MS: Minimalism through intraoperative functional mapping. Clin Neurosurg, 43:324, 1996

13. Smith M: Anaesthesia in epilepsy surgery. p. 794. In Shorvon SD, Dreifuss F, Fish D et al (eds): The Treatment of Epilepsy. Blackwell Science, Oxford, 1996

14. Ojemann GA: Intraoperative electrocorticography and functional mapping. p. 189. In Wyler AR, Hermann BP (eds): The Surgical Management of Epilepsy. Butterworth-Heinemann, Boston, 1994

15. McBride MC, Binnie CD, Janota I et al: Predictive value of intraoperative electrocorticograms in resective epilepsy surgery. Ann Neurol, 30:526, 1991

16. Bronte-Stewart H: Surgical placement of deep brain stimulation leads for the treatment of movement disorders: intraoperative aspects. p. 20. In Marks WJ, Jr (ed): Deep Brain Stimulation Management. Cambridge University Press, Cambridge, 2011

17. Starr PA, Christine CW, Theodosopoulos PV et al: Implantation of deep brain stimulators into the subthalamic nucleus: technical approach and magnetic resonance imaging-verified lead locations. J Neurosurg, 97:370, 2002

18. Starr P: Technical considerations in movement disorders surgery. p. 269. In Schulder M, Gandhi CD (eds): Handbook of Stereotactic and Functional Neurosurgery. Marcel Dekker, New York, 2003

19. Vitek JL, Baron M, Bakay RAE et al: Microelectrode-guided pallidotomy: technical approach and application for medically intractable Parkinson's disease. J Neurosurg, 88:1027, 1998

20. Lozano A, Hutchison W, Kiss Z et al: Methods for microelectrode-guided posteroventral pallidotomy. J Neurosurg, 84:194, 1996

21. Sterio D, Beric A, Dogali M et al: Neurophysiological properties of pallidal neurons in Parkinson's disease. Ann Neurol, 35:586, 1994

22. Vitek JL, Chockkan V, Zhang JY et al: Neuronal activity in the basal ganglia in patients with generalized dystonia and hemiballismus. Ann Neurol, 46:22, 1999

23. Benabid AL, Pollak P, Gao D et al: Chronic electrical stimulation of the ventralis intermedius nucleus of the thalamus as a treatment of movement disorders. J Neurosurg, 84:203, 1996

24. Lenz FA, Normand SL, Kwan HC et al: Statistical prediction of the optimal site for thalamotomy in parkinsonian tremor. Mov Disord, 10:318, 1995

25. Limousin P, Krack P, Pollak P et al: Electrical stimulation of the subthalamic nucleus in advanced Parkinson's disease. N Engl J Med, 339:1105, 1998

26. Deuschl G, Schade-Brittinger C, Krack P et al: A randomized trial of deep-brain stimulation for Parkinson's disease. N Engl J Med, 355:896, 2006

27. Weaver FM, Follett K, Stern M et al: Bilateral deep brain stimulation vs best medical therapy for patients with advanced Parkinson disease: a randomized controlled trial. JAMA, 301:63, 2009

28. Follett KA, Weaver FM, Stern M et al: Pallidal versus subthalamic deep-brain stimulation for Parkinson's disease. N Engl J Med, 362:2077, 2010

29. DeLong MR: Primate models of movement disorders of basal ganglia origin. Trends Neurosci, 13:281, 1990

30. Theodosopoulos PV, Marks WJ, Jr Christine C et al: Locations of movement-related cells in the human subthalamic nucleus in Parkinson's disease. Mov Disord, 18:791, 2003

31. Starr PA: Placement of deep brain stimulators into the subthalamic nucleus or globus pallidus internus: technical approach. Stereotact Funct Neurosurg, 79:133, 2002

32. Starr PA, Theodosopoulos PV, Turner R: Surgery of the subthalamic nucleus: use of movement-related neuronal activity for surgical navigation. Neurosurgery, 53:1146, 2003

Topographic Mapping, Frequency Analysis, and Other Quantitative Techniques in Electroencephalography

MARC R. NUWER and PEDRO COUTIN-CHURCHMAN

Digital electroencephalography (EEG) is the simple recording and interpreting of routine EEG using computer-based technology. Quantitative electroencephalography (QEEG) is the processing of digital EEG with various algorithms and displays. There are many types of QEEG. The EEG can be searched for spikes and seizures. Frequency content can be calculated and compared to prior or normative values. Topographic scalp maps or three-dimensional brain maps can display EEG features, a process often labeled EEG brain mapping.

EEG frequency analysis has been studied for nearly 80 years, and phase and coherence have been studied for more than 50 years. Technical development was slowed by the substantial computer processing required. A routine 20-minute EEG is more than 10 megabytes in size. In the 1970s, there was great enthusiasm for building a computer that could "analyze the EEG" and generate a draft report for each individual clinical record. This goal proved unfeasible. Interpretation still requires expert input from a knowledgeable user. QEEG data can be used to aid in assessing the EEG results. Quantitative analysis acts as a ruler for measuring specific EEG features, which are then presented to a knowledgeable user for further interpretation.

TECHNIQUES

EEG Acquisition and Storage

Routine clinical digital EEG commonly involves recording from all 21 of the electrode locations in the 10–20 system, as well as from several extra artifact-control channels. Digital equipment can record much larger numbers of channels: for example, on epilepsy units, where systems can record from hundreds of channels. Digital EEGs usually are recorded in a referential format with open filter settings, allowing for subsequent review in any montage and with different filter settings.

Digital EEG is stored in public or commercial data formats. The most common public data format is the European data format (edf). Each instrumentation company has its own proprietary format. Some third-party vendors have generic reading stations able to read records from any of several commercial or public formats.

Storage is on digital disks or similar mass storage devices. One problem now is the eventual obsolescence of the data formats and reading hardware. There is no immediate solution for this, and major difficulty may occur with record retrieval in future years. Another problem is reading records run elsewhere on equipment different from that in one's own EEG laboratory. Some companies facilitate such remote reading by providing special reading software that is copied onto discs along with copies of EEGs to be sent elsewhere. This works well because programs often run well on generic office computers.

Display Techniques

Montage reconstruction can be accomplished when the EEG has been recorded and stored in a referential montage. The EEG can be played back in any bipolar or referential montage as long as all needed electrode sites were in the original recording. This technique was developed and used in clinical patient care originally by Williams and Nuwer.[1] Reconstruction is accomplished by subtracting referential channels from each other.

Data are acquired with open filter settings.[2] These settings are adequate as long as the data are not contaminated heavily by artifact. Filter settings can be adjusted during replay to a more restricted setting.[1] For example, a record can be made with filter settings at 0.1 and 100 Hz, and later reviewed at 1.0 and 70 Hz. Similarly, the digital EEG can be replayed with a variety of "paper speeds" or screen compression factors. An interesting segment of record can be replayed on an expanded time scale to look at the timing and phase reversal of spikes and sharp waves in greater detail.

Topographic maps are a controversial way to display some EEG features. EEG voltage or other features are plotted on a scalp map with contour lines or color coding to identify similarly valued regions. Use of color adds an aesthetic touch.

Such EEG brain maps superficially resemble axial cuts of a computed tomography (CT) or magnetic resonance imaging (MRI) scan but, in fact, they differ in a fundamental way. Topographic maps actually represent very few real data points, typically equal to the number of scalp recording electrodes. The remainder of the map, more than 99 percent of the pixels, is nothing more than an interpolation. The interpolation provides no new real data. This is the opposite of the situation with MRI or CT, which has very little redundancy and for which each display pixel corresponds to real data. Color on EEG topographic maps can be helpful or misleading. Sometimes, it points out small differences in data that might otherwise have been overlooked. On other occasions, maps overemphasize meaningless differences.

Low-resolution brain electromagnetic tomography (LORETA) estimates simple EEG sources at superficial or deep sites.[3] Extrapolations from scalp sources suggest the most likely locations of epileptic spike dipoles or frequency component generators. The results are displayed on simulated cerebral topography. These displays more closely resemble CT scan or MR images, but again the data points are mostly extrapolations. The number of actual independent data points underlying LORETA images is the number of scalp electrodes used to record them. The calculations assume simple models for generators, whereas many actual generators may be broad, diffuse, or multifocal.

Analysis Techniques

Many types of analytic and display techniques are available for digital EEG and QEEG.[4,5] Epileptiform spikes and sharp waves, periodic lateralized epileptiform discharges (PLEDs), triphasic waves, and other transients can be viewed most simply on the routine digital EEG. Dipole source localization can aid in estimating generator locations.

Artifacts can be identified best on the routine digital EEG. Artifact identification channels should be run along with the scalp acquisition channels. Digital removal or attenuation of certain artifacts has achieved mixed success through advanced processing techniques.[5–7]

Event detectors can aid in identifying epileptic spikes or subclinical seizures, especially those in long recordings. Ambulatory EEG automated systems can scan 24- to 72-hour EEG recordings in this way.[8,9] Candidate events are detected and presented to a reader for interpretation. False-positive identifications are common.

Frequency analysis involves calculating the amount of EEG in each major frequency band (e.g., the alpha band). Sometimes even smaller bands are used, down to a fraction of a cycle per second. The amount of EEG in each frequency band then is displayed in a numerical table or on a topographic scalp map. Frequencies are usually analyzed for alert subjects but are also used in surgical and critical care monitoring.

The frequency data may be presented as either absolute or relative amounts, and scaled as proportional to either the EEG voltage (amplitude) or the *power*. Power is the square of the voltage, often referred to as the *power spectrum*. *Absolute* voltage scaling corresponds to the EEG amplitudes as observed visually. EEG in each voltage amplitude scaled frequency band is calculated with a root-mean-square (RMS) algorithm, which makes the computer-derived RMS amplitude appear one-third as big as the usual peak-to-peak measurement used in EEG visual analysis (Fig. 8-1). *Relative voltage* or *relative power scaling* also is used commonly. In relative scaling,

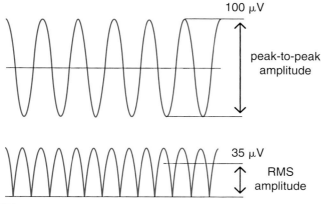

FIGURE 8-1 ■ Illustration of the marked discrepancy between electroencephalographic amplitude as measured by eye (peak-to-peak) and by computer (root-mean-square, RMS). Furthermore, the computer evaluates all time epochs equally, whereas an electroencephalographer often reads amplitudes at times when the waves are seen best (e.g., are largest). As a result, computer measurements of electroencephalographic amplitudes are often only 10 to 15 percent of those scored by ordinary visual review of records. (From Nuwer MR: Quantitative EEG. I. Techniques and problems of frequency analysis and topographic mapping. J Clin Neurophysiol, 5:1, 1988, with permission.)

the amount of EEG in each frequency band is divided by the total voltage or power across all EEG bands for that electrode site. The amount of EEG across all frequency bands totals 100 percent at each site. Such relative EEG values are much less variable than absolute EEG values among the general population. Many systems can display EEG frequency content in both ways.

More complex algorithms are available. A commonly used technique is the subtraction of left from right hemisphere activity, resulting in a display or calculation of the *asymmetry* between the hemispheres. This asymmetry helps to emphasize subtle focal EEG features; however, it makes an asymmetric feature appear farther from the midsagittal plane than it really is. *Coherence* is the tendency of EEG in two different channels to rise and fall in synchrony. Generally, it is calculated within specific frequency bands. If 20 scalp channels are recorded, there can be 20×19 (i.e., 380) individual coherence measurements within each frequency band. Sometimes, this is simplified by looking only at the coherence between homologous channels over the two hemispheres or between frontal-posterior pairs of channels in the same hemisphere. Coherence is still mainly a research tool.

Phase determinations measure which of two coherent channels leads or lags the other. An event or rhythmic activity may be seen earlier in one channel, which is then said to lead the other. Phase relationships are often stated

in degrees of angle that correspond to a complete sinusoidal cycle at a particular frequency.

Multiparametric analysis considers many separate EEG features together. Such analyses include *discriminant analysis*. Dozens or hundreds of EEG features are entered into a predetermined formula. Such a complex calculation can be tuned to look for specific useful traits in EEG signals.[10] Investigators have tried such complex techniques to "diagnose" specific diseases. Some such discriminant features are purported to diagnose specific diseases, including dementia, depression, head injury, and psychiatric and neurobehavioral disorders. These *diagnostic discriminants* remain a highly controversial part of QEEG. Some groups believe strongly in the validity of these techniques, whereas other groups believe that these techniques have not been validated sufficiently yet to allow their use in routine clinical practice.

Statistical techniques have been applied to determine whether individual simple EEG features are "within normal limits" using the z-score method. This assumes that the distribution of a particular EEG feature forms a gaussian or normal bell-shaped curve when sampled in a large population of normal control subjects. The value for an individual patient is compared to this bell-shaped normative distribution with z-score statistics, measuring how much that individual differs from the control group mean. This difference usually is expressed in terms of standard deviations. A patient's EEG feature scored as z = 2.0 (i.e., 2.0 standard deviations above the normative group mean) has a value greater than that seen in 95 percent of normal control subjects. Such z-score techniques can help to highlight areas in which an individual patient differs substantially from an age-matched control group. However, interpretation becomes difficult when a very large number of z-score values are assessed, because chance alone will cause some z-scores to be very high. EEG artifacts, other technical problems, and confounding clinical situations can also cause high z-scores.[4] Even if all possible sources of error are ruled out, statistical "abnormality" does not necessarily mean physiologic abnormality.[11] Therefore z-scores never should be interpreted by themselves, but only in the context of all the other available EEG data.[12]

PROBLEMS

Simple paperless digital EEG recordings can be interpreted in a manner analogous to the interpretation of traditional paper EEGs. Problems are more difficult for the more advanced QEEG techniques. Topographic mapping, frequency analysis, discriminant analysis, and large-scale statistical analysis techniques are often confounded by artifacts, problematic clinical factors, and overinterpretation of statistical variations.

Artifacts

Many artifacts are present in routine digital EEGs. They show up in various, sometimes subtle or confusing ways for advanced QEEG analysis. Artifacts showing up in new and unusual ways make difficult the electroencephalographer's task of interpreting artifact-contaminated data.[4] Some artifacts in QEEG show up in interesting ways (Fig. 8-2).

The only acceptable way of dealing with artifacts is to follow the EEG data carefully through the several steps of the analysis process. A clinical reader must be able expertly to identify and interpret the EEG tracings that form the basis of any analytic QEEG process. Only by understanding such EEG tracings thoroughly can the reader hope to understand the artifacts and problems that occur in any advanced analysis based on those data.[12,13]

There is widespread misunderstanding about the use of automatic "artifact rejection" in QEEG processing. Many users have the mistaken impression that automated digital artifact screening techniques are able to eliminate artifacts from the EEG record, so that the computer-based frequency analysis and topographic maps are free from artifact contamination. Nothing could be further from the truth. Artifact identification techniques are primitive and often identify only high-amplitude transients such as large muscle artifact or eye-blinks. Other kinds of artifacts are detected less easily. Again, the lesson is clear: a reader must evaluate both the EEG tracings and analyzed data together to understand the results of the advanced EEG analysis.

Confounding Clinical Factors

A variety of clinical situations can interfere with QEEG analyses, especially those using normative databases.[4,12,13] Even drowsiness can interfere with normative EEG comparison techniques because the normal control subjects were fully awake. Statistical normative EEG analysis in a drowsy subject therefore is very "abnormal." Medication can affect the EEG; normal control groups are generally medication-free. Other confounding clinical problems include fluid shunting, nystagmus, skull defects, and other problems with the scalp or skull that may not affect brain function. These factors can alter topographic maps, frequency analyses, and statistical

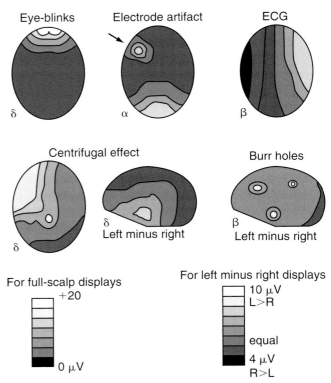

FIGURE 8-2 ▪ Selected examples of artifacts, showing their typical topographic distribution. Eye-blinks and movements (top, left) have stereotypic frontal distributions. Electrode artifacts (top, center) appear as small, geometrically shaped hills or holes, sometimes described as bull's-eyes. Burr holes (bottom, right) can mimic multiple electrode artifacts. Electrocardiogram isopotential contours (top, right) usually run anterior to posterior, with the steepest gradient running downhill from one ear to the other. The centrifugal effect (bottom, left, and center) is a distortion introduced by mapping differences, pushing maxima away from the sagittal midline. The full-scalp and the half-scalp (nose at left) views here are of exactly the same data, but the topographic location has been pushed away from the midsagittal line in the half-scalp display. (From Nuwer MR: Quantitative EEG. I. Techniques and problems of frequency analysis and topographic mapping. J Clin Neurophysiol, 5:1, 1988, with permission.)

analyses substantially, even though they represent no actual cerebral impairment.

The EEG contains phenomena that are of dubious clinical significance: the so-called normal variant waveforms and transients. One example is the mu rhythm in the central region, which is known to have no clear clinical significance. Yet it can affect the statistical calculations and alter the topographic maps of alpha-band activity substantially.

For the reader to be able to understand and evaluate properly the clinical problem at hand, it is necessary to analyze the whole situation, including the clinical problem, medications used, and EEG tracings, as well as the results of QEEG analysis.

Technical Diversity

EEG analytic techniques differ among vendors and among specific analytic programs. Many of these technical differences impact significantly on the results. Because of these differences, the results obtained on one commercial machine are not directly comparable to those obtained on a different machine. Some QEEG techniques are found on certain machines only and are not available on others. Some of this incompatibility is caused by proprietary restrictions or patenting of techniques. In other cases, incompatibility is caused by individual technical decisions made by specific manufacturers. Discriminant or normative comparison studies run using one vendor's program cannot simply be applied to recordings with a different technique using a different program on a different machine. Different techniques used on different machines may each need to be validated clinically.

Statistical Problems

Complex statistical techniques (e.g., z-scores and discriminant analysis) depend on data meeting certain assumptions. In general, data from EEG tests are not distributed in the general population in a gaussian or normal bell-shaped curve.

Because of this, simple parametric statistical analysis is often in error, sometimes by substantial degrees. Such error can be corrected partially by transforming the data in certain mathematical ways. The most common transformations are $\log(x)$ and $\log(x/(1-x))$. Even where transformation corrections are used, the reader or interpreter needs to exercise caution in accepting the results of any purely statistical analysis. In general, the reader might use statistical techniques to help point out features of possible clinical significance but should not make clinical interpretations based on statistical results alone.

Many advanced EEG analytic techniques produce enormous numbers of statistical results, sometimes hundred or thousands of z-score tests. False-positive results are common. Separating the numerous false-positive findings from true-positive findings can be difficult or impossible. This is compounded by the prevalence of artifact contamination and confounding clinical factors previously mentioned.

USE IN CLINICAL SETTINGS

Cerebrovascular Disease

QEEG is more sensitive than routine EEG for detecting cerebral hemispheric abnormalities related to cerebrovascular disease. EEG, whether quantified or routine, can detect abnormalities but cannot differentiate between kinds of pathology; nor does it have the exquisite localizing ability of CT or MRI. Nevertheless, it is inexpensive, noninvasive, reproducible, and sensitive, and it can be done in a variety of settings (e.g., the intensive care unit [ICU] or operating room), even on a continuous monitoring basis.

Routine EEGs are abnormal in about 40 to 70 percent of patients with cerebrovascular accidents (CVAs). In one study, QEEG prospectively classified 64 normal control subjects and 94 patients (54 with stroke and 40 whose symptoms cleared within a week).[14] The classification was abnormal in 90 percent of the patients, compared with only 3 percent false-positive among the normals. This included QEEG abnormalities in 84 percent of patients whose EEGs had been read as normal in routine visual EEG assessment. In three further studies of 15 to 20 patients each, QEEG was abnormal in 85 percent of patients, but no abnormal results were found in control subjects. Routine EEG was abnormal in only one-half of these patients, and often was just diffusely abnormal or poorly localizing. However, QEEG did not do well in precise localization.

QEEG changes correspond well to regional cerebral blood flow, regional oxygen extraction, and metabolism. Relationships are particularly good for relative delta or alpha activity and the ratio of slow to fast rhythms. Several groups have found correlation coefficients of 0.67 to 0.76 relating such EEG features to metabolic parameters.[15,16]

QEEG does not differentiate among types of focal cerebral pathology, e.g., ischemic infarction, intracranial hemorrhages, brain tumors, and head trauma.[17,18] The kinds of EEG changes seen were similar despite obvious differences in the pathology, leading the investigators to conclude that these tests may be sensitive but are nonspecific (Fig. 8-3).

Degree of slowing or loss of fast activity corresponded to National Institutes of Health Stroke Scale (NIHSS) outcome and disability at 30 days and 6 months.[19–21] Degree of QEEG impairment corresponded to the stroke volume, and preserved QEEG cortical function often corresponded to subcortical lacunes as the pathology.[22] Subcortical vascular dementia is more likely to cause a loss of fast activity, which helps to differentiate it on QEEG from Alzheimer dementia, which causes more slowing of the posterior dominant alpha mean frequency.[23]

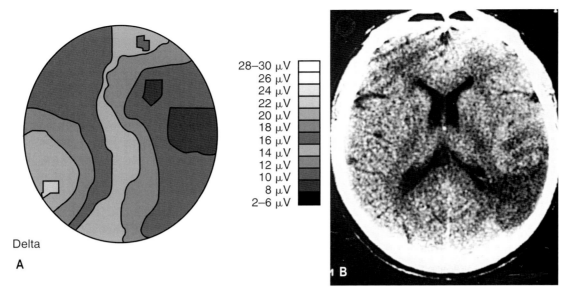

28–30 μV
26 μV
24 μV
22 μV
20 μV
18 μV
16 μV
14 μV
12 μV
10 μV
8 μV
2–6 μV

Delta

A

B

FIGURE 8-3 ■ Comparison of computed tomography (CT) with quantitative electroencephalography (QEEG) in a 57-year-old patient who had sudden onset of fluent aphasia while undergoing balloon angioplasty. **A**, Electroencephalogram (EEG) was being monitored during the procedure, with the use of real-time frequency analysis and topographic mapping. The embolic ischemic change was seen immediately on EEG and indicated in which vessel to look for the errant balloon. **B**, The follow-up CT scan several days later showed a wedge-shaped infarct located very similarly to the changes already localized by QEEG. Note that CT uses a left–right convention opposite to that of EEG topographic maps. (Case and illustrations courtesy of S. Jordan, M.D.)

In most patients, the clinical and MRI findings are already sufficient, and EEG studies provide no useful additional information to help in the care of the patient. In the occasional instance, QEEG is used for patients who cannot obtain imaging.

EEG Monitoring in the Intensive Care Unit

Continuous ICU EEG monitoring has become a commonly used tool for monitoring the brain in certain critically ill patients.[24–27] QEEG measurements are used to display trends of frequency content. Those trends can help to identify changes over time and can measure the variability of the frequencies. Variability is a helpful sign that is not apparent when looking at the routine EEG tracings. *Variability* corresponds to changes in frequency content over long time periods, in contrast to EEG *reactivity*, which corresponds to short-term changes often induced by environmental stimulation. Trends are commonly used in the ICU along with the routine EEG tracings. EEG tracings and trends can be viewed remotely from off-site as well as at the bedside, thereby extending the physician's ability to evaluate the patient.

Monitoring QEEG in the ICU can detect nonconvulsive seizures or unwitnessed convulsive seizures.[24,26,28] They are associated independently with increased midline shift and a poorer overall prognosis. The findings of continuous ICU EEG monitoring result in changes in antiepileptic drug orders in up to half of the patients monitored, based on identification of seizures on EEG.[29,30] Nonconvulsive seizures or nonconvulsive status epilepticus occur in 15 to 25 percent of neurologically critically ill patients.[30–33] Seizures can be identified by trending of QEEG frequency content or by automated seizure detection software, and can be tracked to measure the efficacy of treatment (Fig 8-4).[28,33] Because such seizures sometimes occur only every few hours, a routine 30-minute EEG may miss them. The presence of nonconvulsive seizures in these patients is an independent risk factor associated with poorer outcome and midline shifts. The seizures may provoke secondary damage in marginally compensated brains.

After subarachnoid hemorrhage, trended frequency analysis shows reduced variability and relative alpha during clinical deteriorations. Such an electrographic deterioration precedes overt clinical changes by up to 2 days before an episode of vasospasm. This early warning can prompt early intervention to prevent clinical complications.[34,35]

EEG changes occur within seconds of the onset of ischemia. The QEEG trending can demonstrate dysfunction when the ischemia is severe enough to disrupt function

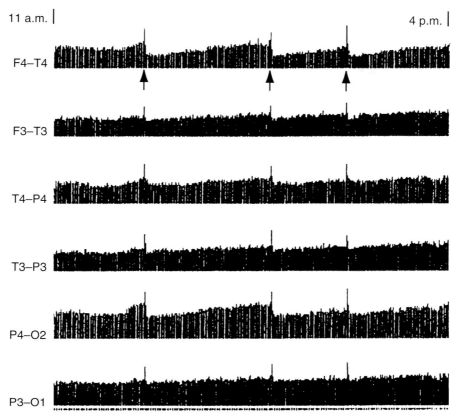

FIGURE 8-4 ▪ Electroencephalographic (EEG) detection of three nonconvulsive seizures. EEG monitoring over 5 hours in a 50-year-old hypertensive man 3 days after a 3-cm left thalamic hemorrhagic stroke. There were no outward signs of seizures on examination of this comatose patient. EEG monitoring detected three nonconvulsive seizures during this 5-hour period. Monitoring trends from six EEG channels are shown. Time is displayed along the horizontal axis, from 11 a.m. to 4 p.m. For each channel, the amount of alpha activity is displayed as vertical bars. Alpha activity is expressed as a percentage of the overall EEG activity from 1 to 30 Hz. The percentage-alpha values range here from approximately 15 percent to 50 percent. Seizures were suspected when an abrupt jump in percentage-alpha was seen, followed by a suppression of alpha activity. The three suspected events are noted here with arrows. Review of the stored polygraph EEG showed that these were generalized electrographic seizure discharges. These nonconvulsive seizures were treated with phenytoin. (Courtesy of UCLA EEG Laboratory.)

but not so severe as to cause infarction such as that associated with decreased perfusion pressure.[36] This immediate feedback makes QEEG trending in the ICU clinically useful for monitoring.

ICU EEG trending has been used to track improvements in ICU patients treated with mannitol or albumin for increased intracranial pressure. The time course of the changes paralleled the several-hour effectiveness of the drugs, suggesting that the QEEG trending techniques effectively monitor reproducible therapeutic effects in lowering intracranial pressure and antiedema effects.[37,38]

In the neonatal ICU, a simplified version of QEEG ICU trending often is used. This measures the total integrated amplitude over minute-long portions of the monitoring for two channels. Goals are similar to those for the adult ICU: identify seizures or other complications and monitor therapy. Normal neonates and infants show age-dependent amplitude and discontinuity features that can be measured on the trending.[39,40] The trending results correspond clinically to the severity of impairment as judged by other means.[41] The trending can detect seizures.[42] Clinical outcome at 15 months corresponds in general to the trending findings.[43]

In surgery, similar trending can assist in measuring frequency content over the hours of a case. Traditional EEG has long been used during carotid endarterectomy to help assess brain function during carotid clamping. In turn, this can be used to help determine whether a vascular shunt is required, or whether any other surgical or anesthetic intervention is needed urgently. Quantified EEG testing can assist in detection of abnormalities with carotid clamping more often than is seen with routine EEG.[18,44]

Epilepsy

Quantitative EEG is used in several ways in evaluating patients with epilepsy. Careful analysis of the scalp voltage fields of epileptiform spikes can shed light on the location of their cortical generators and contribute prognostic information. Automated paradigms may detect spikes and subclinical seizures in prolonged recordings.

THREE-DIMENSIONAL DIPOLE SOURCE LOCALIZATION

Three-dimensional spike generator localization is difficult in routine EEG recordings. Visual inspection can lateralize a spike much better than it can localize its likely generator site. By modeling the epileptic spike generator as a single discrete point source or localized region and quantifying its scalp electrical potential field, the three-dimensional location of the likely epileptic generator can be calculated (Fig. 8-5).[45–51] Averaging together individual occurrences of the epileptic spike reduces background EEG noise. Spikes need to be categorized before processing, so spikes from a single putative generator source are used together, and spikes probably arising from other sites are processed separately.[52] Least square error estimates of scalp potential maps are calculated for various proposed intracranial dipole sources. Some models assume electrical characteristics for brain, cerebrospinal fluid, skull, and scalp. Those models should be adjusted for differences in conductivity through known lesions.[53] Larger numbers of scalp electrodes improve localization accuracy.[54] Deep sources are localized more poorly than are superficial ones, averaging 12-mm error in some studies of deep sources.[55–57] Mesial temporal discharges may not contribute to scalp recordings, so scalp recordings may be measuring regional cortical discharges.[58] All these models have limitations both technically and in the assumptions on which they are based.[59]

Current source density reconstruction of intracranial generators associated with interictal epileptiform activity in temporal lobe epilepsy has been assessed in presurgical patients with temporal lobe epilepsy.[45,60,61] Patients with mesial temporal onsets had epileptic spikes with initial activation maximum in the ipsilateral anterior basal lateral temporal lobe mostly extending up to affected mesial temporal structures. Patients with lateral temporal lesions showed initial activation regions confined to temporal neocortex immediately adjacent to the epileptogenic lesion. Such current density reconstructions are helpful in assessing surgical planning, specifically in helping to determine whether the mesial temporal structures should be considered in the epileptogenic zone.

SPIKE AND SEIZURE DETECTION

Digital EEG analysis can be used to detect spikes and subclinical epileptic seizures in long EEG recordings such as those obtained by ambulatory or inpatient video-EEG monitoring. A variety of seizure and spike detectors have been described[9,62–64]; all have problematic false-positive and false-negative detection rates. They are most successful for large, obvious spikes and for typical, prolonged subclinical epileptic ictal discharges. Such automated detection paradigms help clinicians sort through vast amounts of data. Typical automated paradigms identify candidate spikes or ictal discharges and present them to a human interpreter for evaluation. Seizure detectors may be based on factors such as the tendency for seizures to change their frequency characteristics (e.g., slowing as they develop[65]) or their tendency to involve greatly increased synchrony among channels,[66] whereas the detector avoids simpler rhythmic bursts.[67] Seizures start with simple rhythmic discharges but progress to more complex relationships.[68] Three-dimensional localization paradigms have also been used for spike and seizure detection; these are based on the assumption that spikes and seizures can be constrained to come from reasonable neurologic sites, whereas artifact generators dwell elsewhere.[69,70]

Automated screening can provide statistical summaries of the candidate spikes' location and rates during sleep states, medication challenges, or other events. Such summaries across space and time can be helpful in understanding a patient's clinical seizure disorder. A preponderance of spikes in one location often corresponds to the location of the seizure focus itself.[71] Persistence of epileptiform spiking despite changing sleep state or medication blood levels usually corresponds to the location of the epileptic focus.

Automated screening does detect many events not recognized clinically by the patient. Among 552 records from 502 patients who had ambulatory EEG monitoring, a total of 47 records (8.5 percent) contained focal seizures.[72] Of those 47, 29 (61.7 percent) had electroclinical

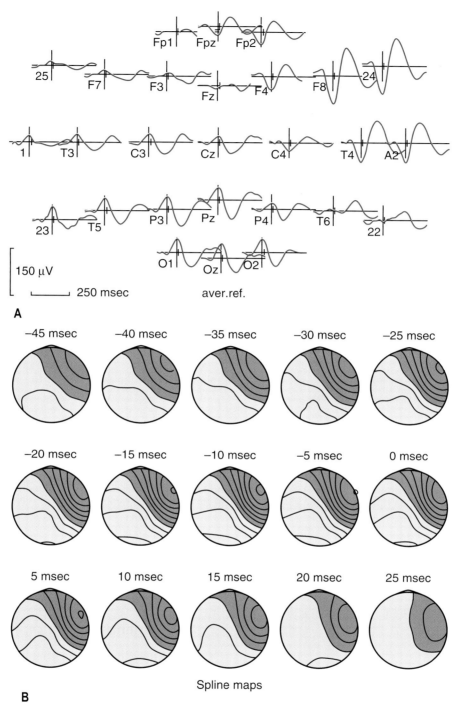

FIGURE 8-5 ▪ **A**, Spatial electroencephalographic display of a right anterior temporal spike. Sites are identified by their International 10–20 System location, along with extra channels in the temporal regions. **B**, A sequence is shown of topographic voltage maps at 5-msec intervals during the same right temporal epileptic spike. In this top-down view of the head, the nose is at the top of each individual topographic map. The field contour isopotential lines are shown. The dark blue regions are of negative electrical activity. Note the stable voltage topography during the course of this spike. Location and contours of the negative spike field remain similar; only the magnitude of the field changes. This particular negative field at right frontal temporal scalp is not accompanied by any other characteristic maximum or minimum, such as a contralateral positive maximum of a voltage dipole.

Continued

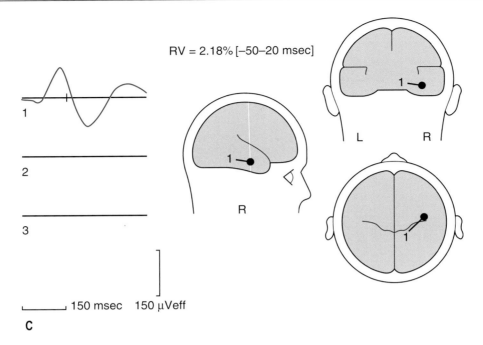

RV = 2.18% [–50–20 msec]

150 msec   150 μVeff

C

FIGURE 8.5—cont'd   C, A temporal and three-dimensional spatial representation of the same epileptic spike as shown in *A* and *B.* Only one simple dipole source appeared, despite the model's freedom to allow a second or third dipole. In the three-dimensional dipole localization, the spike source was found at the deep right temporal region, which is consistent with a localization near the right hippocampus. Such spikes are typical of patients who have right temporal lobe epilepsy caused by mesial temporal sclerosis. Such spike localization has been confirmed by intracranial recordings performed simultaneously with such a scalp dipole localization technique. (From Ebersole JS: Non-invasive localization of the epileptogenic focus by EEG dipole modeling. Acta Neurol Scand Suppl, 152:20, 1994, with permission. ⓒ 1994 Munksgaard International Publishers Ltd., Copenhagen, Denmark.)

seizures identified by patient pushbuttons. Another 18 of 47 records (38.3 percent) had focal seizures that were unrecognized by the patient, including 11 of those 47 records (23.4 percent) recognized only by the computer.

GENERALIZED DISCHARGES

Generalized interictal discharges can be measured with a coherence analysis of bifrontal spike-wave discharges.[73] These spike-wave discharges may represent either primary generalized activity or a secondary bilateral synchrony associated with a unilateral lesion, often frontal. The coherence analysis can distinguish between these two similarly appearing bilateral spike-wave discharges in a way that cannot be accomplished by simple visual analysis (Fig. 8-6). When a bifrontal discharge is driven by a unilateral frontal focus, the coherence analysis reveals that the EEG events occur about 15 msec earlier over the scalp ipsilateral to the focus. Other investigators have also studied the spike-wave discharges of absence

(petit mal) seizures, describing typical details of those EEG events.[74,75]

Dementia and Encephalopathies

EEG traditionally helps to distinguish between dementia and depression. The presence of excessive slowing helps to demonstrate the organic basis of the patient's symptoms, supporting their distinction from depression or normal aging. QEEG techniques may assist when the abnormality is rather borderline or subtle.

Normal elderly persons have gradual changes in EEG frequencies compared with younger normal control subjects. The nature of these changes is still somewhat in dispute. Normal aging is associated with a gradual increase in delta, decrease in beta, and decrease in mean frequency.[76,77]

Patients with Alzheimer disease have increased theta slow activity compared with age-matched normal controls. Their alpha mean frequency is slower and alpha

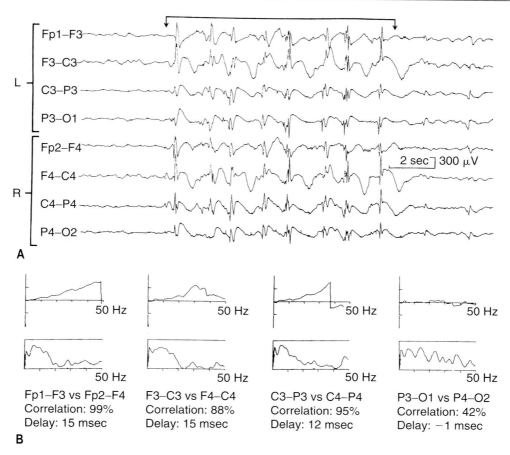

FIGURE 8-6 ■ Measurements of small time differences between spike-wave activity occurring over the two hemispheres. **A**, Burst of slow and irregular spike-wave activity showing apparent synchrony between homologous channels on the left and right scalp. This and similar bursts were subjected to coherence and phase analysis. **B**, Phase and coherence spectra show a linear phase relationship (top graphs) at frequencies for which coherence is high (bottom graphs), except in the posterior electrode pairs. For the three-electrode pairs with positive linear phase slopes, the steepness of the slope reveals that the left hemisphere leads the right by 15, 15, and 12 msec. The patient had a known lesion in the left hemisphere, and these results suggest that the widespread discharges do originate near the lesion. (From Gotman J, Darcey TM, Lieb JP: Commentary: computer analysis of seizure recordings. p. 361. In Engel J, Jr [ed]: Surgical Treatment of the Epilepsies. Raven, New York, 1987, with permission.)

amplitude is reduced.[78] Alpha blocking is impaired or reduced.[79]

Patients with mild cognitive impairment (MCI) who progressed to Alzheimer disease showed decreased QEEG alpha compared with MCI patients who remained stable. Several studies have found a variety of further QEEG abnormalities, sometimes disagreeing with each other about which ones are predictive of Alzheimer disease.[76,77,80-82] In one study, conversion from MCI to Alzheimer disease was predicted by QEEG.[81] At baseline, frontoparietal midline coherence, as well as delta (temporal), theta (parietal, occipital, and temporal), and alpha-1 (central, parietal,

occipital, temporal, and limbic) LORETA sources, were stronger in MCI patients who converted to Alzheimer disease than in patients with stable MCI. Regression modeling showed that low midline coherence and weak temporal LORETA source were associated with a 10 percent annual conversion rate to Alzheimer disease. This conversion rate increased up to 40 to 60 percent when strong temporal delta LORETA sources and high midline gamma coherence were observed. This interesting study awaits replication by others.

A dozen studies have explored the QEEG correlates of response to treatment with acetylcholinesterase inhibitors, many with interesting results.[80,82] Drugs may partially normalize the QEEG findings in persons with mild Alzheimer disease who have responded clinically to treatment with donepezil, an effect that is not seen among treatment nonresponders.[83]

Increased slow-frequency EEG power has been observed in vascular dementia compared to Alzheimer disease; high-frequency power was nearly normal in vascular dementia, but decreased in Alzheimer disease. The increased slow-frequency power with nearly normal high-frequency power in vascular dementia may reflect subcortical pathology, whereas cortical pathology in Alzheimer disease may relate to decreased fast-frequency power.[84] Mean frequency may be the best QEEG feature to differentiate Alzheimer disease from vascular dementia.[23] Furthermore, occipital peak frequency was the QEEG feature best correlated with mini-mental status examination (MMSE) in patients with MCI and Alzheimer disease.[85] These findings were not specific to Alzheimer disease and vascular dementia. Huntington disease and frontotemporal dementia have similar QEEG changes.[86–88] Patients with Parkinson disease showed diffusely increased slowing.[89–92] The amount of frontal QEEG slowing among 32 patients with Parkinson disease did correspond to their decreased executive and motor function.[93,94]

Many investigators have studied only group differences. In contrast, Jordan and associates set forth some specific criteria based on previous publications by others, and prospectively tested how well these criteria could help to evaluate patients with possible early dementia.[95] They selected patients who were presenting for their first visit to a neurologist because of complaints of declining cognitive function. Sixty-four elderly patients with cognitive disturbance were studied, along with age-matched normal control subjects. Quantitative EEG analysis was abnormal in 85 percent of the patients eventually found to have an organic dementia, compared with only 10 percent of patients eventually diagnosed as having depression. The EEG features of relative suppression of alpha activity and suppression of P300 parietal activity were observed in half of the patients with Alzheimer disease, but in only 6 percent of patients with other forms of dementia. Mody and colleagues found that a temporal-parietal-occipital delta plus theta percentage activity score is usually greater than 46 percent in patients with Alzheimer disease.[96] Using that criterion, they were able to distinguish between patients with Alzheimer disease and age-matched normal subjects with a sensitivity of 96 percent.

In a longitudinal study of patients with Alzheimer disease, the EEG worsened in some but not in others over time.[97] It was difficult to predict from the EEG alone which patients would deteriorate clinically or electroencephalographically during the longitudinal follow-up. In one study, a decreased beta activity among normal elderly patients predicted which patients would undergo a longitudinal cognitive decline.[98] EEG plus neurobehavioral abnormalities each were moderately strong predictors of future speed of cognitive decline in Alzheimer disease.[94]

Finally, positron emission tomography (PET) measures of oxygen metabolism correlate well with QEEG frequency analysis in patients with Alzheimer disease.[99] Parietotemporal hypometabolism corresponds to increased frequency content below 8 Hz and to decreased content above 8 Hz (r = 0.65–0.84). This correspondence was seen well, even over individual hemispheres for asymmetric cases.

EEG is well known to slow in the encephalopathies. Similar reports have been published about QEEG in encephalopathy, such as that due to renal failure and solvent exposure.[100,101] The clinical usefulness of such a finding is unclear: for example, the solvent exposure changes did not parallel the degree of exposure.

Hepatic encephalopathy is more amenable to grading using QEEG measurements.[102] QEEG also could be measured in hepatitis C patients who were receiving treatment with interferon.[103]

Medication-induced changes were measured with QEEG in patients starting antiepileptic medications.[104] QEEG occipital channel recordings were measured to assess the effects of therapeutic doses of carbamazepine (CBZ), oxcarbazepine (OXC), valproate, and lamotrigine monotherapy. Measurements were made at predrug baseline and after 8 weeks on the drug. An untreated control group was used for comparison. CBZ and OXC decreased the alpha mean frequency. The other two drugs did not change mean frequency but did reduce total power. CBZ increased theta slowing.

Overall, slowing due to dementia or encephalopathy may be identified, tracked, and localized in patients using QEEG techniques. Many of these tools are of scientific interest in understanding the pathophysiology of dementias and encephalopathies. The clinical yield may be only modest. Alpha mean frequency and amount of slow activity may have the greatest differentiation among the disorders.

Psychiatric and Neurobehavioral Disorders

The role of QEEG in patients with psychiatric and neurobehavioral disorders is controversial. These disorders include learning disabilities and dyslexia,[105–112] schizophrenia,[113,114] depression,[10,115] and neurobehavioral changes following closed head injury.[116–118] Some investigators strongly adhere to beliefs that quantified EEG techniques (e.g., discriminant analysis) have great clinical value. The topics were reviewed by a panel of experts appointed jointly by the American Academy of Neurology and American Clinical Neurophysiology Society.[12] The expert review indicated that QEEG techniques remain investigational in these disorders and are not yet ready for general clinical use.

Some publications have shown diagnostic identification of patients with neuropsychiatric disorders. Many such studies are technically and statistically complex. Most complex techniques have not found general acceptance in the clinical community. Some attempts to replicate these studies have been negative.[119] Ways in which the clinician can use this information at present remain unclear. In one large study of psychiatric, neurologic, and neurobehavioral disorders, no clear common QEEG factors were found that differentiated one diagnosis from another nosologically.[120] Decreased QEEG delta-theta activity was associated with brain atrophy in MRI. Decreased slow activity has been described in several studies, and might be a substantial contribution since, unlike increased slow or fast activity, it cannot be observed by visual inspection of the EEG.[121–123] Its physiologic significance remains unclear. While QEEG features alone cannot differentiate nosological entities, they provide valuable *semiological* data that can help in the overall clinical evaluation.[11] On the other hand, when used in conjunction with LORETA, this decrease in slow bands was found later to be more marked at left temporal regions in alcoholics with associated depression in contrast with nondepressed alcoholics, and was correlated with the severity of depression as measured by the Beck depression inventory, providing further evidence about the possible association of decreased slow-band activity and cortical atrophy or cellular degeneration.[124] A task force of the American Psychiatric Association (APA) concluded that QEEG can help to detect and assess slow activity in organic disorders such as dementia. However, the APA also concluded that these tests are not yet able to aid in the diagnosis of other disorders such as schizophrenia and depression.[125] Observations in children with attention deficit disorders have been very interesting.[99,106–112] In comparison to normal children, patients with attention deficit–hyperactivity disorder (ADHD) show increased theta and decreased beta.[126–135] These observations suggested reduced cortical differentiation and specialization in ADHD. However, some ADHD children show an increased beta, suggesting ADHD does not constitute a homogenous group by QEEG profile.[108] Patients' IQs did not correlate with the QEEG findings.[136] Some have suggested that biofeedback may help ADHD children to overcome this theta-beta imbalance, with the goal of improving their symptoms.[137,138]

Autism is another disorder that may have many contributing causes that present clinically with similar symptoms. QEEG findings have varied. Unmedicated autistic children without comorbidities showed higher EEG amplitudes than normal control children, especially increased amplitude of the beta activity.[139] Children with autism spectrum disorders in one study showed more QEEG delta and less alpha than normal children, whereas in a different study the QEEG showed increased posterior theta, decreased anterior delta, increased midline beta, and various coherence changes.[140,141] These studies were small enough for some reported changes not to be reproducible. Autism may be too heterogeneous and may not have a typical QEEG signature.

The QEEG findings in depression have varied. In one recent study, increased parietal and occipital amplitude across the theta, alpha, and beta bands was found in patients with early stages of depression compared to age-matched controls.[142] An interesting line of investigation examined whether changes in QEEG could predict clinical outcome from starting an antidepressant. To assess changes, Leuchter proposed a QEEG measure he calls *cordance*,[143,144] a sum of the normalized absolute and relative power values, calculated for each recording electrode using nearest-neighbor electrodes as references. In a large multicenter study, QEEG measures were combined to make a treatment response index. The QEEG index was measured at baseline and again after 1 week of antidepressant treatment. The index was a weighted combination of the relative theta and alpha power at week 1, and the difference between alpha-1 power at baseline and alpha-2 power at week 1, scaled to range from 0 (low probability) to 100 (high probability of response). In a study of escitalopram 10 mg,[120,145] the index corresponded to those patients with a good symptomatic response to the drug. Others have reported on findings for other antidepressants.[146,147] More work is needed to evaluate whether this use can be generalized, or how well it could be used for individual patient care treatment decisions.[148]

In alcoholism, the most widely described QEEG feature is increase in beta activity. QEEG beta was increased with benzodiazepine use, as well as with a family history of alcoholism.[149] Decreased QEEG diffuse slow activity was associated with cortical atrophy as seen in MRI, and with hypertension and chronicity of alcohol drinking. Increased QEEG beta was not related to psychiatric features such as anxiety or memory disorders.[149]

Overall, the use of QEEG analysis in these psychiatric and neurobehavioral areas has raised some interesting scientific questions that may facilitate understanding of the underlying pathophysiology of certain disorders once the physiologic significance of the different QEEG alterations is understood adequately. The eventual role of QEEG in the clinical diagnosis of these disorders remains controversial.

Closed Head Injury

After closed head injury, patients with extensive traumatic lesions were reported to have abnormalities on routine EEG, QEEG, and neuroimaging studies, a finding that is not surprising.[116] By 1 year after moderate to severe closed head injury, fast frequencies increased and slow frequencies decreased.[150] Patients in the minimally conscious state without awareness had greater QEEG slowing and less fast activity than patients who were severely impaired neurologically but had signs of awareness.[151]

For mild closed head injury, reports have often been uncontrolled, unblinded, and retrospective, which makes assessment of clinical utility difficult.[116–118,152] Questions have been raised about the accuracy of EEG diagnostic discriminants for closed head injury.[153] Von Bierbrauer and co-workers showed that increased slowing and slowing of the alpha peak frequency occur in the days after a mild closed head injury, but these resolve over weeks (Fig. 8-7).[154] Similarly, McCrea and associates assessed high-school and college football players, 28 with a concussion and 29 without.[155] Players were tested at the beginning of the season and again after a concussion on the day of injury, as well as 8 days and 45 days later. The injured group reported more significant postconcussive symptoms during the first 3 days post-injury, which resolved by days 5 and 8. Injured subjects also performed more poorly than controls on neurocognitive testing on the day of injury, but no differences were evident on day 8 or day 45. QEEG studies revealed significant abnormalities in the injured group on the day of injury and day 8 post-injury, but these had resolved back to normal by day 45. QEEG variables included four variables reflecting changes in interhemispheric (left vs. right) power relationships (asymmetry), one variable associated with interhemispheric coherence relationships (independent of power), and two variables reflecting changes in high and low beta absolute power. It remains to be shown whether any diagnostic QEEG features can be identified after more than a month from a mild closed head injury.

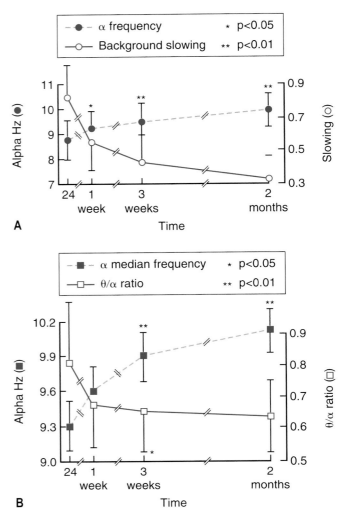

FIGURE 8-7 ■ Changes in the electroencephalogram (EEG) and quantitative electroencephalogram (QEEG) were seen among 31 patients during the 2 months after a mild traumatic brain injury. **A**, In the routine EEG, the posterior dominant alpha frequency gradually increases and the amount of intermixed slowing gradually decreases. **B**, In the QEEG, the median posterior alpha frequency increases and the theta/alpha ratio decreases. (From Nuwer MR, Hovda DA, Schrader LM et al: Routine and quantitative EEG in mild traumatic brain injury. Clin Neurophysiol, 116:2001, 2005, with permission; adapted from von Bierbrauer A, Weissenborn K, Hinrichs H et al: Die automatische (computergestützte) EEG-Analyse im Vergleich zur visuellen EEG—Analyse bei Patienten nach leichtem Schädelhirntrauma (Verlaufsuntersuchung). EEG EMG Z, 23:151, 1992.)

RECOMMENDATIONS

The clinical interpreter of digital EEG studies should have the skills, knowledge, and ability to read routine digital EEG tracings, plus additional experience and understanding of the QEEG techniques.[156] For more complex quantitative analyses, the following recommendations are applicable. This applies especially to techniques such as topographic mapping and frequency analysis.

Quantitative EEG measurements should be run repeatedly, preferably with three separate repetitions of complex types of testing. This would be analogous to the current standard of practice for evoked potential testing. The several repetitions then can be compared with each other, ensuring that the data are reproducible. Routine EEG records should be at least 20 minutes long, whether they are run as routine tracings alone or to serve as a basis for QEEG techniques. Too short a recording may miss optimal segments of fully awake, artifact-free EEG for complex analysis. Good technologic skills are required for noting the behavior of the patient and other events as recordings proceed, as well as for minimizing or eliminating drowsiness, artifacts, and other problems that may arise. QEEG features should not be considered abnormal unless they are reproducible. Even reproducible features are not necessarily caused by cerebral activity but may reflect continuous muscle activity, loose electrodes, or certain other problems. In general, a real EEG feature should show up in at least three adjacent scalp recording sites. Events appearing at just one electrode site should be regarded as artifact until proven otherwise. One also needs to take into account an expectation that many statistical tests will show high z-scores from time to time by random chance alone. This is a substantial problem for the sometimes-encountered shotgun approach to testing of hundreds or thousands of z-scores in one subject.

A QEEG test report should be specific about the techniques used. The report should indicate how much artifact-free EEG was included in the quantitative processing itself, how many data repetitions were run, and whether the results were reproducible across repetitions. A report using statistical testing should estimate the number of separate statistical tests evaluated. The specific criterion used for abnormality should be reported explicitly, describing the affected frequency band, direction of the change (increase or decrease), any accompanying changes in the routine EEG tracings, and the degree to which change was found on statistical testing. For example, rather than simply noting "a statistical abnormality at the left parietal region," the report might describe "a 45 percent increase in theta was seen at left central and parietal regions, which was beyond the normal range for this age; a review of the EEG tracings confirmed this excess slowing."

Statistical changes alone are not sufficient to consider a record abnormal. The change must make sense, must be clinically meaningful, and must reasonably exclude artifact by thorough evaluation of the corresponding EEG tracings. Some EEG changes do not represent pathologic conditions. The reader should expect to encounter artifacts, other technical problems, confounding clinical problems, normal EEG variants, and statistical chance events. This needs to be taken carefully into account whenever one reports on the possible clinical correlations of quantified, digital EEG test results.

CONCLUDING COMMENTS

All community neurologists should be aware of the advantages and limitations of digital and quantitative EEG processing. Even those who do not use these techniques in their own practices will encounter them from time to time. The techniques have promise for furthering the field of EEG in specific ways, but they also bring with them certain problems and disadvantages. Use of these complex, quantified techniques in neurology and psychiatry remains controversial in certain clinical settings. In some situations, these QEEG techniques supplement the routine EEG. This appears to be true in limited settings in the evaluation of cerebrovascular disease, epilepsy, and dementia. The controversial areas include the evaluation of depression, schizophrenia, dyslexia, and neurobehavioral syndromes such as that seen following head trauma. In all these latter settings, further studies are required to clarify the clinical role of such techniques.

REFERENCES

1. Nuwer MR, Engel J, Sutherling WW et al: Monitoring at the University of California, Los Angeles. p. 385. In Gottman J, Ives JR, Gloor P (eds): Long-Term Monitoring in Epilepsy. Elsevier, Amsterdam, 1985
2. Nuwer MR, Comi G, Emerson R et al: IFCN standards for digital recording of clinical EEG. Electroencephalogr Clin Neurophysiol, 106:259, 1998
3. Pascual-Marqui RD, Esslen M, Kochi K et al: Functional imaging with low-resolution brain electromagnetic tomography (LORETA): a review. Methods Find Exp Clin Pharmacol, 24(Suppl C):91, 2002
4. Nuwer MR: Quantitative EEG: I. Techniques and problems of frequency analysis and topographic mapping. J Clin Neurophysiol, 5:1, 1988
5. Scherg M, Ille N, Bornfleth H et al: Advanced tools for digital EEG review: virtual source montages, whole-head mapping, correlation, and phase analysis. J Clin Neurophysiol, 19:91, 2002
6. Picton TW, van Roon P, Armilio ML et al: The correction of ocular artifacts: a topographic perspective. Clin Neurophysiol, 111:53, 2000

7. Ille N, Berg P, Scherg M: Artifact correction of the ongoing EEG using spatial filters based on artifact and brain signal topographies. J Clin Neurophysiol, 19:113, 2002

8. Spatt J, Pelzl G, Mamoli B: Reliability of automatic and visual analysis of interictal spikes in lateralizing an epileptic focus during video-EEG monitoring. Electroencephalogr Clin Neurophysiol, 103:421, 1997

9. Salinsky MC: A practical analysis of computer-based seizure detection during continuous video-EEG monitoring. Electroencephalogr Clin Neurophysiol, 103:445, 1997

10. John ER, Prichep LS, Fridman J et al: Neurometrics: computer-assisted differential diagnosis of brain dysfunctions. Science, 239:162, 1988

11. Coutin-Churchman P, Añez Y, Uzcátegui M et al: Quantitative spectral analysis of EEG in psychiatry revisited: drawing signs out of numbers in a clinical setting. Clin Neurophysiol, 114:2294, 2003

12. Nuwer MR: Assessment of digital EEG, quantitative EEG and EEG brain mapping: report of the American Academy of Neurology and the American Clinical Neurophysiology Society. Neurology, 49:277, 1997

13. Nuwer MR: On the controversies about clinical use of EEG brain mapping. Brain Topogr, 3:103, 1990

14. Jonkman EJ, Poortvliet DCJ, Veering MM et al: The use of neurometrics in the study of patients with cerebral ischemia. Electroencephalogr Clin Neurophysiol, 61:333, 1985

15. Tolonen U, Sulg IA: Comparison of quantitative EEG parameters from four different analysis techniques in evaluation of relationships between EEG and CBF in brain infarction. Electroencephalogr Clin Neurophysiol, 51:177, 1981

16. Nagata K, Tagawa K, Hiroi S et al: Electroencephalographic correlates of blood flow and oxygen metabolism provided by positron emission tomography in patients with cerebral infarction. Electroencephalogr Clin Neurophysiol, 72:16, 1989

17. Mies G, Hoppe G, Hossmann KA: Limitations of EEG frequency analysis in the diagnosis of intracerebral diseases. p. 85. In Pfurtscheller G, Jonkman EJ, Lopes da Silva FH (eds): Brain Ischemia: Quantitative EEG and Imaging Techniques. Elsevier, Amsterdam, 1984

18. van Putten MJ, Tavy DL: Continuous quantitative EEG monitoring in hemispheric stroke patients using the brain symmetry index. Stroke, 35:2489, 2004

19. Finnigan SP, Walsh M, Rose SE et al: Quantitative EEG indices of sub-acute ischaemic stroke correlate with clinical outcomes. Clin Neurophysiol, 118:2525, 2007

20. Sheorajpanday RVA, Nagels G, Weeren AJTM et al: Quantitative EEG in ischemic stroke: correlation with infarct volume and functional status in posterior circulation and lacunar syndromes. Clin Neurophysiol, 122:884, 2011

21. Sheorajpanday RV, Nagels G, Weeren AJ et al: Quantitative EEG in ischemic stroke: correlation with functional status after 6 months. Clin Neurophysiol, 122:874, 2011

22. Sheorajpanday RVA, Nagels G, Weeren AJTM et al: Additional value of quantitative EEG in acute anterior circulation syndrome of presumed ischemic origin. Clin Neurophysiol, 121:1719, 2010

23. Gawel M, Zalewska E, Szmidt-Salkowska E et al: The value of quantitative EEG in differential diagnosis of Alzheimer's disease and subcortical vascular dementia. J Neurol Sci, 283:127, 2009

24. Nuwer MR: EEG and evoked potentials: monitoring cerebral function in the neurosurgical ICU. Neurosurg Clin N Am, 5:647, 1994

25. Friedman D, Claassen J, Hirsch LJ: Continuous electroencephalogram monitoring in the intensive care unit. Anesth Analg, 109:506, 2009

26. Kurtz P, Hanafy KA, Claassen J: Continuous EEG monitoring: is it ready for prime time? Curr Opin Crit Care, 15:99, 2009

27. Guérit JM, Amantini A, Amodio P et al: Consensus on the use of neurophysiological tests in the intensive care unit (ICU): electroencephalogram (EEG), evoked potentials (EP), and electroneuromyography (ENMG). Neurophysiol Clin, 39:71, 2009

28. Vespa PM, O'Phelan K, Shah M et al: Acute seizures after intracerebral hemorrhage: a factor in progressive midline shift and outcome. Neurology, 60:1441, 2003

29. Kilbride RD, Costello DJ, Chiappa KH: How seizure detection by continuous electroencephalographic monitoring affects the prescribing of antiepileptic medications. Arch Neurol, 66:723, 2009

30. Claassen J, Mayer SA, Kowalski RG et al: Detection of electrographic seizures with continuous EEG monitoring in critically ill patients. Neurology, 62:1743, 2004

31. DeLorenzo RJ, Waterhouse EJ, Towne AR et al: Persistent nonconvulsive status epilepticus after the control of convulsive status epilepticus. Epilepsia, 39:833, 1998

32. Hirsch LJ: Continuous EEG monitoring in the intensive care unit: an overview. J Clin Neurophysiol, 21:332, 2004

33. Vespa PM, Nuwer MR, Nenov V et al: Increased incidence and impact of nonconvulsive and convulsive seizures after traumatic brain injury as detected by continuous EEG in the intensive care unit. J Neurosurg, 91:750, 1999

34. Vespa PM, Nuwer MR, Juhasz C et al: Early detection of vasospasm after acute subarachnoid hemorrhage using continuous EEG ICU monitoring. Electroencephalogr Clin Neurophysiol, 103:607, 1997

35. Stuart RM, Waziri A, Weintraub D et al: Intracortical EEG for the detection of vasospasm in patients with poor-grade subarachnoid hemorrhage. Neurocrit Care, 13:355, 2010

36. Diedler J, Sykora M, Bast T: Quantitative EEG correlates of low cerebral perfusion in severe stroke. Neurocrit Care, 11:210, 2009

37. Huang Z, Dong W, Yan Y et al: Effects of intravenous mannitol on EEG recordings in stroke patients. Clin Neurophysiol, 113:446, 2002

38. Huang Z, Dong W, Yan Y et al: Effects of intravenous human albumin and furosemide on EEG recordings in patients with intracerebral hemorrhage. Clin Neurophysiol, 113:454, 2002

39. Niemarkt HJ, Andriessen P, Peters CH: Quantitative analysis of amplitude-integrated electroencephalogram patterns in stable preterm infants, with normal neurological development at one year. Neonatology, 97:175, 2010

40. Niemarkt HJ, Andriessen P, Peters CH: Quantitative analysis of maturational changes in EEG background activity in very preterm infants with a normal neurodevelopment at 1 year of age. Early Hum Dev, 86:219, 2010

41. Hathi M, Sherman DL, Inder T: Quantitative EEG in babies at risk for hypoxic ischemic encephalopathy after perinatal asphyxia. J Perinatol, 30:122, 2010

42. Stewart CP, Otsubo H, Ochi A et al: Seizure identification in the ICU using quantitative EEG displays. Neurology, 75:1501, 2010

43. West CR, Harding JE, Williams CE et al: Cot-side electroencephalography for outcome prediction in preterm infants: observational study. Arch Dis Child Fetal Neonatal Ed, 96:F108, 2011

44. Ahn SS, Youn PY, Jordan SE et al: Computerized EEG topographic brain mapping. p. 170. In Moore W (ed): Surgery for Cerebrovascular Disease. 2nd Ed. Churchill Livingstone, New York, 1996

45. Ebersole JS, Wade PB: Spike voltage topography identifies two types of fronto-temporal epileptic foci. Neurology, 41:1425, 1991

46. Weinberg H, Wong PKH, Crisp D et al: Use of multiple dipole analysis for the classification of benign rolandic epilepsy. Brain Topogr, 3:183, 1990

47. Braga NIO, Manzano GM, Nobrega JAM: Quantitative analysis of EEG background activity in patients with rolandic spikes. Clin Neurophysiol, 111:1643, 2000

48. Yoshinaga H, Amano R, Oka E et al: Dipole tracing in childhood epilepsy with special reference to rolandic epilepsy. Brain Topogr, 4:193, 1992

49. Gotman J: Quantitative measurements of epileptic spike morphology in the human EEG. Electroencephalogr Clin Neurophysiol, 48:551, 1980

50. Grova C, Daunizeau J, Lina JM et al: Evaluation of EEG localization methods using realistic simulations of interictal spikes. Neuroimage, 29:734, 2006

51. Zumsteg D, Friedman A, Wieser HG et al: Source localization of interictal epileptiform discharges: comparison of three different techniques to improve signal to noise ratio. Clin Neurophysiol, 117:562, 2006

52. Flanagan D, Agarwal R, Wang YH et al: Improvement in the performance of automated spike detection using dipole source features for artifact rejection. Clin Neurophysiol, 114:38, 2003

53. Vatta F, Bruno P, Inchingolo P: Improving lesion conductivity estimate by means of EEG source localization sensitivity to model parameter. J Clin Neurophysiol, 19:1, 2002

54. Lantz G, de Peralta RG, Spinelli L et al: Epileptic source localization with high density EEG: how many electrodes are needed? Clin Neurophysiol, 114:63, 2003

55. Cuffin BN, Schomer DL, Ives JR et al: Experimental tests of EEG source localization accuracy in spherical head models. Clin Neurophysiol, 112:46, 2001

56. Kobayashi K, Merlet I, Gotman J: Separation of spikes from background by independent component analysis with dipole modeling and comparison to intracranial recording. Clin Neurophysiol, 112:405, 2001

57. Kobayashi K, Yoshinaga H, Oka M et al: A simulation study of the error in dipole source localization for EEG spikes with a realistic head model. Clin Neurophysiol, 114:1069, 2003

58. Merlet I, Gotman J: Dipole modeling of scalp electroencephalogram epileptic discharges: correlation with intracerebral fields. Clin Neurophysiol, 112:414, 2001

59. Fuchs M, Wagner M, Kastner J: Confidence limits of dipole source reconstruction results. Clin Neurophysiol, 115:1442, 2004

60. Ebersole JS, Wade PB: Spike voltage topography and equivalent dipole localization in complex partial epilepsy. Brain Topogr, 3:21, 1990

61. Huppertz HJ, Hoegg S, Sick C et al: Cortical current density reconstruction of interictal epileptiform activity in temporal lobe epilepsy. Clin Neurophysiol, 112:1761, 2001

62. Wilson SB, Emerson R: Spike detection: a review and comparison of algorithms. Clin Neurophysiol, 113:1873, 2002

63. Gotman J, Flanagan D, Zhang J et al: Automatic seizure detection in the newborn: methods and initial evaluation. Electroencephalogr Clin Neurophysiol, 103:356, 1997

64. Gotman J, Flanagan D, Rosenblatt B et al: Evaluation of an automatic seizure detection method for the newborn EEG. Electroencephalogr Clin Neurophysiol, 103:363, 1997

65. Schiff SJ, Colella D, Jacyna GM et al: Brain chirps: spectrographic signatures of epileptic seizures. Clin Neurophysiol, 111:953, 2000

66. Altenburg J, Vermeulen RJ, Strijers RLM et al: Seizure detection in the neonatal EEG with synchronization likelihood. Clin Neurophysiol, 114:50, 2003

67. Khan YU, Gotman J: Wavelet based automatic seizure detection in intracerebral electroencephalogram. Clin Neurophysiol, 114:898, 2003

68. Bergey GK, Franaszczuk PJ: Epileptic seizures are characterized by changing signal complexity. Clin Neurophysiol, 112:241, 2001

69. Verhellen E, Boon P: EEG source localization of the epileptogenic focus in patients with refractory temporal lobe epilepsy, dipole modelling revisited. Acta Neurol Belg, 107:71, 2007

70. Flanagan D, Agarwal R, Gotman J: Computer-aided spatial classification of epileptic spikes. J Clin Neurophysiol, 19:125, 2002

71. Chauvel P, Buser P, Badier JM et al: The human epileptogenic zone: representation of inter-seizure events by temporospatial maps. Rev Neurol (Paris), 143:443, 1987

72. Tatum WO, Winters L, Gieron M et al: Outpatient seizure identification. J Clin Neurophysiol, 18:14, 2001

73. Gotman J: Interhemispheric relations during bilateral spike-and-wave activity. Epilepsia, 22:453, 1981

74. Blume WT, Lemieux JF: Morphology of spikes in spike-and-wave complexes. Electroencephalogr Clin Neurophysiol, 69:508, 1988

75. Rodin E, Cornellier D: Source derivation recordings of generalized spike-wave complexes. Electroencephalogr Clin Neurophysiol, 73:20, 1989

76. Coben LA, Chi D, Snyder AZ et al: Replication of a study of frequency analysis of the resting awake EEG in mild probable Alzheimer's disease. Electroencephalogr Clin Neurophysiol, 75:148, 1990

77. Besthorn C, Zerfass R, Geiger-Kabisch C et al: Discrimination of Alzheimer's disease and normal aging by EEG data. Electroencephalogr Clin Neurophysiol, 103:241, 1997

78. Czigler B, Csikós D, Hidasi Z et al: Quantitative EEG in early Alzheimer's disease patients—power spectrum and complexity features. Int J Psychophysiol, 68:75, 2008

79. van der Hiele K, Vein AA, van der Welle A et al: EEG and MRI correlates of mild cognitive impairment and Alzheimer's disease. Neurobiol Aging, 28:1322, 2007

80. Jackson CE, Snyder PJ: Electroencephalography and event-related potentials as biomarkers of mild cognitive impairment and mild Alzheimer's disease. Alzheimers Dement, 4:S137, 2008

81. Rossini PM, Del Percio C, Pasqualetti P et al: Conversion from mild cognitive impairment to Alzheimer's disease is predicted by sources and coherence of brain electroencephalography rhythms. Neuroscience, 143:793, 2006

82. Adler G, Brassen S, Chwalek K et al: Prediction of treatment response to rivastigmine in Alzheimer's dementia. J Neurol Neurosurg Psychiatry, 75:292–294, 2004

83. Babiloni C, Cassetta E, Dal Forno G et al: Donepezil effects on sources of cortical rhythms in mild Alzheimer's disease: responders vs non-responders. Neuroimage, 31:1650, 2006

84. Schreiter Gasser U, Rousson V, Hentschel F et al: Alzheimer disease versus mixed dementias: an EEG perspective. Clin Neurophysiol, 119:2255, 2008

85. Kwak YT: Quantitative EEG findings in different stages of Alzheimer's disease. J Clin Neurophysiol, 23:456, 2006

86. Painold A, Anderer P, Holl AK et al: Comparative EEG mapping studies in Huntington's disease patients and controls. J Neural Transm, 117:1307, 2010

87. Passant U, Rosén I, Gustafson L et al: The heterogeneity of frontotemporal dementia with regard to initial symptoms, qEEG and neuropathology. Int J Geriatr Psychiatry, 20:983, 2005

88. Pucci E, Cacchiò G, Angeloni R et al: EEG spectral analysis in Alzheimer's disease and different degenerative dementias. Arch Gerontol Geriatr, 26:283, 1998

89. Serizawa K, Kamei S, Morita A et al: Comparison of quantitative EEGs between Parkinson disease and age-adjusted normal controls. J Clin Neurophysiol, 25:361, 2008

90. Tanaka H, Koenig T, Pascual-Marqui RD et al: Event-related potential and EEG measures in Parkinson's disease without and with dementia. Dement Geriatr Cogn Disord, 11:39, 2000

91. Pezard L, Jech R, Ruzicka E: Investigation of non-linear properties of multichannel EEG in the early stages of Parkinson's disease. Clin Neurophysiol, 112:38, 2001

92. Neufeld MY, Blumen S, Aitkin I et al: EEG frequency analysis in demented and nondemented parkinsonian patients. Dementia, 5:23, 1994

93. Kamei S, Morita A, Serizawa K et al: Quantitative EEG analysis of executive dysfunction in Parkinson disease. J Clin Neurophysiol, 27:193, 2010

94. Morita A, Kamei S, Serizawa K et al: The relationship between slowing EEGs and the progression of Parkinson's disease. J Clin Neurophysiol, 26:426, 2009

95. Jordan SE, Nowacki R, Nuwer M: Computerized electroencephalography in the evaluation of early dementia. Brain Topogr, 1:271, 1989

96. Mody CK, McIntyre HB, Miller BL et al: Topographic brain mapping and EEG frequency analysis in Alzheimer disease: a preliminary report. Bull Clin Neurosci, 53:94, 1988

97. Soininen H, Partanen J, Laulumaa V et al: Serial EEG in Alzheimer's disease: 3 year follow-up and clinical outcome. Electroencephalogr Clin Neurophysiol, 79:342, 1991

98. Williamson PC, Merskey H, Morrison S et al: Quantitative electroencephalographic correlates of cognitive decline in normal elderly subjects. Arch Neurol, 47:1185, 1990

99. Buchan RJ, Nagata K, Yokoyama E et al: Regional correlations between the EEG and oxygen metabolism in dementia of Alzheimer's type. Electroencephalogr Clin Neurophysiol, 103:409, 1997

100. Röhl JE, Harms L, Pommer W: Quantitative EEG findings in patients with chronic renal failure. Eur J Med Res, 12:173, 2007

101. Keski-Säntti P, Kovala T, Holm A et al: Quantitative EEG in occupational chronic solvent encephalopathy. Hum Exp Toxicol, 27:315, 2008

102. Guerit JM, Amantini A, Fischer C et al: Neurophysiological investigations of hepatic encephalopathy: ISHEN practice guidelines. Liver Int, 29:789, 2009

103. Kamei S, Morita A, Tanaka N et al: Relationships between quantitative electroencephalographic alterations and the severity of hepatitis C based on liver biopsy in interferon-alpha treated patients. Intern Med, 48:975, 2009

104. Clemens B, Ménes A, Piros P et al: Quantitative EEG effects of carbamazepine, oxcarbazepine, valproate, lamotrigine, and possible clinical relevance of the findings. Epilepsy Res, 70:190, 2006

105. John ER, Ahn H, Prichep L et al: Developmental equations for the electroencephalogram. Science, 210:1255, 1980

106. Galin D, Raz J, Fein G et al: EEG spectra in dyslexic and normal readers during oral and silent reading. Electroencephalogr Clin Neurophysiol, 82:87, 1992

107. Fein G, Galin D, Yingling CD et al: EEG spectra in dyslexic and control boys during resting conditions. Electroencephalogr Clin Neurophysiol, 63:87, 1986

108. Byring RF, Salmi TK, Sainio KO et al: EEG in children with spelling disabilities. Electroencephalogr Clin Neurophysiol, 79:247, 1991

109. Harmony T, Marosi E, Becker J et al: Longitudinal quantitative EEG study of children with different performances on a reading-writing test. Electroencephalogr Clin Neurophysiol, 95:426, 1995

110. Chabot RJ, Merkin H, Wood LM et al: Sensitivity and specificity of QEEG in children with attention deficit or specific

developmental learning disorders. Clin Electroencephalogr, 27:26, 1996

111. Levy F, Ward PB: Neurometrics, dynamic brain imaging and attention deficit hyperactivity disorder. J Paediatr Child Health, 31:279, 1995

112. Mann CA, Lubar JF, Zimmerman AW et al: Quantitative analysis of EEG in boys with attention-deficit-hyperactivity disorder: controlled study with clinical implications. Pediatr Neurol, 8:30, 1992

113. Merrin EL, Floyd TC, Fein G: EEG coherence in unmedicated schizophrenic patients. Biol Psychiatry, 25:60, 1989

114. John ER, Prichep LS, Alper KR et al: Quantitative electrophysiological characteristics and subtyping of schizophrenia. Biol Psychiatry, 36:801, 1994

115. Pollock VE, Schneider LS: Quantitative, waking EEG research on depression. Biol Psychiatry, 27:757, 1990

116. Wirsén A, Stenberg G, Rosén I et al: Quantified EEG and cortical evoked responses in patients with chronic traumatic frontal lesions. Electroencephalogr Clin Neurophysiol, 84:127, 1992

117. Tebano MT, Cameroni M, Gallozzi G et al: EEG spectral analysis after minor head injury in man. Electroencephalogr Clin Neurophysiol, 70:185, 1988

118. Thatcher RW, Walker RA, Gerson I et al: EEG discriminant analyses of mild head trauma. Electroencephalogr Clin Neurophysiol, 73:94, 1989

119. Yingling CD, Galin D, Fein G et al: Neurometrics does not detect "pure" dyslexics. Electroencephalogr Clin Neurophysiol, 63:426, 1986

120. Leuchter AF, Cook IA, Marangell LB et al: Comparative effectiveness of biomarkers and clinical indicators for predicting outcomes of SSRI treatment in major depressive disorder: results of the BRITE-MD study. Psychiatry Res, 169:124, 2009

121. Prichep L, Alper K, Kowalik SC et al: Neurometric QEEG studies of crack cocaine dependence and treatment outcome. J Addict Dis, 15:39, 1996

122. Wienbruch C, Moratti S, Elbert T et al: Source distribution of neuromagnetic slow wave activity in schizophrenic and depressive patients. Clin Neurophysiol, 114:2052, 2003

123. Saletu-Zyhlarz GM, Arnold O, Anderer P et al: Differences in brain function between relapsing and abstaining alcohol-dependent patients, evaluated by EEG mapping. Alcohol, 39:233, 2004

124. Coutin-Churchman P, Moreno R: Intracranial current density (LORETA) differences in QEEG frequency bands between depressed and non-depressed alcoholic patients. Clin Neurophysiol, 119:948, 2008

125. American Psychiatric Association: Quantitative electroencephalography: a report on the present state of computerized EEG techniques. American Psychiatric Association Task Force on Quantitative Electrophysiological Assessment. Am J Psychiatry, 148:961, 1991

126. Barry RJ, Clarke AR, Johnstone SJ: A review of electrophysiology in attention-deficit/hyperactivity disorder: I.

Qualitative and quantitative electroencephalography. Clin Neurophysiol, 114:171, 2003

127. Snyder SM, Hall JR: A meta-analysis of quantitative EEG power associated with attention-deficit hyperactivity disorder. J Clin Neurophysiol, 23:440, 2006

128. Clarke AR, Barry RJ, McCarthy R et al: Age and sex effects in the EEG: development of the normal child. Clin Neurophysiol, 112:806, 2001

129. Clarke AR, Barry RJ, McCarthy R et al: Age and sex effects in the EEG: differences in two subtypes of attention-deficit/hyperactivity disorder. Clin Neurophysiol, 112:815, 2001

130. El-Sayed E, Larsson JO, Persson HE et al: Altered cortical activity in children with attention-deficit/hyperactivity disorder during attentional load task. J Am Acad Child Adolesc Psychiatry, 41:811, 2002

131. Monastra VJ, Lubar JF, Linden M: The development of a quantitative electroencephalographic scanning process for attention deficit-hyperactivity disorder: reliability and validity studies. Neuropsychology, 15:136, 2001

132. Monastra VJ, Lubar JF, Linden M et al: Assessing attention deficit hyperactivity disorder via quantitative electroencephalography: an initial validation study. Neuropsychology, 13:424, 1999

133. Bresnahan SM, Anderson JW, Barry RJ: Age-related changes in quantitative EEG in attention-deficit/hyperactivity disorder. Biol Psychiatry, 46:1690, 1999

134. Lazzaro I, Gordon E, Li W et al: Simultaneous EEG and EDA measures in adolescent attention deficit hyperactivity disorder. Int J Psychophysiol, 34:123, 1999

135. Lazzaro I, Gordon E, Whitmont S et al: Quantified EEG activity in adolescent attention deficit hyperactivity disorder. Clin Electroencephalogr, 29:37, 1998

136. Clarke AR, Barry RJ, McCarthy R et al: Quantitative EEG in low-IQ children with attention-deficit/hyperactivity disorder. Clin Neurophysiol, 117:1708, 2006

137. Monastra VJ, Lynn S, Linden M et al: Electroencephalographic biofeedback in the treatment of attention-deficit/hyperactivity disorder. Appl Psychophysiol Biofeedback, 30:95, 2005

138. Monastra VJ: Quantitative electroencephalography and attention-deficit/hyperactivity disorder: implications for clinical practice. Curr Psychiatry Rep, 10:432, 2008

139. Chan AS, Leung WW: Differentiating autistic children with quantitative encephalography: a 3-month longitudinal study. J Child Neurol, 21:392, 2006

140. Chan AS, Sze SL, Cheung MC: Quantitative electroencephalographic profiles for children with autistic spectrum disorder. Neuropsychology, 21:74, 2007

141. Coben R, Clarke AR, Hudspeth W et al: EEG power and coherence in autistic spectrum disorder. Clin Neurophysiol, 119:1002, 2008

142. Grin-Yatsenko VA, Baas I, Ponomarev VA et al: EEG power spectra at early stages of depressive disorders. J Clin Neurophysiol, 26:401, 2009

143. Leuchter AF, Cook IA, Lufkin RB et al: Cordance: a new method for assessment of cerebral perfusion and

metabolism using quantitative electroencephalography. Neuroimage, 1:208, 1994

144. Cook IA, O'Hara R, Uijtdehaage SH et al: Assessing the accuracy of topographic EEG mapping for determining local brain function. Electroencephalogr Clin Neurophysiol, 107:408, 1998

145. Leuchter AF, Cook IA, Gilmer WS et al: Effectiveness of a quantitative electroencephalographic biomarker for predicting differential response or remission with escitalopram and bupropion in major depressive disorder. Psychiatry Res, 169:132, 2009

146. Bares M, Brunovsky M, Novak T et al: The change of prefrontal QEEG theta cordance as a predictor of response to bupropion treatment in patients who had failed to respond to previous antidepressant treatments. Eur Neuropsychopharmacol, 20:459, 2010

147. Hunter AM, Muthén BO, Cook IA et al: Antidepressant response trajectories and quantitative electroencephalography (QEEG) biomarkers in major depressive disorder. J Psychiatr Res, 44:90, 2010

148. Iosifescu DV: Prediction of response to antidepressants: is quantitative EEG (QEEG) an alternative? CNS Neurosci Ther, 14:263, 2008

149. Coutin-Churchman P, Moreno R, Añez Y et al: Clinical correlates of QEEG alterations in alcoholic patients. Clin Neurophysiol, 117:740, 2006

150. Alvarez XA, Sampedro C, Figueroa J et al: Reductions in qEEG slowing over 1 year and after treatment with cerebrolysin in patients with moderate-severe traumatic brain injury. J Neural Transm, 115:683, 2008

151. Leon-Carrion J, Martin-Rodriguez JF, Damas-Lopez J et al: Brain function in the minimally conscious state: a quantitative neurophysiological study. Clin Neurophysiol, 119:1506, 2008

152. Moulton RJ, Marmarou A, Ronen J et al: Spectral analysis of the EEG in craniocerebral trauma. Can J Neurol Sci, 15:82, 1988

153. Nuwer MR, Hovda DA, Schrader LM et al: Routine and quantitative EEG in mild traumatic brain injury. Clin Neurophysiol, 116:2001, 2005

154. von Bierbrauer A, Weissenborn K, Hinrichs H et al: Die automatische (computergestützte) EEG-Analyse im Vergleich zur visuellen EEG—Analyse bei Patienten nach leichtem Schädelhirntrauma (Verlaufsuntersuchung). EEG EMG Z, 23:151, 1992

155. McCrea M, Prichep L, Powell MR et al: Acute effects and recovery after sport-related concussion: a neurocognitive and quantitative brain electrical activity study. J Head Trauma Rehabil, 25:283, 2010

156. American Electroencephalographic Society: Standards for practice in clinical electroencephalography. J Clin Neurophysiol, 11:14, 1994

Intraoperative Electroencephalographic Monitoring During Carotid Endarterectomy and Cardiac Surgery

GREGORY D. CASCINO and FRANK W. SHARBROUGH, III

The intraoperative recording of electroencephalographic (EEG) activity began soon after the development and introduction of the EEG as a neurodiagnostic technique. One of the initial clinical applications of the intraoperative recording of cerebral electrical activity was electrocorticography (ECoG) at the time of focal corticectomy for intractable epilepsy.[1-3] This technique was used before the development of extraoperative EEG monitoring to localize the epileptogenic zone in patients with focal seizures.[1-3] ECoG is still used at selected epilepsy centers before and after excision of the epileptic brain tissue. The use of ECoG during epilepsy surgery is addressed in Chapter 7. Other potential indications for intraoperative EEG recordings include the monitoring of cerebral function during carotid endarterectomy and cardiopulmonary bypass surgical procedures.[4-15] The rationale for intraoperative EEG monitoring is the detection of electrophysiologic alterations that are associated intimately with cerebral ischemia or cerebral hypoperfusion before the development of cerebral infarction.[15] Extracranial or scalp-recorded EEG monitoring during carotid endarterectomy has been shown to be a reliable indicator of cerebral ischemia.[15-19] The findings obtained with extracranial EEG monitoring at the time of an endarterectomy may lead to an alteration in operative strategy (i.e., may indicate the need for placement of a carotid artery shunt).[15] Intraoperative EEG recordings have also been performed during cardiac bypass surgery.[7-10] The effect of hypothermia, however, significantly limits the potential utility of EEG monitoring during the latter procedure.[4] Profound hypothermia produces a suppression of EEG activity that reduces the diagnostic yield of intraoperative recordings in identifying alterations resulting from cerebral ischemia.[4,12] Reversible causes of ischemia during cardiac bypass surgery occur much less commonly than during a carotid endarterectomy for carotid artery stenosis.[4]

Intraoperative EEG recordings were the first monitoring technique used during carotid and cardiac surgical procedures to minimize the likelihood of a postoperative neurologic deficit that might affect significantly the individual's quality of life.[4,12] The potential adverse effects of cardiovascular and cerebrovascular surgery include stroke, cognitive impairment, and a postoperative encephalopathy.[12] Importantly, additional neurodiagnostic studies may be used in the operating room to monitor cerebral perfusion and the effect of anesthesia.[4-11,13-15] Transcranial Doppler, carotid ultrasound, and xenon blood flow studies are performed in some centers during carotid endarterectomy and cardiac surgery.[6-11,13-15] The use of transcranial Doppler in selected patients may be predictive of cerebral ischemia in the absence of appropriate EEG changes.[6] Intraoperative carotid ultrasound is being used increasingly to validate the patency of the internal carotid artery after endarterectomy.[11] Monitoring the level of anesthesia by the bispectral index may reduce the hemodynamic changes that occur in some patients undergoing cardiopulmonary bypass.[9]

This chapter provides an overview of some of the aspects of intraoperative EEG monitoring for the identification of changes related to cerebral ischemia during carotid endarterectomy and cardiac surgery. In particular, the clinical applications and potential limitations of such cerebral function monitoring are considered.

CAROTID ENDARTERECTOMY

Carotid endarterectomy is the cerebrovascular surgical procedure most commonly performed to reduce the risk of stroke in patients with symptomatic carotid artery stenosis related to atherosclerosis.[6,12-25] Even before the publication of rigorous scientific studies confirming the efficacy of carotid endarterectomy, the use of this operative technique to protect against ipsilateral stroke had become popular.[22] The increase in the number of operative procedures performed annually in the United States over several years reflects the interest in identifying a protective surgical approach to stroke.[22] Fewer than 15,000 carotid endarterectomies were performed in 1970, but by 1985 an estimated 100,000 carotid endarterectomies had been performed in the United States.[22] The rationale for this operative procedure is the removal of atherosclerotic thrombotic material that may come to restrict flow and lead to either an occlusion of the carotid artery or an artery-to-artery embolus.[21-25] Carotid artery surgery is the direct result of observations in the 1950s that established a relationship between extracranial internal carotid artery disease and stroke.

Studies have indicated that carotid endarterectomy is effective in reducing the risk of ipsilateral stroke in patients with high-grade stenosis (70 to 99 percent) of the internal carotid artery.[21-25] Selected patients with completed strokes may also be candidates for a carotid endarterectomy, depending on their neurologic deficits and the presence of coexistent medical problems. The North American Symptomatic Carotid Endarterectomy Trial (NASCET) demonstrated a significant reduction in the risk of stroke in patients with carotid artery stenosis greater than 70 percent.[24] Ipsilateral stroke occurred at 24 months' follow-up in 26 percent of 328 nonsurgical patients and in 9 percent of 331 patients undergoing a carotid endarectomy.[24] A direct correlation existed between surgical benefit and the degree of carotid artery stenosis. The benefit of carotid artery surgery in the NASCET for patients with 30 to 69 percent stenosis was less clear.[24] The Veterans Affairs Symptomatic Stenosis Trial (VASST) also showed a significant reduction in the risk of stroke in patients with carotid artery stenosis of greater than 50 percent who underwent a carotid endarterectomy.[25] The Asymptomatic Carotid Atherosclerosis Study (ACAS) reported in 1995 that there is an aggregate risk reduction of 53 percent with surgical treatment for asymptomatic carotid artery stenosis.[23] A total of 1,659 patients were entered into this study.[23] All patients had greater than 60 percent carotid artery stenosis and were randomized to surgical or medical therapy.[23] A significant difference was evident between the two treatment groups at 3 years.[23]

The risks of carotid endarterectomy must be considered in any discussion of the putative beneficial effects of this operative procedure. The morbidity of this treatment depends on a number of factors including surgical expertise; degree of carotid artery stenosis; the presence of cerebral infarction; and coexistent medical problems, especially ischemic heart disease. The published morbidity of carotid endarterectomy has ranged from 0 to 20 percent.[22] In one multicenter study, the perioperative morbidity was 2.2 percent and the mortality was 3.3 percent (combined operative complication was 5.5 percent) in "relatively high-risk patients."[25] Importantly, angiography has a reported risk of approximately 1 percent.[22]

The operative procedure is performed with the patient receiving general anesthesia for both comfort and safety. A combination of nitrous oxide and isoflurane is used at the Mayo Clinic. Induction is performed routinely with thiopental.[12] The common carotid artery, internal carotid artery, and carotid bifurcation are exposed at the time of surgery. Atherosclerotic changes are most prominent in the proximal internal carotid artery and the carotid bifurcation. Clamping of the internal carotid artery, common carotid artery, and external carotid artery is necessary for an arteriotomy and endarterectomy to be performed.[4,12] A shunt between the common carotid artery and the internal carotid artery may be placed if the surgical team is concerned that the period of clamping may be associated with cerebral ischemia and perioperative stroke.[4,12] The attitude of neurosurgical teams concerning the use of shunt placement is variable. At the Mayo Clinic, a shunt is placed only if EEG monitoring of cerebral function or cerebral blood flow studies, or both, suggest a hemodynamic insult that may produce a significant reduction in cerebral blood flow.[4,12] The routine use of shunts may be associated with an increased risk of cerebral infarction related to artery-to-artery embolus, and it prolongs the duration of the operation.[12] Importantly, a minority of patients exhibit a significant change in cerebral function monitoring indicative of a hemodynamic insult with a diminished cerebral blood flow.[4,12] The risk of shunt placement in one study was low, with embolism occurring in 2 of 511 patients (0.4 percent).[14]

The introduction of carotid angioplasty and carotid artery stenting for carotid artery stenosis may be an alternative to carotid endarterectomy.[26–28] The methodology for these therapeutic interventions is similar to the techniques introduced for the treatment of cardiovascular disease. Carotid revascularization has also been used in selected patients with restenosis following a carotid endarterectomy.[28] EEG monitoring is not performed routinely during these procedures because the carotid artery is not occluded and there is no consideration of shunt placement. The role for these alternative techniques in the management of asymptomatic or symptomatic carotid artery disease remains under study.[26–28]

INTRAOPERATIVE EEG MONITORING: METHODOLOGY

Intraoperative EEG monitoring is performed commonly during carotid endarterectomy. Computer-assisted digital EEG recordings are now standard during such procedures. There is a diversity of opinion regarding the clinical application of this neurodiagnostic technique in cerebrovascular and cardiac surgery.[4,7,12,16] The "hostile" environment of the operating room often makes intraoperative EEG monitoring technically difficult. Potential problems include electrical interference, which produces significant artifacts; difficulty in ensuring the stable application of the electrodes; and the use of anesthesia and pharmacotherapy that may alter the EEG recording. The technologist and electroencephalographer may also have difficulty in examining the patient and in negotiating their way through the operating room because of the surgical team and the necessary equipment. The technical factors that must be considered during intraoperative extracranial EEG monitoring include proper placement of the scalp electrodes (collodion is used at the Mayo Clinic) before anesthesia induction. Usually, 21 to 23 scalp electrodes are used for intraoperative EEG monitoring.[4,12–15] For appropriate intraoperative recordings, at least 8 channels of EEG should be available. In most instances, 16 or 21 channels for EEG monitoring is strongly

preferred.[4,12,13] Proper grounding is essential for patient safety. The use of a 60-Hz filter is required. The linear frequency is set between 1 and 15 or 30 Hz.[4] Sensitivities of 3 to 5 μV/mm are often necessary for recording the extracranial EEG with the patient under general anesthesia.[6,12–15] A longitudinal bipolar anteroposterior montage is used routinely for intraoperative EEG monitoring.[4,12] The Laplacian montage may also be useful in identifying a focal alteration. Subtle changes in amplitude and frequency related to cerebral ischemia can be visualized easily at the slower recording speeds. The diagnostic yield of the reduced recording speed for identifying reversible alterations associated with cerebral ischemia has been demonstrated.[4,12–15] The recording speed can be restored to 30 mm/sec if a continuous or paroxysmal EEG pattern occurs that cannot be identified.

The use of digital EEG recordings in the operating room has removed concerns regarding paper storage during intraoperative EEG monitoring. The introduction of digital EEG has improved offline analysis and allowed individuals remote from the operating room to review the EEG as it is being acquired (i.e., "real-time" review). The current practice at the Mayo Clinic is to continue to use a recording speed of 5 mm/sec for digital EEG intraoperative recordings because of the amount of data generated. The technologists at our institution are also more familiar with the effects of cerebral ischemia displayed at this slower speed. Computer processing with a compressed spectral array can be used for data interpretation but may have no advantage over visual inspection alone.[4,12,18]

EEG AND ANESTHESIA

It is necessary to review the relationship between anesthesia and the EEG before considering the effects of cerebral ischemia on the intraoperatively recorded EEG. Anesthetic agents may alter the normal background EEG significantly (Fig. 9-1). To some extent, individual anesthetic drugs may have different effects, depending on their concentrations.[4,29] The EEG patterns produced by different anesthetic agents, when used at concentrations below their MAC level (i.e., the minimal alveolar concentration necessary for preventing movement to a painful stimulus in about 50 percent of subjects), are quite similar.[29] Selected anesthetic agents (e.g., thiopental, halothane, enflurane, isoflurane, and nitrous oxide) produce a similar subanesthetic or anesthetic effect associated with a symmetric EEG pattern.[29]

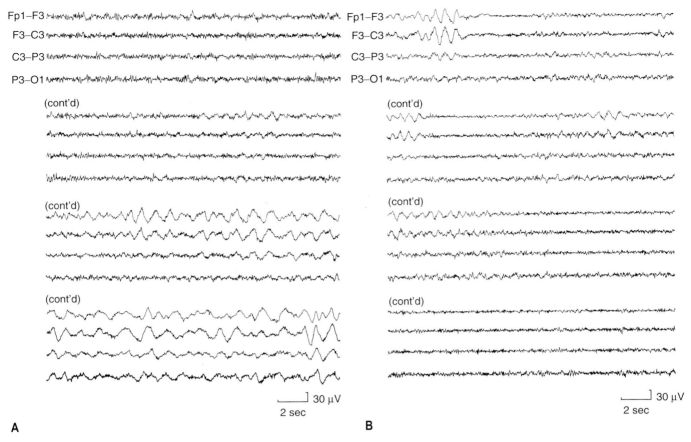

A   **B**

FIGURE 9-1 ■ Electroencephalographic patterns related to **A**, anesthesia induction and **B**, decreasing levels of anesthesia. Note the frontal intermittent rhythmic delta activity that occurs with induction, associated with generalized background slowing.

Symmetric EEG Patterns at Subanesthetic or Minimal Anesthetic Concentrations

Thiopental produces the characteristic drug-induced beta effect at subanesthetic concentrations, which tends to be maximal in the anterior midline distribution.[20,29] Halothane, enflurane, isoflurane, and 50 percent nitrous oxide, administered at subanesthetic concentrations, produce a similar pattern (Fig. 9-2). The drug-induced beta activity is less prominent with these other agents than with thiopental.[20,29]

Symmetric EEG Changes with Induction

Inductions for surgery usually are performed with the rapid administration of thiopental.[4] A characteristic pattern of EEG changes occurs in relation to induction. The drug-induced beta activity noted with thiopental at subanesthetic concentrations becomes distributed

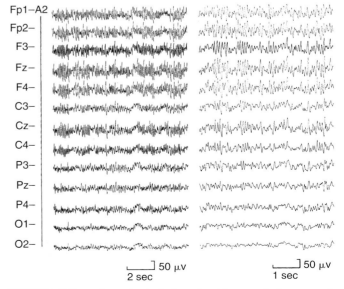

FIGURE 9-2 ■ Anesthesia-induced widespread, but anteriorly predominant, rhythmic fast activity.

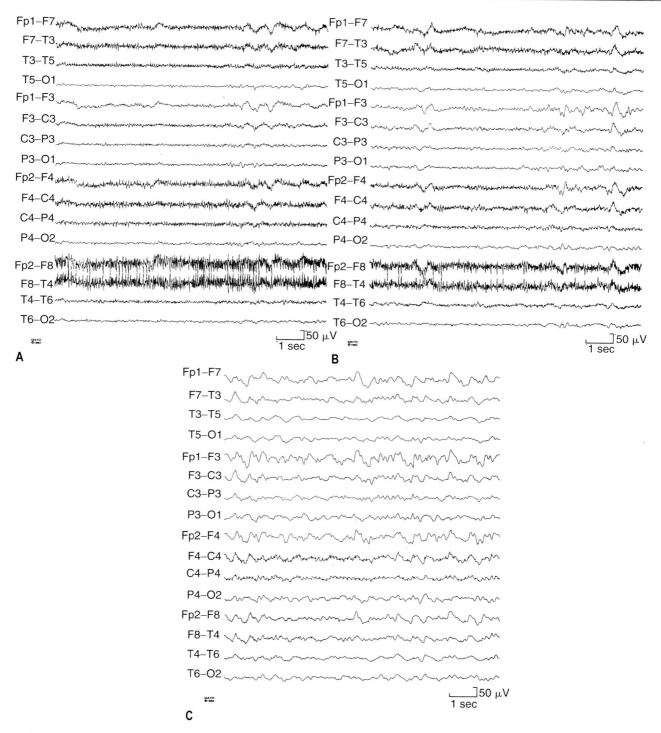

FIGURE 9-3 ■ Electroencephalographic tracings. **A**, Before induction. **B**, 35 seconds after induction. **C**, 70 seconds after induction with fentanyl. Note the posterior alpha activity in the awake electroencephalogram before induction.

more widely, gradually increases in amplitude, and slows in frequency.[12,29] The background frequency ultimately slows from the beta to the alpha range. Paroxysmal bursts of high-amplitude, intermittent slowing occur; these are frontally predominant and resemble frontal intermittent rhythmic delta activity (FIRDA) (see Fig. 9-1; Fig. 9-3).[12] Induction with other anesthetic agents may produce a similar sequence of EEG changes, but with the FIRDA-like pattern being less prominent.[5]

Symmetric EEG Patterns at Sub-MAC Anesthetic Concentrations

The EEG pattern for all anesthetic drugs at a sub-MAC anesthetic concentration consists of generalized background slowing with anteriorly predominant rhythmic fast activity in the beta or alpha frequency range (Fig. 9-4).[4,12,29] Increasing the concentration of anesthetic drug is associated with slowing of the frontal fast activity. The anterior fast activity is nearly continuous in nature and is presumed to represent drug-induced beta activity, which is concentration dependent.

EEG CHANGES UNRELATED TO CAROTID ARTERY CLAMPING

An intraoperative baseline, awake EEG should be obtained before induction to identify any background asymmetry or localization-related abnormality.[4,12] However, one study indicated that a preoperative EEG is not predictive of adverse effects associated with a carotid endarterectomy.[17] The baseline, awake EEG was "highly predictive" of anesthesia-induced EEG changes but not of alterations associated with carotid clamping. This study suggested that the preoperative EEG could be "eliminated."[17] Patients with a history of cerebral infarction may have a persistent or intermittent EEG abnormality (e.g., increased focal slow-wave activity) that should be recognized before carotid clamping. Even in the absence of a history of a cerebral infarction, the baseline EEG is important for comparative purposes. Subtle, lateralized, or localized EEG abnormalities may occur in patients with transient cerebral ischemic attacks and transient monocular blindness that may reflect a significant hemodynamic insult. It is presumed in these patients that diminished cerebral blood flow is sufficient to produce an EEG change in the absence of a persistent neurologic deficit.[4,12] Widely distributed and generalized background alterations are less meaningful and may relate to preoperative medications. The sensitivity of the EEG in patients with stroke depends on the size and pathophysiology of the infarct and the temporal relationship between EEG monitoring and the stroke.

A focal abnormality may also be evident at the time of thiopental induction and usually correlates with that noted in the baseline EEG.[4] The focal abnormality may consist of a unilateral reduction of the anterior, rhythmic fast activity by more than 30 to 40 percent.[4,12] This reduction is associated commonly with an increase in the wavelength and amplitude of any persistent polymorphic slow activity. In most cases, any focal baseline EEG abnormality correlates with preoperative neurologic deficits.[4] Focal anesthetic-related EEG abnormalities usually correlate with those in the preoperative baseline EEG. Rarely, however, the anesthetic effect may obscure an abnormality that was present in the EEG obtained during wakefulness. More commonly, an EEG abnormality develops that was inapparent during the baseline EEG (Fig. 9-5).[12] The EEG recorded during anesthesia may show a major reduction in anterior, rhythmic fast activity and an increase in polymorphic slowing despite a normal baseline EEG with symmetric and reactive posterior alpha activity.[4,12,29] Almost invariably in these instances, the drug-induced beta activity seen during the preanesthetic state is reduced on the side with diminished anterior rhythmic fast activity. Commonly, the EEG during anesthesia shows enhanced abnormalities compared with the baseline recording, especially when the latter contains intermittent rhythmic slowing in the temporal region on the side of the cerebral ischemia. This intermittent abnormality often is converted into a more obvious and persistent focal alteration that is associated with a reduction in the anesthetic pattern.

Finally, it must be noted that a paroxysmal FIRDA-like discharge or continuous generalized background slowing cannot be regarded as abnormal when it occurs during anesthesia; these patterns occur in most patients at some stage of anesthesia.[12]

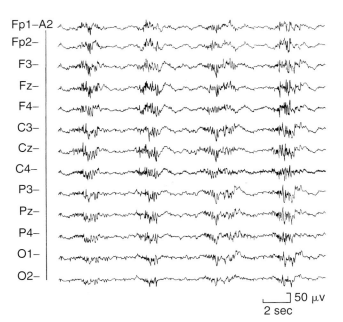

50 μV
2 sec

FIGURE 9-4 ■ Anterior rhythmic fast activity with superimposed anterior triangular slow waves during induction with thiopental.

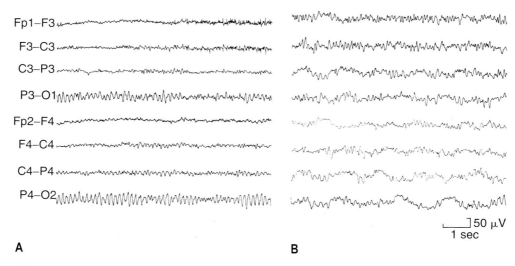

A   **B**

FIGURE 9-5 ▪ The electroencephalogram (EEG) in a patient with a right cerebral infarct. **A**, During wakefulness. **B**. After anesthesia with halothane and nitrous oxide. There is anesthesia-activated right hemisphere slowing. Note the absence of a focal abnormality during the awake EEG.

EEG CHANGES RELATED TO CAROTID ARTERY CLAMPING

The rationale for intraoperative EEG monitoring is to assess the likelihood that the patient will acquire a neurologic deficit related to diminished cerebral blood flow at the time of carotid artery clamping.[4,12–19] The EEG should be recorded for at least 10 minutes with the patient under anesthesia and prior to carotid artery clamping.[12] An alteration in the EEG that is transient or persistent occurs in approximately 25 percent of patients with carotid artery stenosis on clamping of the internal carotid artery, clamping of the common carotid artery, or both.[4,12,13] These changes almost invariably occur within 20 to 30 seconds after clamping and are associated with a reduction of cerebral blood flow to below a critical level (Figs. 9-6 and 9-7).[4,12] The critical level needed to affect the EEG is determined by the specific anesthetic drug. The severity and rapidity of onset of the EEG change vary in proportion to the degree to which blood flow is lowered (Fig. 9-8). Minor changes consist of a 25 to 50 percent reduction in the faster EEG activity and an increase in amplitude and wavelength of slower components (Fig. 9-7).[12–15] Changes seen with more severe reductions in blood flow (i.e., in the range of 6 to 7 ml/100 g/min or less) consist of a greater reduction of anesthetic-induced fast activity and a reduction in amplitude of the slower components, producing a low-amplitude, relatively featureless EEG on the side of clamping (Figs. 9-6, 9-8, 9-9, and 9-10).[4,13] A major change is defined as an attenuation of at least 75 percent of all EEG activity or an increase in

slow activity having a frequency of 1 Hz or less.[12,13] Although approximately 25 percent of EEGs may show some change at the time of carotid artery clamping, only 1 to 3 percent of EEGs show such major alteration.[7] Unilateral changes are more common than bilateral alterations (Figs. 9-6 and 9-9).[4,7] The latter usually reflect a severe compromise in collateral circulation.[6] Focal transient changes, occurring at times other than with clamping, can be seen in as many as 10 percent of patients.[4,12,13] In the majority, this proves to be caused by transient, asymmetric effects of changing levels of anesthesia on a pre-existing focal abnormality and is of no consequence.[13] Some are probably a transient consequence of embolization from the operative site. However, in about 1 percent of endarterectomies, a focal EEG change develops during the course of surgery, is unassociated with carotid clamping, persists throughout the procedure, and ultimately is associated with a new neurologic deficit in the immediate postoperative period.[13] The cause of this EEG change is usually cerebral embolization. An effective way of identifying embolization is to measure cerebral blood flow when a new, persistent focal EEG change develops. Embolization is associated with a change in the EEG in the absence of an alteration in cerebral blood flow.[4,12,13]

The intraoperative EEG in patients undergoing local anesthesia has also been studied.[30] Investigators at the University of Iowa compared the EEG changes in 96 patients receiving local anesthesia and in 121 patients receiving general anesthesia.[30] The two patient groups appeared similar preoperatively. EEG changes were more common in the general anesthesia group (15.7 percent vs. 6.3 percent).[30] The explanation for this difference was not

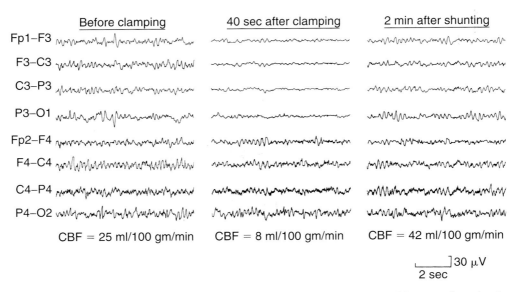

Before clamping	40 sec after clamping	2 min after shunting
CBF = 25 ml/100 gm/min	CBF = 8 ml/100 gm/min	CBF = 42 ml/100 gm/min

30 μV
2 sec

FIGURE 9-6 ▪ Electroencephalographic (EEG) changes related to carotid artery clamping in a patient with high-grade stenosis of the left internal carotid artery. The reduction in cerebral blood flow (CBF) to 8 ml/100 g/min correlates with a marked attenuation of EEG activity on the left. The use of a shunt results in improvement in cerebral blood flow to 42 ml/100 g/min that parallels the improvement in the EEG.

obvious, but the sensitivity and perhaps specificity of intraoperative EEG may be altered by the type of anesthesia.[30] The intraoperative EEG during carotid endarterectomy performed in awake patients using a cervical block was evaluated at the University of Rochester.[16] The EEG findings in 135 such patients were compared with those in 288 patients undergoing endarterectomy under general anesthesia. EEG changes were again more common in the group that was asleep during surgery (15.3 percent vs. 7.4 percent).[16] Global or bihemispheric EEG changes occurred only in the patients receiving general anesthesia.[16] The authors suggested that local anesthesia may be "cerebroprotective," and that variations in blood pressure associated with general anesthesia may be responsible for the global EEG changes.[16]

CEREBRAL BLOOD FLOW

Cerebral blood flow is measured in the operating room at the time of carotid endarterectomy by the xenon-133 intracarotid injection technique.[13] Cerebral blood flow

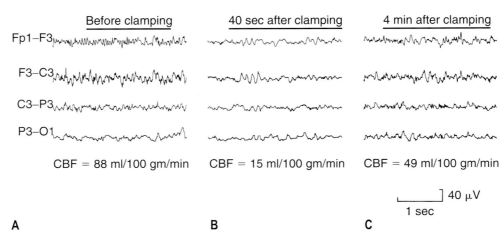

Before clamping	40 sec after clamping	4 min after clamping
CBF = 88 ml/100 gm/min	CBF = 15 ml/100 gm/min	CBF = 49 ml/100 gm/min

40 μV
1 sec

A   **B**   **C**

FIGURE 9-7 ▪ Compared with the electroencephalogram (EEG) before clamping (**A**), the EEG during moderate reduction in cerebral blood flow (CBF) to 15 ml/100 g/min (**B**) reveals a reduction of ipsilateral fast activity with an increase in slowing. Recovery of the anesthetic-induced fast activity occurs with shunting and an improvement in cerebral blood flow (**C**).

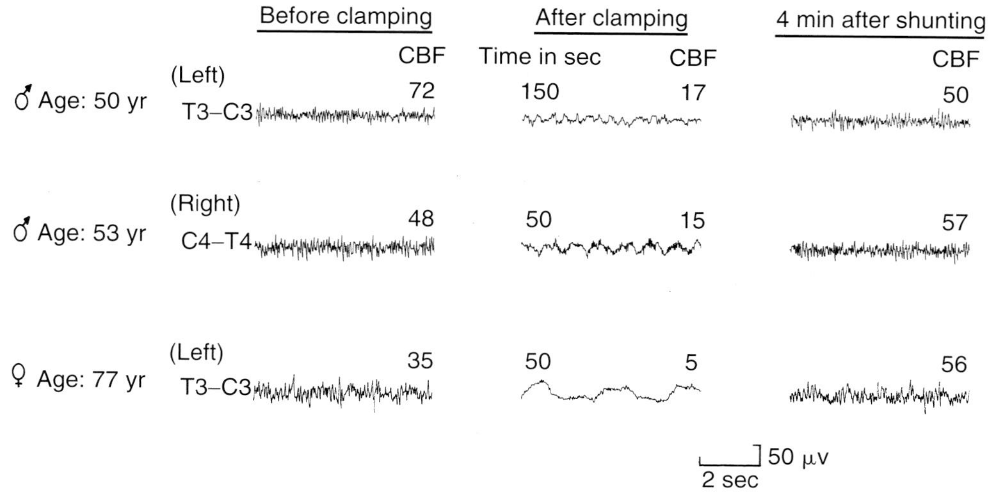

		Before clamping		After clamping		4 min after shunting
			CBF	Time in sec	CBF	CBF
♂ Age: 50 yr	(Left) T3–C3		72	150	17	50
♂ Age: 53 yr	(Right) C4–T4		48	50	15	57
♀ Age: 77 yr	(Left) T3–C3		35	50	5	56

50 µV
2 sec

FIGURE 9-8 ■ Electroencephalographic (EEG) findings in three patients with a significant reduction in cerebral blood flow (CBF) related to carotid clamping. Note that the severity of the EEG alteration correlates with cerebral blood flow measurements. The EEG alterations were reversible, as demonstrated by the recordings obtained after shunting.

measurements are more sensitive than is determination of the "distal stump pressure" obtained by occluding the common carotid and external carotid arteries and measuring the residual pressure in the internal carotid artery.[6] The cerebral blood flow studies are correlated with the EEG findings (cerebral function monitoring)

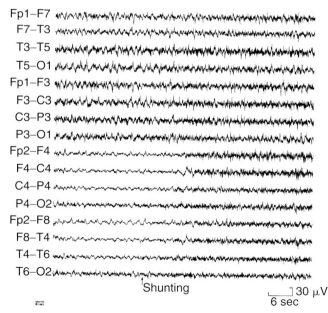

Fp1–F7
F7–T3
T3–T5
T5–O1
Fp1–F3
F3–C3
C3–P3
P3–O1
Fp2–F4
F4–C4
C4–P4
P4–O2
Fp2–F8
F8–T4
T4–T6
T6–O2

Shunting

30 µV
6 sec

FIGURE 9-9 ■ Marked electroencephalographic (EEG) changes related to clamping of the right carotid artery in a patient with left carotid stenosis. There is attenuation of the EEG activity on the right, with an increase in background slowing. Collateral flow was inadequate at the time of the right internal carotid artery occlusion.

to determine the indication for carotid artery shunting at the time of carotid clamping. Xenon is injected into the internal carotid artery above a high-grade stenosis or into the common carotid artery (below the stenosis) with the external carotid artery clamped. A reduction in the cerebral blood flow to 18 ml/100 g/min or less is an indication for shunting.[6] Blood flow is clearly influenced by the $PaCO_2$ level and requires that the xenon be delivered directly to the internal carotid artery while the external carotid artery is clamped. Further, blood flow techniques are intermittent and usually are done before clamping, immediately after clamping, immediately after placement of a shunt (when shunting is necessary), and at the end of the procedure. Xenon intracarotid blood flow studies and EEG monitoring are complementary procedures.[5,12] Focal EEG changes, caused by ischemia brought about by decreased perfusion pressure beyond a clamped carotid artery, are always associated with low blood flow, as measured by the xenon technique. Severe or major EEG changes occur with cerebral blood flow measures below 18 ml/100 g/min, and minor changes occur with values between 18 and 23 ml/100 g/min. No change occurs when the cerebral blood flow is greater than 23 ml/100 g/min.[6,13] An EEG change that persists and is associated with a normal cerebral blood flow is indicative of embolization. The presence of normal blood flow following embolization is explained on the basis of the so-called "look-through phenomenon." If the ischemia results from embolic occlusion of, for example, half the blood vessels to a region, with the other half remaining patent, injection of xenon

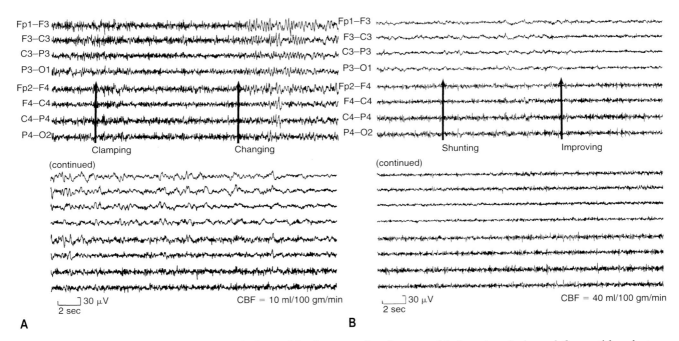

FIGURE 9-10 ■ **A**, Marked electroencephalographic changes related to carotid clamping during a left carotid endarterectomy. Note the rapid attenuation of fast activity and the emergence of increased delta activity at 1 Hz or less, correlating with a significant reduction in cerebral blood flow (CBF). **B**, Shunting increases cerebral blood flow and leads to a gradual increase in fast activity.

results in a normal or, at times, increased flow and washout of xenon through the patent blood vessels, and the totally occluded vessels receive no xenon and therefore do not contribute to the overall measurement of flow.[13]

EEG AND CAROTID ENDARTERECTOMY

The significance of EEG changes during a carotid endarterectomy has been evaluated.[4,12–19] There is conflicting evidence regarding the prognostic importance of cerebral function monitoring.[12] The clinical practice at the Mayo Clinic has been to place a shunt whenever there is an EEG change related to carotid occlusion or when the cerebral blood flow with clamping is less than 18 ml/100 g/min.[12,13] A previous study at the University Hospital in London, Ontario, reported the postoperative outcome in 176 consecutive patients who underwent a carotid endarterectomy without the placement of a shunt.[12,31] No patient without EEG changes or with only minor EEG alterations had a neurologic deficit after surgery. Two of 22 patients (9 percent) with severe EEG changes related to carotid artery clamping had an intraoperative stroke.[7] Some, if not all, of this disagreement may be resolved with an appropriate understanding of the concept of ischemic tolerance of neurologic tissue.[12] The length of time that neural tissue can tolerate ischemia without permanent infarction is related inversely to the severity of the reduction of blood flow

during the time of ischemia. For instance, at zero flow (e.g., with cardiac arrest) it is approximately 4 minutes. At higher levels of flow (approximately 15 ml/100 g/min), laboratory studies suggest that the tolerance may be as long as 1 hour or more. The very low incidence of infarction reported in patients developing EEG changes during occlusion and in whom shunting was not performed probably is related to the fact that only a small percentage of patients (1 to 3 percent) have a severe reduction in cerebral blood flow.[5,12,13] Cerebral infarction may not occur in patients with EEG changes because of the relatively short occlusion time (often less than 20 minutes) that is necessary for the carotid endarterectomy.[12]

The efficacy of intraoperative EEG as a criterion for placement of a shunt was evaluated at one center during 1,661 operations.[32] The overall number of patients with cerebral infarctions was 5. One patient had a "minor" stroke without EEG change. Patients at risk for stroke had an abnormal EEG and contralateral internal carotid artery occlusion (3.3 percent had a cerebral infarction). It was concluded that intraoperative EEG is an excellent predictor for identifying patients who may require placement of a shunt during carotid endarterectomy.[32] The value of intraoperative EEG was confirmed in another study that included 564 patients who underwent a carotid endarterectomy. Again, the EEG was highly predictive of the need for shunt placement, even in individuals with contralateral internal carotid artery occlusion.[33] Bydon and colleagues evaluated the stroke risk in 15 patients with contralateral occlusion without intraoperative shunting.[34] The mean clamp time of the common carotid artery was 18.5 minutes (range, 14 to 30 minutes). None of the patients experienced a cerebral infarct.[34] Therefore controversy remains regarding the primary indication for intraoperative EEG monitoring during carotid endarterectomy and the frequency of adverse effects subsequent to surgery. The divided opinions are the reason that some centers rely on the intraoperative EEG to determine the need for shunt placement, whereas other institutions either use other preoperative or intraoperative data or follow local guidelines.

EVOKED POTENTIALS AND CAROTID ARTERY SURGERY

Somatosensory evoked potentials (SEPs) have been obtained during carotid endarterectomy to demonstrate alterations related to cerebral ischemia.[35,36] The cortical waveforms are altered by a reduction in cerebral blood flow. Persistent SEP abnormalities in one study correlated with the presence of a postoperative neurologic deficit.[36] At present, SEP monitoring has "no advantages" over intraoperative EEG recordings.

EEG MONITORING AND CARDIAC SURGERY

A number of patients undergoing cardiac surgery develop a transient or persistent neurologic deficit (e.g., a cognitive disorder). Several techniques to monitor for the development of such complications have been evaluated, including EEG, transcranial Doppler, cerebral oximetry, and bispectral index monitoring.[7–10]

A reduction in cerebral blood flow may occur during cardiopulmonary bypass for cardiac surgical procedures. EEG monitoring may be useful in detecting significant cerebral ischemia during cardiac surgery.[7,37] EEG monitoring is limited by the use of profound hypothermia, which is associated with increased slowing as the temperature falls below 30°C and a burst-suppression pattern at 20°C. Other potential causes of global EEG changes in patients undergoing heart surgery include hypotension, hemodilution, anesthesia, and air or clot emboli.[7,37] Another cause of a significant EEG change is an obstruction of the pump lines or a low profusion flow and pressure.[37] Significant hypotension may produce generalized EEG changes, including increased background slowing or attenuation. The multifactorial origin of EEG changes during cardiac surgery makes cerebral function monitoring less useful for open-heart surgery than for carotid endarterectomy.[7]

REFERENCES

1. Tripathi M, Garg A, Gaikwad S et al: Intra-operative electrocorticography in lesional epilepsy. Epilepsy Res, 89:133, 2010
2. Gallentine WB, Mikati MA: Intraoperative electrocorticography and cortical stimulation in children. J Clin Neurophysiol, 26:95, 2009
3. Wu JY, Sankar R, Lerner JT et al: Removing interictal fast ripples on electrocorticography linked with seizure freedom in children. Neurology, 75:1686, 2010
4. So EL, Sharbrough FW: Cerebral function monitoring. p. 523. In Daube JR (ed): Clinical Neurophysiology. 2nd Ed. Oxford University Press, Oxford, 2002
5. Guarracino F: Cerebral monitoring during cardiovascular surgery. Curr Opin Anaesthesiol, 21:50, 2008
6. Costin M, Rampersad A, Solomon RA et al: Cerebral injury predicted by transcranial Doppler ultrasonography but not electroencephalography during carotid endarterectomy. J Neurosurg Anesthesiol, 14:287, 2002
7. Edmonds HL, Rodriguez RA, Audenaert SM et al: The role of neuromonitoring in cardiovascular surgery. J Cardiothorac Vasc Anesth, 10:15, 1996
8. Puri GD, Murthy SS: Bispectral index monitoring in patients undergoing cardiac surgery under cardiopulmonary bypass. Eur J Anesthesiol, 20:451, 2003
9. Edmonds HL: Multi-modality neurophysiologic monitoring for cardiac surgery. Heart Surg Forum, 5:225, 2002
10. Lehmann A, Karzau J, Boldt J et al: Bispectral index-guided anesthesia in patients undergoing aortocoronary bypass grafting. Anesth Analg, 96:336, 2003
11. Ascher E, Markevich N, Kallakuri S et al: Intraoperative carotid artery duplex scanning in a modern series of 650 consecutive primary endarterectomy procedures. J Vasc Surg, 39:416, 2004
12. Blume WT, Sharbrough FW: EEG monitoring during carotid endarterectomy and open heart surgery. p. 797. In Niedermeyer E, Lopes da Silva F (eds): Electroencephalography: Basic Principles, Clinical Applications and Related Fields. 4th Ed. Williams & Wilkins, Baltimore, 1999
13. Messick JM, Jr, Casement B, Sharbrough FW et al: Correlation of regional cerebral blood flow (rCBF) with EEG changes during isoflurane anesthesia for carotid endarterectomy: critical rCBF. Anesthesiology, 66:344, 1987
14. Sundt TM, Jr, Sharbrough FW, Piepgras DG et al: Correlation of cerebral blood flow and electroencephalographic changes during carotid endarterectomy. Mayo Clin Proc, 56:533, 1981
15. Tan TW, Garcia-Toca M, Marcaccio EJ, Jr et al: Predictors of shunt during carotid endarterectomy with routine electroencephalography monitoring. J Vasc Surg, 49:1374, 2009

16. Illig KA, Sternbach Y, Zhang R et al: EEG changes during awake carotid endarterectomy. Ann Vasc Surg, 16:6, 2002

17. Illig KA, Burchfiel JL, Ouriel K et al: Value of preoperative EEG for carotid endarterectomy. Cardiovasc Surg, 6:490, 1998

18. Rijsdijk M, Ferrier C, Laman M et al: Detection of ischemic electroencephalography changes during carotid endarterectomy using synchronization likelihood analysis. J Neurosurg Anesthesiol, 21:302, 2009

19. Ballotta E, Saladini M, Gruppo M et al: Predictors of electroencephalographic changes needing shunting during carotid endarterectomy. Ann Vasc Surg, 24:1045, 2010

20. Pasternak JJ, Lanier WL: Neuroanesthesiology update. J Neurosurg Anesthesiol, 22:86, 2010

21. Jacob T, Hingorani A, Ascher E: Carotid artery stump pressure (CASP) in 1135 consecutive endarterectomies under general anesthesia: an old method that survived the test of times. J Cardiovasc Surg (Torino), 48:677, 2007

22. Cohen S: Carotid endarterectomy for asymptomatic disease. J Stroke Cerebrovasc Dis, 6:180, 1997

23. The Asymptomatic Carotid Atherosclerosis Study Group: Endarterectomy for asymptomatic carotid artery stenosis. JAMA, 273:1421, 1995

24. North American Symptomatic Carotid Endarterectomy Trial Collaborators: Beneficial effect of carotid endarterectomy in symptomatic patients with high-grade stenosis. N Engl J Med, 325:445, 1991

25. Mayberg MR, Wilson SE, Yatsu F et al: Carotid endarterectomy and prevention of cerebral ischemia and symptomatic carotid stenosis. JAMA, 266:3289, 1991

26. Brooks WH, McClure RR, Jones MR et al: Carotid angioplasty and stenting versus carotid endarterectomy for treatment of asymptomatic carotid stenosis: a randomized trial in a community hospital. Neurosurgery, 54:318, 2004

27. CARESS Steering Committee: Carotid revascularization using endarterectomy or stenting systems (CARESS): phase I clinical trial. J Endovasc Ther, 10:1021, 2003

28. McDonnell CO, Legge D, Twomey E et al: Carotid artery angioplasty for restenosis following endarterectomy. Eur J Vasc Endovasc Surg, 27:163, 2004

29. Rössel T, Litz RJ, Heller AR et al: Anesthesia for carotid artery surgery. Is there a gold standard? Anaesthetist, 57:115, 2008

30. Wellman BJ, Loftus CM, Kresowik TF et al: The differences in electroencephalographic changes in patients undergoing carotid endarterectomies while under local versus general anesthesia. Neurosurgery, 43:769, 1998

31. Blume WT, McNeill DK, Ferguson GG: EEG during carotid artery clamping at endarterectomy without shunting. Electroencephalogr Clin Neurophysiol, 56:27P, 1983

32. Pinkerton JA: EEG as a criterion for shunt need in carotid endarterectomy. Ann Vasc Surg, 16:756, 2002

33. Schneider JR, Droste JS, Schindler N et al: Carotid endarterectomy with routine electroencephalography and selective shunting: influence of contralateral internal carotid artery occlusion and utility in prevention of perioperative strokes. J Vasc Surg, 35:1114, 2002

34. Bydon A, Thomas AJ, Seyfried D et al: Carotid endarterectomy in patients with contralateral internal carotid artery occlusion without intraoperative shunting. Surg Neurol, 57:325, 2002

35. Markand ON, Dilley RS, Moorthy SS et al: Monitoring of somatosensory evoked responses during carotid endarterectomy. Arch Neurol, 41:375, 1984

36. Horsch S, De Vleeschauwer P, Ktenidis K: Intraoperative assessment of cerebral ischemia during carotid surgery. J Cardiovasc Surg, 31:599, 1990

37. Fedorow C, Grocott HP: Cerebral monitoring to optimize outcomes after cardiac surgery. Curr Opin Anaesthesiol, 23:89, 2010

Magnetoencephalography

WILLIAM W. SUTHERLING

RECORDING TECHNIQUE

LOCALIZATION PROCEDURES

VALIDATION STUDIES OF LOCALIZATION ACCURACY
  Phantom Studies
  Median Somatosensory Evoked Field
  Comparison of Seizure Discharges

CLINICAL STUDIES
  Intractable Focal Epilepsy
  Brain Tumors and Cortical Mapping
    Sensory and Motor Cortex
    Language
CONCLUDING COMMENTS

The term magnetoencephalography (MEG) refers to the recording of the magnetic field of electrocerebral activity. MEG uses specialized equipment and lends itself to source localization using dipole methods and co-registration with magnetic resonance imaging (MRI). Because of the properties of the magnetic field and its lack of interaction with biologic tissues at the frequencies of brain electric currents, the MEG is inherently more accurate and less subject to distortion than is the electroencephalogram (EEG). The co-registration of MEG and MRI is called magnetic source imaging (MSI).

The MEG is generated by the small electric currents set up in neurons during postsynaptic potentials. Because of the symmetry of the magnetic field, MEG records primarily intracellular currents oriented tangentially or parallel to the scalp surface, whereas EEG records extracellular volume currents produced by neurons of all orientations.[1–4] Figure 10-1 shows the MEG and EEG field patterns expected for a tangential source and for two radial sources.

As with the EEG, summation of the activity of a large number of parallel-oriented neurons is necessary to produce a detectable signal outside the head. These conditions are met by the larger pyramidal neurons in cortical layers III to V. The MEG is generated according to the right-hand rule of physics, by which current in a small segment of wire flowing from positive to negative in the direction of the thumb of the right hand will generate a magnetic field in the direction of the curled fingers. The magnetic field map or pattern recorded over the scalp is generated by the electrical current in a small cortical region. This map shows a point of maximum, exiting field-strength or peak; a point of minimum, entering field-strength or valley; and a null point between the peak and valley. This is a "tangential dipolar" pattern and is the usual appearance of the MEG isocontours. This pattern is invariant and easy to model.

RECORDING TECHNIQUE

To record the MEG, two problems had to be solved. First, a sensor with high sensitivity was required to record the very small signal of interest. The MEG is less than one picoTesla (10^{-12} Tesla), or about a billion times smaller than the earth's magnetic field (10^{-4} Tesla). Second, the magnetic fields in the environment create a virtual magnetic storm, and thus a signal-to-noise problem. Magnets used for MRI (about 1 Tesla), fluorescent lights, and cars moving in the street all produce magnetic signals that are much larger than the MEG. This situation is analogous to trying to measure the fluctuating height of a microscopic ripple on a pond while the pond is in the path of a hurricane.

The solutions were ingenious. The problem of sensitivity was solved by the use of a superconducting quantum interference device (SQUID) immersed in liquid helium (at 4° Kelvin, or 4° above absolute zero). Interference devices are very sensitive instruments to measure waves in a wide range of applications. A SQUID is a superconducting ring of metal, with one conducting wire

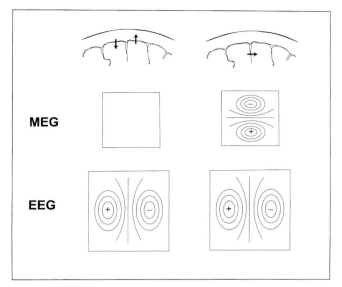

FIGURE 10-1 ▪ The magnetoencephalographic (MEG) and electroencephalographic (EEG) field maps for two radial dipoles and one tangential dipole. At left, two radial dipoles produce a field map in EEG with a maximum and minimum and a null point between. Because a radial dipole produces no magnetic field, the MEG shows no field pattern above noise. At the right, one tangential dipole produces the same basic pattern in the EEG, but now the MEG shows a field map above noise. (Data from Sutherling W, Levesque M, Crandall P et al: Localization of partial epilepsy using magnetic and electric measurements. Epilepsia, 32:29, 1991.)

leading current into the ring and another leading current away from it. The current passes through the metal of the ring by splitting into two halves of current in each of the two semicircles of the ring and then rejoining to flow out of the ring into the exiting conductor wire. There is a "weak link" or segment where the metal is pinched down to a smaller diameter in each of the two parts of the ring, so that much less current can pass through the ring. Each of these weak links has an upper limit of current that can pass through it, called a *critical current*. While the ring is supercooled in liquid helium and superconducting, there is no resistance in the wire. When, however, a change in magnetic field passes through the center hole of the ring, the magnetic field induces a circular current in the ring according to Lenz's law. This increases the current flowing through one of the weak links to above the limit of the critical current. This stops the ring from superconducting, and the ring then has much higher resistance and conducts much less current. There is a very large change in the current passing through the ring in going from a superconducting state, in which there is zero resistance and a very large current, to a normal state, in which there is a large resistance and

much smaller current. This change in current is measured easily at a macroscopic level, so that the MEG, although very small, induces a large change in current in the SQUID.

Two innovations helped to solve the second problem of the signal-to-noise ratio. First, the development of a magnetically shielded room canceled out all environmental noise. Second, a gradiometer coil enabled the magnetic fields from the heart to be canceled out and the magnetic fields to be recorded selectively near the head directly under the sensor. The gradiometer is still needed inside the shielded room to cancel out the heart's magnetic field (MKG), which is one hundred times larger than the MEG. Using a SQUID attached to a gradiometer coil inside a shielded room allows recording of MEG, even in the hostile noise environment of a modern imaging center or hospital.

Figure 10-2 shows a subject having an MEG study under the dewar of a whole-cortex neuromagnetometer inside a magnetically shielded room.

LOCALIZATION PROCEDURES

Although MEG recording equipment is complex and costly, the MEG, once obtained, is easier to analyze than the EEG because of its simpler geometry and invariant field patterns. The first step is reviewing the raw time-series data. This is almost the same as the EEG; the MEG shows alpha rhythm, sleep spindles, evoked responses, and abnormal activity such as spikes.

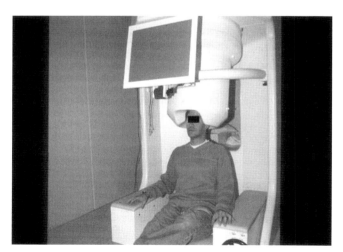

FIGURE 10-2 ▪ Patient undergoing magnetoencephalographic (MEG) recording. The patient's head is placed under the fiberglass dewar. The dewar contains liquid helium, the coils, and superconducting quantum interference device sensors, which record the MEG. The MEG system is inside a magnetically shielded room.

The second step is reviewing the isocontour maps over the head at a single time-point. A map with complementary extrema (maximum and minimum) and a null line between usually indicates an underlying source, which can be modeled as a tangential dipole.

The basic idea of localization by a single dipole model is straightforward. First, a computer program performs a simulation. It places a dipole or infinitesimally small segment of wire with current at a specific location and orientation inside the skull. Then the magnetic field pattern generated by the dipole is compared with the measured MEG field pattern. A goodness-of-fit is calculated using the squared difference between the computed field and the measured field. For that location and orientation, the goodness-of-fit is placed in a table. Then the computer moves the dipole to a new location and new orientation and repeats the whole process, storing the results on the next line of the table. This is repeated many times until the computer finds the location and orientation that has the least squared difference or smallest error between the computed and measured field. The computer then reports that location and orientation as the true location and orientation of the center of the brain electrical activity.

If there were no noise, and if all assumptions of the model were correct, the computed location and orientation would coincide with the actual parameters of the brain activity. Unfortunately, in the real world, there are noises and complexity in the measurements that prevent perfect estimates. The sources of error can be broken down into the parts of the model.

Because of its simpler nature, the MEG lends itself to thorough analysis of the different contributions of noise to its modeling errors. The contributions to localization error arise from several parts of the model, which are best visualized going from the brain to the recording at the SQUID. First, the source of current must be modeled correctly as a single focal region, as multiple regions, or as an extended layer of brain activity. Second, the background activity of the brain or "biologic noise" must be modeled to separate it from the activity of interest, such as an epileptic spike or evoked response. Third, the volume conductor of the head through which the magnetic field travels to get to the sensor must be modeled. Fourth, the sensors must be co-registered to the MRI in correct relation to the brain structures recorded. Fifth, the instrumentation noise of the measurement system, including the inherent noise of the SQUID and the SQUID electronics, must be modeled.

The source model chosen for clinical applications usually is the single dipole discussed earlier. Any type of brain activity usually involves a large ensemble of neurons in a cortical layer of finite extent. However, when the recording sensor is far enough away from a single region of brain activity, the source can be modeled as a point source at the center of the cortical activity. In other applications, the use of two or more dipoles is necessary because there are multiple regions that are simultaneously active. In still other models, no attempt is made to assume a specific type of source, such as a dipole; rather, an estimate is made of the distribution of currents circulating in a wide region. Each of these models has its own advantages and disadvantages; however, the single dipole is useful for most clinical applications.

The signal-to-noise ratio can be improved to detect smaller sources (e.g., sharper initial spikes) using advanced spatiotemporal models such as the recursively applied multiple signal classification algorithm (designated by the acronym RAP-MUSIC), which separates the signal from the noise subspace,[5] increasing the signal-to-noise ratio. More realistic modeling may improve detection sensitivity of MEG. More complex modeling has been used in scientific work by several investigators.[6,7] Propagation is assessed best with the more realistic spatiotemporal dipole model.

The volume conductor for MEG can be modeled simply as a single sphere or local sphere that is homogeneously conducting. Straightforward equations exist that are programmed easily for this application. The EEG, by contrast, arises from volume currents, and the tissue interfaces and conductivities of different brain, cerebrospinal fluid, skull, and scalp layers must be modeled. This is a more difficult problem because these conductivities are not known a priori and are quite variable from patient to patient.[8,9]

The model of the volume conductor significantly affects localization accuracy of dipole and extended source models.[10,11] Several mathematical and geometric models of the human head as a volume conductor have been developed to correlate extracranially measured magnetic fields (i.e., by MEG) and electrical potentials (i.e., by EEG) to their intracranial generators. Models such as multiple concentric spherical shells, the boundary element model, and the finite element model are among the most widely used.[12–19] The boundary element model divides the volume conductor into closed surfaces. The finite element model divides the volume conductor into many small tetrahedrons; it is more realistic but is also computationally intensive. Since exact conductivities are not known in the individual patient, it is also subject to misspecification errors. The boundary element model is a compromise. Skull effects usually dominate in the more complex volume conductor models. Detailed studies of conductivity have revealed the complexity of the skull's electrical properties.[8,9,20]

Inclusion of the results of such studies in the volume conductor model eventually may improve localization from extracranial electrical and magnetic measurements.

The co-registration of sensor sites with the MRI is easier for the MEG than the EEG. The MEG sensors are in a fixed array inside the dewar flask containing the liquid helium. Thus, only the location and orientation of the array center and axis need to be measured, rather than calculating all the locations of each of the electrodes attached to the nonspherical surface of the scalp, as is required for the EEG. This reduces the errors in MEG.

Although, theoretically, EEG is less accurate than MEG for spatial localization,[5,21] and EEG sensors are more difficult to co-register with MRI, EEG has several complementary advantages. It is used routinely in all comprehensive epilepsy centers in the United States. It is less expensive than MEG because it records only the voltage differences between two sites on the head, even though using the recording of this easily obtainable quantity increases the complexity of the volume conductor necessary to analyze it. Recording of epileptic activity usually is easier by EEG, which can be used for long-term studies. The electrodes are attached to the scalp, and the patient can move around while being recorded. This allows the recording of seizures and a large spike sample across wake–sleep states to assess autonomy. The portability of EEG allows recording in the operating room and intensive care unit. EEG measures the same current orientations as intracranial electrographic recordings. EEG also measures more of the cerebral cortex than MEG, concurrently increasing the complexity of the source model required for analysis. The EEG combined with the MEG allows more accurate localization than either MEG or EEG alone.[18,22,23] More realistic volume conductor models are especially important to improve the accuracy of the EEG and are essential to combine the MEG and EEG for localization purposes.[13,24]

VALIDATION STUDIES OF LOCALIZATION ACCURACY

Phantom Studies

MEG localization is accurate. The results from the author's laboratory are reported here as representative of the accumulating literature.[25,26] The localization error in MEG was quantified for a dry dipole phantom for one dipole and two dipoles. It was found that the MEG method, analyzed with realistic modeling, gives accurate localizations for one dipole and for two dipoles overlapping in time.

The dry phantom consisted of two flat plastic semicircular plates fitted together at a right angle along their diameters to mimic a sphere. Small wire current dipoles were embedded in the plastic, tangential to the radii. This is used routinely as a calibration phantom. A single dipole source and a two-dipole source were tested at multiple locations using RAP-MUSIC from National Institutes of Health-funded BrainStorm software, developed as shareware for scientists.[27-29] The phantom was attached mechanically to the bottom of the dewar inside the space for the head in a 100-SQUID 68-sensor channel whole-cortex neuromagnetometer. The neuromagnetometer used 68 sensor first-derivative co-axial gradiometers and 19 reference channels to produce synthetic third-derivative gradiometers, which were flux-transformed to direct-current SQUIDS. Coil parameters were baseline 5 cm and diameter 2 cm. Channel noise was 5 to 7 femtoTesla per root Hz.

For one-dipole activation, mean localization error was 1.0 mm (SEM, 0.4), with 95 percent confidence that the actual location was less than 2 mm from the estimated location. For two dipoles, overlapping in time but offset by 100 msec, mean error was 1.7 mm (SEM, 0.6) for each, with 95 percent confidence that each of the dipoles were within 3 mm of the estimate.

With perfectly synchronous activations of identical waveforms, errors were larger. Such synchrony may not be relevant to human cortex because of delays from finite conduction speed of cortico-cortical association U-fibers.[30] Even in 3-Hz generalized spike-wave activity in primary generalized absence epilepsy (classic "petit mal"), which is the prototype of generalized epileptiform activity, interhemispheric conduction delays are 15 to 20 msec.[31]

Source configurations with two dipoles on the same radius also gave larger errors. This problem, anticipated theoretically, has been approached historically in at least two ways. First, experimental design can help. For instance, the auditory P300 has components from superficial and deep structures that overlap in time and space (e.g., the primary auditory cortex, hippocampus, and lateral neocortex). These structures are in the same temporal lobe and, during some parts of the activity, on similar radii. Investigators have addressed this problem by studying the visual P300, where the primary cortical response is in the occipital lobe and the later response is in the medial temporal lobe.[32] In this case, the fields of the earlier and later responses have less overlap. Thus innovative experimental design helps avoid situations in which larger localization errors result from co-radial sources.

Additional studies showed only slightly larger mean errors of localization when the experiments were repeated in a saline-filled sphere phantom with one dipole.

In that case, the mean localization error was 1.4 mm and the SEM was 0.9 mm.[26]

Combined MEG and EEG methods may help. For instance, comparison of the timing of an EEG component at the deeper sphenoidal electrode with the timing of a component at a lateral scalp electrode may help to distinguish deep and superficial sources.[30,33] The additional sensitivity of an EEG electrode contact recording extracranially but directly under the foramen ovale thus can add complementary sensitivity and spatially specific information to address the problem of temporally overlapping sources that are superficial and deep, with one under the other.

Median Somatosensory Evoked Field

The localizations of the median somatosensory evoked response (SER) have been tested on whole-head neuromagnetometers and replicated between a 68-sensor system (with recordings made in 1998) and a 150-sensor system (localizations made in 2001). The two laboratories were in different cities, about 2,000 miles apart. The electrical stimuli were delivered to the median nerve at the wrist to give a reliable thumb twitch at 3.1 Hz, to avoid 60-Hz line-frequency. The parameters were digitization rate 1,250 Hz, bandpass 0.1 Hz to 300 Hz, and 250-msec sweep with a 50-msec prestimulus baseline, with a subsequent high-pass filter to eliminate low frequencies and later activity, which were not of interest in this study. Localizations from the single moving dipole model were applied to the SER. The latencies of the best-fitting dipoles were slightly different in the two studies but within experimental error for the more stable P30m (P1m). The localization from each laboratory was co-registered on the subject's MRI.

The mean euclidean distance between the co-registered localizations of the two systems was 2.1 mm (standard deviation [SD], 1.84), with the largest error vertically, on the z-axis. This difference is within 1 SD of the localization error in the saline-filled sphere phantom,[25,26] and similar to the 2- to 3-mm error in a phantom study on a 122-channel whole-head system.[34] Thus, within the error limits derived from phantom studies, there was no detectable difference in localization of the early dipolar components of the median SER measured on two different neuromagnetometers many miles apart and over a period of 3 years. This confirms the theoretical predictions of MEG localization accuracy and the lack of a significant difference between 64 and 128 channels for dipole localization of cortical sources.[5]

The comparison of the two studies was facilitated by the ease of data transfer and superimposition in the same programs on the same co-registered MRI. Accurate localization of the superficial focal currents producing the early components of the SER is one of the most difficult tests of a localization method. A superficial source has the highest spatial frequency of topographic map isocontours.[35]

Comparison of Seizure Discharges

The clinical procedure of afterdischarge mapping to determine neocortical epileptogenicity has been used in another test of localization accuracy. Simultaneous MEG and electrocorticogram (ECoG) was recorded for an electrically induced focal afterdischarge seizure in the frontal lobe of a patient undergoing evaluation for epilepsy surgery. In this case the origin of the seizure was known to be in the cortex directly under the stimulating electrode. Dipole localization was applied to the repetitive spiking of the seizure in the ECoG and MEG measured at the same time.

Figure 10-3 shows that the MEG and ECoG localizations were within about 1 cm of the center of the subdural ECoG electrode where the afterdischarge was induced. There was no significant difference between the MEG error (mean 8.5 mm, SEM 1.5) and the ECoG error (mean 10.4 mm, SEM 0.3).[26] In this study, the MEG and ECoG were both able to record the same

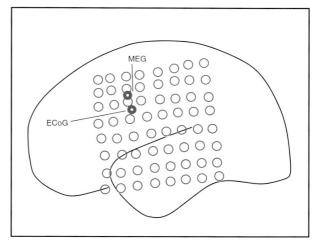

FIGURE 10-3 ■ Localization accuracy of magnetoencephalography (MEG) during a seizure. Cortical stimulation produced a self-limited afterdischarge seizure at the subdural electrode between the two blue dots. The upper dot was the MEG dipole estimate. The lower dot was the electrocorticography (ECoG) dipole estimate. The two show similar error. (Data from Sutherling WW, Akhtari M, Mamelak AN et al: Dipole localization of human induced focal afterdischarge seizure in simultaneous magnetoencephalography and electrocorticography. Brain Topogr, 14:101, 2001.)

event with a similar signal-to-noise ratio, and their localizations were indistinguishable. The ECoG usually has been regarded as superior to noninvasive electrophysiologic methods in both specificity and sensitivity. This study suggests, however, that with similar sensitivities the MEG and ECoG can have equivalent localization specificity for pathologic activity that is the definition of epilepsy (i.e., the seizure itself). This finding is important in suggesting a means to improve noninvasive localization of abnormal activity for focal excisional surgery in epilepsy centers. Many patients now require invasive recording with ECoG or depth electrodes to localize and quantify the zone of seizure origin.[36,37] This study suggested that MEG may provide useful preoperative information to guide electrode placement to avoid sampling error such as edge-of-the-grid effect.

CLINICAL STUDIES

Intractable Focal Epilepsy

Epilepsy occurs in about 1 percent of the population at any one time, and with an incidence of about 3 percent over the lifetime of a patient. About 30 percent of patients with epilepsy have seizures that are uncontrolled by medications[38]; these seizures may be disabling. Most historical studies suggest that about half of the patients with medically intractable epilepsy are good surgical candidates.[39–41] Focal excision abolishes seizures in 70 to 85 percent of these patients with temporal lobe foci and in 40 percent of those with neocortical foci. Localization of the seizure is essential for surgery.[36,40,42,43] Recording from intracranial electrodes allows 36 percent more patients to have surgery compared with those having only scalp recordings.[39] Intracranial recordings have led to improved surgical results[40–42,44] but have the dual disadvantages of invasiveness and sampling error. Epilepsy surgery does not control seizures completely in 15 to 20 percent[39,44] despite intracranial recordings, probably as a result of sampling error in some cases because a spread pattern may be recorded. Sampling error is inherent because of the risk of the procedure, which increases with more electrode coverage. Noninvasive protocols allow about 70 percent of patients with temporal lobe epilepsy to have surgery without intracranial electrodes. Focal temporal-lobe seizure onsets on video-EEG with confirming ipsilateral lesions visualized by positron emission tomography or MRI provide accurate localization, equivalent to recording from intracranial depth electrodes but without the risk.[36,37,41]

Presurgical localization usually is based on seizure recording from inpatient monitoring. Seizure spread can create ambiguity, necessitating invasive recordings for definitive localization. There is more information to be derived from spike discharges than presently is obtained in most surgical centers. Spike discharges may be present on routine outpatient EEG recordings as well as on inpatient monitoring. Spikes help quantify the epileptogenic zone for more effective intracranial sampling and for surgical removal.[45–47]

There are multiple retrospective studies with large-array or whole-head MEG systems that together involve a large number of patients.[48–52] These studies have tested the localization accuracy of MEG in comparison with intracranial electrode recordings. Knowlton and colleagues studied 22 patients with a 37-sensor MEG[48]; Wheless and associates studied 58 patients with two 37-sensor systems[50]; and Lamusuo and co-workers studied 9 patients who had complicated focal epilepsy with a whole-scalp MEG array.[52] Otsubo and Snead studied children with a whole-scalp MEG array.[51,53,54] Mamelak and colleagues studied 23 patients who had MEG and invasive monitoring.[49] All found MEG useful in that it helped to predict seizure zones and improved localization for epilepsy surgery.

Mamelak and colleagues found the MEG useful in guiding invasive recording. This increased the yield of invasive recording in some patients by ensuring that intracranial electrodes were placed correctly to cover the zone of seizure origin. When MEG spike dipoles were clustered tightly with an average distance of 4 mm between spikes, invasive recording successfully localized the seizure zone, leading to surgery. Furthermore, MEG gave nonredundant information. It led to electrode placement near regions that previously were not suspected of being epileptogenic by any other test. Thus, when integrated into a routine presurgical protocol,[36,37,40,55–57] MEG tended to improve the yield of invasive recordings and the yield of the protocol.

The degree of MEG utility has differed between studies. Some found that MEG localized successful surgery in 52 percent of patients,[50] whereas others found accurate MEG localization in 86 percent of patients.[48] This difference is significant. It could be explained by spike propagation or by signal-to-noise ratio. MEG detects ECoG spikes only during synchronous activation of an extended area of cortex when multiple ECoG electrodes are involved; estimates from EEG recorded simultaneous with ECoG strips have indicated an area of about 6 cm.[57,58] Synchronous cortical activity over about 2 cm^2 to 3 cm^2 was required to produce a detectable extracranial spike in the MEG when MEG was compared with simultaneous recording from large ECoG grids where area could be quantified over the cortical surface.[59] This is because of detection sensitivity and signal-to-noise ratio. The MEG is better suited than EEG to extracranial–intracranial correlations because of minimal effect of the volume conductor on MEG,[60] allowing simultaneous MEG and intracranial electrography with grids. The MEG is better in extratemporal than temporal epilepsy,[50] consistent with findings in the EEG for specificity of spikes. These large studies indicated that MEG may

have nonredundant utility compared with routine EEG analysis but remains inferior to invasive intracranial EEG for localization.

MEG in practice is restricted to the recording of interictal spikes; seizures are recorded rarely. The standard of care is to record seizures, which are the single most reliable predictor of the zone of seizure origin and response to focal excisional surgery,[42] indicating that intensive video-EEG inpatient monitoring of seizures remains necessary. Nevertheless, interictal spike discharges

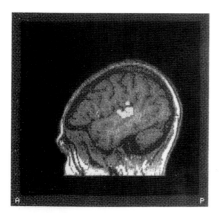
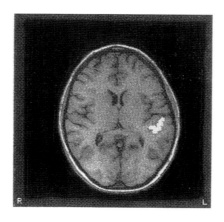
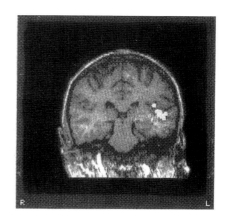

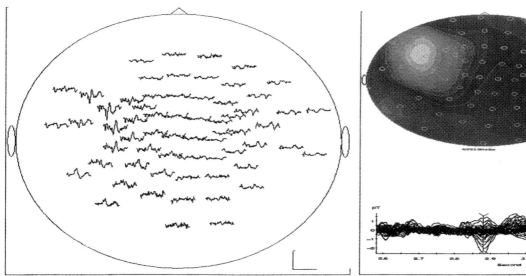
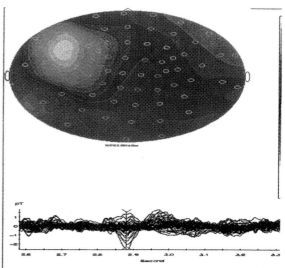

FIGURE 10-4 ■ Magnetic source imaging (MSI) of spikes. This is the standard computer printout of such imaging for epileptic spikes, used in presurgical evaluation. Below at left are the time-series tracings showing spikes over the left temporal lobe. At right are the magnetoencephalography (MEG) field map for the spike and a butterfly plot of the spike, superimposing all channels. Above are the MSIs. In each image the MEG dipoles for each spike recorded are co-registered with the magnetic resonance image. The spikes cluster in the left posterior temporal region, suggesting a left lateral neocortical temporal epileptogenic zone. This study helps guide the placement of a subdural grid centered over the cluster to cover the potential zone of seizure origin completely. Note that the images show the right side on the left, and left side on the right, according to radiologic convention. Calibrations: 3.5 picoTesla and 450 msec.

have unexploited information and are more predictive in neocortical epilepsy, in which MEG appears to be most useful. Near the zone of seizure origin, spike discharges have several characteristics: abundance,[61,62] specific propagation patterns,[63–65] sharpness of the spike,[61,66] and stability of occurrence or constant repetition rate across wake–sleep states. Because MEG is restricted to brief sessions, more prolonged video-EEG monitoring, both outpatient and inpatient, is necessary to assess autonomy, and EEG source localization methods are important.

In light of the different findings in the above studies and the difficulty in comparing their results, two recent

studies are informative. These studies were designed to obtain evidence-based results and enrolled patients considered for intracranial EEG. Knowlton and colleagues used a standard presurgical protocol in 77 patients and found that MEG changed placement of intracranial EEG and improved outcomes.[67] A decision blind to MEG was compared to a decision after the MEG was presented. The authors found that MEG improved outcomes in 8 percent of patients.

Sutherling and colleagues used a similar protocol and method in 69 patients to determine whether MEG influenced decisions for resection, intracranial EEG, or vagal nerve stimulator, and whether MEG improved

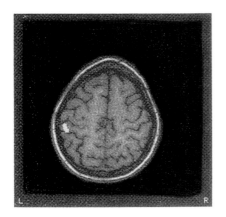
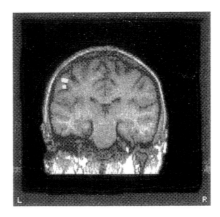
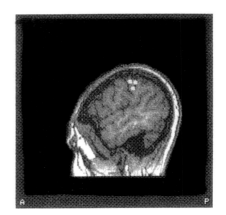

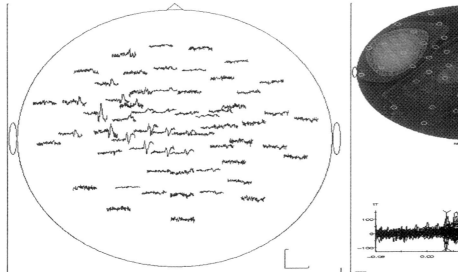
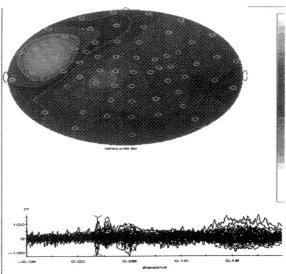

FIGURE 10-5 ■ Magnetic source imaging (MSI) of the somatosensory evoked response. This is a standard computer printout of MSI for locating the central fissure near the hand area, used in preoperative planning for tumors and for epilepsy surgical evaluation. The right median nerve was stimulated, producing activation of the left hand somatosensory region. Note that right and left sides are reversed on these images compared with Figure 10-4, and follow clinical neurophysiologic custom. It is essential to double-check the markings for right and left on all images when reading co-registered images. Calibrations: 200 femtoTesla and 110 msec.

outcomes.[68] They found that MEG added useful information that benefited 9 percent of patients and improved outcomes in 5 percent of the total by intention to treat and in 10 percent of those who actually had surgery.

The similar degree of utility in the two studies is unlikely to be due to chance. The American Academy of Neurology Professional Association has recommended MEG as clinically useful in epilepsy presurgical evaluation.[69]

Figure 10-4 shows a standard computer output of a spike study in a patient with localization-related epilepsy and intractable focal ("complex partial") seizures. The MEG spike dipole cluster suggests that the epileptogenic zone is in the left lateral neocortex, which would require a grid centered on the cluster. Figure 10-5 shows a similar computer output for localization of the right median SER or left somatosensory cortex. This type of imaging is useful both for evaluation before epilepsy surgery and for preoperative surgical planning in resection of tumors.

Brain Tumors and Cortical Mapping

SENSORY AND MOTOR CORTEX

Localization of the central fissure is important to avoid causing hand weakness by surgery. Electrophysiologic techniques are required because visual identification of the central fissure may be inaccurate.[70] Cortical stimulations are usually definitive but require patient cooperation. Intraoperative SERs to median nerve stimulation are accurate but may not identify the central fissure when it is located outside the operative field. MEG reliably localizes the central fissure preoperatively for surgery.[49,71–73] Figure 10-5 shows the SER from MEG. The American Academy of Neurology Professional Association has recommended MEG as clinically useful in presurgical localization of the central fissure in brain tumors and arteriovenous malformations.[69] Furthermore, SER mapping of the thumb may allow more complete resections of epilepsy and tumors below the cortical hand area.[74] Because digit SERs have a smaller signal-to-noise ratio than those of the median nerve, more advanced modeling may also be useful.

LANGUAGE

Some centers have reported that MEG single dipoles lateralize and delimit language cortex in a majority of patients,[75–77] confirmed by the Wada test and cortical stimulation.[78] The Wada test determines the laterality of language and memory. When technically valid, it is a highly specific predictor of the risk of global amnesia from a temporal resection. The MEG is therefore complementary to the Wada test and would be unlikely to replace it. The MEG also appears to be complementary to cortical stimulation and, at this time, there is inadequate evidence for the MEG to replace it. Further evidence-based studies are needed.

CONCLUDING COMMENTS

The MEG is a useful, complementary addition to the EEG in the epileptologist's diagnostic noninvasive armamentarium and is also valuable for the preoperative identification of the central fissure. Present work is focusing on the combination of MEG and EEG to improve source reconstruction methods and on improvement of EEG localization accuracy.

ACKNOWLEDGMENTS

This work was supported by a Public Health Service research grant (RO1 NS20806) from the Epilepsy Branch, National Institute of Neurological Diseases and Stroke, and a shared instrumentation grant (S10 RR13276) from the National Center for Research Resources.

REFERENCES

1. Cohen D, Hosaka H: Magnetic field produced by a current dipole. J Electrocardiol, 9:409, 1976
2. Hamalainen M, Hari R, Ilmoniemi R et al: Magnetoencephalography: theory, instrumentation, and applications to noninvasive studies of the working human brain. Rev Modern Physics, 65:413, 1993
3. Williamson S, Kaufman L: Magnetic fields of the cerebral cortex. p. 353. In Erne S, Hahlbohm H, Lubbig H (eds): Biomagnetism. Walter de Gruyter, Berlin, 1981
4. Williamson S, Kaufman L: Biomagnetism. J Magnetism Magnetic Materials, 22:129, 1981
5. Mosher J, Spencer M, Leahy R et al: Error bounds for EEG and MEG dipole source localization. Electroencephalogr Clin Neurophysiol, 86:303, 1993
6. Dale A, Sereno M: Improved localization of cortical activity by coimaging EEG and MEG with MRI cortical surface reconstruction: a linear approach. J Cogn Neurosci, 5:162, 1993
7. Halgren E, Dhond RP, Christensen N et al: N400-like MEG responses modulated by semantic context, word frequency, and lexical class in sentences. Neuroimage, 17:1101, 2002
8. Akhtari M, Bryant H, Mamelak A et al: Conductivities of three-layer human skull. Brain Topogr, 13:29, 2000
9. Akhtari M, Bryant HC, Mamelak AN et al: Conductivities of three-layer live human skull. Brain Topogr, 14:151, 2002

10. Stinstra JG, Peters MJ: The volume conductor may act as a temporal filter on the ECG and EEG. Med Biol Eng Comput, 36:711, 1998

11. Van den Broek SP, Reinders F, Donderwinkel M et al: Volume conduction effects in EEG and MEG. Electroencephalogr Clin Neurophysiol, 106:522, 1998

12. Buchner H, Knoll G, Fuchs M et al: Inverse localization of electric dipole current sources in finite element models of the human head. Electroencephalogr Clin Neurophysiol, 102:267, 1997

13. Fuchs M, Drenckhahn R, Wischmann HA et al: An improved boundary element method for realistic volume-conductor modeling. IEEE Trans Biomed Eng, 45:980, 1998

14. Yan Y, Nunez P, Hart R: Finite-element model of the human head: scalp potentials due to dipole sources. Med Biol Eng Comput, 29:475, 1991

15. Hamalainen M, Sarvas J: Realistic conductivity geometry model of the human head for interpretation of neuromagnetic data. IEEE Trans Biomed Eng, 36:165, 1989

16. Sarvas J: Basic mathematical and electromagnetic concepts of the biomagnetic inverse problem. Phys Med Biol, 32:11, 1987

17. Stok CJ: The inverse problem in EEG and MEG with application to visual evoked responses. PhD Thesis, State University, Leiden, Netherlands, 1986

18. Stok C: The influence of model parameters on EEG/MEG single dipole source estimation. IEEE Trans Biomed Eng, 34:289, 1987

19. Mejis J, Peters M, Oosterom V: Computation of MEGs and EEGs using a realistically shaped multicompartment model of the head. Med Biol Eng Comput, 23:36, 1985

20. Akhtari M, Bryant HC, Emin D et al: A model for frequency dependence of conductivities of the live human skull. Brain Topogr, 16:39, 2003

21. Cuffin B, Cohen D: Comparison of the magnetoencephalogram and electroencephalogram. Electroencephalogr Clin Neurophysiol, 47:132, 1979

22. Ebersole J, Squires K, Gamelin J: Simultaneous MEG and EEG provide complementary dipole models of temporal lobe spikes. Epilepsia, 34:143, 1993

23. Sutherling W, Crandall P, Engel J et al: The magnetic field of complex partial seizures agrees with intracranial localizations. Ann Neurol, 21:548, 1987

24. Fuchs M, Wagner M, Wischmann HA et al: Improving source reconstructions by combining bioelectric and biomagnetic data. Electroencephalogr Clin Neurophysiol, 107:93, 1998

25. Sutherling W, Arthur D, Mosher J et al: Localization precision of whole cortex neuromagnetometer system for human epilepsy studies. Epilepsia, 42:76, 2001

26. Sutherling W, Akhtari M, Mamelak A et al: Dipole localization of human induced focal afterdischarge seizure in simultaneous magnetoencephalography and electrocorticography. Brain Topogr, 14:101, 2001

27. Mosher J, Leahy R: Source localization using recursively applied and projected (RAP) MUSIC. IEEE Trans Signal Process, 47:332, 1999

28. Mosher JC, Baillet S, Jerbi K et al: MEG multipolar modeling of distributed sources using RAP-MUSIC.

p. 318. In Proceedings of the Thirty-Fourth Asilomar Conference on Signals, Systems and Computers. Vol 1. Asilomar, California, 2000

29. Mosher J, Baillet S, Leahy R: EEG source localization and imaging using multiple signal classification approaches. J Clin Neurophysiol, 16:225, 1999

30. Sutherling W, Barth D: Selective EEG electrode triggering of averaged magnetic data reduces the constraints of the inverse problem of neuromagnetic localization: a principle of relativity in the nervous system due to finite conduction delays. Phys Med Biol, 32:143, 1987

31. Lueders H, Daube J, Johnson J et al: Computer analysis of generalized spike-and-wave complexes. Epilepsia, 21:183, 1980

32. Rogers R, Basile L, Taylor S et al: Laterality of hippocampal responses to infrequent and unpredictable omissions of visual stimuli. Brain Topogr, 9:15, 1996

33. Sutherling WW, Barth DS: Neocortical propagation in temporal spike foci on magnetoencephalography and electroencephalography. Ann Neurol, 25:373, 1989

34. Leahy RM, Mosher JC, Spencer ME et al: A study of dipole localization accuracy for MEG and EEG using a human skull phantom. Electroencephalogr Clin Neurophysiol, 107:159, 1998

35. Romani G, Leoni R: Localization of cerebral sources by neuromagnetic measurements. p. 205. In Weinberg H, Stroink G, Katila T (eds): Biomagnetism: Applications and Theory. Pergamon, New York, 1984

36. Engel J, Levesque M, Crandall P et al: The epilepsies. p. 319. In Grossman R (ed): Principles of Neurosurgery. Raven, New York, 1991

37. Sutherling W, Levesque M, Peacock W et al: Presurgical evaluation: Los Angeles, California, Epilepsy Surgery Program, UCLA. p. 729. In Lueders H (ed): Epilepsy Surgery. Raven, New York, 1992

38. Aicardi J, Shorvon S: Intractable epilepsy. p. 1325. In Engel J, Pedley TA (eds): Epilepsy: A Comprehensive Textbook. Lippincott-Raven, Philadelphia, 1997

39. Spencer S: Depth electroencephalography in section of refractory epilepsy for surgery. Ann Neurol, 9:207, 1981

40. Sutherling W: Identifying and referring patients with epilepsy for surgery. Clin Ther, 7:266, 1985

41. Engel J, Wieser H, Spencer D: Overview: surgical therapy. p. 1673. In Engel J, Pedley TA (eds): Epilepsy: A Comprehensive Textbook. Lippincott-Raven, Philadelphia, 1997

42. Sutherling W, Risinger M, Crandall P et al: Focal functional anatomy of dorsolateral fronto-central seizures. Neurology, 20:87, 1990

43. Wieser H: Selective amygdalohippocampectomy: indications, investigative technique and results. Adv Tech Stand Neurosurg, 13:39, 1986

44. Cahan L, Sutherling W, McCullough M et al: Review of the 20-year UCLA experience with surgery for epilepsy. Cleve Clin Q, 51:313, 1984

45. Sutherling W, Crandall P, Cahan L et al: The magnetic field of epileptic spikes agrees with intracranial localizations in complex partial epilepsy. Neurology, 38:778, 1988

Magnetoencephalography **229**

46. Rose D, Smith P, Sato S: Magneto-encephalography and epilepsy research. Science, 238:329, 1987

47. Nakasato N, Levesque M, Barth D et al: Comparisons of MEG, EEG, and ECoG source localization in neocortical partial epilepsy in humans. Electroencephalogr Clin Neurophysiol, 171:171, 1994

48. Knowlton RC, Laxer KD, Aminoff MJ et al: Magnetoencephalography in partial epilepsy: clinical yield and localization accuracy. Ann Neurol, 42:622, 1997

49. Mamelak AN, Lopez N, Akhtari M et al: Magnetoencephalography-directed surgery in patients with neocortical epilepsy. J Neurosurg, 97:865, 2002

50. Wheless J, Willmore L, Breier J et al: A comparison of magneto-encephalography, MRI, and V-EEG in patients evaluated for epilepsy surgery. Epilepsia, 40:931, 1999

51. Otsubo H, Snead OC III: Magnetoencephalography and magnetic source imaging in children. J Child Neurol, 16:227, 2001

52. Lamusuo S, Forss N, Ruottinen H-M et al: (18F)FDG-PET and whole-scalp MEG localization of epileptogenic cortex. Epilepsia, 40:921, 1999

53. Minassian B, Otsubo H, Weiss S et al: Magnetoencephalographic localization in pediatric epilepsy surgery: comparison with invasive intracranial electroencephalography. Ann Neurol, 46:627, 1999

54. Otsubo H, Sharma R, Elliott I et al: Confirmation of two magnetoencephalographic epileptic foci by invasive monitoring from subdural electrodes in an adolescent with right frontocentral epilepsy. Epilepsia, 40:608, 1999

55. Engel J, Henry T, Risinger M et al: Presurgical evaluation for partial epilepsy: relative contributions of chronic depth-electrode recordings versus FDG-PET and scalp-sphenoidal ictal EEG. Neurology, 40:1670, 1990

56. Henry T, Engel J, Sutherling W et al: Correlation of structural and metabolic imaging with electrographic localization and histopathy in refractory complex partial epilepsy. Epilepsia, 28:601, 1987

57. Risinger M, Engel J, Van Ness P et al: Ictal localization of temporal lobe seizures with scalp/sphenoidal recordings. Neurology, 39:1288, 1989

58. Cooper R, Winter A, Crow H et al: Comparison of subcortical, cortical and scalp activity using chronically indwelling electrodes in man. Electroencephalogr Clin Neurophysiol, 18:217, 1965

59. Baumgartner C, Barth D, Levesque M et al: Detection sensitivity of spontaneous magnetoencephalography spike recordings in frontal lobe epilepsy. Epilepsia, 30:665, 1989

60. Barth D, Sutherling W, Broffman J et al: Magnetic localization of a dipolar current source implanted in a sphere and a human cranium. Electroencephalogr Clin Neurophysiol, 63:260, 1986

61. Lieb J, Engel J, Gevins A et al: Surface and deep EEG correlates of surgical outcome in temporal lobe epilepsy. Epilepsia, 22:515, 1981

62. Blum D: Prevalence of bilateral partial seizure foci and implications for electroencephalographic telemetry monitoring and epilepsy surgery. Electroencephalogr Clin Neurophysiol, 91:329, 1994

63. Buser P, Bancaud J: Unilateral connections between amygdala and hippocampus in man. Electroencephalogr Clin Neurophysiol, 55:1, 1983

64. Barth DS, Sutherling W, Engel J et al: Neuromagnetic evidence of spatially distributed sources underlying epileptiform spikes in the human brain. Science, 223:293, 1984

65. Barth D, Baumgartner C, Sutherling W: Neuromagnetic field modeling of multiple brain regions producing interictal spikes in human epilepsy. Electroencephalogr Clin Neurophysiol, 73:389, 1989

66. Frost J, Kellaway P, Hrachovy R et al: Changes in epileptic spike configuration associated with attainment of seizure control. Ann Neurol, 20:723, 1986

67. Knowlton RL, Elgavish R, Howell J et al: Magnetic source imaging versus intracranial electroencephalogram in epilepsy surgery: a prospective study. Ann Neurol, 59:835, 2006

68. Sutherling WW, Mamelak AN, Thyerlei D et al: Influence of magnetic source imaging for planning intracranial EEG in epilepsy. Neurology, 71:990, 2008

69. American Academy of Neurology Professional Association: Magnetoencephalography (MEG) policy recommended by the AANPA Medical Economics and Management Committee. Approved by the AANPA Board of Directors, St. Paul, Minnesota, on May 8, 2009

70. Wood C, Spencer D, Allison T et al: Localization of human sensorimotor cortex during surgery by cortical surface recordings of somatosensory evoked potentials. J Neurosurg, 68:99, 1988

71. Sutherling WW, Crandall PH, Darcey TM et al: The magnetic and electric fields agree with intra-cranial localizations of somatosensory cortex. Neurology, 38:1705, 1988

72. Sobel D, Gallen C, Schwartz B et al: Locating the central sulcus: comparison of MR anatomic and magnetoencephalographic functional methods. AJNR Am J Neuroradiol, 14:915, 1993

73. Gallen C, Sobel D, Lewine J et al: Neuromagnetic mapping of brain function. Radiology, 187:863, 1993

74. Sutherling WW, Levesque MF, Baumgartner C: Cortical sensory representation of the human hand: size of finger regions and non-overlapping digit somatotopy. Neurology, 42:1020, 1992

75. Breier JI, Simos PG, Zouridakis G et al: Language dominance determined by magnetic source imaging: a comparison with the Wada procedure. Neurology, 53:938, 1999

76. Simos P, Papanicolaou A, Breier J et al: Localization of language-specific cortex by using magnetic source imaging and electrical stimulation mapping. J Neurosurg, 91:787, 1999

77. Merrifield WS, Simos PG, Papanicolaou AC et al: Hemispheric language dominance in magnetoencephalography: sensitivity, specificity and data reduction. Epilepsy Behav, 10:120, 2007

78. Ojemann G, Ojemann J, Lettich E et al: An electrical stimulation mapping investigation in 117 patients. J Neurosurg, 71:316, 1989

Electromyography, Nerve Conduction Studies, and Related Techniques

Clinical Electromyography

MICHAEL J. AMINOFF

The term *electromyography* refers to methods of studying the electrical activity of muscle. Over the years, such methods have come to be recognized as an invaluable aid to the diagnosis of neuromuscular disorders. As is discussed in this chapter, electromyography (EMG) has been used to detect and characterize disease processes affecting the motor units and to provide a guide to prognosis. Electromyographic examination is often particularly helpful when clinical evaluation is difficult or equivocal. The findings commonly permit the underlying lesion to be localized to the neural, muscular, or junctional component of the motor units in question. Indeed, when the neural component is involved, the nature and distribution of EMG abnormalities may permit the lesion to be localized to the level of the cell bodies of the lower motor neurons or to their axons as they traverse a spinal root, nerve plexus, or peripheral nerve. The EMG findings per se are never pathognomonic of specific diseases and cannot provide a definitive diagnosis, although they may be used justifiably to support or refute a diagnosis advanced on clinical or other grounds.

Electromyography is also used in conjunction with nerve conduction studies to obtain information of prognostic significance in the management of patients with peripheral nerve lesions. For example, EMG evidence of denervation implies a less favorable prognosis than otherwise in patients with a compressive or entrapment neuropathy. Again, evidence that some motor units remain under voluntary control after a traumatic peripheral nerve lesion implies a more favorable outlook than otherwise for ultimate recovery, indicating as it does that the nerve remains in functional continuity, at least in part.

The clinical utility of electrodiagnostic testing in patients presenting with a chief complaint of weakness has been examined.[1] The referring diagnosis was compared with the diagnosis immediately after electrophysiologic evaluation, and then with the final diagnosis as recorded 9 months later. This revealed that the testing had resulted in a single correct diagnosis in 73 percent of patients; where it resulted in more than one possible diagnosis, one of them was ultimately confirmed as correct in another 18 percent of patients, to yield an overall diagnostic accuracy of 91 percent. The electrophysiologic diagnosis was unsuspected by the referring physician, regardless of his or her specialty, in approximately one-third of cases.[1]

Over the years, the activity of individual muscles in the maintenance of posture and during normal or abnormal movement has also been studied by EMG. Such studies are of considerable academic interest, and their clinical relevance is considered further in Chapter 20. The interested reader is also referred to a glossary of terms commonly used in electromyography.[2]

PRACTICAL ASPECTS

The electrical activity of muscle is studied for diagnostic purposes by inserting a recording electrode directly into the muscle to be examined. The bioelectric potentials that are picked up by this electrode are amplified, then displayed on a cathode ray oscilloscope for visual analysis and fed through a loudspeaker system so that they can be monitored acoustically. A permanent photographic record of the oscilloscope trace can be made, if desired, or the amplified bioelectric signals can be recorded for retrieval at a later date. Modern, commercially available equipment includes analog-to-digital converters that permit the easy storage of data, advanced signal processing and analysis, and alteration in the display characteristics (e.g., time base and sensitivity) of stored potentials. Signal averaging is possible, and voltage trigger and delay lines facilitate the viewing of potentials.

The concentric needle electrode is a convenient recording electrode for clinical purposes. It consists of a pointed steel cannula within which runs a fine silver, steel, or platinum wire that is insulated except at its tip. The potential difference between the outer cannula and the inner wire is recorded, and the patient is grounded by a separate surface electrode. Alternatively, a monopolar needle electrode can be used. This consists of a solid needle (usually of stainless steel) that is insulated, except at its tip. The potential difference is measured between the tip of the needle, which is inserted into the muscle to be studied, and a reference electrode (e.g., a conductive plate attached to the skin or a needle inserted subcutaneously). The pick-up area of the concentric needle electrode is smaller than that of the monopolar electrode, and it is asymmetric as opposed to the more circular pick-up area of the monopolar electrode. Both concentric and monopolar electrodes are available in disposable or reusable forms. There is no evidence that one type of electrode is more painful to patients than the other.[3]

An electrode exhibits some opposition or impedance to the flow of an electric current, and it is therefore important that it is connected to an amplifier having a relatively high input impedance to prevent loss of the signal. The amplifier, and the recording system to which it is connected, should have a frequency response of 2 or 20 to 10,000 Hz so that signals within this frequency spectrum are amplified uniformly without distortion. When necessary, however, the frequency response of the amplifier can be altered by the use of filters. This allows the attenuation of noise or interference signals that have a frequency different from that of the potentials under study.

Noise, which appears as a random fluctuation of the baseline, is generated within the amplifier and by movement of the recording electrodes or their leads. It can obscure the bioelectric signals to be studied, as can any unwanted interference signals that are picked up by the recording apparatus. Interference signals usually are generated by the alternating-current (AC) power line, by appliances such as radios, or by paging systems; occasionally, however, they are biologic in origin. Technical and safety factors are important when the electrical activity of muscle is to be recorded. They are considered in detail in Chapter 2 and the review by Gitter and Stolov.[4]

Procedure

The patient is examined in a warm, quiet room. The time base of the oscilloscope is allowed to sweep freely from left to right with a speed of 10 msec/cm, or with a slower sweep speed when firing patterns are to be characterized. The gain is set commonly at 50 or 100 μV/cm for examining insertion and spontaneous activity, and at 200 or 500 μV/cm for studying motor unit action potentials. Appropriate filter settings were discussed earlier. Proper grounding is essential, as discussed in Chapter 2. Muscles are selected for examination on the basis of the patient's symptoms and signs, and the diagnostic problem that they raise. A ground lead is attached to the same limb as the muscles that are to be examined. The skin overlying the relaxed muscle to be examined is cleaned with an alcohol swab, allowed to dry, and then held taut while the needle electrode is inserted into the muscle. The presence and extent of any insertion activity are noted. The muscle is then explored systematically with the electrode for the presence of any spontaneous activity. Following this, the parameters of individual motor unit action potentials are defined in different sites during graded muscle contraction, attention being directed not only to the shape and dimensions of the potentials, but also to their initial firing rate and the rate at which they must fire before additional units are recruited. Finally, the interference pattern is compared with the strength of contraction during increasingly powerful contractions, until full voluntary power is being exerted.

Needle EMG is an invasive procedure, and concern has increased about infective complications, involving both patients and electromyographers,[5] especially as regards human immunodeficiency virus (HIV), hepatitis virus, or Creutzfeldt–Jakob disease. It is wise for the physician to wear latex or rubber gloves during the examination and then to discard them in an appropriate receptacle once the procedure is over. Disposable needle electrodes are preferable for patient safety; they must be handled with care and disposed of in proper containers after use. Needles should not be inserted through an infected space.

Other complications are mild or rare. Pain at the site of needle insertion sometimes lasts for 1 or 2 days, and bruising may occur at the site of needle insertion. Pneumothorax is a rare complication of diaphragmatic EMG or of examination of the chest wall, supraspinatus, or cervical or thoracic paraspinal muscles. One patient is reported to have developed an acute compartment syndrome of the leg following needle EMG, probably because of puncture of a small blood vessel by the examining electrode; this necessitated a surgical release procedure.[6] The needle examination carries a small but definite risk of hemorrhagic complications in patients with acquired or inherited coagulopathies and in those patients taking anticoagulants or even antiplatelet agents.[7] When it is required, nevertheless, small electrodes should be used; the advice of a hematologist should be obtained in severe cases. Certain over-the-counter herbal remedies, such as ginkgo biloba and ginseng, may also increase the risk of bleeding.[8] Rare reports of needle electrodes breaking off within a muscle and requiring minor surgery for retrieval have been published.[8]

ELECTRICAL ACTIVITY OF NORMAL MUSCLE

In clinical EMG, electrical activity is recorded extracellularly from muscle fibers embedded in tissue, which is itself a conducting medium. The action potentials that are recorded in this way have a tri- or biphasic configuration. The basis for this is illustrated schematically in Figure 11-1, where the active electrode is shown on the surface of a fiber and the reference electrode is placed at a remote point in the conducting medium. Because there is a flow of current into the fiber (i.e., a current "sink") at the point of excitation, and an outward flow of current in adjacent regions, the propagated impulse can be considered a moving sink of current, preceded and followed by current sources. Accordingly, when an impulse travels toward the active electrode, this electrode becomes relatively more positive as it comes to overlie the current source preceding the action potential (Fig. 11-1, A). A short time later, as the impulse itself arrives, the active electrode registers a negative potential in relation to the distant electrode (Fig. 11-1, B), and then a relatively positive potential as the impulse passes on and is followed by the current source behind it (Fig. 11-1, C). As this too passes on, the electrode comes again to be on a resting portion of the fiber and the potential between the two electrodes returns to the baseline (Fig. 11-1, D). Clearly, the recorded action potential will be biphasic with a negative onset (rather than triphasic with a positive onset) if the active electrode is placed over the region of the fiber where the impulse is initiated.

EMG Activity at Rest

EMG activity usually cannot be recorded outside of the endplate region of healthy muscle at rest, except immediately after insertion or movement of the needle recording electrode. The activity related to electrode movement (i.e., insertion activity) is caused by mechanical stimulation or injury of the muscle fibers and usually stops within about 2 seconds of the movement (Fig. 11-2). After cessation of this activity, spontaneous activity may be found in the endplate region but not elsewhere. This endplate noise, as it is called, consists of monophasic negative potentials that have an irregular, high-frequency discharge pattern; a duration of between 0.5 and 2 msec; and an amplitude that is usually less than 100 μV. The potentials correspond to the miniature endplate potentials that can be recorded with microelectrodes in animals. Biphasic potentials with a negative onset are also a constituent of endplate noise and have a duration of 3 to 5 msec and an amplitude of 100 to 200 μV. They have been held to represent muscle fiber action potentials arising sporadically because of spontaneous activity at the neuromuscular junction or activity in intramuscular nerve fibers.

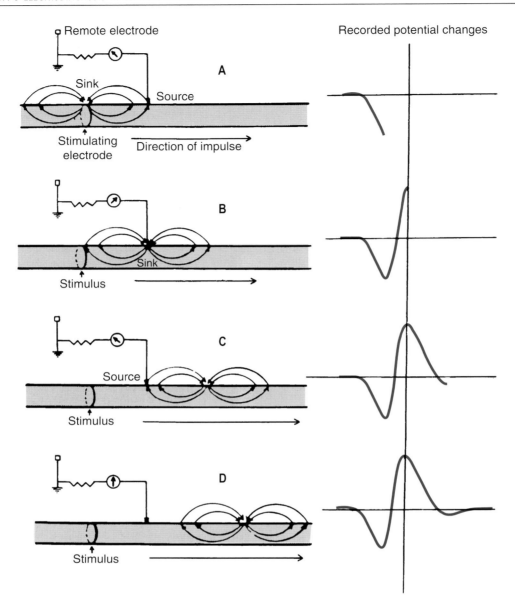

FIGURE 11-1 ■ Schematic diagram of the passage of an action potential along a nerve or muscle fiber in a conducting medium. The active electrode is on the surface of the fiber, and the reference electrode is at a remote point in the conducting medium. (From Brazier MAB: Electrical Activity of the Nervous System. 4th Ed. Pitman Medical, London, 1977, with permission.)

EMG Findings During Activity

MOTOR UNIT ACTION POTENTIALS

Excitation of a single lower motor neuron normally leads to the activation of all of the muscle fibers that it innervates (i.e., those that constitute the motor unit). The motor unit action potential is a compound potential representing the sum of the individual action potentials generated in the few muscle fibers of the unit that are within the pick-up range of the recording electrode. Its *shape* depends on the synchrony of firing of those few muscle fibers.[9] When recorded with a needle electrode, motor unit action potentials are usually bi- or triphasic in shape (Fig. 11-3), but in the limb muscles about 12 percent may have five or more phases and then are described as polyphasic; the actual percentage will vary with the muscle and the age of the patient.[9] The number of phases is calculated by adding 1 to the number of times that the baseline is crossed. The total *duration* of the potentials (i.e., the time taken for the trace to return finally to the baseline after its initial deflection at the beginning of a potential) is normally between 2 and 15 msec,

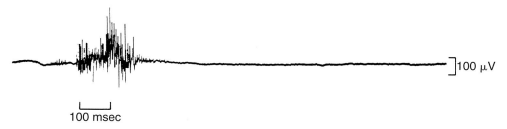

FIGURE 11-2 ▪ Insertion activity evoked in normal muscle. In accordance with convention, an upward deflection in this and subsequent figures indicates relative negativity of the active electrode.

depending on the muscle being examined. The precise value relates to the anatomic scatter of endplates of the muscle fibers in the units under study that are within the pick-up zone of the recording electrode. This is because of the different distances along which the muscle fiber action potentials will have to be conducted from the individual endplates to the recording zone of the electrode. The *amplitude* of the individual motor unit action potentials is measured between the greatest positive and the greatest negative deflections of the potentials. When recorded by a concentric needle electrode, it is usually between 200 μV and 3 mV; this is determined largely by the distance between the recording electrode

and the active fibers that are closest to it, and by the recruitment order. The number of active fibers lying close to the electrode and the temporal dispersion of their individual action potentials also affect the amplitude of the potentials but to a lesser extent. Computer simulations of motor unit action potentials have suggested that amplitude is determined by less than eight fibers situated within 0.5 mm of the electrode.

Other features of individual motor unit action potentials that merit consideration are the rise time, area, and stability. The *rise time* of the negative spike is the interval between the onset and the peak of this component of the motor unit action potential. It reflects the distance between the recording electrode and the muscle fibers that generate the spike, and becomes shorter as this distance is reduced. A rise time of approximately 200 μsec or less is necessary if the other characteristics of the potentials are to be evaluated usefully. The *area* of the negative spike depends on the number and diameter of muscle fibers closest to the recording electrode, and the temporal dispersion of their action potentials. The area of the entire potential provides similar information, but for all of the muscle fibers contributing to the potential. An individual motor unit action potential should show no change in its shape or amplitude in the absence of electrode movement. This *stability* is lost in certain contexts, however, and especially with disorders affecting neuromuscular transmission, when variability of the potentials is seen.

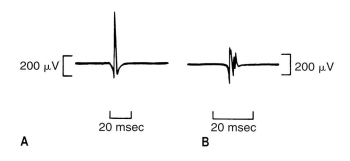

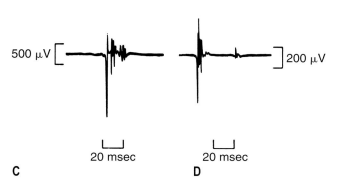

FIGURE 11-3 ▪ Motor unit action potentials. **A**, Normal potential. **B**, Low-amplitude, short-duration, polyphasic potential. **C**, Long-duration, polyphasic potential. **D**, Polyphasic potential with a late component.

Physiologic Factors Influencing Motor Unit Action Potentials

The configuration and dimensions of individual motor unit action potentials are normally constant, provided that the recording electrode is not moved. They are, however, influenced by the characteristics of the recording electrode and apparatus in the electromyograph system; and by physiologic factors such as patient age, intramuscular temperature, the site of the recording electrode within the muscle, and the particular muscle under examination. The potentials recorded with concentric needle electrodes tend to have slightly lower amplitudes and shorter durations than those recorded with monopolar needle electrodes.

With increasing age from infancy to adulthood there is an increase in the mean duration of motor unit action potentials in limb muscles, probably because of growth in width of the territory over which endplates are scattered. Later increases in duration relate to increasing fiber density within motor units as a result of the reduction in muscle volume that occurs in older subjects. Mean duration of motor unit potentials and the number of polyphasic potentials also increase as temperature declines.[10,11] Abnormalities in the parameters of motor unit action potentials occur in neuromuscular diseases, as discussed later.

MOTOR UNIT RECRUITMENT PATTERN

When a muscle is contracted weakly, a few of its motor units begin firing at a low rate. As the force of contraction increases, the firing rate of these active units increases until it reaches a certain frequency, when additional units are recruited. The frequency at which a particular unit must fire before another is recruited (i.e., the recruitment frequency) depends on the muscle and motor unit being studied and on the number of units capable of firing and the tension that they can generate, but it is usually between 5 and 20 times per second. The ratio of the number of active motor units to the firing frequency of individual units is generally less than 5 and is relatively constant for individual muscles. Thus, with a firing frequency of 20, the number of active units will be 4 or more. In general, the units recruited first are smaller in amplitude than those recruited later.

With increasing muscle contraction, so many units are eventually active that the baseline is interrupted continuously by the potentials, and individual potentials cannot be distinguished from each other. The resulting appearance of the oscilloscope trace is referred to as the interference pattern (Fig. 11-4).

Abnormalities of recruitment pattern are discussed on page 243.

EMG ACTIVITY IN PATHOLOGIC STATES

EMG Activity at Rest

INSERTION ACTIVITY

Insertion activity is found only when some muscle tissue remains viable and is therefore absent in the advanced stages of various neuromuscular disorders when muscle

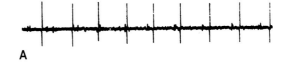

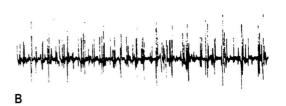

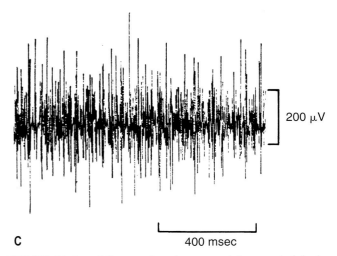

FIGURE 11-4 ■ Motor unit action potentials recorded during (**A**) slight, (**B**) moderate, and (**C**) maximal voluntary contraction of muscle.

has atrophied completely, to be replaced by adipose or connective tissue. It is also reduced or absent when the needle electrode is not situated in muscle, and in certain metabolic disorders (e.g., during the paralysis of hypokalemic periodic paralysis). Insertion activity is prolonged in denervated muscle and may be the first electrophysiologic sign of denervation, occurring within a few days of an acute neurogenic lesion and preceding the development of fibrillation potentials. It is also prolonged in polymyositis, the myotonic disorders, and some of the other myopathies; in these instances, it consists of repetitively firing fibrillation potentials and positive sharp waves. In myotonic disorders, waxing and waning myotonic discharges typically are found (p. 240). Insertion activity consisting of an irregular discharge of variable duration that "snaps, crackles, and pops" and follows normal insertion activity has been described, but it has no particular pathologic significance.

After cessation of all insertion activity, various types of spontaneous activity may be recorded from fully relaxed muscle in patients with a neuromuscular disorder.

FIBRILLATION POTENTIALS AND POSITIVE WAVES

Fibrillation potentials are action potentials that arise spontaneously from single muscle fibers. When they occur rhythmically, their genesis may relate to oscillations of the resting membrane potential of denervated skeletal muscle fibers. Less commonly, they occur irregularly, perhaps relating to random, discrete, spontaneous depolarizations that originate in the transverse tubular system of the muscle fiber. They may occur as spikes or as positive waves. Their density provides a guide to the number of denervated muscle fibers and usually is determined subjectively on a scale of 1+ (a few fibrillations in most areas) to 4+ (profuse fibrillations in all areas, filling the oscilloscope screen)

Spike Form of Fibrillation Potentials

Fibrillation potentials usually have an amplitude of between 20 and 300 μV, a duration of less than 5 msec, and a firing rate of between 2 and 20 Hz (Fig. 11-5). Their amplitude relates to the diameter of type 1 muscle fibers.[12] They have a bi- or triphasic shape, the first phase being positive, except when the potentials are recorded in the endplate region. This positive onset facilitates their distinction from endplate noise. Over the loudspeaker, they give rise to a high-pitched repetitive click, which aids their detection. They are found in denervated muscle, provided that some tissue remains viable and the muscle is warm when examined; however, they may not appear for 3 to 5 weeks after an

acute neuropathic lesion. Once present, they may persist for months or even years, until the muscle fibers have come to be reinnervated or have degenerated. They are not in themselves diagnostic of denervation, however, because they are also seen in primary muscle diseases such as polymyositis, inclusion body myositis, and muscular dystrophy, and in patients with botulism, trichinosis, muscle trauma, or metabolic disorders such as acid maltase deficiency or hyperkalemic periodic paralysis. The presence of fibrillation potentials in myopathic disorders probably relates to isolation of part of the muscle fibers from their endplates, so that they are denervated functionally. Scanty fibrillation potentials occasionally may be found in normal healthy muscle; pathologic significance therefore should not be attributed to them, unless they are detected in at least three separate sites within the muscle being examined.

Positive Waves as Fibrillation Potentials

Positive sharp waves usually are found in association with, and have the same clinical significance as, the spike form of fibrillation potentials. They occur both in denervated muscle and in certain primary disorders of muscle. Indeed, Nandedkar and colleagues have shown the transformation of a fibrillation potential to a positive sharp wave, and vice versa, reinforcing the concept that these potentials are two manifestations of the same phenomenon.[13] They are thought to arise from single muscle fibers that have been injured.[13,14] As viewed on the oscilloscope, they consist of an initial positive deflection, followed by a slow change of potential in a negative direction that may be extended into a small negative phase (see Fig. 11-5). Their amplitude is usually about the same as or slightly greater than that of the spike form

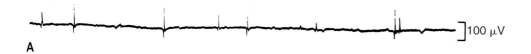

A

]100 μV

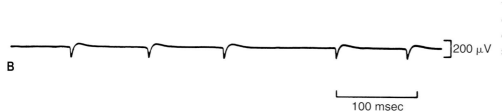

B

]200 μV

100 msec

FIGURE 11-5 ■ Spontaneous activity recorded in relaxed, partially denervated muscle. **A**, Spike form of fibrillation potentials. **B**, Positive sharp waves.

of fibrillation potentials, their duration is often 10 msec or more, and their discharge rate is similar to fibrillation potentials but sometimes can reach values of up to 100 Hz. They may fire regularly or, less commonly, irregularly. Positive sharp waves may occur diffusely in the absence of the spike form of fibrillation,[15] sometimes on a familial basis.

FASCICULATION POTENTIALS

Fasciculation potentials are similar to motor unit action potentials in their dimensions and have been attributed to spontaneous activation of the muscle fibers of individual motor units. They have an irregular firing pattern; an individual potential may occur at a rate that varies from several times per second to less than once per minute. Their detection is aided by the sudden dull "thump" that they produce over the loudspeaker. They may be found in normal persons or in patients with chronic partial denervation, particularly when this is caused by spinal cord pathology, and especially in amyotrophic lateral sclerosis. Benign fasciculations cannot be distinguished from those associated with neuromuscular disorders. Pathologic significance should therefore not be attributed to fasciculations, unless they are accompanied by other evidence of denervation (e.g., fibrillation potentials or changes in motor unit action potentials). Fasciculations also occur in hyperthyroidism, in the cramp-fasciculation syndrome, and with anticholinesterase agents.[9]

In patients with anterior horn involvement, fasciculation potentials can arise at multiple sites along motor axons or the somas of diseased motor neurons; there can be an exclusively distal, exclusively proximal, or a mixed origin, but origin on the distal extremity of the axon seems to be most common. Analysis of the firing pattern of fasciculations in amyotrophic lateral sclerosis using a high-density surface recording technique has shown that potentials of axonal and neuronal origin

can be distinguished and that they may coexist in the same muscle.[16,17]

The basis of fasciculation potentials remains uncertain and may vary in different circumstances. Although widely regarded as representing the activity of muscle fibers in individual motor units, the evidence is conflicting in motor neuron disease and amyotrophic lateral sclerosis.

MYOTONIC DISCHARGES

Myotonic discharges consist of high-frequency trains of action potentials that are evoked by electrode movement or by percussion or contraction of the muscle; they are enhanced by cold and reduced by repeated contractions. The potentials resemble fibrillation potentials or positive sharp waves. Their frequency (20 to 100 Hz) and amplitude (10 μV to 1 mV) wax and wane (Fig. 11-6), and in consequence the trains of potentials produce a sound like that of a dive-bomber on the loudspeaker. They are found in patients with one of the various myotonic disorders, most often in types 1 or 2 myotonic dystrophy (dystrophia myotonica, DM1 or DM2) or in myotonia congenita. They may also be found in hyperkalemic periodic paralysis, and occasionally are found in patients with polymyositis, the myopathy of acid maltase deficiency, chronic axonal polyneuropathies, or neurogenic muscle wasting from other causes, or who have received colchicine or diazocholesterol.

EMG evaluation of 51 patients with chloride, sodium, or calcium channel mutations known to cause myotonia or periodic paralysis has shown differences that generally matched the clinical symptoms. By combining the responses to different exercise tests, five electromyographic patterns were defined that correlated with subgroups of mutations.[18] It is not yet clear whether such techniques can be refined to predict the causal gene reliably in all cases.[19] There are also differences between DM1 and

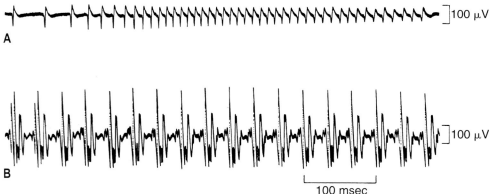

FIGURE 11-6 ■ Spontaneous high-frequency activity. **A**, Myotonic discharge recorded in a patient with myotonia congenita. **B**, Complex repetitive discharges recorded in a partially denervated muscle.

DM2 in the character of the myotonic discharges. In DM1, myotonic discharges wax and wane and their severity correlates with muscle weakness, whereas in DM2 they tend to be waning in character and there is no correlation with weakness.[20] Again, it remains unclear whether such EMG differences can be used to distinguish reliably between these two types of myotonic dystrophy.

Myotonic discharges do not result simply from mechanical irritation because they can be recorded with surface electrodes, and they are not prevented by pharmacologic blockade of neuromuscular transmission. They apparently relate to a disorder of the muscle fiber membrane. Altered chloride channels have been incriminated in myotonia congenita, and altered regulation of sodium channels has been implicated in myotonic dystrophy. Disease of the sodium channels appears to be responsible in hyperkalemic periodic paralysis and paramyotonia congenita.[21]

COMPLEX REPETITIVE DISCHARGES

Trains of high-frequency action potentials are sometimes found in the muscles of patients with muscular dystrophy, inflammatory myopathies, hypothyroid myopathy, or chronic partial denervation. They also occur in patients with metabolic disorders such as hyperkalemic periodic paralysis, hypothyroidism, or certain of the glycogen storage diseases, and are found occasionally in otherwise normal muscles, particularly the iliopsoas. They are often believed to indicate chronicity of the causal disorder, but this probably is not the case.[22] The discharges occur spontaneously and after electrode movement or voluntary contraction. They have a regular firing pattern and an abrupt onset and termination, but unlike myotonic discharges, their amplitude and frequency remain constant (see Fig. 11-6). The individual action potentials are often polyphasic. Their origin is uncertain, but they probably are initiated by a fibrillating muscle fiber which, by ephaptic transmission, depolarizes one or more adjacent hyperexcitable muscle fibers, regardless of whether they are part of the same motor unit. The configuration of the discharges depends on the synchrony of firing of the fibers that contribute to the discharges.[23]

MOTOR UNIT ACTION POTENTIALS

Motor unit activity may occur spontaneously and repetitively, despite full voluntary relaxation of the muscle, in patients with myokymia, muscle cramps, or tetany. Individual action potentials sometimes exhibit a rhythmic, grouped pattern of firing so that double, triple, or multiple discharges are seen (Fig. 11-7). Double discharges also sometimes occur at the beginning of a voluntary contraction in normal subjects and patients with disorders of the anterior horn cells, roots, or peripheral nerves.

Myokymic Discharges

The term *myokymic discharges* is used to refer to spontaneously occurring, grouped action potentials, each group being followed by a period of silence, with subsequent repetition of a grouped discharge of identical action potentials in a semirhythmic manner. The multiplets or grouped motor unit action potentials of tetany may resemble myokymic discharges but are under voluntary control.

Myokymic discharges may occur in the limbs of patients with radiation-induced plexopathy or, less commonly, patients with radiation myelopathy, multiple sclerosis, acute inflammatory polyradiculoneuropathy, chronic radiculopathy or entrapment neuropathy, syringomyelia, or gold intoxication. They also occur in Isaacs syndrome and Morvan syndrome. Myokymic discharges in facial muscles occur in some patients with multiple sclerosis, brainstem neoplasms, or polyradiculoneuropathy, or who have received radiation to the head and neck. The discharges are consistently unilateral when a brainstem neoplasm is responsible, may occur unilaterally or on both sides of the face at different times in multiple sclerosis, and may be bilateral in polyradiculoneuropathy.

The pathophysiologic basis of myokymic discharges is unclear, but suggested mechanisms include abnormal excitability of lower motor neurons or peripheral nerves; ephaptic excitation; and the development of a rhythmic, oscillating, intra-axonal generator of action potentials. It has been suggested that membrane "bistability" of alpha motor neurons is sometimes responsible, the cell membrane having two equilibrium potentials, one at

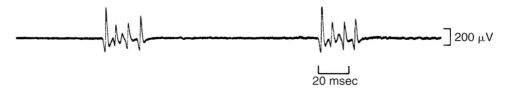

FIGURE 11-7 ▪ Spontaneous repetitive motor unit activity, showing grouped discharges.

the resting potential and a higher one above threshold, generating maintained rhythmic firing.[24]

Cramp Discharges

Cramp discharges consist of the involuntary repetitive firing at high rates (up to 150 Hz) of motor unit action potentials in a large area of muscles, usually associated with painful contraction of the muscle. The discharges typically have an abrupt onset. The number of motor unit action potentials and their discharge frequency increase gradually and then decline as the muscle contraction ceases. Cramps commonly occur in normal people but may also occur with chronic neurogenic disorders, various metabolic disturbances, and in the cramp-fasciculation syndrome.[25]

Neuromyotonic Discharges

Neuromyotonic discharges consist of irregular bursts of high-frequency (up to 300 Hz) discharges of motor unit action potentials as doublets, triplets, or multiplets. The discharges often have an abrupt onset and termination and usually last for a few seconds. Some of the action potentials are very short in duration. The amplitude of the discharges typically wanes. The discharges occur spontaneously or with needle movement, activity, ischemia, or percussion over the nerve, and they do not disappear during sleep. They are abolished by curare. In many instances, the discharges also can be abolished by proximal nerve block, whereas the extent to which more distal nerve block stops the discharges is variable, suggesting that the hyperexcitability sometimes arises in the distal nerve trunk.[26] Neuromyotonic discharges may occur in patients with peripheral neuropathy of the axonal or demyelinative type (e.g., in chronic acquired demyelinating polyneuropathy[27] or multifocal motor neuropathy),[28] and on either a sporadic or a hereditary basis in patients with muscle stiffness and other neuromuscular symptoms (see p. 254) but no evidence of neuropathy (Isaacs syndrome). They have also been described in patients with myasthenia gravis, raised titers of acetylcholine receptor antibodies, or thymoma, with anticholinesterase poisoning, and in those receiving penicillamine.[29] At least in some instances, they appear to relate to the presence of autoantibodies that reduce the number of functional voltage-gated potassium channels and thus lead to hyperexcitability of motor nerves and increased release of acetylcholine; other antigenic targets may also be involved.[26]

A form of these discharges, designated *neurotonic discharges*, occurs with mechanical irritation of nerves at operation. They consist of brief high-frequency discharges of motor unit action potentials. Their recognition is helpful in warning surgeons of possible nerve damage.[9]

EMG Findings During Activity

MOTOR UNIT ACTION POTENTIALS

Any change in the number of functional muscle fibers contained in motor units will affect the parameters of motor unit action potentials. This is exemplified best by the character of the action potentials that are recorded from a muscle when the number of muscle fibers per unit is reduced. The mean duration of the action potentials is shortened because of the loss of some of the distant fibers that previously contributed to their initial and terminal portions, whereas their mean amplitude is reduced because of the loss of some of the fibers lying close to the electrode. If the spikes generated by the surviving muscle fibers of individual units are separated widely in time, there may also be an increased incidence of polyphasic potentials. As might be expected, therefore, the mean duration and amplitude of motor unit action potentials are reduced in patients with *myopathic disorders* (see Fig. 11-3), and there is an increased incidence of polyphasic potentials. This temporal dispersion of spikes may relate to scatter of endplate regions within surviving muscle fibers, variation in diameter of the muscle fibers (so that the conduction velocity in the fibers is more varied), longitudinal fiber splitting, regeneration of muscle fibers, or some combination of these factors.

Similar findings may also be encountered in patients with *disorders of neuromuscular transmission* (e.g., myasthenia gravis or Lambert–Eaton myasthenic syndrome) and during the reinnervation of muscle following severe peripheral nerve injury; however, the characteristic feature in such circumstances is the variability that the action potentials exhibit in their parameters, and especially in their amplitude, during continued activity (Fig. 11-8). A similar variability in amplitude and morphology of motor unit action potentials may be encountered in amyotrophic lateral sclerosis and progressive muscular atrophy, when it signifies active disease and thus a poor prognosis.

In *neuropathic disorders*, it is the number of functional motor units that is reduced, and the average number of muscle fibers per unit actually may be increased if denervated muscle fibers are reinnervated by collateral branches from the nerve fibers of surviving units. The motor unit action potentials recorded in such circumstances are of longer duration than normal and may be polyphasic

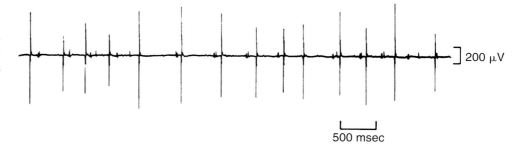

FIGURE 11-8 ▪ Variation in amplitude of a motor unit action potential during continued weak voluntary activity of a reinnervated muscle.

200 µV

500 msec

(see Fig. 11-3). This is because the activity recorded by the electrode is temporally more dispersed than normal, caused primarily by the greater anatomic scatter of endplates in the units but also by the reduced conduction velocity at which immature collateral branches conduct impulses. The action potentials may also have a greater amplitude than normal if the number of muscle fibers lying close to the electrode is increased; such potentials are often particularly conspicuous in patients with involvement of anterior horn cells in the cord.

Polyphasic motor unit action potentials are found in limited numbers in normal muscle, and care must be exercised in attaching any pathologic significance to them, unless they are present in excessive numbers and have abnormal dimensions. Low-amplitude, short-duration polyphasic potentials are seen most characteristically in myopathies and myositis, but are also found during early reinnervation after axonal loss and in disorders of neuromuscular transmission. Similarly, large-amplitude, long-duration polyphasic potentials are typical of disorders characterized by chronic partial denervation with reinnervation (e.g., motor neuron diseases), but may also occur in polymyositis and muscular dystrophies.

Motor unit action potentials sometimes are followed by smaller potentials called *satellite potentials*. These can appear at any point after the termination of the motor unit action potential. Such potentials sometimes occur after an interval of about 15 to 25 msec or more (see Fig. 11-3). These late components may occur in both neurogenic disorders and muscle diseases, such as inflammatory myopathies and muscular dystrophy. They can be explained by the presence of an ectopic endplate or by delayed conduction along unmyelinated collateral nerve sprouts innervating previously denervated muscle

fibers; however, in the latter case a change in the latency of the late component would be expected to occur with sprout myelination. In muscular dystrophy, the denervated fibers probably arise by segmentation of existing muscle fibers or by muscle regeneration.

ABNORMALITIES OF RECRUITMENT PATTERN

When the number of functional motor units is reduced, as in patients with *neurogenic weakness*, there may be a diminution in the density of electrical activity that can be recorded from affected muscles during a maximal voluntary contraction. In severe cases, it may be possible to recognize individual motor unit action potentials (Fig. 11-9). In such circumstances, there is an increase in the rate at which individual units begin to fire and also in the rate at which they must fire before additional units are recruited (i.e., in the recruitment frequency), which, as indicated earlier, is influenced by a number of variables but is usually between 5 and 20 Hz. Firing rates as high as 50 Hz sometimes are encountered.

Reduced recruitment may be the sole EMG abnormality in patients with neurapraxia causing focal conduction block in a peripheral nerve and in patients with an acute axonal lesion if the examination is undertaken early, before fibrillation potentials have had time to develop.

In patients with *myopathic disorders*, the number of functional units remains unchanged until an advanced stage of the disorder, and therefore the interference pattern remains full. Indeed, it may be more complete than normal for a given degree of voluntary activity because there is an increase in the number of units activated to compensate for the reduced tension that individual units (with their reduced fiber content) are able to generate. Motor

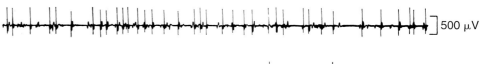

FIGURE 11-9 ▪ Activity recorded during maximal voluntary contraction of a partially denervated muscle.

500 µV

200 msec

unit firing rates tend toward normal unless the myopathy is severe, when the frequency of firing at onset and at recruitment of other units may be increased. In advanced myopathies, however, recruitment is reduced when entire motor units have been lost because of involvement of all of their muscle fibers by the disease process.

When patients are unable to cooperate fully because of limited comprehension or pain, or for psychologic reasons, the interference pattern may be reduced during maximal voluntary effort because only a few units are activated and they fire at low rates (e.g., 10 Hz). The motor unit action potentials, however, are normal in configuration. The distinction of poor activation from the poor recruitment of neurogenic disorders is best made by the rate of firing of individual motor unit action potentials (slow in poor activation and rapid in poor recruitment) and by the ratio of the number of active motor units to the firing frequency of individual units (which is generally less than 5 and is relatively constant for individual muscles).

EMG FINDINGS IN VARIOUS CLINICAL DISORDERS

Myopathic Disorders

The EMG findings in myopathic disorders do not, in themselves, indicate the etiology of the underlying muscle disease. Indeed, the findings do not even establish with certainty that the underlying pathology is a primary disorder of muscle. During the reinnervation of muscle after a severe peripheral nerve lesion, for example, the EMG appearance may be similar to that in a myopathy. Nevertheless, EMG is of undoubted practical usefulness in patients with myopathies.

1. It is helpful in establishing the diagnosis, provided that the clinical context of the examination is borne in mind and the findings are integrated with the results of other laboratory procedures.
2. It is important in providing an indication about the extent and severity of the underlying disease.
3. It permits the course of the disorder and its response to treatment to be followed.
4. It may provide a guide to prognosis.
5. It is helpful in suggesting the best muscle to biopsy. The selected muscle should be homologous to one that, electromyographically, is affected moderately, but should not itself have been examined by a needle electrode because this may lead to histopathologic changes.

The needle examination should involve the sampling of numerous muscles, especially proximal ones (e.g., the iliacus, glutei, spinati, and paraspinal muscles), when a myopathy is suspected. Certain midlimb muscles (e.g., the brachioradialis and tibialis anterior) also have a high yield. It is sensible to examine the muscles on only one side of the body, so that an appropriate muscle on the other side can be used for biopsy if required.

An increased amount of insertion activity may be found in myopathic disorders, and abnormal spontaneous activity is sometimes present, particularly in patients with inflammatory diseases of muscle. Indeed, in the myotonic disorders, the characteristic EMG finding consists of spontaneous high-frequency discharges of action potentials that wax and wane in frequency and amplitude, thereby producing a sound like that of a dive-bomber on the loudspeaker. The features that are most helpful in the EMG recognition of myopathic disorders, however, relate to the character and recruitment pattern of motor unit action potentials. The number of short or small action potentials, or both, characteristically is increased, and many of the potentials are polyphasic. Such action potentials produce a characteristic crackle on the loudspeaker, and this aids in their detection. Because there is a reduction in the tension that individual motor units can generate, an excessive number of units are activated in weak contractions. During strong voluntary contractions a full interference pattern is seen, except at advanced stages, when it may be reduced with loss of all of the muscle fibers in individual units.

In assessing the EMG findings in patients with a suspected myopathic disorder, it must be appreciated that abnormalities may not be detected, despite a meticulous search and quantitative analysis of the data so obtained. It may be, for example, that the pathologic process is patchy in distribution, that only certain types of muscle fibers are affected, or that the electrical properties of the muscle fibers are unaffected by the disease. By contrast, abnormalities sometimes are found when histopathologic studies are normal, so that these two diagnostic approaches are best regarded as complementary procedures.

The findings in various myopathic disorders are discussed in the following sections, with attention directed to the manner in which they may differ from the changes just described. Further details are given elsewhere.[30,31]

MUSCULAR DYSTROPHIES AND OTHER FAMILIAL MYOPATHIES

Electromyography has an important role in determining the distribution and severity of involvement in the muscular dystrophies, and in separating these disorders from others for which they may be mistaken. The usual EMG findings are as described earlier, although abnormalities are sometimes inconspicuous, particularly in the relatively benign forms of muscular dystrophy such as the limb-girdle or facioscapulohumeral varieties. Insertion activity is reduced in areas where muscle has been replaced by fatty tissue, and there are changes in the configuration, dimensions, and recruitment of motor units. Insertion activity sometimes is increased, however, and fibrillation potentials, positive sharp waves, and complex repetitive discharges may be found because of segmental necrosis of muscle fibers or the presence of regenerating fibers. The findings are generally more abnormal in Duchenne than in Becker dystrophy, and may be especially mild in limb-girdle, facioscapulohumeral, scapuloperoneal, ocular or oculopharyngeal, and distal dystrophies. A review of the clinical and genetic aspects of distal myopathies can be found elsewhere.[32] In Emery–Dreifuss dystrophy, the findings sometimes suggest both myopathic and neurogenic processes. Single-fiber EMG (see Chapters 12 and 17) may also be abnormal, revealing increased fiber density and even increased jitter and blocking, especially in Duchenne dystrophy but occasionally also in other varieties such as limb-girdle and facioscapulohumeral dystrophy.[33]

Attempts to identify female carriers of the gene of the sex-linked variety of muscular dystrophy by studying the parameters of motor unit action potentials, the refractory period of muscle fibers, or the pattern of electrical activity of muscle have met with only limited success. Advances in molecular biology now make these electrophysiologic approaches of little practical significance.

In congenital muscular dystrophies, a heterogeneous group of autosomal-recessive neuromuscular disorders, EMG changes of a myopathy are typical and early findings in proximal muscles; an EMG performed at birth may, however, be normal.[34] An associated neuropathy may be evident in patients with a merosin-deficient disorder and sometimes even when merosin expression is normal.

INFLAMMATORY DISORDERS OF MUSCLE

Inflammatory myopathies are characterized clinically by weakness, tenderness, and—in severe cases—wasting of affected muscles. Proximal muscles tend to be affected more severely than distal muscles. Electromyography is helpful in establishing that weakness is myogenic and in distinguishing an underlying inflammatory process from other disorders (e.g., one of the muscular dystrophies) that have no specific treatment. In addition to changes in the configuration and dimensions of motor unit action potentials, abnormal spontaneous activity (fibrillation and positive sharp waves) is often profuse. The EMG abnormalities are patchy in distribution,

however, so that the findings may vary in different muscles or in different parts of the same muscle. Abnormalities are generally more common in proximal than distal muscles, and are especially common in the paraspinal muscles. However, in one large study of 98 patients with myositis, a distal-to-proximal gradient of abnormalities was found in the legs, which might lead to confusion with neurogenic diseases.[35] The EMG findings also vary with the stage of the disease and the activity of the inflammatory process. Determination of muscle-fiber conduction velocity may improve specificity of the electrodiagnostic evaluation, but it is not useful in discriminating inflammatory myopathies from other myopathic disorders, and is not a standard technique at this time.[36]

In *polymyositis*, the character and recruitment pattern of motor unit action potentials are similar to those seen in other myopathic disorders; however, late components are sometimes found, and some polyphasic potentials may be of long duration and large amplitude.[37] Insertion activity is commonly excessive, and spontaneous fibrillation potentials, positive sharp waves, and complex repetitive discharges are found more often and are usually much more conspicuous than in patients with muscular dystrophy. These findings of abnormal spontaneous activity are patchy in distribution but have a high prevalence in the paraspinal muscles and are usually prominent when the disease is in an active phase. The evolution of EMG abnormalities with time is uncertain because virtually all patients receive treatment for the underlying disorder. As the disease progresses from acute to chronic stages, however, there is an increase in the proportion of longer-duration, large-amplitude motor unit action potentials.[38] The long-duration polyphasic potentials in more chronic but less active disease are related to the presence of regenerating muscle fibers on muscle biopsy. Treatment is usually with steroids, but methotrexate, azathioprine, or other immunosuppressive agents have also been used. The presence or absence of abnormal spontaneous activity in the EMG reflects the response to treatment; persisting fibrillation potentials imply a less favorable therapeutic response than otherwise. In patients with increasing weakness that develops during the course of steroid therapy, the EMG findings may help to distinguish between a steroid-induced myopathy and reactivation of the myositis. In the former circumstance, fibrillation potentials are likely to be absent in weak muscles, whereas in the latter context they are likely to be present profusely.

Polymyositis may develop at either an early or a late stage of *HIV infection*. It resembles polymyositis occurring in HIV-negative patients, with slowly progressive, proximal weakness and an elevated serum creatine kinase level.

Its optimal treatment is unclear. Some patients respond well to steroids and can discontinue therapy after 6 to 12 months, but others respond more moderately and are left with persisting weakness. Other immunosuppressive therapies have been used with limited success.[39] Some HIV-infected patients may present with the clinical and electrophysiologic features of a myopathy and are found at muscle biopsy to have selective loss of thick filaments and rod-body formation, with only minor inflammatory changes; benefit may nevertheless follow immunosuppressive or immunomodulating therapies. Certain antiretrovirals may lead to toxic myopathy that has been attributed to impaired mitochondrial function. Treatment of HIV-associated disease with zidovudine may lead to a myopathic disorder that has the EMG features of an inflammatory process, but biopsy reveals ragged-red fibers rather than inflammatory exudates. Stavudine (d4T) may cause HIV-associated neuromuscular weakness syndrome (HANWS), which is characterized by rapidly progressive weakness associated with lactic acidosis, nausea, vomiting, weight loss, abdominal distension, hepatomegaly, and lipoatrophy.[39] Electrodiagnostic and pathologic studies have revealed diverse causes of the weakness: axonal polyneuropathy was the most common, but demyelinating and mixed neuropathies and myopathy also occurred.[40]

Inclusion body myositis, the most common chronic myopathy presenting after the age of 50 years, is an inflammatory disorder that it is without effective treatment[41,42] and is slowly progressive. The quadriceps femoris and forearm muscles (long flexors of the fingers) characteristically are affected early and most severely, but there is some variation in this regard.[43] Diagnosis is made by muscle biopsy. The EMG findings do not distinguish it reliably from the inflammatory myopathies discussed earlier, or from other inflammatory disorders such as trichinosis and toxoplasmosis.[30] In some instances, motor unit action potentials are of increased amplitude, but the concomitant reduction in area or duration is compatible with myopathic remodeling of the motor unit.[44] In patients with *polymyalgia rheumatica*, the EMG findings are usually normal.

ENDOCRINE AND METABOLIC MYOPATHIES

In patients with an endocrine myopathy, the electrophysiologic findings are similar to those of other myopathies, and abnormal spontaneous activity usually is not seen. Abnormalities are often inconspicuous in patients with a steroid-induced myopathy, however, presumably because it is the type 2 muscle fibers that are affected predominantly in this condition.

In thyrotoxicosis, fasciculation potentials may be conspicuous. In hypothyroidism, insertion activity sometimes is increased, and spontaneous fibrillation and fasciculation potentials, together with trains of complex repetitive discharges, may also be found in rare instances. In interpreting findings in patients with endocrine disturbances, it must be remembered that a myopathy may coexist with other types of neuromuscular disorders, and that these may complicate the EMG findings. For example, patients with hypothyroidism are liable to develop peripheral nerve entrapment syndromes, whereas myasthenia gravis sometimes occurs in association with thyrotoxicosis.

The EMG features of a myopathy may also be found in patients with osteomalacia, chronic renal failure, and a number of other less common metabolic disorders. In patients with hypokalemic *periodic paralysis*, the EMG findings between attacks may be normal or, less commonly, suggestive of a proximal myopathy. During the attacks, no abnormality of insertion or spontaneous activity is found, but motor unit action potentials are reduced in duration and number; the interference pattern during attempted voluntary contraction is diminished, and in severe cases there may be complete electrical silence. During attacks of hyperkalemic or normokalemic periodic paralysis, insertion activity is increased; spontaneous fibrillation potentials, myotonic discharges, and complex repetitive potentials may be found; and motor unit action potentials are reduced in duration and number.[30]

In the *glycogen storage diseases* caused by deficiencies of either phosphorylase (McArdle disease) or phosphofructokinase, the EMG of the resting muscle is usually normal but occasionally is suggestive of a myopathy. No electrical activity can be recorded during the contractures that may develop during continued exercise. In patients with acid maltase deficiency (Pompe disease), EMG may reveal increased insertion activity; profuse, spontaneous fibrillation and positive sharp waves; myotonic discharges; and complex repetitive discharges. However, the motor unit action potentials are similar in character to those seen in other myopathies. With deficiency of debrancher enzyme (Cori disease), the electrophysiologic findings may reveal "a mixed pattern," with abnormal spontaneous activity and short, polyphasic motor unit action potentials of normal or reduced amplitude in some patients, and large or long-duration polyphasic potentials in others.

Myopathy is a rare manifestation of primary systemic amyloidosis and usually is diagnosed then by muscle biopsy. Needle EMG reveals findings similar to those of a chronic inflammatory myopathy. Fibrillation potentials are common, most often in the gluteus medius and paraspinal muscles.[45] Motor unit action potentials may be of short duration and low amplitude, especially in proximal muscles; however, long-duration large potentials sometimes are found, and occasionally a mixed population of motor units is encountered. There may also be electrophysiologic evidence of an underlying peripheral neuropathy, which probably accounts for the presence of large-amplitude, long-duration motor unit action potentials.

MYOPATHIES CAUSED BY DRUGS OR ALCOHOL

Changes suggestive of a myopathy may occur in patients taking certain drugs.[46,47] In many instances, however, the clinical or EMG features are more extensive than are those of a simple myopathy. Thus, the presence of abnormal spontaneous activity and the character of the motor unit action potentials suggest that a myositis sometimes is associated with use of cimetidine or D-penicillamine, and the EMG features of a myopathy with increased muscle fiber irritability may also occur with epsilon-aminocaproic acid, emetine, hypokalemic agents, and certain beta-blockers. Colchicine may induce a myopathy, sometimes accompanied by a neuropathy,[48,49] as may chloroquine. Disorders of neuromuscular transmission may occur with certain antibiotics, D-penicillamine, and chloroquine. Among the hypocholesterolemic agents, myopathic changes may occur with clofibrate, the statin group of drugs, gemfibrozil, and niacin. In addition, acute rhabdomyolysis has been associated with the statin drugs and with gemfibrozil, and myotonic discharges are associated with diazocholesterol. Chronic use of steroids sometimes leads to a myopathy, but the EMG findings may be normal.

Among chronic alcoholics with either the acute reversible muscle necrosis that sometimes follows intoxication or the acute hypokalemic myopathy that develops during an alcoholic binge, EMG typically reveals spontaneous fibrillation, positive sharp waves, and motor unit action potentials that are small and of short duration. EMG features of myopathy may also be found in alcoholics developing a more slowly progressive proximal muscle weakness, and sometimes are found in alcoholics without any clinical evidence of myopathy.[30]

CRITICAL ILLNESS MYOPATHY

The occurrence of acute weakness and muscle wasting in the context of fever, sepsis, and treatment with high-dose steroids, nondepolarizing neuromuscular blockers, or both, is now well recognized, and it seems especially common in patients treated for status asthmaticus. Weakness tends to be diffuse in the limbs and may also affect the neck flexors, facial muscles, and diaphragm. The clinical features overlap those of critical illness polyneuropathy or prolonged impairment of neuromuscular transmission, emphasizing the importance of electrodiagnostic evaluation.[50,51] The EMG findings include small, short-duration, polyphasic, motor unit action potentials and early recruitment of motor units; spontaneous fibrillation is sometimes conspicuous and cannot be used to distinguish critical illness neuropathy from myopathy.[52,53] In addition, compound muscle action potentials may be grossly attenuated, sensory nerve action potentials sometimes are reduced, and there may be a decremental response to repetitive nerve stimulation suggestive of a postsynaptic defect of neuromuscular transmission (see Chapter 17). The skeletal muscle may be inexcitable by direct electrical stimulation.[54,55]

CONGENITAL MYOPATHIES OF UNCERTAIN ETIOLOGY

A number of congenital myopathies have been described; these may be associated with specific structural changes that enable distinct entities to be recognized. Appropriate EMG changes may be found in some cases, but in others the findings are normal. In nemaline and centronuclear (myotubular) myopathy, however, abnormal spontaneous activity may be conspicuous. Nemaline myopathy may be manifest by the dropped-head syndrome, other causes of which include polymyositis, isolated neck extensor myopathy, amyotrophic lateral sclerosis, and myasthenia gravis.[56]

MYOTONIC DISORDERS

The differential diagnosis of myotonic disorders is considered elsewhere.[57] The characteristic EMG feature in myotonic dystrophy type 1 (dystrophia myotonica, DM1) or type 2 (DM2, proximal myotonic myopathy, PROMM), the dominant and recessive forms of myotonia congenita, paramyotonia congenita, and Schwartz–Jampel syndrome[58] is the occurrence of myotonic discharges that are evoked by electrode movement and by percussion or voluntary contraction of the muscle being examined. Motor unit potentials are normal in appearance, except in DM1 or DM2 and in the recessive type of myotonia congenita, in which an excess of small, short-duration or polyphasic potentials may be found, as in other myopathic disorders. Myotonic dystrophy is a dominantly inherited disorder, and EMG may reveal abnormalities in the clinically unaffected relatives of patients with the disease. Similarly, brief myotonic discharges may be found in at least one unaffected parent in approximately 67 percent of the families of patients with recessive myotonia congenita.[59]

RIPPLING MUSCLE DISEASE

An autosomal-dominant myopathy characterized by muscle stiffness, hypertrophy, and rippling was described by Torbergsen in 1975.[60] The self-propagating, wave-like rippling of the muscles often can be induced by passive muscle stretch and is electrically silent, thus being a form of muscle contracture. Myalgia is sometimes conspicuous, and mild proximal weakness may be present.[61] Percussion of the muscle may induce a prolonged contraction resembling percussion myotonia and a localized mounding lasting for several seconds. The phenotype may vary within the same family.[62,63] A rare autosomal-recessive form has been described and is associated with severe cardiac disease.[64] Sporadic cases of muscle rippling have also been reported and sometimes resemble familial cases.[61] In other instances, muscle rippling may have a neurogenic basis and has been associated with myasthenia gravis.[65]

Neuropathic Disorders

Immediately after the development of an acute neuropathic lesion, EMG reveals no abnormality other than a reduction in the number of motor unit action potentials under voluntary control in affected muscles. A complete interference pattern is not seen during maximal effort, despite an increase in the firing rate of individual units; in severe cases, there may be no surviving units, so that no electrical activity is recorded during attempted voluntary contraction. The subsequent changes depend on whether denervation has occurred. If it has, the amount of insertion activity increases after several days and abnormal spontaneous activity may be found subsequently, although its appearance may be delayed for up to 5 weeks, depending on the site of the lesion. In particular, fibrillation potentials usually are detected sooner when the lesion is close to the muscle than when a more distant lesion is present. As reinnervation occurs, spontaneous activity becomes less conspicuous and low-amplitude motor unit action potentials are seen. These potentials may exhibit a marked variability in their size and configuration, and some have a complex polyphasic configuration. Initially, the duration of these potentials is quite short, but it increases progressively as more muscle fibers come to be reinnervated; eventually, long-duration polyphasic potentials are found. With time, many potentials regain a normal appearance and the interference pattern becomes more complete, but the extent of any residual EMG abnormality depends on the completeness of recovery.

In patients with chronic partial denervation, insertion activity is increased and spontaneous fibrillation, positive sharp waves, and complex repetitive discharges are found. Fasciculation potentials are often conspicuous in patients with diseases such as motor neuron disease or poliomyelitis, in which the lower motor neurons in the spinal cord are affected, but they may also be found with more peripheral lesions. The mean duration of motor unit action potentials is increased if reinnervation has occurred by collateral sprouting; and there may be an increased incidence of large units, especially in patients with involvement of anterior horn cells. In addition, an excessive number of polyphasic motor unit potentials usually is encountered. There is an increase in the rate at which individual units begin firing and at which they must fire before additional units are recruited, and the interference pattern during maximal contractions is reduced.

The EMG findings may have important medicolegal implications by suggesting the duration of a neuropathic disorder. For example, if a patient claims to have developed a footdrop immediately after a medical or surgical intervention, and needle EMG at that time reveals abnormal spontaneous activity in the weak muscles, the lesion is likely to be at least 1 to 3 weeks old and therefore may have been present before the alleged time of injury. Similarly, the presence of long-duration, large-amplitude polyphasic potentials points to a long-standing lesion because there has been time for reinnervation to occur.

SPINAL CORD PATHOLOGY

Electromyography may help to define the level and severity of lower motor neuron involvement in patients with a cord lesion. Signs of chronic partial denervation are found in the affected muscles of patients with chronic myelopathies if the anterior horn cells are involved. Insertion activity is increased, and spontaneous fasciculations, fibrillation, positive sharp waves, and complex repetitive discharges may be found. The mean duration and amplitude of motor unit action potentials (and the number of polyphasic potentials) are increased, giant potentials may be encountered, and the firing rate and recruitment frequency of individual potentials are increased, whereas the interference pattern is reduced. Upper motor neuron involvement is indicated by poor activation of motor units; the number of units firing and their rate of firing are reduced during maximal volitional activity.

By making it possible to define the precise segmental distribution of a lesion involving lower motor neurons, the EMG examination can aid in the localization of spinal cord lesions. EMG therefore has an important role in distinguishing motor neuron diseases from discrete, surgically remediable conditions affecting the spinal cord. The examination should be continued until it is clear whether the pattern of involved muscles can be accounted for by a restricted cord lesion; proximal and distal muscles supplied by different roots and peripheral nerves are examined, as are muscles in clinically uninvolved limbs. Fibrillation potentials are usually most conspicuous in weak, wasted muscles.

The term *poliomyelitis* is used with regard to an acute flaccid paralysis associated with viral infection. It is not necessarily synonymous with poliovirus infection but may, for example, also embrace infection with West Nile virus as well as enteroviruses, echoviruses, and coxsackieviruses.[66] Recent studies on patients with poliomyelitis have focused particularly on those with West Nile virus infection. There is asymmetric acute denervation of muscles and small or absent compound muscle action potentials of affected muscles. In other instances, patients complain of localized or generalized weakness and of a sense of muscle fatigue, but EMG and other electrodiagnostic studies reveal no abnormality.[66,67]

The diagnosis of *amyotrophic lateral sclerosis* requires clinical evidence of both lower and upper motor neuron involvement, with progressive spread of symptoms or signs within a region or to other regions over time, in the absence of evidence of other disease processes that might explain the findings. When three distinct regions of the body (bulbar, cervical, thoracic, lumbosacral) are affected, the diagnosis is regarded as clinically definite. Less strict criteria have also been proposed. It has also been recommended that electrophysiologic evidence for chronic neurogenic change should be taken as equivalent to clinical information in the recognition of involvement of individual muscles in a limb, and that fasciculation potentials should be regarded as equivalent to fibrillation potentials and positive sharp waves in recognizing denervation.[68]

In amyotrophic lateral sclerosis, then, EMG has an important role in confirming lower motor neuron involvement in clinically affected areas, detecting such involvement in clinically unaffected areas, providing evidence for a slowly progressive disorder, and indicating that abnormalities are too widespread to be explained by a single focal lesion. The EMG abnormalities are typically widespread. Electrophysiologic support of the diagnosis requires evidence of acute and chronic partial denervation in at least two muscles supplied by different roots or spinal nerves and by different cranial or peripheral nerves in at least two distinct anatomic regions (bulbar, cervical, thoracic, lumbosacral). Abnormalities of the facial, tongue, trapezius, or sternocleidomastoid muscles provide evidence of bulbar involvement.[69,70]

Sampling the paraspinal muscles may provide evidence of involvement of the thoracic region and is often rewarding.[71,72] Patients with involvement of the small muscles of the hand sometimes show preferential or greater involvement of the abductor pollicis brevis than the abductor digiti minimi muscle.[73] Fasciculations are often conspicuous. Motor units are recruited abnormally, firing frequency may be increased (except when upper motor neuron involvement predominates), and repetitive or double discharges may occur. Occasionally, when motor units having a high threshold for activation are lost early, apparently normal recruitment may be seen with two or three motor units firing at rates less than 10 Hz, but additional units will not be recruited with increasing effort.[74] An excess of large-amplitude, long-duration polyphasic potentials is characteristic and indicates reinnervation of denervated fibers. In late or rapidly progressive stages, however, low-amplitude, short-duration potentials may be present if reinnervation fails to keep pace with denervation. In advanced cases, a single motor unit may be found in severely affected muscle firing at rates as high as 50 Hz, or there may be no remaining motor units under voluntary control. Marked variation in the configuration of motor unit action potentials from moment to moment sometimes is seen because of impulse blocking or failure of neuromuscular transmission, and single-fiber EMG correspondingly may reveal increased jitter and impulse blocking.[33] Such findings, or EMG evidence of denervation in the diaphragm, indicate a poor prognosis. Serial estimates of motor unit number (Chapter 12) may also have prognostic value.

The findings on needle EMG may help to diagnose amyotrophic lateral sclerosis, but they do not permit distinction of this disorder from other motor neuron diseases (e.g., that occurring with lymphoma,[75] hexosaminidase deficiency, antiganglioside antibodies, or paraproteinemia, and the progressive muscular atrophies) or from disorders simulating an anterior horn cell disease (e.g., multifocal motor neuropathy or organophosphate neurotoxicity).

The *progressive muscular atrophies* are a group of disorders in which disease is confined to the lower motor neurons. They may be hereditary or acquired, and EMG is important in localizing the pathology to the anterior horn cells and in guiding prognosis. The EMG findings are similar to those just described, with evidence of chronic partial denervation and reinnervation, but fasciculations are less common than in amyotrophic lateral sclerosis. In fact, there is overlap of these two disorders because in many adults with progressive muscular atrophy, upper motor neuron involvement becomes apparent later or at autopsy, indicating that the correct diagnosis was amyotrophic lateral sclerosis.[76] In *monomelic amyotrophy* (Sobue disease; Hirayama syndrome), clinical involvement usually is restricted to one of the upper limbs; the EMG findings are restricted correspondingly in distribution, but abnormalities are commonly also present on the clinically unaffected side, suggesting that bilateral involvement is not unusual.

Bulbospinal neuronopathy is an X-linked, recessively inherited, spinal muscular atrophy caused by a CAG repeat expansion in the androgen receptor gene.[77] A characteristic twitching of the chin may occur spontaneously or with voluntary activity such as pursing of the lips. The EMG findings in affected muscles are as described earlier, but the twitching of the chin is associated with grouped discharges of motor units resembling myokymic discharges or with 20- to 40-Hz repetitive discharges of individual motor units that may last for several seconds.[78] In addition, sensory nerve action potentials are often small or absent.

In *syringomyelia*, the electrodiagnostic findings are usually nonspecific, but various types of spontaneous EMG activity may be encountered, including continuous motor unit activity, with the firing frequency of individual potentials ranging from 8 to 13 Hz, respiratory synkinesis (bursts of motor unit action potentials in one or more limb muscles during inspiration), and myokymic discharges in limb or paraspinal muscles.[79] Respiratory synkinesis and myokymia seem to be present only at an advanced stage of the disorder.

Spinal cord disorders usually can be distinguished from peripheral nerve or plexus lesions by the pattern of muscle involvement, but measurement of motor and sensory conduction velocity also may be helpful in this respect. Maximal motor conduction velocity is normal or only slightly slowed with pathology restricted to the cord, although compound muscle action potentials (M waves) may be small, especially when elicited from weak, wasted muscles; sensory conduction studies are normal. Repetitive motor nerve stimulation may yield a small decrement in size of the M wave in amyotrophic lateral sclerosis because of unstable neuromuscular transmission along collateral nerve terminal sprouts; this is held to indicate active disease and a poorer prognosis. It is sometimes hard to distinguish a discrete spinal cord lesion from a root lesion because in both instances EMG abnormalities may have a segmental distribution and changes may be found in the paraspinal muscles. In the former, however, several segments may be involved and bilateral changes usually can be expected. Electromyography in itself does not provide any direct information regarding the pathology of the underlying abnormality.

ROOT LESIONS

Despite the advent of sophisticated imaging techniques, EMG has an important role in the evaluation of patients with suspected root lesions. It detects both compressive and noncompressive radiculopathies, indicates the clinical relevance of structural abnormalities that are a common and often incidental finding,[80] provides a prognostic guide, and can be used to follow the course of the disorder. It therefore complements, rather than substitutes for, imaging studies and has a comparable diagnostic yield. For example, in a study of 47 patients who underwent both EMG and magnetic resonance imaging of the spine within 2 months of each other,[81] Nardin and associates found that 55 percent had an EMG abnormality and 57 percent had an imaging abnormality that correlated with the clinical level of the lesion. The two studies agreed in 60 percent of instances, with both normal in 11 patients and both abnormal in 17; only one study was abnormal in 40 percent of patients, however, indicating the complementary nature of the studies.

In patients with axonal degeneration, EMG signs of partial denervation may be found in muscles supplied by the affected segment. The most helpful sign is the presence of fibrillation potentials. These tend to appear earlier in more proximal muscles, appearing initially in the paraspinal muscles, then in the proximal, and subsequently in the distal limb muscles. They disappear in the same sequence as reinnervation occurs. This generally accepted concept has been questioned by some authors, however, who found no relationship between the presence of abnormal spontaneous activity in the paraspinal muscles and duration of symptoms in patients with cervical radiculopathy.[82] Complex repetitive discharges in a myotomal distribution also may be found in chronic radiculopathies but are rarely the sole abnormality. Similarly, fasciculations are encountered occasionally; when found as the sole abnormality, however, their distribution is widespread and they usually reflect generalized benign fasciculations or motor neuron disease. Motor unit action potentials may be decreased in number and fire at an increased rate, and the incidence of large, long, polyphasic potentials may be increased if the lesion is long-standing. Reliance for diagnosing a radiculopathy must not be placed solely on increased polyphasicity, even when in a myotomal distribution.

The paraspinal muscles should always be examined, and the number of limb muscles examined must be sufficient to distinguish a root lesion from more peripheral (i.e., plexus or peripheral nerve) involvement by the distribution of electrical abnormalities. Radiculopathy may be diagnosed on EMG grounds when abnormalities are present in at least two muscles supplied by the same nerve root but by different peripheral nerves, and abnormalities are not present in muscles supplied by normal roots adjacent to the involved one. It is not necessary for all of the muscles in the myotome to be affected in order to diagnose a radiculopathy. Muscles may be spared electrophysiologically in patients with suspected root involvement because the lesion is only partial, because the muscles are examined at the wrong time (so that changes of denervation have not yet developed or have disappeared with reinnervation), or because the initial diagnosis was incorrect. They also may be spared because of inaccuracies in myotomal charts depicting the segmental innervation of individual muscles. Tsao and colleagues examined the segmental innervation of muscles supplied by the L2–S1 segments by comparing the surgical, imaging, and electrodiagnostic findings in patients with unilevel radiculopathies.[83] They found that the tibialis anterior was innervated predominantly by the L5 segment, both heads of the gastrocnemius by S1, and the two heads of biceps femoris exclusively by S1. Their findings conflict with some earlier studies, as summarized in their report. In a similar study, the pattern of muscle involvement in cervical radiculopathies was examined.[84] With single-level root lesions of C5, C7, and C8, changes were relatively stereotyped. The spinati, deltoid, biceps, and brachioradialis were involved with C5; pronator teres, flexor carpi radialis, triceps, and anconeus with C7; and first dorsal interosseous, abductor digiti minimi, abductor pollicis brevis, flexor pollicis longus, and extensor indicis proprius with C8. The findings with C6 lesions were variable and resembled those in patients with lesions at either the C5 or the C7 level.

Several muscles supplied by the root in question should be examined, and muscles supplied by adjacent roots and by more peripheral structures must also be evaluated. The importance of this is shown most clearly by means of a simple example. Neurogenic weakness of the elbow, wrist, and finger extensors may result from a lesion in any one of several sites, and the examination of a patient with such a deficit must be meticulous for correct localization of the lesion. EMG evidence that flexor carpi radialis (C6, C7) is involved but brachioradialis (C5, C6) is spared would favor a lesion of the C7 root or the middle trunk of the brachial plexus; conversely, involvement of brachioradialis but sparing of flexor carpi radialis would suggest a radial nerve lesion, unless the deltoid (C5, C6) muscle is also affected, in which case the posterior cord of the brachial plexus may well be involved.

It is helpful to examine the *paraspinal muscles*. These are supplied from the spinal roots by their posterior primary rami, whereas the limb plexuses and peripheral nerves are derived from the anterior primary rami. Abnormalities in the paraspinal muscles are therefore common in patients with a radiculopathy, and fibrillation potentials generally are found in them before the limb muscles; they would not be expected in patients with a plexus or peripheral nerve lesion. However, fibrillation potentials will disappear first from these muscles after an acute radiculopathy, as reinnervation occurs. Furthermore, no conclusion should be reached about the level of the lesion from the findings in these muscles because there is a marked overlap in the territory supplied by the posterior primary rami. Finally, paraspinal fibrillation potentials are not specific for compressive radiculopathy. They occur also, for example, with inflammatory or diabetic radiculopathies, myelopathies, arachnoiditis, amyotrophic lateral sclerosis, myopathies, myositis, and malignant disease, and after back surgery, and they become increasingly common in asymptomatic subjects with advancing age.[85]

Diabetic thoracoabdominal radiculopathy presents with gradual onset of severe burning pain that sometimes shows some relation to posture or activity and may be confined to the front of the trunk or involve the back as well. It often involves multiple, usually adjacent, dermatomes. In almost all cases, fibrillation potentials are found in the paraspinal muscles, as well as in the abdominal or intercostal muscles if these are examined. Evidence of a concomitant polyneuropathy may also be found. In most instances, *diabetic amyotrophy* probably is caused by a polyradiculopathy or radiculoplexopathy; painful, progressive, asymmetric wasting and weakness of the thigh muscles are characteristic and may be associated with other neuromuscular complications of diabetes such as a distal polyneuropathy. The EMG findings indicate that the deficit is more extensive than can be attributed to a femoral neuropathy, which once was held responsible for the syndrome. A thoracoabdominal polyradiculopathy has been described in *sarcoidosis* in rare instances. The EMG findings are of active denervation in a pattern consistent with multiple root involvement. *Herpes zoster* also can present with dermatomal pain on the trunk and motor disturbances with fibrillation potentials in paraspinal muscles.

Other electrophysiologic studies are generally not as helpful as needle EMG in patients with root lesions.[86] Motor conduction studies are normal, and M-wave responses usually are not reduced in size unless several adjacent roots are involved (as in cauda equina syndrome following central disc protrusion) or when, as occurs occasionally, the muscle from which the recording is made has atrophied. Sensory conduction studies are normal because the pathology is proximal to the dorsal root ganglia (see Chapter 13). H reflexes (in some S1 radiculopathies) and F-wave responses may be abnormal (see Chapter 18) but provide no indication of the site of the lesion, which can be anywhere along the length of the pathway that is tested. Dermatomal somatosensory evoked potentials (see Chapter 26) are sometimes abnormal but have poor sensitivity and specificity.

PLEXUS LESIONS

The brachial plexus is formed from the anterior primary rami of the C5, C6, C7, C8, and T1 roots, with a variable contribution from C4 (prefixed) and T2 (postfixed plexus) (Fig. 11-10). The C5 and C6 roots combine to form the upper trunk, C7 continues as the middle trunk, and C8 and T1 join to form the lower trunk. The trunks traverse the supraclavicular fossa, and at the upper border

of the clavicle each divides into anterior and posterior divisions. The three posterior divisions then combine to form the posterior cord of the plexus, whereas the anterior divisions of the upper two trunks unite to form the lateral cord and the anterior division of the lower trunk continues as the medial cord. The cords give rise to the main peripheral nerves of the arm.

The lumbar portion of the lumbosacral plexus is derived from the anterior primary rami of the first four lumbar roots, whereas the sacral portion is formed from the lumbosacral trunk (L4 and L5) and the anterior primary rami of the first four sacral roots.

Needle EMG may be helpful in assessing the functional integrity of a nerve plexus, in determining the extent and severity of a plexus lesion, and in distinguishing such a lesion from root or peripheral nerve pathology. The muscles examined should include those supplied by each of the main peripheral nerves and spinal roots in question so that the site of the lesion can be determined by the pattern of involved muscles. The importance of

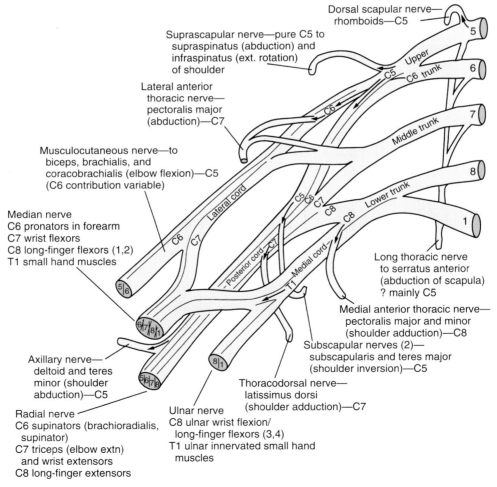

FIGURE 11-10 ■ Anatomy of the brachial plexus. (From Patten JP: Neurological Differential Diagnosis. Springer, New York, 1977, with permission.)

examining the paraspinal muscles when one attempts to distinguish between a root lesion and a plexus lesion has been stressed already. Proximal involvement is indicated further by EMG evidence of denervation in muscles whose nerve supply arises before the brachial plexus (e.g., the rhomboids or serratus anterior muscles). Such a distinction sometimes can also be made by stimulation techniques in which appropriate sensory nerve action potentials are recorded in the extremities (see Chapter 13). These potentials may be small or absent in patients with lesions that are distal to the dorsal root ganglia and have caused afferent fibers to degenerate, but they are preserved in patients with radiculopathy because the lesion is more proximal and peripheral sensory fibers therefore remain intact.

With mild plexopathies, the only electrophysiologic abnormality may be the presence of fibrillation potentials in affected muscles, but not all muscles in the territory supplied by the involved structure necessarily contain them. In more advanced cases, the amplitude of sensory nerve action potentials diminishes, and with increasing severity the amplitude of the M wave to affected muscles also declines.

These principles are exemplified well by the findings in patients in whom the lower trunk of the brachial plexus, or the anterior primary rami of the C8 and T1 nerve roots, are compressed or angulated by a *cervical rib* or band. The muscle wasting that results may be restricted to, or especially conspicuous in, the lateral part of the thenar pad, but careful clinical and EMG examination shows that motor involvement is more extensive than can be accounted for by a median nerve lesion alone, conforming instead to the distribution of muscles supplied by the C8 and T1 segments. Moreover, sensory nerve action potentials may be small or absent when recordings are made from the ulnar nerve at the wrist after stimulation of its digital fibers in the little finger, indicating that the lesion is distal to the dorsal root ganglia, and the latency of the F wave recorded from the hypothenar muscles following ulnar nerve stimulation at the wrist may be increased. The electrophysiologic findings are usually normal in patients with suspected thoracic outlet syndrome when there are no objective neurologic signs.

In *traumatic brachial plexopathy*, EMG is performed to localize the lesion, determine its severity, and guide prognosis. In mild lesions, motor unit recruitment is reduced and sparse fibrillation potentials may be present in affected muscles. With more severe trauma, motor unit recruitment is impaired, motor unit action potentials are lost, and fibrillation potentials are found in the territory supplied by the damaged structures. The axonal dysfunction also may lead to reduced amplitudes of sensory

nerve action potentials and, depending on the severity of the lesion, to small M responses with stimulation of the motor nerves to weak muscles. Conduction velocity usually is not reduced unless only a few fibers remain intact or just a few poorly myelinated regenerating axons are functional. For prognostic purposes, it is important to distinguish a plexopathy from root avulsion. In this regard, EMG abnormalities in the paraspinal muscles and preserved sensory nerve action potentials suggest that the lesion involves the nerve roots, whereas paraspinal abnormalities combined with attenuated sensory nerve action potentials imply a combined lesion. Sufficient time (10 days or so after injury) must be allowed for paraspinal abnormalities to develop before it is concluded that the EMG examination is normal.

In *idiopathic brachial plexopathy* (*neuralgic amyotrophy* or *Parsonage–Turner syndrome*), similar changes are found on needle EMG, and there may be abnormalities of sensory and motor nerve conduction studies indicating single or multiple lesions of peripheral nerves[87] that are not necessarily at the level of the brachial plexus. The musculocutaneous nerve is involved more often than the ulnar and median nerves. EMG abnormalities may be found bilaterally, even though only one side is involved clinically. The pattern of EMG abnormalities sometimes suggests that an individual nerve (e.g., the axillary, radial, or suprascapular) is affected, with little or no involvement of muscles supplied from the same level of the plexus through other nerves. Phrenic neuropathy may occur, leading to unilateral or bilateral diaphragmatic paralysis; needle EMG of the diaphragm then shows abnormal spontaneous activity and reduced numbers of (or absent) motor unit action potentials on inspiration.[88] In *radiation plexopathy*, needle EMG may reveal myokymic discharges, without clinical evidence of myokymia, in addition to signs of denervation.

EMG is probably important as a means of determining the prognosis of *obstetric lesions of the brachial plexus*. Evidence of denervation found during the first week of life does not necessarily indicate an antenatal lesion but may result simply from the short length of the affected axons. Examination at about 3 months of age (when surgical intervention to restore nerve continuity becomes a consideration) may reveal motor unit action potentials in clinically paralyzed muscles, and thus that functional connections already exist between the spinal cord and affected muscles. The cause of this apparent paradox is unclear, but several possible explanations have been proposed.[89]

Lumbar plexopathies often can be distinguished from radiculopathies by examination of the paraspinal muscles and from femoral neuropathy by sampling the thigh adductor muscles, which are supplied by the obturator nerve. *Sacral plexopathies* similarly can be distinguished from multiple lumbosacral radiculopathies by examination of the paraspinal muscles for the presence of fibrillation potentials. Sensory nerve action potentials in the legs are generally small or absent with sacral plexopathies but may also be small in elderly patients.

PERIPHERAL NERVE LESIONS

The EMG distinction of peripheral nerve from other neuropathic lesions has been discussed. In addition to the detection of signs of denervation in muscle supplied by the individual peripheral nerves, motor and sensory conduction can be studied in these nerves; this is discussed in Chapter 13, where the evaluation of polyneuropathies is also considered. In the axonal neuropathies, there may be EMG signs of chronic partial denervation in distal muscles (with or without accompanying evidence of reinnervation), whereas in the demyelinative neuropathies the only or most conspicuous abnormality on the needle examination is reduced recruitment of motor units.

The EMG examination should be part of the electrodiagnostic evaluation of patients with suspected entrapment neuropathies. In some patients with symptoms of carpal tunnel syndrome, for example, the needle examination may suggest another diagnosis (e.g., a proximal median neuropathy) when results of the nerve conduction studies are not definitive.[90] In addition to its diagnostic relevance, EMG may be of prognostic importance in this context.

Needle EMG has an important role in providing a guide to prognosis after peripheral nerve injuries and in following the course of recovery. After injuries in which the function of a nerve is deranged temporarily but its structure remains intact, needle EMG reveals only a reduction in the number of motor units under voluntary control. If the anatomic continuity of nerve fibers is interrupted, however, the amount of insertion activity increases after a few days and abnormal spontaneous activity is found eventually (as described on page 248, where the subsequent changes that occur with regeneration and reinnervation are also considered). In evaluating patients with peripheral nerve injuries, needle EMG may provide evidence that some motor units remain under voluntary control after an apparently complete nerve lesion; this implies a more favorable prognosis than otherwise, provided that the possibility of these units being innervated anomalously has been excluded. Needle EMG is an important method of determining whether denervation has occurred, and this too has prognostic significance. Finally, needle EMG may indicate at an early stage whether recovery is occurring after a complete palsy because voluntary motor unit activity reappears long before any signs of clinical recovery.

Disorders of Neuromuscular Transmission

The EMG findings in patients with disorders of neuromuscular transmission are discussed in Chapter 17. The only point that need be made here is that individual motor unit action potentials may show a marked variation in their dimensions and configuration because of blocking of impulse transmission to individual muscle fibers within the motor unit. Such variability is therefore a common finding in patients with myasthenia gravis, Lambert–Eaton syndrome, congenital myasthenic syndromes, and botulism, and is also encountered as reinnervation occurs after a neuropathic lesion, in inflammatory myopathies, and following muscle trauma. There may also be an increased incidence of short-duration or polyphasic motor unit action potentials in patients with myasthenia gravis, caused by a reduction in the number of functional muscle fibers per unit or by the development of a secondary myopathy. Similar findings may be encountered in Lambert–Eaton syndrome or botulism because of the defect in neuromuscular transmission.

Miscellaneous Disorders

Intermittent bursts of high-frequency, repetitive motor unit discharges are found in different parts of the muscle in patients with cramps. These bursts have an abrupt onset and termination. The number of active motor units and their firing frequency increase as the cramp evolves, declining again as the cramp eases off. In patients with *myokymia*, EMG may reveal prolonged bursts of repetitive motor unit action potentials, or repetitive multiplets containing from 2 to more than 200 action potentials with intervals of about 20 msec between component spikes. Single or double discharges of individual motor units occur spontaneously and regularly at intervals of 100 to 200 msec in patients with *facial myokymia*, or motor units may fire intermittently for up to 900 msec at intervals of 2 to 4 seconds at rates of 30 to 40 Hz. The findings in patients with myotonia or cramps differ from the spontaneous, high-frequency (up to 300 Hz) motor unit action potential discharges (neuromyotonic discharges, p. 242) seen in patients with *Isaacs syndrome*. This disorder is characterized clinically by muscle cramps and stiffness, difficulty in muscle relaxation, muscle twitching, and hyperhidrosis, and may develop spontaneously; on a hereditary basis; or in association with lymphoma,[91] peripheral neuropathy, or certain immunologic disorders such as myasthenia gravis or a thymoma.[26,29] EMG reveals neuromyotonic discharges that may be continuous in severe cases, but there is a marked variability in the configuration and dimensions of the action potentials that are found, some being of particularly low amplitude and short duration. The spontaneous discharges are increased temporarily by voluntary activity, but a brief period of electrical silence may follow strenuous, continuous activity; they commonly disappear after proximal nerve block but may persist despite distal block, disappear after intravenous curare or succinylcholine, and are reduced by phenytoin.

Two types of abnormal movements have been described in patients with *hemifacial spasm*. The first consists of brief twitches that affect several different muscles simultaneously and is accompanied electromyographically by isolated bursts of repetitive, high-frequency motor unit discharges, each burst consisting of discharges from the same unit. The second consists of a prolonged, irregular, fluctuating contraction during which motor units fire irregularly at lower frequencies, although bursts of activity identical to those just described are also seen. The EMG abnormalities of *hemimasticatory spasm* are similar to those of hemifacial spasm, but they are found in the jaw-closing muscles supplied by the trigeminal nerve.[92]

During the spasms of *tetany*, motor unit action potentials may be seen to fire repetitively in doublets, triplets, or multiplets. The number of activated units increases as the spasms intensify, and a full interference pattern eventually may be obtained.

The syndrome of *painful legs and moving toes* is uncommon but well described. The EMG accompaniments of the continuous, involuntary toe movements that typify the disorder are varied, but may include myokymic discharges,[93] normal firing of motor units, and the rhythmic firing of motor units at rates between 0.5 and 3 Hz. Motor unit discharges may alternate in agonist and antagonist muscles or occur synchronously in both groups.

The *stiff person syndrome* (Moersch–Woltman syndrome) is characterized by muscle stiffness and spasms that begin in axial muscles and then become more extensive, involving especially the proximal muscles in the limbs.[94] It has an autoimmune basis and relates to impaired central presynaptic inhibition. EMG reveals continuous motor unit activity that disappears during sleep, with spinal or general anesthesia, and after peripheral nerve block. Nerve conduction studies are normal, but exaggerated and widespread muscle responses follow electrical stimulation.

Contractures are characterized clinically by a painful, involuntary shortening of muscle, and electromyographically by electrical silence.

DIAPHRAGMATIC ELECTROMYOGRAPHY

Needle examination of the diaphragm may be helpful in clarifying the nature of respiratory disturbances in patients with neuromuscular diseases, as discussed in Chapter 34. It is probably best avoided, however, in agitated or uncooperative patients, and in those in whom it may be more hazardous or difficult (e.g., patients with coagulopathies, local infections or neoplasms, hiccoughs, frequent coughing, abdominal distension, or gross obesity).

The reader is referred to the original sources for technical details of the several approaches that have been described. The subcostal approach is safe in that no major complications have followed it, but the examination is technically unsatisfactory in about 10 percent of cases.[95,96] The easier approach favored by Bolton's group involves insertion of a needle electrode through an intercostal space just above the costal margin, but pneumothorax has occurred in a few patients with chronic obstructive pulmonary disease.[97] The substernal approach is an alternative.[98]

The EMG findings should indicate whether a neuropathic or myopathic process is responsible for diaphragmatic weakness, but interpretation may be difficult because the motor unit action potentials of the diaphragm are normally smaller and more abundant than those of the limb muscles. The presence of abnormal spontaneous activity may provide evidence of partial denervation, whereas a reduced interference pattern during inspiration may occur from a demyelinating neuropathy of the phrenic nerve. In amyotrophic lateral sclerosis, the EMG findings may provide a guide to prognosis and planning supportive care.[99]

SPHINCTERIC ELECTROMYOGRAPHY

It is possible to examine the function of the sphincteric muscles by needle EMG, but a variety of other physiologic approaches are also available for this purpose. Further details are provided in Chapter 31.

LARYNGEAL ELECTROMYOGRAPHY

The utility of laryngeal EMG in the diagnosis, prognosis, and treatment of certain laryngeal disorders has been evaluated by an evidence-based review of the voluminous literature that has accumulated.[100] Laryngeal EMG may be useful as an aid to the injection of botulinum toxin into the thyroarytenoid muscle for the treatment of adductor spasmodic dysphonia, but there is only anecdotal evidence about the possible utility of laryngeal EMG for other purposes. The technique usually is undertaken by oto-laryngologists and merits no further discussion here.

SURFACE ELECTROMYOGRAPHY

The recording of myoelectrical signals from sensors on the skin might seem useful as a noninvasive means of studying diseases of muscle and nerve. Simple recordings involve single-channel monopolar and bipolar montages, the former measuring the voltage between an electrode over muscle and one placed more remotely, and the latter measuring the potential difference between two recording electrodes over an individual muscle. Recordings typically are analyzed with the aid of specialized computer software, the data so derived being related to force and duration of muscle contraction. With multichannel recordings, the number of electrodes increases, as does the area of muscle studied. This leads to a reduction in interelectrode distance and recording area, and thus to suppression of far-field activity but greater resolution of individual motor unit or muscle-fiber potentials.

In the last 15 years, various professional societies have evaluated the clinical applicability of surface EMG but concluded that it had no utility as a diagnostic aid or was markedly inferior to conventional needle EMG.[101,102] The most recent review concluded that the data were insufficient to determine its clinical utility in distinguishing between neuropathic and myopathic conditions or for detecting certain more specific neuromuscular disorders, and to compare its diagnostic utility with that of conventional needle EMG.[103]

QUANTITATIVE ASPECTS OF ELECTROMYOGRAPHY

In an endeavor to improve the accuracy, reliability, and speed with which the examination is performed, and to gain further insight into the pathophysiology of neuromuscular disorders, different workers have developed a number of quantitative techniques over the years. These include techniques for measuring the parameters of individual motor unit action potentials, a variety of which are incorporated into newer commercially available equipment. These techniques and others that have been developed for the measurement of motor unit territory, for frequency analysis of the EMG to facilitate the diagnosis of muscle disease, and for estimating the number of motor units in a muscle are discussed in Chapter 12.

REFERENCES

1. Nardin RA, Rutkove SB, Raynor EM: Diagnostic accuracy of electrodiagnostic testing in the evaluation of weakness. Muscle Nerve, 26:201, 2002
2. Caruso G, Eisen A, Stålberg E: Clinical EMG and glossary of terms most commonly used by clinical electromyographers. The International Federation of Clinical Neurophysiology. Electroencephalogr Clin Neurophysiol Suppl, 52:189, 1999
3. Walker WC, Keyser-Marcus LA, Johns JS et al: Relation of electromyography-induced pain to type of recording electrode. Muscle Nerve, 24:417, 2001
4. Gitter AJ, Stolov WG: Instrumentation and measurement in electrodiagnostic medicine. Muscle Nerve, 18:799 and 812, 1995 (two parts)
5. Mateen FJ, Grant IA, Sorenson EJ: Needlestick injuries among electromyographers. Muscle Nerve, 38:1541, 2008
6. Farrell CM, Rubin DI, Haidukewych GJ: Acute compartment syndrome of the leg following diagnostic electromyography. Muscle Nerve, 27:374, 2003
7. Lynch SL, Boon AJ, Smith J et al: Complications of needle electromyography: hematoma risk and correlation with anticoagulation and antiplatelet therapy. Muscle Nerve, 38:1225, 2008
8. Al-Shekhlee A, Shapiro BE, Preston DC: Iatrogenic complications and risks of nerve conduction studies and needle electromyography. Muscle Nerve, 27:517, 2003
9. Daube JR, Rubin DI: Needle electromyography. Muscle Nerve, 39:244, 2009
10. Rutkove S: Effects of temperature on neuromuscular electrophysiology. Muscle Nerve, 24:867, 2001
11. Denys EH: The influence of temperature in clinical neurophysiology. Muscle Nerve, 14:795, 1991
12. Kraft GH: Fibrillation potential amplitude and muscle atrophy following peripheral nerve injury. Muscle Nerve, 13:814, 1990
13. Nandedkar SD, Barkhaus PE, Sanders DB et al: Some observations on fibrillations and positive sharp waves. Muscle Nerve, 23:888, 2000
14. Dumitru D, King JC, Rogers WE et al: Positive sharp wave and fibrillation potential modeling. Muscle Nerve, 22:242, 1999
15. Kraft GH: Fibrillation potentials and positive sharp waves: are they the same? Electroencephalogr Clin Neurophysiol, 81:163, 1991
16. Kleine BU, Stegeman DF, Schelhaas HJ et al: Firing pattern of fasciculations in ALS: evidence for axonal and neuronal origin. Neurology, 70:353, 2008
17. Drost G, Kleine BU, Stegeman DF et al: Fasciculation potentials in high-density surface EMG. J Clin Neurophysiol, 24:301, 2007
18. Fournier E, Arzel M, Sternberg D et al: Electromyography guides toward subgroups of mutations in muscle channelopathies. Ann Neurol, 56:650, 2004
19. Matthews E, Fialho D, Tan SV et al: The non-dystrophic myotonias: molecular pathogenesis, diagnosis and treatment. Brain, 133:9, 2010

20. Logigian EL, Ciafaloni E, Quinn LC et al: Severity, type, and distribution of myotonic discharges are different in type 1 and type 2 myotonic dystrophy. Muscle Nerve, 35:479, 2007

21. Ptacek LJ, Johnson KJ, Griggs RC: Genetics and physiology of the myotonic muscle disorders. N Engl J Med, 328:482, 1993

22. Fellows LK, Foster BJ, Chalk CH: Clinical significance of complex repetitive discharges: a case-control study. Muscle Nerve, 28:504, 2003

23. Daube JR: Electrodiagnosis of muscle disorders. p. 764. In Engel AG, Franzini-Armstrong C (eds): Myology. 2nd Ed. McGraw-Hill, New York, 1994

24. Baldissera F, Cavallari P, Dworzak F: Motor neuron "bi-stability": a pathogenetic mechanism for cramps and myo-kymia. Brain, 117:929, 1994

25. Miller TM, Layzer RB: Muscle cramps. Muscle Nerve, 32:431, 2005

26. Vincent A: Understanding neuromyotonia. Muscle Nerve, 23:655, 2000

27. Meriggioli MN, Sanders DB: Conduction block and continuous motor unit activity in chronic acquired demyelinating polyneuropathy. Muscle Nerve, 22:532, 1999

28. Oleary CP, Mann AC, Lough J et al: Muscle hypertrophy in multifocal motor neuropathy is associated with continuous motor unit activity. Muscle Nerve, 20:479, 1997

29. Newsom-Davis J, Mills KR: Immunological associations of acquired neuromyotonia (Isaacs' syndrome). Report of five cases and literature review. Brain, 116:453, 1993

30. Aminoff MJ: Electromyography in Clinical Practice: Electrodiagnostic Aspects of Neuromuscular Disease. 3rd Ed. Churchill Livingstone, New York, 1998

31. Kimura J: Electrodiagnosis in Diseases of Nerve and Muscle: Principles and Practice. 3rd Ed. Oxford University Press, New York, 2001

32. Saperstein DS, Amata AA, Barohn RJ: Clinical and genetic aspects of distal myopathies. Muscle Nerve, 24:1440, 2001

33. Stalberg E, Trontelj JV: Single Fiber Electromyography. 2nd Ed. Raven, New York, 1994

34. Quijano-Roy S, Renault F, Romero N et al: EMG and nerve conduction studies in children with congenital muscular dystrophy. Muscle Nerve, 29:292, 2004

35. Blijham PJ, Hengstman GJ, Hama-Amin AD et al: Needle electromyographic findings in 98 patients with myositis. Eur Neurol, 55:183, 2006

36. Blijham PJ, Hengstman GDJ, Ter Laak HJ et al: Muscle-fiber conduction velocity and electromyography as diagnostic tools in patients with suspected inflammatory myopathy: a prospective study. Muscle Nerve, 29:46, 2004

37. Uncini A, Lange DJ, Lovelace RE et al: Long-duration polyphasic motor unit potentials in myopathies: a quantitative study with pathological correlation. Muscle Nerve, 13:263, 1990

38. Gilchrist JM, Sachs GM: Electrodiagnostic studies in the management and prognosis of neuromuscular disorders. Muscle Nerve, 29:165, 2004

39. Robinson-Papp J, Simpson DM: Neuromuscular diseases associated with HIV-1 infection. Muscle Nerve, 40:1043, 2009

40. HIV Neuromuscular Syndrome Study Group: HIV-associated neuromuscular weakness syndrome. AIDS, 18: 1403, 2004

41. Griggs RC, Askanas V, Di Mauro S et al: Inclusion body myositis and myopathies. Ann Neurol, 38:705, 1995

42. Amato AA, Barohn RJ: Evaluation and treatment of inflammatory myopathies. J Neurol Neurosurg Psychiatry, 80:1060, 2009

43. Phillips BA, Cala LA, Thickbroom GW et al: Patterns of muscle involvement in inclusion body myositis: clinical and magnetic resonance imaging study. Muscle Nerve, 24:1526, 2001

44. Barkhaus PE, Periquet MI, Nandedkar S: Quantitative electrophysiological studies in sporadic inclusion body myositis. Muscle Nerve, 22:480, 1999

45. Rubin DI, Hermann RC: Electrophysiologic findings in amyloid myopathy. Muscle Nerve, 22:355, 1999

46. Valiyil R, Christopher-Stine L: Drug-related myopathies of which the clinician should be aware. Curr Rheumatol Rep, 12:213, 2010

47. Kuncl RW: Agents and mechanisms of toxic myopathy. Curr Opin Neurol, 22:506, 2009

48. Kuncl RW, Cornblath DR, Avila O et al: Electrodiagnosis of human colchicine myoneuropathy. Muscle Nerve, 12:360, 1989

49. Younger DS, Mayer SA, Weimer LH et al: Colchicine-induced myopathy and neuropathy. Neurology, 41:943, 1991

50. Lacomis D, Zochodne DW, Bird SJ: Critical illness myopathy. Muscle Nerve, 23:1785, 2000

51. Stevens RD, Marshall SA, Cornblath DR et al: A framework for diagnosing and classifying intensive care unit-acquired weakness. Crit Care Med, 37(Suppl):S299, 2009

52. Zochodne DW, Ramsay DA, Saly V et al: Acute necrotizing myopathy of intensive care: electrophysiological studies. Muscle Nerve, 17:285, 1994

53. Gutmann L, Blumenthal D, Gutmann L et al: Acute type II myofiber atrophy in critical illness. Neurology, 46:819, 1996

54. Rich MM, Teener JW, Raps EC et al: Muscle is electrically inexcitable in acute quadriplegic myopathy. Neurology, 46:731, 1996

55. Rich MM, Bird SJ, Raps EC et al: Direct muscle stimulation in acute quadriplegic myopathy. Muscle Nerve, 20:665, 1997

56. Lomen-Hoerth C, Simmons ML, DeArmond SJ et al: Adult-onset nemaline myopathy: another cause of dropped head. Muscle Nerve, 22:1146, 1999

57. Miller TM: Differential diagnosis of myotonic disorders. Muscle Nerve, 37:293, 2008

58. Pascuzzi RM, Gratianne R, Azzarelli B et al: Schwartz–Jampel syndrome with dominant inheritance. Muscle Nerve, 13:1152, 1990

59. Deymeer F, Lehmann-Horn F, Serdaroglu P et al: Electrical myotonia in heterozygous carriers of recessive myotonia congenita. Muscle Nerve, 22:123, 1999

60. Torbergsen T: Rippling muscle disease: a review. Muscle Nerve Suppl, 11:S103, 2002

61. So YT, Zu L, Barraza C et al: Rippling muscle disease: evidence for phenotypic and genetic heterogeneity. Muscle Nerve, 24:340, 2001

62. Sundblom J, Stålberg E, Osterdahl M et al: Bedside diagnosis of rippling muscle disease in CAV3 p.A46T mutation carriers. Muscle Nerve, 41:751, 2010

63. Jacobi C, Ruscheweyh R, Vorgerd M et al: Rippling muscle disease: variable phenotype in a family with five afflicted members. Muscle Nerve, 41:128, 2010

64. Koul RL, Chand RP, Chacko A et al: Severe autosomal recessive rippling muscle disease. Muscle Nerve, 24:1542, 2001

65. Vernino S, Auger RG, Emslie-Smith AM et al: Myasthenia, thymoma, presynaptic antibodies, and a continuum of neuromuscular hyperexcitability. Neurology, 53:1233, 1999

66. Leis AA, Stokic DS, Webb RM et al: Clinical spectrum of muscle weakness in human West Nile virus infection. Muscle Nerve, 28:302, 2003

67. Amer-Shekhlee A, Katirji B: Electrodiagnostic features of acute paralytic poliomyelitis associated with West Nile virus infection. Muscle Nerve, 29:376, 2004

68. de Carvalho M, Dengler R, Eisen A: Electrodiagnostic criteria for diagnosis of ALS. Clin Neurophysiol, 119:497, 2008

69. Li J, Petajan J, Smith G et al: Electromyography of sternocleidomastoid muscle in ALS: a prospective study. Muscle Nerve, 25:725, 2002

70. Sonoo M, Kuwabara S, Shimizu T et al: Utility of trapezius EMG for diagnosis of amyotrophic lateral sclerosis. Muscle Nerve, 39:63, 2009

71. de Carvalho M, Pinto S, Swash M: Motor unit changes in thoracic paraspinal muscles in amyotrophic lateral sclerosis. Muscle Nerve, 39:83, 2009

72. de Carvalho MA, Pinto S, Swash M: Paraspinal and limb motor neuron involvement within homologous spinal segments in ALS. Clin Neurophysiol, 119:1607, 2008

73. Kuwabara S, Sonoo M, Komori T et al: Dissociated small hand muscle atrophy in amyotrophic lateral sclerosis: frequency, extent, and specificity. Muscle Nerve, 37:426, 2008

74. Daube JR: Electrodiagnostic studies in amyotrophic lateral sclerosis and other motor neuron disorders. Muscle Nerve, 23:1488, 2000

75. Younger DS: Motor neuron disease and malignancy. Muscle Nerve, 23:658, 2000

76. Rowland LP: Progressive muscular atrophy and other lower motor neuron syndromes of adults. Muscle Nerve, 41:161, 2010

77. Rhodes LE, Freeman BK, Auh S et al: Clinical features of spinal and bulbar muscular atrophy. Brain, 132:3242, 2009

78. Olney RK, Aminoff MJ, So YT: Clinical and electrodiagnostic features of X-linked recessive bulbospinal neuronopathy. Neurology, 41:823, 1991

79. Nogues MA, Stalberg E: Electrodiagnostic findings in syringomyelia. Muscle Nerve, 22:1653, 1999

80. Jensen MC, Brant-Zawadski MN, Obuchowski N et al: Magnetic resonance imaging of the lumbar spine in people without back pain. N Engl J Med, 14:331, 1994

81. Nardin RA, Patel MR, Gudas TF et al: Electromyography and magnetic resonance imaging in the evaluation of radiculopathy. Muscle Nerve, 22:151, 1999

82. Pezzin LE, Dillingham TR, Lauder TD et al: Cervical radiculopathies: relationship between symptom duration and spontaneous EMG activity. Muscle Nerve, 22:1412, 1999

83. Tsao BE, Levin KH, Bodner RA: Comparison of surgical and electrodiagnostic findings in single root lumbosacral radiculopathies. Muscle Nerve, 27:60, 2003

84. Levin KH, Maggiano HJ, Wilbourn AJ: Cervical radiculopathies: comparison of surgical and EMG localization of single-root lesions. Neurology, 46:1022, 1996

85. Date ES, Mar EY, Bugola MR et al: The prevalence of lumbar paraspinal spontaneous activity in asymptomatic subjects. Muscle Nerve, 19:350, 1996

86. Wilbourn AJ, Aminoff MJ: The electrophysiologic examination in patients with radiculopathies. Muscle Nerve, 21:1612, 1998

87. Cruz-Martinez A, Barrio M, Arpa J: Neuralgic amyotrophy: variable expression in 40 patients. J Peripher Nerv Syst, 7:198, 2002

88. Lahrmann H, Grisold W, Authier FJ et al: Neuralgic amyotrophy with phrenic nerve involvement. Muscle Nerve, 22:437, 1999

89. Van Dijk JG, Pondaag W, Malessy MJA: Obstetric lesions of the brachial plexus. Muscle Nerve, 24:1451, 2001

90. Gnatz SM: The role of needle electromyography in the evaluation of patients with carpal tunnel syndrome: needle EMG is important. Muscle Nerve, 22:282, 1999

91. Lahrmann H, Albrecht G, Drlicek M et al: Acquired neuromyotonia and peripheral neuropathy in a patient with Hodgkin's disease. Muscle Nerve, 24:834, 2001

92. Auger RG, Litchy WJ, Cascino TL et al: Hemimasticatory spasm: clinical and electrophysiologic observations. Neurology, 42:2263, 1992

93. Mitsumoto H, Levin KH, Wilbourn AJ et al: Hypertrophic mononeuritis clinically presenting with painful legs and moving toes. Muscle Nerve, 13:215, 1990

94. Meinck HM, Thompson PD: Stiff man syndrome and related conditions. Mov Disord, 17:853, 2002

95. Saadeh PB, Cristafulli CF, Sosner J: Electrodiagnostic studies of the neuromuscular respiratory system. Phys Med Rehabil Clin N Am, 5:541, 1994

96. Saadeh PB, Cristafulli CF, Sosner J et al: Needle electromyography of the diaphragm: a new technique. Muscle Nerve, 16:15, 1993

97. Bolton CF, Grand'Maison F, Parkes A et al: Needle electromyography of the diaphragm. Muscle Nerve, 15:678, 1992

98. Lagueny A, Ellie E, Saintarailles J et al: Unilateral diaphragmatic paralysis: an electrophysiological study. J Neurol Neurosurg Psychiatry, 55:316, 1992

99. Bolton CF: Clinical neurophysiology of the respiratory system. Muscle Nerve, 16:809, 1993

100. AAEM Laryngeal Task Force: Laryngeal electromyography: an evidence-based review. Muscle Nerve, 28:767, 2003

101. Haig AJ, Gelblum JB, Rechtien JJ et al: Technology assessment: the use of surface EMG in the diagnosis and treatment of nerve and muscle disorders. Muscle Nerve, 19:392, 1996

102. Pullman SL, Goodin DS, Marquinez AI et al: Clinical utility of surface EMG: report of the therapeutics and technology assessment subcommittee of the American Academy of Neurology. Neurology, 55:171, 2000

103. Meekins GD, So Y, Quan D: American Association of Neuromuscular & Electrodiagnostic Medicine evidenced-based review: use of surface electromyography in the diagnosis and study of neuromuscular disorders. Muscle Nerve, 38:1219, 2008

Quantitative Electromyography

MARK B. BROMBERG

The term *quantitative electromyography* (QEMG) refers to a number of different electrodiagnostic techniques and methods of gathering and analyzing data (Table 12-1). No simple definition applies to all aspects of QEMG. QEMG is distinguished from routine electrodiagnostic tests by the continuously variable nature of the data (cardinal data) and by the ability to make statistical inferences and comparisons. The quantitative nature of QEMG is in contrast to the subjective and relative-based data (ordinal data) obtained from most needle EMG studies. For example, data from routine needle EMG studies represent interpretations of motor unit action potential (MUAP) waveforms expressed in relative units based on arbitrary scales that do not have physiologic bases (up and down arrows and gradations noted by plus and minus symbols). In QEMG the same waveform data are expressed in physical and physiologic units (millivolts, milliseconds, milliseconds * millivolts, number of phases and turns), and the averages of such values from a muscle can be presented as summary data. QEMG relies heavily on computers that are integral to modern EMG machines.[1] Computers also allow for the calculation of derived metrics (e.g., MUAP area and area/amplitude ratio, ratio of average number of waveform turns/waveform amplitude, and discharge–discharge waveform component variability). Data can also be viewed in unique displays. The continuously variable nature of QEMG data and its statistical representations (e.g., mean, median, and standard deviation) permit statistically valid comparisons between muscles within a patient and between patients, between serial studies within a patient, and between electrodiagnostic laboratories.[2] Statistical analysis of QEMG data can be used as an expert system when combined with EMG database libraries to provide probabilities of a particular diagnosis.[3]

Of historical note, most principles that underlie the qualitative interpretation of routine needle EMG MUAP waveforms are based on data from early QEMG studies by Buchthal and colleagues in the 1950s. These studies were performed with manual measurements from photographic records and were time-consuming; similar analyses can now be performed in seconds compared to hours, thus making QEMG practical.

The QEMG technique used most commonly is automated extraction of MUAPs. Some QEMG techniques

TABLE 12-1 ■ QEMG Tests, Electrode Requirements, and Unique Information Provided

QEMG Study	Electrode	Information
Individual MUAP analysis	Concentric or monopolar	Quantitative MUAP waveform metrics
Automated MUAP analysis	Concentric or monopolar	Quantitative MUAP waveform metrics
Fiber-density	Single-fiber	Muscle-fiber density
Macro-EMG	Macro single-fiber	Whole motor unit size
Scanning EMG	Concentric	Three-dimensional motor unit view
Motor unit number estimation	Surface	Estimate of number of motor units innervating a muscle
Neuromuscular variability	Single-fiber or small concentric	Quantitative neuromuscular variability (jitter)
CMAP scan	Surface	Estimate of size and excitability of motor units

QEMG, quantitative electromyography; MUAP, motor unit action potential; CMAP, compound muscle action potential.

rely on special electrodes (Fig. 12-1). For routine studies, standard concentric and monopolar electrodes provide comparable information, but MUAP amplitude and duration values are greater with monopolar electrodes.[4]

For MUAP analysis, there are no significant differences between standard- and pediatric-sized concentric electrodes,[5] but the pediatric-sized concentric electrode allows neuromuscular jitter to be measured with results similar to those obtained with a single-fiber electrode. Special electrodes include single-fiber electrodes for assessment of motor unit fiber density and the variability of neuromuscular junction transmission, macro-EMG electrodes to assess the size of the whole motor unit, and a device to slowly withdraw the electrode in scanning EMG to determine the spatial and temporal distribution of the motor unit within a muscle. Special algorithms include plotting of metrics from interference analysis and methods to estimate the number of motor units innervating a muscle by motor unit number estimation (MUNE).

The selection and use of the various QEMG techniques depend on the clinical question to which an answer is sought and on specific computer software programs. The advantage of QEMG is that it is objective. QEMG changes may precede changes observed with routine electrodiagnostic studies. QEMG can also help prevent false-positive interpretations, as the statistical approach

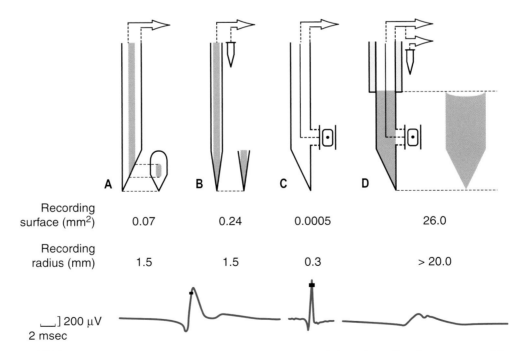

Recording surface (mm²)	0.07	0.24	0.0005	26.0
Recording radius (mm)	1.5	1.5	0.3	> 20.0

200 µV
2 msec

FIGURE 12-1 ■ Configuration and recording characteristics of needle electromyographic (EMG) recording electrodes. **A**, Concentric electrode. The numeric values relate to standard size electrodes; smaller concentric electrodes have a recording surface area of 0.03 mm² and a recording radius of approximately 1.0 mm. **B**, Monopolar electrode. **C**, Single-fiber electrode. **D**, Macro-EMG electrode. (From Bromberg M: Electromyographic [EMG] findings in denervation. Crit Rev Phys Rehabil Med, 5:83, 1993, with permission.)

places less emphasis on rare outlying waveforms and data that may be overweighted in interpretation during qualitative studies.

There are limitations and cautions regarding QEMG. Electrodiagnosis is a tool, and QEMG cannot "deliver" a diagnosis. Results must make sense in the clinical context. Excessive reliance on a numeric value, without considering a broad spectrum of clinical data, may lead to diagnostic errors with QEMG, as with routine electrodiagnostic studies. Most importantly, many QEMG techniques rely on computer-based analysis with waveform markings and values derived automatically from software algorithms.[2] Marking algorithms can result in marking errors, and all QEMG data must be verified by inspection, and errors corrected.[6] Despite the speed of data acquisition, QEMG takes time, perhaps more than routine electrodiagnostic testing, and is not a shortcut to the diagnosis. These issues notwithstanding, certain aspects of QEMG can be incorporated easily into routine studies to enhance the diagnostic process.

MOTOR UNIT ACTION POTENTIAL ANALYSIS

QEMG of MUAPs requires isolation of individual MUAPs from the interference pattern and marking of various portions of the waveforms. Isolation may be accomplished by manual or automated methods. Similarly, marking may be performed manually, but more commonly it is performed automatically, with the ability to make changes.

Manual Motor Unit Isolation

During routine EMG recording (with concentric or monopolar electrodes), a low voluntary effort generates a weak interference pattern with three or four well-defined MUAPs on the screen and a number of less defined motor units in the background (Fig. 12-2). The discharge pattern is viewed in "free run" or in continuous sweep mode, and the sweep speed usually is set to 10 msec/div, resulting in MUAPs that are compressed

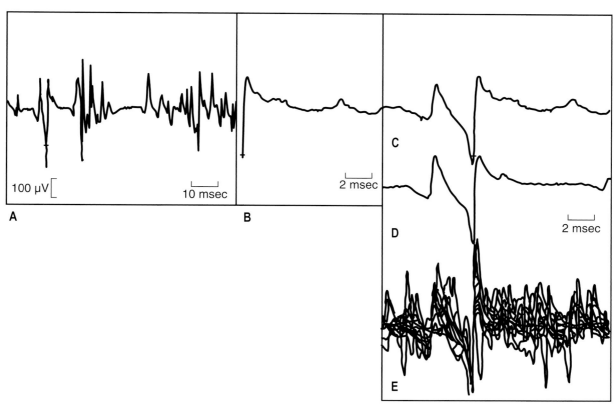

FIGURE 12-2 ■ Motor unit triggering, delay line, and averaging. **A,** Routine electromyographic signal in free-run sweep mode. Horizontal line indicates voltage trigger level for negative-going potentials. **B,** Triggered motor unit action potential (MUAP) with no delay, resulting in loss of waveform segment before the potential crosses the trigger voltage. **C,** Same triggered MUAP but with 4-msec delay, with inclusion of the whole waveform. **D,** Averaged MUAP showing greater clarity of the waveform, facilitating marking of onset and termination points. **E,** Superimposed MUAP waveforms from which the average is extracted.

visually. Motor units discharge independently of each other, resulting in occasional superimposition of MUAPs. Under these conditions, accurate estimates of amplitude, duration, and complexity (phases and turns) are difficult, and only qualitative assessments of these metrics can be made; small MUAP changes are unlikely to be recognized.

Individual MUAPs can be isolated for more accurate analysis. Historically, MUAPs were captured on photographic film, which is very time-consuming and is not feasible for clinical application. Individual MUAPs can be isolated more easily for detailed and accurate observation by the use of a voltage trigger and delay line.[7] With this procedure, the needle electrode is adjusted so that one MUAP has a greater peak amplitude than the others. The trigger voltage level is set so that a negative- or positive-going portion of this MUAP crosses the set voltage level (see Fig. 12-2). The triggered MUAP is viewed on another display screen every time it discharges. This ensures that the same MUAP is captured every time. Triggered motor units may be frozen or averaged to eliminate contamination by background (distant) MUAPs. The sweep speed can be expanded to 2 to 5 msec/div to view MUAPs in greater detail, and quantitative measurements can be made on the isolated MUAPs. The needle then is moved to isolate another MUAP, and the process is repeated.

The delay line takes advantage of the computer-based design of modern EMG machines. Analog waveform signals are converted to digital signals and stored in a short-term memory module. The short-term memory stores a limited duration of the signal, and incoming waveform data displace old data. At the time the waveform crosses the trigger voltage, the computer looks back in time to display the whole MUAP waveform (see Fig. 12-2).

The trigger and delay line can be used easily during routine needle EMG studies in any muscle to obtain detailed views of MUAP waveforms. After obtaining basic data on recruitment and amplitude from the free-run mode, 10 to 20 triggered MUAP waveforms are observed objectively (but qualitatively) at expanded sweep speeds to verify normality or detect subtle pathologic changes such as increased number of turns. A decision then is made about whether to perform QEMG. During examination of triggered MUAP waveforms, the stability of late components can be assessed when successive waveforms are superimposed (Fig. 12-3).[8] Instability viewed in this way represents abnormal transmission at several neuromuscular junctions and is called "jiggle." MUAP instability can represent pathology from reinnervation in denervating disorders or slowed muscle fiber conduction velocities in both denervating and myopathic disorders. With an increase in the low-frequency filter to 1,000 Hz and use of a pediatric-sized electrode or small monopolar electrode, formal measurement of neuromuscular jitter can be made, and will be discussed later.[9]

Automated Motor Unit Isolation

The computer capabilities of EMG machines can be used to extract more MUAPs than by the manual, one-at-a-time method using the trigger and delay line. Automated systems have been developed to identify and measure a number of MUAPs from the same interference pattern.[1]

The digitized interference pattern is analyzed by detection algorithms that can identify individual MUAP waveforms (Fig. 12-4). A variety of algorithms have been developed based on waveform template matching and decomposition; these are available on many EMG

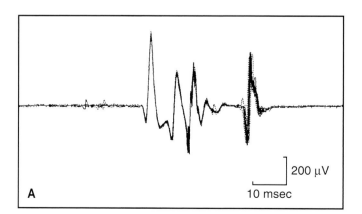

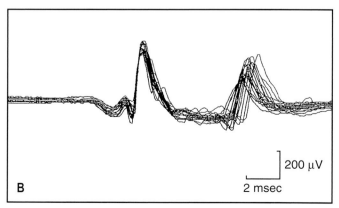

FIGURE 12-3 ■ Qualitative assessment of motor unit action potential (MUAP) waveform instability using the trigger and delay line. **A**, Example of very complex MUAP with long duration (30 msec) but with stable waveform components. **B**, Example of a waveform with instability of late components, called jiggle.

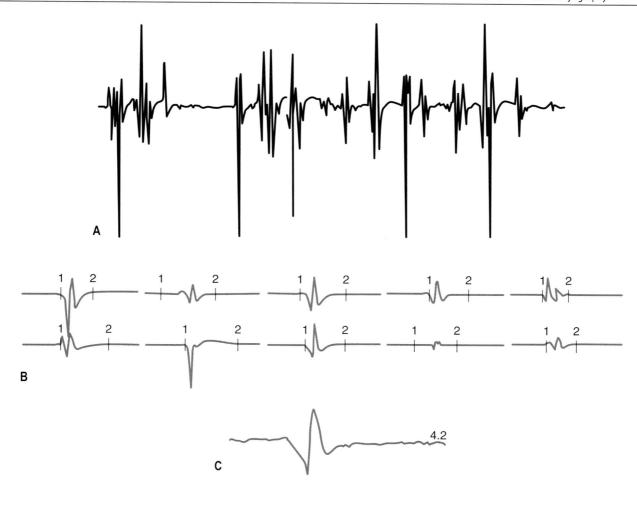

	Amplitude (mV)	Duration (msec)	Area (mVmsec)	Ratio	Phases	Turns
Mean (SD)	1.1 (0.5)	17.8 (3.7)	2.2 (0.9)	2.2 (0.5)	3.6 (0.9)	3.3 (0.8)

FIGURE 12-4 ▪ Automated motor unit action potential (MUAP) analysis. **A**, Sample of mild interference pattern. **B**, Extracted MUAPs from three interference patterns yielding 10 MUAPs (in practice, a sufficient number of interference patterns are obtained to yield 20 to 30 MUAPs). **C**, Individual MUAPs can be viewed for accuracy, adjustment of onset and endpoint markings, and exclusion of questionable potentials. **D**, Summary statistics are generated.

machines.[1] Several terms have been given to the automated process, including *decomposition EMG, multi-motor unit potential (MUP) analysis,* and *multi-MUP analysis.* There have been few comparisons of the accuracy of MUAP extraction algorithms, and not all perform equally.[10]

MUAP data obtained by isolating single MUAPs differ from those obtained by automated systems (Table 12-2). With the former technique, low-threshold motor units are isolated by adjusting the electrode position to achieve a main spike rise-time of 0.5 to 1 msec, thus optimizing

TABLE 12-2 ▪ **Comparison Between Different QEMG Techniques**

	Film	Trigger/Delay Line	Automated
Selection of MUAPs	Manual	Manual	Automated
Investigator bias	Yes	Yes	Minor
Amplitude bias	Above 50 µV	Highest	Above 50 µV
Contraction level	Low	Low	Low–moderate
Time resolution	Low	High	High
Number MUAPs/site	1–2	1	4–8
Analysis time	~1 hr	~20 min	~5 min

QEMG, quantitative electromyography; MUAP, motor unit action potential.

MUAP amplitude. Summary statistics are derived from approximately 20 MUAPs, with no appreciable changes in metric values when more MUAPs are collected.[11] With the automated technique, a more vigorous interference pattern is generated and higher-threshold motor units can be isolated. One automated QEMG program is able to record the surface activity of the muscle under study with a second surface electrode as a root-mean-square signal, which correlates linearly with force.[12,13] By keeping the electrical interference pattern activity within a narrow zone, QEMG data are more consistent. Within the interference pattern, only one or two of the isolated MUAPs have short rise-times and optimized amplitudes, whereas the other extracted MUAPs have longer rise-times and lower amplitudes. Accordingly, the populations of MUAPs differ between the manual and automated techniques. Because of these differences, it is important to obtain reference values in each laboratory for a number of index muscles.[14]

MUAP Metrics

MUAPs isolated by either method must be marked accurately for reliable data. With the manual system, isolated motor unit waveforms may be marked by the operator for duration, amplitude, and number of phases and turns. More commonly, isolated MUAPs are marked automatically by the computer using marking algorithms. Detection of peak amplitudes and baseline crossing is straightforward; however, algorithms for marking MUAP onset and termination points and turns differ among EMG machines (Fig. 12-5). During algorithm development, the various parameters within the algorithm are adjusted until the resultant marks match those set manually by experienced electromyographers.[1] Little information about the marking algorithms accompanies EMG machines, and there is no ability to change marking parameters. Comparisons between EMG machines and their marking algorithms for MUAP duration show clinically significant differences, including those in other

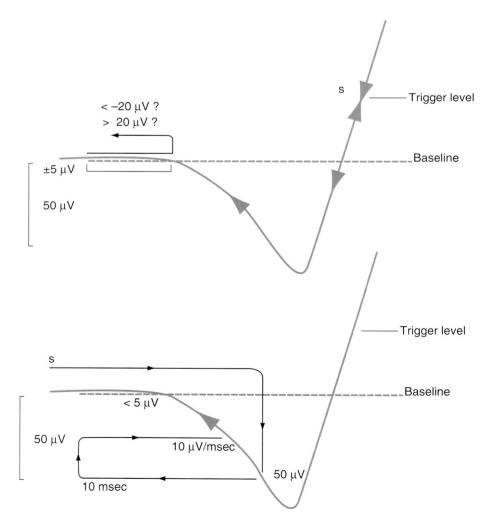

FIGURE 12-5 ■ Automated algorithms for determining motor unit action potential onset and endpoints. Top: Determining the onset: starting from the trigger point, the earlier portion of the signal is inspected to determine the first point that has less than ± 5 μV noise and a value less than ± 20 μV from the baseline. A similar algorithm is applied to determine the endpoint. Bottom: Determining the onset: starting from the trigger point, the earlier portion of the signal is inspected to determine the first point that has less than ± 5 μV noise and a slope that exceeds 10 μV/msec. A similar algorithm is applied to determine the endpoint. (Modified from Stålberg E, Andreassen S, Falck B et al: Quantitative analysis of individual motor unit potentials: a proposition for standardized terminology and criteria for measurement. J Clin Neurophysiol, 3:313, 1986.)

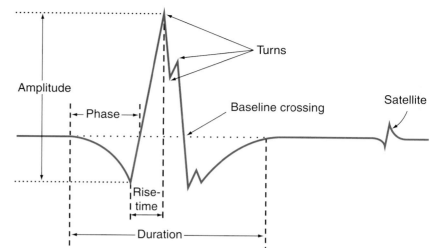

FIGURE 12-6 ■ Motor unit action potential metrics used in quantitative electromyography. Derived metrics include integrated waveform area and area/amplitude ratio.

metrics that are based on duration, such as area and area/amplitude ratio.[6,10] MUAP duration also affects how many phases are counted. Accordingly, it is most important to review each isolated MUAP and adjust markers as necessary.

The MUAP waveform can be analyzed and characterized by a number of metrics, including those based on physiologic features and derived features (Fig. 12-6).

The goal in selecting among various metrics is to distinguish normal from abnormal and, among abnormal, between neuropathic and myopathic disorders. However, only a relatively small number of MUAPs in a diseased muscle have abnormal waveforms and metrics, and there is overlap among traditional metrics of amplitude, duration, and number of phases between normal, neuropathic, and myopathic muscles (Fig. 12-7).[15] Although

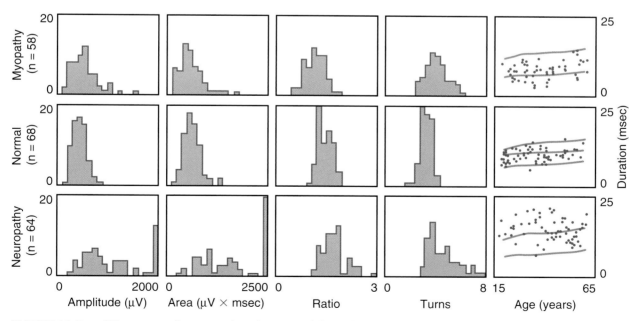

FIGURE 12-7 ■ Histograms of motor unit action potential metrics from biceps-brachialis muscle. Top row: Subjects with myopathic disorders. Middle row: Normal subjects. Lower row: Subjects with neuropathic disorders. First column: Amplitude. Second column: Area. Third column: Area/amplitude ratio. Fourth column: Number of turns. Fifth column: Duration scattergrams with mean value and 95 percent upper and lower limits from normal subjects superimposed on data from myopathic and neuropathic disorders. (From Stewart CR, Nandedkar SD, Massey JM et al: Evaluation of an automatic method of measuring features of motor unit action potentials. Muscle Nerve, 12:141, 1989, with permission.)

MUAP duration traditionally has been used to distinguish between neurogenic and myopathic motor units, determination of the onset and, particularly, the termination of the waveform is problematic. Waveform marking depends on display sensitivity, baseline noise, and marking algorithms. Efforts have been made to develop metrics that better distinguish between these pathologic states and normal. The ratio of the rectified area to the peak-to-peak amplitude has been found to have the least overlap and best discrimination.[15,16] Another approach is to define the range of normal metrics statistically and then assess a muscle to determine whether, among the 20 MUAPs studied, a sufficient number (percentage) of MUAPs have outlying metrics to indicate presence and type of abnormality.[17]

A quite different approach involves pattern discovery in the muscle under investigation based on comparisons with patterns of MUAP waveform features recorded from normal, neuropathic, and myopathic muscles, the latter two confirmed by pathology or genotyping. The pattern discovery is accomplished using Bayesian methods to characterize the muscle.[18,19] This can be used as a decision support aid for QEMG by providing probabilities that a muscle is normal or abnormal and the underlying pathology.

Automated QEMG is available on most commercial EMG machines, although the software may be offered as an option. QEMG can be applied readily during routine EMG studies, and is useful to help distinguish between normal and myopathic states, especially when clinical symptoms and signs are subtle. Familiarity with the particular technique is essential, as is the gathering of reference data from normal subjects in an index muscle. For the analysis of a myopathy, the biceps-brachialis muscle is a reasonable choice for an index muscle because the subject can exert a controlled contraction and it is a proximal muscle that usually is involved. Twenty or more MUAPs can be collected readily and inspected for marking accuracy. The summary statistics for amplitude, duration, area/amplitude ratio, and number of phases and turns can be compared with normal values.

INTERFERENCE PATTERN ANALYSIS

The QEMG methods described above refer to isolation and measurement of individual MUAPs. This must be carried out at low levels of contraction when individual potentials can be isolated and therefore may reflect a biased sample of MUAPs activated at the low end of the recruitment spectrum rather than an estimate of the full spectrum of MUAPs. Analysis of the interference pattern over a range of force levels was developed to discern rapid recruitment of complex MUAPs in myopathic disorders, and in particular to provide a quantitative way to identify MUAP abnormalities when they are of mild degree. Early efforts were semiautomated, with analysis performed offline, and provided data on the number of turns in the interference pattern and the mean amplitude between turns at different levels of force. Later efforts, aided by increasing use of digital computers, explored other metrics, such as integration or spectral analysis of the interference pattern, number of baseline crossings, discharge intervals, and assessment at set levels (forces) of contraction.[20] A robust approach is based on plotting turns/second against mean amplitude/turn at different force levels over the full range of force generation in normal muscle, resulting in a "cloud" of points (Fig. 12-8).[21] Clouds differ with gender, age, muscles, and types of EMG electrodes (concentric or monopolar), and confidence limits enclosing the clouds were derived from these combinations. Abnormal myopathic clouds are defined as more than 10 percent of 20 points below the normal cloud; abnormal neuropathic clouds have more than 10 percent of 20 points above the normal cloud. Later efforts used simulation data to construct interference patterns to identify unique metrics, but such measurements in clinical practice require special software, restricting their use.

SINGLE-FIBER EMG

The term *single-fiber EMG* (SF-EMG) refers to a number of electrodiagnostic techniques that rely on the use of a special needle electrode that has a very small recording surface located on the side of the cannula (see Fig. 12-1). The short recording radius (300 μm) of the electrode allows it to record single muscle fiber action potentials. Single-fiber electrodes can be used to collect several types of data: (1) variability of neuromuscular junction transmission at the level of a single junction or pairs of junctions; (2) fiber density—namely, the relative density of muscle fibers within a motor unit; and (3) macro-EMG, the MUAP representing activity of all muscle fibers in the motor unit by using a modification to a single-fiber electrode. Single-fiber electrodes are expensive but reusable. A special cable is required. Electrodes must be refurbished after 20 or so uses by sharpening the beveled tip and etching the recording surface.[22]

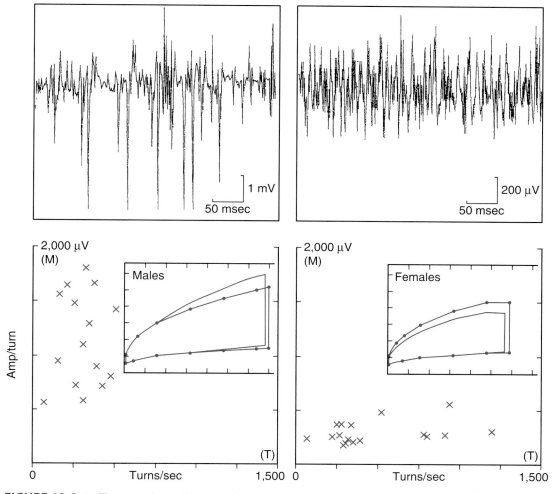

FIGURE 12-8 ▪ Turns and amplitude analysis of the interference pattern. Top panel: Trace of interference pattern. Lower panel: Plotting of average amplitude per turn against average turn per second. Left: Neuropathologic disrders. Right: Myopathic disorders. Insets labeled *Males* and *Females* refer to shapes of normal clouds that differ by gender, electrodes (filled dots outline clouds for concentric and outlines without symbols show clouds for monopolar electrodes), and muscle. (Inset from Stålberg E, Chu J, Bril V et al: Automatic analysis of the EMG interference pattern. Electroencephalogr Clin Neurophysiol, 56:672, 1983, with permission.)

Neuromuscular Jitter

The discharge-to-discharge variability inherent in transmission across the neuromuscular junction can be assessed when single-fiber action potentials are recorded. There are two techniques to activate transmission across the junction: one is to stimulate intramuscular nerve branches and record from single muscle fibers (called stimulation SF-EMG), and the other is to have the patient voluntarily activate motor units and record from pairs of muscle fibers from the same motor unit (called voluntary SF-EMG).[22] A degree of transmission variability is normal, and is called "jitter." Variability relates to several factors: (1) the range of conduction velocities along nerve terminal branches of varying length; (2) time differences in presynaptic mobilization and release of acetylcholine; (3) time differences in opening of postsynaptic acetylcholine receptors; and (4) the threshold for opening voltage-gated sodium channels. Normal jitter values are in the range of microseconds, are determined empirically, and differ by age and among muscles.[23,24] Excess variability reflects altered transmission, but is not specific for site of pathology (presynaptic or postsynaptic), and can be due to abnormalities in any one or a combination of the above sites. SF-EMG recording of jitter is discussed in detail in Chapter 17, but techniques that assess jitter using concentric or monopolar electrodes will be reviewed here.

Fiber Density

The arrangement of muscle fibers within a normal motor unit is not uniform, and few fibers of the same motor unit are contiguous. The number of muscle fibers recorded as a MUAP by an intramuscular electrode depends on the uptake radius of the electrode. Concentric and monopolar EMG needle electrodes have an uptake radius of approximately 1,500 μm and record activity from 7 to 15 fibers of a motor unit (see Fig. 12-1). Single-fiber needle electrodes have a restricted recording uptake radius of approximately 300 μm and record activity from 1 to 3 fibers.[22] The number of fibers in a normal motor unit varies among muscles, but it is estimated to range from 100 to 600 in muscles commonly studied. The routine MUAP waveform therefore reflects less than 10 percent of the total number of fibers of the motor unit. The single-fiber electrode offers a very restricted but detailed view. Advantage can be taken of the short recording radius of the single-fiber electrode to detect small changes in the density of muscle fibers within a motor unit, which thus is a sensitive measure of altered muscle architecture.

The configuration of a single-fiber electrode includes a 0.003-mm^2 active recording surface located in a side port approximately 5 mm from the beveled tip (see Fig. 12-1). The cannula serves as the reference electrode. Fiber density measurements are straightforward to perform on any EMG machine with a trigger and delay line. The low filter is set to 500 Hz, the sweep to 1 msec/div, and the display sensitivity at 100 μV/div. The procedure is to isolate a single-fiber action potential during weak voluntary activation. As an aid to isolation, the low-filter setting is raised to 500 Hz to reduce background slow-wave activity from distant muscle fibers. A voltage trigger and delay line are used to verify that the same index single-fiber action potential is observed from discharge to discharge. To ensure that the recording electrode is reasonably close to the index muscle fiber, the waveform rise-time must be less than 300 μsec and the amplitude greater than 200 μV. When the triggered waveform is stable over approximately 20 sweeps, the waveform is inspected to determine whether other potentials or components are associated with the index potential. Discrete inflections are counted as additional fibers (Fig. 12-9). The number of associated potentials reflects the fiber density of that motor unit. The electrode is moved and another index potential is isolated, and the average of 20 observations is used for the fiber-density value of the muscle.

Fiber density values reflect empiric data on the distribution of muscle fibers within motor units. Any muscle can be studied. Values vary among muscles and increase with age above 65 years, and this has been attributed to subclinical, age-related motor neuron loss (see Fig. 12-9). Tables of normal values reflect 95 percent confidence limits, and averaged values in a muscle that exceed these limits represent pathology (Table 12-3).[23,24]

The utility of fiber density measurement lies in its sensitivity to denervation and reinnervation and to changes in muscle fiber architecture. In neurogenic disorders (e.g., amyotrophic lateral sclerosis and neuropathy), fiber density values rise before other electrodiagnostic tests become abnormal.[25] This is attributed to increases in the number of innervated fibers within a motor unit from collateral reinnervation, and is the electrophysiologic equivalent of histologic fiber-type grouping.[26] Fiber density values are also increased in myopathic conditions. Explanations for these changes in myopathies include fiber splitting and ephaptic transmission between hyperexcitable fibers. Although increased fiber density is a very sensitive marker of neuromuscular disease, it is not specific for the kind of disease and must be considered in the clinical context.

Macro-EMG

The whole motor unit can be included in the recording radius if the cannula of the electrode is used as the active recording surface (see Fig. 12-1). Macro-EMG utilizes a special single-fiber electrode with the distal 15 mm of the cannula left bare as the recording surface and the more proximal segment insulated. The single-fiber port is 7.5 mm from the bevel. Two amplifiers are used (Fig. 12-10). The first amplifier is connected to the single-fiber electrode with the cannula as the reference electrode, as in routine single-fiber EMG. The electrode is adjusted to record an index muscle fiber of a motor unit during a weak voluntary contraction. Care is taken to orient the electrode perpendicular to the direction of muscle fibers in the muscle. The second amplifier is connected to the cannula as the active lead and a second remote electrode as the reference lead. Spike-triggered averaging using the discharge train from the index motor unit is used to extract the associated whole motor unit from background activity that includes many remote motor units. The macro-EMG signal emerges after about 100 averages. The needle is moved to another site, and the index potential is isolated and the cannula potential averaged. Twenty macro-EMG potentials are obtained and averaged.

Macro-EMG can be performed on any EMG machine that has two amplifiers and spike averaging capabilities. A special single-fiber macro-EMG electrode (and cable) is required.

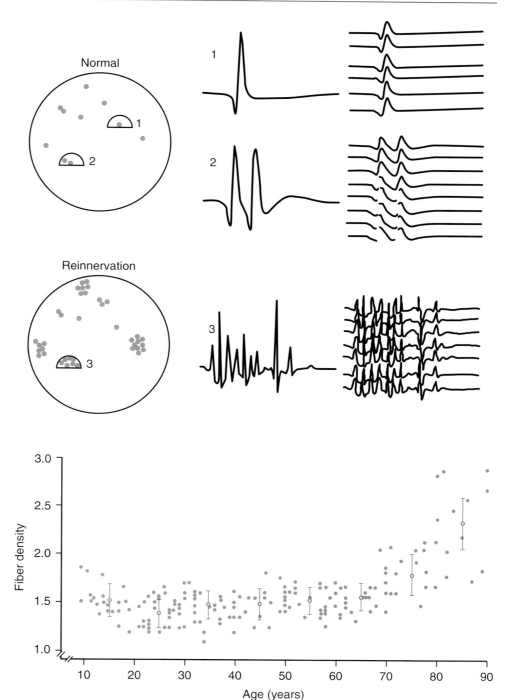

FIGURE 12-9 ■ Fiber density. Top panel: Normal fiber density. The semicircle represents the recording radius of a single-fiber electrode. Middle panel: Increased fiber density due to collateral reinnervation. Lower panel: Fiber density values from normal subjects of varying ages. (Modified from Stålberg E, Trontelj JV: Single Fiber Electromyography. Studies in Healthy and Diseased Muscle. Raven, New York, 1994.)

The macro-EMG waveform has relatively smooth contours, making the onset and termination points difficult to identify and the determination of duration unreliable (Fig. 12-11). Macro-EMG waveform area and amplitude are reported. The distribution of macro-EMG amplitudes may not be gaussian in some muscles, and the median value from 20 observations is used. Individual and median values from normal subjects increase with age, changing at age 65 years (see Fig. 12-11). Normal values reflect empiric data (Table 12-4).

A modification of the single-fiber macro-EMG electrode has been made in the form of a partially insulated concentric needle electrode, and is termed the "conmac electrode."[27] The recording amplifier and averaging techniques are similar to those used for single-fiber macro-EMG (see Fig. 12-10). The recording geometry

TABLE 12-3 ■ Mean Fiber Density Values: 95 Percent Upper Confidence Limit of Normal in Different Age Groups								
	1–10 yr	11–20 yr	21–30 yr	31–40 yr	41–50 yr	51–60 yr	61–70 yr	71–80 yr	81–90 yr
Frontalis	1.67	1.67	1.68	1.69	1.70	1.73	1.76		
Tongue	1.78	1.78	1.78	1.78	1.78	1.79	1.79		
SCM	1.89	1.86	1.90	1.92	1.96	2.01	2.08		
Deltoid	1.56	1.56	1.57	1.57	1.58	1.56	1.60	1.62	1.65
Biceps	1.52	1.52	1.53	1.54	1.57	1.60	1.65	1.72	1.80
EDC	1.77	1.78	1.80	1.83	1.90	1.99	2.12	2.29	2.51
ADQ	1.99	2.00	2.03	2.08	2.16	2.28	2.46		
Quadriceps	1.93	1.94	1.96	1.99	2.05	2.14	2.26	2.43	
Anterior tibial	1.94	1.94	1.96	1.98	2.02	2.07	2.15	2.26	
Soleus	1.56	1.56	1.56	1.57	1.56	1.62	1.66	1.71	

SCM, sternocleidomastoid; EDC, extensor digitorum communis; ADQ, abductor digiti quinti.

Data from: Ad Hoc Committee of the AAEM Special Interest Group on Single Fiber EMG: Single fiber EMG reference values: a collaborative effort. Muscle Nerve, 15:151, 1992; and Bromberg MB, Scott DM, Ad Hoc Committee of the AAEM Single Fiber Special Interest Group: Single fiber EMG reference values: reformatted in tabular form. Muscle Nerve, 17:820, 1994.

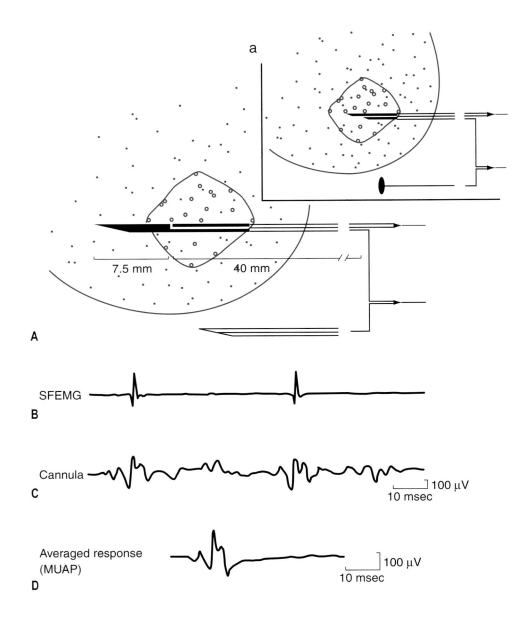

FIGURE 12-10 ■ Macro-electro-myography (EMG) recording arrangement. **A**, Special single-fiber electrode connected to two amplifiers. Single-fiber electrode port is connected to one amplifier with the cannula as the reference. The cannula is connected to the second amplifier with a second needle as the reference. **B**, Trace from single-fiber electrode amplifier showing single action potential. **C**, Trace from cannula electrode amplifier showing complex potential with many motor units. **D**, Averaged cannula potential revealing macro-EMG motor unit action potential. Inset a: Special concentric electrode used to record conmac potentials. (Modified from Stålberg E: Macro EMG. Muscle Nerve, 6:619, 1983.)

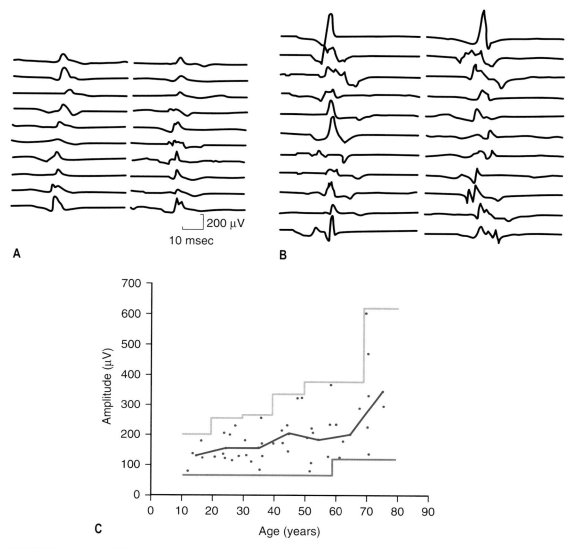

FIGURE 12-11 ■ Macro-electromyography (EMG) potentials. **A**, Normal subject. **B**, Subject with amyotrophic lateral sclerosis. **C**, Increase in macro-EMG with age. The dark line represents median values, and light lines represent limits of normal. (From Stålberg E, Fawcett PR: Macro EMG in healthy subjects of different ages. J Neurol Neurosurg Psychiatry, 45:870, 1982, with permission.)

is different, in that the concentric electrode is at the end of the 15-mm cannula recording surface and isolates an index MUAP with very short rise-times (less than 150 μsec). Despite differences in electrode configuration, data for amplitude and area are comparable between both types of macro-EMG electrodes. The conmac electrode allows comparisons between routine MUAPs recorded with concentric needle electrodes (reflecting the activity of 7 to 15 muscle fibers) and the conmac cannula potential (reflecting the activity of 600 to 1,000 fibers or the whole motor unit).[28] Concentric MUAP area is correlated better than amplitude with corresponding values obtained using the conmac electrode. The better correlation of area than

amplitude is attributed to the fact that MUAP amplitude recorded with a concentric electrode is influenced by the proximity of only 1 to 3 muscle fibers of the motor unit.

The utility of macro-EMG (either type) lies in its reflection of the size of whole motor units. The macro-EMG waveform amplitude is correlated with the number of fibers within the motor unit. Amplitude changes are less informative in myopathies because the low values obtained overlap with values from normal muscles. In denervating disorders, macro-EMG waveform amplitudes generally are increased as a result of collateral reinnervation. Fiber density and macro-EMG values are not always correlated; this is attributed to local variation in denervation–reinnervation

TABLE 12-4 ■ Macro-EMG Values: Median Amplitude of Normal (Based on 20 Observations)

	1–10 yr	11–20 yr	21–30 yr	31–40 yr	41–50 yr	51–60 yr	61–70 yr
Biceps	69	100	99	115	110	122	98
Vastus lateralis	112	163	156	151	166	203	208
Tibialis anterior	132	158	159	207	190	207	351

Data from Stålberg E, Fawcett PR: Macro EMG in healthy subjects of different ages. J Neurol Neurosurg Psychiatry, 45:870, 1982.

and to subsequent motor unit degeneration. Maximal macro-EMG waveform amplitudes reflect the degree of reinnervation and are high in slowly progressive forms of amyotrophic lateral sclerosis (10 to 21 times normal) and highest in static disorders such as old poliomyelitis (25 to 40 times normal).

JITTER MEASURED WITH CONCENTRIC OR MONOPOLAR ELECTRODES

Traditional jitter measurements are made with a single-fiber electrode, but past efforts to use monopolar and small concentric electrodes have been revisited recently due to concerns about transmissible infections with re-usable single-fiber electrodes despite sterilization. A distinction is made in the use of monopolar and small concentric electrodes for qualitative assessment of neuromuscular transmission variability (jiggle) during routine EMG studies and quantitative assessment (jitter). With qualitative assessment, default low-frequency filter settings of 10 to 20 Hz are used; the discharge-to-discharge variability of late MUAP waveform components reflects groups of muscle-fiber action potentials, and a number of neuromuscular junctions contribute to the variability.[8]

For quantitative measurements of jitter with a monopolar or small concentric electrode, the low-frequency filter is raised to 1,000 Hz to reduce the effects of low-frequency components. (In some laboratories it is raised to 2,000 or 3,000 Hz.) Waveforms for measurement must be selected with care, as the spikes for measurement can represent contributions from several muscle-fiber action potentials. Reference values are available and they differ from values obtained by single-fiber electrodes in being slightly lower.[9,29]

Fiber density cannot be measured with a concentric or monopolar electrode as the spike components isolated with these electrodes more often than not reflect a small group of muscle fibers.

The use of small concentric or monopolar electrodes expands the ready availability of QEMG; many studies, including automated motor unit analysis, interference pattern analysis, and measurement of jitter, can be performed rapidly with one electrode. QEMG tests can be selected based on the type of information needed. There are no significant differences in QEMG metrics when recorded with a small rather than a standard concentric electrode.[5]

SCANNING EMG

MUAPs from concentric, monopolar, or macro-EMG electrodes represent two-dimensional views of the motor unit. Scanning EMG is a technique that yields three-dimensional or electrophysiologic cross-sectional views of the motor unit. The procedure is to select a motor unit by recording an index single-fiber action potential with a single-fiber electrode. The single-fiber potential is used to trigger a delay line on another display screen. A concentric electrode is introduced 10 to 20 mm distant from the single-fiber electrode. The concentric electrode is adjusted until it records an MUAP that is time-locked to the single-fiber potential. The concentric electrode is advanced further until it no longer records the time-locked MUAP. It is then withdrawn in uniformly spaced steps and records the changing MUAP waveform configuration along the cross-section of the muscle. The data are processed to provide a three-dimensional display of the MUAP (Fig. 12-12).

The scanning EMG procedure is complex and is facilitated by a stepping motor to pull the electrode through the muscle in 50- to 100-μm steps. A computer is required to collect the 150 to 400 MUAP waveforms generated and to display the data. Data can be displayed as a three-dimensional plot where each waveform is displaced along the y-axis, or as a density or color-coded map (see Fig. 12-12). Although not amenable to routine electrodiagnostic use, scanning EMG provides a unique electrophysiologic view of the whole motor unit. The concept of a motor unit as the alpha motor neuron and all muscle fibers innervated by its terminal branches is straightforward, but it is challenging to view a single motor unit physically. Glycogen-depletion studies are the only anatomic method to determine the number, distribution, and territory of muscle fibers in a motor unit and their changes with denervation. These studies cannot be performed in human subjects. Scanning EMG provides an alternative method to study the distribution and territory of fibers in the motor unit and their changes

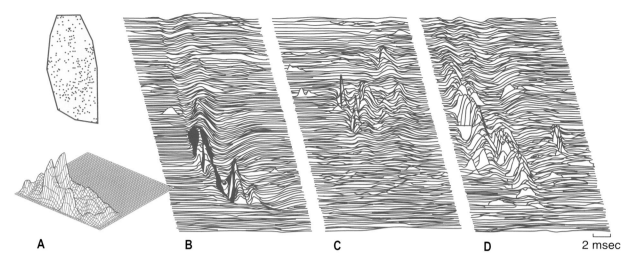

FIGURE 12-12 ■ Scanning electromyography (EMG). **A**, Single motor unit from glycogen depletion study in cat muscle. Upper figure encloses distribution of muscle fibers; lower, contour map based on fiber density. **B**, Scanning EMG from normal subject. **C**, Scanning EMG from subject with polymyositis. **D**, Scanning EMG from subject with amyotrophic lateral sclerosis. (*A*, Modified from Bodine-Fowler S, Garfinkel A, Roy RR, Edgerton VR: Spatial distribution of muscle fibers within the territory of a motor unit. Muscle Nerve, 13:1113, 1990; *B*, *C*, and *D*, Modified from Stålberg E: Single fiber EMG, macro EMG, and scanning EMG. New ways of looking at the motor unit. Crit Rev Neurobiol, 2:125, 1986, with permission.)

with denervation in human subjects. Data from scanning EMG can be compared to data from glycogen-depletion experiments (see Fig. 12-12).[11,30]

Scanning EMG has provided the following data about motor units. The normal motor unit has a cross-sectional diameter of 3 to 10 mm. (It should be noted that the scanning electrode corridor rarely coincides with the true diameter of the motor unit, and diameter values represent cords through the motor unit and underestimate the true diameter.) The three-dimensional plots include peaks and valleys of activity, representing the nonuniform distribution of innervated muscle fibers within the motor unit. In neuropathic disorders, the peaks are higher, reflecting collateral reinnervation (i.e., increased regional fiber densities); they are higher in slowly progressive than in rapidly progressive disorders (because of the greater time for full collateral reinnervation to occur). The overall motor unit diameter does not increase appreciably with reinnervation. There may be jumps in the potential, suggesting the passage of the electrode from a fascicle with innervated fibers to another fascicle without innervated fibers. Fascicular boundaries represent barriers to collateral reinnervation and explain why motor units do not expand their territories. In myopathic disorders, the peaks are of lower amplitude, but the diameter of the motor unit is not changed.

Scanning EMG plots represent MUAPs recorded from concentric or monopolar electrodes, and the larger view of the motor unit from scanning EMG can be used to assess how representative are data from routine EMG studies. During low levels of contraction, the first motor units observed represent the low-threshold motor units for that portion of the muscle only; other motor units in territories distant from the recording electrode may be activated at lower thresholds. The view of the motor unit from the arbitrary position of the electrode in its territory during a routine study may not include "pathologic" portions of the motor unit. Among patients with myopathic disorders (i.e., inflammatory myopathies and dystrophies), only 40 to 60 percent of scans are pathologic. In denervating disorders (e.g., amyotrophic lateral sclerosis), almost all scans include peaks with increased amplitude. These data emphasize the need in routine EMG to sample at least 20 motor units to obtain a representative view of the motor unit and not to miss pathology, especially in muscle disorders.

MOTOR UNIT NUMBER ESTIMATION

MUNE is a physiologic estimate of the number of motor units innervating a muscle or group of muscles. MUNE values are calculated from the ratio:

$$\frac{\text{Maximal CMAP amplitude or area}}{\text{Average SMUP amplitude or area}}$$

with CMAP indicating compound muscle action potential and SMUP the single surface-recorded motor unit potential.

MUNE is unique among QEMG studies in that it is the only electrodiagnostic test that can provide a quantitative estimate of this number; all other electrodiagnostic tests include the effects of collateral reinnervation or assess only a portion of a motor unit.

Principles of MUNE

The concept underlying the MUNE ratio is simple, but there are issues important to understanding and performing MUNE.[31,32]

MUSCLES STUDIED

MUNE is performed most commonly on distal upper-extremity muscles (i.e., median-innervated thenar eminence and ulnar-innervated hypothenar eminence muscles), although lower-extremity muscles can be studied with most techniques, and proximal muscles (e.g., biceps-brachialis and trapezius) can also be studied with certain techniques (Table 12-5).[32,33]

COMPOUND MUSCLE ACTION POTENTIAL

The maximal CMAP is determined by the same techniques used in routine motor nerve conduction studies. Recording electrodes are placed in a belly–tendon arrangement, and the nerve is activated electrically by percutaneous stimulation to achieve the maximal CMAP. Recording electrodes are left in place to record the surface representation of SMUPs. It is preferable that the active recording electrode be positioned optimally over the motor point to record a maximal CMAP amplitude, and this position is associated with a steep waveform rise-time.[34] Variation from the optimal placement of the active recording electrode, with respect to MUNE

estimates, will be manifest equally in CMAP and SMUP waveforms, and MUNE values will not be affected.[35]

SMUP WAVEFORMS

Individual SMUP waveforms vary in size and shape, but typically have an initial negative deflection followed by a terminal positive deflection (Fig. 12-13). Occasional SMUPs are recorded that have almost entirely positive waveforms. These are considered most likely to represent volume-conducted motor units from adjacent muscles, and usually are not included in calculating the average SMUP value.[36] SMUP waveform duration cannot be measured accurately because of difficulties in determining onset and termination points. Peak-to-peak amplitude, negative-peak amplitude, and negative-peak area are measured readily.

The distribution of SMUP amplitudes from normal muscle spans one order of magnitude, from approximately 20 to 200 μV peak-to-peak amplitude.[35] Occasionally, very-low-amplitude SMUPs are recorded, but they are considered likely to represent motor units from distant muscles. Accordingly, SMUPs with negative-peak amplitudes of less than 10 μV, or with negative-peak areas less than 25 μV*msec, are not included in calculating the average SMUP value.[36]

PHASE CANCELLATION

MUNE values can be calculated using a variety of CMAP and SMUP metrics, including peak-to-peak amplitude, negative-peak amplitude, and negative-peak area values. The effects of phase cancellation can result in MUNE value differences of up to 35 percent when different metrics are used (see Fig. 12-13).[37] All metrics of the maximal CMAP incorporate the effects of phase

---

TABLE 12-5 ■ MUNE Techniques: Advantages and Disadvantages

MUNE Technique	Advantages	Disadvantages
Incremental stimulation	Applicable to any EMG machine	Alternation leads to an overestimate of the MUNE
	Passive testing: patient cooperation not necessary	Applicable to distal muscles
Multiple-point stimulation	Applicable to any EMG machine	Applicable to distal muscles
	Avoids alternation	
	Passive testing: patient cooperation not necessary	
F-wave		Difficult to ensure that SMUP waveforms are identified
Statistical	Samples range of nerve fibers	Assumes Poisson statistics
	Passive testing: patient cooperation not necessary	Requires proprietary software
		Applicable to distal muscles
Spike-triggered averaging	Applicable to distal and proximal muscles	Requires intramuscular needle EMG electrode
	Can provide quantitative intramuscular MUAP data	Active testing: requires patient cooperation

MUNE, motor unit number estimation; SMUP, surface-recorded motor unit potential; MUAP, motor unit action potential.

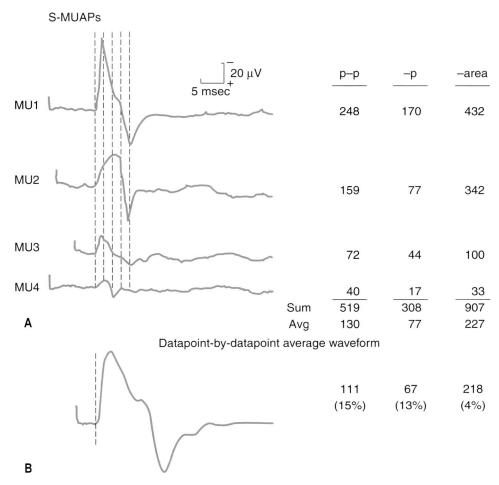

FIGURE 12-13 ■ Effects of phase cancellation on summation of surface-recorded motor unit potential (SMUP) waveforms. Four SMUP waveforms (labeled S-MUAPs) showing an initial negative deflection and later positive deflection. **A**, Waveforms aligned by onset, showing how phase cancellation could affect different methods used to calculate an average value. The table to the right indicates individual and averaged values as calculated from peak-to-peak amplitude (p–p), negative-peak amplitude (–p), and negative-peak (–area) metrics. **B**, Average SMUP waveform calculated by datapoint-by-datapoint averaging. The table to the right indicates averaged SMUP values by using different metrics. Percentages represent differences between simple arithmetic and datapoint-by-datapoint averaging. Note the use of the metric negative-peak area is affected least by phase cancellation. (From Doherty TJ, Stashuk DW, Brown WF: Determinants of mean motor unit size: impact on estimates of motor unit number. Muscle Nerve, 16:1326, 1993, with permission.)

cancellation between the constituent motor units that are caused by differences in conduction velocities of motor units from the site of stimulation to the recording electrode, and differences in the shapes of SMUPs (i.e., relative position of peak negativity and positivity within the waveform. The effect of differences in conduction velocity on phase cancellation will be least problematic if all waveforms, including the CMAP and all SMUPs, are obtained from one nerve stimulation electrode site along the nerve, and most problematic if different stimulation sites are used for the CMAP and SMUPs. One method to

neutralize the effect of different conduction velocities on phase cancellation is to obtain the maximal CMAP from a very distal stimulation site so as to minimize the effect of phase cancellation. With the aid of computer software, individual SMUP waveforms elicited by stimulation at different sites along the nerve can be aligned by onset of the negative deflection before carrying out point-by-point averaging (see Fig. 12-13).[36,37] This, in effect, sets the conduction distance to zero for averaging SMUPs but acknowledges that the CMAP conduction distance is several centimeters.

When manual calculation methods are used, the metric of peak-to-peak amplitude will be affected most by phase cancellation, producing an artificially high average SMUP value and an artificially low MUNE value. Metrics of negative-peak amplitude or negative-peak area are less affected by phase cancellation, but the position of peak negativity within individual SMUP waveforms represents phase cancellation and can affect arithmetic addition in determining the average SMUP.[37]

SMUP Sample Size and Bias

Normal muscles are innervated by different numbers of motor units, ranging from 100 to 600 motor units.[32] A sample of 10 to 20 SMUPs (less than 10 percent of the normal population) is sufficient, with little change in the calculated MUNE values when more than 15 SMUPs are used to determine the SMUP value.[38,39]

Sample bias is potentially more problematic. Most MUNE techniques rely on low-intensity electrical activation of the nerve to evoke SMUPs. Large-diameter axons have lower thresholds to electrical stimulation, suggesting a possible sampling bias to larger-amplitude SMUPs in MUNE techniques that use only low-current strengths. However, investigations comparing SMUP sizes obtained by a variety of MUNE techniques and modeling studies (see below) indicate little bias among them.[39,40] For MUNE techniques that rely on nerve stimulation, the overall geometry of the nerve (including orientation of fascicles and overlying tissue) neutralizes the relationship between axonal size and current intensity.

Test–Retest Reliability

Test–retest reliability has been assessed for most MUNE techniques in normal subjects and in those with denervation. When expressed as correlation coefficients, reliability is 15 to 20 percent. Of note, reliability is higher in denervating conditions when there are reduced numbers of motor units to sample.[38,39]

Independent Verification

There is no independent or anatomic method (i.e., "gold standard") to count motor axons innervating a muscle. MUNE values remain estimates.[32] Animal studies allow some degree of comparison between MUNE and anatomic verification, and show good correlations.[41] Human autopsy studies require assumptions about the percentages of motor efferent and muscle afferent fibers within a motor nerve, but also show good correlations.

MUNE Techniques

A number of MUNE techniques have been developed that differ in how SMUPs are obtained (see Table 12-5). Selection of a MUNE technique is guided by equipment availability, clinical experience, and study objectives. Direct comparisons show good concordance between techniques, with no technique markedly better than another.[39,40,42] Within a study, it is important to have internal validation of the chosen MUNE technique, including measures of test–retest reliability and comparisons with control subjects.

Incremental Stimulation MUNE

This is the original MUNE technique and is based on applying incremental increases in nerve stimulation intensity to generate an envelope of evoked responses. Each step in the envelope is considered to represent the activation of single motor axons that are added serially to the growing evoked response (Fig. 12-14).

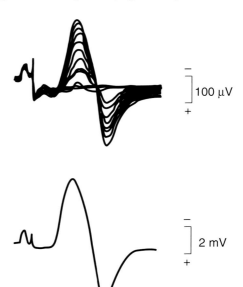

FIGURE 12-14 ■ Original figure of incremental stimulation motor unit number estimation (MUNE) technique. Top trace: Envelope of incremental responses of extensor digitorum brevis muscle following excitation of deep fibular nerve with threshold and slightly suprathreshold stimuli. Bottom trace: Maximal compound muscle action potential (CMAP). Peak-to-peak amplitude of envelope is 440 μV. Dividing by 11 steps in the envelope yields an average surface-recorded motor unit potential (SMUP) of 40 μV. Peak-to-peak amplitude of CMAP is 8,000 μV. Dividing by average SMUP gives an MUNE of 200. (Modified from McComas AJ, Fawcett PR, Campbell M et al: Electrophysiological estimation of the number of motor units within a human muscle. J Neurol Neurosurg Psychiatry, 34:121, 1971, with permission.)

Surface electrodes are placed and a maximal CMAP is recorded. The stimulating electrode remains fixed in the same position on the nerve. The display sensitivity is raised to 100 to 200 µV/div to help visualize low-amplitude steps in the response envelope. The stimulus intensity is lowered to 3 to 10 mA to activate the first axon, indicated by an all-or-none response. By small increases in stimulation intensity, an envelope of responses is obtained, with 8 to 10 discrete steps before the increments in the envelope become indistinguishable. The number of steps is divided into the peak-to-peak amplitude of the envelope to determine the average amplitude of each step. This average value represents the average SMUP, and is used to calculate the MUNE value.

The incremental stimulation technique can be used on any EMG machine. Because the stimulating electrode is fixed in the same position for the maximal CMAP and for determination of the average SMUP, the effects of phase cancellation caused by different axonal conduction velocities will be included in the CMAP and SMUP waveforms.

An axon does not have a discrete threshold current for activation, but activation follows an excitability curve from low probability of activation at lower currents to high probability at higher currents (Fig. 12-15). Thus, at a fixed current intensity within an excitability curve, an axon may or may not be excited with repeated stimuli. When a number of axons have similar and overlapping excitability curves, the steps in the envelope will reflect different combinations of axons being excited and not simply the serial addition of axons. This is termed *alternation* between different combinations of axons in the response. The result is uncertainty in the number of steps that truly are represented in the envelope; a larger number of perceived steps results in a smaller average SMUP and a larger MUNE value.

MULTIPLE-POINT STIMULATION MUNE

This technique was developed to avoid the problem of alternation by activating only single axons, one at a time. Different single SMUPs are obtained by moving the stimulating electrodes to different sites along the nerve.[39] Surface electrodes are placed and a maximal CMAP is recorded. The display sensitivity is raised to 50 to 100 µV/div to record low-amplitude SMUPs. The

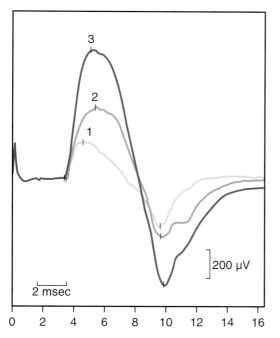
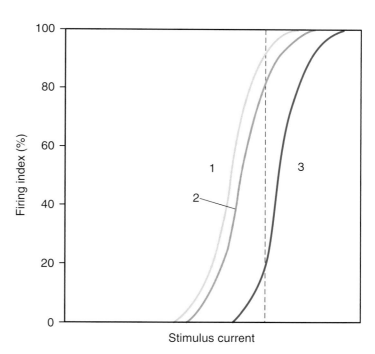

FIGURE 12-15 ▪ The effects of alternation on calculating average surface-recorded motor unit potential. Alternation reflects overlap of axon excitability curves with a different probability that each axon will discharge during a series of constant stimuli. Left: Three waveforms generated by slowly increasing the stimulation current. It is assumed that waveform number 3 represents the sum of responses from axons 1+2+3. Right: Excitability curves of axons 1, 2, and 3, showing that at a constant current intensity (dashed line) the probability of firing for each axon is less than 100 percent. Waveform number 3 elicited at the current intensity indicated by the dashed line could represent the sum of responses from axons 1+2+3, axons 1+3 or 1+2, or axon 3 alone. Uncertainty in the number of axons contributing to the total response affects calculation of the average response.

stimulus intensity is lowered to 3 to 10 mA to activate the first axon. This is verified by an all-or-none response to raising and lowering the stimulation current (Fig. 12-16). The stimulating electrode is moved to a different site along the nerve and another all-or-none response is obtained. Ten to 15 responses are collected and averaged to obtain the average SMUP used to calculate the MUNE value.

The multiple-point stimulation technique avoids the problem of alternation. It can be used on any EMG machine. A suitable number of stimuli must be delivered to ensure that the response represents a single axon; two axons with similar excitability curves could be activated together as a single response most of the time, and fractionation of the response into two SMUPs might become apparent only if a suitable number of stimuli (i.e., greater than 10) are given. Because the stimulating electrode is moved to different sites along the nerve to obtain single SMUPs, alignment of SMUPs by their onset and point-by-point averaging is preferable. With automatic averaging,

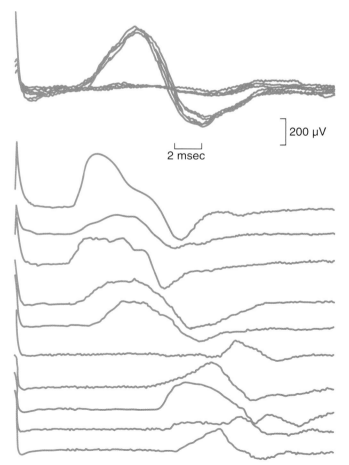

FIGURE 12-16 ■ Multiple-point stimulation technique for motor unit number estimation. Top: All-or-none response. Bottom: surface-recorded motor unit potential waveforms obtained from stimulating at multiple points along the nerve.

the metric of negative-peak area or amplitude is reasonable to reduce the effects of phase cancellation from late-arriving waveforms.

In the multiple-point stimulation technique, SMUPs usually are obtained one at a time, which can be time-consuming, but a technical modification called *adapted multiple-point stimulation* (AMPS) has been developed that combines incremental and multiple-point stimulation techniques.[43] At each site along the nerve, the stimulation intensity is raised to obtain a two- or three-step envelope. Template subtraction is used to separate individual SMUP waveforms to exclude the effects of alternation.

A suitable number of SMUPs can be obtained from five or six stimulation sites along the nerve, reducing the time required for the study. However, the process of template subtraction requires special software. A more simple variant of the AMPS technique is to record an envelope of three steps at three or more stimulation sites along the nerve. The average SMUP at each site is calculated by dividing the third, largest response, by 3; and the overall average SMUP is the average from each stimulation site divided into the CMAP to obtain the MUNE value. As originally proposed, three stimulation sites were recommended. A comparison of MUNE test–retest reproducibility values by using the average SMUP obtained at three to six stimulation sites in normal subjects showed sequentially improved reproducibility with the addition of a fourth stimulation site, but lesser improvements with the inclusion of additional sites.[44]

Another modification of the AMPS technique uses a high-density recording electrode array with up to 120 small electrodes across the muscle.[45,46] The electrode array allows for both temporal and spatial identification of motor unit responses with the ability to detect alternation. This allows for identification of up to 12 motor units within the incremental stimulation envelope, but typically 4 to 5 units can be isolated. MUNE values are higher with this electrode, attributed to the isolation of smaller motor units than with larger recording electrodes. The electrode array and amplifiers represent special equipment.

F-WAVE MUNE

This technique takes advantage of the low probability of antidromic activation of axons to isolate SMUPs.[47] Surface electrodes are placed and a maximal CMAP is recorded. Either the display sensitivity is raised to 200 to 500 µV/div, and the time base increased to 5 or 10 msec/div, or the F-wave program software in the EMG machine is selected (Fig. 12-17). The stimulus

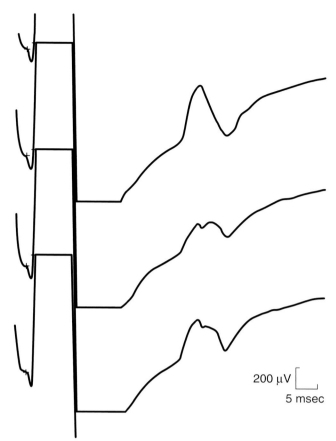

FIGURE 12-17 ■ F-wave technique for motor unit number estimation. Only the first waveform may represent a single surface-recorded motor unit potential (SMUP), whereas the second and third waveforms likely represent several superimposed SMUPs.

200 µV
5 msec

intensity is adjusted to produce a CMAP or M wave of 50 percent or greater of maximum, and a sufficient number of stimuli are delivered to collect 10 to 15 responses that are felt to represent different single F-wave responses.

F-responses occur in 1 to 3 percent of activated axons. If 100 axons or more are activated with nerve stimulation, the F-response waveforms likely represent the simultaneous discharge of more than one axon. Accordingly, it is difficult to be sure that the amplitude or area of an F-response waveform reflects a SMUP rather than the sum of two or more F-responses. The approach to help ensure that individual F-wave responses are identified is to collect a large number of F-responses and search for responses that repeat at least three times. The assumption is that the probability of the same combination of two or more axons being activated antidromically three times is very low, and therefore any identical waveform that occurs three times is more likely to represent the response of a single axon. However, the process of manually comparing a large series of F-wave responses to search for

repeaters is extremely time-consuming. Computer algorithms have been written to match waveform templates, but are not currently available.[48]

STATISTICAL *MUNE*

The statistical technique is a novel approach that uses Poisson statistics to determine the average response based on the variability of the response.[49,50] When multiple stimuli are delivered at a constant stimulation intensity, the evoked response varies from trial to trial (envelope of responses). It can be assumed that this response variability reflects the addition and loss of axons to the response, and thus represents the phenomenon of alternation. Poisson statistics assume that the underlying changes represent discrete steps or axonal responses, and the statistical variance of the amplitude of the response over many trials is equal to the mean value of the change in the response, which is the average value of the SMUP.

Surface electrodes are placed and a maximal CMAP is recorded. The stimulating electrode is fixed and the nerve is "scanned" with a series of 30 stimuli delivered with increasing intensity from just subthreshold to just maximal to generate the total envelope of evoked responses (Fig. 12-18). This scan of the evoked response is used to identify portions of the response envelope that will be sampled. Usually three or four regions are sampled to determine the variance and SMUP amplitude value at each of these regions. The variance of the response in each region is determined by applying sets of 30 stimuli. For each set of 30 stimuli, the variance is calculated and an average SMUP area is determined. Repeated sets of 30 stimuli are performed until the standard error of the different determinations is less than 10 percent. The subject must remain at complete rest to prevent adventitious movement artifacts affecting the amplitude of the envelope.

The average SMUP determined in a region then is used to calculate a MUNE value for that region. The other designated regions are sampled similarly. The regions selected for detailed study from the scan curve include regions with large steps reflecting large-amplitude motor units, and one "average" region considered to represent the unsampled region. The MUNE value then is calculated for the unsampled region using the smallest average SMUP value. Finally, all regional and unsampled MUNE values are combined for a total MUNE value.

Alternation is the major issue in the incremental stimulation MUNE technique, but it is the basis of the statistical technique. The incremental and multiple-point stimulation MUNE techniques rely on electrical

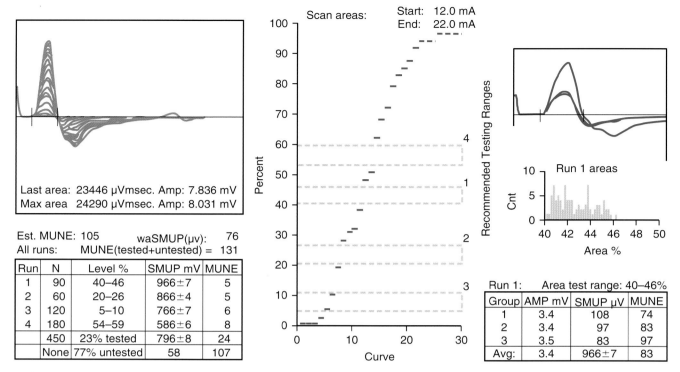

FIGURE 12-18 ■ Statistical technique for motor unit number estimation (MUNE). Upper left panel: compound muscle action potential (CMAP) scan envelope from threshold to supramaximal response evoked by 30 graded stimuli. Middle panel: Same scan, but CMAP amplitudes (small horizontal marks) are displayed as percentage of maximal response. Note four regions selected by the algorithm for determining response variances. Right panel: Top portion shows maximal CMAP and envelope of responses evoked by sets of 30 stimuli at a constant intensity to determine variance in zone 4. Middle plot shows the response in histogram format to determine whether the distribution of responses is skewed appropriately to the left. Lower chart shows calculated variance of the response to sets of 30 stimuli. The variance is equal to the mean change in response amplitude, which is considered to reflect the average surface-recorded motor unit potential (SMUP) amplitude for that region. A corresponding MUNE value is calculated. Three sets (groups) of 30 stimuli were required for the standard error to be less than 10 percent of the mean value (96 ± 7). Lower left panel: Results of testing all four regions (runs). A MUNE value is calculated for each region and summed to give an overall MUNE value for the total percentage of the CMAP tested (23 percent). The untested percentage (77 percent) is assumed to be innervated by the smallest SMUPs, and a MUNE value is calculated accordingly. Tested and untested regions are summed for a final MUNE value of 131. An alternative method is to weigh the tested regions to determine SMUP value (waSMUP). This value is used to calculate an estimated MUNE value. See the text for differences in final MUNE values by the different techniques.

activation of low-threshold axons, whereas in the statistical technique a wide range of axon thresholds and their SMUPs is sampled. Comparison studies between MUNE techniques do not support a significant bias caused by axon diameter because the electrical threshold of an axon has greater dependence on the overall tissue impedance to stimulus current flow around the nerve than the simple axon excitability threshold.[32] A degree of statistical robustness is included in the determination of the average SMUP for each region by applying sets of 30 stimuli repeatedly until the standard error of the response is less than 10 percent of the mean response. The stimulating electrode is fixed for the maximal CMAP and all subsequent determinations, and the

effects of phase cancellation caused by different axonal conduction velocities over different conduction distances are incorporated in the waveforms. Negative-peak area is the metric used in all calculations.

The statistical technique requires proprietary software available on a single brand of EMG machine. SMUP values calculated from the variance of the response represent putative values and not physiologic single motor unit potentials as obtained from the other MUNE techniques. An assumption of Poisson statistics is that the distribution of response amplitudes is skewed to the left, but that does not always occur during the 30 stimuli. Several methods have been used to adjust the stimulus intensity to force a skewed distribution.[50,51] With denervation, there is a reduced number of motor units, and some are enlarged from collateral reinnervation. This appears in the scan curve as large jumps in the amplitude. A number of modifications have been proposed to determine which regions of the scan curve should be tested and the size of the tested regions.[51,52] The proprietary software automatically selects regions to be tested, and each region includes about 6 percent of the total CMAP amplitude. The software also allows the operator to determine regions. One paradigm uses four set regions: (1) 15 to 25 percent; (2) 25 to 35 percent; (3) 35 to 45 percent; and (4) 45 to 55 percent of the total CMAP.[51] There are a number of different methods to calculate average SMUP values that are used to determine the final MUNE. One source of variability in the final MUNE value is reliance on the smallest SMUP value to calculate the MUNE for the untested regions of the CMAP. A modification weights the SMUP values obtained from the tested regions to obtain a more representative average SMUP value (see Fig. 12-18).[53] There are modifications to the original method to calculate the average SMUP to adjust and account for large and small motor units.[42,50] The large number of variables in how data are obtained and calculated with the statistical technique influences the final MUNE calculation, and MUNE values from the same normal subject can vary by more than 30 percent when different calculation methods are used.[50]

Practical experience has accumulated with the statistical technique as a secondary endpoint measurement in several multicenter drug trials in amyotrophic lateral sclerosis.[46,54] A number of subjects with amyotrophic lateral sclerosis were found to have putative SMUP values lower than those in normal subjects, contrary to what would be expected as the consequence of motor unit loss with enlargement of remaining motor units. The lower SMUP values were attributed to amplitude variability from insecure neuromuscular transmission leading to intermittently blocked transmission—the algorithm mistakenly attributed this variability to a small SMUP.[55]

The statistical technique relies upon Poisson statistics to calculate putative SMUP values. However, it is unclear whether the necessary assumptions to use Poisson statistics reliably are met. These include the assumptions that the number of motor units firing probabilistically at a given stimulus intensity has a Poisson distribution and that all motor units have the same size. A new approach has been developed using a Bayesian approach that attempts to incorporate causes of uncertainty before and after data are collected.[56] Areas of uncertainty include the number of motor units and variability between and within motor units, and these uncertainties are expressed as a probability. In the Bayesian approach, biologic knowledge of unknown factors is expressed as a series of prior distributions and acquired data are used to update the distributions.

CMAP Scan

The initial step in the statistical technique is a scan of the nerve under study, produced by increasing stimulating currents in 30 steps from below threshold to maximal, assessing for jumps or gaps in the sigmoid CMAP curve (see Fig. 12-18). The number and size of the gaps are used to set the stimulating currents. By increasing the number of stimulation increments from 30 to 250 or 500, a detailed view of the constituent axons and motor units can be obtained.[57] A scan of 500 stimuli of increasing or decreasing intensity has a smooth sigmoid shape in normal nerves (Fig. 12-19). In contrast, when there are fewer motor units, with subsequent enlargement of units from denervating disease, there are gaps. When motor unit loss is severe (15 to 20 motor units remaining), a MUNE can be made by counting the gaps. Less severe loss can be detected by changes in the shape and width of the curve. Further, differences in axonal excitability from demyelinating neuropathies can be detected by changes in the shape of the curve.

Spike-Triggered Averaging MUNE

The spike-triggered averaging technique is unique in that SMUPs are activated by weak voluntary contraction of the muscle. Surface electrodes are placed and a maximal CMAP is recorded. Two recording channels and electrodes are used, one for an intramuscular electrode and the other for the surface electrode used to record the CMAP and SMUPs. A weak interference pattern is generated and the intramuscular electrode is adjusted to isolate the discharge of one motor unit (Fig. 12-20). A voltage level trigger is set to detect the motor unit's discharge pattern, and the trigger signals from that motor unit are used for spike-triggered averaging of the surface response of the motor unit. The electrode is moved to a different site in the muscle and another SMUP is obtained. Ten to 15 responses are collected and averaged to obtain the average SMUP used to calculate the MUNE value.

This MUNE technique can be applied to proximal muscles because only limited access to the nerve is required to generate a maximal CMAP, whereas longer lengths of nerve are required for the controlled stimulation protocols with the other techniques. Care must be taken to avoid spurious trigger potentials during spike-triggered averaging.[35] There is concern about a sampling bias to early

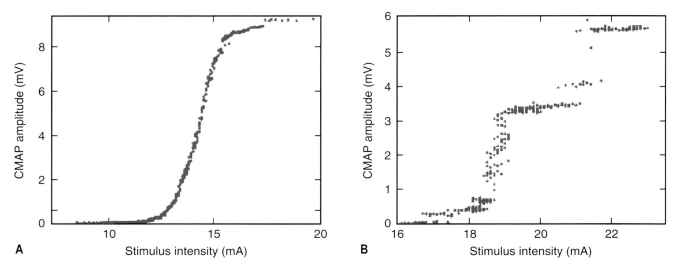

FIGURE 12-19 ▪ Compound muscle action potential (CMAP) scan: curve of growing CMAP amplitude with increasing stimulation intensity from submaximal to maximal. **A**, Normal scan with smooth sigmoid curve and narrow width. **B**, Abnormal scan with reduced numbers of axons causing jumps or gaps due to enlarged motor units and greater curve width. (Modified from Blok JH, Ruitenberg A, Maathuis EM et al: The electrophysiological muscle scan. Muscle Nerve, 36:436, 2007, with permission.)

recruited motor units that might be of lower amplitude than later recruited motor units; however, comparison studies between different MUNE techniques indicate no significant bias.[39,40] The intramuscular electrode can also be used to obtain a full range of MUAP QEMG metrics.

A modification has been made to increase the yield of SMUPs by incorporating decomposition algorithms to isolate 4 to 10 MUAPs from one interference pattern, and their discharge trains are used for spike-trigger averaging to obtain corresponding SMUPs for each MUAP.[58-60] In addition to increasing the yield of SMUPs, decomposition-enhanced spike-triggered averaging includes motor units recruited at higher thresholds than with conventional spike-triggered averaging (Fig. 12-21).

The average SMUP size increases with higher levels of recruitment in normal subjects and should be standardized. As discussed with decomposition MUAP analysis, the root-mean-square of the surface EMG signal can be used to monitor and standardize the level of contraction and motor unit recruitment.[12]

UTILITY OF QEMG

QEMG includes a range of techniques that yield a variety of data about the motor unit that are not available from routine EMG. The availability of QEMG software programs on many EMG machines facilitates its use as an extension of routine EMG studies, particularly in borderline cases in which subjective and qualitative analysis gives equivocal results. Some laboratories incorporate a variety of QEMG techniques in a protocol used to study every muscle.[61] Perhaps the most useful QEMG techniques are automated MUAP analysis and interference pattern analysis. Advantages of automated MUAP analysis include a large sample of MUAPs gathered in a short time, less bias toward particular MUAPs (those with high amplitude or greater complexity), and greater objectivity and reproducibility. Advantages of interference pattern analysis are assessment of the full range of motor units. As with routine electrodiagnostic tests, a basic understanding and experience with the techniques are necessary to interpret QEMG data accurately. Differences among QEMG algorithms result in different MUAP values, and reference values should be obtained for a particular algorithm.[10] There have been no direct comparisons of diagnostic sensitivity between routine and QEMG techniques, but comparisons of data from a variety of QEMG techniques against data in the literature from routine studies indicate good agreement and clarify which metrics are most informative.[62] Expert systems are in the early stages of development but hold promise for accurate classification of MUAP data.

Specialized QEMG tests, such as fiber-density and macro-EMG, have limited applications. Fiber-density measurements can be performed readily when there is a need to determine if there is subtle denervation.

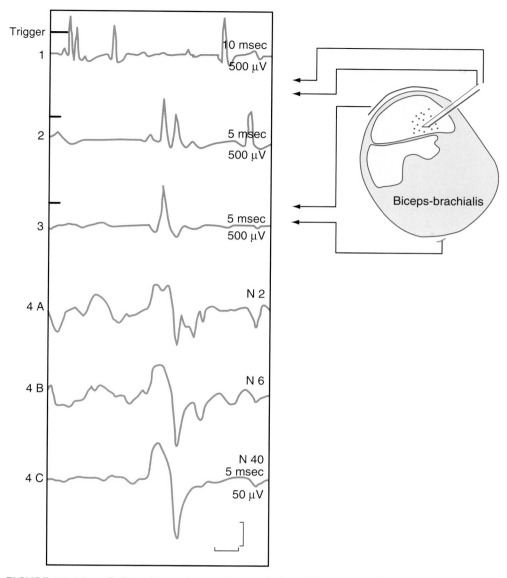

FIGURE 12-20 ▪ Spike-triggered averaging technique for motor unit number estimation. Right figure: Arrangement of intramuscular and surface recording electrodes and amplifiers. Trace 1: Intramuscular needle electromyography (EMG) signal in free-run mode. Trace 2: Intramuscular needle EMG signal with isolation of single motor unit potential (SMUP) by voltage trigger and delay line. Trace 3: Averaged intramuscular motor unit action potential. Trace series 4: Surface recording signal with spike-triggered averaging from intramuscular EMG signal. 4A: averaged 2 times (N : 2) with contamination by background activity. 4B: averaged 6 times (N : 6). 4C: averaged 40 times (N : 40) with clear SMUP waveform.

Macro-EMG is useful if there is need to demonstrate chronic denervation. MUNE is a unique electrodiagnostic technique in its ability to assess the degree of denervation, and is useful in the diagnosis of amyotrophic lateral sclerosis. It is being used as an endpoint measure in clinical drug trials for motor neuron disease, including amyotrophic lateral sclerosis and spinal muscular atrophy.

As a research tool, QEMG provided the foundation data for interpreting all routine EMG tests. Automated MUAP analysis has refined our understanding of motor unit changes with disease, and has pointed out which metrics are most informative.[15] Macro-EMG and scanning EMG have improved our understanding of the structure of the motor unit. QEMG studies have led to computer simulation studies that have expanded our understanding of what elements of the motor unit are recorded with routine and special electrodes, and how they change with disease.

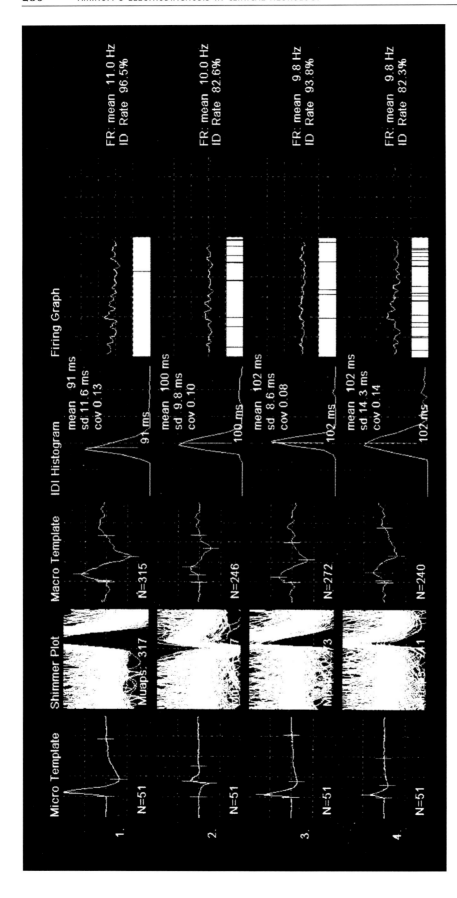

FIGURE 12-21 ■ Decomposition-enhanced spike-triggered averaging technique for motor unit number estimation. "Micro template" panel: Four intramuscular motor unit potentials isolated by the decomposition algorithm and averaged 51 times. "Shimmer plot" panel: Superimposition of all isolated motor unit potentials. "Macro template" panel: Surface motor unit potentials associated with corresponding intramuscular potentials and averaged the indicated number of times. "IDI histogram" panel: Inter-discharge interval (IDI) histogram of each motor unit discharge. "Firing graph" panel: Histogram display of same data. "FR and ID rate" panel: Mean firing rate and identification (ID) rate for isolated motor units.

REFERENCES

1. Stalberg E, Nandedkar SD, Sanders DB et al: Quantitative motor unit potential analysis. J Clin Neurophysiol, 13:401, 1996

2. Stålberg E, Andreassen S, Falk B et al: Quantitative analysis of individual motor unit potentials: a proposition for standardized terminology and criteria for measurement. J Clin Neurophysiol, 3:313, 1986

3. Pino LJ, Stashuk DW, Boe SG et al: Motor unit potential characterization using "pattern discovery". Med Eng Phys, 30:563, 2008

4. Dumitru D, King JC, Nandedkar SD: Motor unit action potential duration recorded by monopolar and concentric needle electrodes. Physiologic implications. Am J Phys Med Rehabil, 76:488, 1997

5. Brownell AA, Bromberg MB: Comparison of standard and pediatric size concentric needle EMG electrodes. Clin Neurophysiol, 118:1162, 2007

6. Bromberg MB, Smith AG, Bauerle J: A comparison of two commercial quantitative electromyographic algorithms with manual analysis. Muscle Nerve, 22:1244, 1999

7. Bromberg M: Electromyographic (EMG) findings in denervation. Crit Rev Phys Rehabil Med, 5:83, 1993

8. Stålberg E, Sonoo M: Assessment of variability in the shape of the motor unit action potential, the "jiggle", at consecutive dishcharges. Muscle Nerve, 17:1136, 1994

9. Stålberg EV, Sanders DB: Jitter recordings with concentric needle electrodes. Muscle Nerve, 40:331, 2009

10. Brownell AA, Ni O, Bromberg MB: Comparison of three algorithms for multi-motor unit detection and waveform marking. Muscle Nerve, 33:538, 2006

11. Engstrom JW, Olney RK: Quantitative motor unit analysis: the effect of sample size. Muscle Nerve, 15:277, 1992

12. Boe SG, Stashuk DW, Brown WF et al: Decomposition-based quantitative electromyography: effect of force on motor unit potentials and motor unit number estimates. Muscle Nerve, 31:365, 2005

13. Boe SG, Rice CL, Doherty TJ: Estimating contraction level using root mean square amplitude in control subjects and patients with neuromuscular disorders. Arch Phys Med Rehabil, 89:711, 2008

14. Bischoff C, Stålberg E, Falck B et al: Reference values of motor unit action potentials obtained with multi-MUAP analysis. Muscle Nerve, 17:842, 1994

15. Stewart CR, Nandedkar SD, Massey JM et al: Evaluation of an automatic method of measuring features of motor unit action potentials. Muscle Nerve, 12:141, 1989

16. Sonoo M, Stålberg E: The ability of MUP parameters to discriminate between normal and neurogenic MUPs in concentric EMG: analysis of the MUP "thickness" and the proposal of "size index". Electroencephalogr Clin Neurophysiol, 89:291, 1993

17. Stålberg E, Bischoff C, Falck B: Outliers, a way to detect abnormality in quantitative EMG. Muscle Nerve, 17:392, 1994

18. Pino LJ, Stashuk DW, Boe SG et al: Probabilistic muscle characterization using QEMG: application to neuropathic muscle. Muscle Nerve, 41:18, 2010

19. Pino LJ, Stashuk DW, Podnar S: Probabilistic muscle characterization using quantitative electromyography: application to facioscapulohumeral muscular dystrophy. Muscle Nerve, 42:563, 2010

20. Fuglsang-Frederiksen A: The utility of interference pattern analysis. Muscle Nerve, 23:18, 2000

21. Stålberg E, Chu J, Bril V et al: Automatic analysis of the EMG interference pattern. Electroencephalogr Clin Neurophysiol, 56:672, 1983

22. Stålberg E, Trontelj JV, Sanders DB: Single Fiber EMG. 3rd Ed. Edshagen, Fiskebackskil, 2010

23. Gilchrist JC: Ad Hoc Committee of the AAEM Special Interest Group on Single Fiber EMG: Single fiber EMG reference values: a collaborative effort. Muscle Nerve, 15:151, 1992

24. Bromberg M, Scott D, Ad Hoc committee of the AAEM Single Fiber Special Interest Group: Single fiber EMG reference values: reformatted in tabular form. Muscle Nerve, 17:820, 1994

25. Stålberg E: Electrodiagnostic assessment and monitoring of motor unit changes in disease. Muscle Nerve, 14:293, 1991

26. Stålberg E, Karlsson L: Simulation of EMG in pathological situations. Clin Neurophysiol, 112:869, 2001

27. Jabre J: Concentric macro electromyography. Muscle Nerve, 14:820, 1991

28. Bauermeister W, Jabre JF: The spectrum of concentric macroEMG correlations. Part 1. Normal subjects. Muscle Nerve, 15:1081, 1992

29. Tutkavul K, Baslo MB: Reference voluntary jitter values using disposable monopolar needle electrodes in the extensor digitorum communis muscle. Clin Neurophysiol, 121:887, 2010

30. Bodine-Fowler S, Garfinkel A, Roy RR et al: Spatial distribution of muscle fibers within the territory of a motor unit. Muscle Nerve, 13:113, 1990

31. Slawnych MP, Laszlo CA, Hershler C: A review of techniques employed to estimate the number of motor units in a muscle. Muscle Nerve, 13:1050, 1990

32. McComas AJ: Motor unit estimation: methods, results, and present status. Muscle Nerve, 14:585, 1991

33. Lewis RA: Motor unit number estimation in the upper trapezius muscle. Suppl Clin Neurophysiol, 60:131, 2009

34. Bromberg MB, Spiegelberg T: The influence of active electrode placement on CMAP amplitude. Electroencephalogr Clin Neurophysiol, 105:385, 1997

35. Bromberg MB, Abrams JL: Sources of error in the spike-triggered averaging method of motor unit number estimation (MUNE). Muscle Nerve, 18:1139, 1995

36. Bromberg MB (ed): Motor Unit Number Estimation (MUNE). Elsevier, Amsterdam, 2003

37. Doherty T, Stashuk D, Brown W: Determinants of mean motor unit size: impact on estimates of motor unit number. Muscle Nerve, 16:1326, 1993

38. Bromberg MB: Motor unit estimation: reproducibility of the spike-triggered averaging technique in normal and ALS subjects. Muscle Nerve, 16:466, 1993

39. Doherty TJ, Brown WF: The estimated numbers and relative sizes of thenar units as selected by multiple point stimulation in young and older adults. Muscle Nerve, 16:355, 1993

40. Stein RB, Yang JF: Methods for estimating the number of motor units in human muscles. Ann Neurol, 28:487, 1990

41. Arasaki K, Tamaki M, Hosoya Y et al: Validity of electromyograms and tension as a means of motor unit number estimation. Muscle Nerve, 20:552, 1997

42. Lomen-Hoerth C, Olney RK: Comparison of multiple-point and statistical motor unit number estimation. Muscle Nerve, 23:1525, 2000

43. Wang FC, Delwaide PJ: Number and relative size of thenar motor units estimated by an adapted multiple point stimulation method. Muscle Nerve, 18:969, 1995

44. Goyal N, Salameh JS, Baldassari LE et al: Added sampling improves reproducibility of multipoint motor unit estimates. Muscle Nerve, 41:114, 2010

45. van Dijk JP, Blok JH, Lapatki BG et al: Motor unit number estimation using high-density surface electromyography. Clin Neurophysiol, 119:33, 2008

46. Shefner JM, Cudkowicz ME, Zhang H et al: The use of statistical MUNE in a multicenter clinical trial. Muscle Nerve, 30:463, 2004

47. Doherty TJ, Komori T, Stashuk DW et al: Physiological properties of single thenar motor units in the F-response of younger and older adults. Muscle Nerve, 17:860, 1994

48. Stashuk DW, Doherty TJ, Kassam A et al: Motor unit number estimates based on the automated analysis of F-responses. Muscle Nerve, 17:881, 1994

49. Daube JR: Estimating the number of motor units in a muscle. J Clin Neurophysiol, 12:585, 1995

50. Daube J: MUNE by statistical analysis. p. 51. In Bromberg M (ed): Motor Unit Number Estimation (MUNE). Elsevier, Amsterdam, 2003

51. Lomen-Hoerth C, Olney RK: Effect of recording window and stimulation variables on the statistical technique of motor unit number estimation. Muscle Nerve, 24:1659, 2001

52. Olney RK, Yuen EC, Engstrom JW: Statistical motor unit number estimation: reproducibility and sources of error in patients with amyotrophic lateral sclerosis. Muscle Nerve, 23:193, 2000

53. Shefner JM, Jillapalli D, Bradshaw DY: Reducing intersubject variability in motor unit number estimation. Muscle Nerve, 22:1457, 1999

54. Shefner JM, Cudkowicz ME, Zhang H et al: Revised statistical motor unit number estimation in the celecoxib/ALS trial. Muscle Nerve, 35:228, 2007

55. Jillapalli D, Shefner J: Single motor unit variability with threshold stimulation in patients with amyotrophic lateral sclerosis and normal subjects. Muscle Nerve, 30:578, 2004

56. Henderson RD, Ridall PG, Hutchinson NM et al: Bayesian statistical MUNE method. Muscle Nerve, 36:206, 2007

57. Blok JH, Ruitenberg A, Maathuis EM et al: The electrophysiological muscle scan. Muscle Nerve, 36:436, 2007

58. Stashuk D: Decomposition and quantitative analysis of clinical electromyographic signals. Med Eng Phys, 21:389, 1999

59. Doherty T, Stashuk D: Decomposition-based quantitative electromyography: methods and initial normative data in five muscles. Muscle Nerve, 28:204, 2003

60. Lawson VH, Bromberg MB, Stashuk D: Comparison of conventional and decomposition-enhanced spike triggered averaging techniques. Clin Neurophysiol, 115:564, 2004

61. Stålberg E, Falck B, Sonoo M et al: Multi-MUP EMG analysis—a two year experience in daily clinical work. Electroencephalogr Clin Neurophysiol, 97:145, 1995

62. Barkhaus P, Nandedkar S, Sanders D: Quantitative EMG in inflammatory myopathy. Muscle Nerve, 13:247, 1990

Nerve Conduction Studies

JASPER R. DAUBE and DEVON I. RUBIN

Nerve conduction studies assist in the evaluation of neuromuscular diseases by providing a physiologic assessment of the peripheral nerve, muscle, neuromuscular junction, dorsal root ganglion cell, and anterior horn cell. They provide the greatest help in assessing peripheral nerve disease. Motor nerve conduction studies assess motor axons by selectively recording muscle responses to nerve stimulation. Sensory nerve conduction studies assess sensory axons by stimulating or recording from peripheral nerves with predominantly sensory axons. Nerve conduction studies most often confirm a clinical diagnosis, but they are also valuable in:

1. Excluding other suspected disorders
2. Identifying unrecognized (subclinical) disorders
3. Localizing focal abnormalities along a nerve
4. Defining severity with objective measurements[1]
5. Characterizing abnormalities, such as conduction block or demyelination
6. Helping to distinguish axonal disorders from anterior horn cell, neuromuscular junction, muscle, and central disorders, and
7. Identifying anomalous innervation.

Motor nerve conduction studies were first described for clinical use in 1948.[2] Subsequent studies defined normal values and the abnormalities seen in clinical disorders.[2] Motor nerve conduction studies have expanded steadily in application since then. Sensory nerve conduction studies initially were demonstrated experimentally by Dawson and Scott in 1949, and were shown to be of clinical value in 1958 by Gilliatt and Sears.[2] Sensory nerve action potentials (SNAPs) are of much lower amplitude than compound muscle action potentials (CMAPs) and are sometimes below the level of noise and artifact in the recordings. Averaging of multiple potentials is often required to record them reliably, particularly at proximal locations.

MOTOR NERVE CONDUCTION STUDIES

The motor axons of any peripheral nerve that innervates somatic muscle can be evaluated by motor nerve conduction studies if the nerve can be stimulated and if the response of one or more muscles innervated by that nerve can be recorded electrically. Standard studies of motor nerve conduction assess the most accessible nerves (i.e., the ulnar and median nerves in the upper extremities and the tibial and fibular [peroneal] nerves in the lower extremities). Reliable motor nerve conduction studies also can be performed on the musculocutaneous, radial, facial, spinal accessory, axillary, suprascapular, femoral, phrenic and spinal nerves, but with increasing technical difficulty.

Stimulation of any of these nerves evokes both an electrical and a mechanical response in the muscles innervated by the nerve distal to the site of stimulation. The mechanical response, or muscle twitch, is not recorded in standard clinical nerve conduction studies, but it may be measured for constructing strength–duration curves or for other special studies. The electrical response is called the compound muscle action potential (Fig. 13-1). It is the summated electrical activity of the muscle fibers that are in the region of the recording electrode and that are innervated by the nerve. The general techniques of stimulating and recording are similar for all motor nerves.

Stimulation

Nerve stimulation is achieved most readily with surface electrodes placed over a nerve where it is relatively superficial, such as over the ulnar nerve at the wrist and elbow. If there is overlying edema or fatty tissue, or if the nerve is deep, a needle electrode permits more precise stimulation with a lower voltage, with only minimal risk of trauma to neighboring structures.

The standard stimulus is a square-wave pulse of current passing between two poles; the cathode (−) depolarizes the underlying axons, while the anode (+) hyperpolarizes

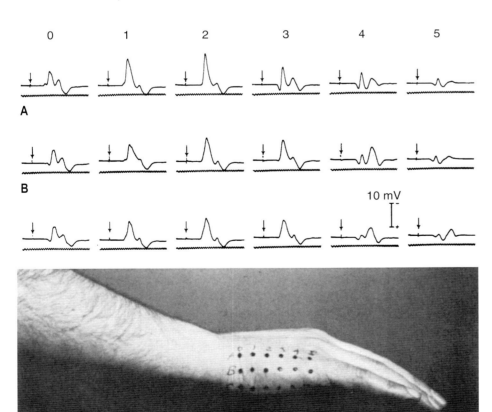

10 mV

FIGURE 13-1 ■ Compound muscle action potentials with ulnar stimulation (top) recorded with different locations of the G1 recording electrode (bottom). (From Carpendale MTF: Conduction Time in the Terminal Portion of the Motor Fibers of the Ulnar, Median and Peroneal Nerves in Healthy Subjects and in Patients with Neuropathy. Thesis, Mayo Graduate School of Medicine, Rochester, MN, 1956, with permission.)

them. Usually, the cathode is closer to the recording electrodes than is the anode to prevent block of axon conduction by hyperpolarization. A gradually increasing stimulus voltage produces a progressive increase in the size of the CMAP as more and more axons in the nerve are activated; the stimulus is increased by 30 percent after the CMAP no longer increases (i.e., the stimulus is supramaximal) to ensure activation of all the motor fibers. A stimulus of 25 mA (100 V) and 0.1 msec in duration is usually sufficient to activate all the large myelinated fibers in a nerve. Although large, low-threshold, fast-conducting axons should be stimulated initially, variations in the location of nerve fascicles and in the patterns of current flow may result in the initial activation of smaller axons with slower conduction. However, for abnormal nerves or for deep nerves, the stimulus may need to be as much as 75 mA (300 V) and 0.5 msec in duration, and it may need to be delivered with a monopolar stimulator (distant anode) or with a near-nerve needle electrode. Nevertheless, it must be remembered that large stimuli may produce errors by stimulating other nearby nerves inadvertently or by activating the nerve at a distance from the stimulating electrode.

Magnetic stimulation of peripheral motor nerves can be less painful and has been suggested as an alternative to electrical stimulation for nerve conduction studies. However, the site of stimulation cannot be defined well enough to permit reliable calculation of velocity, and maximal responses cannot be obtained reliably in diseased nerves.[3–6] Magnetic stimulation at the spinal nerve level does not produce maximal activation of nerve fibers.[7]

Recording

The CMAP is recorded with a pair of electrodes placed over a muscle or group of muscles innervated by the nerve. Recordings are often made from only a subset of all the muscles innervated by the nerve; thus, the recordings assess only the axons innervating those muscles. For instance, recording from the hypothenar muscles is used commonly in tests of ulnar nerve motor conduction. Selective damage to the axons that innervate either the flexor carpi ulnaris muscle or the first dorsal interosseous muscle therefore would not be identified unless recordings were made also from those muscles. Recent studies have shown that recordings from the first dorsal interosseous and the flexor carpi ulnaris muscles can increase the identification of ulnar neuropathies by up to 20 percent.[8] Recording from anterior compartment muscles when no response is obtained distally with fibular (peroneal) nerve stimulation can provide valuable information as well.[9]

Standard anatomic locations of recording electrodes provide reproducible potentials that can be compared with normal values. Measurements of a CMAP are most reliable when recordings are made over the endplate region of the muscle, near the middle of the muscle belly. Recordings are made with a bipolar derivation: an active (G1) electrode over the endplate region and a reference (G2) electrode over the tendon. Larger electrodes result in smaller CMAPs but give greater reproducibility.[10]

Recordings may be made with surface or needle electrodes. Surface electrodes provide the advantage of nontraumatic recordings with less risk of acquired immunodeficiency syndrome (AIDS), hepatitis, and Creutzfeldt–Jakob disease. They can be repositioned more readily to obtain the maximal, initially negative response. Needle electrodes have somewhat higher impedance but can be placed in the subcutaneous tissue immediately adjacent to the muscle to provide a more accurate reflection of the size of the CMAP than do surface electrodes, which may be some distance from deep muscles. Needle electrodes placed within muscle are less reliable because of an unstable configuration and amplitude of the CMAP during muscle movement. However, intramuscular electrodes can record from a more limited area of the muscle and may be of value in assessing individual motor branches of a nerve, atrophic muscle, and anomalous patterns of innervation.

Measurements

The directly evoked CMAP recorded after stimulation of a peripheral nerve is called an M wave. With supramaximal stimulation, all the fibers in a muscle innervated by the nerve contribute to the potential. The earliest component is elicited by the fastest-conducting motor axons. The M wave usually is described by its latency, amplitude, area, and configuration.

Latency is the time in milliseconds from the application of a stimulus to the initial deflection from the baseline, either positive or negative, and is the time required for the action potentials in the fastest-conducting fibers to reach the nerve terminals and activate the muscle fibers (Fig. 13-2). Since the latency of the peak of the CMAP represents activation of different axons at proximal and distal sites of stimulation, peak-latency measurements are not reliable for determining motor conduction velocity. When recording is done over the endplate region of the muscle, the normal configuration of the CMAP is biphasic, negative–positive. If the active electrode is not over the endplate region, the potential is triphasic, with an initial positivity that makes latency measurements less accurate. Since the distal latency

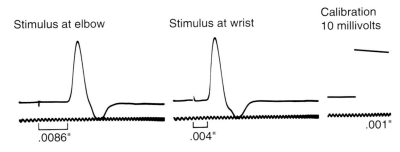

Stimulus at elbow   Stimulus at wrist   Calibration 10 millivolts

.0086"   .004"   .001"

Conduction time, elbow to wrist .0086 − .004 = .0046 sec
Conduction distance, elbow to wrist   .245 m
Conduction velocity   .245 ÷ .0046 = 53 m/sec

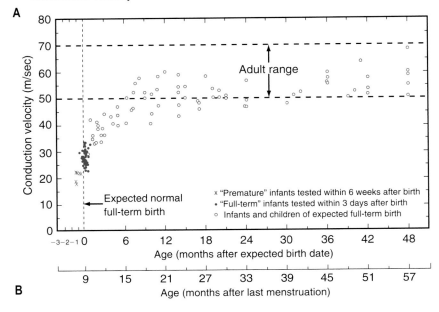

FIGURE 13-2 ■ **A,** Measurement of latency and calculation of conduction velocity in ulnar nerve by recording hypothenar muscle action potential. **B,** The change in conduction velocity with age in children. (From Thomas JE: Conduction Velocity of the Motor Fibers of the Ulnar Nerve in Infants and Children. Thesis, Mayo Graduate School of Medicine, Rochester, MN, 1958. Modified with permission from Mayo Foundation for Medical Education and Research. All rights reserved.)

varies directly with the distance between the stimulating electrode and the muscle, a fixed distal distance improves reliability by eliminating distance differences among individuals.

Normally, only minimal changes in configuration occur with stimulation at proximal sites compared to the responses recorded at distal sites. In some recordings, particularly fibular nerve conduction to the extensor digitorum brevis (EDB), an initial positivity is seen with proximal, but not distal stimulation because of volume conduction of the CMAP from the distal portion of the extensor hallucis longus muscle. The positive component must be ignored in measuring latency since it is not from the EDB. In this case, latency should be measured to where the negative upslope of the CMAP crosses the baseline to become negative.

The distal latency from the most distal site of stimulation includes slowing in the smaller nerve terminals and the neuromuscular transmission time. Thus a conduction velocity cannot be calculated from the distal latency alone. However, an alternate calculation of "residual latency" that compares the expected latency (based on proximal conduction velocity) with the actual latency may be of value in identifying distal demyelinating processes.[11]

If the nerve is accessible, it is stimulated at more than one site along its course to evoke two or more CMAPs from the muscle. The latencies, areas, amplitudes, and configurations of the CMAP at each site are compared. Measurement of the differences in distance and latency between sites of stimulation allows *conduction velocity* calculation in the segment of nerve between the sites of stimulation in meters per second. Accurate distance measurement is of critical importance in calculating velocity. Longer distances improve the reliability of velocity calculation.[12]

Comparison of conduction in selected segments with that in other segments of the nerve and with normal values can localize a lesion along the length of a nerve. Normal conduction velocities are from 40 to 55 m/sec in the legs and from 50 to 70 m/sec in the arms. Conduction is faster in proximal segments of nerves, thus resulting in an inverse relationship between body height and conduction velocity.[13,14]

With supramaximal stimulation, the *area* (in msec.mV) of the negative phase of the action potential measures the number of muscle fibers depolarized and shows only minor change with the distance of the muscle from the stimulating electrodes. Change in CMAP area is the most reliable measure of loss of functioning axons between two points along a nerve and should be measured if the recording equipment permits. Because the contribution of individual motor units to the CMAP is determined by the location of the recording electrodes, they should be applied in standard locations.[15]

If area cannot be measured, *amplitude* can serve the same purpose, provided that the duration of the CMAP does not change between stimulation sites. The amplitude of the CMAP usually is measured as the height in millivolts from the baseline to the peak of the negative phase. The amplitude normally is between 2 and 20 mV, but is somewhat lower in some nerves when more proximal sites are stimulated. The area and amplitude of the CMAP should be measured routinely because they are proportional to the number of muscle fibers activated and provide an estimate of the amount of functioning nerve and muscle. The area and amplitude of the CMAP are affected by a number of variables. The distance between the recording electrode and the muscle has the greatest effect; thus, the presence of edema or excess fat results in CMAPs with small areas and low amplitudes. Fortunately, edema and fatty tissue are recognized easily, so that the low amplitudes are not mistaken for signs of disease.

The area, amplitude, duration, and latency of the CMAP are dependent on a number of factors that must be considered when nerve conduction studies are quantitated. The number of activated axons directly affects the size and shape of the CMAP. For consistency of measurement, supramaximal responses are recorded in standard nerve conduction studies. Submaximal responses have longer latencies, smaller areas, and lower amplitudes. To obtain the maximal response with no initial positivity, the active electrode should be over the endplate region of the main bulk of the muscles innervated by the nerve being tested, with the reference electrode over the tendon of the muscle. The interelectrode distance between the active and the reference electrodes directly affects the area and amplitude of the CMAP and must be standard for each nerve. It must be greater for longer muscles to allow placement of the electrodes over the endplate region and tendon. The CMAP differs when a subcutaneous or an intramuscular needle electrode is used in place of surface electrodes. The temperature of the limb and muscle also affects the CMAP; larger areas, higher amplitudes, and longer latencies are found with lower temperatures.[16,17]

The amplitude and latency of the CMAP change with the site of stimulation. At more proximal sites, the latency increases progressively with increase in distance that the action potential has to travel to the muscle. The amplitude decreases as the synchrony of discharge of the contributing motor units decreases. If all axons conducted at the same velocity, the amplitude would remain unchanged; but because they differ, slower-conducting axons activate the muscle progressively later with more proximal stimulation so that the CMAP becomes longer and lower. Partial CMAP cancellation of negative components by overlapping positive components results in only minimal reduction in area compared to amplitude at more proximal sites of stimulation. A reduction in area or amplitude at a proximal site compared to a distal site of stimulation that is greater than that of a normal nerve is evidence of disease. This reduction can result from diffuse disease with a gradual reduction along the length of the nerve. In contrast, a focal lesion may result in a CMAP reduction over a short distance, called a conduction block. A conduction block is one of the most reliable signs of an acute compression neuropathy. The extent of normal reduction in area and amplitude with more proximal stimulation varies from nerve to nerve; values in individual cases must be compared with normal values for that nerve. In most limb nerves, the reduction in area and amplitude with stimulation between the wrist or ankle and elbow or knee is less than 20 percent.

The *duration* of the response is the time, measured in milliseconds, from the onset to the end of the negative phase of the M wave. Differences in conduction velocity result in the nerve action potentials generated by a single stimulus reaching the muscle slightly dispersed in time. The duration normally increases slightly at more proximal sites of stimulation compared to distal sites. Greater variation in axon velocities results in greater CMAP dispersion with a longer duration. The change in duration of the response provides an approximation of the range of conduction velocities in motor axons. Other methods have been proposed to measure conduction in slower fibers. Paired stimulation (collision) is significantly more time-consuming and seldom provides useful clinical information. F-wave methods can demonstrate more dispersion because of the longer course of nerve traversed (see Chapter 18).

If the action potentials of slower-conducting motor units spread out by dispersion, the CMAP breaks down into an irregular waveform with spike components.[18]

This occurs with the pronounced slowing of conduction velocity in demyelinating disorders and with reinnervation. Dispersion of the CMAP can provide evidence of underlying disease even when the fast-conducting fibers still conduct at normal rates. The most reliable quantitation of a dispersed CMAP is the duration of the negative phase of the CMAP. The increase in duration at proximal sites of stimulation differs for different nerves. Normal values must be defined for each nerve. Identifying the end of the positive phase of the CMAP is more difficult, especially in disease with complex CMAPs having multiple baseline crossings and phases. The duration of such waveforms is best measured to the last baseline crossing.

The *collision and F-wave latency methods* have been reported to measure conduction of slower motor fibers by stimulation of the nerve at proximal and distal sites. In the collision method, two stimuli are applied simultaneously, one at a proximal and the other at a distal site on the nerve. The antidromic CMAP (going up the nerve) from the distal site collides with and cancels the orthodromic (down the nerve) CMAP from the proximal site, so that only the orthodromic CMAP of the distal stimulation is recorded.[19] If the interval between the time of stimulation of the distal and proximal sites is increased gradually, at a certain interval only the more slowly conducting fibers are blocked by collision, because the rapidly conducted potentials already have passed the distal site of stimulation, leaving a CMAP contributed by only the fast-conducting fibers. A plot of the amplitude of the CMAP (elicited by the proximal stimulus) against the interval between the two stimuli provides an estimate of the range of conduction of the fibers in the nerve. In the F-wave method, the range of latencies of F waves is measured with separate stimulation at proximal and distal sites. Comparison of the earliest and latest F-wave latencies at the two sites of stimulation and the distance between them provides a measure of conduction in the fast- and slow-conducting fibers.

With *repetitive stimulation* the area and amplitude of a CMAP are normally constant. In disorders of neuromuscular transmission and in some disorders of nerve and muscle, the area, amplitude, configuration, or latency of consecutive CMAPs may change with repetitive stimulation by either an increment or a decrement in the CMAP. A decrement is measured as a percentage change in the amplitude or area between two CMAPs recorded sequentially on stimulation at the same site. A decrease in amplitude from 10 to 9 mV is a decrement of 10 percent. A decrement at slow rates of stimulation (2 to 5 Hz) usually is caused by disease at the neuromuscular junction. Stimulation (or voluntary activation) at rapid rates (10 to 50 Hz) may result in decrements in normal people or in persons with disease of the neuromuscular junction, nerve, or muscle. Rapid rates of stimulation also may produce an increment in amplitude or area, which also is measured as a percentage change. An increase from 5 to 10 mV is an increase of 100 percent. Area and amplitude changes also may occur slowly after exercise in disorders such as periodic paralysis (Fig. 13-3). Such changes are dependent on the rate of stimulation and are discussed in Chapter 17.

When a peripheral nerve is stimulated, late waveforms may be elicited in addition to the direct M response

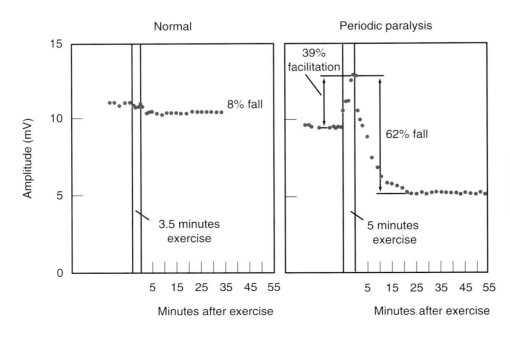

FIGURE 13-3 ▪ Amplitude of a compound muscle action potential after exercise, compared with a resting response in a normal subject and in a patient with periodic paralysis.

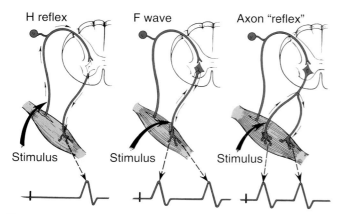

FIGURE 13-4 ▪ Late muscle responses after peripheral nerve stimulation.

(Fig. 13-4). A nerve stimulus normally evokes action potentials that propagate proximally toward the anterior horn cell (antidromic), as well as peripherally (orthodromic) to activate the muscle directly. The antidromic potentials may be blocked by hyperpolarization at the anode, but if the cathode is placed proximally, all the motor axons can be activated antidromically. A small proportion of the anterior horn cells are activated antidromically in either the cell body or the axon hillock; these discharge another action potential orthodromically along the axon. Paired stimuli will block these waves because the second antidromic potential will collide with the recurrent orthodromic potential. These recurrent discharges produce a small muscle potential after a delay of 20 to 50 msec, depending on the distance from the site of stimulation to the spinal cord. These late responses are referred to as F waves (Fig. 13-5) and were first described by Magladery and McDougal.[2]

Individual *F waves* are the action potentials of a single or a few motor units. Although F waves represent only a small sampling of the axons in the nerve, and they have variable latencies as different axons are activated, they can provide an estimate of conduction in the central segments of motor fibers. F-wave latencies are assessed most readily by comparison of the measured latency with normal values at the same distance. F-wave latency values in normal subjects depend on the peripheral conduction velocity and the length to the limb. Estimates of normal values can be obtained readily by doubling the distance from the distal site of stimulation to spinal cord (sternal notch for arm and xiphoid for leg), dividing the result by the peripheral conduction velocity, and adding the distal latency.[20] Values longer than the normal range of F estimates indicate proximal slowing relative to distal, as in a polyradiculopathy; those shorter than the F estimate indicate distal slowing relative to proximal, as in a peripheral neuropathy.

Individual F-wave latencies can be measured to obtain a statistical distribution with a mean, standard deviation, and range.[21] These are time-consuming to collect, but they provide a more accurate measure of the range of velocities in the motor axons and an estimate of conduction in the slower-conducting fibers. Although samples of 20 F waves are needed to provide values of minimum and mean latency within 95 percent of the true value, 8 to 10 responses are sufficient to provide reliable values, and the procedure is tolerated readily by most patients.[22,23] The F-wave amplitudes represent the summated potentials of the muscle fibers of one or more motor units and therefore have different amplitudes and configurations. The amplitude of a group of F waves provides an estimate of the relative amplitudes of the action potential of individual motor units. These also are described best by a combination of means, standard deviation, and maximal and minimal values. If there are only a small number of axons, the F waves of single axons may fire repeatedly to produce identical-appearing F waves from a single motor unit (*repeater F waves*) that are a sign of an underlying neurogenic process with collateral sprouting.[24,25]

FIGURE 13-5 ▪ F waves recorded from abductor hallucis brevis muscle with tibial nerve stimulation at standard (left) and high (right) amplification (multiple traces superimposed).

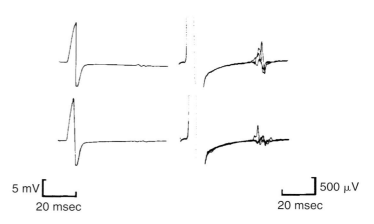

5 mV | 20 msec   500 μV | 20 msec

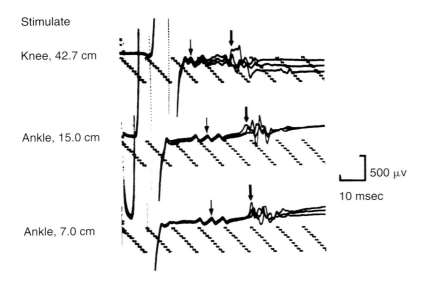

Stimulate

Knee, 42.7 cm

Ankle, 15.0 cm

Ankle, 7.0 cm

500 μV

10 msec

FIGURE 13-6 ■ Late responses in abductor hallucis brevis muscle to tibial nerve stimulation. Broad arrow indicates F waves; narrow arrow indicates axon reflex (A wave).

Other small electrical responses may occur after the M wave. For instance, if a few axons are conducting at a slower rate than the remainder, a small late potential may be seen after and time-locked to the CMAP; this is called an *M-wave satellite*. A second small response that may be confused with an F wave is an *A wave*. This results either from an axon that branches in the peripheral nerve; by spontaneous backfiring of an axon along its length; or by ephaptic activation of one axon by another, called *direct and indirect double-discharges*.[26,27] Electrical stimulation distal to the site of branching produces an antidromic potential that becomes orthodromic at the branch point (see Fig. 13-4; Fig. 13-6).[28] This potential, like the F wave, has a shorter latency as the site of stimulation moves proximally. The axon branch is typically a small, poorly myelinated, high-threshold axon, but a stimulus of sufficiently high intensity may activate the branch and block the A wave by collision. A third type of late response occurs in some diseases of peripheral nerve in which there is unusual irritability. In these diseases, the nerve and muscle discharge repetitively in response to a single stimulus. Each of these discharges must be distinguished carefully from F waves.

The CMAP is the summed response of the potentials of the individual motor units in the muscles activated by the stimulation. In normal people, the individual motor unit potentials are 20 to 200 μV in amplitude when recorded with surface electrodes. These are not recognized in standard nerve conduction studies. However, if a high amplification of the CMAP is combined with fine control of the stimulus intensity near threshold, the individual all-or-none firing potentials of single motor unit potentials can be isolated as step increments in the potential with increased stimulus (Fig. 13-7). The number of motor

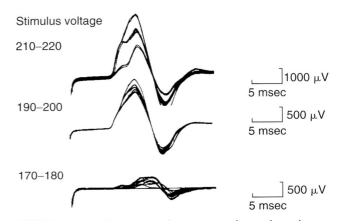

Stimulus voltage

210–220

190–200

170–180

1000 μV
5 msec

500 μV
5 msec

500 μV
5 msec

FIGURE 13-7 ■ Increments in compound muscle action potential of the extensor digitorum brevis muscle with small increases in stimulus to the fibular nerve.

units in a muscle can be estimated by measuring an average size of a single motor unit potential with these increments, then dividing that average into the size of the supramaximal CMAP.[29,30] A number of automated methods have been developed to make this measurement.[31,32] A mean of 320 (100 to 500) motor units is found in thenar and hypothenar muscles, and a mean of 150 (50 to 300) motor units is found in the EDB muscle.[33] These measurements become less reliable with smaller motor units, as in myopathies, but become more reliable and reproducible with neurogenic atrophy. When the motor unit potentials become large, as in amyotrophic lateral sclerosis or after poliomyelitis, motor unit estimate measurements can be used to follow the course of the disorder quantitatively.

Nerve excitability is a more recent development in the testing of peripheral nerve.[34] The method, which is discussed in Chapter 15, is more complicated than standard nerve conduction studies. It measures a number of membrane characteristics related to threshold, including the effect of a test current on the nerve. Automated equipment has been developed for clinical testing. Although still early in its development, it has shown abnormalities in a number of clinical disorders.[35]

SENSORY NERVE CONDUCTION STUDIES

Stimulation and recording directly from a mixed peripheral nerve tests both motor and sensory axons. Evaluation of sensory axons alone requires stimulating and recording from a cutaneous nerve; recording from a cutaneous nerve while a mixed nerve is stimulated; recording from a mixed nerve while a cutaneous nerve is stimulated; or recording from the spinal column or cerebral hemispheres while a cutaneous or mixed nerve is stimulated. Sensory nerve action potentials (SNAPs) are of much lower amplitude than are CMAPs and may be obscured by other electrical activity and artifact. Averaging multiple responses sometimes is needed to provide reliable, measurable sensory potentials. Potentials that are recorded over the spinal column and scalp are called *somatosensory evoked potentials* (SEPs); these are discussed in Chapters 26 and 27. SEPs recorded for the diagnosis of peripheral nerve disease are an extension of sensory nerve conduction studies. Sensory conduction in severe sensory neuropathies in which no SNAP is recordable can sometimes still be measured by recording the SEP.

SNAPs can be recorded readily from the ulnar, median, radial, lateral, and medial antebrachial, fibular, plantar, and sural nerves. SNAPs are also recorded preceding a CMAP at high amplification, if the muscle and overlying skin are innervated by the same nerve (Fig. 13-8).

Sensory recordings from the lateral antebrachial, saphenous, and lateral femoral cutaneous nerves are more difficult to obtain and are rarely of help in routine clinical studies.

Sensory conduction studies can add much to motor conduction studies (e.g., evidence of diffuse sensory fiber involvement, localized lesions involving a cutaneous nerve, or disorders that preferentially damage the sensory fibers in a mixed nerve). Because sensory nerve conduction studies are more sensitive than are motor conduction studies in detecting early or mild disorders, they are a necessary part of any electrophysiologic evaluation of peripheral neuromuscular disease.

Two other techniques, the blink reflex and the H reflex, assess sensory axons of the trigeminal nerve, median nerve, and sciatic nerve; these techniques are discussed in Chapters 18 and 19. In each technique, sensory fibers are stimulated while a recording is made of a reflex motor response mediated by the central nervous system.

Stimulation

Because the speed of conduction in axons is the same orthodromically and antidromically, action potentials may be evoked in either direction for testing sensory conduction (Fig. 13-9). Each has advantages and disadvantages that make it more appropriate for particular clinical situations. Stimulation of a cutaneous nerve at a distal site (e.g., the digital nerves in a digit) produces a small orthodromic nerve action potential that can be recorded over the proximal mixed nerve that it joins.[36] Stimulation also can be applied over a mixed nerve to record a larger antidromic nerve action potential over the cutaneous nerve, but the latter may be associated with a motor response that is difficult to distinguish from the SNAP (Fig. 13-10).

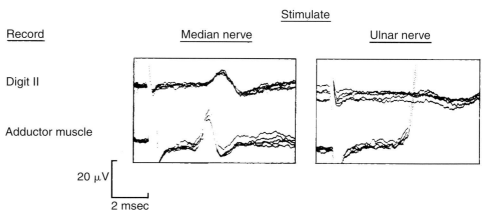

FIGURE 13-8 ■ Cutaneous origin of nerve action potential in amyotrophic lateral sclerosis with no thenar response.

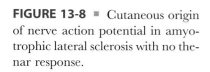

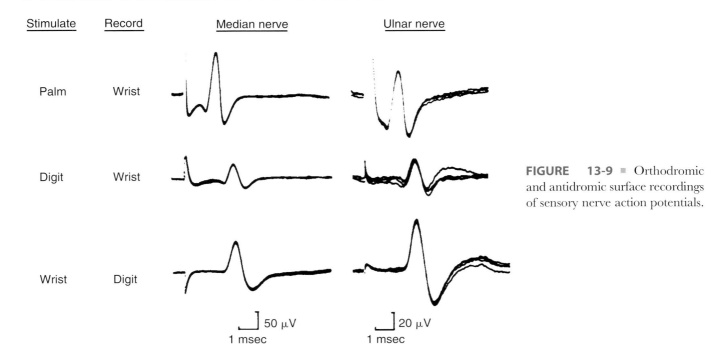

FIGURE 13-9 ■ Orthodromic and antidromic surface recordings of sensory nerve action potentials.

Stimulation parameters for sensory nerve conduction studies are similar to those for motor studies, and stimuli should also be supramaximal. The location and orientation of the stimulating electrodes are important for obtaining artifact-free recordings.

Recording

Recordings of compound SNAPs are technically more difficult to make than are those of CMAPs because of the smaller size of the potentials. Recording electrodes placed on the surface over a mixed or cutaneous nerve (particularly ring electrodes placed over the digits) are most convenient; however, needle recording electrodes placed near the nerve can enhance the amplitude of the response up to fivefold (Fig. 13-11).[37] Small components recorded with needle electrodes are generated by demyelinated or regenerated fibers that may be the only findings in some neuropathies. The nerve action potential is typically triphasic with a positive onset; it has latency proportional to the distance from the stimulating electrodes and an amplitude approximately proportional to the number of active axons, the synchrony of axonal firing, and the distance from the nerve to the recording electrodes. The distance of the electrode from the nerve can be estimated from the rise-time; nearby nerves will have rise-times of less than a millisecond.

The high amplification used for recording makes the stimulus artifact a more common problem. To reduce such artifact, greater attention is required for placement of ground electrodes, elimination of conducting bridges between the ground and the stimulating electrodes, isolation of the stimulating electrodes, and proper orientation of the stimulating and recording electrodes. Another

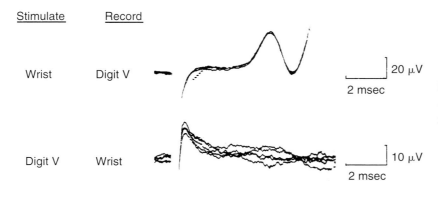

FIGURE 13-10 ■ Volume-conducted motor artifacts with antidromic nerve testing. There is no ulnar nerve sensory potential.

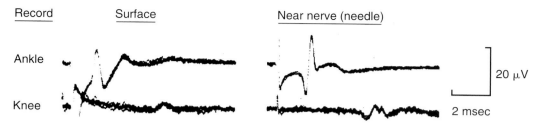

Record   Surface   Near nerve (needle)

Ankle

Knee

20 µV

2 msec

FIGURE 13-11 ▪ Tibial nerve action potentials with medial plantar stimulation recorded by surface and needle electrodes.

common problem in recording sensory potentials is the appearance of background muscle activity, which is reduced most effectively by gentle manipulation of the limb and by providing patients with auditory feedback of their own muscle contractions. Sensory studies require particular attention to temperature because the superficial location of cutaneous nerves makes it more likely that mild slowing in conduction may be caused by low temperature.

Technically, the easiest and most reliable distal SNAP recordings for both the ulnar and the median nerves are obtained by orthodromic activation of axons. Radial and sural nerves, however, are tested more readily with an antidromic volley; recording is performed over a distal branch while the main trunk of the cutaneous nerve is stimulated. Simultaneous recording from more than one distal branch of a cutaneous nerve with antidromic stimulation may enhance sensitivity to localized nerve damage.

The placements of the active electrode and the reference electrode are of critical importance in recording SNAPs. The potential is optimal when the active electrode is immediately adjacent to the nerve and the reference electrode is placed as far away as possible. However, artifacts from intervening muscle or other tissue increase when the reference electrode is moved away. A compromise between optimal SNAP amplitude and an artifact-free signal must be reached. A reference electrode located 4 cm from the active electrode provides almost full representation of the SNAP with a minimum of noise. The reference electrode may be placed either laterally away from the nerve or longitudinally further along the course of the nerve. The latter placement leads to an inverted SNAP (near-field potential) being recorded from the reference electrode. At 4 cm, the inverted reference potential summates with the potential at the active electrode and increases the size of the signal; some distortion results if the active and reference electrodes are too close together.

However, in lateral placement, there is the more difficult problem of recording a far-field potential, which can distort the SNAP in an unpredictable fashion. The far-field potential may be recorded from the reference electrode before the action potential is recorded from the active electrode. The problem of recording far-field potentials from a laterally located reference electrode is less when recording is done with near-nerve needle electrodes because the far-field potential is relatively smaller than is the near-field potential, and it also causes less distortion. Needle electrode recordings also can provide a better representation of the components of the SNAP when the potential is broken up by dispersion. Such apparently dispersed SNAPs with multiple components recorded from either a needle or a surface electrode must be interpreted with caution because they are sometimes artifacts of the recording that are not reflected in either in vitro recordings from whole-nerve biopsy specimens or the distribution of axonal diameters in specimens from nerve biopsies. The multiple components may be artifacts either of stimulation of more than one nerve by an excessively large stimulus (Fig. 13-12) or of recording a far-field potential (Fig. 13-13).

Measurements

Latency, conduction velocity, area, and amplitude are measured for sensory conduction studies, as they are for motor conduction studies, but these are more difficult to measure because of configuration changes and small size. The SNAP is a moving wave recorded in a volume conductor and, therefore, typically has an initial positivity because of current flow ahead of the area of depolarization. The amplitude of the response measured from positive to negative peak provides the best estimate of the total number of fibers activated, although the distance between the recording electrode and the nerve heavily influences the amplitude. Area of the negative spike is a less satisfactory estimate because of the difficulty in defining measurement points.

The latency of the response is related directly to the rate of conduction and the distance between the stimulating and the recording electrodes. Comparisons of

Stimulus:

Supramaximal

Maximal

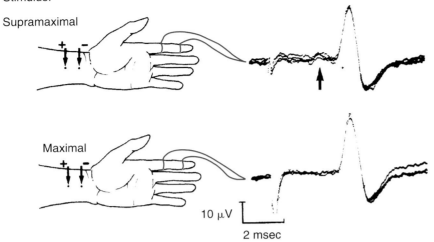

10 μV

2 msec

FIGURE 13-12 ▪ Radial nerve activation by excessive stimulation in median nerve conduction studies.

differences in latency and distance at different sites allow calculations of conduction velocity. Sensory compound nerve action potentials range in amplitude from a few microvolts to 200 μV. Velocities are generally faster than are motor conduction velocities. With distal stimulation, potentials are small when recorded at proximal sites and, at times, this precludes recording them directly without averaging. Larger potentials can be obtained with stimulation of the mixed nerve or by stimulation of unbranched digital nerves (e.g., the median or ulnar nerves in the palm). With palmar stimulation, orthodromic sensory potentials can be recorded at proximal sites without averaging (Fig. 13-14).

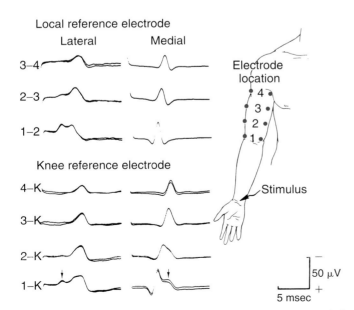

FIGURE 13-13 ▪ Median nerve action potentials recorded with different reference electrodes. Lateral recordings are far-field recordings.

The major problem in measuring the SNAP is its low amplitude, which makes the noise in the recording system a significant percentage of the total waveform. Therefore, the measurement of a single SNAP is unreliable, unless the noise level is very low or the amplitude is greater than 25 μV. Otherwise, averaging is needed. An automatic averager is of major value in measuring the SNAP. The averaged SNAP typically is a triphasic wave. The initial positivity is caused by the current from the potential as it approaches the active electrode, and the late positivity is the current flow of the potential moving away. These positive components are therefore of little diagnostic value. SNAPs have an initial negativity when recorded at the boundary of volume conductors of different sizes (e.g., the potential recorded from the digits).

Latencies of SNAPs are measured to the onset of the negativity, regardless of whether there is an initial positivity. If there is a positivity, the onset of the negativity is taken as the peak of the preceding positive phase. Latency to the onset reflects conduction in the fastest fibers and is used to calculate conduction velocity. Latencies to the negative peak may also be measured because they are defined more easily, especially in noisy recordings. Peak latencies will estimate conduction in the fibers with medium-range velocity. Peak latencies cannot be used to calculate conduction velocity from two points because the axons that produce the peak at the two sites differ as a result of dispersion of the potential. Latencies are measured most precisely with needle electrodes placed near the nerve, but surface measurements are also reliable if the electrode is placed properly to give a fast rise-time.

Conduction velocity in the fast-conducting sensory fibers is measured most accurately (as it is for motor conduction) by using the distance and latency between two points of stimulation. Unlike a motor latency, however, a

Stimulate	Record	Median nerve	Ulnar nerve
Palm	Elbow		
	Wrist		

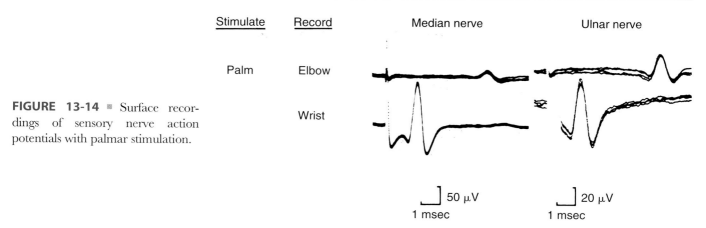

FIGURE 13-14 ■ Surface recordings of sensory nerve action potentials with palmar stimulation.

50 μV
1 msec

20 μV
1 msec

sensory latency does not include the time for neuromuscular transmission, thereby allowing calculation of sensory conduction velocity by the distance and latency with stimulation at a single site. Although it is reliable, one-point velocity calculation still may include some slowing in nerve terminals. A lesion can be localized more precisely by an abrupt change in latency and in waveform of the antidromic sensory potential during "inching" of the stimulus in short increments along the nerve.

Measurements of conduction in the slower-conducting fibers of sensory nerves have been attempted with methods similar to those used in motor conduction studies. The collision method, in which paired stimuli are delivered at two sites along a nerve, gives estimates of conduction in slow sensory fibers. In Figure 13-15, a full-size potential is obtained with intervals greater than 5 msec between stimuli separated by 14 cm. This indicates a minimal conduction velocity of 28 m/sec. All axons are blocked at intervals of less than 3.5 msec between stimuli for a maximal conduction velocity of 40 m/sec. These measurements can be technically

difficult because of the need to average the potentials. A second method that has been used to estimate the conduction in small fibers uses a mathematical analysis of the configuration of the potential. This method has been shown to have some validity when compared with other methods, but it is fraught with unsolved technical problems, such as the distortion caused by the presence of far-field potentials recorded from the reference electrode.

The *amplitude* and *area* of the SNAP are important parameters that provide information about the number of axons and their sizes. They cannot be related directly to the number of axons, however, because the distance of the nerve from the electrode influences them. Surface electrodes can give estimates of the number of axons if they are placed near the nerve, as defined by the rise-time. Responses recorded with needle electrodes are more difficult to interpret because the amplitude, area, and configuration are so heavily dependent on the precise location of the electrode relative to the nerve; however, they can be used if they have fast rise-times. Responses recorded with needle electrodes also show turns, late components, and dispersion in the SNAP that are not seen with surface electrodes. Thus, needle-electrode and surface-electrode recordings of SNAP each have advantages and disadvantages.

The greater range of conduction velocities in sensory axons results in more cancellation of the negative phase of the SNAP by the initial and late positivity as the potential travels longer distances. Therefore, marked reductions in amplitude and area of SNAPs may occur with increased conduction distances, making such measurements less useful, except over distances of 10 cm or less. Decrement in amplitude and area with repetitive stimulation is also less useful because it occurs only with axonal disease and requires rapid rates of stimulation.

Other measures of sensory nerve conduction may be obtained by recording H-wave latency (see Chapter 18) or SEPs (see Chapters 26 and 27).

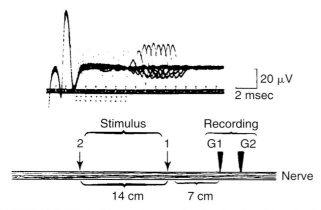

20 μV
2 msec

Stimulus   Recording
2   1   G1   G2

                              Nerve
14 cm   7 cm

FIGURE 13-15 ■ Measuring conduction in slow fibers in the sural nerve by using paired stimuli at two sites to produce collision of potentials. See text for further details.

GENERAL PRINCIPLES OF NERVE CONDUCTION STUDIES

Physiologic Variables

Normal values for latency, area, amplitude, and conduction velocity vary with age, height, temperature, and technique.[14,38] Therefore, each laboratory should determine its own set of normal values. Median and ulnar nerves, and tibial and fibular nerves, have similar conduction velocities to each other and between the limbs for each nerve.[39] Leg nerves conduct 7 to 10 m/sec slower than those in the arms, probably because of slower conduction in longer axons. Conduction in proximal nerve segments is somewhat faster than in distal segments.

Low temperatures result in slower conduction velocities and longer distal latencies; both nerve and muscle action potential amplitudes are higher with lower temperatures. Room temperatures above 70°F (20°C) minimize these changes, but use of a heating lamp or immersion of the hand or foot in water at 40°C before testing may be necessary if they feel cool to the touch. Continuous measurement of skin temperature (above 31°C in the hand and above 29°C in the leg) in the region of a nerve conduction study is necessary to ensure that responses are not altered by temperature.

Conduction velocities change markedly with age between the neonatal period and 6 years, with more gradual subsequent changes up to adulthood. Conduction begins to slow minimally after 40 years of age, but more so after the age of 60 years. Normal value determinations should be age corrected. Conduction velocity in the legs slows with height and should be corrected for heights over 78 inches (198 cm).[14,40,41] Gender differences are caused primarily by differences in height.

Long- and Short-Segment Studies

Motor and sensory nerve conduction studies can be performed over different lengths of nerve. Usually, the length is selected for ease and reliability of testing (e.g., the elbow-to-wrist segment in the arm and the knee-to-ankle segment in the leg). However, both stimulation over short segments and stimulation over long segments have distinct advantages in certain clinical situations. A localized area of abnormality, either slowing or amplitude change, is most apparent if the testing isolates that segment from immediately proximal and distal segments. In longer segments, such local abnormalities may not be apparent because they are averaged with the normal segments.[12] Short-segment testing is best accomplished by "inching" (i.e., stimulation at short intervals of 2 cm along a nerve).[42]

In contrast, recording over long distances that summate abnormalities is the best way to recognize diffuse abnormalities, especially if they are mild. Longer segments also reduce the effect of small errors in distance or latency measurement. F-wave latencies assess the longest segments, and therefore are often more sensitive and accurate in identifying generalized slowing than standard peripheral conduction.

Distinguishing Proximal and Distal Abnormalities

Peripheral nerve disorders may produce slowing in distal segments (peripheral neuropathy), in proximal segments (polyradiculopathy), or in both segments. Distal abnormalities are identified readily with standard nerve conduction studies of limb nerves that involve stimulating and recording conduction velocity and distal latency from distal segments of the nerve. Identification of proximal abnormalities requires stimulating proximal nerves such as the musculocutaneous or facial nerves, or stimulating across plexus segments by percutaneous stimulation of spinal nerves combined with distal nerve stimulation.[43,44] F-wave latency comparisons with F-wave estimates are most efficient for recognizing proximal slowing, as in a polyradiculopathy. Blink reflexes are also important for recognizing proximal slowing.

Various methods of calculation have been devised to obtain estimates of conduction velocities to identify the presence or absence of proximal slowing in combination with peripheral slowing. Comparison of F-wave latency with an estimated F-wave latency that is based on peripheral conduction and length of the nerve to the spinal cord can determine whether conduction slowing is equal proximally and distally, is greater distally than proximally, or is greater proximally than distally (see F-wave section, earlier).[45]

Data Analysis

The analysis and interpretation of the numerical data obtained in nerve conduction studies depend on the reliability of the data and on the normal values with which they are compared. These are ignored too often, leading to erroneous conclusions about the presence or absence of peripheral nerve disease. Reliability is the responsibility of electromyographers, who must define the reproducibility of the data they obtain. This starts with careful attention to eliminating technical errors but then must be assessed formally. Repeating the nerve conduction studies on the same individual a number of times on different days can do this most readily. That variation then defines how to interpret patient data. For example, an ulnar/hypothenar CMAP that is 5 mV, when the lower limit of normal is 6 mV, cannot be considered abnormal unless the reproducibility is less than 1 mV. Amplitude measurements have the poorest reproducibility; distal latency, motor and sensory conduction velocities, and F-wave latency have increasing reproducibility.[46]

A definition of normal values for an individual requires standard nerve conduction testing on a large population of normal subjects whose age, gender, height, and weight are recorded. Automated programs then can give percentiles and normal deviates based on a comparison of the findings in that patient with findings in normal subjects.[47] A percentile analysis provides the percentage of matched normal subjects with that value rather than absolute normal values.[48] In diffuse disorders (e.g., a peripheral neuropathy), the extent of abnormality may be different for different nerves tested. In those situations, assessing the progression of chronic peripheral neuropathies is enhanced by calculating composite scores of the motor or sensory amplitudes or latencies to provide a better picture of the overall status of the disease.[49]

Technical Errors

Technical problems are a common source of error in motor and sensory nerve conduction studies. Any unexpected finding should be assumed to be caused by a technical error until proven otherwise. Spread of current because of excessive stimulation, small responses because of submaximal stimulation when the stimulator is not over the nerve or the nerve is deep, shock artifact, inadequate skin preparation, distance measurement errors, incorrect limb positioning, machine filter settings, inappropriate normal values, and incorrect location of recording electrodes must be watched for and eliminated.

The difficulty of measuring small responses or excessive background noise can lead to errors in measurement of action potentials. Averaging should be used for such signals. Small signals within the noise level of the system require averaging to improve the signal-to-noise ratio. Averaging sums a large series of responses that are time-locked to the stimulus. Random noise will be canceled out, whereas the consistent response becomes more apparent. Averaging is limited to eliminating background noise less than 50 times the signal size.[50]

Risks

Nerve conduction studies are essentially risk-free in normal individuals when using equipment that is grounded properly. Nerve stimulation can be a risk if the current can reach the heart. It is thus relatively contraindicated in patients with catheters inserted directly into the heart. Limb stimulation is safe, but stimulation near the heart, such as phrenic nerve stimulation, should be avoided in patients with pacemakers, cardioverters, and defibrillators.[51,52]

ANOMALIES OF INNERVATION

In standard nerve conduction studies, it is assumed that a patient's nerves follow the normal anatomic patterns. However, as many as 20 percent of people may have anomalous patterns of innervation in the arm or leg; this can result in unusual findings on nerve conduction studies. If these variations are not recognized, they may be mistaken for disorders of peripheral nerves. Two anomalies that are of particular concern in nerve conduction studies are the presence of median–ulnar anastomosis in the forearm (Martin–Gruber anomaly) and a deep accessory branch of the superficial fibular (peroneal) nerve in the leg.

Median–Ulnar Anastomosis

Between 15 and 20 percent of normal people have anomalous axons that pass from the median to the ulnar nerve in the proximal third of the forearm, the so-called Martin–Gruber anastomosis (Fig. 13-16).[53] These axons leave either the main trunk of the median nerve or the anterior interosseous nerve and join the main trunk of the ulnar nerve. Axons leaving or joining a nerve between two sites of stimulation cause an unanticipated change in the size or shape of the CMAP (Fig. 13-17). With ulnar nerve stimulation, the amplitude is lower at more proximal sites of stimulation, whereas with median nerve stimulation, the amplitude is higher at more proximal sites of stimulation. The axons that cross from the median nerve to the ulnar nerve may innervate any of several intrinsic hand muscles, but most commonly they innervate the first dorsal interosseous muscle. For standard nerve conduction studies, the most important sites of innervation are the thenar and hypothenar muscles (Fig. 13-18). Therefore, this anomaly can be particularly confusing in cases of carpal tunnel syndrome, and it can mimic an ulnar neuropathy.[54] The anomaly should be sought whenever the amplitude of the response to median nerve stimulation is higher with elbow than with wrist stimulation, when there is an initial positivity of the median motor response to stimulation at the elbow, or when the response to ulnar stimulation is lower in amplitude at the elbow than at the wrist. Sensory fibers cross in the anastomosis only rarely.[55]

Deep Accessory Branch of Superficial Fibular (Peroneal) Nerve

The other potentially confusing anomaly is the deep accessory branch of the superficial fibular nerve. The axons that innervate the extensor digitorum brevis muscle of the foot

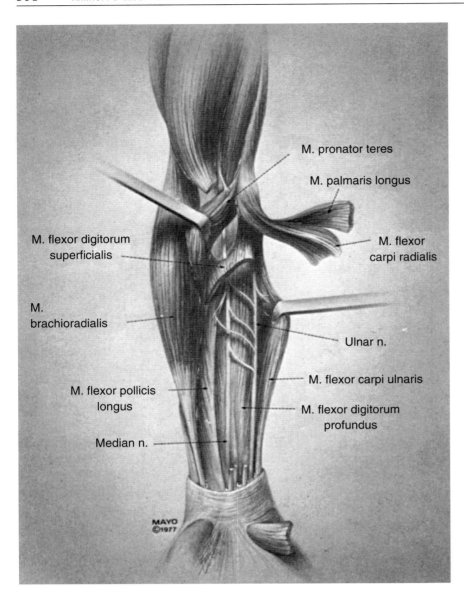

M. pronator teres

M. palmaris longus

M. flexor digitorum superficialis

M. flexor carpi radialis

M. brachioradialis

Ulnar n.

M. flexor carpi ulnaris

M. flexor pollicis longus

M. flexor digitorum profundus

Median n.

MAYO
©1977

FIGURE 13-16 ▪ Sites of anastomotic fibers crossing from median nerve to ulnar nerve. (By permission of Mayo Foundation.)

travel through the superficial rather than through the deep fibular nerve and pass posterior to the lateral malleolus rather than anterior to the ankle.[19] The detour of fibers away from the deep fibular nerve results in a lower-amplitude response with distal than with proximal stimulation of the fibular nerve. This lower amplitude is seen in 15 to 20 percent of normal people and can be especially confusing in the presence of a fibular neuropathy with partial conduction block (Fig. 13-19).

Other Anomalies

In addition to the major ones listed earlier, a number of uncommon anomalies may be encountered during nerve conduction studies. Examples include an anomalous superficial radial sensory branch with Martin–Gruber anastomosis,[56] a radial-innervated extensor digitorum manus

muscle on the dorsum of the hand,[57] an "all-ulnar hand" with lumbrical and thenar muscles innervated by the ulnar nerve, and a fibular-innervated extensor digitorum brevis high on the dorsum of the foot (see Fig. 13-19).

PATHOPHYSIOLOGY

Peripheral nerve disorders produce only a limited number of electrophysiologic alterations; the major types of abnormalities are conduction slowing, conduction block, and reduced or absent motor or sensory potentials.[58] Each of these may be focal or diffuse in distribution. Reduced or absent responses result from Wallerian degeneration after axonal disruption, or from axonal degeneration, as in "dying-back" neuropathies. Slowing of conduction occurs with segmental demyelination or with narrowing of the axons. Conduction block (loss of

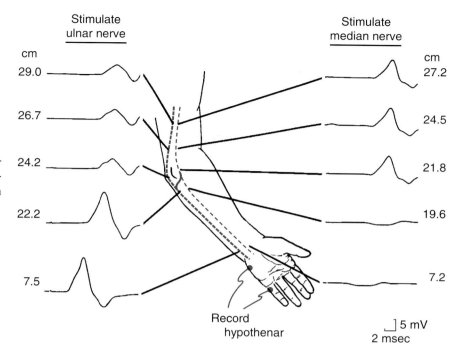

FIGURE 13-17 ▪ Hypothenar muscle evoked responses to ulnar and median nerve stimulation with median-to-ulnar anastomosis in the proximal forearm.

conduction over a short segment of nerve) occurs with a metabolic alteration in the membrane, as with a local anesthetic block, or with a structural alteration in the myelin, as in telescoping or segmental demyelination, and in other multifocal neuropathies such as sarcoid.[59]

Recent reports have described stimulation frequency-dependent conduction block in focal neuropathy.[60]

The hallmark of conduction block is a reduction in amplitude of the response obtained by stimulation proximal to the site of the block, whereas conduction slowing is seen

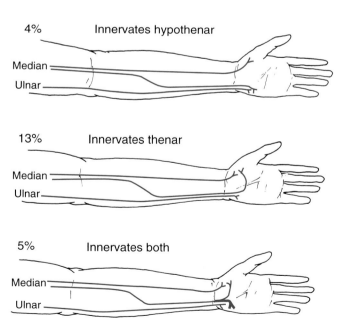

FIGURE 13-18 ▪ Distribution of fibers in three types of median–ulnar forearm anastomosis in 78 normal subjects. (Data from Wilbourn AJ, Lambert E: The forearm median-to-ulnar nerve communication: electrodiagnostic aspects. Neurology, 26:368, 1976.)

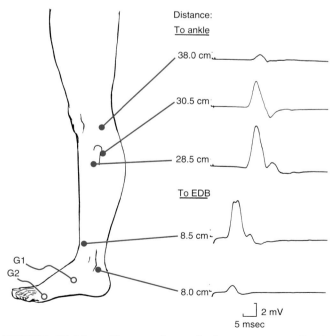

FIGURE 13-19 ▪ Changes in evoked response amplitude from extensor digitorum brevis muscle (EDB) with fibular (peroneal) nerve stimulation in the presence of a localized fibular neuropathy at the head of the fibula and an anomalous deep accessory fibular nerve.

TABLE 13-1 ■ Duration of Deficit After Peripheral Nerve Injury

Injury	Duration of Deficit
CONDUCTION BLOCK (AMPLITUDE CHANGE)	
Metabolic	Seconds to minutes
Myelin loss	Days to weeks
Axonal distortion	Weeks to months
AXONAL DISRUPTION (FIBRILLATION POTENTIALS)	
Few axons	No deficit
Many axons	Weeks to months
All axons	Months to years

as prolonged latency. Although conduction block and slowing may be seen in combination, they often occur independently. Conduction block is more common in rapidly developing disorders and focal conduction slowing is more common in chronic disorders. Lack of function is best identified by an absent or reduced response to stimulation at any site. Amplitude and area can help to categorize nerve damage into broad groups. For instance, in traumatic injuries of a nerve, there is usually either conduction block with an amplitude difference between proximal and distal sites of stimulation, or axonal disruption with low-amplitude responses at all sites of stimulation, and fibrillation potentials in affected muscles. Either process may occur with the other and produce clinical deficits of different durations (Table 13-1).

Thus, no single change in nerve conduction studies is typical of the clinical phenomenon of neurapraxia, in which there is a transient loss of function without atrophy. If neurapraxia is caused by a metabolic alteration, it lasts only a few minutes; however, if caused by axonal distortion with telescoping of internodes, it may persist for weeks or months (Fig. 13-20). The results of nerve conduction studies are a function of the underlying pathologic change and not of the duration of the disorder.

Localized Peripheral Nerve Damage

Localized peripheral nerve damage is characterized by low-amplitude responses, slow conduction, or a change in CMAP amplitude. The CMAP amplitude may be low at all sites of stimulation if the damage is proximal to the sites of stimulation. A lower-amplitude response at proximal sites than at distal sites of stimulation requires a search for a single, localized abnormality along the nerve; reduction in CMAP amplitude localized to a short segment of nerve is called a "conduction block," in which some of the axons are unable to transmit an action potential through the damaged segment but are functioning distal to it. If all axons are blocked in a segment, stimulation proximal to the site of the lesion produces no response distal to the lesion.

Localized nerve damage may also produce a short segment of slow conduction in the nerve that typically is due to chronic, mild compression.[61] Such focal slowing

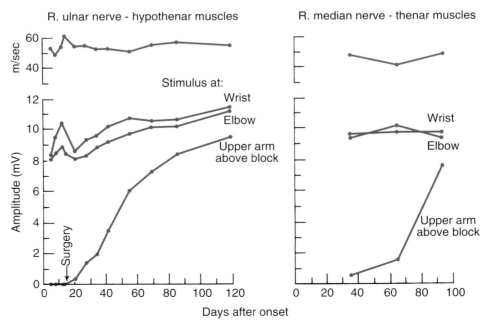

FIGURE 13-20 ■ Evolution of velocity and amplitude changes of hypothenar and thenar evoked responses with ulnar and median neuropathy caused by compression in the upper arm. (By permission of E. H. Lambert, Mayo Clinic, Rochester, MN.)

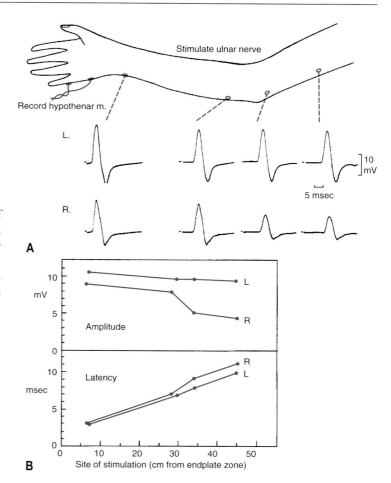

FIGURE 13-21 ▪ Changes in amplitude and latency of hypothenar evoked responses to ulnar nerve stimulation in the presence of a localized right (R) ulnar neuropathy at the elbow. **A**, Tracings. **B**, Plots of evoked responses. Normal responses are present in the left arm (L). (By permission of E. H. Lambert, Mayo Clinic, Rochester, MN.)

of conduction must be distinguished from conduction block, which may also occur with localized nerve damage but is more likely to be due to acute or subacute compression (Fig. 13-21).

Chronic mild compression of a nerve primarily produces slowing of conduction that is proportional to the duration and severity of compression. Selective slowing of nerve conduction in some of the axons in the nerve is associated with a gradual reduction in amplitude on proximal stimulation because of dispersion and increased duration of the response; however, the area of the CMAP remains relatively constant.

Diffuse Peripheral Nerve Damage

Nerve conduction studies can distinguish between general categories of nerve disorders.[62] A disorder associated primarily with axonal destruction (e.g., axonal dystrophies and dying-back neuropathies) is associated predominantly with a reduction in amplitude of the CMAP at all sites of stimulation, with relatively little (or, at the most, up to 30 percent) slowing in conduction velocity. In contrast, a disorder characterized by primary

segmental demyelination is associated with pronounced slowing of conduction (usually to less than 50 percent of normal) and with a progressive, proximal reduction in amplitude of the CMAP caused by dispersion of the response (Fig. 13-22). Although distal latency may increase with low-amplitude CMAPs regardless of their cause, marked slowing of motor conduction generally is sufficient to identify demyelinating neuropathy. Most peripheral nerve disorders produce greater clinical and electrophysiologic changes distally. They commonly are referred to as "length-dependent" neuropathies.

PERIPHERAL NEUROPATHIES

Variations in the distribution and differences in the type of pathologic changes in peripheral neuropathies result in different patterns of abnormality in nerve conduction studies (Table 13-2). Although the location and severity of nerve disease are defined well by nerve conduction studies, the presence of mixed patterns or of mild changes precludes characterization of the pathology of most peripheral neuropathies by nerve conduction

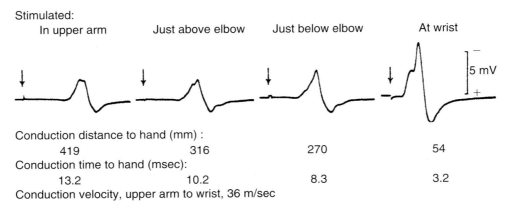

FIGURE 13-22 ■ Dispersion of evoked potentials and reduction of evoked response amplitude from hypothenar muscles in severe neuropathy. (By permission of E. H. Lambert, Mayo Clinic, Rochester, MN.)

studies. Although many patients with neuropathy show mixed findings on nerve conduction studies, some patients may have a predominantly axonal or segmental demyelinating neuropathy (Table 13-3).[62]

Axonal Neuropathies

Axonal neuropathies primarily affect the axon and are characterized by either diffuse degeneration or dying-back of the distal portion of the axon. They are particularly common with toxic and metabolic disorders. The major change on nerve conduction studies is usually a reduction in the amplitude of the SNAP, especially the medial plantar SNAP.[63,64] The CMAP typically is reduced later, but can be lost early in the fibular distribution in predominantly motor axonopathies. This reduction is proportional to the severity of the disease. Some axonal neuropathies (e.g., those associated with vitamin B_{12} deficiency, carcinoma, and Friedreich ataxia) chiefly affect sensory fibers, whereas others (e.g., lead neuropathies) have a greater effect on motor fibers. Sensory axons commonly are involved earlier and more severely than are motor axons.[65] Occasionally, sensory potentials of very low amplitude are associated with only mild sensory symptoms. In contrast to the change in amplitude, there is usually little change in latency or conduction velocity in axonal neuropathies because conduction in individual axons generally remains normal until the axon has degenerated. Therefore, normal conduction velocities should not be considered evidence against the presence of a neuropathy. Often, the only finding will be fibrillation potentials on needle examination of distal muscles (especially intrinsic foot muscles) with or without low-amplitude CMAPs. Collateral sprouting of intact axons can result in normal amplitudes of CMAPs with very low motor unit number estimates.

If many of the large axons are lost, conduction velocity may be reduced slightly but not to less than 70 percent of normal. Axonal neuropathies typically affect the longer

	Motor Nerve Studies				Sensory Nerve Studies		
	Action Potential				**Action Potential**		
Disorder	**Amplitude**	**Duration**	**Conduction Velocity**	**F-Wave Latency**	**Amplitude**	**Duration**	**Conduction Velocity**
Axonal neuropathy	↓	Normal	>70%	Mild ↑	↓↓	Normal	>70%
Demyelinating neuropathy	↓ Proximal	↑ Proximal	<50%	↑	↓	↑ Proximal	<50%
Mononeuropathy	↓	↑	↓	↑	↓↓	↑	↓
Regenerated nerve	↓	↑	↓	↑	↓	↓	↓
Motor neuron disease	↓↓	Normal	>70%	Mild ↑	Normal	Normal	Normal
Neuromuscular transmission defect	(↓)	Normal	Normal	Normal	Normal	Normal	Normal
Myopathy	(↓)	Normal	Normal	Normal	Normal	Normal	Normal

TABLE 13-2 ■ **Patterns of Abnormality in Nerve Conduction Studies of Peripheral Neuromuscular Disorders**

↑, increase; ↓, decrease; ↓↓, greater decrease; (↓) occasionally decreased.

TABLE 13-3 ■ Patterns of Abnormality in Peripheral Neuropathy

PREDOMINANT CHANGES OF AXONAL DEGENERATION

Diabetes (some patients)
Guillain–Barré syndrome (some patients)
Toxic neuropathy (e.g., vincristine, acrylamide)
Alcohol
Uremia
Acute intermittent porphyria
Collagen/vascular diseases
Carcinoma
Amyloid

PREDOMINANT CHANGES OF SEGMENTAL DEMYELINATION

Diabetes (some patients)
Guillain–Barré syndrome (some patients)
Déjerine–Sottas disease
Diphtheritic neuropathy
Chronic inflammatory neuropathy
Refsum disease
Leukodystrophies
Neuropathy with monoclonal protein

axons earlier and therefore are seen first in the lower extremities; typically, they are more severe distally (length-dependent neuropathy). Nerves that are more susceptible to local trauma because of their superficial location are also more sensitive. Accordingly, these disorders are often manifested electrophysiologically first as fibular neuropathies with low-amplitude or absent responses, whereas other motor nerves remain intact. Axonal neuropathies may be associated with a change of the refractory period of the nerve and with a relative resistance to ischemia.

Patients with acute- or subacute-onset neuropathy usually have acute inflammatory demyelinating polyradiculoneuropathy or, less commonly, a toxic neuropathy.[65] A subset of patients with rapid-onset, generalized neuropathies have acute motor axonal neuropathy (AMAN) with low-amplitude CMAPs, normal sensory potentials and F-wave latencies, and prominent fibrillation potentials.[66,67] If the low amplitude is caused by severe, proximal axonal destruction, the prognosis for recovery is poorer. In some patients with AMAN, especially after *Campylobacter* infection, the process attacks the intramuscular nerve terminals with loss of amplitude, small motor unit action potentials, and fibrillation potentials. The electrodiagnostic findings may resemble a myopathy, but rapid recoveries can occur.[68]

Segmental Demyelinating Neuropathies

The Guillain–Barré syndrome, or acute inflammatory demyelinating polyradiculoneuropathy (AIDP), has a spectrum of electrophysiologic changes. There may

be no abnormalities on nerve conduction studies, or the abnormalities may be limited to proximal slowing with prolongation of the F-wave or H-reflex latency.[69] Although some nerve conduction findings are more commonly abnormal early in the disorder (i.e., F waves, low CMAPs, an abnormal upper-extremity SNAP combined with a normal sural response, and multiple indirect discharges), any one or more of them may be abnormal in individual patients.[70,71] The occurrence of multiple late waves likely is related to the occurrence of myokymia in some patients. Thus, a subacute neuropathy with marked slowing or dispersion in more than one nerve is highly suggestive of AIDP. Sensory fibers are less involved than are motor ones; when the former are affected, it is primarily by axonal loss, in contrast to the prominent demyelination that occurs in motor fibers. The responses recorded distally with stimulation at proximal sites (e.g., a spinal nerve or the brachial plexus) also may be abnormal. More commonly, however, the disorder is associated with prolonged distal latencies of a mild or moderate degree in many separate nerves and with variable slowing of conduction velocities, which may be symmetric or asymmetric. The facial nerves or other cranial nerves may be involved, with abnormalities on blink-reflex testing or on facial nerve stimulation (Fig. 13-23).

Segmental demyelinating neuropathies are usually subacute inflammatory disorders such as AIDP, chronic

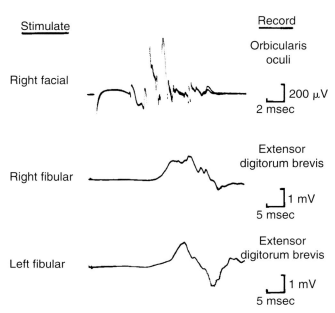

FIGURE 13-23 ■ Dispersion of compound muscle action potentials with needle and surface electrode recordings in Guillain–Barré syndrome.

inflammatory demyelinating polyradiculoneuropathy (CIDP), and diphtheritic neuropathies. However, similar patterns may be seen in hypertrophic neuropathies such as Déjerine–Sottas disease and hereditary motor sensory neuropathy (Charcot–Marie–Tooth type 1, or CMT1).[72] Demyelinating neuropathies typically are associated with prolonged latencies and with a pronounced slowing of conduction, often in the range of 10 to 20 m/sec. Commonly, the CMAP is relatively preserved in amplitude on distal stimulation but is reduced and dispersed on proximal stimulation (see Fig. 13-22). Long-duration (greater than 9 msec) CMAPs are a characteristic of CIDP that is not seen in localized neuropathies, even with markedly prolonged distal latencies.[73] The proximal increase in duration typically is associated with CMAP dispersion with an irregular waveform. These characteristics are important in distinguishing long-duration CMAPs in demyelinating neuropathies from the long-duration CMAPs of criticial illness myopathy (see later). In some hereditary disorders (e.g., Déjerine–Sottas disease) the velocity may be only a few meters per second.[74] Acquired demyelinating neuropathies commonly affect sites of nerve compression early, producing asymmetric neuropathies of the fibular, ulnar, or median nerves at the knee, elbow, or wrist, respectively. The refractory period in demyelinating neuropathies is reduced, often to the extent that repetitive stimulation at rates as low as 5 Hz causes a decrement, although the decrement most commonly does not appear until rates of 10 or 20 Hz are used. One form of demyelinating neuropathy with multifocal motor conduction block may resemble amyotrophic lateral sclerosis superficially, but it often has other widespread changes including focal conduction blocks on nerve conduction studies.[75,76]

At times, the pattern of nerve conduction abnormality in demyelinating neuropathies helps to differentiate an acquired process from a hereditary one. The former typically has scattered areas of slowing, with some areas being much more abnormal than others, whereas hereditary disorders generally have uniform, symmetric patterns of abnormality. Thus, a single normal motor nerve conduction study can serve to exclude CMT1, but several nerves need to be tested when one attempts to demonstrate uniformity in CMT1.[77]

Hereditary neuropathy with pressure palsies (HNPP or tomaculous neuropathy) shows an unusual combination of mild generalized slowing of conduction with multifocal conduction block at sites of common compression, such as the median nerve at the wrist, ulnar nerve at the elbow, or fibular nerve at the knee.[78]

Acquired demyelinating disorders often show more dispersion with proximal stimulation than do hereditary disorders. This latter distinction is not always reliable, however, because some patients who have a hereditary demyelinating neuropathy with a low-amplitude CMAP may have pronounced dispersion at proximal sites of stimulation (Fig. 13-24).[79] Because of the varied nature of the disorder, attempts have been made to develop consensus criteria or other defining criteria for the diagnosis of CIDP. A recent one had sensitivity around 60 percent.[80] Criteria in another recent publication attempted to increase the sensitivity by defining the number of nerves with conduction block or temporal dispersion.

Similar consensus criteria have been developed for multifocal motor neuropathy.[81] Criteria for a definite diagnosis include the following:

1. Weakness in multifocal distribution with normal sensation
2. Definite conduction block in two nerves, excluding common sites of compression
3. Normal sensory conduction across the same segment
4. Normal sensory conduction in three nerves, and
5. Absence of signs of upper motor neuron involvement.

A probable diagnosis requires probable conduction block in two or more nerves, or definite conduction block in one nerve and probable block in another.

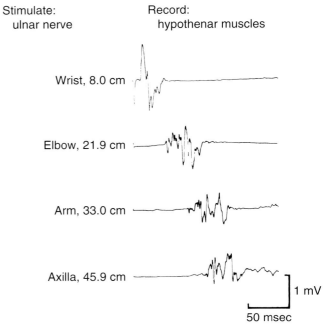

FIGURE 13-24 ■ Dispersion of compound muscle action potentials in hereditary motor and sensory neuropathy.

Mixed Axonal and Demyelinating Neuropathies

Diabetes is the most common cause of a peripheral neuropathy, and may show either axonal, demyelinating, or mixed features.[82] In diabetes, small vascular lesions in a multifocal distribution result in a variety of patterns of abnormality on nerve conduction studies. Among the most common patterns in diabetes are a mild, generalized distal neuropathy caused by multiple small additive lesions; and mononeuropathies of the median nerve at the wrist, ulnar nerve at the elbow, or fibular nerve at the knee. Often, the focal mononeuropathies are superimposed on mild, diffuse change, with generalized reduction in amplitudes of the CMAP and mild slowing of conduction. Needle examination often shows only mild changes, usually distally. However, some patients with diabetes have a lumbosacral polyradiculopathy manifested primarily by diffuse fibrillation potentials in the L2 to L4 paraspinal muscles. This pattern may be associated with prolongation of F-wave latencies as a result of proximal slowing of conduction. F waves are the most sensitive measure of the lumbosacral polyradiculopathy and generalized neuropathy of diabetes.[83] Nerve conduction studies show a high correlation with clinical findings. Threshold electrotonus measurements have demonstrated unique findings in diabetes, suggesting an abnormal inward rectification that may provide insights into the pathophysiology of diabetic neuropathy.[84]

FOCAL NEUROPATHIES

The electrophysiologic changes found by nerve conduction studies in mononeuropathies vary with the rapidity of development, the duration of damage, and the severity of damage, as well as with the underlying disorder. With a chronic compressive lesion, localized narrowing or paranodal or internodal demyelination produces localized slowing of conduction. Narrowing of axons distal to a chronic compression causes a slowing of conduction along the entire length of the nerve. Telescoping of axons with intussusception of one internode into another distorts and obliterates the nodes of Ranvier and blocks conduction. Moderate segmental demyelination and local metabolic alterations are often associated with conduction block. Such conduction blocks are manifested as a lower-amplitude CMAP with stimulation proximal, rather than distal, to the site of damage. Such localized damage without axonal disruption may take up to 3 months to recover.[85] A segment of nerve distal to complete disruption of the axons after an acute lesion may continue to function normally for as many as 5 days. Then, as the axons undergo Wallerian

TABLE 13-4 ▪ Compound Action Potential Amplitude to Supramaximal Stimulation After Peripheral Nerve Injury

Injury	Amplitude		
	0–5 Days	After 5 Days	Recovery
CONDUCTION BLOCK			
Proximal stimulation	Low	Low	Increases
Distal stimulation	Normal	Normal	Normal
AXONAL DISRUPTION			
Proximal stimulation	Low	Low	Increases
Distal stimulation	Normal	Low	Increases

degeneration, their conduction ceases and the amplitude of the CMAP diminishes and finally disappears. One week after an acute injury, the amplitude of the evoked response can be used as an approximation of the number of intact, viable axons (Table 13-4).

An evolution of electrophysiologic changes after peripheral nerve injury is also seen on needle examination and is an aid in characterizing mononeuropathies (Table 13-5). Therefore, adequate assessment of a peripheral nerve injury should include both needle examination and nerve conduction studies. The significance of changes with time after injury is outlined in Table 13-6. The sequence of changes shows that nerve conduction studies can be important in the assessment of nerve injury within the first few days after injury.

Whereas electrophysiologic testing can aid in identifying, localizing, and characterizing a neuropathy, these tests are commonly of particular value in the assessment of the median, ulnar, and fibular nerves.

Median Neuropathies

The most common focal mononeuropathy is the carpal tunnel syndrome, in which the median nerve is compressed in the space formed by the wrist bones and the carpal ligament. Early or mild compression of the median nerve

TABLE 13-5 ▪ Findings on Needle Examination After Peripheral Nerve Injury

Injury	0–15 Days	After 15 Days	Recovery
CONDUCTION BLOCK			
Fibrillation potentials	None	None	None
Motor unit potentials	↓ Recruitment	↓ Recruitment	↑ Recruitment
AXONAL DISRUPTION			
Fibrillation potentials	None	Present	Reduced
Motor unit potentials	↓ Recruitment	↓ Recruitment	"Nascent"

TABLE 13-6 ■ **Interpretation of Electrophysiologic Findings After Peripheral Nerve Injury**

Finding	Interpretation
0–5 DAYS	
Motor unit potentials present	Nerve intact, functioning axons
Fibrillations present	Old lesion
Low compound action potential	Old lesion
5–15 DAYS	
Compound action potential distal only	Conduction block
Low compound action potential	Amount of axonal disruption
Motor unit potentials present	Nerve intact
AFTER 15 DAYS	
Compound action potential distal only	Conduction block
Motor unit potentials present	Nerve intact
Fibrillation potentials	Amount of axonal disruption
	Distribution of damage
RECOVERY	
Increasing compound action potential	Block clearing
Increasing number of motor unit potentials	Block clearing
Decreasing number of fibrillation potentials	Reinnervation
"Nascent" motor unit potentials	Reinnervation

in the carpal tunnel may not lead to any electrophysiologic abnormalities; however, more than 90 percent of symptomatic patients have localized slowing of conduction in sensory fibers.[86] Median nerve conduction abnormalities may be detected with a number of different techniques, each of which has advantages and disadvantages. The sensory latency through the carpal tunnel is the most sensitive measurement. The sensitivity can be enhanced by comparison of the wrist segment with a more distal segment, or by comparison of the median palm-to-wrist latency with the ulnar palm-to-wrist latency (Fig. 13-25).[87] Wrist-to-palm motor conduction may also enhance detection.[88] At times, selective damage to individual fascicles may make recording from single digits important. Comparison of median with radial distal latency is also quite sensitive in identifying carpal tunnel syndrome but is less specific because of its lower sensitivity to other forms of peripheral nerve damage.[89] Summation of the differences in latency between median and radial latencies to the thumb, median and ulnar midpalmar orthodromic latencies, and median and ulnar latencies to the ring finger ("combined sensory index") may demonstrate signs of median neuropathy at the wrist when single measurements do not do so.[90]

More severe nerve compression reduces the amplitude of the SNAP and prolongs the latency to a greater extent and over a longer distance. Severe median neuropathy at the wrist also increases the distal motor latency to the thenar muscles and eventually can reduce the thenar CMAP (Fig. 13-26). Reduction of the CMAP is often associated with mild slowing of motor conduction velocity in the forearm, primarily caused by the loss of faster-conducting axons.[91] When the thenar CMAP is absent, lumbrical responses are often still preserved and permit local slowing to be recognized; comparison of lumbrical to interosseous latencies has been shown to match standard studies in recognition of carpal tunnel syndrome.[92,93] Severe abnormalities on nerve conduction studies are associated with fibrillation potentials or large motor unit action potentials on needle electromyography (EMG) with a predictive accuracy of 50 to 70 percent.[94]

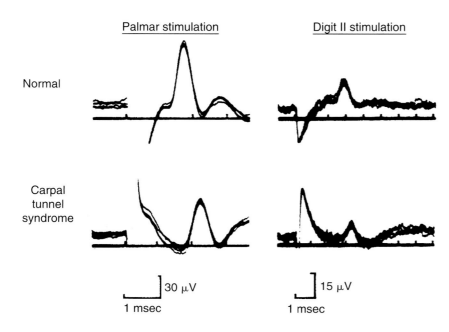

Palmar stimulation   Digit II stimulation

Normal

Carpal tunnel syndrome

30 μV   15 μV
1 msec   1 msec

FIGURE 13-25 ■ Sensory nerve action potentials in carpal tunnel syndrome. Palmar latency is prolonged (2.4 msec), whereas digital latency is still in the normal range (3.3 msec).

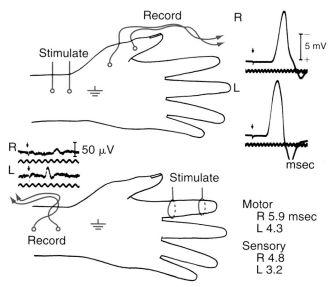

FIGURE 13-26 ■ Prolonged motor and sensory latencies with carpal tunnel syndrome on the right. (From Department of Neurology, Mayo Clinic and Mayo Foundation: Clinical Examinations in Neurology. 6th Ed. Mosby-Year Book, St. Louis, 1991, with permission.)

EMG thus can often add information to the assessment of carpal tunnel syndrome. Patients with chronic carpal tunnel syndrome have a higher incidence of anomalous innervation of the thenar muscles, with the amplitude of the response then being higher on elbow stimulation than on wrist stimulation or with an initial positivity of the CMAP with elbow stimulation (Fig. 13-27). Surgical outcomes are significantly poorer with both normal and severely abnormal nerve conduction studies, compared to patients with mild to moderately abnormal studies.[95]

Many patients with carpal tunnel syndrome have bilateral abnormalities on nerve conduction studies, even though symptoms may be unilateral. Therefore, conduction in the opposite extremity should be measured if a median neuropathy at the wrist is identified. A few patients have a normal sensory response and a prolonged distal motor latency. This may have a number of causes. For instance, there may be slowing with a chronic neurogenic atrophy because of a more proximal lesion (e.g., a C8 radiculopathy or anterior horn cell disease); or a radial sensory response may be evoked inadvertently by high-voltage stimulation of the median nerve and recorded as an apparent median sensory potential. Occasionally, patients have sensory branches to one or more fingers that are separated anatomically from the motor fibers and are relatively spared. Moreover, the severity of compression may not be the same for all fascicles of the median nerve, so that there is greater slowing in the axons to some digital nerves than to others. A median neuropathy may be an early finding in patients with more diffuse neuropathies, and it is therefore

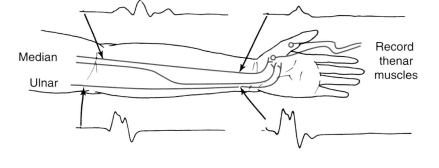

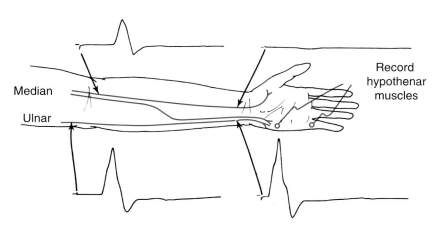

FIGURE 13-27 ■ Carpal tunnel syndrome with anomalous median-to-ulnar anastomosis. Thenar response with median nerve stimulation at the elbow is larger and more complex than that with stimulation at the wrist, and has too short a latency.

necessary to assess other nerves to exclude this possibility in patients with clinical evidence only of carpal tunnel syndrome. However, comparison of median conduction with conduction in other upper-limb nerves should be interpreted with caution in identifying carpal tunnel syndrome in patients with diabetes and neuropathy, who often have more prominent prolongation of median latencies than of other nerves.[96] It is safest to require moderate or marked relative median distal latency prolongation compared to other nerves to identify carpal tunnel syndrome in the presence of generalized peripheral neuropathy.[97] Indeed, segmental conduction including the most distal segment of the median nerve may be more reliable in identifying carpal tunnel syndrome superimposed on a peripheral neuropathy.[98,99]

Median neuropathies in the forearm are much less common and only rarely show abnormality on nerve conduction studies other than slightly low-amplitude sensory responses, motor responses, or both. Anterior interosseous neuropathy and pronator syndrome usually are manifested by fibrillation potentials in the appropriate muscles. Rarely, patients have localized slowing of conduction in the damaged segment of nerve.

Ulnar Neuropathies

The electrophysiologic alteration in ulnar neuropathies varies with the severity and location of the lesion. Rarely, a patient with compression of the ulnar nerve in the hand has a prolonged latency only in the branch to the first dorsal interosseous muscle or to the lumbrical muscle. In such a patient, the hypothenar muscles should not be the only recording site for ulnar nerve conduction studies. In most patients with an ulnar neuropathy, the abnormality is at the elbow and can be identified by recordings from the hypothenar muscle (see Figs. 13-20 and 13-21). As in the carpal tunnel syndrome, sensory fibers are more likely to be damaged than are motor fibers, so that the compound sensory action potential commonly is lost early. In some patients, focal slowing in ulnar sensory fibers across the elbow can be demonstrated. The most common localizing finding in ulnar neuropathy of recent onset is conduction block or, less likely, slowing at the elbow (see Fig. 13-21). Amplitude of the response is normal with stimulation at the wrist and below the elbow, but is lower by 30 percent or more with stimulation at sites above and proximal to the elbow. Precise localization of the site of damage is sometimes possible by stimulation at short intervals (inching) and may be

improved by near-nerve recording.[100,101] The conduction block may be associated with local slowing. Chronic ulnar neuropathy usually results in slowing of conduction, which typically is localized to the elbow, but in long-standing ulnar neuropathies may extend distal to the elbow. Conduction slowing of greater than 10 m/sec in the across-elbow segment compared to the forearm segment is seen with focal demyelination at the elbow. Although an occasional patient has slowing of conduction to the flexor carpi ulnaris, this muscle usually shows little or no change on nerve conduction studies and needle examination. In ulnar and median neuropathies, the F-wave latency is prolonged in proportion to the slowing in the peripheral segments. Because ulnar neuropathies commonly are bilateral, when an ulnar neuropathy is evident on one side, the opposite extremity should also be tested. Local sensitivity to mechanical stimulation at the elbow may be shown with electromyographic recordings in the absence of changes on nerve conduction studies.[102] Damage to the ulnar nerve distally in the deep ulnar branch in the palm can also be identified on nerve conduction studies.[92]

Fibular (Peroneal) Neuropathies

Neuropathy of the fibular nerve at the head of the fibula is another common focal lesion. Neuropathy of recent onset caused by compression is associated most often with a conduction block that can be localized precisely by stimulation at short intervals along the nerve to identify the area where the CMAP decreases (Fig. 13-28). Neuropathy without conduction block is not infrequently due to ganglion cyst damage to the nerve; ultrasound or magnetic resonance imaging (MRI) of the knee should always be considered in these patients.[103] Conduction across this segment generally is not slowed, although in lesions of longer standing the slowing becomes more prominent in adults and children.[104]

Nerve conduction studies of the superficial fibular nerve may be of value in localizing damage to fibular fibers along their length. A localized fibular neuropathy usually shows loss of the sensory response, as do lesions of the sciatic nerve, lumbar plexus, and spinal nerve distal to the dorsal root ganglion. In an L5 radiculopathy with sensory loss and some motor slowing, the superficial fibular sensory nerve is normal in most patients if the damage is proximal to the dorsal root ganglion.[105,106] Some patients with a moderately severe fibular neuropathy may lose the response from the extensor digitorum brevis, the most common site of recording. In such

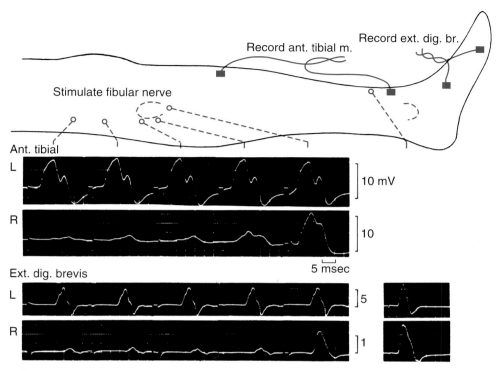

FIGURE 13-28 ■ Localized conduction block at head of fibula in "crossed-leg" fibular neuropathy. (By permission of E. H. Lambert, Mayo Clinic, Rochester, MN.)

circumstances, recordings from the anterior tibial muscle and other anterior compartment muscles on stimulation at the head of the fibula and the knee may still demonstrate a block or slowing of conduction in the nerve. F-wave latencies may aid in distinguishing between fibular neuropathies and L5 root lesions if they show proximal slowing. Anomalous innervation of the extensor digitorum brevis muscle by a deep accessory branch of the superficial fibular nerve may make it more difficult to recognize a fibular neuropathy. Because sciatic nerve lesions may present as fibular neuropathies without localized slowing of conduction, the short head of the biceps femoris muscle should be tested for fibrillation potentials to exclude a more proximal lesion.[107]

Other Neuropathies

A few other neuropathies, such as those of the radial and tibial nerves, are localized less commonly by nerve conduction studies, whereas evaluation of many others is not aided by nerve conduction studies because the neuropathies do not show localized slowing. In facial neuropathies such as Bell palsy, stimulation cannot be applied proximally and distally to the site of the lesion. The usual findings in Bell palsy with neurapraxia are normal amplitudes and latencies of CMAPs; in axonal degeneration, the amplitude of the CMAP is decreased in proportion to the axonal destruction. Blink reflexes can be used to measure conduction across the involved segment, but they are commonly absent in Bell palsy. Conduction studies can help to differentiate hemifacial spasm from other facial movements by demonstrating ephaptic activation of lower facial muscles during periods of spasm (i.e., the "lateral spread response"). The normal early-response blink reflex occurs only in the ocular muscles on the stimulated side. After aberrant reinnervation in patients with Bell palsy and in patients with hemifacial spasm, an early response can be recorded over the perioral muscles on stimulation of the first division of the trigeminal nerve.

Most brachial plexus lesions are traumatic and nerve conduction studies are of limited value. In general, the amplitude of the CMAP is reduced and sensory responses are absent in the distribution of the damaged fibers. In patients with lower-trunk lesions, the ulnar sensory response and medial antebrachial cutaneous responses are reduced or absent; in those with upper-trunk lesions, the median sensory response of the thumb and the lateral antebrachial cutaneous response are reduced or absent; and in middle-trunk lesions, the median sensory

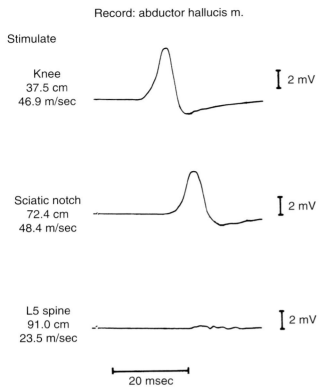

Record: abductor hallucis m.

Stimulate

Knee
37.5 cm
46.9 m/sec

$\biguplus$ 2 mV

Sciatic notch
72.4 cm
48.4 m/sec

$\biguplus$ 2 mV

L5 spine
91.0 cm
23.5 m/sec

$\biguplus$ 2 mV

20 msec

FIGURE 13-29 ■ Responses of the abductor hallucis muscle to stimulation of its nerve supply at the knee, at the sciatic notch, and at the root level. There is conduction block caused by sacral plexus compression.

response to the third digit is reduced.[108] Phrenic nerve conduction studies may show abnormality in C5-level damage.[109] In patients with slowly evolving or compressive lesions of the plexus (e.g., tumors), a localized slowing of conduction of motor or sensory fibers and, occasionally, conduction block may be identified on stimulation at the supraclavicular or nerve root level (Fig. 13-29). In the neurogenic thoracic outlet syndrome, there may be a reduction in amplitude of ulnar sensory action potentials, but there is no slowing of nerve conduction unless there has been axonal damage and regeneration.

Nerve conduction studies in lumbosacral plexus lesions show reduction in motor and sensory response amplitudes. Proximal stimulation with needle electrodes may help to localize slowing or conduction block to the plexus.[110]

Radiculopathies

Cervical and lumbosacral radiculopathies usually are not associated with changes in nerve conduction studies; however, if there is sufficient destruction of axons and Wallerian degeneration in the distribution of the nerve

being tested, the amplitude of the CMAP may be reduced.[111] For instance, in an L5 radiculopathy, the response of the extensor digitorum brevis muscle to fibular nerve stimulation often is either reduced in amplitude or absent. In the presence of atrophy and a small CMAP, there may be mild slowing of conduction in the motor axons innervating the atrophic muscle. In mild lumbosacral radiculopathy, measurements of H-reflex latencies have been reported to aid in identifying proximal slowing of conduction, but F-wave latencies and dispersion (chronodispersion) are not of help in identifying lumbar radiculopathies. Because most lesions of the spinal nerve and nerve root are proximal to the dorsal root ganglion, the sensory potentials typically are normal, even in the distribution of a sensory deficit. This phenomenon is valuable in identifying avulsion of a nerve root, in which there is total anesthesia and loss of motor function with normal sensory potentials.

SYSTEM DEGENERATIONS

Degenerative diseases of the central nervous system may involve either dorsal root ganglion or anterior horn cells. Because the peripheral axons of the anterior horn cells and dorsal root ganglion cells are assessed in nerve conduction studies, both groups show abnormalities on electrophysiologic testing.

Motor System

Motor system degenerations include motor neuron disease such as amyotrophic lateral sclerosis, spinal muscular atrophy, the neuronal form of Charcot–Marie–Tooth disease, Kugelberg–Welander disease, and Werdnig–Hoffmann disease. Each of these disorders is associated with degeneration of the anterior horn cells and loss of peripheral motor axons. The individual axons conduct normally until they cease to function.[112] Therefore, nerve conduction does not become slow unless there is a significant loss of large axons. The conduction measured from the whole nerve after large, fast-conducting axons are lost does not fall below 70 percent of the lower limit of normal, but ion dysfunction has been demonstrated.[113,114] F-wave latencies show little or no slowing but the responses are often of large amplitude from collateral sprouting.[115]

The most striking change found in nerve conduction studies of motor neuron diseases is a reduction in the amplitude of the CMAP.[116] This reduction is related to the loss of innervation of the muscle but varies with the rate of progression of the disease. In slowly progressive disorders, if collateral sprouting and reinnervation compensate for loss of the anterior horn cells, the amplitude of the CMAP may remain normal, with a slight slowing of conduction. In these cases, motor unit number estimates will demonstrate the loss of motor units.[117–119] Usually, mild slowing of motor conduction is not seen until the action potential amplitude has decreased below normal. Occasionally, a patient with motor neuron disease will have a decrement on repetitive stimulation, particularly when responses are of low amplitude. Low-amplitude CMAPs and a decrement on repetitive stimulation indicate a poor prognosis in motor neuron disease. In motor neuron diseases, sensory fibers generally are not involved and sensory conduction studies are usually normal.

Sensory System

Afferent axons may undergo mild degeneration in disorders such as Friedreich ataxia, adrenomyeloneuropathy, and vitamin B_{12} deficiency (carcinomatous sensory neuropathy may have a similar picture), and in a number of toxic or infectious disorders.[120,121] The degeneration seen in the axons in the posterior and lateral columns of the spinal cord in these disorders is caused by degeneration of their cells of origin in the dorsal root ganglia. These cell bodies also give rise to the large sensory fibers in the peripheral nerves that are the source of the largest proportion of the compound nerve action potentials recorded in sensory nerve conduction studies. Therefore, in this group of disorders, the amplitude of the compound sensory action potential typically is reduced, and SNAPs often cannot be recorded with surface electrodes. There also may be mild changes in motor nerve conduction studies in these patients, but to a much lesser extent than those in sensory studies.

PATTERNS OF ABNORMALITY

Although most nerve conduction studies involve either mononeuropathies or diffuse neuropathies that do not suggest specific etiologies, some patterns of abnormality can suggest a possible etiology or pathologic process. The following summary and Tables 13-2, 13-4, 13-5, and 13-6 summarize the significance of patterns of abnormality that have been discussed earlier in the chapter.

1. Markedly reduced CMAP amplitudes with normal sensory responses can occur with motor polyradiculopathies, but they are seen more commonly with amyotrophic lateral sclerosis.
2. Demyelinating disorders with comparable diffuse abnormalities in most nerves are more likely to

be inherited than acquired; acquired processes are more likely to be asymmetric with variable involvement along the course of nerves.
3. The medial plantar and sural SNAP are the most sensitive sensory responses, and are abnormal in most large-fiber neuropathies. They show a greater reduction in amplitude than the sensory response of the median nerve; the reverse is true in demyelinating neuropathies.[122]
4. Dense sensory loss with normal sensory potentials in that distribution most likely is caused by damage at or proximal to the dorsal root ganglion, whereas more distal damage results in low-amplitude sensory potentials.[123]
5. Interpretation of findings with focal nerve damage is time-dependent. Change in response amplitude with conduction block or axonal disruption can localize the site of a lesion immediately after injury. Thus, the common belief that nerve conduction studies are without clinical value until 2 weeks after an injury is erroneous.
6. The amplitude of responses distal and proximal to a nerve injury beyond 5 days can define the extent of axonal disruption and the prognosis for spontaneous recovery.
7. Weakness solely due to conduction block recovers in 1 to 12 weeks, depending on the type of damage.

DISORDERS OF THE NEUROMUSCULAR JUNCTION

Of the disorders of neuromuscular transmission, the myasthenic syndrome and *Clostridium botulinum* intoxication are most likely to show changes on nerve conduction studies, with low-amplitude CMAPs. In both of these conditions, the rate of release of acetylcholine from nerve terminals is very low, and neuromuscular transmission is blocked to a large proportion of the muscle fibers. Therefore, a single stimulus usually elicits small CMAPs (Fig. 13-30).[124] Patients with a clinical history of weakness who have low CMAPs should always be tested further with slow, repetitive stimulation and exercise to search for evidence of a decrement and facilitation, the usual signs of a defect of neuromuscular transmission (see Chapter 17). In myasthenia gravis, the CMAP amplitude may be lower than normal, but most patients have amplitudes that are in the normal range. Motor nerve conduction velocities and sensory nerve conduction studies are normal. Congenital myasthenic syndromes may show repetitive firing of the CMAP.

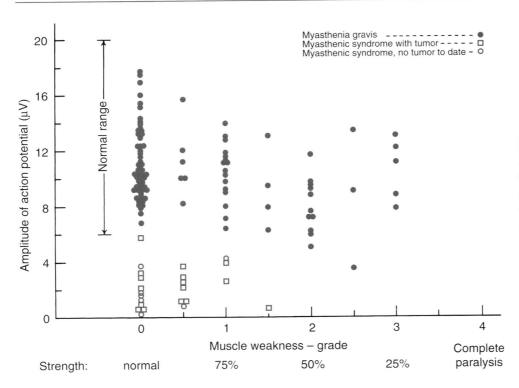

FIGURE 13-30 ◾ Amplitudes of hypothenar compound muscle action potentials in myasthenia gravis and myasthenic syndrome at different grades of muscle weakness. (By permission of E. H. Lambert, Mayo Clinic, Rochester, MN.)

PRIMARY MUSCLE DISORDERS

Most myopathies affect the proximal muscles that are not tested on routine nerve conduction studies; therefore, routine studies show little change from normal. However, with proximal nerve conduction studies or in patients with myopathies involving distal muscles, the CMAP often is reduced in proportion to the amount of muscle atrophy (Fig. 13-31). Motor and sensory conduction velocities and latencies are normal. In some myopathies, particularly those associated with myotonia, such as periodic paralysis and myotonic dystrophy, the excitability of the muscle fiber membrane varies. The CMAP may change with repetitive stimulation or change slowly during a period of 30 to 60 minutes at rest. After prolonged exercise, the amplitude may decrease to 50 percent of normal before slowly returning to normal (Fig. 13-32). If a patient with a myotonic disorder has been physically active just before nerve conduction studies are performed, the CMAP may be of low amplitude initially and then return gradually to normal levels. Some patients with myotonic dystrophy have mild slowing of motor conduction velocity in the lower extremities.

Critical illness myopathy is characterized by low-amplitude, very-long-duration CMAPs without the proximal dispersion seen in demyelinating neuropathies.[125] The broad response with a minimum of late positivity is missed easily on standard nerve conduction studies unless the CMAP duration is compared specifically with normal (Fig. 13-33). Muscle fibers in critical illness myopathy, unlike critical illness neuropathy, are inexcitable.[126,127]

DISORDERS ASSOCIATED WITH INVOLUNTARY ACTIVITY OF PERIPHERAL NERVE ORIGIN

A small group of disorders are manifested as stiffness of muscles, myokymia, and cramping as a result of excessive discharges in peripheral axons. In these disorders, there are many clinical patterns and a wide variation in electrical manifestations. The disorders can be subdivided into four categories: (1) those associated with clinical and pathologic evidence of peripheral nerve disease; (2) those associated with disorders of calcium, such as tetany and hypocalcemia; (3) those of unknown origin, which have been called continuous muscle fiber activity, neuromyotonia, cramp-fasciculation syndrome, and Isaacs syndrome; and (4) those that are hereditary. EMG in each of these disorders reveals characteristic findings that can help to identify them and distinguish between the groups. Conduction velocities and amplitudes of evoked responses are normal in both motor and sensory nerves except in diseases with clinical and

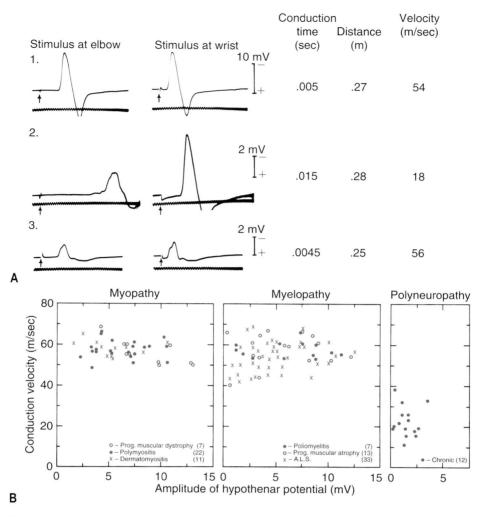

FIGURE 13-31 ■ Ulnar nerve conduction velocity and amplitude measurements in (1) a normal person, (2) peripheral neuropathy, and (3) myopathy. **A**, Traces from individual subjects. **B**, Plots of grouped data. ALS, amyotrophic lateral sclerosis. (From Department of Neurology, Mayo Clinic and Mayo Foundation: Clinical Examinations in Neurology. 6th Ed. Mosby-Year Book, St. Louis, 1991, with permission.)

pathologic signs of nerve damage. However, motor nerve stimulation typically produces a repetitive discharge of the muscle. Instead of a single CMAP after a single stimulus, a group of two to six potentials of decreasing amplitude occurs at regular intervals.[128]

MONITORING DURING SURGICAL PROCEDURES

Nerve conduction studies have proved useful in the operating room as a means of assisting the surgeon in localizing nerve involved in tumor and in identifying and defining the site and nature of localized nerve lesions, and also as a means of detecting potential nerve damage during surgical procedures.[129,130] Surgical procedures performed in or around peripheral nerves in the limbs, the plexus, and the cranial nerves may warrant intraoperative nerve conduction studies. These surgical procedures include ulnar nerve transposition, pronator syndrome release, shoulder reconstruction, resections of tumors involving the brachial plexus, brachial plexus reconstruction following injury, resection of sciatic nerve and other peripheral nerve tumors, hip reconstruction, and operations on tumors in the posterior fossa.

The methods of stimulation and recording used for intraoperative monitoring are similar to those used for standard nerve conduction studies, including the

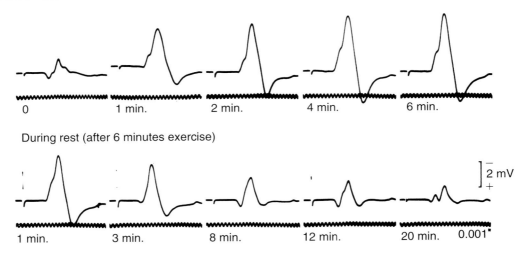

During rest (after 6 minutes exercise)

FIGURE 13-32 ■ Amplitude of the hypothenar evoked response with supramaximal ulnar nerve stimulation in a patient with hypokalemic periodic paralysis. (By permission of E. H. Lambert, Mayo Clinic, Rochester, MN.)

measurement of amplitude and latency of compound muscle and compound nerve action potentials with direct stimulation of the nerve in the surgical field. Intraoperative monitoring often requires specially designed stimulating and recording electrodes, and it always requires special techniques to maintain sterility in the surgical field. The clinical neurophysiologist must be familiar with the problems unique to the operating room. Response alterations caused by the activities of the anesthesiologist and surgeon are common. Electrical artifacts are always present, and they are more diverse than under standard testing conditions.

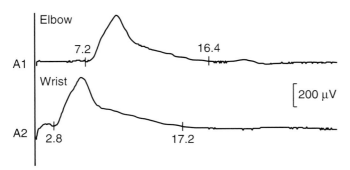

FIGURE 13-33 ■ Compound muscle action potentials (CMAP) in critical illness myopathy. Ulnar motor CMAP recorded from hypothenar muscles with wrist and elbow stimulation. Onset and termination of the CMAP is marked by cursors, with time indicated. Note low-amplitude, markedly prolonged CMAP duration (normal < 9.0 msec) without dispersion, and the minimum of late positivity.

Peripheral Nerve

Any motor, sensory, or mixed peripheral nerve can be monitored during a surgical procedure. Appropriate selection of recording or stimulating sites can isolate the motor or sensory axons, just as it does for diagnostic studies in the laboratory. To provide maximal information and back-up in case of technical problems, multiple stimulation and recording sites are typical. Monitoring of each of the cervical nerve roots with SEPs and motor evoked potentials (MEPs), in addition to direct recording of nerve action potentials, has become a major aid to reconstructive surgery of the brachial plexus.[115] Ulnar nerve monitoring is among the more common intraoperative peripheral monitoring procedures. Direct nerve action potentials are obtained from electrodes placed on the nerve, or CMAPs are recorded from peripheral muscles. In each case, stimulation or recording is obtained from multiple sites at short intervals along the nerve to define precisely the areas of major damage (Figs. 13-34 and 13-35).

Cranial Nerve

Intraoperative monitoring of cranial motor nerves is used primarily during resection of acoustic neuromas or meningiomas, but it is also useful during microvascular decompression procedures and surgery on tumors at the petrous ridge.[56] Cranial nerves III, V, VI, VII, X, XI, and XII can be monitored singly or simultaneously, as

1 cm latency differences, msec

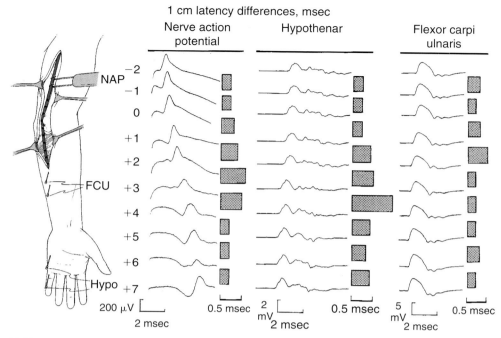

FIGURE 13-34 ▪ Compound nerve and muscle action potentials recorded distally during direct stimulation of the ulnar nerve at operation. (From Daube JR, Harper CM, Litchy WJ et al: Intraoperative monitoring. p. 739. In Daly DD, Pedley TA [eds]: Current Practice of Clinical Electroencephalography. 2nd Ed. Raven, New York, 1990, with permission.)

dictated by the surgical needs. Recordings are made with surface electrodes or fine wire electrodes placed in individual muscles. It is best to perform nerve conduction studies in combination with electromyographic

monitoring during surgical dissection. Irritation or damage to the nerve can be recognized by the presence of neurotonic discharges or changes in amplitude of the CMAP (Figs. 13-36 and 13-37).

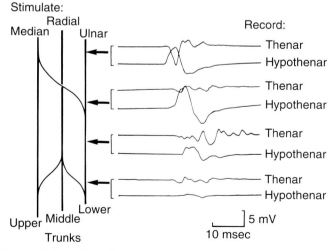

FIGURE 13-35 ▪ Compound muscle action potential recorded directly during direct stimulation of the brachial plexus at operation. (From Daube JR, Harper CM, Litchy WJ et al: Intraoperative monitoring. p. 739. In Daly DD, Pedley TA [eds]: Current Practice of Clinical Electroencephalography. 2nd Ed. Raven, New York, 1990, with permission.)

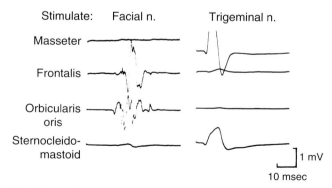

FIGURE 13-36 ▪ Compound muscle action potentials recorded from cranial muscles during direct stimulation of cranial nerves in the surgical field. (From Daube JR, Harper CM, Litchy WJ et al: Intraoperative monitoring. p. 739. In Daly DD, Pedley TA [eds]: Current Practice of Clinical Electroencephalography. 2nd Ed. Raven, New York, 1990, with permission.)

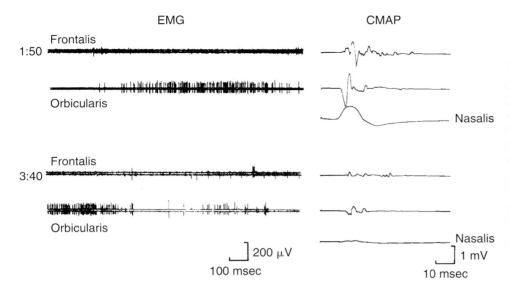

FIGURE 13-37 ▪ Electromyographic and compound muscle action potential recordings from facial muscles during an operation in the posterior fossa for removal of acoustic neuroma. (From Daube JR, Harper CM, Litchy WJ et al: Intraoperative monitoring. p. 739. In Daly DD, Pedley TA [eds]: Current Practice of Clinical Electroencephalography. 2nd Ed. Raven, New York, 1990, with permission.)

REFERENCES

1. Dyck PJ, Karnes JL, O'Brien PC et al: The Rochester Diabetic Neuropathy Study: reassessment of tests and criteria for diagnosis and staged severity. Neurology, 42:1164, 1992

2. Daube JR: Nerve conduction studies. p. 285. In Aminoff MJ (ed): Electrodiagnosis in Clinical Neurology. 5th Ed. Elsevier, Philadelphia, 2005

3. Olney RK, So YT, Goodin DS et al: A comparison of magnetic and electrical stimulation of peripheral nerves. Muscle Nerve, 13:957, 1990

4. Evans BA, Litchy WJ, Daube JR: The utility of magnetic stimulation for routine peripheral nerve conduction studies. Muscle Nerve, 11:1074, 1988

5. Cros D, Day TJ, Shahani BT: Spatial dispersion of magnetic stimulation in peripheral nerves. Muscle Nerve, 13:1076, 1990

6. Ono S, Oishi M, Du CM: Magnetic stimulation of peripheral nerves. Comparison of magnetic stimulation with electrical stimulation. Electromyogr Clin Neurophysiol, 35:317, 1995

7. Troni W, Bianco C, Moga MC: Improved methodology for lumbosacral nerve root stimulation. Muscle Nerve, 19:595, 1996

8. Lo YL, Ratnagopal P, Leoh TH et al: Clinical and electrophysiological aspects of distal ulnar neuropathy. Acta Neurol Scand, 105:390, 2002

9. Lee HJ, Bach JR, DeLisa JA: Peroneal nerve motor conduction to the proximal muscles. Am J Phys Med Rehabil, 76:197, 1997

10. Ferdjallah M, Wertsch JJ, Harris GF: Effects of surface electrode size on computer simulated surface motor unit potentials. Electromyogr Clin Neurophysiol, 39:259, 1999

11. Radziwill AJ, Steck AJ, Renaud S: Distal motor latency and residual latency as sensitive markers of anti-MAG polyneuropathy. J Neurol, 250:962, 2003

12. Landau ME, Diaz MI, Barner KC: Optimal distance for segmental nerve conduction studies revisited. Muscle Nerve, 27:367, 2003

13. Zwarts MJ, Guechev A: The relation between conduction velocity and axonal length. Muscle Nerve, 18:1244, 1995

14. Stetson DS, Albers JW, Silverstein BA: Effects of age, sex, and anthropometric factors on nerve conduction measures. Muscle Nerve, 15:1095, 1992

15. McGill KC, Lateva ZC: The contribution of the interosseous muscles to the hypothenar compound muscle action potential. Muscle Nerve, 22:6, 1999

16. Rutkove SB, Kothari MJ, Shefner JM: Nerve, muscle, and neuromuscular junction electrophysiology at high temperature. Muscle Nerve, 20:431, 1997

17. Kimura J: Kugelberg lecture: principles and pitfalls of nerve conduction studies. Electroencephalogr Clin Neurophysiol, 106:470, 1998

18. Schulte-Mattler WJ, Muller T, Georgiadis D et al: Length dependence of variables associated with temporal dispersion in human motor nerves. Muscle Nerve, 24:527, 2001

19. Sander HW, Quinto C, Chokroverty S: Accessory deep peroneal neuropathy: collision technique diagnosis. Muscle Nerve, 21:121, 1998

20. Daube JR: Compound muscle action potentials. p. 371. In Daube JR, Rubin DI (eds): Clinical Neurophysiology. Oxford University Press, New York, 2009

21. Panayiotopoulos CP, Chroni E: F waves in clinical neurophysiology. Electroencephalogr Clin Neurophysiol, 101:365, 1996

22. Chroni E, Taub N, Panayiotopoulos CP: The importance of sample size for the estimation of F wave latency parameters in the peroneal nerve. Electroencephalogr Clin Neurophysiol, 101:375, 1996

23. Fisher MA, Hoffen B, Hultman C: Normative F wave values and the number of recorded F waves. Muscle Nerve, 17:1185, 1994

24. Dengler R, Kossev A, Wohlfahrt K et al: F waves and motor unit size. Muscle Nerve, 15:1138, 1992

25. Pastore C, Gonzalez O, Geijo E: A study of F-waves in patients with unilateral lumbosacral radiculopathy. Eur J Neurol, 16:1233, 2009

26. Magistris MR, Roth G: Motor axon reflex and indirect double discharge: ephaptic transmission? A reappraisal. Electroencephalogr Clin Neurophysiol, 85:124, 1992

27. Roth G, Soichot P, Egloff-Baer S: Clinical Motor Electroneurography: Evoked Responses Beyond the M-Wave Ectopic Activity. Elsevier, Amsterdam, 2000

28. Bischoff C: Neurography: late responses. Muscle Nerve Suppl, 11:S59, 2002

29. Daube JR: Estimating the number of motor units in a muscle. J Clin Neurophysiol, 12:585, 1995

30. Shefner JM, Gooch CL: Motor unit number estimation. Phys Med Rehabil Clin N Am, 14:243, 2003

31. Simmons Z, Epstein DK, Borg B et al: Reproducibility of motor unit number estimation in individual subjects. Muscle Nerve, 24:467, 2001

32. Olney RK, Yuen EC, Engstrom JW: Statistical motor unit number estimation: reproducibility and sources of error in patients with amyotrophic lateral sclerosis. Muscle Nerve, 23:193, 2000

33. Lomen-Hoerth C, Slawnych MP: Statistical motor unit number estimation: from theory to practice. Muscle Nerve, 28:263, 2003

34. Kiernan MC, Burke D, Andersen KV et al: Multiple measures of axonal excitability: a new approach in clinical testing. Muscle Nerve, 23:399, 2000

35. Kuwabara S, Ogawara K, Sung JY et al: Differences in membrane properties of axonal and demyelinating Guillain–Barré syndromes. Ann Neurol, 52:180, 2002

36. Aprile I, Stalberg E, Tonali P et al: Double peak sensory responses at submaximal stimulation. Clin Neurophysiol, 114:256, 2003

37. Park KS, Lee SH, Lee KW et al: Interdigital nerve conduction study of the foot for an early detection of diabetic sensory polyneuropathy. Clin Neurophysiol, 114:894, 2003

38. Phillips LH: Pitfalls in nerve conduction studies: temperature and distance measurement. In Kimura J, Shibasaki H (eds): Recent Advances in Clinical Neurophysiology. Elsevier, Amsterdam, 1996

39. Bromberg MB, Jaros L: Symmetry of normal motor and sensory nerve conduction measurements. Muscle Nerve, 21:498, 1998

40. Salerno DF, Franzblau A, Werner RA et al: Median and ulnar nerve conduction studies among workers: normative values. Muscle Nerve, 21:999, 1998

41. Rivner MH, Swift TR, Malik K: Influence of age and height on nerve conduction. Muscle Nerve, 24:1134, 2001

42. Azrieli Y, Weimer L, Lovelace R et al: The utility of segmental nerve conduction studies in ulnar mononeuropathy at the elbow. Muscle Nerve, 27:46, 2003

43. Rajabally YA, Jacob S: Proximal nerve conduction studies in chronic inflammatory demyelinating polyneuropathy. Clin Neurophysiol, 117:2079, 2006

44. Aranye Z, Szabo G, Szepesi-Folyovich A: Proximal conduction abnormality of the facial nerve in Miller Fisher syndrome. Clin Neurophysiol, 117:821, 2006

45. Daube J: Compound muscle action potentials. p. 245. In Daube JR (ed): Clinical Neurophysiology. Oxford University Press, New York, 2002

46. Kohara N, Kimura J, Kaji R et al: F-wave latency serves as the most reproducible measure in nerve conduction studies of diabetic polyneuropathy: multicentre analysis in healthy subjects and patients with diabetic polyneuropathy. Diabetologia, 43:915, 2000

47. Benatar M, Wuu J, Peng L: Reference data for commonly used sensory and motor nerve conduction studies. Muscle Nerve, 40:772, 2009

48. Dyck PJ, O'Brien PC, Litchy WJ et al: Use of percentiles and normal deviates to express nerve conduction and other test abnormalities. Muscle Nerve, 24:307, 2001

49. Dyck PJ, Litchy WJ, Daube JR et al: Individual attributes versus composite scores of nerve conduction abnormality: sensitivity, reproducibility, and concordance with impairment. Muscle Nerve, 27:202, 2003

50. Normand NM, Daube JR: Interaction of random electromyographic activity with averaged sensory evoked potentials. Neurology, 42:1605, 1992

51. Nora LM: American Association of Electrodiagnostic Medicine Guidelines in Electrodiagnostic Medicine: Implanted cardioverters and defibrillators. Muscle Nerve, 19:1359, 1996

52. Schoeck AP, Mellion MN, Gilchrist JM et al: Safety of conduction studies in patients with implanted cardiac devices. Muscle Nerve, 35:521, 2007

53. Amoiridis G, Vlachonikolis IG: Verification of the median-to-ulnar and ulnar-to-median nerve motor fiber anastomosis in the forearm: an electrophysiological study. Clin Neurophysiol, 114:94, 2003

54. Marras C, Midroni G: Proximal Martin–Gruber anastomosis mimicking ulnar neuropathy at the elbow. Muscle Nerve, 22:1132, 1999

55. Simonetti S: Electrophysiological study of forearm sensory fiber crossover in Martin–Gruber anastomosis. Muscle Nerve, 24:380, 2001

56. Leis AA, Stetkarova L, Wells KJ: Martin–Gruber anastamosis with anomalous superficial radial innervation. Muscle Nerve, 41:313, 2010

57. McManis PG, Daube JR: Electromyographic evaluation of an accessory hand muscle. Muscle Nerve, 12:460, 1989

58. Krarup C, Moldovan M: Nerve conduction and excitability studies in peripheral nerve disorders. Curr Opin Neurol, 22:460, 2009

59. Sawai S, Misawa S, Kobayashi K et al: Multifocal conduction blocks in sarcoid peripheral neuropathy. Intern Med, 49:471, 2010

60. Watson BV, Doherty TJ: Localization of frequency-dependent conduction block in carpal tunnel syndrome. Muscle Nerve, 42:120, 2010

61. Normand MM, Daube JR: Cranial nerve conduction and needle electromyography in patients with acoustic neuromas. Muscle Nerve, 17:1401, 1994

62. Logigian EL, Kelly JJ, Adelman LS: Nerve conduction and biopsy correlation in over 100 consecutive patients with suspected polyneuropathy. Muscle Nerve, 17:1010, 1994

63. An J, Park M, Kim J et al: Comparison of diabetic neuropathy symptoms score and medial plantar sensory nerve conduction studies. Intern Med, 47:1395, 2008

64. Hemmi S, Inoue K, Murakami T et al: Novel method to measure distal sensory nerve conduction in the medial plantar nerve. Muscle Nerve, 36:307, 2007

65. Krarup C, Trojaborg W: Sensory pathophysiology in chronic acquired demyelinating neuropathy. Brain, 119:257, 1996

66. McKhann GM, Cornblath DR, Griffin JW et al: Acute motor axonal neuropathy: a frequent cause of acute flaccid paralysis in China. Ann Neurol, 33:333, 1993

67. Visser LH, Van der Meche FG, Van Doorn PA: Guillain–Barré syndrome without sensory loss (acute motor neuropathy). Brain, 118:841, 1995

68. Hsieh TW, Nachamkin ST, Willison HJ et al: Motor nerve terminal degeneration provides a potential mechanism for rapid recovery in acute motor axonal neuropathy after *Campylobacter* infection. Neurology, 48:717, 1997

69. Kiers L, Clouston P, Cros D: Quantitative studies of F responses in Guillain–Barré syndrome. Electroencephalogr Clin Neurophysiol, 93:255, 1994

70. Gordon PH, Wilbourn AJ: Early electrodiagnostic findings in Guillain–Barré syndrome. Arch Neurol, 58:913, 2001

71. Roth G, Magistris MR: Indirect discharges as an early nerve conduction abnormality in the Guillain–Barré syndrome. Eur Neurol, 42:83, 1999

72. Ammar N, Nelis E, Merlini L et al: Identification of novel GDAP1 mutations causing autosomal recessive Charcot–Marie–Tooth disease. Neuromuscul Disord, 13:720, 2003

73. Cleland JC, Logigian EL, Thaisetthawatkul P et al: Dispersion of the distal compound muscle action potential in chronic inflammatory demyelinating polyneuropathy and carpal tunnel syndrome. Muscle Nerve, 28:189, 2003

74. Gabreels-Festen A: Dejerine–Sottas syndrome grown to maturity: overview of genetic and morphological heterogeneity and follow-up of 25 patients. J Anat, 200:341, 2002

75. Chaudry V, Corse AM, Cornblath DR: Multifocal motor neuropathy: electrodiagnostic features. Muscle Nerve, 17:198, 1994

76. Katz JS, Wolfe GI, Bryan WW et al: Electrophysiologic findings in multifocal motor neuropathy. Neurology, 48:700, 1997

77. Kaku DA, Parry GJ, Malamut R: Uniform slowing of conduction velocities in Charcot–Marie–Tooth polyneuropathy type 1. Neurology, 43:2664, 1993

78. Li J, Krajewski K, Shy ME et al: Hereditary neuropathy with liability to pressure palsy: the electrophysiology fits the name. Neurology, 58:1769, 2002

79. Saperstein DS, Katz JS, Amato AA et al: Clinical spectrum of chronic acquired demyelinating polyneuropathies. Muscle Nerve, 24:311, 2001

80. Nevo Y, Topaloglu H: 88th ENMC International Workshop: childhood chronic inflammatory demyelinating polyneuropathy (including revised diagnostic criteria), Naarden, The Netherlands, December 8–10, 2000. Neuromuscul Disord, 12:195, 2002

81. Olney RK, Lewis RA, Putnam TD et al: Consensus criteria for the diagnosis of multifocal motor neuropathy. Muscle Nerve, 27:117, 2003

82. Feki I, Lefaucheur JP: Correlation between nerve conduction studies and clinical scores in diabetic neuropathy. Muscle Nerve, 24:555, 2001

83. Andersen H, Stalberg E, Falck B: F-wave latency, the most sensitive nerve conduction parameter in patients with diabetes mellitus. Muscle Nerve, 20:1296, 1997

84. Horn S, Quasthoff S, Grafe P et al: Abnormal axonal inward rectification in diabetic neuropathy. Muscle Nerve, 19:1268, 1996

85. Montoya L, Felice KJ: Recovery from distal ulnar motor conduction block injury: serial EMG studies. Muscle Nerve, 26:145, 2002

86. Padua L, Monaco LO, Valente EM: A useful electrophysiologic parameter for diagnosis of carpal tunnel syndrome. Muscle Nerve, 19:48, 1996

87. Kuntzer T: Carpal tunnel syndrome in 100 patients: sensitivity, specificity of multi-neurophysiological procedures and estimation of axonal loss of motor, sensory and sympathetic median nerve fibers. J Neurol Sci, 127:221, 1994

88. Chang MH, Wei SJ, Chiang HL et al: Comparison of motor conduction techniques in the diagnosis of carpal tunnel syndrome. Neurology, 58:1603, 2002

89. Cifu DX, Saleem S: Median-radial latency difference: its use in screening for carpal tunnel syndrome in twenty patients with demyelinating peripheral neuropathy. Arch Phys Med Rehabil, 74:44, 1993

90. Imada M, Misawa S, Sawai S et al: Median-radial sensory nerve comparative studies in the detection of median neuropathy in diabetic patients. Clin Neurophysiol, 118:1405, 2007

91. Chang MH, Liao KK, Chang SP: Proximal slowing in carpal tunnel syndrome. J Neurol, 240:287, 1993

92. Kothari MJ, Preston DC, Logigian EL: Lumbrical-interossei motor studies localize ulnar neuropathy at the wrist. Muscle Nerve, 19:170, 1996

93. Loscher WN, Auer-Grumbach M, Trinka E et al: Comparison of second lumbrical and interosseus latencies with standard measures of median nerve function across the carpal tunnel: a prospective study of 450 hands. J Neurol, 247:530, 2000

94. Werner RA, Albers JW: Relation between needle electromyography and nerve conduction studies in patients with carpal tunnel syndrome. Arch Phys Med Rehabil, 76:246, 1995

95. Bland JD: Do nerve conduction studies predict the outcome of carpal tunnel decompression? Muscle Nerve, 24:935, 2001

96. Kim WK, Kwon SH, Lee SH et al: Asymptomatic electrophysiologic carpal tunnel syndrome in diabetics: entrapment or polyneuropathy. Yonsei Med J, 41:123, 2000

97. Perkins BA, Olaleye D, Bril V: Carpal tunnel syndrome in patients with diabetic polyneuropathy. Diabetes Care, 25:565, 2002

98. Hansson S: Segmental median nerve conduction measurements discriminate carpal tunnel syndrome from diabetic polyneuropathy. Muscle Nerve, 18:445, 1995

99. Sheu JJ, Yuan RY, Chiou HY et al: Segmental study of the median nerve versus comparative tests in the diagnosis of mild carpal tunnel syndrome. Clin Neurophysiol, 117:1249, 2006

100. Azrieli Y, Weimer L, Lovelace R et al: The utility of segmental nerve conduction studies in ulnar mononeuropathy at the elbow. Muscle Nerve, 27:46, 2003

101. Odabasi Z, Oh SJ, Claussen GC et al: New near-nerve needle nerve conduction technique: differentiating epicondylar from cubital tunnel ulnar neuropathy. Muscle Nerve, 22:718, 1999

102. Kingery WS, Park KS, Wu PB et al: Electromyographic motor Tinel's sign in ulnar mononeuropathies at the elbow. Am J Phys Med Rehabil, 74:419, 1995

103. Young NP, Sorenson EJ, Spinner RJ et al: Clinical and electrodiagnostic correlates of peroneal intraneural ganglia. Neurology, 72:447, 2009

104. Jones HR, Felice KJ, Gross PT: Pediatric peroneal mononeuropathy. Muscle Nerve, 16:1167, 1993

105. Oh SJ, Demirci MD, Dajani B et al: Distal sensory nerve conduction of the superficial peroneal nerve: new method and its clinical application. Muscle Nerve, 24:689, 2001

106. Levin KH: L5 radiculopathy with reduced superficial peroneal sensory responses: intraspinal and extraspinal causes. Muscle Nerve, 21:3, 1998

107. Katirji B, Wilbourn AJ: High sciatic lesion mimicking peroneal neuropathy at the fibular head. J Neurol Sci, 121:172, 1994

108. Ferrante MA, Wilbourn AJ: The utility of various sensory nerve conduction responses in assessing brachial plexopathies. Muscle Nerve, 18:879, 1995

109. Chen ZY, Xu JG, Shen LY et al: Phrenic nerve conduction study in patients with traumatic brachial plexus palsy. Muscle Nerve, 24:1388, 2001

110. Menkes DL, Hood DC, Ballesteros RA et al: Root stimulation improves the detection of acquired demyelinating polyneuropathies. Muscle Nerve, 21:298, 1998

111. Fisher MA: Electrophysiology of radiculopathies. Clin Neurophysiol, 113:317, 2002

112. Theys PA, Peeters E, Robberecht W: Evolution of motor and sensory deficits in amyotrophic lateral sclerosis estimated by neurophysiological techniques. J Neurol, 246:438, 1999

113. de Carvalho M, Swash M: Nerve conduction studies in amyotrophic lateral sclerosis. Muscle Nerve, 23:344, 2000

114. Bostock H, Sharief MK, Reid G et al: Axonal ion channel dysfunction in amyotrophic lateral sclerosis. Brain, 118:217, 1995

115. Ibrahim IK, el-Abd MA: Giant repeater F-wave in patients with anterior horn cell disorders. Am J Phys Med Rehabil, 76:281, 1997

116. Daube JR: Electrodiagnostic studies in amyotrophic lateral sclerosis and other motor neuron disorders. Muscle Nerve, 23:1488, 2000

117. van Dijk JP, Schelhaas HJ, Van Schaik IN et al: Monitoring disease progression using high-density motor unit number estimation in amyotrophic lateral sclerosis. Muscle Nerve, 42:239, 2010

118. She ME: MUNE and progression of CMT1A. Eur J Neurol, 17:997, 2010

119. Suzuki K, Katsuno M, Banno H et al: The profile of motor unit number estimation (MUNE) in spinal and bulbar muscular atrophy. J Neurol Neurosurg Psychiatry, 81:567, 2010

120. Chaudry V, Moser HW, Cornblath DR: Nerve conduction studies in adrenomyeloneuropathy. J Neurol Neurosurg Psychiatry, 61:181, 1996

121. Rubin DI, Daube JR: Subacute sensory neuropathy associated with Epstein–Barr virus. Muscle Nerve, 22:1607, 1999

122. Killian JM, Foreman PJ: Clinical utility of dorsal sural nerve conduction studies. Muscle Nerve, 24:817, 2001

123. Levin KH: L5 radiculopathy with reduced superficial peroneal sensory responses: intraspinal and extraspinal causes. Muscle Nerve, 21:3, 1998

124. Hatanaka T, Owa K, Yasunaga M et al: Electrophysiological studies of a child with presumed botulism. Childs Nerv Syst, 16:84, 2000

125. Goodman BP, Harper CM, Boon AJ: Prolonged compound muscle action potential duration in critical illness myopathy. Muscle Nerve, 40:1040, 2009

126. Rich MM, Bird SJ, Raps EC et al: Direct muscle stimulation in acute quadriplegic myopathy. Muscle Nerve, 20:665, 1997

127. Allen DC, Arunachalam R, Mills KR: Critical illness myopathy: further evidence from muscle-fiber excitability studies of an acquired channelopathy. Muscle Nerve, 37:14, 2008

128. Kiernan MC, Hart IK, Bostock H: Excitability properties of motor axons in patients with spontaneous motor unit activity. J Neurol Neurosurg Psychiatry, 70:56, 2001

129. Crum BA, Strommen JA: Peripheral nerve stimulation and monitoring during operative procedures. Muscle Nerve, 35:159, 2007

130. Pondaag W, van der Veken LP, van Someren PJ et al: Intraoperative nerve action and compound motor action potential recordings in patients with obstetric brachial plexus lesions. J Neurosurg, 109:946, 2008

Microneurography and its Potential Clinical Applications

DAVID BURKE

Microneurography was developed by Karl-Erik Hagbarth and Åke Vallbo in Uppsala, Sweden in the early 1960s, and the first definitive papers were published in 1968 (on cutaneous and muscle afferents).[1,2] With this invasive technique it is possible to study how receptors in muscle, skin, and joints behave under natural conditions and how the sympathetic innervation of skin and muscle normally behaves. A number of authoritative reviews of the technique and the information obtained thereby have been published.[3–13]

Microneurography has generated many data that illuminate normal neural mechanisms and the disorders that occur in a wide variety of disease processes. The development of conduction block in single axons has been studied in microneurographic recordings, as has the ectopic activity responsible for paresthesias. It is also possible, for example, to record compound sensory action potentials containing identifiable deflections due to large and small, myelinated and unmyelinated axons. However, this can be done almost as readily and less invasively using near-nerve needle recordings.

Overall, microneurography seems to be of limited diagnostic value. There are four main reasons. First, it takes skill and perseverance to obtain satisfactory recordings. Second, only a few satisfactory recordings from single axons can be obtained in any one session, too few for meaningful statistical comparisons against control values while, with population responses involving many axons, the recorded activity varies with the position of the microelectrode within the nerve fascicle. As a result, the intensity of neural activity can vary greatly from experiment to experiment. Third, if pathology leads to a loss of activity (rather than activity that is preserved but abnormal), as in autonomic failure, no activity will be recorded. This then begs the question of whether the absence of activity is due to technical failure or the pathologic process. Finally, the trauma of the study is a consideration, not because of discomfort, but because, conceivably, the microelectrode could damage the few surviving axons in a patient with, for example, amyotrophic lateral sclerosis, or exacerbate the pain of a patient with a complex pain syndrome.

While microneurography has resulted in major changes in thought about the nature of the feedback that the nervous system receives from peripheral receptors and how it uses that feedback for perception and for movement, this chapter will focus on findings that shed light on clinical phenomena. The reader is referred to previously published reviews for more comprehensive treatises on normal physiology.

RECORDING TECHNIQUE

The basic technique has changed little since first described.[3,4] Most authorities use a microelectrode made from tungsten with a shaft diameter of approximately 200 μm, insulated to the tip. The greater the diameter, the more that penetration of a fascicle hurts; a diameter of less than 200 μm is not sufficiently rigid. The experimenter inserts the microelectrode manually through the skin to impale the peripheral nerve. Commonly, weak electrical stimuli are delivered through the electrode and the experimenter hones in on an appropriate nerve fascicle, guided by the evoked paresthesias (when seeking a cutaneous fascicle) or the twitch contraction (when seeking a motor fascicle). Vallbo and colleagues initially insert a low-impedance electrode to locate an appropriate fascicle and then use its location to guide the insertion of the recording microelectrode, the impedance of which has been decreased to near-optimal levels. Others rely on the passage through the skin and the subcutaneous and perineural tissue to remove insulation and reduce the impedance to a satisfactory level. When in place, the optimal impedance of the electrode is perhaps 50 kΩ for multi-unit recordings and some 100 to 150 kΩ for single-unit recordings (though higher impedances may assist single-unit C fiber recordings).

Once the experimenter has manipulated the tip into the fascicle, afferents in that fascicle can be activated, for example by tapping on the muscle tendon or scraping the skin (Fig. 14-1). The activation of mechanoreceptors creates an auditory signal that can be used to guide further small adjustments of the electrode. The electrode is not fixed securely because external fixation leads to electrode dislodgement when minor movements inevitably occur. It is stabilized at its proximal end by a coiled insulated copper wire to the preamplifier and at the recording end by the rigidity of the tissue into which the electrode has been inserted. Nevertheless, minor movements—particularly those that displace skin at the recording site—can jeopardize the recording. This creates an issue for motor control studies because the range of movement that can be studied is small, and consequently it is prudent not to generalize too far about, for example, the role of the fusimotor system in normal motor behavior (see below).

The insulation created by the tissue that surrounds a nerve fascicle is very effective. It is virtually impossible to record the activity of single axons if the microelectrode tip is just outside a fascicle, even if the discharge of that axon is used to trigger averages of many sweeps. Once the microelectrode is within a fascicle, axonal activity can be recorded readily, and it is then possible for the

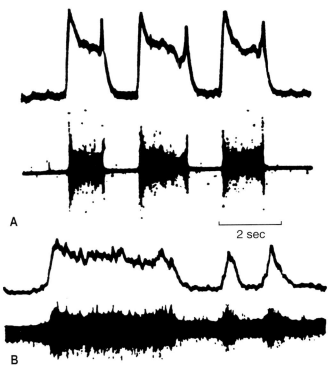

FIGURE 14-1 ■ Multi-unit responses to cutaneous stimuli (median nerve). **A,** Responses to moderately heavy touch stimuli. Note the "on" and "off" responses. **B,** Responses to scraping the skin with sandpaper. Lower traces illustrate the raw neurogram and upper traces the "integrated" neurogram. In *A*, the amplitude discriminator has been used to eliminate most of the noise, while in *B* the neurographic activity is not so treated. (From Burke D, Mackenzie RA, Skuse NF et al: Cutaneous afferent activity in median and radial nerve fascicles: a microelectrode study. J Neurol Neurosurg Psychiatry, 38:855, 1975, with permission.)

experimenter to focus on spontaneous neural discharges (e.g., the bursts of activity that occur in sympathetic efferent axons innervating skin or muscle) or the neural discharge evoked by mechanical stimuli, such as tapping on the muscle belly or tendon (with a motor fascicle) or stroking the skin (with a cutaneous fascicle).

Obtaining stable recordings from single axons requires skill and patience. It is helpful if the axon has a background discharge because, unless the discharge of the axon can be heard, it may be difficult to know that the electrode is close to it. This means that the recordings inevitably will be biased toward axons that maintain a background discharge, and this is probably the main reason that there are fewer recordings from group Ib afferents from Golgi tendon organs than from group Ia afferents from primary spindle endings. In addition, because action potential amplitude is a function of the cross-sectional area of the axon, the potentials of large axons will be distinguished more readily from the background noise—perhaps explaining why

FIGURE 14-2 ■ Three types of action potential morphology. **A**, "Positive single-peaked" (23 percent). **B**, "Negative" (1.4 percent). **C**, "Positive double-peaked" (75 percent): six examples. **D**, Explanation for positive double-peaked units. If the microelectrode tip impaled the myelin sheath, the current fluctuations at the nodes of Ranvier on each side of the recording microelectrode would contribute to the recorded action potential. If internodal conduction is prolonged, two distinct "positive peaks" would occur (see Figs. 14-3 and 14-16).(From Inglis JT, Leeper JB, Burke D et al: Morphology of action potentials recorded from human nerves using microneurography. Exp Brain Res, 110:308, 1996, with permission.)

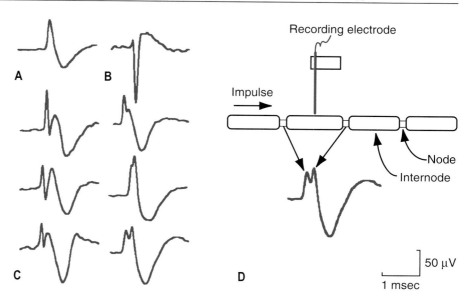

there are few recordings from cutaneous Aδ axons. Paradoxically, it is relatively easy to obtain recordings from unmyelinated C fibers. This is because they occur in clusters of approximately six or more axons within the cytoplasm of a Schwann cell (the so-called Remak bundle) containing C fibers with different properties, so that a recording from this group of axons can be made quite readily, particularly if they are sympathetic and have a background discharge. The action potentials from myelinated axons commonly have a bifid appearance (in about 75 percent of units, Fig. 14-2, *C*). The two peaks represent action potentials at nodes of Ranvier on either side of the impalement of the axon by the microelectrode (Fig. 14-2, *D*). That two peaks are discernible implies that conduction across the internode is slow (see later, in section on Conduction Block). When the action potential has a simple biphasic morphology (as in Fig. 14-2, *A*), it could be "normal" or one in which conduction across the impaled internode is blocked.

The technique has been developed to allow stimulation through the intrafascicular microelectrode (often referred to as *microstimulation*). With myelinated axons, activation is likely to occur at the nodes of Ranvier on either side of impalement (as in Fig. 14-2, *C* and *D*). In studies of the perceptual correlates of afferents, this effectively then would be the proximal node because any action potential from the distal node will occur during the refractory period for the proximal node, even when internodal conduction is delayed (see later). With afferents, intrafascicular stimulation has allowed (1) the cortical evoked potentials produced by the stimulated afferents or their reflex effects to be defined, and (2) the perceptual responses associated with activity in single afferent axons to be documented. With efferents, intrafascicular stimulation has been used (1) to produce the twitch contraction of the receptor-bearing muscle to differentiate spindle endings from Golgi tendon organs, as discussed later, and (2) to document the contraction properties of single motor units.[7]

The critical step with single units is to identify the axon. This can be done for afferents by locating the receptor in skin or muscle and characterizing its responses to a variety of stimuli: mechanical, thermal, nociceptive. With α motor axons, the axon will be active only if there is a deliberate, inadvertent, or involuntary contraction of the innervated muscle involving that motor unit, and the neural spike can then be used to spike-trigger average the ongoing electromyographic activity (Fig. 14-3). This then should allow the motor unit action potential to be defined at a latency appropriate for direct conduction from the stimulating site to the muscle. It has been claimed that γ motor axons (which innervate the intrafusal muscle of the muscle spindle) can be identified on discharge characteristics alone, but it would be prudent to retain reservations about such claims because there are scant data on how γ motor neurons discharge in natural acts in animals, and no such data for human subjects. Accurate identification can be time-consuming, and may require maneuvers that displace the skin at the recording site (e.g., a twitch contraction), so that recordings are lost before meaningful data can be obtained from that axon.

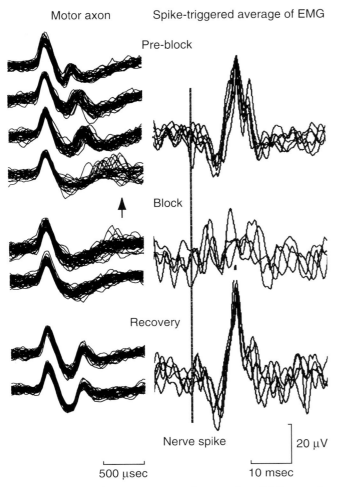

Motor axon — Spike-triggered average of EMG

Pre-block

Block

Recovery

Nerve spike — 20 µV

500 µsec — 10 msec

FIGURE 14-3 ■ An α-motor axon innervating tibialis anterior undergoing activity-dependent conduction block. The traces on the left represent superimposed consecutive nerve action potentials recorded at different stages during the development of conduction block and, after rest, recovery therefrom, for a motor axon discharging in a voluntary contraction. The traces on the right represent spike-triggered averages of surface electromyogram (EMG) of tibialis anterior, each trace consisting of approximately 32 sweeps, corresponding to the neural spikes on the left. The timing of the nerve action potential is indicated by the vertical line. In the top left panel a second positive peak was seen in each recording, though the interpeak interval gradually increased and became highly unstable in the fourth trace. The EMG potential was consistently recordable. In the middle panel (*Block*), the second positive peak was present only in a few sweeps in the upper set of traces. There was no consistent EMG potential. Following rest for a few minutes, a further contraction was performed; the second positive peak was again present in the nerve action potential, and the EMG potential had reappeared (*Recovery*). Note the difference in time base for the nerve action potential and the EMG potential. The longest interpeak interval (fourth set of traces under *Pre-block*) was 1.43 msec (indicated by vertical arrow). (From Inglis JT, Leeper JB, Wilson LR et al: The development of conduction block in single human axons following a focal nerve injury. J Physiol, 513:127, 1998, with permission.)

MUSCLE AFFERENTS

The motor control literature has focused on large myelinated axons innervating the muscle spindle and the Golgi tendon organ, which are well-defined encapsulated receptors. Such axons are termed group I (Ia afferents from the primary ending of the muscle spindle; Ib from the Golgi tendon organ) or group II (slightly smaller axons from the secondary ending of the muscle spindle and also from nonspindle receptors). Given conduction velocities of approximately 60 m/sec for human group I afferents and approximately 40 m/sec for human group II afferents,[13] the diameter of group II afferents can be estimated as 9.8 to 16 µm if group I axons have diameters of 12 to 20 µm. However, there are many more afferents with small myelinated or unmyelinated axons that arise as free nerve endings, and they are responsive to mechanical stresses, and chemical, thermal, and nociceptive stimuli. There have been only a few studies on slowly conducting human muscle afferents and their correlation with muscle pain, and they will not be addressed further.

The primary ending of the muscle spindle is exquisitely sensitive to small perturbations, arguably more so than any sensor that we can devise to detect the perturbation. Characteristically, the endings are said to respond to the extent of stretch and to its velocity (Fig. 14-4, *B*), and their responsiveness can be altered by producing (nonpropagated) contractions of the modified muscle fibers ("intrafusal fibers", i.e., muscle fibers within the fusiform muscle spindle) which they encircle. These focal contractions are produced by γ motor axons (which innervate only the muscle spindle) and/or β motor axons (which innervate both the muscle spindle and nearby muscle fibers, so-called "extrafusal" muscle). Two types of γ efferent are recognized: those with predominantly "dynamic" effects on the discharge of the primary ending and those with predominantly "static" effects.

The secondary ending of the muscle spindle has little sensitivity to the derivatives of length, and it operates more as a length transducer (see Fig. 14-4, *B*; 14-5, *D*). Each spindle gives rise to a number of group II afferents but only a single group Ia afferent. Only static γ motor axons will affect the discharge of the secondary ending.

The muscle spindle lies in parallel with surrounding muscle fibers so that their contraction will shorten the spindle and relaxation will stretch it. However, some muscle fibers insert directly into the capsule of the spindle and there may be fascial interconnections between spindle and muscle fibers, so that contraction of the relevant motor units may activate spindle endings directly rather than unload them. Primary and secondary endings on the muscle spindle behave similarly, with the

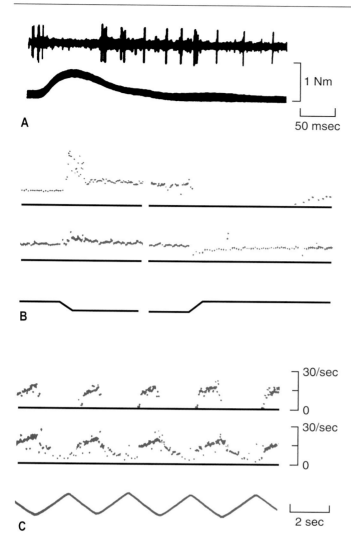

FIGURE 14-4 ■ Identification of spindle endings. **A**, Twitch test showing afferent potentials in the original neurogram (upper trace) and the torque produced by contraction of the receptor-bearing muscle (lower trace). Five superimposed sweeps. Note that an early discharge occurs before torque starts to rise. Spindle discharge pauses as torque rises. **B**, "Instantaneous" frequency plots of spindle responses to ramp stretch and shortening of 3 to 4° at 7.5°/sec for a primary ending (upper trace) and a secondary ending (middle trace). Calibrations as in **C**. **C**, "Instantaneous" frequency plots of responses to alternating movements at 7.5°/sec for primary ending (upper trace) and secondary ending (middle trace). In both B and C, the movement of the ankle joint is shown in the lower trace, but for simplicity, the goniometer record for the primary ending has been omitted. The imposed movements for the two endings in C were very similar, but not quite identical in amplitude, so that occasionally the discharge of the primary ending appears slightly out of phase. A downward deflection represents stretch of the receptor-bearing muscle in this figure and in Figures 14-5 and 14-6. (From Burke D, Hagbarth K-E, Löfstedt L et al: The responses of human muscle spindle endings to vibration of non-contracting muscles. J Physiol, 261:673, 1976, with permission.)

exception that any change in discharge of the primary ending contains a dynamic component. The term "Golgi tendon organ" is a misnomer because few tendon organs lie within the tendon itself. Tendon organs occur where muscle fibers insert into fascia or tendon and, in most muscles, tendon organs are located mainly within the anatomic confines of the muscle belly. Between 5 and 15 muscle fibers insert into the capsule of any one tendon organ, and these fibers generally come from different motor units, so a single tendon organ samples the activity of a subset of motor units but only those that are anatomically close. These receptors are exquisitely sensitive to force applied directly to them, and the contraction of a single muscle fiber may be sufficient if it inserts into the tendon organ capsule. Under isometric conditions, the summed activity of a number of tendon organs accurately reflects overall contraction force. Tendon organs are, however, much less sensitive to the forces produced by muscle stretch, even though they are grouped together with spindle endings as "stretch receptors." In noncontracting muscles, tendon organs usually have no background discharge and, given that most microneurographic studies are performed with the subjects initially at rest, it is not surprising that the responses of tendon organs are less well documented than those of muscle spindles.

The differentiation of Ia, II, and Ib afferents depends on the use of a twitch test to distinguish a spindle ending from a tendon organ, the variability of any discharge that is present at rest (spindle endings only), and the responses of the ending to a variety of stimuli (stretch and shortening, contraction, vibration). The most popular methods for producing the twitch contraction involve stimulation of the innervating nerve trunk or stimulating maximally within the selected motor fascicle. The former will produce a larger twitch contraction, thereby risking dislodging the microelectrode, and may activate other muscles so that the twitch contraction is not confined to the receptor-bearing muscle, risking that the afferent might be unloaded by a dominant contraction of an unintended muscle. The latter method restricts the contraction to the receptor-bearing muscle, but requires a special amplifier which can be switched off transiently to allow the stimulus to be delivered through the microelectrode and then switched back on, with a gap of only some tens of milliseconds or less. A third method involves stimulating through surface or needle electrodes inserted over or into the receptor-bearing muscle, surface electrodes being suitable only with superficial muscles.

The typical unloading/reloading ("in-parallel") responses of muscle spindle endings in the twitch test are shown in Figures 14-4, *A* and 14-5, *E*. Typically the primary ending may resume firing on the falling phase of

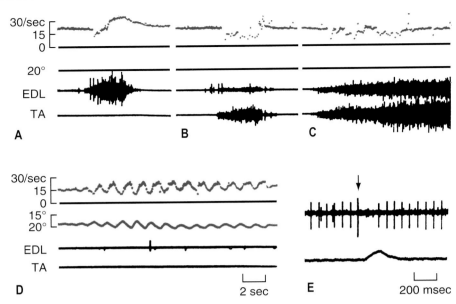

FIGURE 14-5 ■ The effects of isometric voluntary contractions on the discharge rate of a secondary ending in extensor digitorum longus (EDL). In **A**, **B**, **C**, and **D**, traces are: instantaneous frequency; joint angle; electromyogram (EMG) of EDL; EMG of tibialis anterior (TA). In **E**, an electrically induced twitch delivered at the arrow produces a twitch contraction, recorded by the myograph (lower trace), and a typical pause in spindle discharge, seen in the original neurogram (upper trace). In *D*, the close parallelism between imposed joint movement and discharge rate suggests that the ending is a secondary ending. Stretch of EDL is indicated by a downward movement of the joint angle trace. In *A*, contraction of EDL accelerates the spindle (after a brief unloading). In *B*, contraction of predominantly TA decreases discharge rate. In *C*, contraction of both muscles, the opposing effects largely cancelling out. (From Burke D, Hagbarth K-E, Löfstedt L et al: The responses of human muscle spindle endings to vibration during isometric contraction. J Physiol, 261:695, 1976, with permission.)

the twitch contraction with a high-frequency burst of impulses (see Fig. 14-4, *A*). By contrast, tendon organs are activated on the rising phase of the twitch, and this produces a loading ("in-series") response. With muscle stretch and shortening, the Ib response is minimal, that of Ia afferents characterized by a dynamic response to the movement with a steady discharge at an adapted level to maintained stretch, and a pause in discharge on shortening (see Fig. 14-4, *B*). Typically, group II afferents lack the dynamic response to stretch and the pause on shortening. Dependent on muscle length, many spindle afferents and all Ib afferents are silent in relaxed EMG-silent muscles, but for those that are active, the variability of discharge of Ia afferents is higher than that of group II afferents. Both tendon organs and muscle spindles may be activated during a voluntary contraction, the former stimulated directly by the muscle contraction, the latter because fusimotor neurons are activated along with α motor axons by voluntary effort.

Clinically Relevant Insights

Recordings from muscle spindle afferents can provide insight into the role of the γ efferent (fusimotor) system. However, this insight is quite indirect, and only as good as the controls used to ensure that any change in spindle behavior is not due to inadvertent stretch or contraction of the receptor-bearing muscle.[14] Using rigid controls creates a dilemma because the constraints may well change the subject's mental set and thereby the way in which fusimotor neurons behave. In addition, the risk of jeopardizing recordings limits the types of movement that can be studied. It would be surprising if the recordings so far reported for humans are truly representative of the full motor repertoire at our disposal but, even allowing for this, it is clear that the human fusimotor system behaves differently from that of the awake behaving cat.[4,13,15,16] This should not be surprising, given that there are major species differences: size, length of conduction pathways, conduction velocities, morphology of spindle endings, and differences in motor skill. For example, the quadrupedal digitigrade stance and locomotion of the cat differ from the more unstable bipedal plantigrade stance and locomotion of humans, in whom there seems to be greater reliance on anticipatory and feedforward control mechanisms than on feedback adjustments.[13]

If one accepts these reservations, recordings from spindle afferents do allow a number of conclusions to be put forward.

SENSORY ROLE OF MUSCLE SPINDLES

Microstimulation of single spindle afferents produces no discernible sensation, but activation of a population of afferents by electrical stimulation or tendon vibration can evoke sensations of movement or a change in position. These illusory movements can be quite strong, sufficient to move a limb or joint to an anatomically impossible position. However, muscle afferents are not the sole source of proprioceptive cues, and the responses to microstimulation are not unlike those with stimulation of cutaneous SA2 afferents (see below).

FUSIMOTOR FUNCTION AT REST

There seems to be general agreement that the level of γ_s drive (i.e., drive from γ-static neurons) directed to noncontracting muscles is low, if it exists at all—certainly too low to have a significant effect on spindle function.

The extent to which this applies to γ_d activity (i.e., activity of γ-dynamic neurons) is uncertain.[4] There have been intermittent reports of spindles behaving as if they do receive some background γ_d drive, even in relaxed muscles, but nevertheless any such background drive is not a prerequisite for a tendon jerk. De-efferenting spindles by injection of local anesthetic around the nerve does not alter their responses to changes in muscle length (Fig. 14-6) or their responses to tendon percussion.

For the clinician, absence of a tendon jerk is more likely to be due to a loss of afferent input to the spinal cord or to low central excitability than to a low level of fusimotor drive to spindles in the percussed muscle.

FUSIMOTOR FUNCTION DURING VOLUNTARY CONTRACTIONS

There is some evidence that γ_d fusimotor neurons are activated during voluntary contractions, but there are few insights into the patterns of γ_d activity or precisely what such activity achieves (other than speculation that it might serve to help smooth out irregularities in movement). There is also no unequivocal evidence that the γ_d activity overflows to adjacent muscles. On the other hand, there is clear evidence that γ_s fusimotor neurons innervating the contracting muscle are activated along with and in proportion to the activation of α motor neurons. Indeed, the activation of group II afferents during voluntary contractions is cogent evidence that there was an increase in γ_s fusimotor drive to the contracting

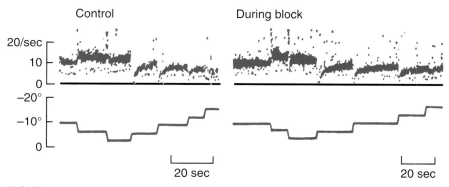

FIGURE 14-6 ■ The effect of de-efferentation on the response to stretch and shortening of a primary ending in the relaxed fibularis (peroneus) longus muscle. De-efferentation was achieved by complete nerve block with lidocaine (2 percent) injected proximal to the recording site at the fibular head. The block produced distal anesthesia and complete paralysis of muscles innervated by the deep and superficial fibular (peroneal) nerve branches. *Upper trace*: "Instantaneous" frequency plot. *Lower trace*: Joint position. There was no change in the discharge rate of the responses to stretch and shortening of the de-efferented primary ending. A downward deflection indicates stretch of the receptor-bearing muscle. (From Burke D, Hagbarth K-E, Löfstedt L et al: The responses of human muscle spindle endings to vibration during isometric contraction. J Physiol, 261:695, 1976, with permission.)

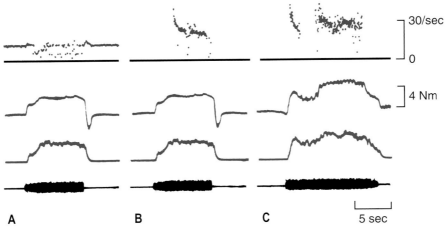

FIGURE 14-7 ■ Simultaneous recordings from two spindle endings in tibialis anterior. **A**, Recording from an initially active ending during an isometric voluntary contraction below threshold for the ending. **B**, Recording from an initially silent ending which was activated in the same contraction. **C**, A second isometric contraction, the initially silent ending being activated at the same effort (torque) level as in *B*. Traces are: instantaneous frequency plot; contraction torque; integrated electromyogram (EMG) of tibialis anterior (time constant 0.2 sec); and EMG of tibialis anterior. (From Burke D, Hagbarth K-E, Skuse NF: Recruitment order of human spindle endings in isometric voluntary contractions. J Physiol, 285:101, 1978, with permission.)

muscle. The γ_s activation does not precede the α activation and appears to be directed to the contracting muscle only, such that spindle endings in noncontracting muscles may be unloaded (see Fig. 14-5, *B*). Note that the increase in spindle discharge during voluntary contractions seen in Figures 14-5, 14-7, and 14-8 starts after the onset of EMG and occurs despite the muscle fiber shortening which would have unloaded the spindle but for the heightened fusimotor drive, and that the increase in fusimotor drive to a muscle may be insufficient to increase the discharge of all spindle endings in that muscle (compare Fig. 14-7, *A* and *B*).

The efficacy of this increase in fusimotor drive is commonly overestimated and said to be sufficient to maintain a coherent spindle discharge during movement, but this view is unproven hypothesis not established fact. In free unloaded movements, the drive is usually *insufficient* to maintain spindle discharge in the face of the unloading produced by muscle shortening. This will be even more so when the extent of movement is faster and greater than can be studied using microneurography. However, during eccentric contractions, spindles respond strongly to the combined inputs of fusimotor drive and muscle stretch.

The value of the enhanced spindle discharge during isometric contractions should not be underestimated; manipulative skill is not innate. It requires learning, and movements commonly are then slow and involve quasi-isometric contractions producing small movements, if any, with movement proceeding by adjustment of a co-contraction of antagonists. There is evidence of greater fusimotor drive to a co-contracting muscle than to a muscle producing the same EMG but contracting by itself.[17] Perhaps, then, in humans, an important role for the fusimotor system is motor learning and skill acquisition. This does not mean that in all learning tasks the level of fusimotor drive is disproportionately high; indeed, Vallbo's group have produced evidence that it is not. It could imply that the dependence on fusimotor drive is smaller when one has gained sufficient skill to perform a task without thinking about it. Then movement may be so rapid that any reflex support available through fusimotor/spindle mechanisms would be counterproductive because it occurred too late.

FUSIMOTOR FUNCTION DURING CONTRACTIONS OF REMOTE MUSCLES, MOTOR IMAGERY, AND PREPARATION FOR A CONTRACTION

Can fusimotor drive be activated by mental effort, without also activating α motor neurons? Intuitively, it would be unreasonable to have retained a separate control of α and γ motor neurons and of γ_d and γ_s fusimotor neurons if that served no real purpose. Defining precisely what is that

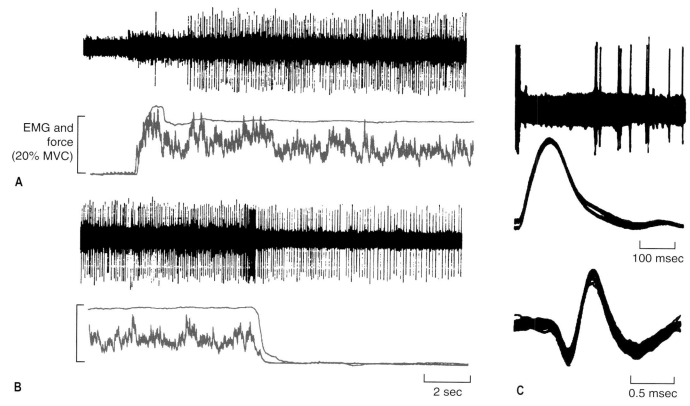

FIGURE 14-8 ▪ Muscle spindle ending in tibialis anterior. **A** and **B** show the start and end of a 1-minute submaximal contraction of ankle dorsiflexors (approximately 20 percent maximal voluntary force [MVC]). There are 30 seconds between *A* and *B*. The raw neurogram, force, and integrated tibialis anterior electromyogram (EMG) are shown. Spindle discharge was maintained throughout the 60-second contraction at approximately 12 Hz; there was a high-frequency burst of impulses on relaxation of the contraction, but discharge continued at approximately 8 Hz in the absence of EMG following the contraction. **C**, The upper two panels show the twitch test for the unit (three traces superimposed). The lowest panel shows superimposed action potentials from the unit (on a faster time base). The continued discharge of the afferent following relaxation of the contraction is due to the thixotropic properties of intrafusal fibers, not evidence of continuing fusimotor drive (see Wilson LR, Gandevia SC, Burke D: Increased resting discharge of human spindle afferents following voluntary contractions. J Physiol, 488:833, 1995). (From Macefield G, Hagbarth K-E, Gorman R et al: Decline in spindle support to α-motoneurones during sustained voluntary contractions. J Physiol, 440:497, 1991, with permission.)

purpose has proved elusive, with many statements in the literature based on unproven theories of little relevance to how human subjects actually move. Perhaps the focus on the control of movement has been a distraction, ignoring the fact that the spindle is a sensory receptor and that its afferents project to cerebellum and to cortex, and are critically involved in the programming and elaboration of movement on the one hand, and on the awareness of where one's limbs are in space on the other hand.

Motor imagery and provision of cues to movement have formed the basis of many studies of motor cortical excitability using transcranial magnetic stimulation and functional imaging. Often, such studies ignore the fact that the excitability of the cortex is influenced by input from the spinal cord, and that cortical excitability commonly is tested using a motor evoked potential from a limb muscle, which involves transmission through complicated spinal

circuits. There is no evidence for a significant enhancement of spindle input to the spinal cord under such circumstances, but there is clear evidence for enhanced spinal reflex excitability (Fig. 14-9, *A* and *B*). Nevertheless, it remains possible that modulation of corticofugal control of the background activity at the relays in Clarke's column, nucleus Z, or thalamus leads to enhanced spindle feedback to cortex. It also needs to be ensured that the enhanced spinal reflex excitability[4] seen in Figure 14-9 is not responsible for any change in the motor evoked potential.[18]

There is debate about whether spindle endings can be activated when a remote muscle is contracted[13,14] Nevertheless, even if there is heightened γ_d drive to noncontracting muscles, this is not responsible for the reinforcement of the tendon jerk or H reflex by maneuvers such as the Jendrassik maneuver (Fig. 14-9, *C* and *D*). Nor, for that matter, is the reflex enhancement

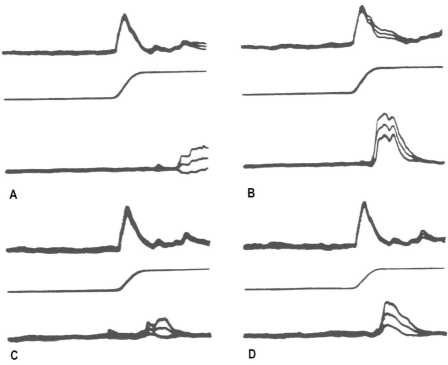

FIGURE 14-9 ■ Responses to a visual warning (*A*, *B*) and during the Jendrassik maneuver (*C*, *D*). **A**, Test sequences for which the subject opposed a stretching perturbation, having received no warning. **B**, Test sequences for which a visual warning preceded the perturbation. Traces are: average multi-unit muscle afferent neural activity from tibialis anterior (TA), average joint position, and average "integrated" electromyogram (EMG), each with 95 percent confidence limits. In the joint position trace, an upwards movement indicates stretch of TA. There is no significant short-latency change in the EMG response to the stretch in *A* but there is in *B*. However, there is no significant change in the neural activity generated by the stretch. Each sweep is the average of 15 responses; sweep duration, 500 msec; bin width, 1 msec; joint movement from 14° to 16° plantar flexion. **C** and **D**, Displays of neural activity, joint position, and "integrated" EMG from the same experiment for tests in which the subject was instructed to make no active response to the perturbation. Some perturbations were preceded by the auditory warning, in response to which he performed a Jendrassik maneuver. *C*, Control sequences (without reinforcement). *D*, Test sequences during which the reinforcement maneuver was performed. Note the potentiation of the reflex EMG burst in the absence of any effect on the neural activity responsible for the reflex activity. Each sweep is the average of 12 sequences; sweep duration, 500 msec; bin width, 1 msec; joint movement from 14° to 16° plantar flexion. (From Burke D, McKeon B, Skuse NF et al: Anticipation and fusimotor activity in preparation for a voluntary contraction. J Physiol, 306:337, 1980, with permission.)

due to a decrease in presynaptic inhibition of Ia afferents from the test muscle.[13]

FUSIMOTOR FUNCTION IN MOTOR DISORDERS

Hyporeflexia is not due to depressed fusimotor drive.[19] For it to be so, normal muscle tone would be dependent on an active stretch reflex. In fact, many normal subjects can relax completely, and in them reflex mechanisms will not contribute to muscle tone. Moreover, as discussed earlier, there is little, if any, fusimotor drive to relaxed muscles to be withdrawn. *Hyperreflexia* is not caused by overactivity of the fusimotor system. At most, this would enhance the spindle input to the nervous system and, when the nervous system is normal, subjects do not become spastic or rigid when the spindle input to the spinal cord is enhanced. The question then arises as to whether fusimotor dysfunction might contribute to the disability in these disorders.

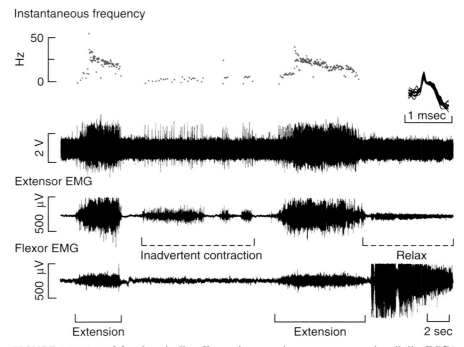

FIGURE 14-10 ■ Muscle spindle afferent innervating extensor carpi radialis (ECR) during deliberate isometric wrist extension in a patient suffering from hemiplegic spasticity (extensor strength was 68 percent of that of the contralateral side). The afferent did not maintain a background discharge when truly at rest. During voluntary efforts to contract the muscle ("*Extension*"), the spindle ending was activated together with the electromyogram (EMG) of ECR. Between the deliberate contractions, the ending was activated unintentionally during inadvertent contractions, but again with EMG. The ending in ECR was not activated during an unintentional contraction of the forearm flexors that occurred when the patient was told to relax ECR. *Inset* (top right) shows action potential morphology (multiple superimposed discharges). (From Wilson LR, Gandevia SC, Inglis JT et al: Muscle spindle activity in the affected upper limb after a unilateral stroke. Brain, 122:2079, 1999, with permission.)

Hemiplegic Spasticity

The discharge rates of spindle endings in triceps surae and in the forearm extensor muscles of patients are not abnormal, and neither are their responses to stretch or other maneuvers (Fig. 14-10).[20]

Spinal Spasticity

Spasticity due to conditions such as spinal cord injury, multiple sclerosis, and hereditary spastic paraplegia remains "*terra incognita*." There have been no reports of spindle recordings in these conditions. However, it is intuitively reasonable for there to be disordered spindle function due to disinhibited cutaneous and other exteroceptive reflexes operating on γ motor neurons.

Parkinson Disease

The data on Parkinson disease consist of single-unit recordings in parkinsonian tremor and multi-unit recordings of fluctuating afferent activity in parallel with fluctuating rigidity. These data are insufficient to establish whether the supraspinal control of fusimotor neurons is normal or abnormal, and further studies are indicated.

CUTANEOUS AND JOINT AFFERENTS

A neural discharge can be recorded as an evoked compound action potential, with the recording sweep triggered by an electrical or mechanical stimulus to skin (Fig. 14-11) or muscle, or the innervating nerve distal to the recording site. As with the compound sensory action potentials recorded with near-nerve electrodes, components in the evoked activity separate out by latency, but again the potentials of pathologically slow large axons may be difficult to distinguish from those of normal, slowly conducting axons. The intrafascicular recording provides little more than can be obtained with near-nerve recordings, with one exception: the ability to define potentials of unmyelinated axons, conducting at 0.5 to 2 m/sec (not illustrated with the time base of Fig. 14-11).

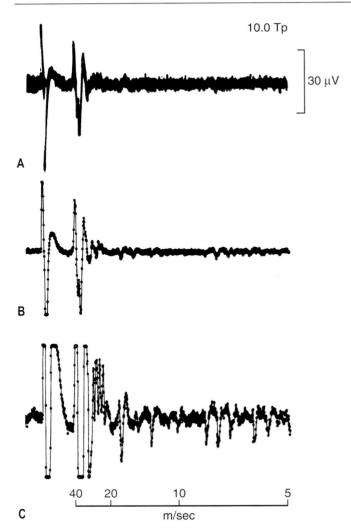

10.0 Tp

30 µV

A

B

40   20   10   5

C   m/sec

FIGURE 14-11 ■ Myelinated A-fiber activity recorded from the superficial (cutaneous) branch of the radial nerve. **A,** Five sweeps have been superimposed. A few slow potentials can be discerned but signal-to-noise ratio is poor. **B,** Average of 100 sweeps. Slow myelinated potentials are more obvious. **C,** Average of 100 sweeps after increasing the input gain. Multiple slow potentials in the Aδ range are visible but the voltage of the fast potentials exceeds the input levels of the averager so that their details are lost. (From Burke D, Mackenzie RA, Skuse NF et al: Cutaneous afferent activity in median and radial nerve fascicles: a microelectrode study. J Neurol Neurosurg Psychiatry, 38:855, 1975, with permission.)

Large Myelinated Cutaneous Afferents

The best-characterized recordings have been from the median nerve at the wrist. The glabrous skin of the hand is innervated by four different types of fast-conducting (group Aα/β) afferents, each representing a different encapsulated mechanoreceptor; fast-adapting type 1 (FA1) afferents probably innervate Meissner corpuscles (which have a small receptive field), fast-adapting type 2 (FA2)

afferents innervate Pacinian corpuscles (large receptive field), slowly adapting type 1 (SA1) afferents innervate Merkel endings (small receptive field), and slowly adapting type 2 (SA2) afferents innervate Ruffini endings (responsive to skin stretch and often directionally sensitive). Hairy skin possesses these same receptors, but in addition a rapidly adapting hair follicle receptor, responsive to movements of hair without contact with skin. Hairy skin is also innervated by non-nociceptive mechanosensitive C fibers. The sensations experienced by healthy volunteers have been correlated with natural activation of the relevant receptor and the discharge pattern of the afferent, and it has been found that each receptor type produces a unique sensation. These conclusions have been confirmed using intrafascicular microstimulation of individual afferents—a sensation of "flutter" or "vibration" with FA1 and FA2 (Meissner or Pacinian corpuscles, respectively), dependent on frequency, "pressure" with SA1 (Merkel discs), and no specific sensation with SA2 (Ruffini endings). It is notable that, when attention is focused on the receptive field, a single impulse may evoke a sensation referred to the site of the receptor (though not with SA2 receptors). Microstimulation of single SA2 units produces no defined percept. The situation with SA2 afferents is reminiscent of muscle spindles which, individually, produce no detectable sensation (although activation of a population of group Ia spindle afferents, whether naturally or electrically, can evoke a movement-related sensation). This difference is logical; tactile acuity depends on the ability to localize and discriminate the inputs in different afferent channels, a feature not required of proprioceptive afferents (spindle afferents and cutaneous SA2 afferents). With proprioception, discordant information in a single channel is unlikely to outweigh the information from the many afferents from all muscles operating on the joint.

Cutaneous Afferent C Fibers

The majority of these afferents respond to moderate or intense thermal (heat), mechanical, and nociceptive stimuli (hence "polymodal nociceptors"), though specific mechanosensitive and "warm" units have been described (and even some selectively responding to cold). Polymodal nociceptors may have extensive and complex receptive fields, with a number of areas of heightened sensitivity. Interest has revolved mainly around their role in nociception, and the general conclusion is that most, if not all, of the characteristics of the pain percept can be explained by the pattern of input to the spinal cord. Sensitization of receptors and of previously silent ("sleeping")

C-fiber terminals can account for many of the features of pain,[12] such as hyperalgesia (an excessive perceptual response to a stimulus that is normally painful) and allodynia (pain due to a stimulus that does not normally provoke pain). In healthy subjects, silent C fibers can be sensitized by the application of pain-producing substances such as mustard oil or capsaicin to the skin.

Pain is an emotive experience, and so too is research into its pathophysiology and management. The role of central mechanisms in the elaboration and maintenance of pain is not denied,[21] but microneurographic findings point to the importance of a disturbed afferent C-fiber input as a central mechanism. Based on nerve blocks, microneurographic findings, use of placebos, and clinical judgment, advocates such as Ochoa and colleagues have argued forcefully that the terms "*reflex sympathetic dystrophy*" and "*sympathetically maintained pain*" may well have constrained thinking about the underlying pathophysiology of the pain reported by the patient.[22] These views are not supported universally.[12,23,24] However, studies of sympathetic function, including microneurographic recordings of skin sympathetic activity, indicate that these conditions cannot be explained by either an abnormal sympathetic drive to skin or some as yet undefined sympathetic effect on sensitized C-fiber terminals.[25]

The sensation of "*itch*" is encoded by C afferents, but apparently not those mediating nociceptive sensations. Instead, it seems to involve histamine sensitization of mechanically insensitive afferents.

The perceptual correlates of an individual axon (or group of axons) depend on whether they can conduct impulses past the microelectrode, and this they cannot always do (see Conduction Block, later). However, microstimulation can bypass any block effectively and has confirmed the correlates for both A and C afferents. "[The] sensations elicited by a train of impulses in a single afferent unit are remarkably distinct and well characterized in a number of respects."[26]

Joint Afferents

These afferents are largely detectors of stresses placed on a joint when it is moved into extreme positions (Fig. 14-12) or when the joint is distended or inflamed. They do not provide a coherent signal of joint position (and it would be appropriate to eschew the term "joint position sense" in favor of "kinesthesia"). Similarly, microstimulation of single joint afferents can produce a sense of joint rotation but not of movement or a change in position. The senses of position and movement are indicated better by the convergent input from muscle

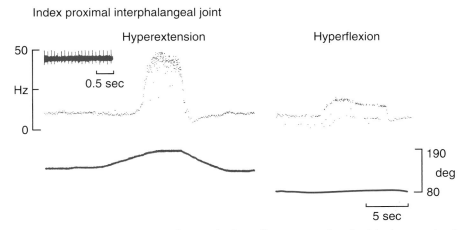

FIGURE 14-12 ▪ Behavior of an articular afferent, associated with the proximal interphalangeal joint of the index finger (median innervation), during passive rotation in the flexion–extension axis. The afferent did not respond in either the abduction–adduction or extorsion–intorsion axes. *Upper trace,* An example of the afferent's tonic discharge when the interphalangeal joint was in the rest position. *Middle trace,* Instantaneous frequency record. *Lower trace,* Goniometer record. Note in the left panel the sustained high-frequency discharge when the joint was moved into the limits of extension and no change in background discharge when moved into flexion, and in the right panel the sustained discharge when forced into extreme flexion. (From Burke D, Gandevia SC, Macefield G: Responses to passive movement of receptors in joint, skin and muscle of the human hand. J Physiol, 402:347, 1988, with permission.)

spindle and cutaneous mechanoreceptors, supplemented when moving by knowledge of the motor command.

Clinically Relevant Insights

The evoked compound action potential of cutaneous A fibers can be recorded readily using an intrafascicular microelectrode, but the recordings provide few advantages and no novel insights into pathophysiology that cannot be obtained using near-nerve electrodes, perhaps with the exception that fewer responses need be averaged. However, the potentials of unmyelinated axons (orthodromic afferent C fibers and antidromic sympathetic efferents) can be recorded more readily with microelectrodes, though whether this is of clinical value is not established conclusively.

Recordings of the natural activity of single afferents and stimulus-evoked compound action potentials have been made in patients with different forms of neuropathy, but these provide few novel insights into the underlying disease processes, and have little diagnostic value in the individual patient. In part, this is because only a few axons can be studied fully in any one experiment.

Local anesthetics must diffuse to the target nerve trunk to block axons in that nerve. They tend to block small before large afferents, but microneurographic recordings indicate that the sequence is not invariant, probably because of unequal or irregular diffusion. Pressure will block large axons before small preferentially, but it is difficult to control the block and differentiation between myelinated axons of different size may be difficult, though afferent and efferent C fibers are not susceptible.

Disordered sympathetic function or even normal sympathetic driving of sensitized C endings in the skin probably is not responsible for pain in the majority of patients considered to suffer from "reflex sympathetic dystrophy" or "sympathetically maintained pain." The role of the sympathetic nervous system in driving these syndromes still remains unclear. However, sensitization of C-fiber endings and of previously silent ("sleeping") endings contributes to many of the features of these syndromes, such as hyperalgesia and allodynia. "Itch" involves a specific subpopulation of mechanically insensitive C afferents that are sensitive to histamine.

Joint afferents make little contribution to "joint position sense."

SYMPATHETIC EFFERENT ACTIVITY

Sympathetic activity occurs in apparently spontaneous bursts in nerve fascicles innervating skin (skin sympathetic activity, SSA) and muscle (muscle sympathetic activity, MSA). SSA occurs irregularly, with bursts of variable duration, often modulated by respiration, and readily provoked by arousal stimuli, whereas MSA occurs in a pulse-synchronous pattern (Fig. 14-13), with more discrete bursts that show little overt response to unexpected arousal stimuli, and are more frequent and stronger when diastolic blood pressure is falling.

Most SSA serves a thermoregulatory role, and sympathetic bursts contain specific subpopulations of efferent C fibers that have sudomotor or vasomotor functions and, in hairy skin, pilomotor functions. The vasomotor fibers may be vasoconstrictor or vasodilator, activity in the latter becoming apparent only as temperature is increased, when sudomotor fibers are also active (and they may, in fact, be the same axons). SSA may be particularly strong when the ambient temperature is low and the subject feels cold, and the bursts then are correlated with cutaneous vasoconstriction. There may be minimal SSA at approximately 24°C, but sudomotor/vasodilator bursts increase and become dominant as temperature increases further. Although their responses to temperature are the opposite, arousal stimuli produce activity in both

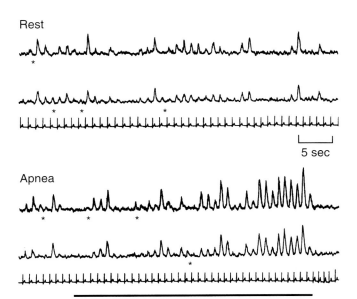

FIGURE 14-13 ▪ Bilateral recordings of muscle nerve sympathetic activity from the right and left fibular (peroneal) nerves showing the similarity of the integrated neurograms. In each panel the upper trace is the neurogram from the right leg, the second trace the neurogram from the left leg, and the third trace the electrocardiogram. Bursts which appear only on one side are indicated by asterisks. In the lower panel, the subject was apneic for the period indicated by the horizontal bar. (From Wallin BG, Burke D, Gandevia SC: Coherence between the sympathetic drives to relaxed and contracting muscles of different limbs of human subjects. J Physiol, 455:219, 1992, with permission.)

subpopulations of SSA. Thus the recorded activity depends on the experimental conditions, and on the temperature of the patient and that of the environment. The "sympathetic skin response" is a stimulus-triggered, arousal-related galvanic skin response reflecting the resultant change in skin conductance. As such, it is an end-organ response, measures sudomotor function only, and is dependent on temperature and the integrity of skin and sweat glands. It is subject to habituation and has the same need for controls over patient and environmental conditions as SSA. It is discussed further in Chapter 21.

Muscle constitutes the largest vascular bed in the body, and MSA is vasoconstrictive. It is regulated by inhibitory feedback to the brainstem from arterial baroreceptors in the aortic arch and carotid body, and this imposes the pulse-synchronous pattern (see Fig. 14-13) that waxes and wanes with fluctuations in diastolic blood pressure. There is no short-term response to arousal stimuli or to changes in ambient temperature. In addition, low-pressure volume receptors in the thorax can influence MSA. It increases with voluntary apnea (see Fig. 14-13) and with changes in posture from lying, to sitting, to standing, when there is a need for greater MSA to maintain blood pressure in the face of a decreased cardiac return (Fig. 14-14). In normal subjects at rest, there is a wide range in incidence of MSA bursts (from approximately 5/100 heart beats to over 90/100 beats) but there is remarkable homogeneity in the outflow to different limbs (see Fig. 14-13). However, this homogeneity is not inviolate; mild to moderate exercise appears to decrease MSA to the exercising muscle but not to other muscles. On the contrary, with contraction of upper-limb muscles (e.g., an isometric hand grip), there is an increase in MSA to nonexercising leg muscles. It is not known whether the "dissociation" of the drives is programmed centrally or depends on local mechanisms overriding a common central program.

Clinically Relevant Insights

Autonomic failure is associated with a loss of recordable sympathetic activity. However, if SSA or MSA can be recorded in patients with autonomic dysfunction, it has a normal pattern, whether the dysfunction is central or peripheral. The abnormality consists of inability to record SSA more often than might occur in healthy subjects. MSA with the normal pulse synchrony may be increased in patients with Guillain–Barré syndrome suffering attacks of hypertension, possibly because of involvement of the afferent limb of the baroreflex with loss of feedback from intrathoracic and perhaps also arterial baroreceptors (although, despite this, the MSA generally retains its pulsatile pattern).

The *sympathetic skin response*, discussed in Chapter 21, is an end-organ response, reflects only the sudomotor component of SSA, and is critically dependent on recording conditions and ambient temperature.

Vasovagal syncope is associated with withdrawal of sympathetic outflow to muscle (and possibly other beds) resulting in peripheral vasodilatation (Fig. 14-15), despite progressive bradycardia (that is evidence of vagal overactivity). The bradycardia and decline in blood pressure normally would be associated with a compensatory intensification of MSA.

The inter-individual differences in the extent of MSA are great, and any increase in MSA in the hypertensive patient is quite modest. Joyner and colleagues conclude that, although most studies have found evidence for increased sympathetic activity directed to muscle, kidneys, and heart in *essential hypertension*, high levels of MSA do not cause hypertension.[11] However, MSA increases with obesity and ageing, both of which are associated with an increased incidence of hypertension, and it was also concluded that there are circumstances in which "high levels of MSNA [muscle sympathetic nerve activity]

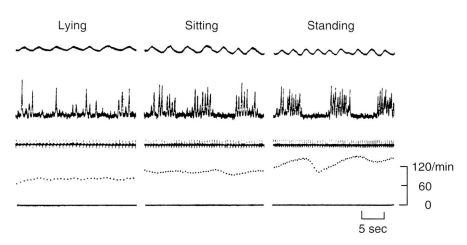

FIGURE 14-14 ▪ Differences between mean voltage records of muscle sympathetic activity (MSA) in lying, sitting, and standing postures in a single experimental session. Traces are, from above: respiratory movements (as in Fig. 14-15, inspiration upwards); mean voltage MSA (time constant 0.05 sec); electrocardiogram; instantaneous heart rate. (From Burke D, Sundlöf G, Wallin BG: Postural effects on muscle nerve sympathetic activity in man. J Physiol, 272:399, 1977, with permission.)

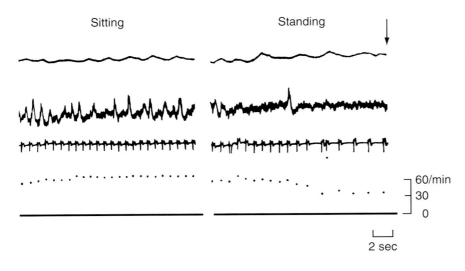

FIGURE 14-15 ■ Vasovagal syncope. Muscle sympathetic activity and heart rate during fainting. Left panel obtained when sitting 2 to 3 minutes before standing up. Right panel on standing, starting just when stable stance had been achieved and ending with the subject collapsing (arrow). Records photographed from oscilloscope on alternating-current mode. Traces as in Figure 14-14. In the right panel, note that the disappearance of sympathetic bursts (apart from a single burst in the middle of the trace) is accompanied by bradycardia (to 30/min). (From Burke D, Sundlöf G, Wallin BG: Postural effects on muscle nerve sympathetic activity in man. J Physiol, 272:399, 1977, with permission.)

clearly contribute to increases in blood pressure. We expect sympathetically mediated hypertension to be an important pathophysiological phenomenon as the developed world and the developing world gets both older and fatter." *Obesity* is associated with hypertension, and obese subjects and those with type 2 diabetes have greater MSA than nonobese controls, even if normotensive. Certainly, in *obstructive sleep apnea* there are clear increases in MSA, even during the day when patients are not hypoxemic.

Resting MSA is increased greatly in *cardiac failure*, in patients with unstable *angina*, and for several months following *myocardial infarction*, particularly if patients are hypertensive beforehand. It is unchanged in those who have suffered a remote infarct.

CONDUCTION BLOCK AND ECTOPIC IMPULSE ACTIVITY

Recordings from axons as they developed conduction block following impalement by the recording microelectrode provide some clinically relevant insights into activity-dependent conduction block.[27] In axons that have been impaled by a microelectrode, it is often possible to recognize components of the single unit potential generated at the nodes immediately proximal and distal to the site of microelectrode damage (see Fig. 14-2, *D*). Internodal conduction time is normally approximately 30 μsec for large myelinated axons, but these damaged axons could conduct long impulse trains with reasonable stability when internodal conduction time was less than 500 μsec. When over 600 μsec, activity could precipitate a gradual increase in internodal conduction time with the development of instability, intermittent conduction failure, and finally complete conduction block. Figures 14-3 and 14-16 illustrate these findings for an

α motor axon and a group Ia afferent, respectively. Importantly, the conduction failure could recover when the activity driving the conduction block ceased, only to recur if it resumed. For all units, the longest internodal conduction time recorded just prior to complete conduction failure was, on average, 1.12 msec (range, 0.8 to 1.4 msec). The unit shown in Figure 14-16 was a group Ia afferent that underwent reversible conduction block when pressure on the receptor increased its discharge.

Ectopic activity in cutaneous A fibers has been recorded in the peripheral nerves of healthy subjects following release of ischemia, following prolonged high-frequency tetanization of cutaneous afferents, and during hyperventilation, in patients with polyneuropathy, and in a variety of patients having paresthesias associated with focal lesions (e.g., ulnar neuropathy; S1 root compression; probable thoracic outlet syndrome; and multiple sclerosis with Lhermitte symptom, precipitated by neck flexion).[28] Whether induced by a maneuver in healthy subjects or by a disease process in patients, axonal dysfunction can produce excitability changes that result in "spontaneous" discharges in previously silent axons, commonly bizarre, repetitive, high-frequency bursts of action potentials, which are felt as paresthesias. Pain and dysesthesias, by contrast, are associated with ectopic activity in nociceptive afferents, and this has been recorded directly in patients with phantom limb pain associated with a neuroma and in others with neuropathic pain, of various etiologies, including diabetes.

Clinically Relevant Insights

The ability of a damaged axon that is just managing to conduct can be impaired further by conduction of normally arising impulse trains. This is presumably because

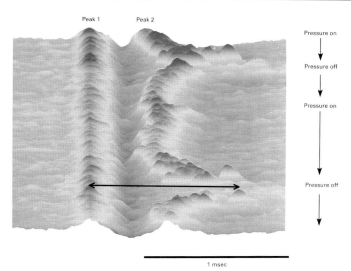

Peak 1   Peak 2

Pressure on

Pressure off

Pressure on

Pressure off

1 msec

FIGURE 14-16 ■ Activity-dependent conduction block. Raster display of action potentials of a muscle spindle afferent developing conduction block during a discharge that was maintained by pressure over the receptor. The action potential had two positive (upward) peaks (as in Figs. 14-2C, 14-2D, and 14-3) indicating marked prolongation of internodal conduction time. Muscle spindle afferent from extensor pollicis longus. It had no background discharge, but maintained an irregular discharge at approximately 3 Hz due to light pressure on the ending. When the pressure was increased (*"Pressure on"*), 10 minutes after the onset of the recording, the discharge rate of the afferent increased to approximately 20 Hz, and the second positive peak became unstable and disappeared. When pressure was relaxed (*"Pressure off"*), the second peak reappeared, only to disappear 2 minutes later when pressure was again increased. The longest interpeak intervals were 975 μsec in the first episode and 1.02 msec immediately after the second episode, the latter indicated by the horizontal arrow. The illustrated sequence contains 891 consecutive action potentials. (From Inglis JT, Leeper JB, Wilson LR et al: The development of conduction block in single human axons following a focal nerve injury. J Physiol, 513:127, 1998, with permission.)

of a normal phenomenon; conducting a train of impulses causes axons to hyperpolarize so that they are more dependent on the size of the driving current at the distal node. If this occurs on a background of pathology (injury or demyelination) that has impaired the safety margin for impulse conduction, conduction block may ensue.

In routine nerve conduction studies, latency prolongation of less than 0.5 msec is often sufficient to produce diagnostic changes indicating abnormality. Such delays need not involve more than a single internode and may not jeopardize impulse conduction (unless some other factor intervenes).

Ectopic discharges in disturbed or diseased cutaneous A and C afferents in the peripheral nerve underlie the sensations of paresthesias and dysesthesias, respectively.

REFERENCES

1. Vallbo ÅB, Hagbarth K-E: Activity from skin mechanoreceptors recorded percutaneously in awake human subjects. Exp Neurol, 21:270, 1968
2. Hagbarth K-E, Vallbo ÅB: Discharge characteristics of human muscle afferents during muscle stretch and contraction. Exp Neurol, 22:674, 1968
3. Vallbo ÅB, Hagbarth K-E, Torebjörk HE et al: Somatosensory, proprioceptive, and sympathetic activity in human peripheral nerves. Physiol Rev, 59:919, 1979
4. Gandevia SC, Burke D: Does the nervous system depend on kinesthetic information to control natural limb movements? Behav Brain Sci, 15:614, 1992
5. Hagbarth K-E: Microelectrode recordings from human peripheral nerves (microneurography). Muscle Nerve Suppl, 11:S28, 2002
6. Burke D, Gandevia SC, Macefield VG: Microneurography and motor disorders. p. 153. In Hallett M (ed): Movement Disorders. Handbook of Clinical Neurophysiology. Vol. 1, Elsevier, Amsterdam, 2003
7. McNulty PA, Macefield VG: Intraneural microstimulation of motor axons in the study of human single motor units. Muscle Nerve, 32:119, 2005
8. Macefield VG: Physiological characteristics of low-threshold mechanoreceptors in joints, muscle and skin in human subjects. Clin Exp Pharmacol Physiol, 32:135, 2005
9. Mano T, Satoshi Iwase S, Toma S: Microneurography as a tool in clinical neurophysiology to investigate peripheral neural traffic in humans. Clin Neurophysiol, 117:2357, 2006
10. Wallin BG, Charkoudian N: Sympathetic neural control of integrated cardiovascular function: insights from measurement of human sympathetic nerve activity. Muscle Nerve, 36:595, 2007
11. Joyner MJ, Charkoudian N, Wallin BG: A sympathetic view of the sympathetic nervous system and human blood pressure regulation. Exp Physiol, 93:715, 2008
12. Namer B, Handwerker HO: Translational nociceptor research as guide to human pain perceptions and pathophysiology. Exp Brain Res, 196:163, 2009
13. Pierrot-Deseilligny E, Burke D: The Circuitry of the Human Spinal Cord: Spinal and Corticospinal Mechanisms of Movement. Cambridge University Press, Cambridge, in press, 2011
14. Hagbarth K-E, Wallin G, Burke D et al: Effects of the Jendrassik manoeuvre on muscle spindle activity in man. J Neurol Neurosurg Psychiatry, 38:1143, 1975
15. Prochazka A, Hulliger M: Muscle afferent function and its significance for motor control mechanisms during voluntary movements in cat, monkey, and man. Adv Neurol, 39:93, 1983

16. Taylor A, Gladden MH, Durbaba R (eds): Alpha and Gamma Motor Systems. Plenum, New York, 1995

17. Nielsen J, Nagaoka M, Kagamihara Y et al: Discharge of muscle afferents during voluntary co-contraction of antagonistic ankle muscles in man. Neurosci Lett, 170:277, 1994

18. Burke D, Pierrot-Deseilligny E: Caveats when studying motor cortex excitability and the cortical control of movement using transcranial magnetic stimulation. Clin Neurophysiol, 121:121, 2010

19. Burke D: Spasticity as an adaptation to pyramidal tract injury. Adv Neurol, 47:401, 1988

20. Wilson LR, Gandevia SC, Inglis JT et al: Muscle spindle activity in the affected upper limb after a unilateral stroke. Brain, 122:2079, 1999

21. Koltzenburg M, Torebjörk HE, Wahren LK: Nociceptor modulated central sensitization causes mechanical hyperalgesia in acute chemogenic and chronic neuropathic pain. Brain, 117:579, 1994

22. Ochoa JL: The irritable human nociceptor under microneurography: from skin to brain. Clin Neurophysiol Suppl, 57:15, 2004

23. Schattschneider J, Binder A, Siebrecht D et al: Complex regional pain syndromes: the influence of cutaneous and deep somatic sympathetic innervation on pain. Clin J Pain, 22:240, 2006

24. Naleschinski D, Baron R: Complex regional pain syndrome type I: neuropathic or not? Curr Pain Headache Rep, 14:196, 2010

25. Elam M, Olausson B, Skarphedinsson JO et al: Does sympathetic nerve discharge affect the firing of polymodal C-fibre afferents in humans? Brain, 122:2237, 1999

26. Torebjörk HE, Vallbo ÅB, Ochoa JL: Intraneural microstimulation in man. Its relation to specificity of tactile sensations. Brain, 11:1509, 1987

27. Inglis JT, Leeper JB, Wilson LR et al: The development of conduction block in single human axons following a focal nerve injury. J Physiol, 513:127, 1998

28. Nordin M, Nyström B, Wallin U et al: Ectopic sensory discharges and paresthesiae in patients with disorders of peripheral nerves, dorsal roots and dorsal columns. Pain, 20:231, 1984

Nerve Excitability: A Clinical Translation

MATTHEW C. KIERNAN and CINDY SHIN YI LIN

Over the past 30 years there have been few significant changes to the neurophysiologic investigation of patients with suspected neuromuscular disorders. Motor and sensory nerve conduction studies, in combination with needle electromyography, have remained the method of choice for the clinician investigating peripheral nerve function. Although routine nerve conduction studies can document the presence of a neuropathy, they do not provide further insight into disease pathophysiology. Measurements of action potential amplitude and latency are limited indices of function, providing information only on the number of conducting fibers and the conduction velocity of the fastest.

Measurements of nerve excitability by threshold tracking provide complementary information to conventional nerve conduction studies. Nerve excitability is determined by the activity of a variety of ion channels, energy-dependent pumps, and ion exchange processes activated during the process of impulse conduction.[1,2] In recent years, threshold tracking methods have been used increasingly as research tools for investigating physiologic and pathophysiologic mechanisms, such as the mechanisms of ectopic discharges, and the biophysical basis for functional differences between motor and

sensory axons. More recently, these excitability techniques have been introduced into the clinical investigation of patients with neurologic disorders, and have yielded novel insight into disease mechanisms and treatment strategies. As such, the present chapter aims to provide a broad overview of current excitability techniques as employed in a clinical setting.

FUNCTIONAL INSIGHTS DERIVED FROM AXONAL STRUCTURE

The traditional view of impulse propagation has been that most electrical activity develops at nodes of Ranvier, through specific Na$^+$ and K$^+$ channels and leakage currents, whereas the internodal axolemma and myelin function as a passive isolated cable. It was not known whether there was homogenous distribution of ion channels along the axon's length or whether, in contrast, there was specialization of the nodal and internodal membrane structures. However, relatively recent microelectrode studies in intact myelinated axons and voltage clamp studies on demyelinated axons have identified multiple channel types, distributed differently between

345

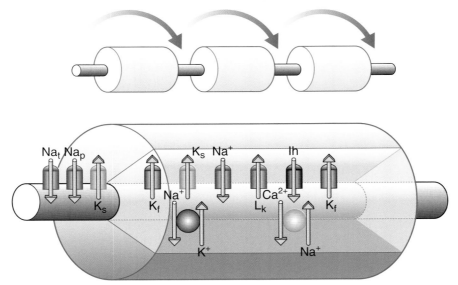

FIGURE 15-1 ■ Saltatory conduction (upper panel) is dependent on the specialized structure of the axonal membrane (lower panel). Different channels are distributed unevenly along the axonal membrane; sodium (Na^+) channels are found in high concentrations at the node, as are slow potassium (K^+) channels (Ks). Fast potassium channels (Kf) are almost exclusively paranodal. Inward rectifier channels (I_H), permeable to both K^+ and Na^+ ions, act to limit axonal hyperpolarization, whereas the Na^+/K^+ pump serves to reverse ionic fluxes that may be generated through activity. Two classes of Na^+ channels are found at the node: transient (Na_t) and persistent channels (Na_p). Under physiologic conditions, the Na^+–Ca^{2+} exchanger assists in the restoration of the membrane potential by extruding Na^+ and Ca^{2+} ions. The action potential is terminated by closure of the Na_t with the Na^+/K^+ pump restoring the resting membrane potential by extruding 3 Na^+ ions for 2 K^+ ions.

nodal, paranodal, and internodal regions, which interact electrically.[3,4] This, in turn, has led to new concepts in the understanding of nerve excitation and impulse propagation. Differences have been shown to exist in the specialized organization of ion channels across axons, suggesting that although the function of axons remains to transmit impulses faithfully from end to end, different patterns of impulse activity call for different patterns of membrane organization.

From a human axonal perspective, there are several critically important neuronal ion channels involved in impulse conduction.

Axonal Na⁺ Channels

These membrane-spanning protein molecules contain a pore through which Na^+ ions can diffuse almost freely in the open state. In myelinated axons from peripheral nerve, voltage-sensitive Na^+ channels are clustered at high densities (up to $1,000/\mu m^2$) in the nodal axon, compared to the internodal region ($25/\mu m^2$).[5] The high density of Na^+ channels at the node reflects the need of saltatory conduction for a large inward current at the node (Fig. 15-1).

When the nodal membrane is depolarized, an inward current is established, carried by Na^+ ions. This current is voltage-sensitive and regenerative; it increases with depolarization, and this in turn leads to depolarization of the next node. This potentially explosive process would end with the whole axon becoming depolarized, were it not for the fact that Na^+ channels immediately start closing again, due to channel inactivation.

Two functionally distinct types of Na^+ current can be distinguished. Classic *transient* Na^+ conductances account for about 98 percent of the total current[1,6]. *Persistent* or non-inactivating Na^+ current is activated equally rapidly but at membrane potentials that are up to 20 mV more negative. At the most negative potentials over which these conductances operate, inactivation is minimal, giving rise to a persistent inward leak of Na^+ ions at resting potential, a potentially destabilizing property. This non-inactivating Na^+ current appears to have a greater expression in sensory axons than motor axons, likely to underlie the greater susceptibility for sensory nerves to become spontaneously active when damaged or diseased, leading to the sensation of paresthesias, dysesthesias, and pain.

Axonal K$^+$ Channels

Discussion of K$^+$ channels similarly may be simplified based on channel kinetics. Fast K$^+$ channels, found almost exclusively in the paranodal region, are responsible for limiting the re-excitation of the node that occurs following conduction of an action potential.[7] Blockade of these channels by 4-aminopyridine, a treatment used to counter fatigue and weakness in patients with demyelinating neurologic diseases such as multiple sclerosis, may result in patients experiencing paresthesias as a result of removing the stabilizing influence of fast K$^+$ channels.

In contrast, slow K$^+$ channels are found in high density at the node.[7,8] This nodal localization has been inferred from studies using tetraethylammonium, a selective K$^+$ channel blocker. Although slow K$^+$ channels are present at the node, they are not responsible for repolarization after conduction of single action potentials because of their slow activation time. However, these channels are open at resting membrane potential and so may contribute to its maintenance, whilst also acting to limit repetitive firing.

Inward Rectification (I_h)

In addition to conventional K$^+$ channels, axons possess inwardly rectifying channels, permeable to K$^+$ ions and Na$^+$ ions. Inward rectification is widespread in excitable cells and is the basis, for instance, of cardiac rhythmicity, and consequently is referred to as the pacemaker current.[9] This conductance is activated by membrane hyperpolarization, and attempts to limit excessive hyperpolarization. It seems likely that this conductance functions to maintain impulse transmission when the axon is hyperpolarized, as may occur following conduction of trains of impulses.

Axonal Na$^+$/K$^+$ Pump

The Na$^+$/K$^+$ pump, termed electrogenic because it generates a net outward flow of cations, is present on the axonal membrane. As initially demonstrated by Hodgkin and Huxley,[10] the electrogenic Na$^+$/K$^+$ pump drives three Na$^+$ ions out in exchange for two K$^+$ ions pumped in, with the process requiring metabolic energy from the

hydrolysis of adenosine triphosphate. As the coupling ratio for Na$^+$/K$^+$ exchange is unequal, a transmembrane current is produced by the operation of the pump. At rest and during activity, Na$^+$ ions enter the cell and K$^+$ ions leave by flowing down their concentration gradients. The axonal membrane Na$^+$/K$^+$ pump may serve to reverse these fluxes and so maintain transmembrane ionic gradients. The role of restoring gradients of Na$^+$ and K$^+$ in axons is of particular importance following high-frequency impulse activity. The pump also participates in the regulation of the resting membrane potential.[11] When the pump is blocked by cooling or application of a specific blocking agent such as ouabain or digitalis, the result is membrane depolarization.

THRESHOLD AND AXONAL MEMBRANE POTENTIAL

Measurements of peripheral nerve excitability using threshold tracking protocols are sensitive to membrane potential at the site of stimulation and thereby may provide complementary information to conventional nerve conduction studies. With the refinement of threshold tracking techniques and the development of automatic testing protocols, evaluation of axonal excitability has been employed in a number of clinical settings.[1,2,12] A set of useful indices of axonal excitability collectively may provide insights into the mechanisms responsible for membrane polarization, ion channel function, and activity of ionic pumps to help understanding of the pathophysiology of human neuropathies. The measurement and implications of these excitability indices are described in detail in the following section.

Although it is not possible to measure membrane potential directly in intact human axons, it is possible to obtain indirect evidence about membrane potential through the identification of coherent changes in a number of excitability indices. In this setting, the stimulus intensity required to produce a compound potential of a fixed size of maximal response may be defined as *threshold*, as used in the context of nerve excitability studies. Consequently, when the membrane depolarizes, the threshold current required to elicit the target potential decreases, and conversely increases when the membrane hyperpolarizes. Therefore, threshold is often used as a surrogate marker of membrane potential. However, there are circumstances when axonal excitability does not precisely parallel membrane potential and, particularly in these cases, ambiguity may be resolved by measuring other indices of axonal excitability. The measurement of these excitability indices and subsequent interpretation are provided in the following sections.

NERVE EXCITABILITY INDICES

Stimulus–Response Curve

Excitability testing is determined essentially by the stimulus–response properties of the axon. As the stimulus intensity increases, the size of the compound action potential will increase until it reaches a maximum peak response (Fig. 15-2). Subsequently, the amount required to change the stimulus, following a change in the response, then can be predicted from the response error (i.e., the difference between the actual and target responses) and the *slope of the stimulus–response curve* (see Fig. 15-2). Therefore the stimulus–response relationship is integral in setting the target submaximal response (i.e., the steepest part of the curve) for threshold tracking, and the slope of this relationship then may be used in conjunction with the tracking error to optimize the subsequent threshold tracking.

Strength–Duration Properties

As the *duration* of a test stimulus increases, the *strength* of the current required to activate a single fiber or a specified fraction of a compound action potential decreases. Strength–duration time constant (or chronaxie) and rheobase are parameters that describe the strength–duration curve, i.e., the curve that relates the intensity of a threshold stimulus to its duration. *Strength–duration time constant* (SDTC) is an apparent membrane time constant inferred from the relationship between threshold

current and stimulus duration, and provides a measure of the rate at which threshold current increases as the duration of the test stimulus is reduced to zero. In human peripheral nerve, the strength–duration relationship is described remarkably well by Weiss's empirical law:[13]

$$Q = I \cdot t = I_{rh} \, (t + SDTC)$$

where Q = stimulus charge; I = stimulus current of duration t; I_{rh} = rheobasic current.

Weiss's formula is used widely to calculate SDTC.[14,15] In this formulation, SDTC equates to *chronaxie* (the stimulus duration corresponding to a threshold current that is twice rheobase). *Rheobase* is the threshold current (or estimated threshold current in mA) required if the stimulus is of infinitely long duration. Because there is a linear relationship between stimulus charge and stimulus duration, rheobase and SDTC can be calculated from a charge–stimulus duration plot with four different stimulus widths (0.2, 0.4, 0.8, and 1 msec).[15,16] SDTC is derived from the x-intercept of the straight line fitted to the points representing different stimulus widths, whereby the slope of this relationship equates to the rheobase (Fig. 15-3). Rheobase and SDTC are both properties of the nodal membrane. SDTC averages 0.46 msec in human motor axons and 0.67 msec in sensory axons of peripheral nerve.[15] These values are much longer than the passive time constant of the nodes of Ranvier (approximately 50 μsec) because the effects of subthreshold current pulses are prolonged by the local response of low threshold Na$^+$ channels, particularly by persistent Na$^+$ channels.[17] These channels are

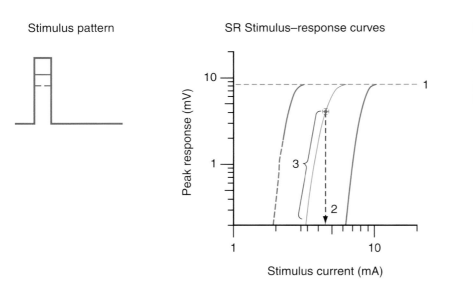

Stimulus pattern

SR Stimulus–response curves

Derived excitability parameters

1. Supramaximal peak response (mV)
2. Stimulus (mA) for 50% max response
3. Stimulus–response slope

FIGURE 15-2 ■ Stimulus–response behavior of the axonal membrane: derivation of the stimulus–response curve, with the stimulus pattern depicted on the left. Middle: Stimulus–response curve plotted as the current required to achieve peak response. The responses to hyperpolarization are shifted to the right (higher stimulus strength), and with depolarization are shifted to the left (lower stimulus intensity).

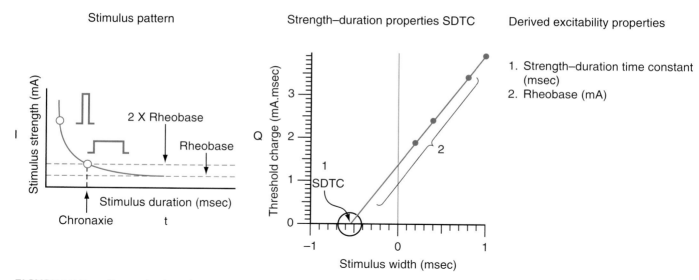

FIGURE 15-3 ▪ Strength–duration properties derived from plots of stimulus strength versus stimulus duration, illustrating rheobase as the threshold current required for a stimulus of infinite duration, and chronaxie as the stimulus duration at which the threshold current is twice rheobase (left). Plot of threshold charge versus stimulus width, illustrating the determination of strength–duration time constant using Weiss's Law (middle). Strength–duration time constant can be determined as the negative intercept on the x-axis of the line determined by only two stimulus widths.

also important in determining repetitive and spontaneous activity, and this is the reason that SDTC is a clinically important excitability parameter.

Recovery Cycle of Excitability

Following conduction of a single nerve impulse, an axon undergoes a well-characterized and reproducible sequence of excitability changes before returning to its resting state, a process termed the recovery cycle (Fig. 15-4). Initially, there is an *absolute refractory* period during which the axon is completely inexcitable and a propagated action potential cannot be generated, regardless of the strength of the stimulus. Subsequently, the axon becomes *relatively refractory*, during which period an action potential may be generated, but only if a stronger than normal stimulus is used. In human large myelinated axons the relative refractory period (RRP) is generally short, lasting less than 3 msec in most human studies. Adrian and

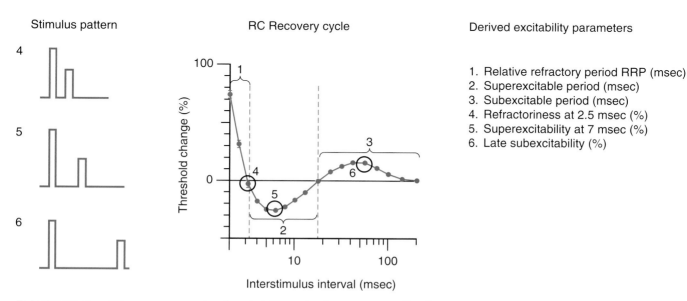

FIGURE 15-4 ▪ The recovery cycle of excitability: stimulus patterns utilized to generate the recovery cycle waveforms (left) numbered to correspond to the relevant points on the recovery cycle curve. Recovery cycle plot illustrating the relative refractory period, superexcitability and subexcitability.

Lucas in 1912 first observed that, following the relative refractory period, axons become excited more easily (*superexcitable period*) and also conduct impulses at a greater velocity than in the resting state.[18] Following the superexcitable period, there is an additional period of decreased excitability (*subexcitable period*), before membrane potential settles back to its resting state.

The mechanisms responsible for both the absolute and relative refractory periods are now well established; absolute refractoriness is due to inactivation of transient Na^+ channels, and the RRP is due to the gradual recovery of Na^+ channels from inactivation.[10] The RRP increases with membrane depolarization and decreases with membrane hyperpolarization.[19,20] Because of its sensitivity to polarization, refractoriness can be used as an indicator of membrane potential. However, the RRP is also sensitive to temperature and may be prolonged by cooling[21–23] because of slowed channel kinetics at lower temperatures.

Superexcitability is due to a depolarizing afterpotential. During the action potential, there is a large influx of Na^+ ions at the node, which is not offset by an equal efflux of K^+ ions, so the axon as a whole is left with a net depolarizing charge, spread over nodal and internodal axolemma. During the action potential, the node depolarizes the internode, as the internode helps repolarize the node, both ending depolarized by a few millivolts.[24] After the action potential, the large capacitance of the internode enables it to keep the node depolarized for tens of milliseconds. In myelinated axons, the superexcitability is strongly dependent on membrane potential; background depolarization reduces Na^+ influx and increases K^+ efflux, thus reducing the charge imbalance during the action potential; also, the opening of paranodal and internodal K^+ channels at rest short-circuits the afterpotential and reduces its duration.[24–26] Conversely, hyperpolarization increases and prolongs the depolarizing afterpotential and superexcitability. Superexcitability therefore can also be used as an indicator of membrane potential.

Finally, the long-lasting phase of late subexcitability reflects hyperpolarization of the membrane potential, due to current through slow K^+ channels at the nodes of Ranvier. The channels are activated during the action potential (and also during the depolarizing afterpotential) and deactivate slowly.[4,27] If an axon conducts a brief train of impulses, this late subexcitability becomes accentuated, producing the H_1 phase of activity-dependent hypoexcitability,[28,29] a hyperpolarization that therefore is also due to nodal slow K^+ channels. Late subexcitability is not simply sensitive to resting membrane potential (E_R), but to the electrochemical gradient for K^+ ions,

i.e., to the difference between E_R and the potassium equilibrium potential (E_K), which is normally on the hyperpolarized side of E_R. This means that if axons are depolarized by polarizing currents (i.e., without changing E_K), then the electrochemical gradient for K^+ ions is increased and subexcitability is increased. On the other hand, if axons are depolarized by raising extracellular K^+, as occurs during ischemia, E_K is depolarized towards or beyond E_R, and late subexcitability is abolished.[20] Late subexcitability is therefore not such a good indicator of membrane potential as superexcitability, but it can provide information about extracellular K^+ levels.

Threshold Electrotonus

Changes in potential of the nodal membrane spread into the internode, but slowly because of the resistance of the myelin sheath and consequently the slow charging of the internodal capacitance. This process results in slow activation and deactivation of voltage-dependent channels on the internodal membrane. Although Na^+ channel density is insufficient for the internodal membrane to generate an action potential, the changes in resistance of the internodal membrane and in the current stored on it will affect the behaviour of the node.[30]

The only physiologic method available to examine the behavior of internodal conductances in living patients is the technique of threshold electrotonus (TE) (Fig. 15-5). The term *electrotonus* refers to changes in membrane potential evoked by subthreshold depolarizing or hyperpolarizing current pulses. The technique of threshold electrotonus measures the threshold changes produced by prolonged depolarizing or hyperpolarizing currents, which are too weak to trigger action potentials (subthreshold currents). The term *threshold electrotonus* reflects the fact that, under most circumstances, the threshold changes parallel the underlying electrotonic changes in membrane potential.[31,32] The changes in threshold were produced by 100-msec polarizing currents with intensities set to 40 percent of the unconditioned threshold, using 1-msec test pulses. In contrast to the recovery cycle, threshold changes conventionally are plotted as threshold reductions, with depolarizing responses upwards, to match the conventional way of plotting changes in membrane potential induced by such currents (i.e., electrotonus).

There are different phases of threshold electrotonus. In response to depolarizing current pulses, there is an initial fast phase that corresponds to the applied current (the "F" phase). A polarizing current 40 percent of threshold unsurprisingly reduces threshold by 40 percent. This is

Stimulus pattern

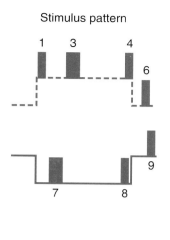

TE threshold electrotonus

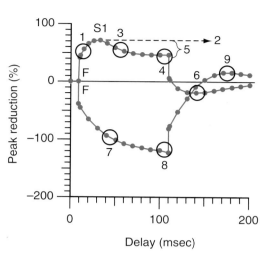

Derived excitability parameters

1. TEd (10–20 msec)
2. TEd peak
3. TEd (40–60 msec)
4. TEd (90–100 msec)
5. S2 accomodation
6. TEd (undershoot)
7. TEh (20–40 msec)
8. TEh (90–100 msec)
9. TEh (overshoot)

FIGURE 15-5 ■ The current utilized to produce the threshold electrotonus waveform, with numbered bars reflecting the corresponding points on the threshold electrotonus curve (left panel). Threshold electrotonus waveform (depolarizing direction plotted upwards, hyperpolarizing direction plotted downwards) illustrating the response of the axon to 100 msec subthreshold polarizing currents ($\pm$ 40 percent of threshold). Fast (F) phases in response to initial polarization and slow (S1) phases due to the gradual spread of current into the internode are indicated on the figure.

followed by further depolarization that develops slowly over some tens of milliseconds, measured as TEd (10 to 20 msec), as the current spreads to and depolarizes the internodal membrane (the "S1" phase). The threshold decrease (i.e., the extent of depolarization) reaches a peak—TEd(peak)—about 20 msec after the onset of the current pulses, dependent on its strength, and threshold then starts to return slowly towards the control level, TEd (90 to 100 msec). This reduction in excitability is termed S2 *accommodation*, and is due to activation of a hyperpolarizing conductance with slow kinetics. The use of K^+ channel blocking agents indicates that the slow accommodative process is due to activation of slow K^+ channels, which are located on both the node and the internode.[27,31,32] When the direct-current (DC) pulse is terminated, threshold increases rapidly and there is then a slow undershoot—TEd(undershoot)—before it gradually recovers to control level. This is due to persistence of the increase in slow K^+ conductance, which deactivates slowly.

With long-lasting hyperpolarizing DC pulses, there is a fast increase in threshold, proportional to the applied current, and analogous to the comparable phase with depolarizing currents (the "F" phase). Then threshold continues to increase as the hyperpolarizing spreads to the internode: TEh(10 to 20 msec). This "S1" phase starts as a mirror image of the S1 phase with depolarizing current but soon diverges, because hyperpolarization closes K^+ channels (slow nodal, and fast and slow internodal K^+ channels), and this increases the amplitude and

time constant of S1, the TEh(90 to 100 ms). On termination of the hyperpolarizing DC pulses, threshold rapidly decreases and then undergoes a slow, depolarizing overshoot—the TEh(overshoot)—as I_H slowly deactivates and the slow K^+ conductance is reactivated.

Current–Voltage Relationship and Slope

Just as the activation of different voltage-dependent channels in a cell can be identified by plotting a current–voltage (I/V) relationship, it can be convenient to plot the threshold changes at the ends of a series of long current pulses (i.e., 200-msec) of different amplitudes as a current–threshold relationship. This is done conventionally with threshold increase (hyperpolarization) to the left, threshold decrease (depolarization) to the right, depolarizing current to the top and hyperpolarizing current to the bottom, to correspond to a conventional I/V plot.[12,32] This current–threshold relationship therefore reflects the rectifying properties of the axon (both nodal and internodal axolemma).

Outward rectification due to K^+ channel activation causes a steepening of the curve in the top right quadrant, and the steepening of the relationship in the bottom left quadrant indicates inward rectification due to activation of I_H. The slope (i.e., hyperpolarizing I/V slope) of

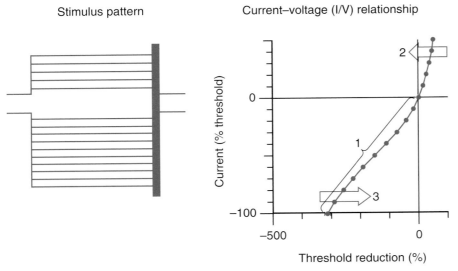

FIGURE 15-6 ■ Stimulus pattern required to generate the current–voltage relationship (left). The currents utilized to produce the current–voltage relationship represent 200 msec polarizing stimuli, ranging from +50 to −100 percent of threshold current. The current–voltage relationship, with response to depolarizing current depicted in the upper right quadrant and response to hyperpolarizing current in the lower left quadrant (middle). Outward rectification shifts the upper curve to the left, related to the activity of K^+ channels. Inward rectification occurs in response to hyperpolarization, related to the activity of the cation conductance I_H and shifting the lower curve to the right.

this curve can be used to provide an estimate of the threshold analog of input conductance (Fig. 15-6). The two parameters, resting I/V slope and minimum I/V slope, are derived from the current–threshold plot. If I/V slope is shifted to the left, the threshold analog of the conductance changes to more negative potentials, consistent with axonal depolarization.

DEVELOPMENT OF PROTOCOLS FOR EXCITABILITY TESTING IN PATIENTS

Stimulus–response behavior, strength–duration time constant, threshold electrotonus to 100-msec polarizing currents, a current–threshold relationship, and the recovery of excitability following supramaximal activation can now be investigated using recently developed protocols for clinical investigation.[12,32,33] These protocols begin by recording a stimulus–response curve to set the target submaximal response (approximately 40 percent of peak) for threshold tracking. Four stimuli of different widths are used to estimate the strength–duration time constant and rheobase for axons of different threshold. As mentioned earlier, the voltage-dependence of these parameters is due to a nodal persistent Na^+ current.[14,15]

The protocols then use prolonged subthreshold currents to alter the potential difference across the internodal axonal membrane in order to measure threshold electrotonus.[32] Threshold tracking is used to record the changes in threshold induced by subthreshold polarizing currents, 100 msec in duration, set to +40 percent (depolarizing) and −40 percent (hyperpolarizing) of the control threshold current. Three stimulus combinations typically are tested in turn: test stimulus alone (to measure the control threshold current), test stimulus in conjunction with a depolarizing conditioning current, and test stimulus combined with a hyperpolarizing conditioning current. Similar to threshold electrotonus, the current–threshold relationship typically is tested using 1-msec pulses at the end of subthreshold polarizing currents lasting 200 msec. The polarizing current is altered in a ramp fashion from +50 percent (depolarizing) to −100 percent (hyperpolarizing) of the control threshold in steps of 10 percent.

Finally, the clinical excitability protocols record the recovery cycle of excitability, using a supramaximal conditioning stimulus. Changes are recorded at 18 conditioning–test intervals, decreasing from 200 to 2 msec in approximately geometric progression. Recordings are analyzed during the absolute and relative refractory periods (measures of Na^+ channel inactivation and recovery), the superexcitable period (a sensitive measure of membrane potential dependent on paranodal fast K^+ channels), and the late subexcitable phase (determined by nodal slow K^+ conductances).

COHERENT PATTERNS OF CHANGE IN EXCITABILITY INDICES

Although changes in a single excitability parameter may reflect changes in a specific ionic conductance, certain patterns of change in multiple parameters may reflect change in resting membrane potential.[20] Membrane depolarization, as occurs with nerve ischemia or alterations in extracellular electrolyte concentrations,[20,34] produces an increase in axonal excitability, with an increase in the slope of the current–threshold relationship, a fanning in of TE, a decrease in superexcitability, and increases in both refractoriness and strength–duration time constant. Changes in the opposite direction would be expected with membrane hyperpolarization, as may occur following conduction of a train of impulses or after the remission of nerve ischemia.[16,35]

The acute effects of Na^+ channel blockade on nerve excitability also have been studied in patients. Nerve excitability parameters were assessed in four patients who had ingested puffer fish, containing tetrodotoxin, which blocks the outer pore of the Na^+ channel and prevents passage of Na^+ ions through the pore of the channel.[36] In these patients, axons were of higher threshold, latency was prolonged, and there was a reduction in SDTC. Refractoriness, superexcitability, and late subexcitability were reduced. There was a reduction in depolarizing threshold electrotonus (TEd) and an increase in hyperpolarizing threshold electrotonus (TEh). The changes in excitability were reproduced in a mathematical model by reducing Na^+ permeabilities by 50 percent. The study demonstrates the utility of nerve excitability techniques in detecting Na^+ channel abnormalities in vivo.

NERVE EXCITABILITY FINDINGS IN NEUROLOGIC DISEASE

Excitability techniques have now been translated into the clinical setting to examine a range of inherited and acquired neuropathies. An outline of clinical nerve excitability findings in neuropathy is summarized in Table 15-1. To cover all of these studies is beyond the scope of this chapter. However, illustrative examples of the ability of excitability techniques to provide novel insight into disease pathophysiology, and the scope for its use as a clinical tool to provide early identification of presymptomatic patients and to monitor the impact of therapy, are provided in the following sections.

Chemotherapy-Induced Neurotoxicity

Chemotherapy-induced neuropathy typically presents as a predominantly sensory or mixed sensorimotor axonal neuropathy with prominent symptoms of distal paresthesias, numbness, and pain.[37,38] In severe cases, neuropathic symptoms may lead to significant disability with deficits in balance and fine motor skills.[39] There are currently no identified preventative approaches or treatments for chemotherapy-induced neuropathy. Many of the chemotherapies associated with risk of neurotoxicity are used in the adjuvant setting as a preventative measure in patients with completely cured disease. Patients with excellent long-term survival prospects thus may be left with severe and permanent nerve damage due to their chemotherapy.

The pathogenesis of chemotherapy-induced neuropathy remains unclear, making it difficult to develop rational neuroprotective approaches and effective treatments. The most commonly hypothesized targets include the sensory cell bodies in the dorsal root ganglia (DRG), damage to axoplasmic transport systems, or Wallerian degeneration[37,38] (Fig. 15-7, A). As the DRG neurons are not well protected by the blood–nerve barrier, they may be more vulnerable to toxic compounds, leading to neuronal cell death. Microtubule-related structures such as tubulin may also provide a target for chemotherapy-induced neurotoxicity, as microtubules are key in axonal transport processes and in ensuring that the distal axon is supplied with energy, organelles, and trophic factors.[40] Classic Wallerian degeneration also represents a putative mechanism for chemotherapy-induced neuropathy, involving damage to the distal axon and subsequent degeneration. In order to provide greater information about the pathogenic basis for chemotherapy-induced neuropathy, axonal excitability techniques have been utilized to assess patients receiving neurotoxic chemotherapies.

Oxaliplatin has been utilized extensively in both early and advanced colorectal cancer. It is a platinum-based compound, derived from cisplatin, which exerts cytotoxicity via cross-linking DNA complexes to inhibit DNA synthesis.[41] Oxaliplatin treatment produces two forms of neurotoxicity—an acute neurotoxicity that develops immediately following infusion and a chronic sensory neuropathy that follows increasing cumulative exposure.[42] Acute oxaliplatin-induced neurotoxicity is characterized by both sensory and motor manifestations triggered by cold exposure, including paresthesias, fasciculations, and cramps.[43] These symptoms occur in 95 percent of patients and typically resolve within several days.[41,42] At higher doses, oxaliplatin produces an axonal sensory neuropathy with distal paresthesias and numbness leading to functional disability.[42]

TABLE 15-1 ■ **Summary of Nerve Excitability Studies in Neurologic Disorders**

Neurologic disorder	Nerve Excitability Parameters			Clinical Interpretation	References
	SDTC	Threshold Electrotonus	Recovery Cycle		
I. ACQUIRED					
Metabolic Conditions					
Diabetes mellitus	↓	Fanning in	↓ in all RC parameters	↓ Na$^+$ conductances Na$^+$/K$^+$ pump dysfunction	74–87
Hypokalemia	↓	Fanning out	↓ Refractoriness ↑ Superexcitability ↑ Late subexcitability	Membrane hyperpolarization	88, 89
Uremic neuropathy	↑	Fanning in	↑ Refractoriness ↓ Superexcitability ↓ Late subexcitability	Membrane depolarization	90–96
Hepatic failure	N	Fanning in	↓ Superexcitability	Membrane depolarization	97
Critical illness neuropathy	N	Fanning in	↑ Refractoriness ↓ Superexcitability ↓ Late subexcitability	Membrane depolarization	98
Immune-mediated					
Guillain–Barré syndrome/AMAN	N	N	↑ Refractoriness	Distal conduction failure	99–101
Chronic inflammatory demyelinating polyneuropathy	↓	N	↓ in all RC parameters	Morphological changes	70, 102–107
Multifocal motor neuropathy	N	Fanning out	↑ Superexcitability	Membrane hyperpolarization	107–110
Neuromyotonia	N	Overshoot	↑ Late subexcitability	Upregulation of slow K$^+$ conductance	111–113
Multiple sclerosis	N	↓ TEd	↓ Superexcitability ↑ Late subexcitability	↑ Slow K$^+$ channel activity	114
Drug or Toxins					
Chemotherapy-induced					
Acute sensory neuropathy (oxaliplatin)	N	N	↓ in all RC parameters	Acute Na$^+$ channelopathy	44–48
Chronic sensory neuropathy (oxaliplatin)	–	Fanning out	↓ Refractoriness ↑ Superexcitability	Early detection of sensory neuropathy	48, 115
Shellfish, marine toxins					
Puffer fish tetrodotoxin poisoning	↓	↓ TEd, ↑ TEh	↓ in all RC parameters	Blockade of Na$^+$ channel	116, 117
Camphor poisoning	N	↑ TEh	N	↓ Inward rectifying conductance I_H	118
Tick paralysis	N	N	↑ Refractoriness		119
Mexiletine	↓	N	↓ Refractoriness	↓ Persistent Na$^+$ conductance	120, 121
Entrapment					
Carpal tunnel syndrome	↑	N	↑ Refractoriness	Activity-dependent conduction block	122–124
Trauma					
Spinal cord injury	↓	Fanning in	↑ Refractoriness ↓ Superexcitability ↓ Late subexcitability	Decentralization and consequent inactivity	72, 73
Neurodegenerative					
Amyotrophic lateral sclerosis	↑	↑ TEh	↑ Superexcitability	↑ Persistent Na$^+$ ↓ K$^+$ conductance	125–135
Hirayama disease	↑	Fanning out	↑ Refractoriness ↑ Superexcitability	Membrane depolarization	136
II. HEREDITARY					
Acute intermittent porphyria	N	↑ TEh	N	↓ Inward rectifying conductance I_H at resting state	61
Charcot–Marie–Tooth disease	N	Fanning out	↓ Refractoriness ↓ Superexcitability	↑ Fast K$^+$ conductances	137

Continued

TABLE 15-1 ■ **Summary of Nerve Excitability Studies in Neurologic Disorders—cont'd**

Neurologic disorder	Nerve Excitability Parameters			Clinical Interpretation	References
	SDTC	Threshold Electrotonus	Recovery Cycle		
II. HEREDITARY—Cont'd					
Episodic ataxia (EA) type 1	N	Fanning out	↓ Refractoriness ↑ Superexcitability ↑ Late subexcitability	Differentiate EA type 1 from normal controls	138
Episodic ataxia type 2	N	↓ Early TE	↑ Refractoriness ↓ Late subexcitability	Effects on KCNQ channels	139
Fabry disease	–	Fanning in	↓ Superexcitability	Membrane depolarization	140
MELAS	↑	Fanning in	↑ Refractoriness ↓ Superexcitability	Membrane depolarization	141
Kennedy disease	↑	↑ TEd	N	Membrane hyperpolarization	142
Myotonic dystrophy	N	Fanning in	↑ Refractoriness	Membrane depolarization	143, 144
Machado–Joseph disease	↑	N	N	↑ Persistent Na$^+$ conductance	145
SCN1B mutation–GEFS	↓	↑ TEh	↓ Refractoriness	↓ Nodal Na$^+$ conductances	146

N, normal; SDTC, strength–duration time constant; TEd, depolarizing threshold electrotonus; TEh, hyperpolarizing threshold electrotonus; RC, recovery cycle; AMAN, acute motor axonal neuropathy; MELAS, mitochondrial myopathy, encephalopathy, lactic acidosis, and stroke-like episodes; GEFS, generalized epilepsy febrile seizures; KCNQ, voltage-gated potassium channel.

To examine the pathophysiology underlying these two forms of neurotoxicity, large-scale axonal excitability studies have been undertaken in oxaliplatin-treated patients. Because of the immediate onset of neuropathic symptoms following oxaliplatin infusion, it has been suggested that acute oxaliplatin-induced neurotoxicity reflects a functional change in axonal excitability and ion-channel function rather than structural damage. To examine this hypothesis, patients were assessed before and after oxaliplatin infusion. Following oxaliplatin infusion, changes developed in Na$^+$ channel-associated parameters in both motor and sensory axons (Fig. 15-7, *B*).[44-48] These changes developed primarily in recovery cycle parameters associated with inactivation properties (refractoriness) and suggested that an acute Na$^+$ channelopathy underlies the development of acute oxaliplatin-induced neurotoxicity. These clinical findings were supported by experimental evidence that suggested oxaliplatin modulated Na$^+$ channel function in vitro.[49-53]

In contrast, a different pattern emerged in longitudinal studies across 6 months of oxaliplatin treatment. In sensory axons, progressive and step-wise change in several excitability parameters, including threshold electrotonus and recovery cycle, developed across treatment (Fig. 15-7, *C*).[48] Importantly, these longitudinal changes did not occur in motor axons in the same patients, reflecting the purely sensory symptoms of oxaliplatin-induced neuropathy. In addition, these changes occurred significantly earlier than reductions in peak sensory amplitudes and were able to predict severity of neuropathy at long-term follow-up, suggesting that they may provide an early biomarker of axonal dysfunction in oxaliplatin-induced neurotoxicity.

Another commonly used chemotherapy associated with neuropathy is paclitaxel, a taxane derived from the Pacific yew tree and used extensively in the treatment of solid tumors, including ovarian and breast cancers. Paclitaxel-induced neuropathy typically presents as a distal sensory neuropathy at higher cumulative doses.[54] It has been hypothesized that paclitaxel leads to microtubule dysfunction and, accordingly, disruption of axonal transport as a mechanism of neurotoxicity.[55,56] While the symptoms of chronic paclitaxel-induced neuropathy may have appeared subjectively similar to those in chronic oxaliplatin-treated patients, axonal excitability studies revealed a different mechanistic pattern. Over 12 weeks of paclitaxel treatment, there were significant early reductions in sensory amplitudes and increases in stimulus threshold, indicating early and progressive disruption of axonal function consistent with symptoms of sensory neuropathy.[57] In contrast to this early reduction in sensory amplitudes observed with paclitaxel, a substantially different time course of sensory amplitude decline occurred with oxaliplatin, and amplitudes were not reduced until later

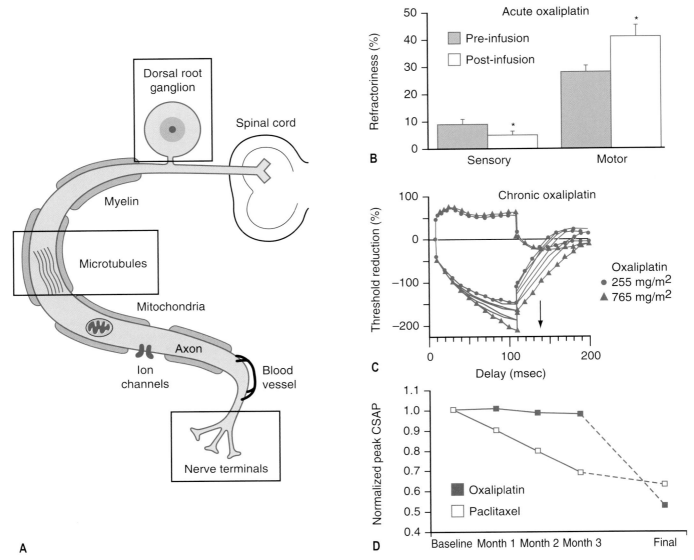

FIGURE 15-7 ■ **A**, Potential targets of chemotherapy-induced neurotoxicity in the peripheral nervous system, with major hypothesized sites including dorsal root ganglia, microtubule-associated structures, and axonal degeneration from the distal nerve terminals. **B**, Acute oxaliplatin-induced neurotoxicity: changes in refractoriness acutely following oxaliplatin infusion in motor and sensory axons in a cohort of oxaliplatin-treated patients. **C**, Chronic oxaliplatin-induced neurotoxicity: Progressive and step-wise changes in threshold electrotonus waveforms in sensory axons demonstrated in a single patient with increasing cumulative oxaliplatin dosage from 255 mg/m^2 (circles) to 765 mg/m^2 (triangles). **D**, Comparison of reduction in peak compound sensory action potential (CSAP) amplitude between patients treated with paclitaxel (open squares) and oxaliplatin (filled squares), normalized to baseline values, demonstrating reduction in amplitude of the CSAP across 3 months of chemotherapy treatment and at final treatment.

treatment cycles (Fig. 15-7, *D*). In addition, there was no evidence of changes in specific membrane conductances or generalized excitability in paclitaxel-treated patients, in sharp contrast to oxaliplatin-treated patients. These findings suggested a different underlying mechanism of neurotoxicity in paclitaxel- and oxaliplatin-induced neuropathy.

In summary, these studies of chemotherapy-induced neuropathy utilizing axonal excitability techniques demonstrated new insights into the pathophysiologic mechanisms of axonal dysfunction in toxic neuropathy. Despite subjective symptomatic similarities between paclitaxel- and oxaliplatin-induced chronic neuropathy, the mechanisms underlying the development of axonal damage were very different, indicating that a different approach to neuroprotection would be required.

Porphyric Neuropathy

There are four types of acute hepatic porphyria which may produce the neuropathy that develops in 40 percent of patients.[58] Of these, the most common is acute intermittent porphyria (AIP), resulting from an inherited deficiency in the third heme pathway enzyme, porphobilinogen deaminase.[59] In patients with AIP, porphyric neuropathy develops in the context of an acute porphyric crisis involving severe abdominal pain, neuropsychiatric manifestations, and autonomic and motor neuropathy. Although the main hypotheses regarding the pathogenesis of neuropathy in acute porphyria relate it to the effects of heme deficiency on axonal energy supply or direct neurotoxicity by accumulated porphyrin precursors,[60] the exact cause of porphyric neuropathy remains unclear.

In asymptomatic patients with AIP who previously had experienced acute porphyric attacks, differences have been found in the response to hyperpolarizing currents (current–threshold relationship) of motor axons.[61] These findings suggest that changes in nerve function persisted between acute attacks in AIP patients (Fig. 15-8).

Subsequently, these changes identified by excitability techniques were modeled using a mathematical model of a human axon. An underlying reduction by 27 percent in inwardly rectifying conductances (I_H) was found,[61]

suggesting that alterations in I_H may be an early subclinical sign of metabolic distress in AIP patients. In support, there was experimental evidence to suggest that the I_H current was regulated by metabolic stimuli,[62] and that metabolic disturbance and subsequent hypoxia resulted in a reduction in I_H current.[63,64]

During an acute attack of porphyric neuropathy, a different pattern of change was identified, consistent with the development of axonal membrane depolarization. Membrane depolarization could result from dysfunction of the Na^+/K^+ pump, which remains strongly energy-dependent. In the context of an acute porphyric attack, Na^+/K^+ pump dysfunction and reduced energy availability are likely to be responsible for the development of peripheral neuropathy.

Inflammatory Neuropathy and its Treatment

The mechanisms underlying the development of inflammatory neuropathy have not been defined, with proposed involvement of both humoral and cellular immune systems, auto-antibodies, and inflammatory mediators.[65,66] Acquired inflammatory neuropathies comprise several

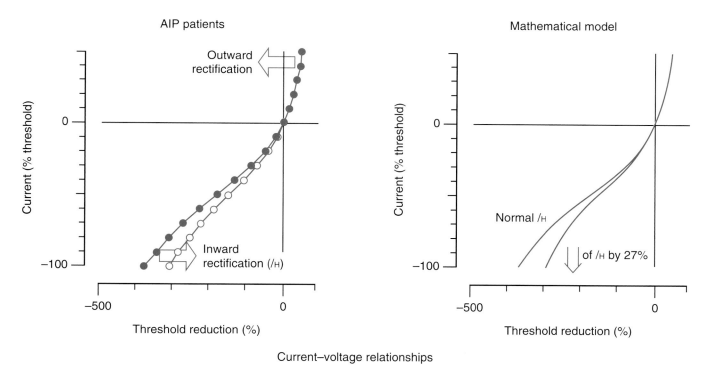

FIGURE 15-8 ■ Left: Current–threshold (I/V) relationship recordings from patients with acute intermittent porphyria (AIP) without neuropathy (open circles), with normal control recordings (filled circles). Right: Mathematical modeling of the human motor axon established that a 27 percent reduction in inwardly rectifying conductances was required to produce the excitability profile of AIP patients.

different forms, including chronic inflammatory demyelinating polyneuropathy (CIDP), an immune-mediated sensory and motor neuropathy with a variable course and a prevalence of 2 to 7 per 100,000.[65,67]

Immunomodulatory treatments such as plasmapheresis and intravenous immunoglobulins (IVIg) are most successful for treating acquired inflammatory neuropathies.[68] However, the high demand, side-effect profile, and extreme cost of such treatments mandate difficult choices about which patients will most benefit from them.[69] There remains a need for disease biomarkers to be developed in order to select populations likely to be responsive to different lines of therapy.

Axonal excitability studies have been utilized in patients with CIDP to examine the changes in axonal function in relation to immunomodulatory treatment.[70] Within 1 week of IVIg infusion, patients demonstrated a pattern of excitability change consistent with stabilization of axonal membrane potential, potentially providing an environment necessary to promote axonal recovery (Fig. 15-9). This modulatory effect of IVIg within the period of a single infusion suggested that the immediate role of IVIg was to stabilize and prevent further axonal degeneration. Importantly, a similar pattern was observed in CIDP patients longitudinally across treatment, suggesting that long-term IVIg treatment acted to modify axonal accommodation over time.

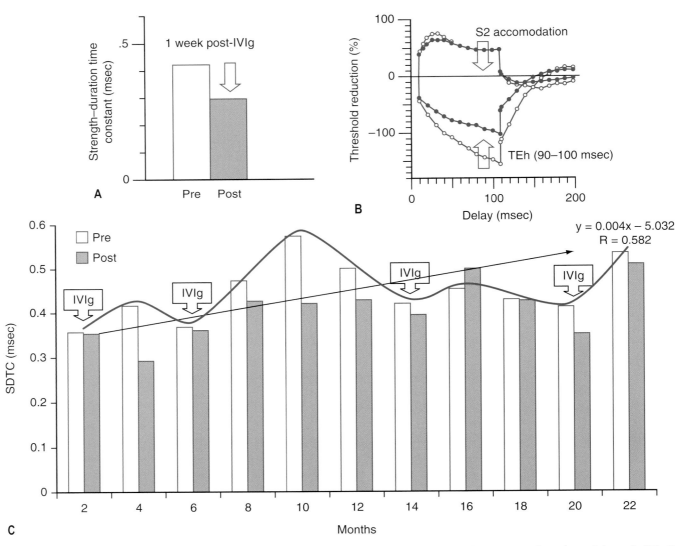

FIGURE 15-9 ■ Motor excitability recordings pre-intravenous immunoglobulin (IVIg) treatment (open), and 1 week (filled) post-IVIg treatment in a single representative chronic inflammatory demyelinating polyneuropathy patient **A**, Changes in strength–duration time constant (SDTC). **B**, Changes in threshold electrotonus. **C**, Changes in SDTC within the same infusion; and longitudinally (22 months) in the same patient.

Spinal Cord Injury

While treatment strategies for spinal cord injury (SCI) typically have focused on neuronal recovery and protection, there has been increasing awareness over recent years of the importance of maintaining function below the level of the lesion.[71] In addition, preservation of peripheral nerve function will be critically important to the success of future strategies aimed at regenerating the spinal cord at the site of injury. With this perspective, initial axonal excitability studies in SCI patients have established that peripheral axons have a high threshold and that amplitudes of motor responses (M waves) are reduced.[72] In addition, a complex pattern of peripheral axonal excitability changes was identified, perhaps related

to the influence of decentralization and inactivity in such patients.

In order to examine the development of these abnormalities, axonal excitability studies subsequently were undertaken in patients during the acute phase of treatment following SCI, within 15 days of hospitalization.[73] Significant functional changes were identified in peripheral axons, coinciding with the period of spinal shock (Fig. 15-10). These changes evolved over the course of hospital admission, with peripheral nerve function and depolarization-like changes reaching a nadir before normalizing to some extent prior to hospital discharge. In total, these findings confirmed that negative downstream effects developed early during spinal shock. They further suggested that methods to preserve or maintain

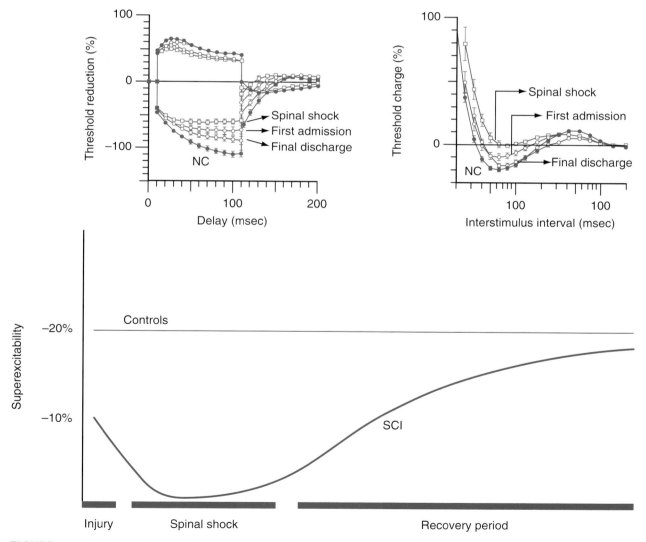

FIGURE 15-10 ■ Top: Threshold electrotonus (left) and recovery cycle (right) recorded from tibialis anterior in patients with spinal cord injury, demonstrating changes from first admission (open circle), to period of spinal shock (open square), and final discharge (open diamond). Data for healthy controls are depicted as filled circles. Bottom: Demonstration of changes in superexcitability from the period of first admission to the recovery period.

peripheral nerve function are warranted after acute SCI to improve the prognosis for rehabilitation and functional therapies.

CONCLUDING COMMENTS

Clinical excitability techniques are now being adopted to complement diagnostic nerve conduction studies. As demonstrated by the illustrative examples presented in this chapter, measurement of nerve excitability by threshold tracking provides complementary information to conventional nerve conduction studies and may be used to infer the activity of a variety of ion channels, energy-dependent pumps, and ion exchange processes activated during the process of impulse conduction. Although routine nerve conduction studies will remain the gold standard investigation to document the presence of a neuropathy, these traditional studies do not provide further insight into pathophysiology. There is now growing evidence to support the use of excitability studies to provide novel insights into the pathophysiologic mechanisms involved in neuropathic disease states; as a functional biomarker of disease progression; and as an objective measure of treatment effect.

REFERENCES

1. Burke D, Kiernan MC, Bostock H: Excitability of human axons. Clin Neurophysiol, 112:1575, 2001
2. Krishnan AV, Lin CSY, Park SB et al: Axonal ion channels from bench to bedside: a translational neuroscience perspective. Prog Neurobiol, 89:288, 2009
3. Arroyo EJ, Scherer SS: On the molecular architecture of myelinated fibers. Histochem Cell Biol, 113:1, 2000
4. Schwarz JR, Reid G, Bostock H: Action potentials and membrane currents in the human node of Ranvier. Pflugers Arch, 430:283, 1995
5. Ritchie JM, Chiu SY: Distribution of sodium and potassium channels in mammalian myelinated nerve. Adv Neurol, 31:329, 1981
6. Crill WE: Persistent sodium current in mammalian central neurons. Annu Rev Physiol, 58:349, 1996
7. Roper J, Schwarz JR: Heterogeneous distribution of fast and slow potassium channels in myelinated rat nerve fibres. J Physiol, 416:93, 1989
8. Devaux JJ, Kleopa KA, Cooper EC et al: KCNQ2 is a nodal K^+ channel. J Neurosci, 24:1236, 2004
9. Pape HC: Queer current and pacemaker: the hyperpolarization-activated cation current in neurons. Annu Rev Physiol, 58:299, 1996
10. Hodgkin AL, Huxley AF: A quantitative description of membrane current and its application to conduction and excitation in nerve. J Physiol, 117:500, 1952
11. Rakowski RF, Gadsby DC, De Weer P: Stoichiometry and voltage dependence of the sodium pump in voltage-clamped internally dialyzed squid giant axon. J Gen Physiol, 93:903, 1989
12. Kiernan MC, Burke D, Andersen KV et al: Multiple measures of axonal excitability: a new approach in clinical testing. Muscle Nerve, 23:399, 2000
13. Weiss G: Sur la possibilité de rendre comparables entre eux les appareils servant à l'excitation électrique. Arch Ital Biol, 35:413, 1901
14. Bostock H: The strength–duration relationship for excitation of myelinated nerve: computed dependence on membrane parameters. J Physiol, 341:59, 1983
15. Mogyoros I, Kiernan MC, Burke D: Strength–duration properties of human peripheral nerve. Brain, 119:439, 1996
16. Bostock H, Bergmans J: Post-tetanic excitability changes and ectopic discharges in a human motor axon. Brain, 117:913, 1994
17. Bostock H, Rothwell JC: Latent addition in motor and sensory fibres of human peripheral nerve. J Physiol, 498:277, 1997
18. Adrian ED, Lucas K: On the summation of propagated disturbances in nerve and muscle. J Physiol, 44:68, 1912
19. Burke D, Mogyoros I, Vagg R et al: Quantitative description of the voltage dependence of axonal excitability in human cutaneous afferents. Brain, 121:1975, 1998
20. Kiernan MC, Bostock H: Effects of membrane polarization and ischaemia on the excitability properties of human motor axons. Brain, 123:2542, 2000
21. Burke D, Mogyoros I, Vagg R et al: Temperature dependence of excitability indices of human cutaneous afferents. Muscle Nerve, 22:51, 1999
22. Kiernan MC, Cikurel K, Bostock H: Effects of temperature on the excitability properties of human motor axons. Brain, 124:816, 2001
23. Stys PK, Ashby P: An automated technique for measuring the recovery cycle of human nerves. Muscle Nerve, 13:750, 1990
24. Barrett EF, Barrett JN: Intracellular recording from vertebrate myelinated axons: mechanism of the depolarizing afterpotential. J Physiol, 323:117, 1982
25. David G, Barrett JN, Barrett EF: Evidence that action potentials activate an internodal potassium conductance in lizard myelinated axons. J Physiol, 445:277, 1992
26. David G, Modney B, Scappaticci KA et al: Electrical and morphological factors influencing the depolarizing afterpotential in rat and lizard myelinated axons. J Physiol, 489:141, 1995
27. Baker M, Bostock H, Grafe P et al: Function and distribution of three types of rectifying channel in rat spinal root myelinated axons. J Physiol, 383:45, 1987
28. Miller TA, Kiernan MC, Mogyoros I et al: Activity-dependent changes in impulse conduction in normal human cutaneous axons. Brain, 118:1217, 1995
29. Taylor JL, Burke D, Heywood J: Physiological evidence for a slow K^+ conductance in human cutaneous afferents. J Physiol, 453:575, 1992

30. Baker MD: Axonal flip-flops and oscillators. Trends Neurosci, 23:514, 2000

31. Bostock H, Baker M: Evidence for two types of potassium channel in human motor axons *in vivo*. Brain Res, 462:354, 1988

32. Bostock H, Cikurel K, Burke D: Threshold tracking techniques in the study of human peripheral nerve. Muscle Nerve, 21:137, 1998

33. Kiernan MC, Lin CSY, Andersen KV et al: Clinical evaluation of excitability measures in sensory nerve. Muscle Nerve, 24:883, 2001

34. Kiernan MC, Guglielmi J-M, Kaji R et al: Evidence for axonal membrane hyperpolarization in multifocal motor neuropathy with conduction block. Brain, 125:664, 2002

35. Vagg R, Mogyoros I, Kiernan MC et al: Activity-dependent hyperpolarization of human motor axons produced by natural activity. J Physiol, 507:919, 1998

36. Kiernan MC, Isbister GK, Lin CSY et al: Acute tetrodotoxin-induced neurotoxicity after ingestion of puffer fish. Ann Neurol, 57:339, 2005

37. Hausheer FH, Schilsky RL, Bain S et al: Diagnosis, management, and evaluation of chemotherapy-induced peripheral neuropathy. Semin Oncol, 33:15, 2006

38. Park SB, Krishnan AV, Lin CSY et al: Mechanims underlying chemotherapy-induced neurotoxicity and the potential for neuroprotective strategies. Curr Med Chem, 15:3081, 2008

39. Quasthoff S, Hartung HP: Chemotherapy-induced peripheral neuropathy. J Neurol, 249:9, 2002

40. Conde C, Cáceres A: Microtubule assembly, organization and dynamics in axons and dendrites. Nat Rev Neurosci, 10:319, 2009

41. Grothey A: Oxaliplatin-safety profile: neurotoxicity. Semin Oncol, 30:5, 2003

42. Gamelin E, Gamelin L, Bossi L et al: Clinical aspects and molecular basis of oxaliplatin neurotoxicity: current management and development of preventive measures. Semin Oncol, 29:21, 2002

43. Wilson RH, Lehky T, Thomas RR et al: Acute oxaliplatin-induced peripheral nerve hyperexcitability. J Clin Oncol, 20:1767, 2002

44. Kiernan MC, Krishnan AV: The pathophysiology of oxaliplatin-induced neurotoxicity. Curr Med Chem, 13:2901, 2006

45. Krishnan AV, Goldstein D, Friedlander M et al: Oxaliplatin-induced neurotoxicity and the development of neuropathy. Muscle Nerve, 32:51, 2005

46. Krishnan AV, Goldstein D, Friedlander M et al: Oxaliplatin and axonal Na^+ channel function *in vivo*. Clin Cancer Res, 12:4481, 2006

47. Park SB, Goldstein D, Lin CSY et al: Acute abnormalities of sensory nerve function associated with oxaliplatin-induced neurotoxicity. J Clin Oncol, 27:1243, 2009

48. Park SB, Lin CSY, Krishnan AV et al: Oxaliplatin-induced neurotoxicity: changes in axonal excitability precede development of neuropathy. Brain, 132:2712, 2009

49. Adelsberger H, Quasthoff S, Grosskreutz J et al: The chemotherapeutic oxaliplatin alters voltage-gated $Na(+)$ channel kinetics on rat sensory neurons. Eur J Pharmacol, 406:25, 2000

50. Benoit E, Brienza S, Dubois JM: Oxaliplatin, an anticancer agent that affects both Na^+ and K^+ channels in frog peripheral myelinated axons. Gen Physiol Biophys, 25:263, 2006

51. Grolleau F, Gamelin L, Boisdron-Celle M et al: A possible explanation for a neurotoxic effect of the anticancer agent oxaliplatin on neuronal voltage-gated sodium channels. J Neurophysiol, 85:2293, 2001

52. Webster RG, Brain KL, Wilson RH et al: Oxaliplatin induces hyperexcitability at motor and autonomic neuromuscular junctions through effects on voltage-gated sodium channels. Br J Pharmacol, 146:1027, 2005

53. Wu S-N, Chen B-S, Wu Y-H et al: The mechanism of the actions of oxaliplatin on ion currents and action potentials in differentiated NG108-15 neuronal cells. Neurotoxicology, 30:677, 2009

54. Rowinsky EK, Donehower RC: Paclitaxel (taxol). N Engl J Med, 332:1004, 1995

55. Nakata T, Yorifuji H: Morphological evidence of the inhibitory effect of taxol on the fast axonal transport. Neurosci Res, 35:113, 1999

56. Theiss C, Meller K: Taxol impairs anterograde axonal transport of microinjected horseradish peroxidase in dorsal root ganglia neurons in vitro. Cell Tissue Res, 299:213, 2000

57. Park SB, Lin CSY, Krishnan AV et al: Early, progressive, and sustained dysfunction of sensory axons underlies paclitaxel-induced neuropathy. Muscle Nerve, 43:267, 2011

58. Albers JW, Fink JK: Porphyric neuropathy. Muscle Nerve, 30:410, 2004

59. Grandchamp B: Acute intermittent porphyria. Semin Liver Dis, 18:17, 1998

60. Thunell S: Porphyrins, porphyrin metabolism and porphyrias. I. Update. Scand J Clin Laborator Invest, 60:509, 2000

61. Lin CSY, Krishnan AV, Lee M-J et al: Nerve function and dysfunction in acute intermittent porphyria. Brain, 131:2510, 2008

62. Wahl-Schott C, Biel M: HCN channels: structure, cellular regulation and physiological function. Cell Mol Life Sci, 66:470, 2009

63. Duchen MR: Effects of metabolic inhibition on the membrane properties of isolated mouse primary sensory neurones. J Physiol, 424:387, 1990

64. Zhang K, Peng B-W, Sanchez RM: Decreased I_H in hippocampal area CA1 pyramidal neurons after perinatal seizure-inducing hypoxia. Epilepsia, 47:1023, 2006

65. Vallat J-M, Sommer C, Magy L: Chronic inflammatory demyelinating polyradiculoneuropathy: diagnostic and therapeutic challenges for a treatable condition. Lancet Neurol, 9:402, 2010

66. Vucic S, Kiernan MC, Cornblath DR: Guillain–Barré syndrome: an update. J Clin Neurosci, 16:733, 2009

67. Rajabally YA, Simpson BS, Beri S et al: Epidemiologic variability of chronic inflammatory demyelinating polyneuropathy

with different diagnostic criteria: study of a UK population. Muscle Nerve, 39:432, 2009

68. Lunn MPT, Willison HJ: Diagnosis and treatment in inflammatory neuropathies. J Neurol Neurosurg Psychiatry, 80:249, 2009

69. Griffin JW, Hughes RAC: Intravenous immunoglobulin for neuromuscular disease: costs, benefits and reimbursement. Nat Clin Pract Neurol, 5:119, 2009

70. Lin CS, Krishnan AV, Park SB et al: Modulatory effects on axonal function following intravenous immunoglobulin therapy in CIDP. Arch Neurol, 68:862, 2011

71. Hubli M, Bolliger M, Dietz V: Neuronal dysfunction in chronic spinal cord injury. Spinal Cord, 49:582, 2011

72. Lin CS-Y, Macefield VG, Elam M et al: Axonal changes in spinal cord injured patients distal to the site of injury. Brain, 130:985, 2007

73. Boland RA, Lin CS-Y, Engel S et al: Adaptation of motor function after spinal cord injury: novel insights into spinal shock. Brain, 134:495, 2011

74. Horn S, Quasthoff S, Grafe P et al: Abnormal axonal inward rectification in diabetic neuropathy. Muscle Nerve, 19:1268, 1996

75. Kikkawa Y, Kuwabara S, Misawa S et al: The acute effects of glycemic control on nerve conduction in human diabetics. Clin Neurophysiol, 116:270, 2005

76. Kitano Y, Kuwabara S, Misawa S et al: The acute effects of glycemic control on axonal excitability in human diabetics. Ann Neurol, 56:462, 2004

77. Krishnan AV, Kiernan MC: Altered nerve excitability properties in established diabetic neuropathy. Brain, 128:1178, 2005

78. Krishnan AV, Lin CSY, Kiernan MC: Activity-dependent excitability changes suggest Na^+/K^+ pump dysfunction in diabetic neuropathy. Brain, 131:1209, 2008

79. Kuwabara S: Shortened refractory periods in human diabetic neuropathy. Clin Neurophysiol, 114:169, 2003

80. Kuwabara S, Ogawara K, Harrori T et al: The acute effects of glycemic control on axonal excitability in human diabetic nerves. Intern Med, 41:360, 2002

81. Misawa S, Kuwabara S, Kanai K et al: Axonal potassium conductance and glycemic control in human diabetic nerves. Clin Neurophysiol, 116:1181, 2005

82. Misawa S, Kuwabara S, Kanai K et al: Nodal persistent Na^+ currents in human diabetic nerves estimated by the technique of latent addition. Clin Neurophysiol, 117:815, 2006

83. Misawa S, Kuwabara S, Kanai K et al: Aldose reductase inhibition alters nodal Na^+ currents and nerve conduction in human diabetics. Neurology, 66:1545, 2006

84. Misawa S, Kuwabara S, Ogawara K et al: Strength–duration properties and glycemic control in human diabetic motor nerves. Clin Neurophysiol, 116:254, 2005

85. Misawa S, Kuwabara S, Ogawara K et al: Hyperglycemia alters refractory periods in human diabetic neuropathy. Clin Neurophysiol, 115:2525, 2004

86. Misawa S, Sakurai K, Shibuya K et al: Neuropathic pain is associated with increased nodal persistent Na^+ currents in human diabetic neuropathy. J Peripher Nerv Syst, 14:279, 2009

87. Bae JS, Kim OK, Kim JM: Altered nerve excitability in subclinical/early diabetic neuropathy: evidence for early neurovascular process in diabetes mellitus? Diabetes Res Clin Pract, 91:183, 2011

88. Krishnan AV, Colebatch JG, Kiernan MC: Hypokalemic weakness in hyperaldosteronism: activity-dependent conduction block. Neurology, 65:1309, 2005

89. Kuwabara S, Kanai K, Sung JY et al: Axonal hyperpolarization associated with acute hypokalemia: multiple excitability measurements as indicators of the membrane potential of human axons. Muscle Nerve, 26:283, 2002

90. Bostock H, Walters RJ, Andersen KV et al: Has potassium been prematurely discarded as a contributing factor to the development of uraemic neuropathy? Nephrol Dial Transplant, 19:1054, 2004

91. Krishnan AV, Kiernan MC: Uremic neuropathy: clinical features and new pathophysiological insights. Muscle Nerve, 35:273, 2007

92. Krishnan AV, Phoon RK, Pussell BA et al: Altered motor nerve excitability in end-stage kidney disease. Brain, 128:2164, 2005

93. Krishnan AV, Phoon RK, Pussell BA et al: Neuropathy, axonal Na^+/K^+ pump function and activity-dependent excitability changes in end-stage kidney disease. Clin Neurophysiol, 117:992, 2006

94. Krishnan AV, Phoon RK, Pussell BA et al: Ischaemia induces paradoxical changes in axonal excitability in end-stage kidney disease. Brain, 129:1585, 2006

95. Krishnan AV, Phoon RK, Pussell BA et al: Sensory nerve excitability and neuropathy in end-stage kidney disease. J Neurol Neurosurg Psychiatry, 77:548, 2006

96. Kiernan MC, Walters RJ, Andersen KV et al: Nerve excitability changes in chronic renal failure indicate membrane depolarization due to hyperkalaemia. Brain, 125:1366, 2002

97. Ng K, Lin CS, Murray NMF et al: Conduction and excitability properties of peripheral nerves in end-stage liver disease. Muscle Nerve, 35:730, 2007

98. Z'Graggen WJ, Lin CSY, Howard RS et al: Nerve excitability changes in critical illness polyneuropathy. Brain, 129:2461, 2006

99. Kuwabara S, Bostock H, Ogawara K et al: The refractory period of transmission is impaired in axonal Guillain–Barré syndrome. Muscle Nerve, 28:683, 2003

100. Kuwabara S, Nakata M, Sung JY et al: Hyperreflexia in axonal Guillain–Barré syndrome subsequent to *Campylobacter jejuni* enteritis. J Neurol Sci, 199:89, 2002

101. Kuwabara S, Ogawara K, Sung JY et al: Differences in membrane properties of axonal and demyelinating Guillain–Barré syndromes. Ann Neurol, 52:180, 2002

102. Cappelen-Smith C, Kuwabara S, Lin CS et al: Activity-dependent hyperpolarization and conduction block in chronic inflammatory demyelinating polyneuropathy. Ann Neurol, 48:826, 2000

103. Cappelen-Smith C, Kuwabara S, Lin CS et al: Membrane properties in chronic inflammatory demyelinating polyneuropathy. Brain, 124:2439, 2001

104. Cappelen-Smith C, Lin CS, Kuwabara S et al: Conduction block during and after ischaemia in chronic inflammatory demyelinating polyneuropathy. Brain, 125:1850, 2002

105. Kuwabara S, Nakajima Y, Hattori T et al: Activity-dependent excitability changes in chronic inflammatory demyelinating polyneuropathy: a microneurographic study. Muscle Nerve, 22:899, 1999

106. Sung J-Y, Kuwabara S, Kaji R et al: Threshold electrotonus in chronic inflammatory demyelinating polyneuropathy: correlation with clinical profiles. Muscle Nerve, 29:28, 2004

107. Boërio D, Créange A, Hogrel J-Y et al: Nerve excitability changes after intravenous immunoglobulin infusions in multifocal motor neuropathy and chronic inflammatory demyelinating neuropathy. J Neurol Sci, 292:63, 2010

108. Cappelen-Smith C, Kuwabara S, Lin CS et al: Abnormalities of axonal excitability are not generalized in early multifocal motor neuropathy. Muscle Nerve, 26:769, 2002

109. Kaji R, Bostock H, Kohara N et al: Activity-dependent conduction block in multifocal motor neuropathy. Brain, 123:1602, 2000

110. Kiernan MC, Guglielmi JM, Kaji R et al: Evidence for axonal membrane hyperpolarization in multifocal motor neuropathy with conduction block. Brain, 125:664, 2002

111. Burke D: Excitability of motor axons in neuromyotonia. Muscle Nerve, 22:797, 1999

112. Kiernan MC, Hart IK, Bostock H: Excitability properties of motor axons in patients with spontaneous motor unit activity. J Neurol Neurosurg Psychiatry, 70:56, 2001

113. Maddison P, Newsom-Davis J, Mills KR: Strength–duration properties of peripheral nerve in acquired neuromyotonia. Muscle Nerve, 22:823, 1999

114. Ng K, Howells J, Pollard JD et al: Up-regulation of slow K^+ channels in peripheral motor axons: a transcriptional channelopathy in multiple sclerosis. Brain, 131:3062, 2008

115. Park SB, Lin CSY, Krishnan AV et al: Oxaliplatin-induced Lhermitte's phenomenon as a manifestation of severe generalized neurotoxicity. Oncology, 77:342, 2009

116. Isbister GK, Son J, Wang F et al: Puffer fish poisoning: a potentially life-threatening condition. Med J Aust, 177:650, 2002

117. Kiernan MC, Isbister GK, Lin CS et al: Acute tetrodotoxin-induced neurotoxicity after ingestion of puffer fish. Ann Neurol, 57:339, 2005

118. Jankelowitz S, Mohamed A, Burke D: Axonal effects of camphor poisoning. J Clin Neurosci, 16:1639, 2009

119. Krishnan AV, Lin CS, Reddel SW et al: Conduction block and impaired axonal function in tick paralysis. Muscle Nerve, 40:358, 2009

120. Isose S, Misawa S, Sakurai K et al: Mexiletine suppresses nodal persistent sodium currents in sensory axons of patients with neuropathic pain. Clin Neurophysiol, 121:719, 2010

121. Kuwabara S, Misawa S, Tamura N et al: The effects of mexiletine on excitability properties of human median motor axons. Clin Neurophysiol, 116:284, 2005

122. Cappelen-Smith C, Lin CS, Burke D: Activity-dependent hyperpolarization and impulse conduction in motor axons in patients with carpal tunnel syndrome. Brain, 126:1001, 2003

123. Han SE, Boland RA, Krishnan AV et al: Ischaemic sensitivity of axons in carpal tunnel syndrome. J Peripher Nerv Syst, 14:190, 2009

124. Mogyoros I, Kiernan MC, Burke D: Strength–duration properties of sensory and motor axons in carpal tunnel syndrome. Muscle Nerve, 20:508, 1997

125. Bostock H, Sharief MK, Reid G et al: Axonal ion channel dysfunction in amyotrophic lateral sclerosis. Brain, 118:217, 1995

126. Kiernan MC, Burke D: Threshold electrotonus and the assessment of nerve excitability in amyotrophic lateral sclerosis. p. 359. In Eisen A (ed): Handbook of Clinical Neurophysiology: Clinical Neurophysiology of Motor Neuron Diseases. Elsevier, Amsterdam, 2004

127. Kanai K, Kuwabara S, Misawa S et al: Altered axonal excitability properties in amyotrophic lateral sclerosis: impaired potassium channel function related to disease stage. Brain, 129:953, 2006

128. Kuwabara S, Kanai K: Altered axonal ion channel function in amyotrophic lateral sclerosis. Brain Nerve, 59:1109, 2007

129. Mogyoros I, Kiernan MC, Burke D et al: Ischemic resistance of cutaneous afferents and motor axons in patients with amyotrophic lateral sclerosis. Muscle Nerve, 21:1692, 1998

130. Mogyoros I, Kiernan MC, Burke D et al: Strength–duration properties of sensory and motor axons in amyotrophic lateral sclerosis. Brain, 121:851, 1998

131. Nakata M, Kuwabara S, Kanai K et al: Distal excitability changes in motor axons in amyotrophic lateral sclerosis. Clin Neurophysiol, 117:1444, 2006

132. Vucic S, Kiernan MC: Axonal excitability properties in amyotrophic lateral sclerosis. Clin Neurophysiol, 117:1458, 2006

133. Vucic S, Kiernan MC: Abnormalities in cortical and peripheral excitability in flail arm variant amyotrophic lateral sclerosis. J Neurol Neurosurg Psychiatry, 78:849, 2007

134. Vucic S, Krishnan AV, Kiernan MC: Fatigue and activity dependent changes in axonal excitability in amyotrophic lateral sclerosis. J Neurol Neurosurg Psychiatry, 78:1202, 2007

135. Vucic S, Kiernan MC: Upregulation of persistent sodium conductances in familial ALS. J Neurol Neurosurg Psychiatry, 81:222, 2010

136. Nodera H, Bostock H, Kuwabara S et al: Nerve excitability properties in Charcot–Marie–Tooth disease type 1a. Brain, 127:203, 2004

137. Tomlinson SE, Tan SV, Kullmann DM et al: Nerve excitability studies characterize Kv1.1 fast potassium channel dysfunction in patients with episodic ataxia type 1. Brain, 133:3530, 2010

138. Krishnan AV, Bostock H, Ip J et al: Axonal function in a family with episodic ataxia type 2 due to a novel mutation. J Neurol, 255:750, 2008

139. Tan SV, Lee PJ, Walters RJL et al: Evidence for motor axon depolarization in Fabry disease. Muscle Nerve, 32:548, 2005

140. Sawai S, Misawa S, Kanai K et al: Altered axonal excitability properties in juvenile muscular atrophy of distal upper extremity (Hirayama disease). Clin Neurophysiol, 122:205, 2011

141. Farrar MA, Lin CS-Y, Krishnan AV et al: Acute, reversible axonal energy failure during stroke-like episodes in MELAS. Pediatrics, 126:e734, 2010

142. Vucic S, Kiernan MC: Pathophysiologic insights into motor axonal function in Kennedy disease. Neurology, 69:1828, 2007

143. Krishnan AV, Kiernan MC: Axonal function and activity-dependent excitability changes in myotonic dystrophy. Muscle Nerve, 33:627, 2006

144. Boërio D, Hogrel J-Y, Bassez G et al: Neuromuscular excitability properties in myotonic dystrophy type 1. Clin Neurophysiol, 118:2375, 2007

145. Kanai K, Kuwabara S, Arai K et al: Muscle cramp in Machado–Joseph disease: altered motor axonal excitability properties and mexiletine treatment. Brain, 126:965, 2003

146. Kiernan MC, Krishnan AV, Lin CS et al: Mutation in the Na^+ channel subunit SCB1b produces paradoxical changes in peripheral nerve excitability. Brain, 128:1841, 2005

APPENDIX

15-1

Glossary

Accommodation The tendency of membrane potential to return towards the resting level conditioning with a sustained depolarizing or hyperpolarizing stimulus.

Activation The time-dependent growth of a voltage-dependent membrane conductance after a change in membrane potential.

Chronaxie The stimulus duration for which the threshold current is twice the rheobase. Chronaxie is equal to the strength–duration time constant when Weiss's Law is obeyed.

Conductance The conductance G_X of a channel permeable to the ion X is given by $G_X = I_X/(E_m-E_X)$, where E_m is the membrane potential and E_X the equilibrium (Nernst) potential for the ion. The term is also used in the sense of an ionic pathway or channel.

Depolarization A change in the membrane potential, which becomes less negative.

Electrotonus Changes in membrane potential evoked by subthreshold depolarizing or hyperpolarizing current pulses.

Fanning-in Threshold electrotonus waveforms in which the responses to depolarizing and hyperpolarizing currents are less than normal and come closer together with time. Typically occurs with axonal depolarization with time.

Fanning-out Threshold electrotonus waveforms deviating more than usual from baseline with time during the polarizing currents. Typically occurs with axonal hyperpolarization.

Hyperpolarization A change in the membrane potential, which becomes more negative.

I_H Hyperpolarization-activated cation current.

Inward rectification The passing of more current in the inward than the outward direction. This term sometimes is used for the I_H conductance, but more often for a potassium channel K_{IR}.

Membrane potential Voltage difference across the axonal membrane (inside–outside).

Refractoriness The decrease in excitability during the relative refractory period after a nerve impulse. It may be expressed quantitatively as the percentage increase in threshold when a test stimulus is preceded by a conditioning stimulus at an interval within the relative refractory period (e.g., 2 msec).

Absolute refractory period The period immediately after a nerve impulse during which an axon cannot be excited, however great the stimulus.

Relative refractory period (RRP) The period between the end of the absolute refractory period and the start of the superexcitable period, when an axon may be excited but its threshold is increased.

Rheobase (I$_{rh}$)   The threshold current (or estimated threshold current) for a stimulus of infinitely long duration.

Strength–duration time constant (SDTC)   An apparent membrane time constant inferred from the relationship between threshold current and stimulus duration.

Subexcitability (late)   A decrease in excitability (increase in threshold) occurring after the superexcitability following an impulse.

Subthreshold   Below the threshold to trigger an action potential.

Superexcitability   An increase in excitability (or reduction in threshold current) commonly observed shortly after a nerve impulse. It may be expressed quantitatively as the percentage change in threshold when a test stimulus is preceded by a conditioning stimulus at an interval within the superexcitable period (e.g., 7 msec).

Threshold (current)   The stimulus current required to excite a single unit, or to evoke a compound potential that is a defined fraction of the maximum.

Threshold electrotonus   Threshold changes produced by prolonged subthreshold depolarizing or hyperpolarizing currents, normally corresponding to the induced change in membrane potential (i.e., electrotonus).

Threshold tracking   Adjustment of stimulus intensity (usually by computer) to produce a test potential of specified size.

Weiss's Law   An empirical formula for the strength–duration relationship, which is followed closely by myelinated fibers: the stimulus charge [Q, i.e., the product of stimulus current (I) and the duration (t)] at threshold is directly proportional to stimulus duration.

Neuromuscular Ultrasound as a Complement to the Electrodiagnostic Evaluation

FRANCIS O. WALKER and MICHAEL S. CARTWRIGHT

Over the last three decades, ultrasound technology has evolved such that clinicians working in small laboratories can now use it to image nerve and muscle routinely. Growing evidence has established its diagnostic utility in neuromuscular disease.

Electrophysiologic and ultrasonographic studies are complementary. Whereas electromyography (EMG) and nerve conduction studies capture electrophysiologic alterations in neuromuscular disease, ultrasound captures anatomic pathology and functional changes in terms of size, movement, and blood flow. Both electrodiagnostic and ultrasound studies involve real-time technologies that can explore limited sections of the neuromuscular system sequentially. It follows that the physician who performs the clinical and electrodiagnostic examination and who thereby knows the likely site of pathology is probably the individual best suited to conduct the ultrasound examination. This chapter will review the basic principles of neuromuscular ultrasound and the manner in which it can be used to enhance the diagnosis and care of patients.

THEORETICAL AND TECHNICAL ASPECTS OF ULTRASONOGRAPHY

The principles of ultrasound technology are considered in detail elsewhere.[1-3] The use of the oscilloscope in ultrasonography lagged behind its use in EMG because of the need to develop a suitable transducer that could send pulses of sound energy into tissue and reconvert returning echoes into electrical signals for display.[4] It was this step that made ultrasound practical for routine diagnostic use and which eventually led to the conversion of graphic displays of time and amplitude into real-time images.[1-3]

Piezoelectricity

The bulky electromagnets and diaphragms traditionally used for interconverting sound and electrical energy (e.g., in microphones and speakers) are not well suited to the study of human tissue. However, piezoelectric crystals fit perfectly the size and power requirements for ultrasound examinations. Initially, these were quartz (silicon dioxide) crystal chips that had an asymmetric molecular conformation and charge. When a small current was applied across them, it predictably would excite atoms in each molecule into different orbits, slightly altering the shape of the chip. This abrupt shift generated a brief sound pulse. Perhaps of even greater importance was the reverse property. When struck by a returning echo, the same crystal chip would respond by generating a small electrical current that correlated in its size to the intensity of the echo. Using this type of piezoelectric crystal, it became possible for a transducer to send sound energy into tissue, and then to record the latency of the returning echoes and their respective intensities.[1-3]

Modern piezoelectric materials are lead zirconate ceramics that are more conducive to the shapes required to create modern multi-element, multifrequency ultrasound probes.

Display Modes

The initial ultrasound recordings involved a single crystal chip generating a single ultrasound pulse into tissue and a subsequent recording of the echoes that returned over time. These simple recordings displayed latency on the x-axis and amplitude on the y-axis, similar to a standard electrodiagnostic recording. This basic ultrasound method is termed amplitude or A-mode recording. This type of recording was capable of measuring the distance between parietal bones in a developing fetus or assessing a midline shift in a calcified pineal gland in an adult, but it was a far cry from modern ultrasound capabilities.[1-3,5]

However, even simple A-mode recordings could be complicated by problems such as the profound loss of sound energy as it travelled through and was reflected by tissue. This meant that echoes from deeper structures were predictably much smaller in intensity than those from near structures, even if they occurred at similar types of tissue interfaces, because of the attenuation of sound energy over distance. To adjust for this, attenuation estimates of normal tissues were calculated and a correction factor applied automatically to enhance distant (later) echoes so that they would be comparable in displayed amplitude to near (sooner) echoes.[1-3] This process is called time–gain compensation and is an automatic adjustment in all ultrasound instruments subject to manual override. In most instruments there is a small set of levers on the control panel that allows the operator to adjust the degree of time–gain compensation at different layers of an image (Fig. 16-1).

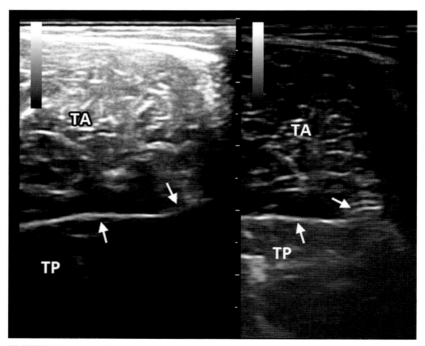

FIGURE 16-1 ■ Two identical axial sections of the same tibialis anterior (TA) muscle shown with different time–gain compensation adjustments. The left image has amplified near echoes, providing greater brightness display of the more superficial portions of the muscle. In the right image there is greater brightness display of the deeper structures, the interosseus membrane (upward-pointing arrow) and its attachment to the fibula (downward-pointing arrow), and the tibialis posterior muscle (TP).

Once the problems of generating sound, recording echoes, and adjusting for the loss of sound energy over distance in human tissues were addressed with piezoelectric transducers and time–gain compensation, useful A-mode displays could be obtained reliably and still are used in some ophthalmic circumstances.[6] But the numerical measurements they generated proved to be of limited diagnostic capacity. Because A-mode images contained only one line of data which varied considerably with variations in the angle of incidence, ultrasound was viewed primarily as an internal caliper useful for measuring distances between a small set of distinct tissue interfaces.[5,6]

It subsequently became apparent that data from multiple transducers (or one transducer moving from side to side), if coordinated reliably together, could help provide a broader assessment of more tissue. However, in a two-dimensional display, it was not possible to superimpose multiple A-mode traces to create an informative image because of the clutter involved. The next key advance in ultrasound was the development of brightness-mode (B-mode) display. This is also known as gray-scale ultrasound. B-mode display is a way of compressing an A-mode display into a single line of data that codes amplitude not as a variation on a different axis, but as brightness.[1-3] The amplitude of a returning echo therefore is coded as brightness, with the strength of the brightness correlating with the intensity of the echo. When multiple lines of B-mode from an array of transducers are stitched together, it creates a single, spatial image, in the same way a television creates an image from multiple parallel lines of data that can be updated many times per second. With this display, the bright edges of tissue interfaces are visualized and tracked easily, and their changes in real time observed. A quick glance at this type of image display, one that can be checked against anatomic specimens or magnetic resonance images, provides a self-evident display of the intuitive validity and reliability of the technique.

Few currently available instruments display A-mode images. However, an image similar to A-mode can be inferred from an M-mode display. In M-mode imaging, a single line of gray-scale data is recorded, but this information is updated over time, in a display in which time is on the horizontal axis and depth on the vertical axis (Fig. 16-2). This view, although not used often, is helpful for measuring temporal events, such as intervals between tremor bursts or the duration of fasciculation potentials.

Ultrasound Probes

Modern probes used in neuromuscular ultrasonography have more than 100 individual transducer elements arranged in a linear array. The long footprint of the probe is determined by the number of transducer elements and

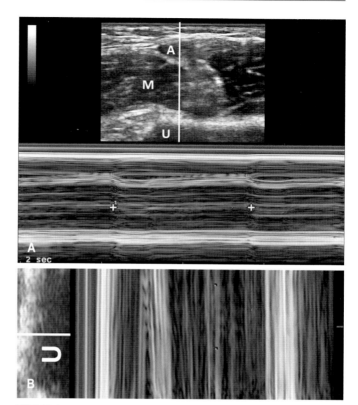

FIGURE 16-2 ▪ **A**, M-mode display from an axial image of the brachial artery (A) in the antecubital fossa, showing the proximal portion of the pronator teres muscle (M) and the ulna (U). A single line of ultrasound data, corresponding to the line shown bisecting the artery, is displayed below over a total of 2 seconds. The pulsations of the artery are captured by the two small crosses on the figure, showing an interpulse interval of 849 msec or a pulse rate of 71 per minute. **B**, Small section of the same image displayed after rotating it 90 degrees. This rotated image provides an idea of how original A-mode views were obtained. In A-mode, the y-axis would display the amplitude of the brightness shown in this B-mode section, and the latency would be presented on the x-axis, as is more typical of a standard oscilloscope tracing.

determines the number of lines of data and the width of the displayed image. Probes with smaller footprints (e.g., hockey stick design) have correspondingly smaller displays. The thick cord attached to the base of the transducer reflects the amount of wiring required for all of the individual elements. The casing of the transducer is designed to help match tissue impedance to enhance transmission of sound into tissue, and to dampen the reverberations of the piezoelectric elements and reduce the duration of the sound pulse. Given the complexity of this device, the ultrasound probe is expensive but, because it addresses the wiring needs of the patient in a single simple device, it significantly reduces the time required to complete a study.

The thickness of the transducer element determines the emitted frequency, and the instrumentation that drives the probe determines the duty factor, which is the percentage of time that the probe is emitting sound pulses. The emission of sound pulses is typically less than 1 percent of the time, with the remaining 99 percent being used to record returning echoes. (With color Doppler, the duty factor increases, leading to more tissue insonation and potential tissue heating.) The instrument controls a number of other functions of the probe, and these can be explored in greater detail in other sources.[1-3]

Sound and Echoes in Tissue

The speed of sound is determined by the medium through which it passes. Harder or stiffer substances conduct sound faster than softer or looser structures, so the speed of sound in air is much slower than that in steel. This is why an approaching train is detected better by listening on the rail than through air. Most human tissues conduct sound between 1,450 m/sec (fat) and 1,585 m/sec (muscle). By convention, all ultrasound instruments base their displays on the assumption that sound travels at 1,540 m/sec, which is an average speed of sound in human soft tissues. The displayed depth of a tissue that generates an echo is based on this estimate of the speed of sound. However, because some tissues conduct sound faster or slower than this, there is a subtle but unflattering bias in that ultrasound tends to overestimate slightly the thickness of fat (by about 6 percent) and underestimate the thickness of muscle (by about 3 percent). These changes may account for subtle differences between magnetic resonance imaging (MRI) and ultrasound estimates of tissue volumes but otherwise have a negligible impact on side-to-side comparisons or serial ultrasound measurements.[1-3]

The key to ultrasound lies in the tendency for a small amount of an emitted sound pulse to be reflected back from a tissue interface and for a large part of it to be transmitted through the interface to reach deeper structures. The physics of this relationship are fairly straightforward, in that the percentage of reflected sound is directly proportional to the difference in acoustic impedance of the two interfacing tissues (where acoustic impedance is related directly to the speed of sound in each tissue). As such, the subtle variation in sound speed found in human tissues is ideal for echo-based imaging, allowing for small detectable echoes at tissue interfaces and continued penetration of most sound energy to deeper structures. Problems, however, do arise with air-filled structures (e.g., lungs, 331 m/sec) and bone (4080 m/sec), which have markedly different conduction speeds than human soft tissue. For both air and bone, most sound is reflected at the interface, leaving virtually none for transmission and imaging of deeper structures. Ultrasound

probes are designed with several impedance-matching layers covering the actual transducer elements and require imaging gel to couple them to the skin in order to avoid the profound loss of insonated energy that would otherwise occur between a bare transducer element and the skin.[1-3]

Of course, not all sound is reflected or transmitted in tissue; some sound energy is absorbed as well. For every centimeter of depth, a certain amount of sound energy is lost (attenuation). Unlike the speed of sound in tissue, which is unrelated to the frequency of sound, attenuation is related directly to sound frequency. Higher frequencies attenuate more than lower frequencies, a property true not only in tissue but also in air. This is the reason that the low-pitched rumble of lightning as thunder is audible for miles, whereas the high-pitched and ominous crack of a lightning strike is audible only to those nearby. The degree of sound attenuation correlates with the degree of sound energy absorption and therefore with the heating of tissue. This property is of some therapeutic use, as ultrasound can be used to heat tissue. Because it is absorbed preferentially by deeper structures such as tendons, ligaments, and bones, ultrasound can deliver therapeutic heating to deep musculoskeletal structures without requiring excessive heat at the surface.[1,3]

As is the case with the speed of sound in tissue, the degree of attenuation of sound in tissue is assumed to be constant by the ultrasound instrument and is corrected for automatically by a time–gain compensation algorithm. However, the degree of attenuation of sound in tissue is not constant and varies with the type of tissue and the presence or absence of pathology. Manual override of the time–gain compensation is possible on almost all machines, and this can be used to correct the image display more accurately.

Two common ultrasound artifacts result from tissues that cause either too much or too little attenuation. Calcifications in tissue, from atherosclerosis, inflammation, or trauma, reflect almost all the incident sound, casting what appears to be a shadow on the image display (Fig. 16-3). Sometimes, because of directional backscattering, enhanced reflection is not readily apparent, but whenever shadowing is seen, it typically points to something that does not permit the transmission of sound, such as bone, air, or calcium. In contrast, sometimes a tissue, such as a fluid-filled cyst, causes minimal attenuation of sound. As a result, structures immediately deep to a cyst appear brighter than normal, because more sound energy is available to generate echoes. The presence of acoustic enhancement is evidence of a superficial structure that has reduced sound attenuation (Fig. 16-4).[1-3]

A third ultrasound artifact results from another sound reflection property of soft tissue, known as anisotropy.

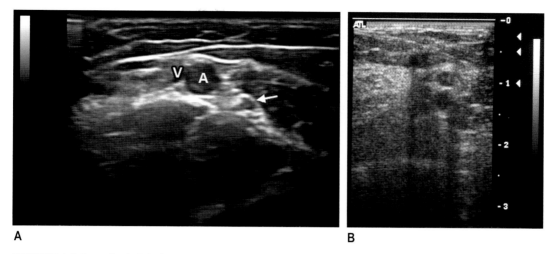

A   **B**

FIGURE 16-3 ▪ **A**, Axial view of a normal neurovascular bundle just distal to the antecubital fossa, showing the brachial artery (A), vein (V), and median nerve (arrow), with normal visualization of tissue deep to these structures. **B**, Axial image from the middle of the upper arm in a patient with vasculitis, myositis, and intravascular calcifications. Note the significant shadowing of distal tissues from the intravascular calcifications.

Some tissues backscatter reflected sound in all directions, whereas others tend to reflect insonated sound more like the way a mirror reflects light, in a defined ray or beam that forms an angle of reflection equal to the angle of incidence. The more a tissue approximates an acoustic mirror, the more it is said to have anisotropy. Tendons have high anisotropy and therefore appear very bright when the angle of incident sound is at 90 degrees to the transducer, but very dark when the probe angle changes just a few degrees. Nerves have much less anisotropy, and therefore show little difference in echogenicity when the probe angle changes from the perpendicular. Since anisotropy is tissue dependent, varying the probe angle helps distinguish different tissues from one another (Fig. 16-5).

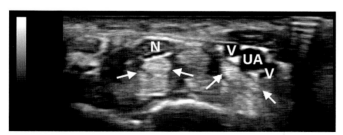

FIGURE 16-4 ▪ Axial view of the wrist. Note that, deep to the median nerve (N) and the ulnar artery (A) and vein (V), the tendons (arrows) appear brighter than the tendons between these structures. This acoustic enhancement results from less than expected attenuation of the ultrasound beam by the nerve or blood vessels, a finding more commonly seen deep to fluid-filled cysts (not shown).

Table 16-1 summarizes the ultrasound physics discussed in this section.

NORMAL AND DISEASED MUSCLE

Ultrasound of Normal Muscle

Normal muscle has a characteristic appearance on ultrasound (Fig. 16-6). On axial images, it consists of a largely hypoechoic (dark) matrix with interspersed bright small curvilinear elements.[7–10] On sagittal images, these bright intrusions are seen to be the fibrous supporting tissues of muscle, primarily epimysium and perimysium. Sometimes a prominent aponeurosis is apparent and is continuous with a muscle's tendinous attachment. Patients can contract their muscles on request, which leads to focal bulging and movement, making muscle recognition simple. Muscle has a modest degree of anisotropy, so small adjustments in the angle of insonation of the probe change the brightness of muscle. As such, by rotating the probe to show the difference between axial and sagittal views, moving the probe distal and proximal to show the belly of the muscle versus its tendinous insertions, asking the patient to contract and relax, and by changing the angle of incidence of the probe, the identification of muscle and its distinction from other nearby tissues is relatively straightforward. During an examination, sonographers constantly move the probe and change the angle of insonation as they interrogate human tissue. These movements, and sometimes maneuvers by the

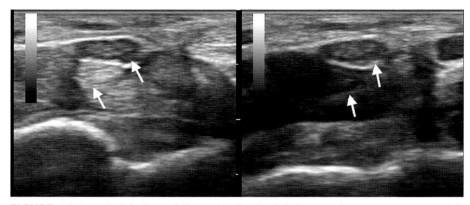

FIGURE 16-5 ■ Axial view of the wrist. In the left image, the nerve (top arrow) is much darker than the tendon (lower arrow). However, if the probe is tilted slightly forward (right image) so that the nerve is bisected by the plane of the image in a slightly oblique fashion, the tendon becomes much darker than the nerve, which shows little change in brightness. The nerve has a greater tendency to backscatter sound in multiple directions, whereas the tendons, which have greater anisotropy, reflect sound away from the probe unless it is directly perpendicular to them.

patient, enable examiners to recognize tissues of interest and their relationships to nearby structures.

For clinical neurophysiologists, electrodiagnostic studies are an extension of the physical examination. In like manner, ultrasound allows for detailed exploration of specific components of the physical examination. Ultrasound provides basic information regarding the location, depth, and extent of nerve and muscle—items of particular interest in evaluating patients with dysmorphic features, anatomic variants, surgical re-attachments, or congenital abnormalities—but it also provides valuable additional information about the surrounding anatomy and systemic vascular supply to these tissues.

Reference values for the thickness of normal human muscles, adjusted for age and sex, have been published, including significant side-to-side differences.[7,11] In addition, there are both qualitative and quantitative data about the echogenicity of normal human muscles, and the values vary from muscle to muscle. For example, the triceps tends

to be hypoechoic and the tibialis anterior hyperechoic compared to each other[8] (see Fig. 16-6).

Relatively little has been published on normal imaging of muscle contraction and relaxation. Using M-mode, the mechanical contraction of normal human muscle in response to supramaximal nerve stimulation can be recorded. This highlights the differences between the compound muscle action potential (CMAP), which is a recording of the surface membrane potential of muscle, and the actual mechanical contraction, including the phases of shortening and relaxation that follow (Fig. 16-7). The kinesiology of muscle contraction can also be studied with ultrasound. For example, ultrasound can depict differences in the relative activation of vastus intermedius and rectus femoris with different leg movements (Fig. 16-8).

Another aspect of ultrasound imaging that provides useful physiologic information about muscle is blood flow. Even a modest amount of exercise significantly increases

	Tissue-Specific Value	Transducer Frequency	Acoustic Impedance Difference at Tissue Interfaces	Ultrasound Power	Sensitivity (gain)
Speed of sound in tissue	Y	U	U	U	U
Tissue attenuation	Y	P	U	U	U
Degree of anisotropy	Y	U	U	U	U
Display: tissue echogenicity	Y	U	U	P	P
Display: tissue interface echogenicity	N	U	P	P	P
Angle of through transmission	N	U	P	U	U

TABLE 16-1 ■ **The Physics of Ultrasound**

Y, yes; N, no; U, unrelated; P, proportional.

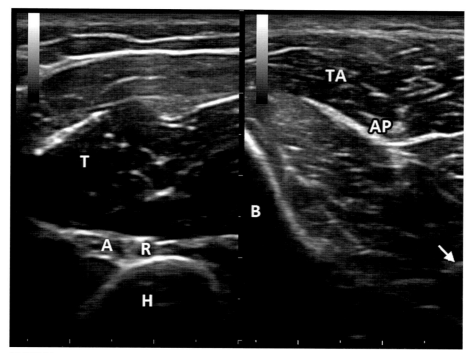

FIGURE 16-6 ▪ Axial images of the triceps (T) on the left and the tibialis anterior (TA) on the right at about the mid-level of the muscle belly. Both images show the normal appearance of skeletal muscle, which is mostly dark with bright interspersed fibrous septa providing a stark contrast, most apparent in the aponeurosis (AP). Bone shows an interface of stronger echogenicity compared to fibrous tissue in muscle, as shown by the tibia (B) and humerus (H). The radial nerve (R) and a small associated artery (A) are also apparent in these images at the level of the spiral groove.

muscle blood flow, as detected by power Doppler ultrasound.[7] With ultrasound contrast agents, this increase is even more apparent. Nerve blood flow is an area of increasing interest as well.[12] Preliminary studies suggest that blood-flow changes may provide useful information about certain types of inflammatory or compressive disorders.

Ultrasonographic Changes in Muscle Disease

The earliest reports of ultrasound in muscle disease were in muscular dystrophy, and the original observations by Heckmatt and colleagues some 30 years ago are still applicable.[13] Muscle disease typically causes: (1) increased echogenicity of muscle; (2) loss of heterogeneity in muscle (which is the loss of ability to distinguish between muscle tissue and areas of fibrous tissue within muscle); (3) atrophy (although rarely hypertrophy is also seen); and (4) loss of bone shadow deep to muscle (acoustic shadowing). These findings are the result of disruption of the normal architecture of muscle and correlate with the degree of histopathologic change in muscle.[14] As normal muscle fibers become necrotic or inflamed and are replaced by fat

or fibrosis, more tissue interfaces that reflect sound are created. In consequence, more sound is reflected, increasing echogenicity, and more is absorbed, leading to relative acoustic shadowing of bone.[7,9,10,13] The findings are seen in both myopathy and in neurogenic causes of muscle loss (Fig. 16-9). Ultrasound changes are not characteristic of a specific etiology, but in general neurogenic disorders tend to cause a more moth-eaten and irregular pattern, and myopathic disorders a more diffuse, homogeneous change (a generalized smudge).[6,7] More helpful, often, is the distribution of ultrasound findings. For example, in inclusion-body myositis the changes are most pronounced in forearm flexors and quadriceps, whereas in generalized neuropathies abnormalities are conspicuous in the most distal muscles.[7,8,15] A few rare disorders have characteristic findings, such as Bethlehem myopathy, in which there is a characteristic "outside-in" pattern.[8,16]

A simple global impression scale based on the Heckmatt and Dubowitz observations is an accurate indicator of muscle disease in childhood myopathies, with over 80 percent specificity and sensitivity.[17–19] Ultrasound is less helpful in children younger than 3 years of age or in those with mitochondrial myopathies.[7,8]

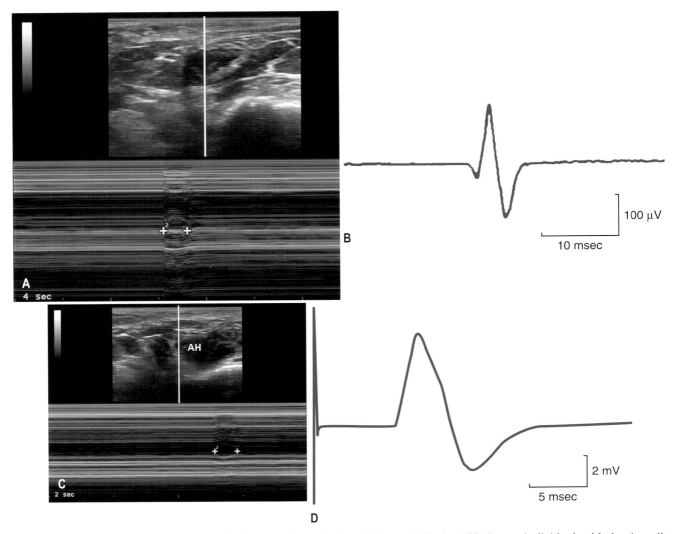

FIGURE 16-7 ■ **A** and **C**, Axial M-mode images through the abductor hallucis (AH) in an individual with benign distal fasciculations. **B** and **D**, Surface-electrode recordings from the same muscle. **A**, Image of the muscle contraction that results from a single supramaximal stimulation of the tibial nerve at the ankle. **B**, Tracing of the compound muscle action potential (CMAP) from this same muscle. **C,** Image of a fasciculation in the muscle. **D**, Surface electromyographic (EMG) recording of the fasciculation potential. Note the significantly longer duration of the mechanical contractions on ultrasound than on the EMG recording (247 msec vs. 12 msec for the CMAP, and 174 msec vs. 8 msec for the fasciculation potential). Whereas EMG records the electrical membrane potential of a muscle contraction, ultrasound demonstrates its mechanical properties. Note that the supramaximal contraction, which involves the entire muscle, differs from the fasciculation that spares the most superficial and deep layers of muscle in this image.

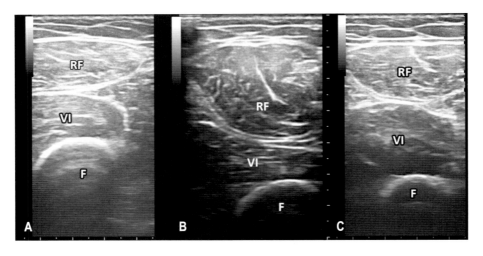

FIGURE 16-8 ■ Axial images of the quadriceps muscle at mid-femur (F) in an individual at rest (**A**), isometrically extending the knee from a joint angle of 90 degrees (**B**), and isometrically locking the knee in a fully extended position (**C**). Note the relative activation of the more superficial rectus femoris (RF) in *B*, and the vastus intermedius (VI) in *C*, as these agonist muscles contribute in different ways to stabilize and move the knee.

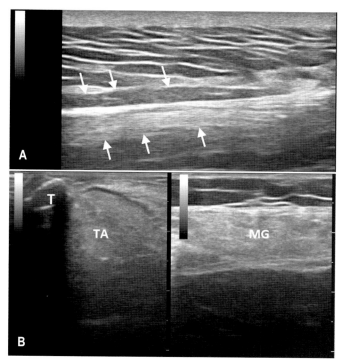

FIGURE 16-9 ▪ **A**, Sagittal view of the paraspinal muscles in a patient with severe myopathy. The superficial layer of muscle (downward arrows) is normal by ultrasound and electromyography (EMG); however, the deeper layer (upward arrows) is markedly echogenic, and on EMG showed profuse fibrillation potentials and small-amplitude short-duration polyphasic motor unit action potentials with early recruitment. Biopsy confirmed the presence of myopathy in this patient with Parkinson disease and dropped-head syndrome, initially referred for botulinum toxin injections with suspected antecollis from cervical dystonia. **B**, Axial images from the distal lower extremity showing end-stage muscle disease in a 72-year-old man with limb-girdle dystrophy. Note the marked homogenous increase in echogenicity of the tibialis anterior (TA) and medial gastrocnemius (MG); the bony edge of the tibia is obscured almost completely, and the soleus, deep to medial gastrocnemius, is shadowed almost completely because of the intense reflections from medial gastrocnemius. This type of image is nonspecific and could be seen in the end stage of a variety of nerve or muscle disorders.

Ultrasonography and Pathologic Movements in Muscle

Ultrasound is quite sensitive for identifying fasciculations in muscle (see Fig. 16-7).[20] These appear as focal perturbations in muscle, and when seen in the axial view they often have a rotational component. They last in the order of a few hundred milliseconds and occur randomly interspersed throughout muscle tissue. Their duration is significantly longer than the duration of EMG-recorded fasciculation potentials, which is a measure of the compound surface action potential of the motor unit.

Ultrasound captures its actual mechanical duration. It has been suggested that ultrasound is even more sensitive than EMG in fasciculation detection because EMG only records from one point at a time, whereas ultrasound scans a muscle one plane at a time.[20] Other movements may resemble fasciculations, such as arterial pulsations in muscle (see Fig. 16-2), but these are regular, localized perturbations that coincide with a palpated pulse.

Ultrasound can be used to measure the frequency and amplitude of tremors (Fig. 16-10). The technique is sometimes more informative than EMG for this purpose. With action tremors, for example, due to background EMG noise and difficulty in localizing specific muscles related to an observed movement, it can be difficult to identify EMG bursts in synchrony with the movements. For those wanting to quantify the duration of episodic movements such as tics or myoclonus, ultrasound measures mechanical perturbations and may be better able to correlate with direct visual observations of movement compared to electrical recordings, which only capture electrical signaling in muscle. Little has been published in this area.

The most interesting recent finding in muscle is the ability of ultrasound to detect fibrillations.[21,22] Using a very high frame-rate (which requires limiting the focal zone of an instrument and removing high-resolution averaging features for still images) with a high-resolution transducer, fibrillation in muscle appears as random small movements in muscle tissue. The ability to detect these movements is enhanced by warming the tissue. Although not as sensitive as needle EMG for detecting fibrillation potentials, ultrasound shows potential as a screening tool for these indicators of muscle pathology.

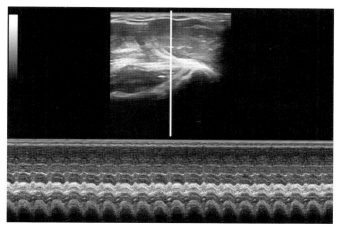

FIGURE 16-10 ▪ Axial M-mode image through the lateral neck in a patient with essential tremor of the head. Note the regular sinusoidal movements of the neck muscles, which correspond to a 5-Hz tremor based on the 4-second epoch recorded below.

Muscle Ultrasound in the Electrodiagnostic Laboratory

Ultrasound is complementary to EMG in evaluating a variety of neuromuscular disorders. In situations where needle examination is tolerated poorly, such as in young children, ultrasound can be used to recognize atrophy. A corresponding increase in muscle echogenicity suggests that the process is long-standing and associated with chronic histopathologic changes, such as fatty infiltration and fibrosis. If needed in such cases, EMG can be useful to determine whether there are large-amplitude, long-duration motor unit action potentials of reduced recruitment characteristic of spinal muscular atrophy, or early recruiting small-amplitude motor unit potentials of short and long duration, more characteristic of muscular dystrophy. If muscle echogenicity is normal, EMG can be used to determine whether any ongoing pathologic process is acute with normal EMG findings (suggestive of disuse atrophy) or subacute, such as recent denervation with fibrillation potentials and positive waves. If there is hypertrophy and normal echogenicity by ultrasound, EMG can determine whether there is an underlying myotonic disorder or dystonia; if there is pseudohypertrophy, as sometimes seen in the gastrocnemius muscles of patients with dystrophinopathies, the ultrasound will show increased echogenicity. As in the case of EMG, the distribution of findings by ultrasound is often informative as well, and careful correlation with clinical examination and laboratory testing may obviate the need for electrodiagnosis in some individuals.[7,8]

In adult patients with suspected bulbar amyotrophic lateral sclerosis, where clinical manifestations in the extremities may be limited, it may take an extensive needle EMG examination to identify extremity or truncal muscles with pathologic findings. Ultrasound is a useful screening tool for identifying muscles with fasciculations, which often are muscles with other manifestations of motor neuron loss. Thus, the time and discomfort of the examination can be limited by pre-EMG ultrasound muscle screening.

Ultrasound almost always is also abnormal in patients with decreased insertional activity, which is typically a sign that there is a long-standing process, one often associated with major changes in muscle histopathology.[14] Ultrasound can determine whether the process is a focal one from scar tissue or local ischemia to muscle,[23] limited to a single muscle, or involves a group of muscles sharing common innervation, vascular supply, or pathologic susceptibility (Figs. 16-9 and 16-11).

Much of the literature on muscle ultrasound has focused on pediatric indications. Although most clinical neurophysiologists consider EMG innocuous, pediatricians

and surgeons often disagree. The extent to which this limits diagnostic referrals of children (and occasional adults) that might benefit from studies or follow-up is unknown. Ultrasound offers a valuable window into muscle pathology that is quick, simple, and painless. Even if needle EMG examination is needed in such patients, the use of ultrasound can limit the number and extent of electrodiagnostic tests. Furthermore, for an examiner skilled in both ultrasound and EMG, who recognizes the relationship between electrodiagnostic and ultrasound findings in a given patient, ultrasound may lead to shorter examinations and make it possible for follow-up to involve imaging alone.

ULTRASOUND OF NERVE

Compression Neuropathies

The most substantial advance in nerve ultrasound came in the early 1990s with Buchberger's reports on the ability of ultrasound to identify the presence of carpal tunnel syndrome.[24,25] These studies recognized several key findings associated with the median nerve at the wrist in carpal tunnel syndrome, specifically that it is focally enlarged, hypoechoic (reduced echogenicity), and flattened. Subsequent studies have shown that the most consistent and reliable of these findings is nerve enlargement as measured by cross-sectional area, a finding that is perhaps quite counterintuitive.[26] Traditionally, the notion had been that nerves were "pinched" at sites of anatomic compression. In fact, Tachibana and associates showed that the median nerve invariably is enlarged in carpal tunnel syndrome, but that there may be slightly less enlargement at the site of maximal compression, with the nerve being larger both distal and proximal to this.[26] Although relative hourglass changes may be encountered occasionally, most routine imaging of nerve entrapments do not show an hourglass effect.

The cause of nerve enlargement in compressive neuropathies is understood poorly. In animal models of chronic compression, the nerve is known to develop endoneurial edema and Schwann cell proliferation in response to a compressing cuff over the nerve.[27–30] Researchers have speculated that edema results from damming of axoplasmic and venous flow. Since nerves lack lymphatics, excess fluid is not resorbed readily. A cascade of other events has been postulated to occur as well.[31] In humans, a recent study has shown that carpal tunnel syndrome is associated with increased vascularity of the nerve as demonstrated by power Doppler imaging.[12] In the authors' experience, the increased vascularity is recognized more easily in larger nerves, and it

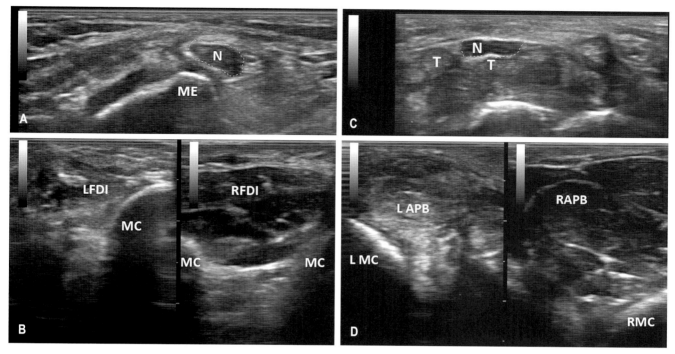

FIGURE 16-11 ■ **A**, Axial image of the left ulnar nerve (N) adjacent to the medial epicondyle (ME). The nerve is hypoechoic and twice the normal size at 17 mm². **B**, Axial image of the left first dorsal interosseus (LFDI) muscle showing that it is hyperechoic and atrophic compared with the corresponding but normal muscle on the right (RFDI), adjacent to the metacarpals (MC). **C**, Axial image of the left median nerve (N) at the wrist that shows it is particularly hypoechoic compared to the tendons (T) and is twice the normal size at 20 mm². **D**, Axial images of the right and left abductor pollicis brevis (APB) muscles in which the affected (left) muscle is hyperechoic and atrophic compared to the normal side. This patient sustained a severe burn injury to the left arm and had evidence of both direct trauma to the muscles and compression neuropathies.

rapidly dissipates after local injection of steroids.[32] As steroid injections also lead to a rapid measurable loss of nerve size, it seems likely that increased vascularity is part of the process that leads to nerve enlargement. It may also explain, in part, why the nerve is hypoechogenic in carpal tunnel syndrome, as increased blood flow likely would be associated with fewer reflections or echoes from the nerve. Subsequent studies of other focal neuropathies have shown that nerve enlargement at the site of entrapment is a common ultrasound finding irrespective of location.[9,10,31,33–38]

Ultrasound has also been informative regarding the mobility of peripheral nerves. Nerves traditionally have been thought of as relatively static structures, but ultrasound of the median nerve at the wrist shows the nerve is particularly mobile at this site. In the axial plane, with simultaneous flexion of the fingers and the wrist, the median nerve moves freely between different tendons in the carpal tunnel and sometimes loses contact with the roof of the tunnel completely (Fig. 16-12).[9,10,39] In the sagittal plane, the nerve slides distal and proximal with extension and flexion of the fingers—not as much as the digital tendons

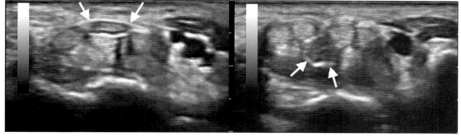

FIGURE 16-12 ■ Axial images of the median nerve (arrows) at the wrist, with the wrist in a neutral position (left panel) and the wrist and fingers fully flexed (right panel). Notice the shift in the position of the median nerve relative to the tendons and the roof of the carpal tunnel.

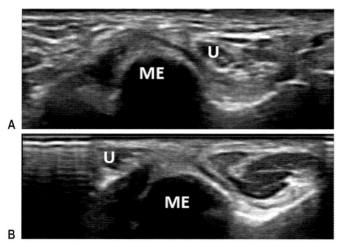

FIGURE 16-13 ■ **A**, Axial image of the ulnar nerve with the elbow flexed to 90 degrees. The ulnar nerve (U) is located lateral to the medial epicondyle (ME), its normal position. **B**, Ulnar nerve in the same individual with the elbow flexed to its extreme at 150 degrees. Note the subluxation of the ulnar nerve (U) with a shift to the medial side of the medial epicondyle.

but perhaps fully one-third as much. Nerves are somewhat elastic, and at rest there is always a slight tension on them. If the nerve is transected, this tension results in a gap between the distal and proximal ends, but the elastic nature of a nerve also allows for some distal and proximal movement with maneuvers of the extremity.[40] Ulnar nerve subluxation with extreme elbow flexion exemplifies resting nerve tension in that this dislocation reduces the distance the nerve has to stretch in order to accommodate this maneuver (Fig. 16-13).[41]

The relationship of nerve mobility to compression neuropathies is not well understood. In the authors' experience, limited mobility of the nerve is associated with carpal tunnel syndrome, but it is not clear whether this is simply a consequence of nerve enlargement or evidence of a distinct predisposing or contributing factor to the disorder. In a somewhat similar manner, it has long been believed that subluxing ulnar nerves at the elbow are more prone to injury or entrapment, but this is not well substantiated, given the absence of a routinely applied test for this process. Ultrasound will make it easier to investigate the interrelationship of nerve mobility and compressive neuropathies.

Nerve mobility also has an effect on determining how best to measure nerve enlargement in compression neuropathies. One of the problems with ultrasound as it has evolved is the operator dependence of the procedure. To minimize this effect, sonographers have tended to measure structures at sites related to bony anatomic landmarks in order to ensure reliability if measures are taken by different examiners or over time. However, this may not be the best way to measure the degree of abnormality of a structure. In the case of an aneurysm, for example, it is best to measure its cross-sectional area at the point of greatest enlargement rather than at an arbitrary junction of the artery with an underlying structure. In tubular structures with a relatively constant bore over a distance, such as a blood vessel, it proves to be quite straightforward to identify the point of maximal swelling. Nerves show a similar tendency to be of relatively constant cross-sectional area throughout most of an extremity,[42] and given the relatively fusiform enlargement of nerve in compression neuropathies, it is simplest to measure their cross-sectional area at the point of maximal enlargement. Although measurement of nerve enlargement at a consistent anatomic site may help to standardize the measure for comparative purposes, it may underestimate the maximum nerve enlargement. As the pathology in nerve compression seems related to nerve enlargement, precedence should perhaps be given to quantifying pathologic change. In a study of patients with ulnar neuropathy, for example, the site of maximal enlargement varied over the course of several centimeters around the elbow in different individuals.[34] Because of the mobility of nerves, it is unlikely that maximal nerve swelling will be localized consistently to a specific anatomic landmark.

In reviewing the literature, it is important to consider the technique used to determine nerve enlargement. Some authors measure nerves at predetermined anatomic sites; others scan the nerve for several centimeters distal and proximal to identify the site where the nerve shows greatest enlargement. At this point, the nerve area can be measured in two ways that are highly correlated. In the first, an on-screen cursor, manipulated by a trackball on the control panel, is moved around the inner edge of a nerve to calculate cross-sectional area; the second technique fits an oval, which can be stretched and compressed using the control panel trackball, to approximate the shape of the nerve outline. Some authors have elected to measure nerve thickness; however, this technique does not necessarily capture the cross-sectional area of a nerve, particularly if it is asymmetric or flattened. The use of the "trace method" to determine the nerve area at the site of maximal nerve enlargement seems most accurate, followed by the oval approximation method; measurement of cross-sectional area at a predetermined anatomic site is less reliable, and unidimensional measures of nerve thickness are even less helpful.

At this time, measurement of echogenicity of the nerve is done only by inspection. The potential usefulness of a more quantifiable measure of this parameter is as yet unknown. Similarly, measures of blood flow in the nerve are still largely descriptive. Over time, more sophisticated engineering of ultrasound instruments may allow for quantitative measures of these parameters.

Entrapment Syndromes

Nerve ultrasound shows its greatest utility in the assessment of entrapment syndromes, which are among the most common disorders routinely evaluated in electrodiagnostic laboratories. For that reason, additional detail is provided regarding the use of ultrasound in the evaluation of carpal tunnel syndrome, ulnar neuropathy at the elbow, fibular (peroneal) neuropathy at the fibular head, and radial neuropathy at the spiral groove.

Carpal Tunnel Syndrome

Ultrasound of the median nerve in the carpal tunnel syndrome is both specific and sensitive for the diagnosis of the disorder. There are too few direct comparisons of ultrasound with nerve conduction studies to determine which technique is superior, but nerve conduction studies currently are better accepted and somewhat more sensitive than ultrasound. However, ultrasound still may reveal abnormalities when nerve conduction studies are normal, and it provides information not available by electrophysiologic techniques, such as whether a bifid nerve, persistent median artery, or other local pathology is present (e.g., ganglion cyst).[38,43,44] It is particularly helpful in cases in which the findings on nerve conduction studies are normal or fail to identify an entrapment neuropathy clearly; focal nerve enlargement is then suggestive of focal compression.

Imaging the nerve is best done first at the distal wrist crease, initially in the axial plane (see Figs. 16-5, 16-11, 16-12). The transducer then is moved slowly into the palm and back up the wrist to determine the site where the nerve has its maximal cross-sectional area, and the nerve area is measured and its relative echogenicity noted at this point. Using trace mode, the cursor is moved just inside the boundary of the nerve. If there are questions about nerve size, the probe can be repositioned, the nerve measured three times, and the results averaged. Nerve cross-sectional area of 12 mm^2 or greater is typically abnormal. For comparison, the probe then can be moved up the forearm, following the median nerve as it wraps around the flexor digitorum sublimis, and cross-sectional area measured about midway between the elbow and wrist. In normal subjects, the ratio of the measurement at the wrist

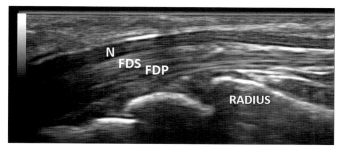

FIGURE 16-14 ■ Sagittal image of the median nerve (N) diving into the carpal tunnel to the left; the flexor digitorum sublimis tendon (FDS) and deeper flexor digitorum profundus tendon (FDP) are below the nerve, and deeper is the distal end of the radius and carpal bones.

and the elbow is less than 1.5. In normal subjects, nerve size is slightly greater in larger individuals, whether measured by weight, height, or body mass index. The ratio method helps to address the relative bias that this may cause in very large or very small individuals.

The nerve should also be imaged in the sagittal plane (Fig. 16-14), and power Doppler used to assess for the presence of low-velocity blood flow. Sliding of the nerve proximally and distally should be observed with slow flexion and extension of the digits. The nerve should be imaged again in the axial plane at the wrist, with the hand in the neutral position. Then, the fingers should be flexed into the palm, followed by maximal wrist flexion to look at the mobility of the nerve. Typically, it rotates 90 degrees, and sometimes is engulfed by the surrounding tendons (see Fig. 16-12). The intrusion of either lumbrical muscles with finger flexion or flexor digitorum muscles with finger and wrist hyperextension should be noted, as it occurs almost 80 percent of the time. Carpal tunnel syndrome sometimes has been attributed to excessive muscle intrusion into the tunnel, and muscle debulking during surgery then has been felt to contribute to clinical improvement. Imaging of the abductor pollicis brevis muscle also can be performed if there is concern about distal atrophy. Side-to-side comparisons of nerve or muscle are possible, but the tendency of carpal tunnel syndrome to occur bilaterally limits the value of this approach.

In patients who have undergone recent decompressive surgery, the nerve should be smaller in cross-sectional area compared to its preoperative size. When possible, the transverse carpal ligament should be studied to determine whether it is divided across its length. Evidence of incomplete surgical repair or other anomalous findings of significance sometimes are revealed by ultrasound.

The comparison of ultrasound with electrodiagnostic evaluation in carpal tunnel syndrome is complicated by the lack of a gold standard for the diagnosis, and the lack of a single metric for diagnosis with either modality. Experienced clinical neurophysiologists look at a number of electrodiagnostic parameters when evaluating patients for suspected carpal tunnel syndrome. In ultrasound, it is not only the cross-sectional area of the nerve at the wrist that is relevant, but its cross-sectional area more proximally, its echogenicity, the presence or absence of vascularity and mobility, changes seen on muscle ultrasound of the abductor pollicis brevis, and the presence of other anatomic abnormalities. It seems likely that a combination of electrodiagnostic and imaging techniques is more likely to be helpful in diagnosis than sole reliance on either approach alone.

Ulnar Neuropathy at the Elbow

The ulnar nerve is palpable and imaged easily in the ulnar groove in an axial view, where it is closely approximated to the medial epicondyle (see Figs. 16-11 and 16-13). From there, it can be followed several centimeters distally and proximally to determine the site of maximal enlargement. In some patients, the nerve is enlarged in more than one site (e.g., at the medial epicondyle and the humero-ulnar arcade distally), in which case more than one set of measurements should be made. Typically, the nerve cross-sectional area is 10 mm^2 or less. As in the case of the median nerve, a ratio can be determined with the ulnar nerve in the forearm (near where it is joined by the ulnar artery); the ulnar nerve at the elbow should not be more than 1.5 times the area of the nerve distally or proximally. Side-to-side comparisons are of somewhat limited value because of the tendency of the disorder to be bilateral. The ulnar nerve in healthy individuals typically has decreased echogenicity, so it can be difficult to rate this parameter, but, in general, enlarged ulnar nerves tend to be less echogenic than normal. A small artery sometimes follows the nerve, and is a normal variant unless obviously enlarged. The nerve should be viewed in the sagittal plane and power Doppler used to look for abnormal vascularity within the nerve. The nerve again should be viewed in the axial plane and the arm passively flexed to its maximum to see whether nerve subluxation occurs during the process (see Fig. 16-13).

Imaging of the first dorsal interosseus muscle or other ulnar-innervated muscles in the forearm can be informative in cases with chronic compression or evidence of distal muscle involvement (see Fig. 16-11, *B*). Even if atrophy or increased echogenicity is not present, localized fasciculations may provide a clue to possible chronic reinnervation in this muscle.

Too few direct comparison studies have been performed to determine whether there is a clear superiority between nerve conduction studies and ultrasound. It is of value, however, to perform ultrasound in patients in whom nerve conduction studies are normal, given the fairly high rate of false-negative studies with ulnar neuropathy at the elbow (sometimes for technical reasons[41]).

Fibular (Peroneal) Neuropathy at the Fibular Head

The fibular nerve tends to be more echogenic than either the median nerve at the wrist or the ulnar nerve at the elbow, making it somewhat more difficult to recognize on ultrasound. Furthermore, the nerve, as it wraps around the fibular head, often is not perfectly parallel to the surface, which may complicate imaging and measurements. When there is doubt, tracing the nerve to where it joins the tibial nerve proximal to the knee to form the sciatic nerve ensures that localization is correct. Like many motor nerves, the nerve is difficult to follow once it begins branching into muscular nerves, in this case, distal to the fibular head.

The cross-sectional area of this nerve tends to be more variable in normals than upper-extremity nerves, so that the upper limit of normal is 18 mm^2 and the side-to-side difference should not exceed 5 mm^2. Normal values for distal–proximal ratios have not yet been established. Imaging of the tibialis anterior can be performed, as well as other muscles innervated by the nerve. Although fibular neuropathies commonly are associated with chronic leg crossing or weight loss, in subjects without obvious risk factors there is a fairly high incidence of intraneural cysts that can compress this nerve.[45–47] Such lesions are identified easily by ultrasound.

Radial Neuropathy at the Spiral Groove

The radial nerve may be compressed against the humerus at the spiral groove (see Fig. 16-6). The nerve can be imaged here in the axial plane, but it is simpler to identify the nerve just lateral to the antecubital fossa, where it often stands out as an echogenic structure, sometimes with two distinct fascicles, surrounded by hypoechoic muscle. Once identified, it can be followed proximally to the spiral groove, or distally, where the two fascicles can be seen to split into the posterior interosseus nerve which can be followed to the supinator and sometimes more distally, and the superficial radial sensory nerve, which can be followed to the wrist.

A single episode of acute compression (Saturday night palsy) may not lead to chronic enlargement of the nerve, but imaging is particularly informative in fractures or suspected fractures of the humerus, especially where the nerve may be involved intimately.[38] In patients with complications following correction of humeral fractures, imaging may reveal unexpected and sometimes correctable pathology at this site.[48] Side-to-side comparison and study of distal muscles may also be informative. The cross-sectional area just distal to the spiral groove should not exceed $14 \, mm^2$ and the side-to-side difference should not exceed $5 \, mm^2$.

OTHER COMPRESSION NEUROPATHIES

The sonographic appearance of a number of other compression neuropathies has been described in small case series or case reports; decreased echogenicity and increased nerve cross-sectional area are typical manifestations. Additional literature is available.[38,49]

Generalized Neuropathies

Ultrasound has shown characteristic changes in neuropathies known to be associated with hypertrophic nerves, perhaps easiest to demonstrate in demyelinating forms of Charcot–Marie–Tooth disease.[50,51] In this disorder, the enlargement seems to be diffuse, with significant enlargement of individual fascicles. It is not clear whether the enlargement is seen in a distal–proximal gradient, changes over time with age, is associated with changes in nerve blood flow, or affects some nerves more than others. Cranial nerve enlargement has been seen.[51] In chronic inflammatory demyelinating neuropathy, nerves commonly are enlarged, but little is known about the time course or distribution of findings. Localized conduction block may be associated with focal enlargement, and nerve enlargement may recede with effective treatment, but it is also clear that conduction block and response to therapy may occur without changes in nerve size.[50,52] In acute inflammatory demyelinating neuropathy, nerve enlargement occurs,[52] but its presence at an early stage, when diagnosis is most challenging, is not well studied. Multifocal motor neuropathy is known to be associated with significant enlargement of nerves in the brachial plexus.[53] This finding might be quite helpful in the differential diagnosis of this disorder, since such changes have never been described in motor neuron disease.

Leprosy, a common cause of neuropathy in some parts of the world, is associated with significant nerve enlargement that is detected easily by ultrasound.[54–56] The presence of blood flow may provide some evidence of active inflammation. Further studies are needed.

OTHER USES OF ULTRASOUND

Whereas it has taken over two decades for ultrasound to influence practice patterns in electrodiagnostic and neuromuscular medicine, it has had a revolutionary impact on the practice of regional anesthesia over a much shorter time. Once it was discovered that ultrasound could be used to help administer local anesthetic injections around peripheral nerves or plexuses and to observe the distribution of the injectate, ultrasonography rapidly replaced needle stimulation or use of superficial landmarks for needle guidance. Compared to these approaches, ultrasound guidance improves accuracy and minimizes local anesthetic dose required—findings relevant to patient safety.[57–62] Moreover, ultrasound guidance significantly reduces the wait time in the surgical suite for the effect of blockade.

The experience of regional anesthesiologists has been a considerable boost to the development of diagnostic applications of neuromuscular ultrasound, in that it has shown the practicality of imaging multiple nerves and provided a detailed description of the normal anatomy of nerves, particularly the brachial plexus.[63] Furthermore, regional anesthesiologists have documented the ease of placing needles in close approximation to anatomic structures of interest, an observation of particular relevance to the practicality of near-nerve recordings. This work has highlighted the development of needle guidance techniques for procedures of neurologic interest, such as steroid injections for carpal tunnel syndrome,[64] injection of chemodenervating agents into muscle,[65,66] and the use of phenol for the treatment of spasticity.[67] A detailed description of the technique of ultrasound-guided injections is beyond the scope of this chapter, but ultrasound offers a practical alternative to EMG guidance for those unfamiliar with EMG, or to ensure the drug is delivered to targets without insertional activity, such as the salivary glands.[66,68]

An underused application of ultrasound is as a direct adjunct to electrodiagnosis. Near-nerve needle stimulation and recording techniques can provide a great deal of information about nerve function but they have been underutilized, in part from concern about placing needles close to nerves of interest because of the risks to adjacent structures. Cervical spinal roots are identified easily with ultrasound, as are superior and inferior portions of the brachial plexus,[63] the phrenic nerve,[69] and the lateral femoral cutaneous nerve of the thigh,[70] facilitating needle placement. Ultrasound also enhances the feasibility and safety of studies of the diaphragm.[23,71] Diaphragmatic EMG is often avoided because of the perceived risk of pneumothorax, so ultrasound guidance may increase its use and accuracy.

Finally, ultrasonography may well have a role in the investigation of the autonomic nervous system, although this requires further study and evaluation.[72]

CONCLUDING COMMENTS

Ultrasonography is a valuable, accessible technology for diagnosing a variety of neuromuscular disorders, such as myopathies, compression neuropathies, and various polyneuropathies, and for the guidance of injections of steroids or botulinum toxin. It may also assist in the performance of certain types of near-nerve electrodiagnostic studies and in the evaluation of cranial nerves and small muscles in ways that have yet to be explored fully. Its role in the evaluation of the autonomic nervous system is unclear and awaits study. As ultrasound technology continues to develop in pace with other advances in computerization, it is likely the technology will become more accurate, sensitive, portable, and available.

REFERENCES

1. Kremkau FW: Diagnostic Ultrasound: Principles and Instruments. WB Saunders, St. Louis, 2002
2. Brandt WE: The Core Curriculum. Ultrasound. Lippincott Williams & Wilkins, Philadelphia, 2001
3. Walker FO: Basic principles of ultrasound. p. 1. In Walker FO, Cartwright MS (eds): Neuromuscular Ultrasound. Elsevier, Philadelphia, 2011
4. Walker FO: The four horsemen of the oscilloscope: dynamic ultrasound, static ultrasound, electromyography and nerve conduction studies. Clin Neurophysiol, 118:1177, 2007
5. Willocks J, Donald I, Duggan TC et al: Foetal cephalometry by ultrasound. J Obstet Gynaecol Br Commonw, 71:11, 1964
6. Gerding MN, Prummel MF, Wiersinga WM: Assessment of disease activity in Graves' ophthalmopathy by orbital ultrasonography and clinical parameters. Clin Endocrinol (Oxf), 52:641, 2000
7. Zwarts MJ, Alfen NV, Pillen S: Ultrasound of muscle. p. 23. In Walker FO, Cartwright MS (eds): Neuromuscular Ultrasound. Elsevier, Philadelphia, 2011
8. Zaidman CM: Ultrasound of muscular dystrophies, myopathies and muscle pathology. p. 131. In Walker FO, Cartwright MS (eds): Neuromuscular Ultrasound. Elsevier, Philadelphia, 2011
9. Walker FO, Cartwright MS, Wiesler ER et al: Ultrasound of nerve and muscle. Clin Neurophysiol, 115:495, 2004
10. Walker FO: Neuromuscular ultrasound. Neurol Clin, 22:563, 2004
11. Arts IM, Pillen S, Schelhaas HJ: Normal values for quantitative muscle ultrasonography in adults. Muscle Nerve, 41:32, 2010
12. Mallouhi A, Pülzl P, Trieb T et al: Predictors of carpal tunnel syndrome: accuracy of gray-scale and color Doppler sonography. AJR Am J Roentgenol, 186:1240, 2006
13. Heckmatt JZ, Dubowitz V, Leeman S: Detection of pathological change in dystrophic muscle with B-scan ultrasound imaging. Lancet, 1:1389, 1980
14. Reimers K, Reimers CD, Wagner S et al: Skeletal muscle sonography: a correlative study of echogenicity and morphology. J Ultrasound Med, 12:73, 1993
15. Adler RS, Garolfalo G, Paget S et al: Muscle sonography in six patients with hereditary inclusion body myopathy. Skeletal Radiol, 37:43, 2008
16. Bönnemann CG, Brockmann K, Hanefeld F: Muscle ultrasound in Bethlem myopathy. Neuropediatrics, 34:335, 2003
17. Aydinli N, Baslo B, Caliskan M et al: Muscle ultrasonography and electromyography correlation for evaluation of floppy infants. Brain Dev, 25:22, 2003
18. Maurits NM, Bollen AE, Windhausen A et al: Muscle ultrasound analysis: normal values and differentiation between myopathies and neuropathies. Ultrasound Med Biol, 29:215, 2003
19. Zaidman CM, Holland MR, Anderson CC et al: Calibrated quantitative ultrasound imaging of skeletal muscle using backscatter analysis. Muscle Nerve, 38:893, 2008
20. Walker FO, Donofrio PD, Harpold GJ et al: Sonographic imaging of muscle contraction and fasciculations: a correlation with electromyography. Muscle Nerve, 13:33, 1990
21. van Baalen A, Stephani U: Fibration, fibrillation, and fasciculation: say what you see. Clin Neurophysiol, 118:1418, 2007
22. Alfen NV, Nienhuis M, Zwarts MJ et al: Detection of fibrillations using muscle ultrasound: diagnostic accuracy and identification of pitfalls. Muscle Nerve, 43:178, 2011
23. Boon AJ, Harper MC: Ultrasound as a complement to electrodiagnostic studies. p. 166. In Walker FO, Cartwright MS (eds): Neuromuscular Ultrasound. Elsevier, Philadelphia, 2011
24. Buchberger W, Judmaier W, Birbamer G et al: Carpal tunnel syndrome: diagnosis with high-resolution sonography. Am J Roentgenol, 159:793, 1992
25. Buchberger W, Schön G, Strasser K et al: High-resolution ultrasonography of the carpal tunnel. J Ultrasound Med, 10:531, 1991
26. Nakamichi KI, Tachibana S: Enlarged median nerve in idiopathic carpal tunnel syndrome. Muscle Nerve, 23:1713, 2000
27. Gupta R, Steward O: Chronic nerve compression induces concurrent apoptosis and proliferation of Schwann cells. J Comp Neurol, 461:174, 2003

28. Gupta R, Rowshan K, Chao T et al: Chronic nerve compression induces local demyelination and remyelination in a rat model of carpal tunnel syndrome. Exp Neurol, 187:500, 2004

29. Olmarker K, Rydevik B, Holm S et al: Effects of experimental graded compression on blood flow in spinal nerve roots. A vital microscopic study on the porcine cauda equina. J Orthop Res, 7:817, 1989

30. Prinz RA, Nakamura-Pereira M, De-Ary-Pires B et al: Experimental chronic entrapment of the sciatic nerve in adult hamsters: an ultrastructural and morphometric study. Braz J Med Biol Res, 36:1241, 2003

31. Visser LH, Beekman R: Ultrasound of peripheral nerves. p. 23. In Walker FO, Cartwright MS (eds): Neuromuscular Ultrasound. Elsevier, Philadelphia, 2011

32. Cartwright MS, White DL, DeMar S: Median nerve changes following steroid injection for carpal tunnel syndrome. Muscle Nerve, 44:25, 2011

33. Martinoli C, Bianchi S, Gandolfo N et al: US of nerve entrapments in osteofibrous tunnels of the upper and lower limbs. Radiographics, 200:S199, 2000

34. Yoon JS, Walker FO, Cartwright MS: Ultrasonographic swelling ratio in the diagnosis of ulnar neuropathy at the elbow. Muscle Nerve, 38:1231, 2008

35. Visser LH: High-resolution sonography of the superficial radial nerve with two case reports. Muscle Nerve, 39:392, 2009

36. Lo YL, Fook-Chong S, Leoh TH et al: Rapid ultrasonographic diagnosis of radial entrapment neuropathy at the spiral groove. J Neurol Sci, 271:75, 2008

37. Martinoli C, Bianchi S, Pugliese F: Sonography of entrapment neuropathies in the upper limb (wrist excluded). J Clin Ultrasound, 32:438, 2004

38. Cartwright MS: Ultrasound of focal neuropathies. In Walker FO, Cartwright MS (eds): Neuromuscular Ultrasound. Elsevier, Philadelphia, 2011

39. Cartwright MS, Shin HW, Passmore LV et al: Ultrasonographic reference values for assessing the normal median nerve in adults. J Neuroimaging, 19:47, 2009

40. Cartwright MS, Chloros GD, Walker FO et al: Diagnostic ultrasound for nerve transection. Muscle Nerve, 35:796, 2007

41. Kim BJ, Koh SB, Park KW et al: Pearls & oysters: false positives in short-segment nerve conduction studies due to ulnar nerve dislocation. Neurology, 70:e9, 2008

42. Cartwright MS, Passmore LV, Yoon JS et al: Cross-sectional area reference values for nerve ultrasonography. Muscle Nerve, 37:566, 2008

43. Visser LH, Smidt MH, Lee ML: High-resolution sonography versus EMG in the diagnosis of carpal tunnel syndrome. J Neurol Neurosurg Psychiatry, 79:63, 2008

44. Beekman R, Visser LH: Sonography in the diagnosis of carpal tunnel syndrome: a critical review of the literature. Muscle Nerve, 27:26, 2003

45. Young NP, Sorenson EJ, Spinner RJ et al: Clinical and electrodiagnostic correlates of peroneal intraneural ganglia. Neurology, 72:447, 2009

46. Lo YL, Fook-Chong S, Leoh TH et al: High-resolution ultrasound as a diagnostic adjunct in common peroneal neuropathy. Arch Neurol, 64:1798, 2007

47. Visser LH: High-resolution sonography of the common peroneal nerve: detection of intraneural ganglia. Neurology, 67:1473, 2006

48. Bodner G, Buchberger W, Schocke M et al: Radial nerve palsy associated with humeral shaft fracture: evaluation with US—initial experience. Radiology, 219:811, 2001

49. Peer S, Bodner G: High-Resolution Sonography of the Peripheral Nervous System. Springer, Berlin, 2003

50. Hobson-Webb LD: Ultrasound of polyneuropathy. p. 106. In Walker FO, Cartwright MS (eds): Neuromuscular Ultrasound. Elsevier, Philadelphia, 2011

51. Cartwright MS, Brown ME, Eulitt P et al: Diagnostic nerve ultrasound in Charcot–Marie–Tooth disease type 1B. Muscle Nerve, 40:98, 2009

52. Zaidman CM, Al-Lozi M, Pestronk A: Peripheral nerve size in normals and patients with polyneuropathy: an ultrasound study. Muscle Nerve, 40:960, 2009

53. Beekman R, van den Berg LH, Franssen H et al: Ultrasonography shows extensive nerve enlargements in multifocal motor neuropathy. Neurology, 65:305, 2005

54. Elias J, Jr, Nogueira-Barbosa MH, Feltrin LT et al: Role of ulnar nerve sonography in leprosy neuropathy with electrophysiologic correlation. J Ultrasound Med, 28:1201, 2009

55. Jebaraj I, Rao A, NK S et al: Imaging of tender neuropathy in leprosy. Indian J Lepr, 77:51, 2005

56. Martinoli C, Derchi LE, Bertolotto M et al: US and MR imaging of peripheral nerves in leprosy. Skeletal Radiol, 29:142, 2000

57. Marhofer P, Harrop-Griffiths W et al: Fifteen years of ultrasound guidance in regional anaesthesia: Part 2: Recent developments in block techniques. Br J Anaesth, 104:673, 2010

58. Marhofer P, Harrop-Griffiths W, Kettner SC et al: Fifteen years of ultrasound guidance in regional anaesthesia: Part 1. Br J Anaesth, 104:538, 2010

59. Tsui BC, Pillay JJ: Evidence-based medicine: assessment of ultrasound imaging for regional anesthesia in infants, children, and adolescents. Reg Anesth Pain Med, 35:Suppl S47, 2010

60. Liu SS, Ngeow J, John RS: Evidence basis for ultrasound-guided block characteristics: onset, quality, and duration. Reg Anesth Pain Med, 35:Suppl S26, 2010

61. McCartney CJ, Lin L, Shastri U: Evidence basis for the use of ultrasound for upper-extremity blocks. Reg Anesth Pain Med, 35:Suppl S10, 2010

62. Neal JM, Brull R, Chan VW et al: The ASRA evidence-based medicine assessment of ultrasound-guided regional anesthesia and pain medicine: executive summary. Reg Anesth Pain Med, 35:Suppl S1, 2010

63. Weller RS: Ultrasound of the brachial plexus. p. 91. In Walker FO, Cartwright MS (eds): Neuromuscular Ultrasound. Elsevier, Philadelphia, 2011

64. Smith J, Wisniewski SJ, Finnoff JT et al: Sonographically guided carpal tunnel injections: the ulnar approach. J Ultrasound Med, 27:1485, 2008

65. Py AG, Zein Addeen G, Perrier Y et al: Evaluation of the effectiveness of botulinum toxin injections in the lower limb muscles of children with cerebral palsy. Preliminary prospective study of the advantages of ultrasound guidance. Ann Phys Rehabil Med, 52:215, 2009

66. Ellies M, Laskawi R, Rohrbach-Volland S et al: Botulinum toxin to reduce saliva flow: selected indications for ultrasound-guided toxin application into salivary glands. Laryngoscope, 112:82, 2002

67. Lee J, Lee YS: Percutaneous chemical nerve block with ultrasound-guided intraneural injection. Eur Radiol, 18:1506, 2008

68. Walker FO: Interventional ultrasound. p. 150. In Walker FO, Cartwright MS (eds): Neuromuscular Ultrasound. Elsevier, Philadelphia, 2011

69. Canella C, Demondion X, Delebarre A et al: Anatomical study of phrenic nerve using ultrasound. Eur Radiol, 20:659, 2010

70. Damarey B, Demondion X, Boutry N et al: Sonographic assessment of the lateral femoral cutaneous nerve. J Clin Ultrasound, 37:89, 2009

71. Boon AJ, Alsharif KI, Harper CM et al: Ultrasound-guided needle EMG of the diaphragm: technique description and case report. Muscle Nerve, 38:1623, 2008

72. Walker FO: Autonomic testing. p. 487. In Kimura J (ed): Peripheral Nerve Diseases. Elsevier, New York, 2010

Electrophysiologic Study of Disorders of Neuromuscular Transmission

DONALD B. SANDERS

Tests of neuromuscular transmission are used most often to detect the abnormalities characteristic of myasthenia gravis. Although myasthenia is not a common disease, it is often included in the differential diagnosis of patients with symptoms of weakness and fatigue who are referred for electrodiagnostic studies. Much less common diseases with abnormal neuromuscular transmission are Lambert–Eaton myasthenic syndrome (LEMS) and botulism. Neuromuscular transmission may also be abnormal in primary nerve or muscle disease and may be demonstrated by sensitive electrodiagnostic tests, such as single-fiber electromyography (EMG). Electrophysiologic tests of neuromuscular transmission require experience and careful attention to detail. Information from these tests complements that from tests of nerve conduction and needle electromyography.

NORMAL NEUROMUSCULAR TRANSMISSION

The neuromuscular junction consists of the motor nerve terminal, a bulbous structure at the end of the motor nerve; the muscle endplate, with its folded postsynaptic membrane; and the synaptic cleft, which separates these two structures. In most human muscles, there is one endplate on each muscle fiber, located approximately halfway along the length of the fiber. Synaptic transmission from nerve to muscle involves a complex series of electrical and chemical reactions (Fig. 17-1).

The neuromuscular transmitter acetylcholine (ACh) is synthesized in the motor nerve and stored within vesicles in the nerve terminal. The amount of ACh in a vesicle constitutes a basic unit or "quantum" of transmitter.

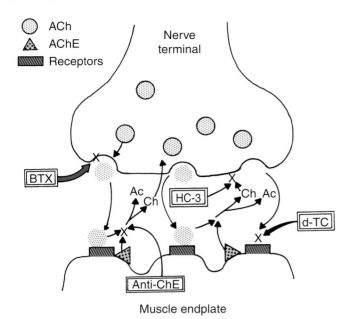

FIGURE 17-1 ■ The neuromuscular junction and some agents that interfere with synaptic transmission. Neuromuscular transmission takes place when discrete "quanta" of acetylcholine (ACh) are released from the nerve terminal and cross the synaptic cleft to interact with specific receptors on the muscle endplate. ACh is then broken down by acetylcholinesterase (AChE) into acetate (Ac) and choline (Ch). The release of ACh is blocked by botulinum toxin (BTX). *d*-Tubocurarine (d-TC) blocks the interaction of ACh with the receptors. Anticholinesterase (Anti-ChE) blocks the action of AChE. Hemicholinium (HC-3) prevents the uptake of choline into the nerve for synthesis into ACh.

When the motor nerve is activated voluntarily or by electrical stimulation, a wave of depolarization travels distally to the nerve terminal from which, via a complex mechanism that requires the presence of calcium in the extracellular fluid, there is near-simultaneous release of many ACh vesicles into the synaptic cleft. The neurotransmitter crosses the synaptic cleft to interact with specific receptors on the tips of the folded postsynaptic muscle membrane. Ion channels in the endplate membrane are opened by the interaction of ACh and receptor, allowing Na^+ to move into the muscle. This produces a local depolarization at the endplate, the endplate potential (EPP). If the EPP is sufficiently large, depolarization spreads to the periendplate region and then radially to both ends of the muscle fiber, with subsequent excitation-contraction coupling and muscle contraction. After interaction with the receptor, the ACh is broken down to choline and acetate by acetylcholinesterase (AChE) on the endplate membrane. The choline is taken up by the nerve and incorporated into newly synthesized ACh.

During stimulation of the motor nerve, the number of ACh quanta released from the nerve terminal varies.

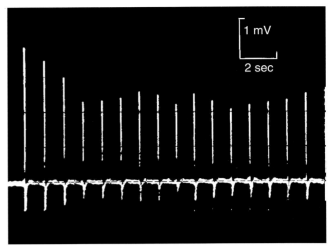

FIGURE 17-2 ■ Endplate potentials recorded with an intracellular electrode in an intercostal muscle biopsy from a patient with myasthenia gravis. The intramuscular nerve was stimulated at 1 Hz. The amplitude progressively decreases until the fourth response; thereafter, the amplitude fluctuates because of variations in the number of acetylcholine quanta released. (From Sanders DB: Electrodiagnosis of myasthenia gravis: recent techniques. p. 275. In Albuquerque EX, Eldefrawi AT [eds]: Myasthenia Gravis. Chapman & Hall, London, 1983, with permission.)

At stimulation rates greater than 0.1 Hz, progressively fewer quanta are released by the first four or five nerve discharges of a train ("depression"), after which the mean amount of ACh released per impulse becomes relatively constant, with some variation around the mean value (Figs. 17-2 and 17-3).

Following muscle activation, there is a period of "facilitation," during which each nerve impulse releases more ACh than before activation. Facilitation lasts for 30 to 60 seconds and is followed by a period of "postactivation exhaustion," during which less ACh is released by each nerve impulse. Exhaustion is maximal 2 to 5 minutes after the end of activation.

The ratio of the EPP amplitude to the threshold for action potential initiation is called the "safety factor" of neuromuscular transmission. In normal muscle, the safety factor is great enough to ensure that each nerve impulse is followed by muscle contraction (see Fig. 17-3).

The amount of ACh released by a nerve impulse depends on the interplay among these different processes, which have no clinical or electromyographic manifestations unless the safety factor is reduced. When neuromuscular transmission is impaired, however, the action potential threshold in some muscle fibers may be exceeded only by the first few impulses of a train of stimuli, and transmission of the later impulses fails (see Fig. 17-3). This manifests electromyographically as a decrementing

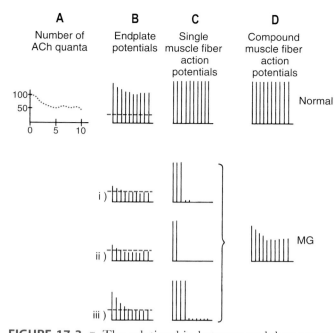

A
Number of ACh quanta

B
Endplate potentials

C
Single muscle fiber action potentials

D
Compound muscle fiber action potentials

Normal

MG

FIGURE 17-3 ■ The relationship between endplate potentials, muscle fiber action potentials, and compound muscle action potentials. **A**, The number of quanta of acetylcholine (ACh) released from a motor nerve during a train of low-frequency stimuli. **B**, Endplate potentials produced by a train of nerve stimuli decrease in a pattern reflecting the number of ACh quanta, as in *A*. The broken line represents the threshold for action potential generation, and the ratio between the endplate potential amplitude and this threshold is the safety factor of neuromuscular transmission. In normal muscle, all endplate potentials exceed threshold and produce action potentials (**C**) and compound muscle action potentials (CMAPs) of constant amplitude (**D**). When the safety factor for neuromuscular transmission is reduced, as in myasthenia gravis (MG), the threshold is not reached by the later stimuli of a train (*B i, ii,* and *iii* represent responses from different fibers within the muscle), and action potentials are not produced by these endplate potentials. The summated effect of these changes in individual muscle fibers produces a decrementing pattern in CMAPs (*D*).

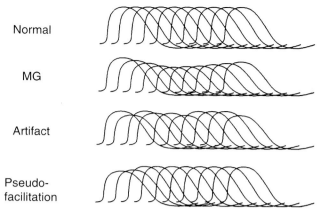

Normal

MG

Artifact

Pseudo-facilitation

FIGURE 17-4 ■ Representative patterns of response to low-frequency repetitive nerve stimulation. Normally, there is no significant change in the size of compound muscle action potentials (CMAPs). In myasthenia gravis (MG), the CMAP size falls initially, then returns toward the original size, producing a "U-shaped" envelope. Irregular patterns of response indicate the presence of artifacts. Pseudofacilitation can be recognized when the amplitude of CMAPs increases during the initial responses while the area of the responses remains relatively constant (see Fig. 17-10).

muscle response to repetitive nerve stimulation (Fig. 17-4). Postactivation exhaustion also may be seen when neuromuscular transmission is abnormal (Fig. 17-5). Postactivation facilitation is seen most dramatically when there is a presynaptic block, as in LEMS (Fig. 17-6).

Neuromuscular transmission may be blocked at many sites (see Fig. 17-1). For example, hemicholinium blocks the uptake of choline necessary for the synthesis of ACh and leads to depletion of ACh stores in the nerve terminal; botulinum toxin blocks the release of ACh from the nerve terminal; curare interferes with the interaction of ACh and receptor; and cholinesterase inhibitors block the action of acetylcholinesterase, causing ACh to accumulate at the endplate, producing depolarization block.

FIGURE 17-5 ■ An "activation" cycle, characteristic of myasthenia gravis, demonstrating changes in the decrement induced by repetitive nerve stimulation before and at indicated intervals after activation by maximum voluntary contraction for 20 seconds. The percentage change in compound muscle action potential amplitude decrement of the fourth response of each train is noted for each train.

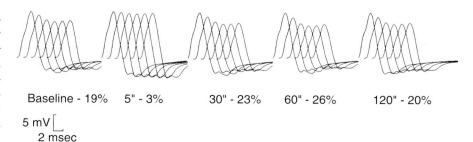

Baseline - 19%   5" - 3%   30" - 23%   60" - 26%   120" - 20%

5 mV
2 msec

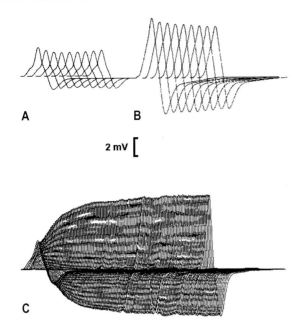

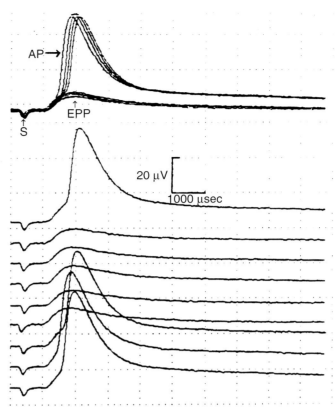

FIGURE 17-6 ■ Repetitive nerve stimulation studies in the abductor digiti minimi muscle of a patient with Lambert–Eaton myasthenic syndrome. Responses to 3-Hz stimulation before (**A**) and immediately after (**B**) maximum voluntary contraction of the muscle for 10 seconds. Before activation, the initial compound muscle action potential (CMAP) is small (3.5 mV), and there is a 15-percent decrement. After activation, the amplitude of the initial CMAP is 100 percent greater than before activation. **C**, Stimulation at 20 Hz for 6 seconds. After an initial decrement, the CMAP amplitude increases to become 160 percent greater than the initial CMAP. (From Sanders DB: Lambert–Eaton myasthenic syndrome: clinical diagnosis, immune-mediated mechanisms and update of therapies. Ann Neurol, 37:Suppl 1, S63, 1995, with permission.)

FIGURE 17-7 ■ Neuromuscular jitter and blocking. Recordings made with an intracellular microelectrode in a muscle fiber from an intercostal muscle biopsy of a patient with myasthenia gravis, during stimulation (S) of the intramuscular nerve. Variations in latency from stimulus to action potentials (AP) result from variations in the time required for endplate potentials (EPP) to reach threshold. Blocking occurs when EPPs do not reach threshold. Nine traces are shown superimposed (above) and rastered (below).

Variation in the amplitude of endplate depolarizations causes the EPPs to reach threshold at slightly different times (Fig. 17-7). This variation in time between nerve impulse and generation of the muscle action potential is called the neuromuscular jitter. When the safety factor of neuromuscular transmission is reduced for any reason, be it a presynaptic abnormality of quantal release or postsynaptic block of the receptors, the neuromuscular jitter increases; thus, jitter is a reflection of the safety factor of neuromuscular transmission.

Release of ACh from the motor nerve and the response of the muscle to known amounts of this transmitter have been measured in biopsied muscle to define the pathophysiology of diseases in which neuromuscular transmission is abnormal (e.g., myasthenia gravis and LEMS). Microelectrodes are inserted near the endplate to measure intracellular potentials. Single quanta of ACh constantly are being released spontaneously from nerve terminals,

and these produce transient depolarizations of the muscle endplate called miniature endplate potentials (MEPPs). The MEPP amplitude is a measure of the amount of ACh in each quantum. Intracellular recordings in muscle biopsies have shown that MEPP amplitude is reduced in myasthenia gravis because of decreased sensitivity of the postjunctional muscle membrane to applied ACh. In LEMS, such studies have demonstrated that the endplate responses to ACh are normal, but fewer quanta are released from the nerve.

In the developing neuromuscular junction, clustering of ACh receptors (AChRs) is dependent upon muscle-specific tyrosine kinase (MuSK) and rapsyn.[1] In response to agrin, a glycoprotein secreted from motor nerve terminals, MuSK induces clustering of AChR on the postjunctional membrane. In mature, innervated muscle MuSK is essential in maintaining normal AChR clustering. Circulating antibodies to MuSK have been found in up to 50 percent of patients with generalized myasthenia gravis who do not have antibodies to the AChR. (See the section on myasthenia gravis later in the chapter.)

REPETITIVE NERVE STIMULATION

The most commonly used electrodiagnostic test of neuromuscular transmission is repetitive nerve stimulation. Progressive reduction or disappearance of visible muscle contraction during faradic stimulation in myasthenia gravis was described by Jolly in 1895.[2] He called this a "myasthenic reaction." Harvey and Masland described the decrementing muscle electrical response to repetitive nerve stimulation that is the basis of the test in current use.[3,4]

In this test, compound muscle action potentials (CMAPs), which reflect the number of activated muscle fibers, are recorded during repetitive stimulation of the motor nerve. Repetitive nerve stimulation produces a decrementing pattern in a train of CMAPs if progressively fewer muscle fibers respond to nerve stimulation (see Fig. 17-3). This is the typical finding when the number of blocked endplates increases during repetitive nerve stimulation as a result of depletion of the readily releasable transmitter stores. However, a decrement may not be seen if many endplates are blocked at rest or if the total number of blocked endplates does not change during repetitive nerve stimulation.[5]

Recording Technique

Technically excellent recordings are necessary for minimizing artifacts. The recording electrodes should be placed so that there is an initially sharp negative (upward-going) deflection of the CMAP, indicating that the active (G1) electrode is over the motor point of the muscle. The reference (G2) electrode should be over a distal point where minimal activity is recorded. It may be necessary to immobilize the appropriate joints if movement artifact interferes with measurements of the CMAP. The stimulating and ground electrodes should be positioned to minimize stimulus artifact. The low-frequency filter should be 10 Hz or lower for most muscles, but testing of proximal muscles (e.g., biceps or deltoid) requires settings as low as 2 Hz. The high-frequency filter should be 5 kHz or higher. The stimulus duration should be no longer than is necessary for ensuring maximal stimulation during the entire testing session. A setting of 0.1 msec is usually adequate when surface electrodes are used for stimulation, but this is determined

empirically for each stimulation site. If stimulation is performed with needle electrodes inserted near the nerve, shorter-duration, lower-intensity stimulation pulses are adequate and are less painful. With either type of stimulating electrode, the stimulus intensity should be 10 to 25 percent greater than that necessary for activating all muscle fibers. This helps to ensure that all responses are maximal during trains of stimuli.

Muscle Temperature

The decremental response in myasthenia gravis and LEMS is less when the muscle is cool (Fig. 17-8). In myasthenia gravis, it is common to see a normal response to repetitive nerve stimulation when the surface temperature over the muscle is below 30°C (which is common in unwarmed hand muscles) and then to find a significant decrement after the muscle has been warmed. Hand or foot muscles should be warmed to a surface temperature of at least 34°C. Cooling is not a factor in proximal or facial muscles, which need not be warmed. In myasthenia gravis, the decrement is greater at a surface temperature of 44°C than at 32°C,[6] but it is

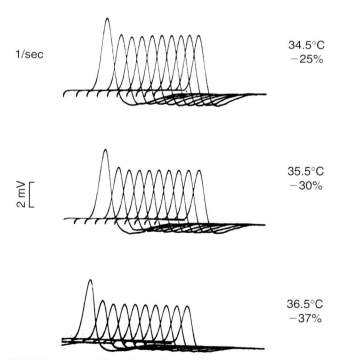

FIGURE 17-8 ■ The effect of temperature on repetitive stimulation studies in the hypothenar muscles of a patient with myasthenia gravis. The intramuscular temperature and change in amplitude of the fifth response of each train are noted at right. (From Sanders DB: Acquired myasthenia gravis. p. 275. In Brumback RA, Gerst J [eds]: The Neuromuscular Junction. Futura, Mt. Kisco, NY, 1984, with permission.)

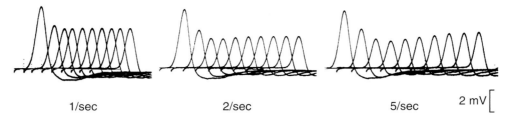

1/sec   2/sec   5/sec   2 mV

FIGURE 17-9 ■ Repetitive stimulation studies performed at different stimulation rates in the hypothenar muscles of a patient with myasthenia gravis. There is a decrement, which is maximal in the fourth response, and a subsequent reversal of the decrement, at all three stimulation rates, but more marked at the highest rate. (From Sanders DB: Acquired myasthenia gravis. p. 275. In Brumback RA, Gerst J [eds]: The Neuromuscular Junction. Futura, Mt. Kisco, NY, 1984, with permission.)

not clear that heating above physiologic temperatures increases the sensitivity of repetitive nerve stimulation testing.

Stimulation Technique

A decremental response in myasthenia gravis is demonstrated best at stimulation rates of 3 to 5 Hz, and the decrement increases with the stimulation rate, up to 10 Hz (Fig. 17-9). At higher stimulation rates, artifacts caused by movement are common and decrements up to 50 percent have been reported in normal muscle at rates greater than 10 Hz.[7]

The CMAP size may increase during high-frequency nerve stimulation or after voluntary activation. This is called *potentiation*. Potentiation may result from an increase in the number of activated muscle fibers (facilitation) or in the amplitude or summation of action potentials of individual muscle fibers (pseudofacilitation) (see Figs. 17-4 and 17-10). Each nerve depolarization releases calcium into the periterminal space, which increases the local concentration of calcium for 100 to 200 msec. If another depolarization occurs during this time, the higher calcium concentration increases the number of ACh quanta released. When neuromuscular transmission is impaired, this greater ACh release may improve synaptic transmission briefly, producing facilitation. Marked facilitation is characteristic of presynaptic blockade, but is also seen occasionally in myasthenia and during poisoning with curare, which has a predominantly postsynaptic action. Thus, facilitation in itself does not always indicate a presynaptic abnormality.

Pseudofacilitation has been attributed to increased synchronization of propagation velocities of muscle fiber action potentials or to shortening of muscle fiber length, particularly when the muscle is tested without fixation. In normal muscle, pseudofacilitation may increase the CMAP amplitude by as much as 50 percent during

stimulation at rates up to 50 Hz.[8] This can mask a decrementing response or may be mistaken for true facilitation. The duration of the CMAP decreases during pseudofacilitation, and the area of the waveform therefore remains relatively constant (see Fig. 17-10). Measuring the duration of the CMAP will determine how much the waveform has shortened during activation, and will indicate whether pseudofacilitation has contributed to at least some of any potentiation.

Measurement Technique

The size of the CMAP may be assessed by measuring the peak-to-peak or negative-peak amplitude. Many technical problems that arise during repetitive nerve stimulation can be detected if the CMAP waveforms are

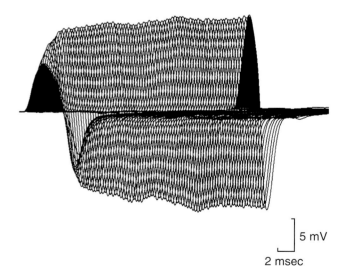

5 mV

2 msec

FIGURE 17-10 ■ Pseudofacilitation during repetitive nerve stimulation at 10 Hz in a normal hand muscle. The area of the negative peak of the compound muscle action potential waveform (filled) remains constant, but the peak amplitude increases and the duration decreases. (From Stålberg EV, Trontelj JV, Sanders DB: Single Fiber Electromyography. Edshagen, Fiskebäckskil, 2010, with permission.)

observed at a display setting of 50 to 100 msec per screen during stimulation. Movement of the stimulating electrode or the joint may produce changes in CMAP size that do not correspond to patterns expected in disease (see Fig. 17-4). In myasthenia gravis, the typical pattern is a progressive decrement from the second through the fourth or fifth response, with some return toward the initial CMAP size during the subsequent responses (see Figs. 17-4 and 17-5).

Changes in CMAP size are quantified by calculating the percentage change in amplitude between the first and the fourth (or fifth) responses of a train of stimuli, using the following formula:

$$D_{4 \text{ (or 5)}} = \frac{V_{4 \text{ (or 5)}} - V_1}{V_1} \times 100$$

where V is the amplitude of the CMAP. At stimulation rates of 3 to 5 Hz, the CMAP amplitude may decline by up to 8 percent in normal muscle, probably as a result of artifacts. If artifacts can be excluded, a decrement greater than 8 percent indicates that neuromuscular transmission is abnormal. The following criteria are useful in determining whether a measured decrement is caused by abnormal neuromuscular transmission:

1. *Reproducibility*. The same decrement should be seen when the stimulation is repeated after a period of rest.
2. *Envelope shape*. Changes in CMAP amplitude during a train of stimuli should conform to a pattern seen in disease, without sudden or irregular variations between consecutive responses (see Fig. 17-4).
3. *Activation cycle*. The changes induced by activation (discussed in the following section) should conform to an acceptable pattern (see Fig. 17-5).
4. *Response to edrophonium (Tensilon)*. Administration of intravenous edrophonium usually reduces or obliterates the decrement in myasthenia gravis.

Measurements of the CMAP amplitude during high-frequency stimulation may give variable and inconsistent results, and it has been recommended by some that the CMAP area, rather than amplitude, be measured to assess facilitation.[9] However, area measurements are affected by the position of the reference electrode, repolarization, and muscle fiber fatigue, and are markedly dependent on filter settings. In most cases, the results from area and amplitude measurements are concordant; any discrepancy should lead to a search for technical problems.

Activation

Facilitation may be induced either by high-frequency nerve stimulation (20 to 50 Hz) for 10 seconds or by a brief maximal voluntary contraction of the tested muscle. The latter is much less painful. Trains of low-frequency stimuli are given at the end of activation to demonstrate facilitation and then every minute or, later, every other minute for up to 10 minutes to demonstrate postactivation exhaustion. Voluntary muscle contraction is maintained for 10 seconds to demonstrate facilitation, as when testing for LEMS, or for 60 to 90 seconds to demonstrate exhaustion. In LEMS, the postactivation stimulus must be given as soon as possible after the end of activation because facilitation persists for only a short time.[10]

Muscle Selection

In myasthenia gravis, proximal muscles usually are affected earlier and more severely than are distal muscles, and there is usually a higher diagnostic yield with repetitive nerve stimulation studies of proximal or facial muscles.[11-15] To obtain the maximal diagnostic yield, it is necessary to test several muscles, including those most likely to be involved in the individual patient.

HAND MUSCLES

Hand muscles are the most convenient to test. Recordings usually are made from the hypothenar muscles while the ulnar nerve is stimulated or from the thenar muscles while the median nerve is stimulated. The hand can be immobilized by specially designed clamps or straps, but it is usually adequate for the examiner to hold the patient's hand firmly on the examining table. Activation is produced by having the patient contract the tested muscle against resistance. The temperature should always be monitored in these muscles.

BICEPS

The biceps is tested by stimulating the musculocutaneous nerve in the axilla with the patient supine and the arm supinated on the examining table or armrest. Recording electrodes are placed on the belly and tendon of the muscle in a position that gives a monophasic CMAP. Stimulation can be performed with surface electrodes pressed firmly against the posterior border of the short head of the biceps within 1 inch of the inferior edge of the axillary fold. Care should be taken to avoid stimulating other nerves in the axilla. The position of the stimulating electrode must be kept constant while trains of stimuli are applied. The arm must be restrained to prevent movement, which can produce artifacts in the recordings and can dislodge the stimulating electrode. Immobilization can be achieved by the examiner holding the forearm firmly against the supporting surface. Activation is produced by having the patient flex the elbow against resistance. This test is uncomfortable, especially if prolonged or high-frequency stimulation is used. Stimulation with a needle electrode inserted near the nerve reduces discomfort, and the needle electrode is less likely than a surface electrode to be dislodged during stimulation and activation.

ANCONEUS

This muscle is examined with the patient seated or lying supine, the pronated forearm resting on the examining table or armrest (Fig. 17-11). The active recording electrode is placed over the belly of the muscle, approximately three fingerbreadths distal to the olecranon, at the apex of an isosceles triangle with its base formed by the olecranon and the lateral epicondyle. It may be necessary to move the electrode slightly more anteriorly toward the lateral border of the ulna to record a monophasic CMAP. The reference electrode is placed on the posterior surface of the forearm. The radial nerve is stimulated in the lateral intermuscular septum, 1 to 2 cm proximal to the lateral epicondyle. Supramaximal stimulation is usually possible with relatively low-intensity stimulation. Activation of the muscle is achieved by the patient extending the elbow against resistance, although it may be difficult to keep the stimulating electrode in place during this maneuver. In patients with generalized myasthenia gravis, repetitive stimulation of the anconeus was found to be more sensitive than a hand muscle and equally as sensitive as the deltoid.[11]

DELTOID

The deltoid muscle is tested with the patient seated, the active recording electrode being placed on the belly of the muscle and the reference electrode on the acromion. The arm is held adducted against the side. Activation is produced by the patient abducting the arm against resistance. Stimulation at Erb's point is performed with a surface electrode pressed firmly behind the clavicle. With this positioning of the electrode, the patient is uncomfortable and it is not possible to avoid stimulating other muscles. Comparison studies suggest that a decremental response is found in the deltoid slightly more often than in the trapezius in myasthenia gravis.[12,13]

TRAPEZIUS

The trapezius is the easiest shoulder muscle to test.[14] The patient is examined while seated on a chair (Fig. 17-12). The arm is immobilized by having the patient grip the bottom of the chair. The active recording electrode is placed on the belly of the trapezius at the angle between the neck and the shoulder, and the reference electrode is placed on the acromion. The spinal accessory nerve is stimulated at the posterior border of the sternocleidomastoid muscle where it is superficial and can be stimulated maximally with low-intensity pulses; this minimizes discomfort and avoids stimulating other muscles. Activation of this muscle is produced by the patient shrugging the shoulder while holding the bottom of the chair or while the examiner pushes down on the top of the shoulder.

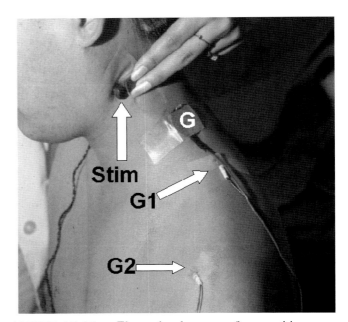

FIGURE 17-12 ■ Electrode placement for repetitive nerve stimulation studies of the trapezius muscle. Stim, stimulating electrode; G, ground electrode; G1, active recording electrode; G2, reference electrode. Copyright D. B. Sanders.

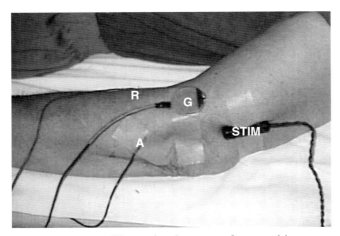

FIGURE 17-11 ■ Electrode placement for repetitive nerve stimulation studies of the anconeus muscle. STIM, stimulating electrode; G, ground electrode; A, active recording electrode; R, reference electrode. See text for details.

FACIAL MUSCLES

Facial nerve responses may be tested by recording from any of several facial muscles. Responses from the nasalis muscle usually have a predominantly monophasic waveform, which makes it easier to measure changes in CMAP size.[15] The active recording electrode is placed over the nasalis and the reference electrode is placed lateral to the eye (Fig. 17-13). The facial nerve is stimulated percutaneously below the ear or with a monopolar needle inserted near the zygomatic branch of the facial nerve, anterior to the ear. Movement artifacts limit the evaluation of responses from facial muscles, and some patients do not tolerate the stimulation. Facial muscles most often show a decremental response when myasthenia affects the ocular or facial muscles.[16,17]

The platysma can be studied by recording signals between subcutaneous needle electrodes placed near the endplate region and below the clavicle, then stimulating the facial nerve below the angle of the jaw.[18] Although studies in this muscle have a high diagnostic yield, an elaborate apparatus is necessary for immobilizing the head and preventing movement artifacts.

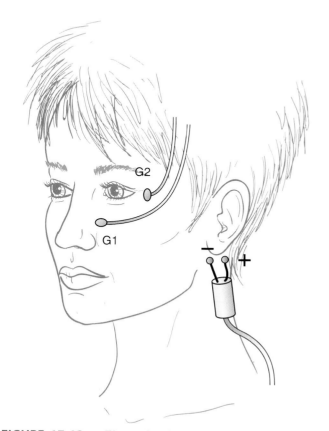

FIGURE 17-13 ■ Electrode placement for repetitive nerve stimulation studies of the nasalis muscle. G1, active recording electrode; G2, reference electrode.

MASSETER

The masseter muscle is tested easily and is commonly abnormal in myasthenic patients with oropharyngeal weakness.[19] The masseteric branch of the mandibular nerve is stimulated with a monopolar needle inserted to a depth of 2 to 3 cm at a point between the mandibular incisure and the zygomatic arch that is approximately 2 cm anterior to the ear (Fig. 17-14). If the stimulating needle is too superficial, the facial nerve will be stimulated. The active recording electrode is placed over the belly of the masseter, and the reference is placed under the jaw at a site selected to produce a predominantly monophasic CMAP. With appropriate electrode positioning, supramaximal stimulation of the masseteric nerve can be achieved with very low-intensity pulses, and movement artifact is negligible. The muscle is activated by clenching the jaw.

DIAPHRAGM

Repetitive stimulation studies of the diaphragm have been shown to correlate with respiratory muscle weakness in myasthenia gravis, and they may be useful in evaluating patients with undiagnosed respiratory failure.[20,21] Recordings are made with surface electrodes, the active electrode over the sternum, 5 cm superior to the xiphoid tip, and the reference on the costal margin, 16 cm from the active electrode.[22] The phrenic nerve is stimulated percutaneously in the supraclavicular fossa.

LOWER-LIMB MUSCLES

Muscles in the lower limb are studied primarily when weakness is limited to the legs.[23] The extensor digitorum brevis is tested easily, with the active electrode over the belly of the muscle and the reference distally over the lateral aspect of the base of the little toe. The fibular nerve is stimulated over the dorsum of the ankle, and the muscle is activated by dorsiflexing the toes. The tibialis anterior is tested with the active electrode over the belly of the muscle, the reference a few centimeters distally, and by stimulating the fibular nerve at the fibular head. The muscle is activated by dorsiflexing the ankle. It is difficult to avoid movement artifact when testing the quadriceps, and supramaximal repetitive stimulation of the femoral nerve is painful. The patient may be seated, with the lower leg restrained by straps around the leg of the chair, or lying supine, with straps around the thigh. The active recording electrode is placed on the anterior thigh in a position that gives the simplest monophasic waveform, and the reference is positioned over the patellar tendon. The femoral nerve is stimulated in the groin just lateral to the femoral artery.

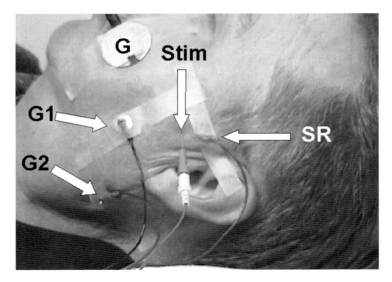

FIGURE 17-14 ▪ Electrode placement for repetitive nerve stimulation studies of the masseter muscle. G1, active recording electrode; G2, reference recording electrode; Stim, stimulating monopolar needle electrode; SR, stimulation reference electrode; G, ground electrode. See text for details. Copyright D. B. Sanders.

Methods for Enhancing or Provoking a Decrementing Response

Before single-fiber EMG (SF-EMG) was generally available as a test for neuromuscular transmission, a number of techniques were developed to increase the sensitivity of repetitive nerve stimulation. These enhancing techniques have been supplanted largely by jitter measurements; they are presented here for their historical interest.

If no significant decrement was seen before or after activation, mild abnormalities in myasthenia gravis sometimes could be detected by prolonged stimulation at slow rates (3 Hz for 4 to 5 minutes). The sensitivity of this technique in hand muscles could be enhanced further by producing ischemia in the tested muscle during the period of prolonged stimulation and subsequent exhaustion. A blood pressure cuff was placed around the upper arm and inflated above systolic pressure. The median or ulnar nerve then was stimulated repetitively, and the responses recorded from an appropriate muscle in the hand. This procedure could be used only for distal muscles, was painful, and was not tolerated by some patients.

Mild abnormalities of neuromuscular transmission could also be detected by repetitive nerve stimulation after regional infusion of small doses of curare. For this, a blood pressure cuff was placed around the upper arm and inflated above systolic pressure, and 0.2 mg of *d*-tubocurarine was injected into a distal vein. Stimulation then was performed distal to the cuff. This technique was reported to increase the diagnostic yield by about 20 percent over more conventional repetitive nerve stimulation testing. In a modification of this technique, perfusion of the drug was delimited further by placing a second cuff below the elbow, injecting the curare solution into a vein

at the elbow, and then stimulating the nerve to the biceps. These techniques are no longer used, jitter measurements being much more sensitive and safer.

Repetitive CMAPs

Repetitive CMAPs after nerve stimulation occur when excess ACh accumulates at the endplate, as in congenital endplate acetylcholinesterase deficiency, or with acetylcholinesterase inhibition by drugs such as edrophonium, pyridostigmine, or organophosphates.[24,25] Repetitive CMAPs are also seen in the slow channel congenital myasthenic syndrome, in which endplate potentials are prolonged beyond the refractory period for the muscle fiber action potential (Fig. 17-15).

In most cases, the initial CMAP is followed within 5 to 8 msec by a single, smaller CMAP. During trains of repetitive nerve stimulation, consecutive repetitive CMAPs are smaller than the preceding ones (see Fig. 17-15), even at rates as low as 0.5 Hz, and they may not be apparent after the first 3 or 4 stimuli. Exercise will also abolish the repetitive CMAPs, and they can be missed easily unless single stimuli are delivered at 5- to 10-second intervals in well-rested muscle. Repetitive CMAPs can be difficult to see when the CMAP waveform is broad.[26]

Repetitive Nerve Stimulation in Children

Many children older than 8 to 10 years can be examined using the same technique of repetitive nerve stimulation as for adults, with appropriate adjustments for limb size. Shorter limb length requires great attention to stimulus artifacts. Stimulating electrodes with a shorter

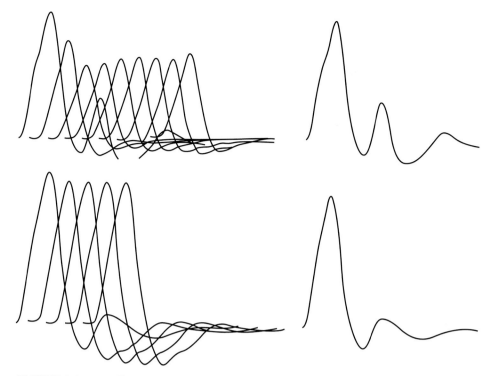

FIGURE 17-15 ■ Repetitive nerve stimulation in a hand muscle of a patient with congenital endplate acetylcholinesterase deficiency, performed before (top) and immediately after (bottom) a maximal voluntary contraction for 30 seconds. The initial response in each train is shown at right. The compound muscle action potential (CMAP) decrement and the amplitude of the repetitive CMAP are less after activation. Copyright D. B. Sanders.

interelectrode distance (1.5 to 2 cm) should be used in infants and small children, but standard recording disk electrodes are suitable. In young and uncooperative children, conscious sedation or general anesthesia is required; the technique of sedation is determined by institutional policy. The tested limb should be immobilized with appropriate restraints in unconscious children, and care should be taken to maintain a suitable temperature in the tested muscle.

There are no well-established normative data for repetitive nerve stimulation in neonates, in whom the neuromuscular junction is immature. Decrementing responses up to 25 percent may be seen in normal neonates at stimulation rates greater than 20 Hz, and increments of 10 percent or more are common at 5 Hz to 10 Hz. Stimulation rates of 3 Hz to 5 Hz are thus best to demonstrate abnormal neuromuscular transmission in this age group.

NEEDLE ELECTROMYOGRAPHY

In patients suspected of having myasthenia gravis, needle-electrode EMG is performed primarily to exclude other diseases that may resemble or occur concomitantly with myasthenia (e.g., inflammatory or ocular myopathy). When neuromuscular transmission is impaired

and there is blocking of impulses to the muscle fibers, the motor unit action potential (MUAP) recorded by the EMG needle electrode may vary in shape and amplitude among consecutive discharges (Fig. 17-16). Blocking of neuromuscular transmission, when severe, can produce MUAPs that are smaller than normal and may be misinterpreted as evidence of myopathy. Fibrillations and positive sharp waves may be seen, especially in the paraspinal muscles and when myasthenia gravis is severe and rapidly progressive.

SINGLE-FIBER ELECTROMYOGRAPHY

Single-fiber electromyography (SF-EMG) is a selective EMG recording technique that allows measurement of neuromuscular transmission in individual endplates in situ.[27] The selectivity of SF-EMG results from the use of a specially constructed concentric needle electrode with a very small recording surface that permits identification of action potentials from individual muscle fibers. When action potentials are recorded from two muscle fibers in the same voluntarily activated motor unit, the time interval between the two potentials varies from discharge to discharge, a manifestation of the neuromuscular jitter (Fig. 17-17). SF-EMG recordings can

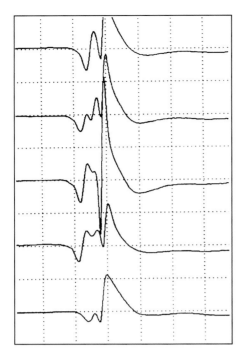

FIGURE 17-16 ■ Motor unit action potentials recorded with a concentric electromyographic electrode from a single motor unit in the biceps muscle of a patient with Lambert–Eaton myasthenic syndrome, demonstrating a varying waveform caused by abnormal neuromuscular transmission. Calibration: 1 msec/div, 0.5 mV/div. (From Sanders DB: Lambert–Eaton myasthenic syndrome: clinical diagnosis, immune-mediated mechanisms and update of therapies. Ann Neurol, 37:Suppl 1, S63, 1995, with permission.)

also be made with axonal stimulation via a monopolar needle electrode placed near the nerve.[28] This can be particularly useful in patients who cannot cooperate (e.g., young children) or have a tremor, and in demonstrating the effect of firing rate on the jitter.

Jitter is quantified as the mean difference between consecutive intervals (MCD), using the formula:

$$\text{MCD} = \frac{|\text{Int}_1 - \text{Int}_2| + |\text{Int}_2 - \text{Int}_3| + \ldots + |\text{Int}_{n-1} - \text{Int}_n|}{n-1}$$

where *Int* is the interpotential interval measured during voluntary activation or the stimulus–response interval measured during axonal stimulation. The normal mean MCD value varies from 10 to 50 μsec among different muscles. Jitter is increased when neuromuscular transmission is disturbed by any process. With more pronounced disturbances, impulses to individual muscle fibers intermittently fail to occur (Fig. 17-18), producing neuromuscular blocking. Only when blocking occurs is there clinical weakness or a decrement on repetitive nerve stimulation.

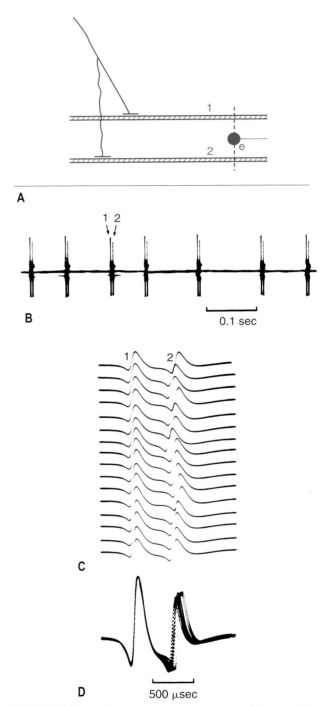

FIGURE 17-17 ■ Single-fiber electromyographic recordings. **A**, The electrode recording surface (e) is positioned to record from two muscle fibers innervated by the same motor nerve. **B**, Paired potentials from the two fibers during slight voluntary contraction of the muscle. **C**, At a faster sweep speed, with the oscilloscope sweep triggered by the rising phase of the first potential, the potential pairs are delayed electronically and displayed in a rastered mode. **D**, Ten oscilloscope sweeps, as obtained in *C*, are superimposed, demonstrating the variations in interpotential intervals (the neuromuscular jitter). (Adapted from Stålberg E, Trontelj J: Single-Fibre Electromyography. Mirvalle, Old Woking, Surrey, UK, 1979, with permission.)

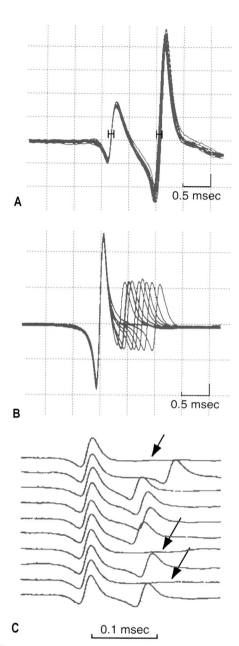

FIGURE 17-18 ■ Representative single fiber electromyographic recordings during voluntary muscle activation. **A**, Ten superimposed discharges of a pair of potentials with normal jitter. **B**, Ten superimposed discharges of a pair of potentials with increased jitter. **C**, Ten discharges of a pair of potentials in which the second potential intermittently blocks (arrows). Copyright D. B. Sanders.

The typical finding in myasthenia gravis is that, within a single muscle, jitter is normal in some motor endplates and increased in others, some of which will have intermittent blocking.[29] To demonstrate the overall degree of abnormality, at least 20 fiber pairs or 30 endplates should be studied in each muscle. The results can be expressed as the mean or median MCD of all fiber pairs

or endplates studied, the percentage of fiber pairs or endplates with blocking, and the percentage with normal jitter. The degree of abnormal jitter correlates with the severity of weakness in the muscle being examined, but jitter usually is increased, even in clinically unaffected muscles.

Measuring Jitter with Concentric Needle Electrodes

By increasing the low-frequency filter settings, it is possible, to some extent, to identify action potentials from single muscle fibers in MUAPs recorded with conventional concentric needle (CN) electrodes. However, because of the larger recording surfaces, it is not possible to determine whether spikes recorded with these electrodes are produced by single action potentials or superimposed potentials from two or more fibers. To make this clear, simple spikes recorded with CN electrodes have been referred to as "apparent single-fiber action potentials" (ASFAPs).[30,31] The following steps should be followed if CN electrodes are used for jitter measurements:[31,32]

1. Use a small CN electrode (pediatric or facial needle).
2. Use a low-frequency (high-pass) filter setting of 1 kHz.
3. Measure jitter during voluntary activation.
4. Exclude spikes with a notch or "shoulder," as they are produced by more than one action potential, and jitter measured from such spikes is influenced unpredictably by the interaction of the comprised action potentials.
5. Measure jitter only between spikes separated by a clear baseline if a voltage level algorithm is used. If a peak detection algorithm is used, jitter can be measured between clearly defined spikes, even if there is no baseline between them.
6. Use reference values specific for CN electrodes.

Jitter values obtained with CN electrodes are usually lower than those obtained with a single-fiber electrode and the difference depends on the jitter measurement algorithm used—that is, on whether it is a voltage level or peak detection algorithm.[32] Using a peak detection algorithm, reference values for jitter obtained with a CN electrode are about 5 μsec lower than those obtained with a single-fiber electrode.[31] Increased jitter detected with CN electrodes indicates abnormal neuromuscular transmission, but mild jitter abnormalities are not detected as well as with single-fiber electrodes. The higher high-pass filter settings reduce the amplitude of the recorded signals; thus spikes as low as 50 μV are acceptable for measurement if they have a rise time less than 300 μsec.

A study of a small number of normal and myasthenia gravis subjects found similar jitter values and equal diagnostic sensitivity of jitter measurements made with CN and single-fiber electrodes when normative values obtained with single-fiber electrodes were used.[30] In a study of 56 patients with myasthenia gravis, jitter measured during voluntary activation with CN electrodes in the orbicularis oculi and extensor digitorum communis (EDC) was abnormal in 96 percent using normative data from 20 control subjects.[33] This sensitivity approximates that reported for recordings made with single-fiber electrodes.

More reference values must be collected from multicenter studies, after agreement on filter settings, signal definitions, and analysis methods. The criteria for acceptable signals for analysis must be well defined, and this is more difficult than the precise definition used in SF-EMG. More extensive studies, including in other neuromuscular diseases, are necessary to determine the specificity of CN jitter studies.

The most accurate jitter measurements require a well-maintained single-fiber electrode but, if this is not available, jitter analysis can be made with a small CN electrode. Because of their larger pickup area, monopolar needle electrodes are even more likely to record superimposed action potentials and should not be used for jitter measurements. Axonal stimulation studies using CN electrodes have more technical pitfalls than those performed with voluntary activation, and the results of such studies should be interpreted with caution.

DISEASES WITH ABNORMAL NEUROMUSCULAR TRANSMISSION

Myasthenia Gravis

Acquired myasthenia gravis is an autoimmune disease that can begin at any age, with a modal age at onset in the third decade of life and a later secondary peak. The diagnosis is made by demonstrating fluctuating weakness, commonly of the ocular and oropharyngeal muscles, that improves after the administration of cholinesterase inhibitors such as edrophonium. Weakness varies greatly among patients and from time to time in the same patient. In some patients, weakness is confined to the ocular muscles.

Circulating antibodies to the AChR are found in the serum of most patients with acquired myasthenia gravis. The abnormality of neuromuscular transmission in these patients is caused by complement-mediated disruption of the postsynaptic muscle membrane, reduced

AChR concentration on the muscle endplate, and a direct blocking effect of antibodies on these receptors.

Antibodies to MuSK are found in approximately 40 percent of patients with generalized acquired myasthenia gravis who do not have antibodies to the acetylcholine receptor,[34] and in occasional patients with ocular myasthenia. These antibodies are found predominantly in women, and weak muscles may be atrophic. In many of these patients, weakness predominates in facial or neck and shoulder muscles in patterns that differ from most patients with non-MuSK myasthenia gravis.[35] Jitter measurement is the most sensitive electrodiagnostic procedure in these patients, at least in part because repetitive nerve stimulation may be normal in unaffected limb muscles and may be impossible to perform in the most severely involved muscles, such as neck extensors. Jitter may be normal in limb muscles but markedly abnormal in facial muscles, or abnormal only in muscles that are weak (Fig. 17-19). Thus, electrodiagnostic testing should focus on proximal limb and facial muscles, as well as clinically weak muscles.

Antibodies to the acetylcholine receptor or MuSK confirm the diagnosis of myasthenia gravis, but these antibodies are not found in about half of patients with purely ocular myasthenia or in 10 percent of patients with generalized myasthenia. Electrodiagnostic tests are of great value in patients who do not have these antibodies.

The electrodiagnostic approach in patients suspected of having myasthenia gravis is determined by the tests available to the electrodiagnostic consultant and by the clinical presentation of the patient. One approach is to begin with repetitive nerve stimulation studies. If there is weakness in limb muscles, a hand muscle can be tested first. If there is no decrement in this muscle, a proximal shoulder muscle can be tested. We have found a decrementing response to 3-Hz repetitive nerve stimulation of a hand or shoulder muscle in 76 percent of untreated patients with generalized myasthenia (Fig. 17-20). If there is no decrement in either of these muscles, jitter measurements can be performed at this point. If SF-EMG is not readily available, repetitive nerve stimulation of a facial muscle is performed.

Repetitive nerve stimulation shows a decrement in only about 50 percent of patients with purely ocular weakness (see Fig. 17-20). In these patients, testing may begin with jitter measurements of a facial muscle.

In our experience, jitter is increased in the EDC in almost 90 percent of myasthenic patients who have weakness in any limb muscle or in the oropharyngeal muscles. Thus, it is reasonable to examine the EDC first in patients with more than ocular muscle symptoms. If jitter is normal in that muscle, a facial muscle is tested. We usually test the frontalis at that point because most

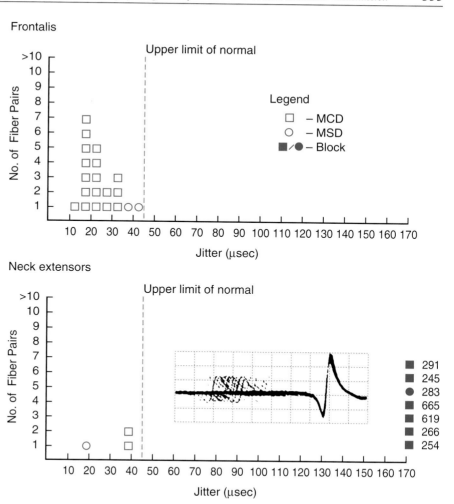

FIGURE 17-19 ■ Histograms of jitter measurements made during voluntary activation in the frontalis and neck extensor muscles in a patient with myasthenia gravis and muscle-specific tyrosine kinase (MuSK) antibody. Weakness was maximum in neck extensor muscles. Vertical lines indicate the upper limit of normal for the tested muscle. Filled symbols indicate that blocking was present. In the bottom panel, superimposed discharges of one pair of potentials with marked jitter are displayed. Jitter was also normal in the extensor digitorum communis in this patient (not shown). MCD, mean difference of consecutive interpotential intervals; MSD, mean difference of sorted interpotential intervals. Copyright D. B. Sanders.

patients can activate it easily and because jitter is increased in this muscle in most patients with myasthenia. If the frontalis is normal, the orbicularis oculi is examined.[36] Jitter is increased in at least one of these muscles in almost all myasthenic patients.

In patients with weakness limited to a few muscles, it may be necessary to examine a weak muscle to demonstrate abnormal jitter. This is particularly true in patients with MuSK-positive myasthenia who have weakness mainly in shoulder or neck muscles (see Fig. 17-19[35,37]) or in

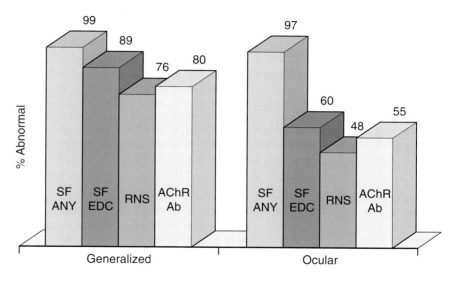

FIGURE 17-20 ■ Sensitivity of diagnostic tests in 844 patients with generalized or ocular myasthenia gravis, performed before thymectomy or immunosuppression. SFANY, increased jitter in any tested muscle; SFEDC, increased jitter in extensor digitorum communis; RNS, abnormal decrement in a hand or shoulder muscle; AChR Ab, elevated acetylcholine receptor antibody level. (Sanders DB, Massey JM, Juel VC et al: unpublished data)

others in whom weakness is most prominent in or limited to facial muscles.[38]

There is a strong correlation between change in clinical status and change in jitter measurements in patients with myasthenia gravis.[29] Jitter measurements may be of value in predicting change in disease severity. For example, when the jitter in a muscle has been constant for several months, a subsequent increase in jitter usually accompanies or heralds clinical deterioration.

In patients with myasthenia gravis, jitter increases during sustained muscle activity, with increasing temperature, and during ischemia. In patients who are not receiving cholinesterase inhibitors, jitter and blocking decrease after the administration of edrophonium.[39] In patients receiving cholinesterase inhibitors, jitter may increase in some endplates after injection of edrophonium, indicating cholinergic overdose in those endplates. The diagnostic sensitivity of SF-EMG usually is not affected by ongoing treatment with cholinesterase inhibitors. If jitter measurements are normal in a patient taking these medications, however, testing should be repeated after they have been discontinued.[40] If serial studies are performed on patients taking cholinesterase inhibitors, these medications should be withheld for at least 12 hours before testing, or follow-up studies should be performed at a constant time after a dose of medication.

Most patients, including children older than 7 years, can cooperate for jitter studies with voluntary activation, although it may not be possible to make recordings from distal limb muscles in patients with a tremor. A facial or proximal limb muscle usually can be studied successfully in such patients, or jitter can be measured with axonal stimulation.

COMPARISON OF ELECTRODIAGNOSTIC TECHNIQUES IN MYASTHENIA GRAVIS

Repetitive nerve stimulation is the most commonly used electrodiagnostic test of neuromuscular transmission. It has the major advantage of being relatively simple and easy to perform. Several muscles must be tested to obtain the best diagnostic yield. Studies of hand muscles are well tolerated by most patients and present few technical problems, but the findings are normal in many patients with myasthenia. Studies in proximal or facial muscles detect abnormalities in most myasthenic patients with moderate or severe weakness, but are normal in many patients with mild or restricted ocular weakness. A decremental response to repetitive nerve stimulation may also be seen in diseases of nerve or muscle (Fig. 17-21), and these conditions should be excluded

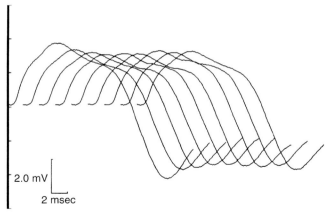

FIGURE 17-21 ■ Repetitive nerve stimulation studies at 3 Hz in the biceps muscle of a patient with rapidly progressive motor neuron disease. There is a 12 percent decrement in the fourth response, and thereafter the compound muscle action potentials return toward the initial size, producing a "U-shaped" envelope.

by appropriate electrodiagnostic tests whenever a decrement is found.

SF-EMG is the most sensitive electrodiagnostic test of neuromuscular transmission; it demonstrates increased jitter in virtually all myasthenic patients if the muscles most likely to be involved are examined. SF-EMG requires extensive training and experience. Because it is so sensitive, SF-EMG can be especially useful in demonstrating abnormalities in patients with mild or ocular myasthenia. SF-EMG is particularly valuable in excluding myasthenia; if jitter is normal in a weak muscle, the weakness is not caused by abnormal neuromuscular transmission. Because of its great sensitivity, however, SF-EMG also demonstrates increased jitter in nerve or muscle diseases, which must be excluded by appropriate nerve conduction and electromyographic tests before it is concluded that the patient has myasthenia gravis.

Nerve conduction velocity measurements are normal in myasthenia. The size of the resting CMAP is normal, although the average CMAP amplitude is below the normal average.

Genetic Forms of Myasthenia

Several forms of myasthenia arise from genetic defects and have no immunologic basis. AChR antibodies are not found in patients with these conditions. Some forms of genetic myasthenia have characteristic clinical features and electrodiagnostic findings.[25]

Congenital myasthenia is a clinical term used to describe patients with one of several genetic neuromuscular defects who have ophthalmoparesis and ptosis at birth or shortly thereafter.[41] Mild facial paresis may be present, and mild generalized weakness sometimes develops as well, but major dysfunction usually is limited to the eye muscles. Edrophonium usually produces transient improvement in ocular motility. Intracellular recordings demonstrate reduced MEPP amplitude and normal quantal release in some patients, as in acquired myasthenia gravis. In others, however, MEPP amplitude is not reduced, indicating that the pathophysiology is not the same in all patients with congenital myasthenia. The electrodiagnostic findings are similar to those of the acquired disorder; repetitive nerve stimulation demonstrates a decremental response that is corrected by edrophonium, and SF-EMG shows increased jitter. Intracellular recordings of biopsied muscle or molecular studies must be performed to determine the physiologic abnormality and the specific diagnosis in each patient.

Familial infantile myasthenia (also known as congenital myasthenic syndrome with episodic apnea; CMS-EA) has characteristic clinical and electrophysiologic features that differ from those of congenital myasthenia. Affected children are hypotonic at birth and have severe and repeated bouts of respiratory insufficiency and feeding difficulty. Fluctuating ptosis may occur, but otherwise ocular muscle function is usually normal. Edrophonium provides transient clinical benefit. Improvement occurs after a few weeks, but episodes of weakness and life-threatening apnea recur throughout infancy and childhood, sometimes even into adult life. Physiologic studies demonstrate findings consistent with an abnormality of ACh resynthesis or mobilization. In weak muscles, repetitive nerve stimulation may demonstrate a decremental response, but in strong muscles a decremental response

may be seen only after sustained voluntary muscle activity or prolonged nerve stimulation. In particular, the nerve is stimulated at 3 to 5 Hz for 5 minutes, after which brief trains of 3- to 5-Hz stimuli are delivered. These trains demonstrate a decrementing pattern that clears over a 20- to 30-minute period (Fig. 17-22) and can be corrected with edrophonium. Progressive neuromuscular blockade can also be demonstrated with SF-EMG, which shows increasing jitter during prolonged nerve stimulation (Fig. 17-23).

Slow channel syndrome may not become symptomatic until adult life, which makes it difficult to distinguish this condition from acquired myasthenia gravis. The physiologic abnormality is a prolonged open time of the ACh channel. Symptoms always begin after infancy, sometimes as late as the third decade. Slowly progressive weakness selectively involves the arm, leg, neck, and facial muscles, and the symptomatic muscles may be atrophic. The disease is transmitted by autosomal-dominant inheritance, and a family history of similar illness is often obtained. Repetitive nerve stimulation produces a decremental response. Repetitive CMAPs are seen in most, but not all, muscles,[26] and are similar to those seen with AChE inhibitor toxicity and congenital endplate AChE deficiency (see Fig. 17-15). Cholinesterase inhibitors cause an increase in the number and size of repetitive CMAPs in slow channel syndrome but have no effect in congenital endplate AChE deficiency[25]; this difference can be used to distinguish these conditions.

In congenital endplate AChE deficiency, weakness of facial, oropharyngeal, neck, and limb muscles is apparent in the neonatal period or shortly thereafter.

FIGURE 17-22 ■ Repetitive nerve stimulation tests in the hypothenar muscles of a patient with congenital myasthenic syndrome with episodic apnea. The ulnar nerve was stimulated at the wrist with five 1-minute 3-Hz trains separated by rest for 5 seconds. **A,** No decrement occurs during the first two trains, but the amplitude began to fall during the third train. **B,** Immediately after the end of continuous stimulation, there was a greater than 30 percent decrement between the first and the fourth volleys. The decrement returned toward baseline values during the ensuing 20 minutes. (From Stålberg EV, Trontelj JV, Sanders DB: Single Fiber Electromyography. Edshagen, Fiskebäckskil, 2010, with permission.)

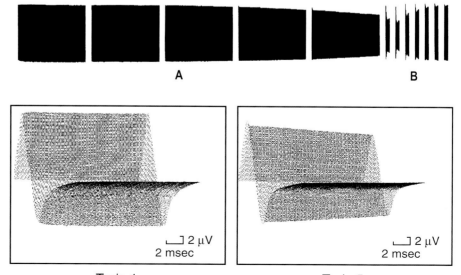

A   B

⌐ 2 µV
2 msec

⌐ 2 µV
2 msec

Train 1   Train 5

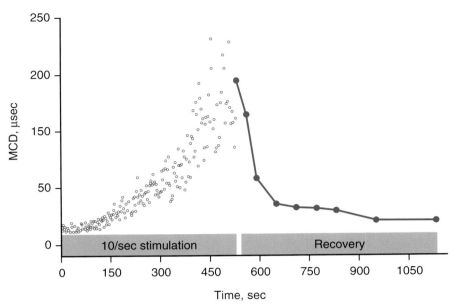

FIGURE 17-23 ▪ Congenital myasthenic syndrome with episodic apnea. Jitter measured in action potentials from one muscle fiber in the extensor digitorum communis during intramuscular axonal stimulation at 10 Hz. Open circles, mean difference between consecutive intervals (MCD) calculated from consecutive groups of 50 responses during continuous stimulation. Filled circles, MCD calculated from 50 responses during intermittent stimulation for 5 seconds at intervals after the end of continuous stimulation. Jitter was 20 μsec in this endplate initially. After 2 minutes of continuous stimulation, the jitter began to increase. Blocking was first seen after 6 minutes, when jitter had increased to 50 μsec. After 8 minutes of stimulation, jitter was greater than 100 μsec and 50 percent of responses were blocked. After continuous stimulation ceased, jitter fell rapidly and there was no blocking after 2 minutes. After 7 minutes, jitter had returned to initial values. (From Stålberg EV, Trontelj JV, Sanders DB: Single Fiber Electromyography. Edshagen, Fiskebäckskil, 2010, with permission.)

The pupillary light response is sluggish, and there is variable ptosis and ophthalmoparesis. Weakness progresses slowly, and patients develop postural, then fixed spinal column deformity. There is no response to AChE inhibitors. A decrement is seen during 2-Hz repetitive nerve stimulation, and there are repetitive CMAPs similar to those seen in slow channel syndrome.

Limb-girdle myasthenia typically becomes apparent during the teenage years, with proximal muscle weakness that improves after treatment with AChE inhibitors but slowly progresses otherwise. Repetitive nerve stimulation demonstrates a decremental pattern, and there are EMG and biopsy findings of a myopathy.

Lambert–Eaton Myasthenic Syndrome

The Lambert–Eaton myasthenic syndrome (LEMS) is a rare condition in which weakness results from a presynaptic abnormality of ACh release at the neuromuscular junction. It was described first as a paraneoplastic syndrome in patients with lung cancer, but about one-half of patients with LEMS do not have cancer. The clinical picture is usually quite different from that of myasthenia gravis: patients commonly have symmetric proximal weakness, autonomic dysfunction, and hypoactive or absent

tendon reflexes. Strength may improve with repeated effort, but this is not always seen. Dry mouth is a common complaint. The response to AChE inhibitors is usually poor. There is an exaggerated response to neuromuscular blocking agents, and some cases are recognized when prolonged apnea follows exposure to these drugs during surgery. Defective release of ACh from motor nerve terminals in LEMS is caused by an autoimmune attack directed against calcium channels on the presynaptic nerve terminal.

ELECTROMYOGRAPHIC FINDINGS

The following findings on repetitive nerve stimulation are highly characteristic of LEMS and constitute the most definitive electrodiagnostic features (see Fig. 17-6):

1. CMAPs are usually small, often as low as 10 percent of normal.
2. There is a decrementing response to stimulation at 3 to 5 Hz.
3. CMAP amplitude increases at least 100 percent after activation or during stimulation at rates greater than 20 Hz.

Virtually all patients with LEMS have a decrementing response to 3-Hz stimulation in a hand or foot muscle, and almost all have low-amplitude CMAPs.[42] Facilitation exceeding 100 percent is not seen in all muscles, and it may therefore be necessary to examine several muscles to demonstrate this abnormality. These various abnormalities may be masked partially by low muscle temperature, and muscles should be warmed before testing. In proximal muscles, the CMAP amplitude is usually normal, there is usually a decrementing pattern, and the amount of facilitation is variable.

Facilitation greater than 50 percent in any muscle suggests LEMS, but may also be seen in myasthenia gravis. If facilitation exceeds 50 percent in most muscles tested or is greater than 400 percent in any muscle, the patient almost certainly has LEMS. If facilitation is less than 50 percent in all muscles tested, the patient still may have LEMS, especially if weakness has been present for only a short time or the patient has been partially treated.

To demonstrate the characteristic findings of LEMS, the following tests are performed in the abductor pollicis brevis or abductor digiti minimi muscles, with stimulation of the median or ulnar nerve, respectively, at the wrist:

1. The amplitude of the CMAP elicited by a single supramaximal nerve stimulus is measured in the warmed, rested muscle (Fig. 17-24).
2. The patient is asked to contract the tested muscle maximally for 10 seconds and then completely relax it. A single supramaximal nerve stimulus is delivered within 5 seconds after the end of activation. The amplitude of the CMAP is compared with that obtained before activation. This sequence is repeated three times, and the average change in amplitude is used

to assess facilitation. Alternatively, nerve stimulation at 20 Hz may be used to activate the muscle (see Fig. 17-6). The amplitude of the maximum CMAP after 5 to 10 seconds of continuous stimulation is compared with that of the initial response. Pseudofacilitation may contribute significantly to amplitude changes produced by high-frequency stimulation and may be indistinguishable from facilitation (see Fig. 17-10). High-frequency stimulation is also painful.

3. After several minutes of relaxation, a train of low-frequency (2- to 5-Hz) stimuli is delivered to the nerve, and the decrement in the fourth or fifth response is measured.
4. When a decrement exceeds 10 percent and facilitation is between 35 percent and 100 percent, steps 1 to 3 are repeated in the other muscle in the same hand. If facilitation is between 35 percent and 100 percent in both hand muscles, steps 1 to 3 are repeated in the extensor digitorum brevis muscle in the foot, with stimulation of the fibular (peroneal) nerve at the ankle.

LEMS may be suspected initially when needle EMG demonstrates markedly unstable MUAPs (see Fig. 17-16), a typical finding in this condition.

Jitter is increased markedly in all tested muscles in patients with LEMS, with frequent blocking. In many endplates, the jitter and blocking decrease as the firing rate increases; however, this is not seen in all endplates or in all patients with LEMS.[43,44] Moreover, jitter and blocking may also improve at higher firing rates in some endplates in myasthenia gravis; thus improvement of jitter and blocking at higher rates, unless dramatic, does not necessarily indicate a presynaptic abnormality.

Nerve conduction velocity measurements are usually normal in LEMS unless there is a coincident peripheral neuropathy.

Overlap Syndrome

No single clinical or electromyographic feature distinguishes between myasthenia gravis and LEMS in all patients. Facilitation of as much as 100 percent at high stimulation rates has been reported in patients with clinically typical myasthenia gravis. Conversely, patients with LEMS may have EMG features more characteristic of myasthenia gravis at some time during their illness.[45] In other patients, mixed clinical and EMG features make it impossible to distinguish between the two diseases. A true overlap syndrome, with antibodies against both voltage-gated calcium channels and ACh receptors, has

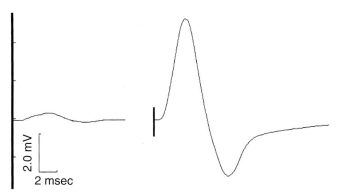

FIGURE 17-24 ▪ Compound muscle action potentials recorded from a hand muscle in a patient with Lambert–Eaton myasthenic syndrome, before (left) and immediately after (right) maximum voluntary contraction of the muscle for 10 seconds.

been confirmed in a small number of reports,[46–49] and the author has seen one such case among 1,200 patients with acquired myasthenia gravis and 102 with LEMS.

Botulism

Botulism results from a toxin produced by an anaerobic bacterium, *Clostridium botulinum*. Major symptoms of botulism include blurred vision, dysphagia, and dysarthria. Pupillary responses to light are impaired, and tendon reflexes are reduced variably. The weakness progresses for several days and then reaches a plateau. Fatal respiratory paralysis may occur rapidly. Most patients have autonomic dysfunction (e.g., dry mouth, constipation, or urinary retention). In patients who survive, recovery may take many months but is usually complete. The edrophonium (Tensilon) test is positive in only about one-third of patients and does not distinguish botulism from other causes of neuromuscular blockade.[50]

Food-borne botulism results from ingestion of botulinum toxin in incompletely sterilized canned foods. Neuromuscular symptoms usually begin 12 to 36 hours after ingestion of contaminated food.

The most common form of botulism in the United States today is wound botulism, which occurs predominantly in drug abusers following subcutaneous injection of heroin.[51] *Clostridium* bacteria colonize the injection site and release toxin that produces local and patchy systemic weakness. The diagnosis of wound botulism is confirmed by wound cultures and serum assay for botulinum toxin.

Infant botulism results from the growth of *C. botulinum* in the infant gastrointestinal tract and the elaboration of small quantities of toxin over a prolonged period. Symptoms of constipation, lethargy, poor suck, and weak cry usually begin at about 4 months of age. Examination reveals weakness of the limb and oropharyngeal muscles, poorly reactive pupils, and hypoactive tendon reflexes. Most patients require ventilatory support. The diagnosis of infant botulism is confirmed by demonstrating botulinum toxin in the stool or by isolating *C. botulinum* from stool culture.

ELECTROPHYSIOLOGIC FINDINGS

Electrophysiologic abnormalities in botulism tend to evolve with time and may not be present early in the disease. The EMG findings in botulism include the following[52]:

1. Reduced CMAP amplitude in at least two muscles
2. At least 20 percent facilitation of CMAP amplitude during tetanic stimulation
3. Persistence of facilitation for at least 2 minutes after activation
4. No postactivation exhaustion.

Not all patients with botulism meet the first criterion. If none of these criteria is met, the diagnosis of botulism is unlikely. If all four are met, only hypermagnesemia is in the differential diagnosis.

SF-EMG demonstrates markedly increased jitter and blocking, and has been abnormal in all reported cases with food-borne or wound botulism.[53] Jitter and blocking may decrease as the firing rate increases, but this is not a consistent finding.[54]

Other Conditions with Disturbed Neuromuscular Transmission

Neuromuscular transmission may be abnormal in diseases other than those that affect the neuromuscular junction primarily.

Fluctuating weakness that responds to AChE inhibitors is common in patients with *amyotrophic lateral sclerosis* (ALS). A decrement on repetitive nerve stimulation has been described in two-thirds of patients with ALS, and increased jitter and blocking on SF-EMG are seen in most patients with this disease. Various manifestations of abnormal neuromuscular transmission have also been reported in syringomyelia, poliomyelitis, peripheral neuropathy, and inflammatory myopathy. The distinction between myasthenia gravis and these diseases is made clinically and by other electrophysiologic techniques. In oculocraniosomatic myopathy, the distribution of weakness may resemble ocular myasthenia, but the course is slowly progressive and the weakness does not fluctuate or improve after edrophonium. Increased jitter, especially in the facial muscles, has been found in patients with this condition.[55] Most of these patients have myopathic features on EMG of shoulder muscles, and muscle biopsy usually shows characteristic "ragged-red fibers."

Many drugs have neuromuscular blocking actions. These effects usually are clinically apparent only in patients with renal or hepatic disease, electrolyte disturbance, or abnormal neuromuscular transmission secondary to myasthenia gravis or LEMS; or after administration of neuromuscular blocking agents during general anesthesia. The aminoglycoside antibiotics (e.g., streptomycin, neomycin, kanamycin, gentamicin, tobramycin, and amikacin), ciprofloxacin, erythromycin, polymyxin, colistin, and colistimethate are the most common offenders. Others are quinine, quinidine, and procainamide, and beta-adrenergic blocking agents (e.g., propranolol, oxyprenolol, and timolol). For a comprehensive account of this subject, the reader is referred to reviews by Howard[56] and Wittbrodt.[57]

Magnesium blocks neuromuscular transmission by interfering with the action of calcium in the release of

ACh from the motor nerve terminal. *Hypermagnesemia* occurs in patients with renal insufficiency who receive oral magnesium (e.g., laxatives) and in women who receive magnesium for pre-eclampsia. Severe weakness develops when the serum level of magnesium exceeds 10 mEq/liter, but symptoms may appear at lower levels, especially if the patient has an underlying disease affecting neuromuscular transmission. The clinical manifestations of hypermagnesemia resemble LEMS: proximal muscle weakness that may progress to respiratory insufficiency in severe cases, relative sparing of ocular muscles, and depressed tendon reflexes. The diagnosis is made by demonstrating elevated serum magnesium levels and by observing the return of tendon reflexes as the serum magnesium level declines. Edrophonium may improve strength in some patients. The response to repetitive nerve stimulation resembles that in botulism: low-amplitude CMAP responses, a decremental response to low-frequency stimulation, prolonged facilitation after muscle activation, and no postactivation exhaustion.

Organophosphates irreversibly inhibit AChE, producing neuromuscular blockade as well as autonomic and central nervous system dysfunction. They are used as insecticides and as chemical warfare agents. EMG studies can be of great value in making a diagnosis and in following the course of intoxication by these agents. When AChE has been blocked, excess ACh accumulates at the neuromuscular junction and impairs neuromuscular transmission by depolarizing the postjunctional muscle membrane. Receptors on the presynaptic nerve are also activated by the excess ACh, producing repetitive discharges when the nerve is activated. Repetitive nerve stimulation produces a decrementing pattern. The combination of repetitive discharges and a decrement to repetitive stimulation is seen within hours after ingestion of organophosphates and resembles findings in slow channel syndrome and congenital AChE deficiency. A distinctive "decrement-increment" pattern of response to repetitive stimulation is seen in the early stages of organophosphate intoxication and again later as the intoxication resolves.[58] At the peak of intoxication, neuromuscular blockade may be so severe that no response is seen after the first few stimuli in a train.

Neuromuscular block is the primary effect of envenomation by cobras, kraits, and some other poisonous snakes. Toxins of snakes such as the cobra and death adder, which act postsynaptically and bind competitively to the receptor, produce a pattern of weakness identical to that of myasthenia gravis. In such cases, EMG demonstrates a decrementing response and weakness is reversed by AChE inhibitors.

REFERENCES

1. Liyanage Y, Hoch W, Beeson D et al: The agrin/muscle-specific kinase pathway: new targets for autoimmune and genetic disorders at the neuromuscular junction. Muscle Nerve, 25:4, 2002
2. Jolly F: Ueber myasthenia gravis pseudoparalytica. Berl Klin Wochenschr, 32:1, 1895
3. Harvey AM, Masland RL: A method for the study of neuromuscular transmission in human subjects. Bull Johns Hopkins Hosp, 68:81, 1941
4. Harvey AM, Masland RL: The electromyogram in myasthenia gravis. Bull Johns Hopkins Hosp, 69:1, 1941
5. Sonoo M, Ueseugi H, Mochizuki A et al: Single fiber EMG and repetitive nerve stimulation of the same extensor digitorum communis muscle in myasthenia gravis. J Clin Neurophysiol, 112:300, 2001
6. Rutkove SB: The effects of temperature in neuromuscular electrophysiology. Muscle Nerve, 24:867, 2002
7. Oh SJ, Eslami N, Nishihira T et al: Electrophysiological and clinical correlation in myasthenia gravis. Trans Am Neurol Assoc, 12:348, 1982
8. Oh SJ: Repetitive nerve stimulation in various diseases. p. 140. In Oh SJ (ed): Electromyography and Neuromuscular Transmission Studies. Williams & Wilkins, Baltimore, 1988
9. Aiello I, Sau GF, Bissakou M et al: Standardization of changes in M-wave area to repetitive stimulation. Electromyogr Clin Neurophysiol, 26:529, 1986
10. Tim RW, Sanders DB: Repetitive nerve stimulation studies in the Lambert–Eaton syndrome. Muscle Nerve, 17:995, 1994
11. Kennett RP, Fawcett PR: Repetitive nerve stimulation of anconeus in the assessment of neuromuscular transmission disorders. Electroencephalogr Clin Neurophysiol, 89:170, 1993
12. Schady W, MacDermott N: On the choice of muscle in the electrophysiological assessment of myasthenia gravis. Electromyogr Clin Neurophysiol, 32:99, 1992
13. Yiannikas C, Sheean GL, King PJL: The relative sensitivities of the axillary and accessory nerves in the diagnosis of myasthenia gravis. Muscle Nerve, 17:561, 1994
14. Schumm F, Stohr M: Accessory nerve stimulation in the assessment of myasthenia gravis. Muscle Nerve, 7:147, 1984
15. Ruys-Van Oeyen AE, van Dijk JG: Repetitive nerve stimulation of the nasalis muscle: technique and normal values. Muscle Nerve, 26:279, 2002
16. Oey PL, Wieneke GH, Hoogenraad TU et al: Ocular myasthenia gravis: the diagnostic yield of repetitive nerve stimulation and stimulated single fiber EMG of orbicularis oculi muscle and infrared reflection oculography. Muscle Nerve, 16:142, 1993
17. Niks EH, Badrising UA, Verschuuren JJ et al: Decremental response of the nasalis and hypothenar muscles in myasthenia gravis. Muscle Nerve, 28:236, 2003
18. Krarup C: Electrical and mechanical responses in the platysma and in the adductor pollicis muscles: in patients with myasthenia gravis. J Neurol Neurosurg Psychiatry, 40:241, 1977

19. Pavesi G, Cattaneo L, Tinchelli S et al: Masseteric repetitive nerve stimulation in the diagnosis of myasthenia gravis. Clin Neurophysiol, 112:1064, 2001

20. Zifco UA, Nicolle MW, Griswold W et al: Repetitive phrenic nerve stimulation in myasthenia gravis. Neurology, 53:1083, 1999

21. Mier A, Brophy C, Moxham J et al: Repetitive stimulation of phrenic nerves in myasthenia gravis. Thorax, 47:640, 1992

22. Chen R, Collins S, Remtulla H et al: Phrenic nerve conduction study in normal subjects. Muscle Nerve, 18:330, 1995

23. Oh SJ, Head T, Fesenheimer J et al: Peroneal nerve repetitive nerve stimulation test: its value in diagnosis of myasthenia gravis and Lambert-Eaton myasthenic syndrome. Muscle Nerve, 18:867, 1995

24. van Dijk JG, Lammers GJ, Wintzen AR et al: Repetitive CMAPs: mechanisms of neural and synaptic genesis. Muscle Nerve, 19:1127, 1996

25. Harper CM: Congenital myasthenic syndromes. p. 1687. In Brown WF, Bolton CF, Aminoff MJ (eds): Neuromuscular Function and Disease. WB Saunders, Philadelphia, 2002

26. Bedlack RS, Bertorini TE, Sanders DB: Hidden afterdischarges in slow channel congenital myasthenic syndrome. J Clin Neuromusc Dis, 1:186, 2000

27. Stålberg EV, Trontelj JV, Sanders DB: Single Fiber EMG. 3rd Ed. Edshagen, Fiskebäckskil, 2010

28. Stålberg E, Trontelj JV: The study of normal and abnormal neuromuscular transmission with single fibre electromyography. J Neurosci Methods, 74:145, 1997

29. Stålberg EV, Trontelj JV, Sanders DB: Myasthenia gravis and other disorders of neuromuscular transmission. p. 218. In Single Fiber EMG. Edshagen, Fiskebäckskil, 2010

30. Ertas M, Baslo MB, Yildiz N et al: Concentric needle electrode for neuromuscular jitter analysis. Muscle Nerve, 23:715, 2000

31. Stålberg EV, Sanders DB: Jitter recordings with concentric needle electrodes. Muscle Nerve, 40:331, 2009

32. Stålberg EV, Trontelj JV, Sanders DB: Measuring jitter with concentric electrodes. p. 267. In Single Fiber EMG. Edshagen, Fiskebäckskil, 2010

33. Sarrigiannis PG, Kennett RP, Read S et al: Single fiber EMG with a concentric needle electrode: validation in myasthenia gravis. Muscle Nerve, 33:61, 2006

34. Guptill JT, Sanders DB: Update on MuSK antibody positive myasthenia gravis. Curr Opin Neurol, 23:530, 2010

35. Stickler DE, Massey JM, Sanders DB: MuSK-antibody positive myasthenia gravis: clinical and electrodiagnostic patterns. Clin Neurophysiol, 116:2065, 2005

36. Valls-Canals J, Povedano M, Montero J et al: Stimulated single-fiber EMG of the frontalis and orbicularis oculi muscles in ocular myasthenia gravis. Muscle Nerve, 28:501, 2003

37. Sanders DB, Juel VC: MuSK-antibody positive myasthenia gravis: Questions from the clinic. J Neuroimmunol, 85:201–202, 2008

38. Evoli A, Tonali PA, Padua L et al: Clinical correlates with anti-MuSK antibodies in generalized seronegative myasthenia gravis. Brain, 126:2304, 2003

39. Stålberg EV, Trontelj JV, Sanders DB: Pharmacological studies. p. 180. In Single Fiber EMG. Edshagen, Fiskebäckskil, 2010

40. Massey JM, Sanders DB, Howard JF, Jr: The effect of cholinesterase inhibitors on SFEMG in myasthenia gravis. Muscle Nerve, 12:154, 1989

41. Engel AG: Congenital myasthenic syndromes. p. 285. In Engel AG (ed): Neuromuscular Junction Disorders. Elsevier, Edinburgh, 2008

42. Tim RW, Massey JM, Sanders DB: Lambert–Eaton myasthenic syndrome. Electrodiagnostic findings and response to treatment. Neurology, 54:2176, 2000

43. Trontelj JV, Stålberg E: Single motor end-plates in myasthenia gravis and LEMS at different firing rates. Muscle Nerve, 14:226, 1991

44. Sanders DB: The effect of firing rate on neuromuscular jitter in Lambert–Eaton myasthenic syndrome. Muscle Nerve, 15:256, 1992

45. Scoppetta C, Casali C, Vaccario ML et al: Difficult diagnosis of Eaton Lambert myasthenic syndrome. Muscle Nerve, 7:680, 1984

46. Oh SJ, Sher E: MG and LEMS overlap syndrome: case report with electrophysiological and immunological evidence. Clin Neurophysiol, 116:1167, 2005

47. Newsom-Davis J, Leys K, Vincent A et al: Immunological evidence for the co-existence of the Lambert–Eaton myasthenic syndrome and myasthenia gravis in two patients. J Neurol Neurosurg Psychiatry, 54:452, 1991

48. Katz JS, Wolfe GI, Bryan WW et al: Acetylcholine receptor antibodies in the Lambert–Eaton myasthenic syndrome. Neurology, 50:470, 1998

49. Kanzato N, Motomura M, Suehara M et al: Lambert–Eaton myasthenic syndrome with ophthalmoparesis and pseudoblepharospasm. Muscle Nerve, 22:1727, 1999

50. Burningham MD, Walter FG, Mechem C et al: Wound botulism. Ann Emerg Med, 24:1184, 1994

51. Anonymous: Wound botulism—California, 1995. MMWR, 44:889, 1995

52. Gutierrez AR, Bodensteiner J, Gutmann L: Electrodiagnosis of infantile botulism. J Child Neurol, 9:362, 1994

53. Padua L, Aprile I, Lo Monaco M et al: Neurophysiological assessment in the diagnosis of botulism: usefulness of single-fiber EMG. Muscle Nerve, 22:1388, 1999

54. Mandler RN, Maselli RA: Stimulated single-fiber electromyography in wound botulism. Muscle Nerve, 19:1171, 1996

55. Krendel DA, Sanders DB, Massey JM: Single fiber electromyography in chronic progressive external ophthalmoplegia. Muscle Nerve, 10:299, 1987

56. Howard JF, Jr, Sanders DB: Drugs and other toxins with adverse effects on the neuromuscular junction. p. 369. In Engel AG (ed): Neuromuscular Junction Disorders. Elsevier, Edinburgh, 2008

57. Wittbrodt ET: Drugs and myasthenia gravis—an update. Arch Intern Med, 157:399, 1997

58. Besser R, Gutmann L, Dillmann U et al: End-plate dysfunction in acute organophosphate intoxication. Neurology, 39:561, 1989

H-Reflex and F-Response Studies

MORRIS A. FISHER

H reflexes and F waves are commonly recorded electrophysiologic responses (Figs. 18-1, 18-2, and 18-3). H reflexes are reflexes that are produced by afferent conduction in large afferent fibers and by efferent conduction in alpha motor neurons. By contrast, F waves are produced by antidromic activation ("backfiring") of the alpha motor neurons. Despite their differences (Table 18-1), they commonly are discussed together. H reflexes and F waves are studied for similar clinical problems, are found at comparable latencies, reflect conduction to and from the spinal cord, and involve motor neuron activation.

H REFLEX

Physiology

In 1918, Hoffman described a reflex response in calf muscles that followed stimulation of the posterior tibial nerve and was comparable in latency to the Achilles reflex.[1,2] In recognition of Hoffman's original contribution, the response was named the H reflex by Magladery and McDougal.[3]

Because H reflexes involve conduction from the periphery to and from the spinal cord, they occur at latencies considerably longer than the latency of a direct motor response. A necessary condition for establishing an H reflex is that this "late" response must be larger than the preceding direct motor response. This condition can occur only with central amplification of the motor response caused by reflex activation of motor neurons. Careful observation of H reflexes as they increase in amplitude often reveals a decrease in latency. This decrease is consistent with the orderly activation of smaller and then larger motor neurons, with an associated increase in axonal conduction velocities, as would be expected in a reflex response.

The arc of the H reflex includes conduction in large, fast-conducting Ia fibers. In that sense, the H reflex is similar to the phasic myotatic ("deep tendon") reflex produced by muscle stretch. Although the phasic myotatic reflex generally is considered monosynaptic and there is a monosynaptic component to the H reflex, evidence exists that the H reflex also has oligosynaptic components.[4,5] These include contributions from spindle afferents, as well as inhibitory Ib effects from Golgi tendon organs. Achilles and calf H reflexes are generally present together, and calf H-reflex amplitudes have been correlated positively with prominence of the Achilles reflex.[6] Unlike the phasic myotatic reflex, however, the H reflex does not involve muscle spindle activation. This difference at times may explain the presence of calf H reflexes in the absence of Achilles reflexes.

H reflexes are inhibited as the stimulus intensity is increased from submaximal to that required for eliciting a maximal direct (M) response. This relationship has been explained by "collision" of orthodromic impulses with impulses conducted antidromically in motor axons. In fact, this mechanism has little or no role in the inhibition of H reflexes that occurs with increasing stimulus intensity. To be complete, such collision must occur distal to the motor neurons. Allowing for rise times for motor neuron excitatory postsynaptic potentials (EPSPs) of at

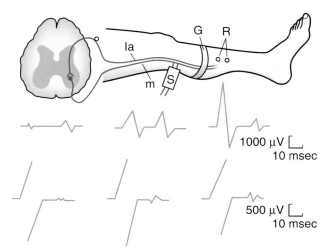

FIGURE 18-1 ■ Drawings of H reflexes (upper) and F responses (lower) recorded (R) from calf muscles. Stimulation (S) of the tibial nerve in the popliteal fossa activates Ia fibers with a resultant reflex discharge of motor (m) axons. H reflexes are present at low levels of stimulation, when the M wave may be absent or lower in amplitude than the H reflex, and are inhibited with increasing stimulus intensity. With supramaximal stimulation, low-amplitude, variable F responses are produced by antidromic activation of motor neurons. G, ground. (From Fisher MA: H reflexes and F waves: physiology and clinical indications. Muscle Nerve, 15:1223, 1992, with permission.)

least 3 msec, as well as for at least one synapse, the differences in afferent and efferent conduction in H reflexes necessary for collision inhibition have not been established. Large H reflexes are obtained from calf muscles, even with supramaximal stimulation, if the stimuli are timed appropriately with phasic contractions of the muscles.[7] This indicates that H-reflex inhibition does not depend on peripheral collision of afferent and efferent impulses. Experimental studies in normal and spastic subjects are consistent with central inhibition of H reflexes occurring as stimulus intensities are increased.[8]

Inhibitory mechanisms present in the spinal cord can explain H-reflex inhibition. Inhibitory interneurons (Renshaw cells) are activated by antidromic stimulation, are distributed widely throughout the motor neuron pool, and discharge more strongly and with shorter latency as stimulus intensity increases. H reflexes may be monosynaptic, whereas H-reflex inhibition by Renshaw cells would involve two synapses. Any resulting difference in the onset of inhibitory and excitatory effects may be as brief as 0.3 msec[9] and therefore well within a reasonable physiologic range given motor neuron EPSP rise times. Direct connections between motor neurons are also present and could contribute to H-reflex inhibition. Single-fiber electromyographic (EMG) studies

of H reflexes support a process of active inhibition involving inhibitory synapses with stimuli of increasing intensity.[10]

In infants younger than 2 years, H reflexes are distributed widely. Beyond infancy, H reflexes are found regularly in calf muscles (primarily the soleus) and homologous forearm flexors. They are also commonly present in the quadriceps and occasionally in plantar foot muscles. This restricted distribution of H reflexes with age is caused by changes associated with physiologic maturation of the central nervous system (CNS).

The fraction of the soleus motor neuron pool activated in an H reflex is usually about 50 percent but can be as high as 100 percent. The ratio of the peak-to-peak maximum H-reflex to maximum M-wave amplitude (H/M ratio) provides a measure of motor neuron pool activation and therefore excitability. The H/M ratio for calf H reflexes is normally less than 0.7 but there is considerable variation. A recent study has recommended evaluating M responses and H reflexes over the entire stimulus range in order to standardize H-reflex responses better, not only between studies and subjects but also from the same subject. This method allows not only for normalization of the H reflex itself but also for the relative stimulus intensity needed to elicit a response.[11]

H reflexes involve the activation of a portion of the segmental motor neuron pool and therefore are enhanced by maneuvers that increase excitability of the motor neuron pool. H reflexes can be produced by facilitation maneuvers (e.g., contraction or post-tetanic potentiation) in muscles where they are not otherwise present, such as the small hand muscles. H reflexes, particularly those of low amplitude, are depressed by prior stimulation.[12] This is related to homosynaptic depression rather than presynaptic inhibition from flexor afferents.[13]

H reflexes have been used to explore the physiology of the CNS. A recent review has emphasized the problems with equating H-reflex responsiveness with motor neuron excitability.[5] Such equating of these two phenomena is limited, for example, by the effects of presynaptic inhibition and postactivation depression on H reflexes. In general, H reflexes are subject to a complex of segmental and suprasegmental influences related to both the physical and mental state of the individual. With these limitations, H reflexes remain an important tool for investigating the central control of movement.[14,15]

H reflexes have been used to study patterns of central reflex organization, as reviewed elsewhere.[4,5] Studies have shown changes in H reflexes consistent with an influence on the reflex of both group Ia and group II afferents. H reflexes have been used to analyze patterns of reciprocal inhibition. The methodology for this in the

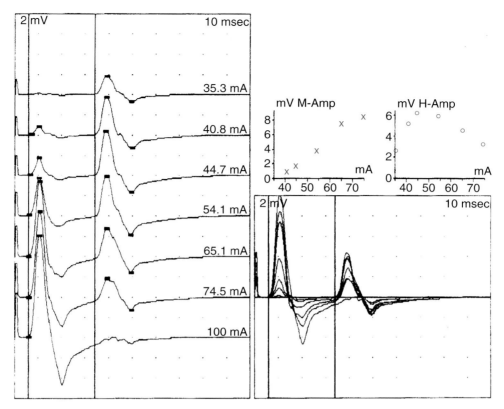

FIGURE 18-2 ■ H reflexes with increasing stimulus intensity shown in a raster mode (left) and superimposed (right). The inserts show in graphic form that, as the M-wave amplitude increases, the H-reflex amplitude initially increases and then decreases. At the highest level of stimulation (last response in the raster mode), the H reflex has disappeared and is replaced with an F wave. (Calibration per division, 2 mV and 10 msec.)

forearm has been well described.[16] Myotatic arcs between proximal and distal muscles also affect H reflexes. Activation of the quadriceps, for example, inhibits the soleus H reflex.[17] Presynaptic inhibition of Ia afferent fibers is decreased on fibers projecting on motor neurons of contracting muscles, but it is increased on afferents to motor neurons supplying muscles that are not involved in the contraction.[18] Passive cyclic movements of the legs produce inhibition of H reflexes; this is probably because of presynaptic inhibition that can be integrated at the spinal cord level.[19]

Characteristic changes in H-reflex amplitude can be defined if test stimuli are given at varying intervals after a conditioning stimulus. These excitability or recovery curves vary with the level of stimulation (Fig. 18-4) and are not established clearly until 1 year of age.

H reflexes are inhibited by vibration as a result of vibration-induced activation of large afferent fibers with consequent peripheral "busy line" interference, presynaptic inhibition of afferent input, and activation of spindles in antagonist muscles. Vibration of the tibialis anterior muscle has been used to assess the degree of

presynaptic inhibiton of Ia projections from the quadriceps to soleus motor neurons.[4,5]

Technique of Recording H Reflexes

H reflexes are obtained readily with percutaneous stimulation and surface recording techniques. Responses are stable, but only under similar conditions of stimulation and recording. The stimulating cathode should be proximal to avoid anodal block. Stimulus pulses of long duration (1 msec) are used to activate the large sensory fibers preferentially.[20,21] Stimulus frequency should be 0.2 Hz or less to allow recovery of postactivation depression of the H reflex from a prior stimulus.

A series of responses should be obtained. Starting with submaximal stimuli and increasing to supramaximal stimulation, one should verify whether the "late" response can be larger than the preceding direct motor response, determine which H reflex has the largest amplitude, and demonstrate that inhibition of the H reflex occurs with increasing stimulus intensity. Latencies should be measured to the onset of the responses (either negative

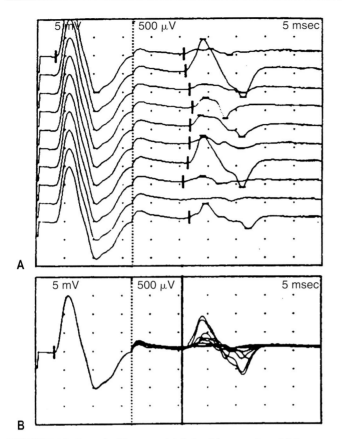

FIGURE 18-3 ▪ **A,** F waves (right) with associated M waves (left) recorded from the abductor pollicis brevis muscle following supramaximal stimulation at the wrist. The inherent variability of F waves is emphasized in the superimposed recordings (**B**). The chronodispersion is the difference between the shortest and longest F-wave latencies. The persistence in this series of 10 recordings is 90 percent, because in one an F wave is absent. The two largest responses are repeater waves. (Calibration per division, 5 mV for M waves, 500 μV; 5 msec.) (From Fisher MA: Normative F-wave values and the number of recorded F waves. Muscle Nerve, 17:1185, 1994, with permission.)

TABLE 18-1 ▪ H Reflexes and F Waves		
Feature	H Reflexes	F Waves
Response	Reflex	Antidromic firing of motor neurons
Afferent fibers	Ia afferents	Alpha motor fibers
Efferent fibers	Alpha motor fibers	Alpha motor fibers
Distribution	Restricted	Ubiquitous
Stimulus intensity	Low	High
Increasing stimulus intensity	Inhibits response	Facilitates response
Amplitude	Large	Small
Morphology	Stable	Variable
Motor units	Different from M wave	Same as in M wave

or positive), and amplitudes should be measured from peak to peak.

For calf H reflexes, the posterior tibial nerve is stimulated in the popliteal fossa. Bipolar stimulation is usually adequate. Use of an anode with a large surface area at the patella can decrease stimulus artifact and may provide more discrete cathodal excitation of the nerve in the popliteal fossa. Recordings are made from the soleus muscle. Although techniques vary, a standard and convenient location for the active electrode is medial to the tibia at a point that is half the distance between the stimulation site and the medial malleolus, with the indifferent electrode placed on the Achilles tendon. H reflexes in the forearm are recorded readily from the flexor carpi radialis muscle.[22] The recording electrode is placed at the junction of the upper one-third and lower two-thirds of the distance between the medial epicondyle and the radial styloid. The median nerve is stimulated percutaneously in the cubital fossa. At times, H reflexes in normal subjects can be recorded from the quadriceps with stimulation of the femoral nerve in the femoral triangle and from the abductor hallucis with stimulation of the tibial nerve at the ankle.[23]

H reflexes are recorded routinely with the muscle at rest. Contraction of the recording muscle will enhance H reflexes by facilitating the motor neuron pool. Such contraction can help to identify H reflexes in muscles in which H reflexes are normally present, as well as elicit H reflexes in muscles where they are not normally found.[24] This facilitation of H reflexes by contraction is sometimes clinically useful and demonstrates that the normal distribution of H reflexes is based on physiologic, not structural, factors.

Uses of H-Reflex Studies

The upper limit of normal latency for the H reflex of the soleus is 35 msec, and that of the flexor carpi radialis is 21 msec. H-reflex latencies are related directly to leg or arm length, height, and, to a lesser degree, age (see Fig. 18-4). For clinical purposes, it is best to use regression equations including height and age as variables. Normal values for infants and children are available.[25,26] With careful technique, the upper limits of normal for side-to-side latency differences have been reported to be as low as 1.5 msec for calf muscles (mean, 0.09 ± 0.70 standard deviation [SD]) and 1.0 msec for forearm flexor muscles (mean, 0.002 ± 0.42 SD). For routine clinical work and consistent with a criterion of 3 SD from the mean, 2 msec should be allowed for side-to-side differences with recordings from the calf, and 1.5 msec allowed for recordings from the forearm.

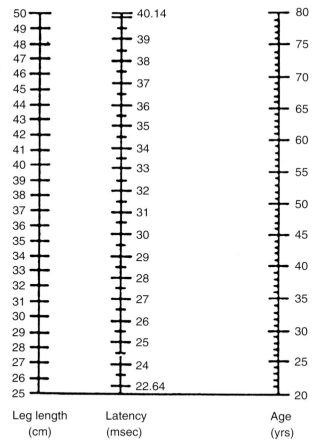

Leg length   Latency   Age
(cm)   (msec)   (yrs)

FIGURE 18-4 ▪ Nomogram of the regression of H-reflex latency on leg length and age. (From Braddom RI, Johnson EW: Standardization of the H reflex and diagnostic use in S1 radiculopathy. Arch Phys Med Rehabil, 55:161, 1974, with permission.)

Side-to-side latency differences may be larger in the elderly.[27] The upper limit of normal for the interside ratio of H-reflex amplitudes for calf muscles has been reported as 2,[28] but a preferable figure for general clinical work is probably 3. This is similar to the interside ratio for H-reflex amplitudes in the forearm.

Calf and forearm H reflexes are usually present in normal subjects. As with phasic myotatic reflexes, however, this is not always true, and symmetrically absent H reflexes are not necessarily abnormal. The percentage of absent responses increases in the elderly.[29]

Disorders of the Peripheral Nervous System

H reflexes are a sensitive test for polyneuropathies and may be abnormal even in mild neuropathies. H reflexes involve conduction in proximal as well as distal fibers. These studies, therefore, can define proximal nerve injury and may be abnormal even when studies of distal function are unremarkable. Absent H reflexes are

characteristic of acute inflammatory demyelinating polyneuropathy (Guillain–Barré syndrome). This loss of H reflexes occurs early and may be an isolated finding in patients studied within several days after onset of illness. H reflexes may be abnormal in asymptomatic patients with possible neuropathic dysfunction,[30] and in plexopathies and radiculopathies. H reflexes in the forearm flexor muscles may be abnormal with C6 or C7 root injury,[31] and calf H reflexes may be abnormal with S1 radiculopathies. H reflexes are affected by injury to either the posterior or anterior roots. Examination of these reflexes therefore can be important in the electrodiagnostic evaluation of radiculopathies by documenting nerve injury, even when needle EMG is unrevealing owing to sparing of the anterior roots. Eliciting the H reflex by direct stimulation of the S1 root may enhance their utility for detecting an S1 radiculopathy.[32] Increase in the stimulus threshold has been noted in patients with neurogenic claudication when studied after reproduction of their symptoms with walking.[33]

Disorders of the Central Nervous System

H reflexes are a recognized probe for noninvasive study of the reflex organization of the CNS and of motor control in general, as reviewed elsewhere.[4,15] H-reflex studies have also been used to monitor spinal cord plasticity.[34]

The H reflexes may be abnormally widespread in patients with CNS lesions and upper motor neuron signs. The presence in adults of H reflexes in muscles where they are not normally present (e.g., in the tibialis anterior or small hand muscles) may be clinically useful for documenting dysfunction of the central motor system.

Patients with even mild hemiparesis have decreased potentiation of H reflexes with muscle contraction, and this finding is consistent with decreased background facilitation of motor neurons. At the same time, H/M ratios tend to be increased in patients with CNS lesions and upper motor neuron signs, and recruitment curves are altered in a manner consistent with increased excitability of the central motor neuron pool.[35] Conversely, H reflexes may be depressed when excitability of the central motor neuron pool is decreased. As mentioned previously, however, a simplistic relation between motor neuron excitablity and H reflexes cannot be assumed, given the complexity of influences affecting the H reflex, including pre- and postsynaptic events.[5]

Changes in H reflexes after CNS lesions are time dependent. H reflexes are depressed acutely after spinal cord injury. Increased H/M ratios develop during the weeks to months following a cerebrovascular lesion associated with the appearance of features of the upper motor neuron syndrome (e.g., increased tone, brisk reflexes, and extensor plantar responses). In patients with chronic upper motor neuron lesions, vibratory inhibition of H reflexes is less than expected, possibly because of decreased presynaptic inhibition. In contrast, vibratory inhibition of H reflexes may be enhanced in patients with acute cerebral lesions. H reflexes are preserved relatively well acutely after spinal shock, at a time when both Achilles reflexes and H-reflex recovery curves are depressed.[36] Alterations in soleus H reflexes have been related to specific features of the upper motor neuron syndrome: in particular, decreased vibratory inhibition of H reflexes with hypertonia, increased H/M ratios with increased reflexes, and late facilitation of the recruitment curve with clonus.[37]

Within several months after a central injury, H-reflex excitability curves can show an abnormally rapid pattern of recovery (Fig. 18-5) associated with increased H/M ratios. These patterns differ from those in patients with parkinsonian rigidity or cerebellar hypotonia.

Studies of recovery curves and patterns of reciprocal inhibition of forearm flexor H reflexes have revealed abnormalities in patients with various types of dystonia, even in clinically normal parts of the body.[38,39] Analyses of H-reflex recovery curves may distinguish between focal and generalized dystonia.[40] Altered patterns of reciprocal reflex activity have been found in hereditary hyperekplexia ("startle disease").[41] In patients with chronic long-tract motor dysfunction, H reflexes have been used to analyze altered patterns of reflex activity between flexor and extensor muscles.[42,43] These findings have included increased reciprocal inhibition of flexor muscles by extensors.

H-reflex studies have been helpful for understanding the specific pathophysiology of CNS dysfunction. For example, H-reflex studies have supported the idea that spasticity (i.e., a velocity-sensitive increase in tone) is related to reduction in spinal inhibitory mechanisms, particularly disynaptic inhibition.[44]

F RESPONSE

Physiology

F waves are produced by antidromic activation ("backfiring") of motor neurons. They are low-amplitude, ubiquitous responses inherently variable in amplitude, latency, and configuration. Because of this variability and their dependence on motor neuron discharge, meaningful evaluation of F waves requires an approach different from that for other, commonly used electrodiagnostic variables.

F waves originally were recorded in small foot muscles,[45] hence their name. The initial concept that these responses were reflexes was challenged, particularly by the observation that motor units were present only in F waves if they were also present in the direct motor response.[46] The antidromic origin of F waves has been confirmed by the presence of F waves in deafferented animals and humans and by single-fiber EMG analysis, which has indicated that an F wave requires activation of the motor axon producing that particular response.[47] For an individual motor unit, the size and shape of the motor unit in the direct motor (M) and F waves should be the same.

Motor neurons are activated by depolarization at the low-threshold initial segment and subsequent invasion of the soma. The available evidence would indicate that this is true, regardless of whether the stimulus is orthodromic or antidromic. The shortest F-wave latencies

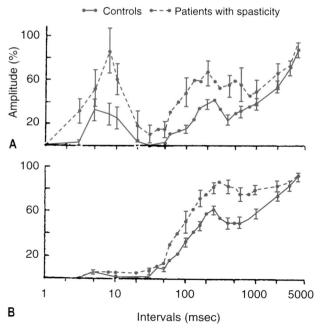

FIGURE 18-5 ■ H-reflex recovery curves recorded from calf muscles. Note the less pronounced inhibition in patients with spasticity in comparison to control subjects for stimuli near threshold (**A**), as well as at levels producing maximal H reflexes (**B**). Abscissa, time between conditioning and test stimuli (logarithmic scale); ordinate, test reflex amplitudes as percentages of conditioning reflex amplitudes. The vertical bars denote mean errors. (Modified from Olsen PZ, Diamantopoulos E: Excitability of spinal motor neurones in normal subjects and patients with spasticity, parkinsonian rigidity, and cerebellar hypotonia. J Neurol Neurosurg Psychiatry, 30:325, 1967, with permission.)

are comparable to H-reflex latencies, but they may be 1 to 2 msec shorter. In contrast to H reflexes, F waves are most prominent when elicited by stimuli of high intensity. F-wave impulses must pass orthodromically through an axonal initial segment that has been discharged by a preceding antidromic impulse. Therefore, the effect of altered motor neuron excitability on F waves is variable. If a motor neuron is at a high level of excitability (i.e., already relatively depolarized), neuronal activation will occur rapidly and the resultant orthodromic axonal discharge may present at the initial segment at a time when it is still refractory. Increased excitability of the motor neuron pool could then result in decreased prominence of F waves.[47] As a result, the effects of agonist and antagonist contraction are less predictable with F waves than with H reflexes and are dependent on the physiologic organization of a particular muscle.[48]

Individual motor neurons are activated infrequently with antidromic stimulation, and F waves usually have no more than several motor unit action potentials.[49] As a result, F waves may not appear after each stimulus, are variable in configuration, and are low in amplitude (see Fig. 18-3). An important area of controversy is whether the range of F-wave latencies reflects the full range of conduction in motor axons. Several reports have suggested an absence of bias of motor unit discharge in F waves.[50,51] Circumstantial and direct evidence, however, is consistent with a selective discharge of larger motor neurons in the generation of F waves.[52-55] All studies supporting an absence of selection in motor unit discharge in F waves have been performed using submaximal stimulation, whereas F waves clinically are recorded using supramaximal stimuli. Renshaw cells inhibit large motor neurons less than small ones. Activation of these inhibitory interneurons by antidromic nerve discharges therefore provides a physiologic model for the selective firing of larger motor neurons in the generation of F waves.

The time between the start of antidromic activation and subsequent orthodromic discharge (i.e., the central "turnaround" time) is uncertain. Based on a statement by Eccles,[56] the turnaround time commonly is estimated to be 1 msec, but this figure has never been demonstrated directly. In invertebrates, these central delays can be orders of magnitude greater. In humans, identical F waves have been recorded from foot muscles with latency variations of 3 msec.[57] Whatever the uncertainties, the variation in F-wave latencies is neither so random nor so large as to preclude their clinical use.

Because of the inherent variability of F waves, the number of F waves used for analyses in clinical studies has varied from 50 or greater to as few as 3. A consensus

has developed in the literature that analysis of 10 to 20 F waves is a reasonable balance between feasibility (including patient tolerance) and adequate data. Studies of the abductor pollicis brevis muscle, however, have indicated that evaluation of 16 to 20 F waves (20 stimuli) is needed for accurate measurement of "true" latencies based on an analysis of responses following up to 100 stimuli.[54,58-60] Whatever the uncertainties, the normal variability of latencies in a series of F waves is about 10 percent. This is comparable to the range of error for measurements of other commonly used electrophysiologic responses. The clinical importance of defining "true" latency values varies. For example, it is important when clinical evaluation depends on small latency differences between sides (e.g., for radiculopathies) but less important when latency prolongation may be profound (e.g., in demyelinating neuropathies). Even in the latter circumstance, however, accurate measurements are important if comparisons are to be made over time.

Latencies are the most commonly reported variables of F waves. F-wave latencies are directly related to height; limb length; and, to a lesser degree, age. Considering these variables when defining normal F-wave latency values increases the clinical sensitivity of individual F-wave latency measurements. F-wave latencies are reported most often as minimal latencies, a practice that has been recommended by certain professional organizations.[61] F waves often arise from an unstable baseline and A waves may be superimposed on them, making accurate measurement of individual F-wave latencies problematic at times. The use of minimal latencies to define abnormality implies that F-wave latency values would be considered as normal even when—in a series of F waves—a single F wave has a normal latency but all the others are abnormal. Expressing F-wave latencies as mean values minimizes the errors inherent in a single latency measurement, provides some measure of the normality or abnormality of the range of F-wave latencies, and produces results that are more reproducible. This has been the consistent finding of studies that have examined this question for over 25 years.[62-65] There is no justification for using minimal rather than mean latencies based on the investigative literature. Median latency values have been suggested as a more statistically correct way of defining F-wave latencies. This approach, however, requires more complex analyses and may add little if, indeed, F-wave latencies are distributed normally.[54]

Proximal conduction can be compared with distal conduction by comparing the latencies of F waves and M waves. F-wave latencies have been used to estimate conduction in limited portions of proximal nerves. F-wave latencies have been converted into conduction velocities using measurements of limb length and an estimate of the F-wave "turnaround" time. It has been argued that this methodology is a sensitive method for detecting mild nerve dysfunction and has the further advantage of allowing comparison of conduction velocity in subjects with differing limb lengths.[59] However, F-wave conduction velocities are less accurate than latency values alone because additional errors of measurement may be introduced, and F-wave latencies can be normalized readily to a particular arm or leg length.

Analysis of F-wave parameters other than latency has clinical utility and may at times be more important than latency measurements. The difference between minimal and maximal latencies in a series of F waves (i.e., F chronodispersion) provides a measure of the range of conduction velocities in the axons contributing to the recorded F waves. F-wave duration and amplitude are related to both the size and the number of motor units contributing to a particular F wave. F-wave persistence refers to the percentage of measurable F responses that follow a series of stimuli and is related to the antidromic excitability of a particular motor neuron pool. The recurrence of individual motor units in a series of F waves measures the selectivity of F-wave discharge. The ratio of F-wave amplitudes to those of the associated M waves (i.e., F/M ratios) is a measure of the proportion of a motor neuron pool activated by antidromic stimulation. As with latency measurements, given the F-wave variability, mean F-wave rather than maximum F-wave amplitudes are preferable for calculating F/M ratios.

F-wave recovery curves have been defined by measuring F-wave amplitude or persistence following conditioning stimuli that precede the test stimulus at varying intervals. As with H reflexes, there is an early depression of the response, followed by a later facilitation from about 80 to 300 msec.[66]

F waves have helped to define normal CNS physiology. As with H reflexes, F waves have been used to define patterns of spinal cord interactions. In resting individuals, F-wave studies have shown a relatively increased central excitability of the antigravity calf muscle in comparison to the antagonist tibialis anterior muscles. With isometric contraction, the central excitability of the tibialis anterior muscle increases relative to that of calf muscles so that statistically significant differences in F-wave persistence are no longer present.[49] In contrast to the situation at rest, these results are consistent with a more balanced central excitability state between flexor and extensor muscles with activity. In general, F waves reflect motor neuron excitability, possibly more so for inhibition than facilitation.[67] There is evidence that central drive affects

F waves. F-wave amplitudes and persistences reportedly decrease over hours when muscles are volitionally inactivated,[68] and motor imagery without voluntary contraction is said to have the reverse effect.[69]

Technique of Recording F Waves

F waves are recorded in a manner similar to that used for direct motor responses. Although the importance of anodal block has been questioned,[70] the standard methodology is for the stimulating cathode to be proximal to the anode. Unlike for H reflexes, a long stimulus duration is not required because there is no reason to activate preferentially the large afferent fibers. The author stimulates at rates less than 0.5 Hz to avoid the effects of an earlier stimulus on a subsequent response. In contrast to H reflexes, F waves are enhanced by stimulation at high intensity because of increased amplitude and persistence. High stimulus intensities also block axon reflexes that may be confused with F waves, as well as limiting contamination by H reflexes. The conventional stimulus intensity is 25 percent above maximal for eliciting a direct response. This provides a consistent physiologic environment for eliciting F waves. F waves are present at submaximal stimulation. This has the advantage of increased patient comfort and may provide adequate information in situations in which the only question is whether F-wave latencies are markedly prolonged. There has been interest in eliciting F waves using low-intensity stimulation since this could lessen patient discomfort. Submaximal stimulation does not affect F-wave latency or duration, but does affect all other F-wave parameters and would require more stimuli for accurate data. To date, all normative F-wave data are based on supramaximal stimulation. This therefore should be used until it is established that submaximal stimulation can produce meaningful, reproducible information for all F-wave parameters, and the number of stimuli required for such values has been determined.

Adequate display of F waves usually requires an amplifier gain of 200 or 500 μV per division and a sweep of 5 or 10 msec per division. As such, different recording parameters usually are required to evaluate fully the associated larger M wave. To be clearly identifiable, F waves should be at least 20 μV in peak-to-peak amplitude.

As discussed earlier, the number of F waves required to permit measurement of different F-wave parameters has been examined.[54,59,60] Data from 8 to 10 identifiable, sequential F waves can provide a reasonable estimate of persistence. Accurate F-wave latency measurement requires 16 to 20 F waves and is expressed best as a mean rather than a minimal value. The same number of F waves is adequate for measuring F/M ratios and the percentage of responses in a series of F waves that are the same (i.e., repeater waves). F waves usually are recorded from antigravity muscles with high persistences, so that the use of 20 stimuli is recommended for routine purposes. Even two F waves may define an abnormal chronodispersion if the two latencies are dispersed sufficiently, but determination of a truly representative value requires 45 to 55 F waves (50 to 60 stimuli). Accurate determination of the number of individual waves that repeat may require more than 90 F waves. When there is low persistence, more stimuli than usual may be needed to obtain adequate data.

Muscle belly–tendon recordings are standard for hand and foot muscles, with the recording cathode placed over the motor point. For calf F responses, muscle belly recordings often are preferred because the effects of extraneous muscle activity are decreased when recording the low-amplitude F waves. The active electrode is placed as for H reflexes.

F waves are recorded routinely with the muscle relaxed. Slight voluntary contraction will enhance F waves. This is sometimes helpful clinically, but the contraction will alter F-wave parameters such as amplitude and will increase the possibility of contamination by H reflexes.

F waves are ubiquitous in distribution. Recording from proximal muscles, however, is difficult because the low-amplitude F waves are superimposed on the associated M wave. F waves therefore are recorded routinely only from muscles of the hand, foot, and leg, with standard stimulation sites at the wrist, ankle, and knee respectively. F waves can be recorded in hand muscles with stimulation in the axilla if collision techniques are used so that the orthodromic M wave from the axilla is blocked by collision with antidromic impulses from the wrist.

F waves usually are recorded in a raster fashion so that individual responses and the associated maximum M waves are available for analysis. Standard protocols include measurement of minimal and mean F-wave latency, F-wave chronodispersion, F-wave persistence, and the F/M amplitude ratio. The latter is calculated as the mean of the amplitudes of the F waves divided by the M-wave amplitude, with both measured from peak to peak.

Clinical Application of F-Wave Studies

The upper limits of normal for minimal F-wave latencies in the author's laboratory are 33, 36, and 64 msec when recording from hand, calf, and foot muscles, respectively.

Mean latencies are about 2 to 3 msec longer. Side-to-side differences exceeding 2 msec are regarded as abnormal for both minimal and mean values in recordings from the hand; 3 msec in recordings from the calf; and 4 msec in recordings from the foot. Detailed tables have been published of normal minimal and mean F-wave latencies related to height for hand and foot muscles.[71–74] Regression equations relating minimal or mean latencies to age and height (or limb length) for the abductor pollicis brevis, abductor digiti minimi, calf, and abductor hallucis muscles are also available.[75,76] In recordings from hand muscles, values that exceed by 3 msec or more the predicted value based on regression equations are abnormal, and those between 2 and 3 msec are borderline; comparable values for the soleus are 4 and 3 msec. Minimal and mean F-wave latency data have been reported for the radial nerve, recording from the extensor indicis,[77] and for the facial nerve, recording from the nasalis.[78]

Based on the literature, upper normal limits for chronodispersion (mean plus 2 SD) are 6.2 msec for the abductor pollicis brevis, 5.5 msec for the abductor digiti minimi, 7 msec for the soleus, 9.5 msec for the extensor digitorum brevis, and 9.3 msec for the abductor hallucis. Normal F/M ratios in the author's laboratory, based on mean F-wave amplitudes, are 2.2 ± 1.0 percent for the abductor pollicis brevis and 2.5 ± 1.2 percent for the soleus, equivalent to an upper limit of normal of about 5 percent. Mean values for F-wave persistence recording from the abductor pollicis brevis, abductor digiti minimi, soleus, and abductor hallucis are about 0.8 to 0.9, whereas in the antigravity antagonist tibialis anterior, extensor digitorum brevis, and extensor digitorum communis muscles these values are about 0.3 to 0.4, but the range of normal is high for individual measurements. When recording from the extensor digitorum brevis, for example, only 55 percent of normal subjects would be expected to have a persistence of 0.5 or greater,[74] whereas this might be expected in 96 percent of subjects when recording from the abductor hallucis.[73] The low persistence in antigravity antagonist muscles (e.g., the extensor digitorum brevis) argues against the routine recording of F waves from these muscles. The normal maximum frequency of an individual response in a series of F waves from hand muscles is about 10 percent, but the percentage of responses in which repeater waves are seen is higher because there may be more than one repeater wave and each individual repeater wave may be present more than twice. A frequency of an individual repeater wave as high as 58 percent has been noted in recordings from the extensor digitorum brevis of normal subjects (mean, 21.5 percent).[57]

DISORDERS OF THE PERIPHERAL NERVOUS SYSTEM

Prolonged F-wave latencies are a sensitive indicator in polyneuropathies and may be found even when other measures of distal motor nerve conduction are unremarkable. They may be more sensitive than standard motor conduction studies in injury to motor axons, perhaps because F-wave studies monitor nerve dysfunction along the entire course of the nerve. F-wave recordings are the most reliable and reproducible conduction study for monitoring patients with neuropathies,[79,80] and F-wave latencies are reportedly the most sensitive measure for defining nerve injury in patients with diabetes mellitus.[81] Markedly prolonged F waves—120 percent of the upper limit of normal if the M-wave amplitude exceeds 80 percent of the lower limit of normal, or 150 percent if the M wave is smaller—are thought to be supportive of demyelinating injury. Absent F waves with normal M-wave amplitudes suggest conduction block.[82] Using a nonparametric methodology, recent studies have supported the idea that F waves may be helpful in providing a meaningful physiologic classification of neurogenic injury.[83]

Prominent slowing of proximal F-wave conduction in comparison to distal motor nerve conduction studies has been found in patients with Guillain–Barré syndrome, thus confirming the importance of proximal nerve lesions in these patients. F-wave studies have been abnormal in 92 percent of nerves in patients with Guillain–Barré syndrome and in 95 percent of nerves in those patients with chronic inflammatory demyelinating polyneuropathy.[84] In about 20 percent of these nerves, motor conduction studies were unremarkable. F-wave abnormalities consisted not only of prolonged latencies or absent responses, but also decreased persistence and increased chronodispersion. Indeed, abnormal F waves are so common in acquired demyelinating neuropathies that the diagnosis, at least, should be questioned in the absence of such findings. F-wave latencies may also be prolonged in plexus injury and in syringomyelia, but proximally predominant abnormalities have not been found in patients with uremia, diabetes mellitus, or Charcot–Marie–Tooth disease.

F-wave chronodispersion may be prolonged in polyneuropathies.[82,84,85] Chronodispersion tends to be larger in nerves with demyelinating, rather than axonal, injury,[82] and is relatively decreased with conduction block.[85]

The number of identical responses in a series of F waves may be increased in patients with neurogenic atrophy, consistent with a decrease in the number of motor neurons capable of responding to antidromic stimulation.[57] Increased repeater waves have been found in patients with amyotrophic lateral sclerosis, cervical myeloradiculopathies, and certain entrapment neuropathies such as carpal tunnel syndrome.

The value of F-wave latency studies in detecting injury to proximal nerve segments (e.g., as occurs with radiculopathies) is controversial.[86] Concerns have included overlapping root innervation in muscles, as well as the limited information available from F-wave studies in a situation in which needle EMG also evaluates injury to motor fibers. There has also been concern that F-wave latency abnormalities may be masked because the effect of the conduction slowing is "diluted" by the long course of the pathway being tested. Modeling of proximal injury affecting F waves, however, indicates that the important issue is the variance of the recordings, not the distance over which the impulses travel.[87]

Studies of patients with possible nerve root injury usually have been limited by a failure to examine a sufficient number (16 to 20) of F waves or to evaluate F-wave variables other than latency. Such analyses may add to the sensitivity of F-wave studies. Some studies have indicated a sensitivity of F-wave studies in L5 or S1 radiculopathies comparable to that of needle EMG, with the F-wave abnormalities often providing complementary information.[88–92] F-wave abnormalities may be prominent in patients with spinal stenosis, possibly because of the multiple roots involved, and F-wave variables may change following exercise in such patients.[93,94] In sum, there is considerable evidence that F waves can be useful in the evaluation of patients with lumbosacral root injury, particularly if relevant F-wave variables are analyzed. This is not surprising, given the focal demyelination and biophysical changes associated with root injury.

There is little evidence that F waves are clinically useful in the evaluation of cervical radiculopathies. This is probably because most cervical root lesions involve the C5, C6, or C7 roots, whereas the muscles commonly used for F-wave recordings are innervated by the C8 or T1 roots.

Abnormal F-wave chronodispersion and persistence in the legs may be conspicuous in patients with axonal injury due to chronic peripheral arterial disease,[95] especially in studies performed after exercise.[96] In amyotrophic lateral stenosis (ALS), decreased F-wave persistence has been associated with the degree of neurogenic weakness.[97,98] In addition, the F-wave latency may be prolonged and the amplitude and chronodispersion increased. An ALS neurophysiologic index has been proposed based on recordings from the abductor digiti minimi of M waves, distal motor latencies, and F persistence. This index has been correlated strongly with weakness in the recording muscle.[99]

DISORDERS OF THE CENTRAL NERVOUS SYSTEM

F-wave analyses to define increased central excitability states are more complicated than analyses of H reflexes. Single-fiber studies in patients with upper motor neuron syndromes indicate that antidromically activated motor neurons fire more frequently than do those in normal individuals.[47] At the same time, a frequently backfired motor neuron will discharge less frequently with activation by muscle contraction, whereas motor neurons that discharge infrequently will increase their firing rate. At times, therefore, increased central excitability results in decreased discharge of larger motor neurons in an F wave, owing to blockage at the still refractory initial segment of the motor neuron. Despite this complexity, analyses of F waves are a valuable technique for monitoring central motor neuron excitability.

In patients with CNS lesions, the normal, relatively increased prominence of F waves in resting extensor muscles compared with flexor muscles may be disrupted. F-wave amplitudes and persistence are decreased in clinically involved limbs, and this finding is compatible with decreased central excitability in patients studied early after unilateral cerebrovascular lesions, a period when decreased tone and reflexes are common findings.[65] However, decreased movement itself can decrease the prominence of F waves.[68] F waves are absent in patients with spinal shock and are decreased in prominence in patients with acute spinal cord injury without spinal shock.[36] Clinical improvement has been associated with increased F-wave amplitudes and persistence in serial studies.[100]

F-wave persistence, durations, amplitudes, and latencies, and F/M ratios may be increased in patients with long-standing "spasticity" or upper motor neuron syndromes,[65] sometimes even when there is little or no motor deficit.[101] These data are consistent with the discharge of a greater number of smaller, slower-conducting motor units owing to increased central excitability while larger motor neurons are blocked because of too rapid activation.

Knowledgeable use of F waves requires an understanding that these responses originate at the interface between the central and the peripheral nervous systems. F-wave studies can provide physiologic insight into that interface. F/M amplitude ratios, for example, are increased in patients with polyneuropathy, as well as in those with spastic hyperreflexia. Log F/M values are normally correlated directly with neuromuscular efficiency as defined by twitch tension/M-wave amplitudes. This relationship is disturbed most prominently in patients with CNS abnormalities, but is also disturbed in patients with peripheral nerve dysfunction.

REFERENCES

1. Hoffman P: Über die Beziehungen der Sehnenreflexe zur willkurlichen Bewegung zum Tonus. Z Biol, 68:351, 1918
2. Hoffman P: Untersuchungen über die Eigenreflexe [Sehnenreflexe] menschlicher Muskeln. Springer, Berlin, 1922
3. Magladery JW, McDougal DB: Electrophysiological studies of nerve and reflex in normal man. I: Identification of certain reflexes in the electromyogram and the conduction velocity of peripheral nerve fibers. Bull Johns Hopkins Hosp, 86:265, 1950
4. Pierrot-Deseilligny E, Mazevet D: The monosynaptic reflex: a tool to investigate motor control in humans. Interest and limits. Neurophysiol Clin, 30:67, 2000
5. Misiaszek JE: The H-reflex as a tool in neurophysiology: its limitations and uses in understanding nervous system function. Muscle Nerve, 28:144, 2003
6. Katirji B, Weissman JD: The ankle jerk and the tibial H-reflex: a clinical and electrophysiological correlation. Electromyogr Clin Neurophysiol, 34:331, 1994
7. Fisher MA: H-reflexes and F-waves: physiology and clinical indications. Muscle Nerve, 15:1223, 1992
8. Hilgevoord AA, Rour LJ, Koehlman JH et al: Soleus H-reflex inhibition in controls and spastic patients: ordered occlusion or diffuse inhibition? Electroencephalogr Clin Neurophysiol, 97:402, 1995
9. Eccles JC, Fatt P, Koketsu K: Cholinergic and inhibitory synapses in a pathway from motor-axon collaterals to motor neurons. J Physiol, 126:524, 1954
10. Stålberg E, Tronetlj J: Reflex studies. p. 226. In Single Fiber Electromyography: Studies in Healthy and Diseased Muscle. Raven, New York, 1994
11. Brinkworth RSA, Tuncer M, Tucker KJ et al: Standardization of H-reflex analyses. J Neurosci Methods, 162:1, 2007
12. Floeter MK, Kohn AF: H-reflexes of different sizes exhibit differential sensitivity to low frequency depression. Electroencephalogr Clin Neurophysiol, 105:470, 2007
13. Kohn AF, Floeter MK, Hallett M: Presynaptic inhibition compared with homosynaptic depression as an explanation for soleus H-reflex depression in humans. Exp Brain Res 116:375, 1997
14. Pierrot-Deseilligny E, Mazevet D: The monosynaptic reflex: a tool to investigate motor control in humans. Interest and limits. Neurophysiol Clin, 30:67, 2000
15. Knikou M: The H-reflex as a probe: pathways and pitfalls. J Neurosci Methods, 171:1, 2008
16. Fuhr P, Hallett M: Reciprocal inhibition of the H-reflex in the forearm: methodological aspects. Electroencephalogr Clin Neurophysiol, 93:202, 1994
17. Meunier S, Mogyoros I, Kiernan MC et al: Effects of femoral nerve stimulation on the electromyogram and reflex excitability of tibialis anterior and soleus. Muscle Nerve, 19:1110, 1996
18. Pierrot-Deseilligny E: Assessing changes in presynaptic inhibition of Ia afferents during movement in humans. J Neurosci Methods, 74:189, 1997

19. Misiaszek JE, Brooke JD, Lafferty KB et al: Long-lasting inhibition of the human soleus H-reflex pathway after passive movement. Brain Res, 677:69, 1995

20. Panizza M, Nilsson J, Hallett M: Optimal stimulus for the H-reflex. Muscle Nerve, 12:576, 1989

21. Lagerquist O, Collins DF: Stimulus pulse-width influences H-reflex recruitment but not H_{max}/M_{max} ratio. Muscle Nerve, 37:483, 2008

22. Christie AD, Inglis JG, Boucher JP et al: Reliability of the FCR H-reflex. J Clin Neurophysiol, 22:204, 2005

23. Vresino M, Candeloro E, Tavazzi E et al: The H reflex from the abductor brevis hallucis muscle in healthy subjects. Muscle Nerve, 36:39, 2007

24. Burke D, Adams RW, Skuse NF: The effect of voluntary contraction on the H-reflex of human limb muscle. Brain, 112:417, 1989

25. Miller RG, Kunz N: Nerve conduction studies in infants and children. J Child Neurol, 1:19, 1986

26. Bryant PR, Eng GD: Normal values for the soleus H-reflex in newborn infants 31–45 weeks post conceptual age. Arch Phys Med Rehabil, 72:28, 1991

27. Falco FJ, Hennessey WJ, Goldberg G et al: H-reflex latency in the elderly. Muscle Nerve, 17:161, 1994

28. Nishida T, Kompoliti A, Janssen I et al: H-reflex in S-1 radiculopathy: latency versus amplitude controversy revisited. Muscle Nerve, 19:915, 1996

29. Weintraub JR, Madalin K, Wang M et al: Achilles tendon reflex and the H response. Muscle Nerve, 11:972, 1988

30. Trujillo-Hernández B, Huerta M, Trujillo X et al: F-wave and H-reflex alterations in recently diagnosed diabetic patients. J Clin Neurosci, 12:763, 2005

31. Eliaspour D, Sanati E, Hedayati Moquadam MR et al: Utility of flexor carpi radialis H-reflex in diagnosis of cervical radiculopathy. J Clin Neurophysiol, 26:458, 2009

32. Jin X, Shu Y, Lu FZ et al: H-reflex to S1-root stimulation improves utility for diagnosing S1 radiculopathy. Clin Neurophysiol, 121:1329, 2010

33. Pastor P, Valls-Sole J: Recruitment curve of the soleus H reflex in patients with neurogenic claudication. Muscle Nerve, 31:985, 1998

34. Wolpow JR: Spinal cord plasticity in acquisition and maintenance of motor skills. Acta Physiol, 189:155, 2007

35. Hilgevoord AAJ, Koelman JHTM, Bour LJ et al: Normalization of H-reflex recruitment curves in controls and a population of spastic patients. Electroencephalogr Clin Neurophysiol, 93:202, 1994

36. Leis AA, Kronenberg MF, Stětkárová I et al: Spinal motoneuron excitability after acute spinal cord injury in humans. Neurology, 47:231, 1996

37. Koelman JHTM, Bour LJ, Hilgevoord AAJ et al: Soleus H-reflex test and clinical signs of the upper motor neuron syndrome. J Neurol Neurosurg Psychiatry, 56:776, 1993

38. Panizza M, Hallett M, Nilsson J: Reciprocal inhibition in patients with hand cramps. Neurology, 39:85, 1989

39. Panizza M, Lelli S, Nilsson J et al: H-reflex recovery curve and reciprocal inhibition of H-reflex in different kinds of dystonia. Neurology, 40:824, 1990

40. Sabbahi M, Etnyre B, Al-Jawayed I et al: Soleus H-reflex measures in patients with focal and generalized dystonia. Clin Neurophysiol, 114:288, 2003

41. Floeter MK, Andermann F, Andermann E et al: Physiological studies of spinal inhibitory pathways in patients with hereditary hyperekplexia. Neurology, 46:766, 1996

42. Arteida J, Quesada P, Obeso JA: Reciprocal inhibition between forearm muscles in spastic hemiplegia. Neurology, 41:286, 1991

43. Yang JF, Fung J, Edamura M et al: H-reflex modulation during walking in spastic paretic subjects. Can J Neurol Sci, 18:443, 1991

44. Nielsen JB, Crone C, Hultborn H: The spinal pathophysiology of spasticity—from a basic science point of view. Acta Physiol, 189:171, 2007

45. Magladery JW, McDougal DB, Stoll J: Electrophysiological studies of nerve and reflex activity in normal man. II: The effects of peripheral ischemia. Bull Johns Hopkins Hosp, 86:291, 1950

46. Thorne J: Central responses to electrical activation of the peripheral nerves supplying the intrinsic hand muscles. J Neurol Neurosurg Psychiatry, 28:482, 1965

47. Stålberg E, Trontelj JV: Single Fiber Electromyography. Raven, New York, 1994

48. Fisher MA: Relative changes with contraction in the central excitability state of the tibialis anterior and calf muscles. J Neurol Neurosurg Psychiatry, 43:243, 1989

49. Fisher MA: F waves. p. 473. In Brown WF, Bolton CF, Aminoff MJ (eds): Neuromuscular Function and Disease. Vol 1, Philadelphia, WB Saunders, 2003

50. Dengler R, Kossev A, Wohlfahrt K et al: F waves and motor unit size. Muscle Nerve, 15:1138, 1992

51. Doherty TJ, Komori T, Shahsuk DW et al: Physiological properties of single thenar motor units in the F-response of younger and older single adults. Muscle Nerve, 17:860, 1994

52. Fisher MA: Evidence for selective activation of faster conducting motor fibers in F waves. Muscle Nerve, 11:983, 1988

53. Guiloff RJ, Modarres-Sadeghi H: Preferential generation of recurrent responses by groups of motor neurons in man. Brain, 114:1771, 1991

54. Fisher MA, Hoffen B, Hultman C: Normative F waves and the number of recorded F waves. Muscle Nerve, 17:1185, 1994

55. Vatine JJ, Gonen B: Behavior of F-response and determination of actively involved motor neurons. Electromyogr Clin Neurophysiol, 36:349, 1996

56. Eccles JC: The central action of antidromic impulses in motor nerve fibers. Pflugers Arch, 260:385, 1955

57. Petajan JH: F-waves in neurogenic atrophy. Muscle Nerve, 18:690, 1985

58. Chroni E, Taub N, Panayiotopoulos CP: The importance of sample size for the estimation of F wave latency parameters in the peroneal nerve. Electroencephalogr Clin Neurophysiol, 101:375, 1996

59. Payiotoupoulos CP, Chroni E: F-waves in clinical neurophysiology: a review, methodological issues and overall

value in peripheral neuropathies. Electroencephalogr Clin Neurophysiol, 101:365, 1996

60. Raudino F: F-wave: sample size and normative values. Electromyogr Clin Neurophysiol, 37:107, 1997

61. Jablecki CK, Busis NA, Brandstater MA et al: Reporting the results of needle EMG and nerve conduction studies. Muscle Nerve, 32:682, 2005

62. Taniguchi MH, Hayes J, Rodriguez AA: Reliability determination of F mean response latency. Arch Phys Med Rehabil, 74:1139, 1993

63. Panayiotopoulos CP, Chroni E: F-waves in clinical neurophysiology: a review, methodological issues and overall value in peripheral neuropathies. Electroencephalogr Clin Neurophysiol, 101:365, 1996

64. Nobrega JAM, Pinheiro DS, Manzano GM et al: Various aspects of F-wave values in a healthy population. Clin Neurophysiol, 115:2336, 2004

65. Fisher MA: F-waves—physiology and clinical uses. Scientific World Journal, 7:144, 2007

66. Mastaglia FL, Carroll W: The effects of conditioning stimuli on the F-response. J Neurol Neurosurg Psychiatry, 48:182, 1985

67. Lin JZ, Floeter MK: Do F-wave measurements detect changes in motor neuron excitability. Muscle Nerve, 30:289, 2004

68. Taniguchi S, Kimura J, Yanagisawa R et al: Rest-induced suppression of anterior horn cell excitability as measured by F waves: comparison between volitionally inactivated and control muscles. Muscle Nerve, 37:343, 2008

69. Hara M, Kimura J, Walker D et al: Effect of motor imagery and voluntary muscle contraction on the F wave. Muscle Nerve, 42:208, 2010

70. Kirschblum S, Cai P, Johnston MV et al: Anodal block in F-wave studies. Arch Phys Med Rehabil, 79:1059, 1998

71. Buschbacher RM: Median nerve F-wave latencies recorded from the abductor pollicis brevis. Am J Phys Med Rehabil, 78:Suppl, S32, 1999

72. Buschbacher RM: Ulnar nerve F-wave latencies recorded from the abductor digiti. Am J Phys Med Rehabil, 78: Suppl, S38, 1999

73. Buschbacher RM: Tibial nerve F-wave latencies recorded from the abductor hallucis. Am J Phys Med Rehabil, 78: Suppl, S43, 1999

74. Buschbacher RM: Peroneal nerve F-wave latencies recorded from the extensor digitorum brevis. Am J Phys Med Rehabil, 78:Suppl, S48, 1999

75. Fisher MA: F response latency determination. Muscle Nerve, 6:730, 1982

76. Puksa L, Stålberg E, Falck B: Reference values of F wave parameters in healthy subjects. Clin Neurophysiol, 114:1079, 2003

77. Papathanasiou ES, Zamba E, Papacostas SS: Radial nerve F-waves: normative values with surface recording from the extensor indicis muscle. Clin Neurophysiol, 112:145, 2001

78. Wedekind C, Stauten W, Klug N: A normative study on human facial F waves. Muscle Nerve, 24:900, 2001

79. Pinheiro DS, Monzano GM, Nóbrega JAM: Reproducibility in nerve conduction studies and F-wave analysis. Clin Neurophysiol, 119:2070, 2008

80. Kihara N, Kimura J, Kaji R et al: Multicenter analysis on intertrial variability of nerve conduction studies: healthy subjects and patients with diabetic neuropathy. p. 809. In Kimura J, Shibasaki H (eds): Recent Advances in Clinical Neurophysiology. Elsevier, Amsterdam, 1996

81. Andersen A, Stålberg E, Falck B: F-wave latency, the most sensitive nerve conduction parameter in patients with diabetes mellitus. Muscle Nerve, 20:1296, 1997

82. Fraser JL, Olney RK: The relative diagnostic sensitivity of different F wave parameters in various neuropathies. Muscle Nerve, 14:912, 1991

83. Patil VK, Gordon J, Keller A et al: Characterization of F-waves by recurrence quantification analysis. Muscle Nerve, 42:684, 2010

84. Kiers L, Clouston P, Zuniga G et al: Quantitative studies of F responses in Guillain–Barré syndrome and chronic inflammatory demyelinating polyneuropathy. Electroencephalogr Clin Neurophysiol, 93:255, 1994

85. Shivde AJ, Fisher MA: F chronodispersion in polyneuropathy. Muscle Nerve, 11:960, 1988

86. Fisher MA: F-wave studies: clinical utility. Muscle Nerve, 21:1098, 1998

87. Gozani SN, Kong X, Fisher MA: Factors influencing F-wave latency detection of lumbosacral root lesions using a detection theory based model. Clin Neurophysiol, 117:1449, 2006

88. Scelsa SN, Herskovitz S, Berger AR: The diagnostic utility of F waves in L5/S1 radiculopathy. Muscle Nerve, 18:1496, 1995

89. Toyojura M, Murakami K: F-wave study in patients with lumbosacral radiculopathies. Electromyogr Clin Neurophysiol, 37:19, 1997

90. Weber F, Albert U: Electrodiagnostic examination of lumbosacral radiculopathies. Electromyogr Clin Neurophysiol, 40:231, 2000

91. Wells MG, Meyer AP, Emley M et al: Detection of lumbosacral root compression with a novel composite nerve conduction measurement. Spine, 27:2811, 2002

92. Fisher MA, Bajwa R, Somashekar KN: Routine electrodiagnosis and a multiparameter technique in lumbosacral radiculopathies. Acta Neurol Scand, 118:99, 2008

93. Adamova R, Vohanka S, Dusek L: Dynamic electrophysiological examination in patients with lumbar spinal stenosis: is it useful in clinical practice? Eur Spine J, 14:269, 2005

94. Wallbom AS, Geissner ME, Haig AJ et al: Alterations of F wave parameters after exercise in symptomatic spinal stenosis. Am J Phys Med Rehabil, 87:270, 2008

95. Weber F, Ziegler A: Axonal neuropathy in chronic peripheral arterial occlusive disease. Muscle Nerve, 26:471, 2002

96. Argyriou AA, Tsolakis I, Papadoulas S: Dynamic F wave study in patients suffering from peripheral arterial occlusive disease. Acta Neurol Scand, 115:84, 2007

97. Drory VE, Kovach I, Groozman GB: Electrophysiologic evaluation of upper motor involvement in amyotrophic lateral sclerosis. Amyotroph Lateral Scler Other Motor Neuron Disord, 2:147, 2001

98. Argyriou A, Panagiotis P, Talelli P et al: F wave study in amyotrophic lateral sclerosis: assessment of balance between upper and lower motor neuron involvement. Clin Neurophysiol, 117:1260, 2006

99. de Carvalho M, Swash M: Nerve conduction studies in amyotrophic lateral sclerosis. Muscle Nerve, 23:344, 2000

100. Kim J, Takafumi A, Hiromoto I: Evaluation of parameters of serially monitored F-waves in acute spinal cord injury. J Nippon Med Sch, 74:106, 2007

101. Blicher JU, Nielsen JF: Evidence of increased motoneuron excitability in stroke patients without clinical spasticity. Neurorehabil Neurol Repair, 23:14, 2009

The Blink Reflex and Other Cranial Nerve Reflexes

JOSEP VALLS-SOLÉ

Blinking is one of the most frequent motor actions that humans perform every day. It involves the rapid activation of the orbicularis oculi muscle and relaxation of the levator palpebrae muscle. Simply counting the rate of spontaneous blinking and recording the electromyographic (EMG) activity and eyelid movement with EMG electrodes can furnish very relevant information that is of value in the diagnosis of neurologic disorders.[1] However, for neurophysiologic testing, it is customary to induce blinking by applying a sensory stimulus. The most typical method is to apply an electric shock to the supraorbital nerve. Unilateral stimuli give rise to bilateral blink reflexes in the orbicularis oculi muscles. This permits separate assessment of the afferent and the efferent arms of the reflex circuit. The blink reflex, together with other cranial nerve reflexes, such as the jaw jerk and the masseteric silent period, permits the neurophysiologic evaluation of many disorders affecting the cranial nerves and brainstem. Additionally, the blink reflex can be used to examine various functions that are either integrated in, or mediated by, the brainstem. The physiology and clinical utility of the blink reflex are reviewed in this chapter. Other brainstem reflexes, such as the jaw jerk and the masseter inhibitory reflex, are also considered briefly.

BLINK REFLEX

Physiologic Aspects

Blinking is a frequent human action that occurs spontaneously or in response to various sensory inputs. Blink and corneal reflexes are elicited by finger tap on the forehead or light touch of the cornea, and the resulting response can be observed clinically. Recording the EMG activity from the orbicularis oculi provides for a more complete evaluation of the reflex circuit. The most commonly used sensory stimulus for eliciting the blink reflex in the laboratory is a brief electrical shock applied to the supraorbital nerve. The reflex response to that stimulus consists of two separate components: an early ipsilateral R1 and a later bilateral R2 (Fig. 19-1, A). The two responses have a different afferent circuit in the brainstem (Fig. 19-1, B), based on observation of the abnormalities generated with various focal disorders.[2–5] The afferent input goes to facial motor neurons in the facial nucleus in the pons.

The R1 response relates to an oligosynaptic pontine reflex, whereas R2 is relayed through a more complex route including many interneurons in the pons and lateral medulla. R1 serves as a more reliable measure of nerve conduction along the cranial nerves and reflex pathways, with only one or two interneurons between the trigeminal input and the responding facial motor neurons.[6] Analysis of the ipsilateral and contralateral R2 components helps to localize any lesion to the afferent or efferent reflex arc.[7] Involvement of the trigeminal nerve causes an afferent pattern of abnormality, which consists in a delay or diminution of R2 bilaterally after stimulation on the affected side. Diseases of the facial nerve give rise to an efferent pattern with alteration of R2 only on the affected side, regardless of the side of stimulation. A pattern of abnormality not reflecting either an afferent or efferent lesion often indicates the presence of a lesion in the brainstem.[8]

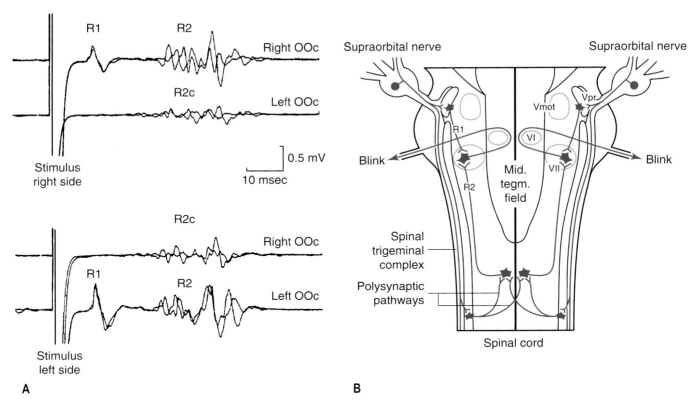

FIGURE 19-1 ▪ **A**, Responses of the orbicularis oculi of both sides to electrical stimulation of the supraorbital nerve of either side. R1 refers to the ipsilateral early response whereas R2 and R2c refer to the late bilateral (ipsilateral and contralateral) responses. **B**, Schematic representation of the brainstem circuit of the blink reflex. The input from the supraorbital nerve reaches the brainstem through the trigeminal root and Gasserian ganglion. It influences two circuits that impinge on facial motor neurons after some delay: an oligosynaptic one at the pontine level, which leads to the R1 response, and a polysynaptic one through the bulbopontine reticular formation, which leads to the bilateral R2 responses. VI, sixth cranial nerve; VII, seventh cranial nerve; Vmot, motor nucleus of the Vth cranial nerve; Vpr, principal nucleus of the Vth cranial nerve. (From Valls-Solé J: Electrodiagnostic studies of the facial nerve in peripheral facial palsy and hemifacial spasm. Muscle Nerve, 36:14, 2007, with permission.)

Blink reflexes can be obtained by electrical stimulation of cranial nerves other than the supraorbital nerve. Stimulation of the infraorbital nerve evokes R1 in some cases and R2 in most subjects, with similar latencies to those elicited by supraorbital nerve stimulation. Shocks applied to the mental nerve elicit R1 or R2 inconsistently and with variable latency. When electrically induced, the blink reflex is believed to result from activation of cutaneous type II afferents. However, the blink reflex can also be induced by activation of other nerve fibers using specific stimuli. This is the case for nociceptive trigeminal afferents. Ellrich and co-workers first pointed out the possibility that some components of the blink reflex were elicited by nociceptive inputs.[9,10] Katsarava and colleagues, using a specially designed electrical stimulator to activate selectively or preferentially small nociceptive fibers of the trigeminal nerve, induced a nociceptive blink reflex response consisting of a bilateral R2 response at a latency of about 50 msec.[11] Other authors subsequently confirmed that the blink reflex can be induced by activation of nociceptive trigeminal afferents by using laser or contact heat stimulators.[12–14] A mechanical tap over the supraorbital notch or to the glabella also elicits a blink reflex of similar characteristics as the one evoked by electrical stimulation. However, although the stimulus is a gentle tap, the response is considered an exteroceptive reflex rather than a stretch reflex; it probably is relayed via the same polysynaptic reflex pathways as the electrically elicited blink reflex. Magnetic stimulation over the supraorbital nerve or at various scalp sites where it can activate trigeminal skin afferents can be used as an alternative in patients who cannot tolerate electrical stimulation.[15]

The blink reflex may also occur as a response to auditory stimuli. The response can be limited to the orbicularis oculi, the so-called auditory blink reflex (ABR). Alternatively, depending on the intensity of the sound and the subject's reactivity, the response can be part of a more generalized startle reaction. The auditory blink reflex and the startle response follow two different brainstem

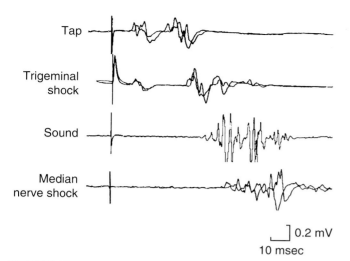

Tap

Trigeminal shock

Sound

Median nerve shock

0.2 mV
10 msec

FIGURE 19-2 ■ Blink reflexes recorded in the orbicularis oculi to the various types of stimuli indicated on the left of each trace. The R1 is seen only with mechanical or electrical stimuli at the forehead

circuits.[16–18] Nevertheless, many similarities exist between these two types of response. The same is probably true for the responses of the orbicularis oculi to electrical stimuli applied to peripheral nerves in the limbs.[19,20] In this case, the orbicularis oculi response is known as the somatosensory blink reflex but it also could be part of a startle reaction to the somatosensory stimuli.[21] Figure 19-2 shows the blink response recorded in the orbicularis oculi to various types of stimuli.

The blink reflex is a powerful tool to measure the excitability of the trigemino-facial reflex arc and, through that, the physiologic correlates of certain functions (and the pathophysiology of dysfunctions) that are either integrated in, or mediated by, the brainstem. There are two main techniques for using the blink reflex to measure excitability of brainstem interneurons or their modulation by rostral inputs: the blink reflex excitability recovery curve (BRER) and blink reflex inhibition by a prepulse (BRIP).

BRER is examined using the double-shock technique.[22] The first stimulus (conditioning) induces a transient change in the excitability of reflex circuits, and the second stimulus (test), delivered at varying interstimulus intervals with respect to the first, is used as a probe stimulus. The BRER curve is obtained by plotting the size of the response elicited by the test stimulus as a percentage of the response to the conditioning stimulus for all intervals tested (usually between 100 and 1000 msec). With paired supraorbital nerve electrical stimuli, R1 is affected little by the conditioning shock, whereas R2 usually is abolished completely from 0 to 200 or 300 msec, and then slowly recovers to reach about 30 to 50 percent at the 500-msec interval and 70 to 90 percent at the 1500-ms interval. Since the same facial motor neurons

subserve both R1 and R2, the different behavior of R1 and R2 is attributed commonly to differences in the interneuronal net. Because interneuronal excitability is under the control of rostral structures, including the basal ganglia, patients with disorders such as parkinsonian syndromes and many forms of dystonia show an enhancement of the R2 excitability recovery curve. The circuits by which the basal ganglia influence the excitability of brainstem interneurons are not understood completely. A pathway comprising the nucleus raphe magnus and the superior colliculus has been suggested[23–25] on the basis of the relationship between saccades and gaze shifts.[26]

BRIP is examined using methods described mainly in regard to the prepulse effect on the startle reaction. A prepulse is any low-intensity stimulus that is unable to cause a recordable response by itself but that induces changes in the response to a subsequent suprathreshold stimulus.[27–29] This effect is considered to be due to the attentional shift required to process the information brought about by the prepulse. Healthy subjects probably are able to integrate at the subcortical level impulses generated by the environmental conditions of daily life, such as visual, acoustic, or somatosensory impulses. These environmental impulses may adopt the role of prepulse stimuli and cause inhibition of undesired motor reactions, which otherwise would interfere with sensory processing of relevant inputs. A prepulse leads to inhibition of the R2 component in the blink reflex to supraorbital stimuli, and also to an increase in the amplitude of the R1 component at a relatively short interstimulus interval between prepulse and supraorbital nerve stimuli.[30] This effect on R1 is not obvious with other stimuli. The dissociation of the prepulse effects on the R1 and R2 components of the blink reflex suggests that the effects of a prepulse take place in sensory integration centers at a pre-motor neuronal level.

The circuit mediating prepulse inhibition is not well known but it is likely related to the pedunculopontine tegmental nucleus. Using the electrodes inserted in the subthalmic nucleus for repetitive deep brain stimulation in patients with Parkinson disease, Costa and coworkers[31] found that the latency of the prepulse effect on the blink reflex was between 0 and 5 msec, suggesting that the effect was mediated by a nearby structure. Since the electrical stimulus first depolarizes axons that are perpendicular to the electrical field, the authors suggested that a likely site of the prepulse effect is the fiber bundle that links the globus pallidus internus with the pedunculopontine tegmental nucleus. It is also possible that some neuronal groups in the subthalamic nucleus projecting to the pedunculopontine nucleus were influenced by the electrode. The excitability of the prepulse circuit can

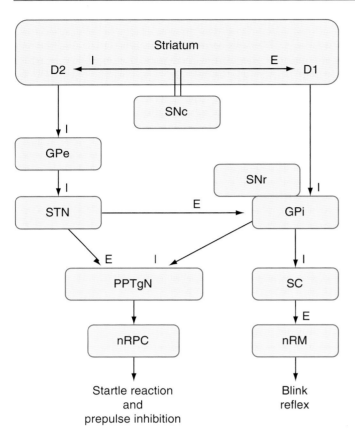

FIGURE 19-3 ■ Schematic circuit through which the basal ganglia can influence the excitability (E) of brainstem interneurons and modify the blink reflex and the prepulse inhibition (I). D1/D2, dopaminergic receptors; SNc, substantia nigra pars compacta; GPe, globus pallidus externus; STN, subthalamic nucleus; SNr, substantia nigra pars reticulata; GPi, globus pallidus internus; PPTgN, pedunculopontine tegmental nucleus; nRPC, nucleus reticularis pontis caudalis; SC, superior colliculus; nRM, nucleus raphe magnus.

be modulated by inputs from the basal ganglia through the output connections from the globus pallidus internus to the pedunculopontine tegmental nucleus, and from this to the nucleus reticularis pontis caudalis. Disorders of the basal ganglia can affect both the BRER and BRIP through these specific circuits. Figure 19-3 shows a hypothetical schematic explanation of the circuits engaged in the basal ganglia modulation of BRER and BRIP.

Methods and Normative Data

Subjects should be resting on a bed or comfortable chair. Surface electrodes are used for both stimulation of the nerve and recording of the response from the orbicularis oculi muscle. Electrical shocks can have a duration of 0.1 or 0.2 msec and an intensity 2 to 3 times above perception threshold (usually ranging between 50 and 100 V or 5 to 10 mA, assuming a skin resistance of 10 kOhm). The

R1 response is usually present with these stimulation parameters but, if not, a good strategy is to request a mild voluntary contraction or apply paired shocks with interstimulus intervals of 3 to 5 msec. The R2 response is habituated easily and, therefore, it is best to give single stimuli with enough separation between them to provide for full recovery of excitability in the circuit. Stimuli applied unexpectedly may be more effective for eliciting the R2 responses. The active recording electrode is placed on the lower aspect of the orbicularis oculi muscle and the reference electrode is placed 2 to 3 cm laterally. Careful placement of the electrodes helps reduce the stimulus artifact that may be bothersome with supraorbital nerve stimulation. An optimal frequency response ranges from 10 Hz to 10 kHz for the recording of either the R1 or R2 component. Increasing the low-frequency cutoff to 100 Hz or even more may be helpful in sharpening the contrast of the responses against baseline, but cutting low frequencies may diminish response amplitude and delay the onset latency. The ground electrode can be placed on the chin or the ears or in another position in the body where it does not interfere with the recordings. Impedance should be checked and electrode placement adjusted if artifacts are problematic.

Normative values for latency of the responses should be obtained in each neurophysiologic laboratory before any patients are studied. The reference values used in the author's laboratory, obtained using a standard technique, are summarized in Table 19-1. The R2 response of the side ipsilateral to the stimulus is usually of larger amplitude and duration than that obtained contralaterally (see Fig. 19-1 and data in Table 19-1). The ratio between R2 responses generated in the same orbicularis oculi after ipsilateral and contralateral stimulation is thus larger than 1.[32] Interestingly, latency values for R1 obtained in infants are usually longer than in adults, despite a considerably shorter reflex arc. In contrast to adults, an R2 response is present in only two-thirds of neonates, mostly on the side ipsilateral to the stimulus, and rarely in premature babies.[33]

TABLE 19-1 ■ **Normative Data for Blink Reflexes to Supraorbital Nerve Stimulation, Obtained in the Author's Laboratory**

	R1	R2	R2c
Mean latency (msec)	11.7 (0.4)	35.1 (2.3)	35.3 (2.4)
Amplitude (mV)	0.7 (0.6)	0.9 (0.7)	0.7 (0.4)
Duration (msec)	5.4 (0.5)	22.1 (17.2)	18.7 (14.9)
Latency upper limit (msec)	13.0	42.2	43.1
Latency difference between sides (msec)	0.5 (0.1)	3.2 (2.2)	3.5 (2.8)

Numbers in parentheses are standard deviations.

JAW JERK AND MASSETERIC SILENT PERIOD

Physiologic Aspects

The mandibular reflex, or jaw jerk, is the only monosynaptic reflex available for electrophysiologic testing in the cranial muscles. It is elicited by a mechanical tap over the mandible with a tendon reflex hammer. The jaw jerk is difficult to evaluate simply by inspection. It is impossible to discern whether there are any abnormalities restricted to one side, or even whether the reflex is present at all in patients who show a response of the lips as well. EMG monitoring of the masseter or temporalis muscle response is of paramount importance in the evaluation of suspected brainstem lesions.[34] The mandibular reflex circuit is also unusual regarding the location of the involved cell bodies. In contrast to those of all other muscles in the body, the proprioceptive neurons of the jaw muscles lie within the neuraxis, protected by the blood–brain barrier from peripheral circulating agents.[35] This is important regarding the diagnosis of certain disorders due to immunologic involvement of the sensory neurons of the Gasserian ganglia.

Stimulation of the stretch receptors induces not only the jaw jerk but also an inhibitory response in the contracting masseter muscles. This is known as the masseter silent period and may correlate with the reaction that occurs when there is an unexpected pinch of our tongue or lips, as while eating. However, in patients with ill-fitting dentures, this silent period may not be reliable.[36,37] A standardized way of measuring the inhibitory masseteric reflexes is to apply an electrical shock to the mentalis nerve. This gives rise to a long-duration silent period, also called the masseter inhibitory reflex (MIR), which is divided into two phases by a burst of EMG activity.[37] Afferent impulses reach the pons via the sensory mandibular or maxillary root of the trigeminal nerve. The first inhibitory period (MIR1; 10- to 13-msec latency) probably is mediated by inhibitory interneurons located close to the ipsilateral trigeminal motor nucleus and projecting onto jaw-closing motor neurons bilaterally. The whole circuit lies in the mid-pons. The afferents for the second inhibitory period, the MIR2 (40- to 50-msec latency), descend in the spinal trigeminal tract and connect to a polysynaptic chain of excitatory interneurons, probably located in the medullary lateral reticular formation. The last interneuron of the chain is inhibitory and gives rise to ipsilateral and contralateral collaterals that ascend to the spinal trigeminal complexes of both sides, to reach the trigeminal motor neurons.[38] Masseter inhibitory reflexes cannot be tested by clinical procedures alone.

The MIR is also consensual—that is, a unilateral stimulus gives rise to bilateral responses. The MIR can provide information on the functional state of the trigemino-trigeminal inhibitory circuits. The MIR also can be elicited by stimulation of the infraorbital nerve with similar characteristics to that obtained by stimulation of the mentalis nerve. Other stimuli, such as magnetic stimulation over the scalp[39,40] or laser stimulation to the face,[41] can give rise to a transient inhibition of masseter muscle contraction.

Methods and Normative Data

The EMG evaluation of the jaw jerk requires use of a reflex hammer that electronically triggers the oscilloscopic sweep. The reflex responses are recorded simultaneously from the right and left masseter muscles using pairs of surface electrodes, the active one placed over the muscle belly at the angle of the mandible, and the reference one placed over the mastoid process or ear lobe. Mean latency of the reflex response is variable on both sides, depending on the strength of the tap and whether the masseter muscle is at rest or tonically contracted. If the reflex response is not obtained at rest, a good strategy is to request the subject to close the mouth slowly while the mandible is tapped. Since reflex latencies vary with successive trials, comparison of simultaneously recorded right-sided and left-sided responses is more meaningful than absolute values, which are of the order of 6 to 8 msec in normal subjects.[34]

Mandibular tapping induces a silent period with a latency of between 10 and 14 msec, which duration is rather variable, depending in part on the strength of the tap and the level of activity in the masseter muscles. The MIR usually is obtained by electrical stimulation of the mentalis nerve. If the MIR is to be used for electrodiagnostic purposes, the subject must exert a steady background voluntary contraction, and the amount of inhibition should be quantified (e.g., the area of suppression). To do that, the signals must be either full-wave rectified and averaged, or examined by superimposing several trials. As with the blink reflex, the MIR can provide information on the site of the lesion by analyzing whether the pattern of abnormality is afferent, mixed, or efferent.[38] Some subjects may not be able to activate their masseter muscles in isolation and contract, instead, the perioral muscles.[42,43] In these cases, no suppression of the EMG activity can be elicited with either a tap to the chin or an electrical stimulus, because there is no silent period in most facial muscles. This should not be mistaken for an abnormal MIR.

TABLE 19-2 ■ **Normative Data for the Jaw Jerk, the Masseteric Silent Period to Chin Taps and the Masseteric Inhibitory Reflex (MIR), Obtained in the Author's Laboratory**

	Side 1	Side 2	Maximum Interside Difference
Jaw jerk mean latency (msec)*	5.6 (1.1)	5.6 (1.1)	0.7
Masseteric silent period latency (msec)*	11.8 (1.2)	11.8 (1.2)	0.8
Masseteric silent period duration (msec)*	18.7 (7.1)	18.7 (7.1)	6.8
MIR1 latency (msec)	14.5 (2.1)	14.5 (2.1)	0.8
MIR1 duration (msec)	19.8 (5.5)	20.1 (5.7)	3.8
MIR2 latency (msec)	44.6 (2.8)	44.9 (3.2)	4.1
MIR2 duration (msec)	22.6 (9.1)	22.2 (9.3)	7.4

Numbers in parentheses are standard deviations.
*Both sides usually have the same response characteristics in healthy subjects.

MIRs cannot be tested by clinical procedures alone and, in some patients, testing the MIR may be the only way of revealing trigeminal or brainstem dysfunction. For the reflex responses of the masseter muscles to have clinical relevance, standardized methods of stimulation and recording should be used. Again, normative values should be obtained in every neurophysiologic laboratory. Table 19-2 provides the reference values obtained in the author's laboratory and Figure 19-4 shows an

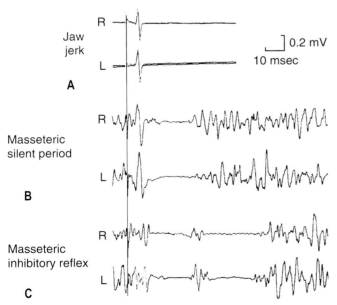

FIGURE 19-4 ■ Trigemino-trigeminal reflexes. **A,** Jaw jerk. **B,** Silent period of the masseter muscles induced by a mechanical tap to the chin. **C,** Masseteric inhibitory reflex induced by electrical stimuli to the mentalis nerve. Note the two phases of the masseteric inhibitory reflex, whereas the silent period to taps shows only one phase.

example of the jaw jerk, the masseter silent period induced by a chin tap, and the MIR induced by electrical stimuli to the mentalis nerve.

CLINICAL APPLICATIONS

The study of the blink reflex to supraorbital nerve stimulation helps in the assessment of many disorders involving the trigeminal and facial nerves and the brainstem. Latency and amplitude of the responses are the most clinically useful parameters but a study of excitability might be important in some central nervous system (CNS) disorders.

Trigeminal Nerve Lesions

The R1 response of the blink reflex is relatively stable with repeated trials and therefore is better suited for assessing nerve conduction through the trigeminal and facial nerves. Analysis of R2, however, helps in localizing the lesion in the trigeminal nerve or nuclei. In these cases, R2 is slowed, diminished, or absent bilaterally when the affected side of the face is stimulated (afferent delay), whereas the responses are normal to stimulation of the unimpaired nerve.

Selective lesions of trigeminal sensory branches are relatively infrequent. They may occur as a result of traumatic nerve injuries or ischemia in relation to arteritis or inflammation in connective tissue diseases. The ophthalmic branch of the trigeminal nerve may be involved together with the oculomotor nerve in the wall of the cavernous sinus and in the Tolosa–Hunt syndrome. The infraorbital and mental branches of the trigeminal nerve can be damaged at the infraorbital foramen or the mental foramen, when the nerves cross the skull, in the so-called numb-cheek or numb-chin syndrome. These syndromes typically are associated with metastatic infiltration of bone in patients with cancer of various types, but the most common causes are lesions resulting from dental procedures or bone infection.[44] The appropriate tests should be chosen according to lesion localization. While the blink reflex can be used to assess the ophthalmic and infraorbital branches, the MIR can provide evidence for involvement of the mentalis branch or infraorbital branches. In fact, the MIR is a trigemino-trigeminal reflex. Testing the MIR may be the only way in some patients of revealing trigeminal or brainstem dysfunction. As in blink reflex studies, the pattern of abnormality (afferent, mixed, or efferent) provides information on the site of the lesion. However, the efferent pattern of lesion is extremely rare except in conditions such as a purely motor trigeminal neuropathy and hemimasticatory spasm.[38]

Involvement of the trigeminal nerve is relatively frequent in patients with Sjögren syndrome. These patients may have a focal or multifocal axonal lesion of the trigeminal nerve or an antigen-mediated immunologic neuronopathy involving neurons in the Gasserian ganglion.[45] Even though both types of lesions have certain clinical similarities, the underlying pathophysiology is quite different. Brainstem reflex testing ideally should indicate the site of the damage. In lesions involving the Gasserian ganglion, the jaw jerk is preserved but the cutaneous-mediated reflex responses are abnormal. In focal or multifocal lesions of the trigeminal nerve or its branches, a branch-compatible distribution of the abnormalities is seen when various brainstem reflexes are studied in combination.[46,47] A variable pattern of lesions may also be found in other disorders—for instance, in systemic sclerosis, where the damage may include both intra- and extra-axial lesions.[48]

No abnormalities usually are detected with the study of brainstem reflexes in patients with idiopathic trigeminal neuralgia. In contrast, R1 was abnormal on the affected side of the face in 10 of 17 patients with tumor, infection, or other demonstrable causes of facial pain.[7] Lesions may be induced in neurons of the Gasserian ganglion following therapeutic thermocoagulation or compression.[49] In accordance with the fact that thermocoagulation predominantly affects small fibers while compression affects large fibers, Cruccu and associates found that patients with thermocoagulation had predominant impairment of corneal reflexes whereas patients treated with compression had predominantly abnormal jaw jerks.[49]

Brainstem vascular lesions may cause injuries in many sites involving the nuclei and tracts of the trigeminal nerve.[34] The most frequent and also the most studied of them is Wallenberg syndrome, which involves the nucleus ambiguus, the spinothalamic tract, and the spinal trigeminal nucleus. Depending on the exact location of the lesion, patients with Wallenberg syndrome may present with a slightly different picture regarding clinical, imaging, and electrophysiologic abnormalities.[50] Again, an afferent pattern of lesion is observed in the R2 responses of the blink reflex but it is important to note that the R1 response, which is integrating in the upper brainstem, is spared (Fig. 19-5).

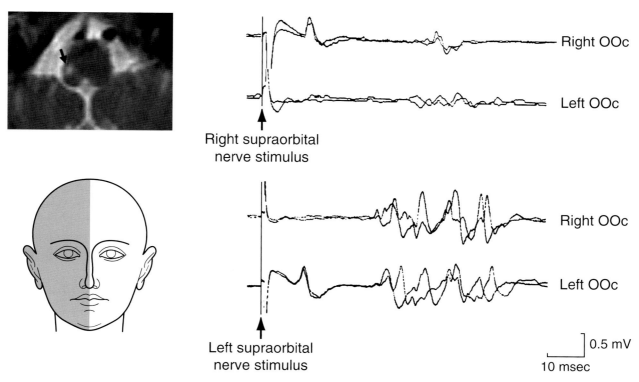

FIGURE 19-5 ■ Blink reflexes obtained in the orbicularis oculi of both sides (right OOc and left OOc) to supraorbital nerve stimuli in a patient with right-sided Wallenberg syndrome (arrowhead in the magnetic resonance image of the brainstem at the upper left side of the figure). The patient complained of right hemifacial hypesthesia (lower left side of the figure). Note the latency delay and amplitude reduction of the R2 and R2c responses, with sparing of R1, to the right supraorbital nerve stimulus.

Facial Nerve Lesions

Facial nerve lesions involving the upper part of the face exhibit an efferent pattern of abnormality in the blink reflex. Responses are abnormal on the affected side and normal on the unimpaired side, regardless of the side where stimuli are applied. Most facial nerve lesions occur in the proximal segments of the nerve. As a consequence, nerve conduction studies using nerve stimulation distal to the lesion site (at the tragus or over a peripheral nerve branch) give rise to a normal compound motor action potential in the nasalis or the orbicularis oculi muscles, provided that no axonal degeneration has occurred, as is usually the case during the first few days after onset of the lesion. However, at this time, the blink reflex already may show nerve conduction abnormalities in proximal segments. In mild cases, there is a partial conduction block with a moderate increase in latency of the

R1 response compared to the other side (Fig. 19-6). The delay is less conspicuous in the R2 responses, which usually are of reduced amplitude if present on the affected side.

In mild cases, patients with idiopathic facial palsy (Bell palsy) are likely to recover motor function within a few days or weeks. However, in some patients (about 10 percent in the author's experience), motor disturbances persist for longer and may be permanent. This is the case in patients with secondary axonal degeneration after Bell palsy or with direct axonal damage in herpetic neuropathy, trauma, or ischemic nerve injury. Substantial axonal degeneration leads to a delayed and usually incomplete recovery associated with synkinesis.[51]

The blink reflex does not differentiate between causes of peripheral facial palsy. Although the most frequent cause is an inflammatory reaction within the petrosal

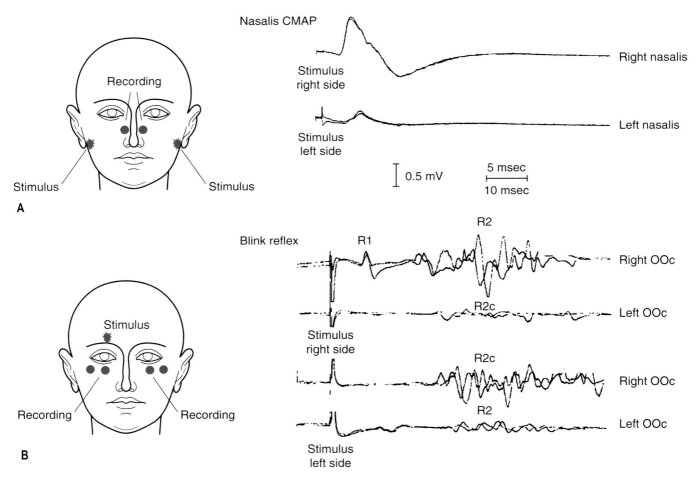

FIGURE 19-6 ▪ **A**, Nasalis compound muscle action potential (CMAP) and **B**, blink reflex responses of the orbicularis oculi (right OOc and left OOc) to stimulation of the supraorbital nerve in a patient with idiopathic peripheral left facial palsy of mild severity. Horizontal calibration bar is 5 msec for the nasalis CMAP and 10 msec for the blink reflex. Note the decrease in the CMAP to about 20 percent of that of the healthy side and the delay of the R1, R2, and R2c responses recorded in the left OOc (efferent pattern of abnormality). This case would be judged as having a relatively good prognosis.

canal from unknown causes or herpes virus infection, hypothetical compression of the nerve by a tumor may give rise to a similar pattern of abnormalities. Neuroimaging may be helpful when the etiology is uncertain.

In patients with Guillain–Barré syndrome, bilateral facial nerve paralysis is common. In such instances, the blink reflex demonstrates a delay in the R1 and R2 responses that occurs relatively early in the course of the disorder and sometimes indicates subclinical involvement of the trigeminal and facial nerves.[52,53] The blink reflex usually is spared in Miller Fisher syndrome unless there is an accompanying peripheral facial palsy that delays R1 on the affected side.

The trigeminal and facial nerves are also involved in hereditary peripheral neuropathies. In hereditary motor and sensory neuropathy type I (HMSN-I), the blink reflex shows a marked delay of R1 and R2.[54] This does not occur in patients with HMSN-II.

Chronic renal failure often causes an abnormal blink reflex that improves after hemodialysis. Exposure to trichloroethylene, known to have specific toxic effects on the trigeminal nerve, also delays R1 latency.[55] It is remarkable that, in most disorders involving the cranial nerves, the latencies of R2 show just a moderate delay that may not differ from normal in individual cases. By contrast, the R1 may be absent or so markedly delayed and temporally dispersed that the response is unrecognizable.

If the facial nerve undergoes axonal degeneration, the first signs of reinnervation may take 3 months or longer to develop, depending on the regeneration distance from the lesion site. However, before then, small polyphasic motor unit action potentials may be recorded from the orbicularis oris of the affected side with a needle inserted lateral and caudal to the oral commissure.[56–59] Interestingly, these action potentials cannot be activated by stimulation of the ipsilateral facial nerve but, instead, they respond to stimuli applied to the contralateral facial nerve. This is, therefore, a good example of reinnervation activity triggered in a healthy nerve by damage to a neighboring nerve.[60] Two mechanisms have been suggested to explain contralateral reinnervation in peripheral facial palsy. One possibility is that terminal axons growing from the facial nerve of the unimpaired side cross the midline and reinnervate denervated perioral muscle fibers on the affected side.[58,59] Another possibility is that reinnervation takes place at the unaffected side in semicircular muscle fibers that had their motor endplates in the affected side.[56,57] These newly formed synapses may interfere with the subsequent growth of axons from the damaged facial nerve and contribute to abnormal muscle function.

After about 3 months or more, axons in the ipsilateral facial nerve will have regenerated to reach and innervate the denervated muscle fibers, and more motor unit action potentials can be detected with a needle electrode in the orbicularis oris or orbicularis oculi. However, electrical stimulation of the ipsilateral facial nerve still is unable to produce direct short-latency activation of those motor units. Instead, they are activated via reflex circuits after stimulation of the trigeminal nerve (either cutaneous afferent branches adjacent to the site of intended facial nerve stimulation at the tragus or the supraorbital nerve). Responses are remarkably similar at all stimulation sites, occurring in both the orbicularis oculi and the orbicularis oris (Fig. 19-7). This observation has been taken as evidence for axonal hypoexcitability combined with motor neuronal hyperexcitability during the reinnervation period.[51] It also indicates that reinnervation abnormalities occur from the very beginning of reinnervation. It is difficult to know whether such abnormalities result from changes at the motor neuronal level or from aberrant axonal branching or ephapsis.

Reinnervation can lead to *synkinesis*, in which any attempt to move a specific facial muscle causes unwanted activation of other facial muscles. In the full-blown postparalytic facial syndrome, patients exhibit myokymia, synkinesis, and hemifacial mass contractions that sometimes may resemble those seen in essential hemifacial spasm.[51] Such uncomfortable mass contractions are triggered by automatic or emotional facial movements and may be very distressing. Disturbing hemifacial mass contractions were reported by 5 of 23 patients with postparalytic facial syndrome following Bell palsy suffered 1.5 to 16 years earlier.[61] These 5 patients experienced not just hemifacial synkinesis, but severe episodes of muscular pain, tension, and spasms induced by common maneuvers such as eating, smiling, kissing, or singing.

Synkinetic movements develop in nearly all cases after an axonal lesion of the facial nerve, unless only a very distal branch was involved.[7] They can be documented by obtaining the two components of the blink reflex not only in the orbicularis oculi but also in the orbicularis oris when the supraorbital nerve is stimulated. Synkinesis is also a typical feature of essential hemifacial spasm, which goes together with lateral spread, autoexcitation, and ephaptic transmission.[62,63]

Although the exact mechanism for the generation of *hemifacial spasm* is not known, it is believed that chronic compression by a vascular structure impinging over the nerve at the level of root entry in the posterior fossa causes irritation of the nerve with generation of ectopic discharges, autoexcitation, ephapsis, and lateral spread of excitation among nerve fibers, giving rise to the

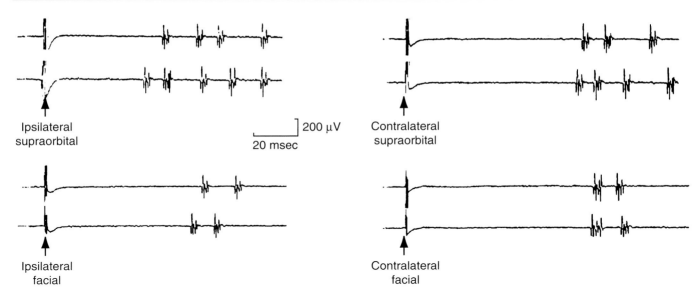

FIGURE 19-7 ■ Responses to nerve stimulation recorded by needle electromyography from the orbicularis oris in a patient with facial paralysis, at onset of reinnervation (about 3 months after onset of symptoms). Two response traces are shown for each stimulation site (arrowhead). Note that the responses are made of action potentials of similar shape, firing repeatedly. In this case, response latency is about 60 msec for all stimulation sites except for the ipsilateral supraorbital nerve stimulation, which is about 40 msec. The observation is compatible with reflex generation of abnormal synkinetic responses in the orbicularis oris at a time when direct responses are not yet obtained.

involuntary muscle twitching and spasms. In essential hemifacial spasm, activity in one branch of the facial nerve generates impulses in adjacent branches.[62,63] For instance, stimulation of the zygomatic branch results in the expected response in the orbicularis oculi muscle but also a simultaneous response in the mentalis muscle. In the damaged nerve zone, ectopic activity may be triggered by mechanical irritation or flow of extracellular current during passage of nerve impulses.

The constant bombardment of antidromic inputs to the facial motor neurons may also cause secondary motor neuronal hyperexcitability that contributes to abnormal hyperactivity of the facial nerve-innervated muscles.[64] In idiopathic hemifacial spasm, synkinetic responses are more variable in latency and waveform than those in the postparalytic facial syndrome. Moreover, in the former, the involuntary twitches of the muscles of one side of the face are not necessarily triggered by voluntary or automatic muscle contraction but may occur apparently spontaneously. This is a crucial difference to the mass contractions of the postparalytic facial syndrome, which always are started by intended muscular contraction. In essential hemifacial spasm, the abnormal contraction is usually paroxysmal and consists of rapid, irregular clonic bursts of EMG activity, involving the lower and upper facial muscles simultaneously. In some instances there may also be long-lasting tonic contractions. The twitching may be induced by 2 to 3 minutes

of hyperventilation, which presumably causes respiratory alkalosis and decreases the calcium level, triggering ectopic excitation.[62]

A feature common to both entities is synkinesis. This may occur even in patients who underwent a surgical anastomosis between the XII nerve and the facial nerve. This has been attributed to plastic changes in the connectivity between nuclei of the hypoglossal and facial nerves. However, another more parsimonious explanation relates to the fact that facial motor nerve terminals are excitable at the site where the stimulus intended for the supraorbital nerve is applied.[65] In this circumstance, the antidromically conducted impulse can reach a site of branching or ephaptic transmission and give rise to axo-axonal responses in distant facial muscles (Fig. 19-8). This makes it unnecessary to hypothesize the occurrence of plastic changes in connectivity in the brainstem.

Intra-Axial Lesions

The blink reflex may be used to document brainstem lesions involving the reflex arc. A thorough neurophysiologic study of blink, jaw, and masseteric inhibitory reflexes may be valuable for the topographic diagnosis of neurologic lesions. This may be important for disorders that can affect both peripheral nerves and intra-axial sites, such as a vasculitis or other inflammatory processes. Detailed neurophysiologic study in such cases

FIGURE 19-8 ■ Schematic representation of the two circuits by which an electrical stimulus in the supraorbital region could lead to synkinetic responses of the orbicularis oculi and orbicularis oris in a patient with a lesion inducing ephaptic responses in the facial nerve. The electrical stimulus can induce depolarization of supraorbital nerve axons, leading to trans-synaptic activation of facial motor neurons and an orthodromically propagated volley in the facial nerve. Also, the electrical stimulus can lead to depolarization of facial nerve axon terminals of muscles below the electrode. The volley in this case will be conducted antidromically until the site of ephapsis.

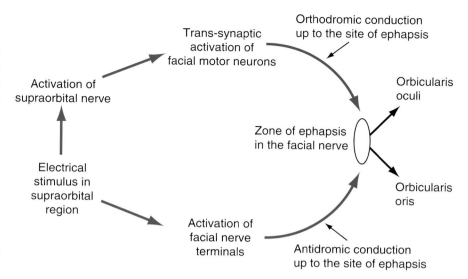

may complement the neuroimaging findings and sometimes will reveal functional lesions with no clear structural correlate.[5,66]

The R1 of the blink reflex to supraorbital nerve stimulation may be delayed or absent in intra-axial brainstem lesions, as well as with extra-axial lesions that compress or displace the cranial nerves or brainstem.[7] Preservation of R1 with impairment of R2 of the blink reflex is the archetypical pattern of intra-axial lesions involving the lower part of the brainstem, such as in Wallenberg syndrome.[50,67] Wallenberg syndrome results from a selective infarction of the lateral medulla.[50] In these patients, the R2 can be absent, of low amplitude, or delayed on both sides to stimulation of the supraorbital nerve of the side on which the infarct occurred. In contrast, stimulation on the normal side of the face evokes a normal R2 bilaterally. Stimulation of the infraorbital nerve or mental nerve gives rise to a similar afferent pattern of abnormality. The preservation of R1 indicates normal afferent conduction in the trigeminal nerve and normal efferent conduction in the facial nerve after normal integration at the pontine level, whereas abnormal ipsilateral and contralateral R2 responses indicate the involvement of circuits or centers mediating those responses in the reticular formation level before the facial nucleus is reached. Different types of blink reflex findings seen in Wallenberg syndrome reflect variations of the infarcted area of the brainstem within the lateral medulla.[68,69]

An efferent pattern of abnormalities in the blink reflex as a result of intra-axial lesions is markedly less frequent than the afferent pattern. A mixed pattern, not characteristic of either type, may suggest either combined involvement of the trigeminal and facial nerves or a relatively widespread brainstem lesion.

Patients with hemispheric lesions may also develop an afferent delay of R2 when the affected side of the face is stimulated. This abnormality, sometimes indistinguishable from that found in Wallenberg syndrome, is seen commonly, although not exclusively, in patients with substantial sensory disturbances of the face. The MIR is of similar value to the blink reflex in the evaluation of the infraorbital and mentalis branches of the trigeminal nerve. The first MIR period appears to be insensitive to peripheral conditioning and suprasegmental modulation; its latency varies little, and it probably is mediated by a small number of afferents. For these reasons it is the best available response for assessing function of the maxillary and mandibular afferents, in focal and generalized diseases. The latency of the first MIR period can be delayed significantly in patients with demyelinating polyneuropathies or severe diabetic polyneuropathy.[37] In patients with symptomatic trigeminal neuralgia or focal lesions within the pons, it has a diagnostic sensitivity similar to that of the R1 of the blink reflex.

Apart from the blink reflex induced by supraorbital nerve stimulation, studying the somatosensory blink reflex may be of interest for the evaluation of brainstem lesions. Miwa and associates reported enhanced responses of the orbicularis oculi to median nerve stimuli in patients with Miller Fisher syndrome.[20] It has been found that this reflex response was abolished in patients with progressive supranuclear palsy.[70] Interestingly, another facial reflex elicited by median nerve stimulation, a mentalis muscle response that could be a correlate of the palmomental reflex,[71] was preserved in the same patients that had an absent somatosensory blink reflex. It was therefore concluded that the abnormality was not in the afferent or efferent arms of the reflex but in a brainstem structure where the sensory inputs were integrated on their way to activate facial motor neurons of the orbicularis oculi. A similar pattern of abnormalities has since been noted in a patient medicated with clebopride, a prokinetic drug with central antidopaminergic effects,[72] and in patients with vascular or immune-mediated upper brainstem lesions.[73] Remarkably, the blink reflex to supraorbital nerve stimuli is normal in these patients and in patients with progressive supranuclear palsy.[70] Therefore, the circuits mediating the somatosensory blink reflex seem to be affected separately from those of the blink reflex induced by trigeminal afferents. These findings make the somatosensory blink reflex an interesting technique for the neurophysiologic assessment of patients with mesencephalic lesions.

The blink reflex is frequently abnormal in patients with multiple sclerosis.[74,75] However, the incidence of abnormalities varies greatly, depending on the selection of patients (i.e., the longer the history of clinical symptoms, the higher is the probability of brainstem lesions). A conspicuous delay of the R1 has been reported in lesions involving the pons in multiple sclerosis.[7] However, the delay was always less than in patients with Guillain–Barré syndrome or HMSN. Consecutive evaluations of the blink reflex and, especially, the R1 latency may help in localizing a subclinical lesion to the pons and, therefore, establishing spatial dissemination of lesions.[75]

Impairment of Brainstem Interneuronal Excitability

The late blink reflex responses are mediated by many interneurons, the excitability of which has an important role in the prevalence and size of the R2 and R2c responses. Many disorders may cause a change in the excitability of groups of brainstem interneurons. One of the hypothesized control mechanisms of the excitability of trigeminal interneurons is the input that these interneurons receive from the basal ganglia.[23,24] Another circuit of control links the basal ganglia with the nuclei of the reticular formation through the pedunculopontine tegmental nuclei (see Fig. 19-3). Therefore, disorders of the basal ganglia are likely to cause an impairment in the excitability of the brainstem circuits mediating the blink reflex and other reflex responses. The methods used to test brainstem interneuronal excitability through the blink reflex are mainly two: BRER and BRIP.

Paired conditioning and test stimulation at short interstimulus intervals can document the dysfunction of brainstem interneurons. This was one of the earliest contributions of brainstem reflex studies to the assessment of CNS abnormalities in patients with parkinsonism.[22] Abnormally enhanced trigemino-facial reflex excitability can be demonstrated with a decrease in the habituation of the R2 response, while the R1 response is not affected. This suggests that the disturbance lies in the interneurons rather than in the motor neurons.

Since the first publication by Kimura on the relevance of the technique of paired stimulation in demonstrating the alterations of trigemino-facial interneuron excitability in parkinsonism,[22] many authors have studied the blink reflex excitability recovery curve to paired stimuli, by dividing the size of the response to the test stimulus by that of the response to the conditioning stimulus. An abnormal blink reflex excitability recovery curve has been reported not only in almost all diseases presenting with parkinsonism, but in many other disorders as well.[76,77] It is therefore of little use for differential diagnosis between degenerative disorders. In clinical practice, the assessment of enhanced trigemino-facial reflex excitability may be of interest for documenting abnormal function of brainstem interneurons in patients in whom clinical assessment is dubious or at early stages of their disease. Similarly to the R2 blink reflex, the second period of the MIR shows a strongly enhanced recovery cycle in patients with extrapyramidal disorders such as Parkinson disease and dystonia, and conversely, increased habituation in hemiplegia. The excitability of the second period of the MIR is a focus of research in patients with headache.

The blink reflex can be inhibited also by a preceding weak stimulus, as discussed earlier. Such prepulse inhibition is a ubiquitous phenomenon that has been used only occasionally in clinical studies.[78] Prepulse effects reveal sensorimotor integration at the subcortical level, offering the possibility of evaluating the function of relatively complex reflex circuits in the characterization of various psychologic conditions or neurologic diseases. Healthy subjects probably are able to integrate at the subcortical level impulses generated by the environmental conditions of daily life, such as visual, acoustic, or somatosensory impulses. These environmental impulses may adopt the role of prepulse stimuli and effectively suppress unwanted attentional shifts or reactions. This seems not to be the case in patients with schizophrenia.[79] Prepulse inhibition has been reported as abnormal in certain neurologic disorders such as Parkinson disease,[80,81] Huntington disease,[82,83] and cranial dystonia.[84] The author has also found prepulse abnormalities in other syndromes presenting with parkinsonism, such as progressive supranuclear palsy (Fig. 19-9).

FIGURE 19-9 ■ Examples of prepulse inhibition in a healthy control subject (**A**) and in a patient with parkinsonism (**B**). Responses were recorded in the right and left orbicularis oculi muscles (OOc). In the upper traces, only a supraorbital nerve stimulus was applied at the thick arrowhead, and the typical R1, R2, and R2c responses were obtained. In the lower traces, the same supraorbital nerve stimulus was preceded by a prepulse stimulus, a low-intensity electrical stimulus to the third finger that did not generate any reflex response by itself. Note the inhibition of the R2 and R2c responses in the healthy subject, and their preservation (abnormally reduced inhibition) in the patient.

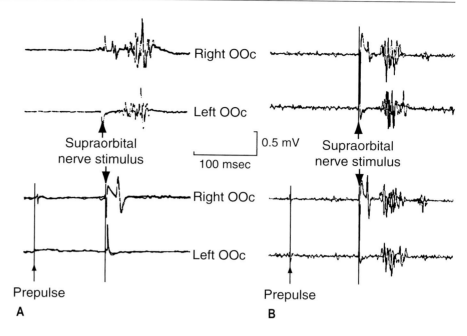

CONCLUDING COMMENTS

The blink reflex is useful for the study of trigeminal, facial, or brainstem disorders. Techniques range from simply counting the occurrence of spontaneous blinking to analyzing complex phenomena of excitability control. They are not demanding in terms of technical complexity or equipment and, therefore, they are relatively cheap in comparison to other investigative techniques. The only requirement is a basic knowledge of physiology and anatomy, as well as neurophysiologic skills to ensure the correct execution of the tests and a sufficient knowledge of clinical neurology to be able to fit the results into their clinical context. The information thus provided should be relevant for the interpretation of symptoms, differential diagnosis, and prognosis of many neurologic disorders involving brainstem functions.

REFERENCES

1. Valls-Solé J: Neurophysiology of motor control and movement disorders. p. 7. In Jankovic J, Tolosa E (eds): Parkinson's disease and Movement Disorders. Lippincott Williams & Wilkins, Philadelphia, 2007
2. Kimura J, Lyon LW: Orbicularis oculi reflex in the Wallenberg syndrome: alteration of the late reflex by lesions of the spinal tract and nucleus of the trigeminal nerve. J Neurol Neurosurg Psychiatry, 35:228, 1972
3. Ongerboer de Visser BW, Goor C: Electromyographic and reflex study in idiopathic and symptomatic trigeminal neuralgias: latency of the jaw and blink reflexes. J Neurol Neurosurg Psychiatry, 37:1225, 1974
4. Aramideh M, Ongerboer de Visser BW: Brainstem reflexes: electrodiagnostic techniques, physiology, normative data, and clinical applications. Muscle Nerve, 26:14, 2002
5. Cruccu G, Iannetti GD, Marx JJ et al: Brainstem reflex circuits revisited. Brain, 128:386, 2005
6. Trontelj MA, Trontelj JV: Reflex arc of the first component of the human blink reflex: a single motoneurone study. J Neurol Neurosurg Psychiatry, 41:538, 1978
7. Kimura J: Electrodiagnosis in Diseases of Nerve and Muscle. Principles and Practice. 3rd Ed. Oxford University Press, New York, 2001
8. Aramideh M, Ongerboer de Visser BW, Koelman JH et al: The late blink reflex response abnormality due to lesion of the lateral tegmental field. Brain, 120:1685, 1997
9. Ellrich J, Hopf HC: The R3 component of the blink reflex: normative data and application in spinal lesions. Electroencephalogr Clin Neurophysiol, 101:349, 1996
10. Ellrich J, Bromm B, Hopf HC: Pain-evoked blink reflex. Muscle Nerve, 20:265, 1997
11. Katsarava Z, Ellrich J, Diener HC et al: Optimized stimulation and recording parameters of human "nociception specific" blink reflex recordings. Clin Neurophysiol, 113:1932, 2002
12. Romaniello A, Valls-Solé J, Ianetti G et al: Nociceptive quality of the laser-evoked blink reflex in humans. J Neurophysiol, 87:1386, 2002
13. Romaniello A, Iannetti GD, Truini A et al: Trigeminal responses to laser stimuli. Neurophysiol Clin, 33:315, 2003
14. Truini A, Galeotti F, Pennisi E et al: Trigeminal small-fibre function assessed with contact heat evoked potentials in humans. Pain, 132:102, 2007
15. Bischoff C, Liscic R, Meyer B-U et al: Magnetically elicited blink reflex: an alternative to conventional electrical stimulation. Electromyogr Clin Neurophysiol, 33:265, 1993

16. Davis M, Gendelman DS, Tischler MD et al: A primary acoustic startle circuit: lesion and stimulation studies. J Neurosci, 2:791, 1982

17. Hori A, Yasuhara A, Naito H et al: Blink reflex elicited by auditory stimulation in the rabbit. J Neurol Sci, 76:49, 1986

18. Brown P, Rothwell JC, Thompson PD et al: New observations on the normal auditory startle reflex in man. Brain, 114:1891, 1991

19. Gokin AP, Karpukhina MV: Reticular structures of the cat brain participating in startle reflexes in response to somatic stimuli of different modalities. Neurofiziologia, 17:380, 1985

20. Miwa H, Nohara C, Hotta M: Somatosensory-evoked blink response: investigation of the physiological mechanisms. Brain, 121:281, 1998

21. Alvarez-Blanco S, Leon L, Valls-Solé J: The startle reaction to somatosensory inputs: different response pattern to stimuli of upper and lower limbs. Exp Brain Res, 195:285, 2009

22. Kimura J: Disorders of interneurons in parkinsonism. The orbicularis oculi reflex to paired stimuli. Brain, 96:87, 1973

23. Basso MA, Powers AS, Evinger C: An explanation for reflex blink hyperexcitability in Parkinson's disease. I. Superior colliculus. J Neurosci, 16:7308, 1996

24. Basso MA, Evinger C: An explanation for reflex blink hyperexcitability in Parkinson's disease. II. Nucleus raphe magnus. J Neurosci, 16:7318, 1996

25. Rothwell JC: Physiology and anatomy of possible oscillators in the central nervous system. Mov Disord, 13(Suppl 3):24, 1998

26. Evinger C, Manning KA, Pellegrini JJ et al: Not looking while leaping: the linkage of blinking and saccadic gaze shifts. Exp Brain Res, 100:337, 1994

27. Graham FK: The more or less startling effects of weak prestimulation. Psychophysiology, 12:238, 1975

28. Hoffman HS, Ison JR: Reflex modification in the domain of startle. I. Some empirical findings and their implications for how the nervous system processes sensory input. Psychol Rev, 87:175, 1980

29. Ison JR, Hoffman HS: Reflex modification in the domain of startle. II. The anomalous history of a robust and ubiquitous phenomenon. Psychol Bull, 94:3, 1983

30. Ison JR, Sanes JN, Foss JA et al: Facilitation and inhibition of the human startle blink reflexes by stimulus anticipation. Behav Neurosci, 104:418, 1990

31. Costa J, Valls-Solé J, Valldeoriola F: Single subthalamic nucleus deep brain stimuli inhibit the blink reflex in Parkinson's disease patients. Brain, 129:1758, 2006

32. Manca D, Munoz E, Pastor P: Enhanced gain of blink reflex responses to ipsilateral supraorbital nerve afferent inputs in patients with facial nerve palsy. Clin Neurophysiol, 112:153, 2001

33. Hatanaka T, Yasuhara A, Kobayashi Y: Electrically and mechanically elicited blink reflexes in infants and children—maturation and recovery curves of blink reflex. Electroencephalogr Clin Neurophysiol, 76:39, 1990

34. Hopf HC: Topodiagnostic value of brainstem reflexes. Muscle Nerve, 17:475, 1994

35. Graus F, Santamaría J, Obach J et al: Sensory neuropathy as remote effect of cancer. Neurology, 37:1266, 1987

36. Cruccu G, Frisardi G, Pauletti G et al: Excitability of the central masticatory pathways in patients with painful temporomandibular disorders. Pain, 73:447, 1997

37. Cruccu G, Ongerboer de Visser BW: The jaw reflexes. In IFCN Recommendations for the Practice of Clinical Neurophysiology. Electroencephalogr Clin Neurophysiol Suppl, 52:243, 1999

38. Cruccu G, Deuschl G: The clinical use of brainstem reflexes and hand-muscle reflexes. Clin Neurophysiol, 111:371, 2000

39. Cruccu G, Inghilleri M, Berardelli A: Cortical mechanisms mediating the inhibitory period after magnetic stimulation of the facial motor area. Muscle Nerve, 20:418, 1997

40. Jaberzadeh S, Sakuma S, Zoghi M: Focal transcranial magnetic stimulation of motor cortex evokes bilateral and symmetrical silent periods in human masseter muscles. Clin Neurophysiol, 119:693, 2008

41. Cruccu G, Romaniello A: Jaw-opening reflex after CO_2 laser stimulation of the perioral region in man. Exp Brain Res, 118:564, 1998

42. Valls-Solé J: Neurophysiological assessment of trigeminal nerve reflexes in disorders of central and peripheral nervous system. Clin Neurophysiol, 116:2255, 2005

43. Valls-Solé J, Deuschl G: Reflex responses, silent period and long latency reflexes. p. 237. In Kimura J (ed): Peripheral Nerve Diseases. Elsevier, Amsterdam, 2006

44. Liguori R, Cevoli S, Montagna P: Electroneurographic investigation of the mandibular nerve in lingual neuropathy. Muscle Nerve, 21:410, 1998

45. Font J, Ramos-Casals M, De la Red G et al: Pure sensory neuropathy in primary Sjögren's syndrome. Longterm prospective follow-up and review of the literature. J Rheumatol, 30:1552, 2003

46. Valls-Solé J, Graus F, Font J et al: Normal proprioceptive trigeminal afferents in patients with Sjögren's syndrome and sensory neuronopathy. Ann Neurol, 28:786, 1990

47. Aramideh M, Valls-Solé J, Ongerboer de Visser BW: Electrophysiological investigations in cranial hyperkinetic syndromes. p. 559. In Hallett M (ed): Handbook of Clinical Neurophysiology. Elsevier, Amsterdam, 2003

48. Casale R, Frazzitta G, Fundaro C et al: Blink reflex discloses CNS dysfunction in neurologically asymptomatic patients with systemic sclerosis. Clin Neurophysiol, 115:1917, 2004

49. Cruccu G, Inghilleri M, Fraioli B: Neurophysiologic assessment of trigeminal function after surgery for trigeminal neuralgia. Neurology, 37:631, 1987

50. Valls-Solé J, Vila N, Obach V et al: Brainstem reflexes in patients with Wallenberg's syndrome. Muscle Nerve, 19:1093, 1996

51. Valls-Solé J: Electrodiagnostic studies of the facial nerve in peripheral facial palsy and hemifacial spasm. Muscle Nerve, 36:14, 2007

52. Kimura J: Conduction abnormalities of the facial and trigeminal nerves in polyneuropathy. Muscle Nerve, 5(9S): S139, 1982

53. Vucic S, Cairns KD, Black KR et al: Neurophysiologic findings in early acute inflammatory demyelinating polyradiculoneuropathy. Clin Neurophysiol, 115:2329, 2004

54. Ishpekova BA, Christova LG, Alexandrov AS et al: The electrophysiological profile of hereditary motor and sensory neuropathy-Lom. J Neurol Neurosurg Psychiatry, 76:875, 2005

55. Feldman RG, Niles C, Proctor SP et al: Blink reflex measurement of effects of trichloroethylene exposure on the trigeminal nerve. Muscle Nerve, 15:490, 1992

56. Trojaborg W, Siemssen SO: Reinnervation after resection of the facial nerve. Arch Neurol, 26:17, 1972

57. Trojaborg W: Does cross-innervation occur after facial palsy? J Neurol Neurosurg Psychiatry, 40:712, 1977

58. Gilhuis HJ, Beurskens CHG, Marres HA et al: Contralateral reinnervation of midline muscles in facial paralysis. Muscle Nerve, 24:1703, 2001

59. Gilhuis HJ, Beurskens CHG, de Vries J et al: Contralateral reinnervation of midline muscles in nonidiopathic facial palsy. J Clin Neurophysiol, 20:151, 2003

60. Valls-Solé J, Castillo CD, Casanova-Molla J et al: Clinical consequences of reinnervation disorders after focal peripheral nerve lesions. Clin Neurophysiol, 122:219, 2011

61. Cossu G, Valls-Solé J, Valldeoriola F: Reflex excitability of facial motoneurons at onset of muscle reinnervation after facial nerve palsy. Muscle Nerve, 22:614, 1999

62. Nielsen VK: Pathophysiology of hemifacial spasm: I. Ephaptic transmission and ectopic excitation. Neurology, 34:418, 1984

63. Nielsen VK: Pathophysiology of hemifacial spasm: II. Lateral spread of the supraorbital nerve reflex. Neurology, 34:427, 1984

64. Möller AR: The cranial nerve vascular compression syndrome: II. A review of pathophysiology. Acta Neurochir, 113:24, 1991

65. Montero J, Junyent J, Calopa M: Electrophysiological study of ephaptic axono-axonal responses in hemifacial spasm. Muscle Nerve, 35:184, 2007

66. Marx JJ, Iannetti GD, Thömke F et al: Somatotopic organization of the corticospinal tract in the human brainstem: a MRI-based mapping analysis. Ann Neurol, 57:824, 2005

67. Ongerboer de Visser BW, Kuypers HGJM: Late blink reflex changes in lateral medullary lesions: an electrophysiological and neuroanatomical study of Wallenberg's syndrome. Brain, 101:285, 1978

68. Sacco RL, Freddo L, Bello JA et al: Wallenberg's lateral medullary syndrome. Clinical-magnetic resonance imaging correlations. Arch Neurol, 50:609, 1993

69. Kim JS, Lee JH, Lee MC: Patterns of sensory dysfunction in lateral medullary infarction. Neurology, 49:1557, 1997

70. Valls-Solé J, Valldeoriola F, Tolosa E et al: Distinctive abnormalities of facial reflexes in patients with progressive supranuclear palsy. Brain, 120:1877, 1997

71. Dehen H, Bathien N, Cambier J: The palmo-mental reflex. An electrophysiological study. Eur Neurol, 13:395, 1975

72. Campdelacreu J, Kumru H, Tolosa E et al: Progressive supranuclear palsy syndrome induced by clebopride. Mov Disord, 19:482, 2004

73. Leon L, Casanova-Molla J, Lauria G et al: The somatosensory blink reflex in upper and lower brainstem lesions. Muscle Nerve, 43:196, 2011

74. Khoshbin S, Hallett M: Multimodality evoked potentials and blink reflex in multiple sclerosis. Neurology, 31:138, 1981

75. Kiers L, Carroll WM: Blink reflexes and magnetic resonance imaging in focal unilateral central trigeminal pathway demyelination. J Neurol Neurosurg Psychiatry, 53:526, 1990

76. Smith SJ, Lees AJ: Abnormalities of the blink reflex in Gilles de la Tourette syndrome. J Neurol Neurosurg Psychiatry, 52:895, 1989

77. Eekhof JL, Aramideh M, Bour LJ et al: Blink reflex recovery curves in blepharospasm, torticollis spasmodica, and hemifacial spasm. Muscle Nerve, 19:10, 1996

78. Valls-Solé J, Valldeoriola F, Molinuervo JL et al: Prepulse modulation of the startle reaction and the blink reflex in normal human subjects. Exp Brain Res, 129:49, 1999

79. Campanella S, Guerit JM: How clinical neurophysiology may contribute to the understanding of a psychiatric disease such as schizophrenia. Neurophysiol Clin, 39:31, 2009

80. Nakashima K, Shimoyama R, Yokoyama Y et al: Auditory effects on the electrically elicited blink reflex in patients with Parkinson's disease. Electroencephalogr Clin Neurophysiol, 89:108, 1993

81. Lozza A, Pepin JL, Rapisarda G et al: Functional changes of brainstem reflexes in Parkinson's disease. Conditioning of the blink reflex R2 component by paired and index finger stimulation. J Neural Transm, 104:679, 1997

82. Swerdlow NR, Paulsen J, Braff DL: Impaired prepulse inhibition of acoustic and tactile startle response in patients with Huntington's disease. J Neurol Neurosurg Psychiatry, 58:192, 1995

83. Muñoz E, Cervera A, Valls-Solé J: Neurophysiological study of facial chorea in patients with Huntington's disease. Clin Neurophysiol, 114:1246, 2003

84. Gomez-Wong E, Marti MJ, Tolosa E et al: Sensory modulation of the blink reflex in patients with blepharospasm. Arch Neurol, 55:1233, 1998

Electrophysiologic Evaluation of Movement Disorders

MARK HALLETT

The electrophysiologic evaluation of movement disorders is not used as widely as traditional electromyography (EMG) and nerve conduction studies, but it can contribute to clinical management.[1,2] Physiologic analysis can be useful in the classification of difficult involuntary movements by providing information that is impossible to obtain by clinical observation alone. Physiologic studies can also be valuable for guiding therapy and for increasing our understanding of the pathophysiology of movement disorders. Additionally, physiologic analysis permits the quantification of involuntary movements, which is particularly valuable for research purposes such as in drug trials.

ANALYSIS OF MOVEMENT

Measurement of Movement

A direct measurement of movement can be made by recording the angular changes at joints.[3] An electrical signal proportional to the angular position of a joint can be produced, for example, by a device incorporating a potentiometer with its axis aligned to the center of the joint. Velocity and acceleration can be obtained by differentiation. Movement also can be measured with video systems; these are used commonly for complex movement such as gait. Movement of the hand in two dimensions can be assessed with a data tablet. Acceleration can be determined directly with an accelerometer. Accelerometers in common use measure movement only in one axis, so they must be oriented carefully in the direction of movement. Also available are triaxial accelerometers that measure movement in three orthogonal axes and permit three-dimensional description of movement. Accelerometers are used most commonly for the analysis of tremor. Less commonly used are gyroscopic devices that measure rotations. There are also triaxial gyroscopes, and even devices with both triaxial accelerometers and triaxial gyroscopes that then permit a complete description of translations and rotations.

The output of an accelerometer is a time-varying analog signal proportional to instantaneous acceleration (Fig. 20-1).[4] In the case of tremor, the signal can be processed in several ways to get a number (or numbers) to characterize the waveform. The root-mean-square (RMS) amplitude calculated over a period (e.g., 20 to 30 seconds) is the best measure of the "average" amplitude. A more complete analysis of the waveform can be made by calculating the Fourier transform (usually accomplished by computer using a fast Fourier transformation, or FFT). This produces a plot of power in the signal as a function of frequency. If the signal has one major frequency component, the plot will have a single major peak; the power of that peak will be proportional to the RMS amplitude. The acceleration signal can be double-integrated to produce the total distance moved; if only the portion of the signal in the tremor peak is processed in this way, the result is the distance moved by virtue of tremor.

Electromyographic Activity

Another measure of movement is the electromyogram of the muscles producing the movement.[5] Because EMG is a direct measure of alpha motor neuron activity, it provides information about the central nervous system command that generates the movement. Numerous muscles act on each joint; it is necessary to record from at least two muscles with antagonist actions. EMG is used occasionally as a measure of force, even though the relationship between EMG amplitude and force is only approximate. The timing information from the EMG signal is much more accurate.

EMG data can be measured with surface, needle, or wire electrodes.[1,5] The advantages of surface electrodes are that they are not painful and record from a relatively large volume of muscle. The advantage of needle electrodes is that they are more selective; this is sometimes a necessity when recording from small or deep muscles. Traditional needle electrodes are stiff, and it is best to use them when recording from muscles during movements that are close to isometric. Pairs of fine wire electrodes have the advantage of selectivity similar to that of needle electrodes and are also flexible, permitting free movement with only minimal pain. In any case, it is important to avoid movement artifact, which can contaminate the EMG signal. Wire movement should be limited. Low-frequency content of the EMG signal can be restricted with filtering. Impedance of surface electrodes should be reduced.

Inspection of the EMG signal of an involuntary movement reveals, first, whether the movement is regular (usually a tremor) or irregular. There are sometimes surprises in such an analysis. Rhythmic EMG activity can appear irregular clinically if the amplitude varies; irregular EMG activity sometimes will appear rhythmic clinically if it is rapid. The duration of the EMG burst

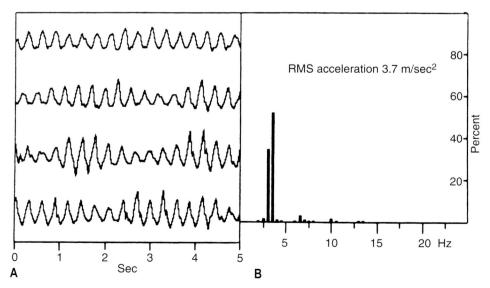

FIGURE 20-1 ■ Accelerometer recording of tremor. **A**, The direct signal in four successive segments of 5 seconds each. **B**, Frequency analysis of the same 20 seconds of recording with a scale of percentage of total power.

associated with an involuntary movement can also be measured; specific ranges of duration are associated with different types of movements. Specification of duration in the range of 30 to 300 msec merely by clinical inspection is virtually impossible because of the relative slowness of the mechanical events compared with the electrical events. Finally, antagonist muscle relationships can be specified as synchronous or asynchronous (reciprocal) by inspection of the EMG signal. In a tremor, asynchronous activity would be described as alternating.

Assessment of Voluntary Movement

As with involuntary movements, it is possible to measure voluntary joint movement directly. Movement can be analyzed at a single joint or at several joints at the same time. Measurements can be made of the movement time (i.e., time from initiation to completion of a movement) and accuracy. If the movement is triggered by a stimulus, then the reaction time (i.e., time from stimulus to initiation of movement) also can be measured.

EMG patterns with voluntary movement also provide valuable information. Normal patterns vary with the speed of movement (Fig. 20-2).[6] A slow, smooth movement is characterized chiefly by continuous activity in the agonist. A movement made as rapidly as possible (a so-called ballistic movement) has a triphasic pattern with a burst of activity in the agonist lasting 50 to 100 msec; a burst of activity in the antagonist lasting 50 to 100 msec; and return of activity in the agonist, often in the form of a burst.

TREMOR

Tremors can be divided into two types: those at rest and those seen with action. "Rest" is only relative; some slight tonic postural maintenance often is required. Action tremors must be subdivided into those seen just with postural maintenance (postural or static tremor) and those requiring goal-directed movement (intentional or kinetic tremor). A third division of action tremors is those seen only with specific types of kinetic movement, such as handwriting, and is called task-specific tremor.

The physiology differs in different forms of human tremor.[7-9] Tremors may come from mechanical oscillations, mechanical-reflex oscillations (EMG activity is entrained with a mechanical oscillation), normal central oscillators, and pathologic central oscillators (Fig. 20-3). An excellent method for determining the physiology consists of combined accelerometry and EMG using spectral analysis and study of the tremor with and without weighting of the body part. This allows separation of

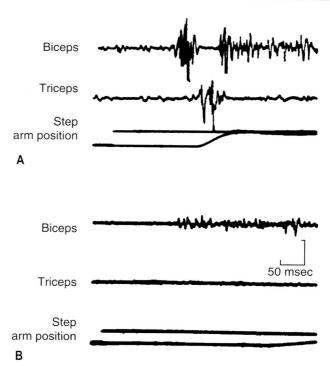

FIGURE 20-2 ▪ Electromyographic activity in biceps and triceps during **A**, fast flexion of the elbow and **B**, slow, smooth flexion. *Step* indicates the target to be tracked and *arm position* is the actual elbow angle; reaction time and movement time information can be obtained from these records. The vertical calibration line corresponds to 500 μV for *A* and 20 μV for *B*. (Modified from Hallett M, Shahani BT, Young RR: EMG analysis of stereotyped voluntary movements in man. J Neurol Neurosurg Psychiatry, 38:1154, 1975, with permission.)

tremors of mechanical and mechanical-reflex origin from those brought about by central oscillators because mechanical and mechanical-reflex tremors have a slower frequency with limb weighting.

Parkinsonian Tremor at Rest

The most common tremor at rest is that seen with Parkinson disease or other parkinsonian states, such as that produced by neuroleptics.[10] The tremor usually is seen in the context of other basal ganglia symptoms, but on rare occasions it can be the sole clinical finding. It is present at rest and disappears with action, but it may resume with a static posture, particularly late in the disease. The frequency is 3 to 7 Hz. EMG studies show antagonist muscles to be active alternately (Fig. 20-4). The tremor frequency is not altered by weighting and hence has its origin in a central oscillator, but its location is not known. Postural tremors may occur in Parkinson disease, as well as a rest tremor.[11]

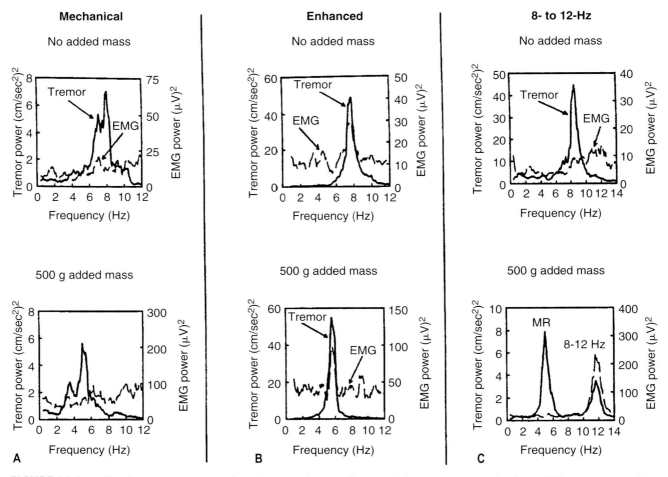

FIGURE 20-3 ■ Fourier power spectra of accelerometric recordings and electromyograms for three different tremors. For each tremor, the top panel shows the recording with no added mass and the bottom shows the recording with 500 g. **A**, Physiologic tremor with pure mechanical nature. **B**, Enhanced or exaggerated physiologic tremor that has a mechanical-reflex (MR) nature. **C**, Physiologic tremor with an 8- to 12-Hz central oscillator component as well as an MR component. (From Elble RJ: The pathophysiology of tremor. p. 405. In Watts RL, Koller WC (eds): Movement Disorders. Neurologic Principles and Practice. McGraw-Hill, New York, 1997, with permission.)

Exaggerated Physiologic Tremor

Physiologic tremor is a normal postural action tremor. In certain circumstances (e.g., anxiety, fatigue, thyrotoxicosis, and excessive use of caffeine), the tremor can be increased in magnitude and may be symptomatic. The frequency usually is in a range from 5 to 12 Hz, varying in part because of the weight of the tremulous body part. The EMG in mild cases may look just like a normal interference pattern without well-defined bursting. In more severe cases, bursting may appear; it is usually synchronous in antagonist muscles. The accelerometric and EMG spectral peaks will be the same and will shift together with weighting. There may also be a component from an 8- to 12-Hz central oscillator in this condition.[8]

Essential Tremor

Essential tremor is a common neurologic disorder that often runs as an autosomal-dominant trait in families.[12,13] It may appear in childhood or late in life and runs a slowly progressive course. Typically, it is a postural tremor; in some patients there is some increase in tremor with intention (kinetic movement), and in others the tremor occurs primarily with goal-directed movement (intentional essential tremor). Rarely, it appears to persist with rest. In most circumstances it is seen as the sole neurologic abnormality; there are pathologic changes in the cerebellum in many patients, but the pathophysiology is not clear. The frequency ranges from 4 to 12 Hz. EMG studies commonly show synchronous activity in antagonist muscles (Fig. 20-5), but alternating

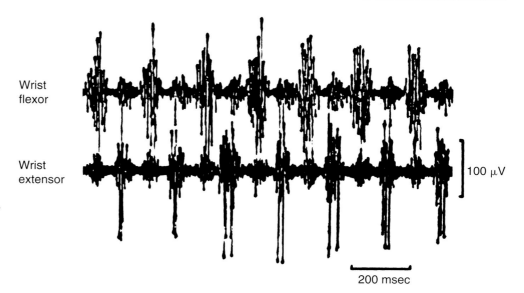

FIGURE 20-4 ■ Electromyographic recording of a parkinsonian tremor. Note the predominant alternating activity of antagonist muscles. There are also small co-contraction bursts that may be confusing by suggesting that the tremor is a synchronous tremor at twice the frequency. Accelerometric recording can help if necessary.

activity is also possible. Sometimes it is clinically difficult to separate exaggerated physiologic tremor from essential tremor. Using accelerometry and EMG, there is a constant frequency with weighting, which is usually different from that seen with exaggerated physiologic tremor.[8] This observation indicates that essential tremor originates from a generator in the central nervous system. The cerebellum and cerebellar circuits seem involved,[14] and one commonly considered candidate is the inferior olivary nucleus.

Cerebellar Tremor

Tremor with cerebellar lesions can be postural, as well as the better-known kinetic tremor. Postural cerebellar tremor can be separated into two groups designated as mild and severe. The more characteristic is severe postural cerebellar tremor, which may be present also at rest, persists or worsens with goal-directed movement, and is associated with dysmetria. It has been called rubral tremor, an inaccurate term because the responsible lesion is often in the superior cerebellar peduncle. More frequently, it is referred to as Holmes tremor.[15] Typically, it has a frequency of 2.5 to 4 Hz, affects proximal muscles more than distal muscles, waxes and wanes, and has a tendency to increase progressively in amplitude with prolonged posture. EMG studies show bursts of activity lasting 125 to 250 msec and alternation of activity in antagonist muscles. The most common etiology in general neurologic practice may be multiple sclerosis, but there are other causes such as stroke, head trauma, or tumors.

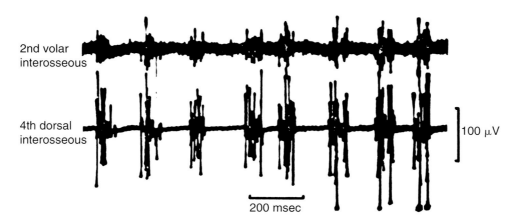

FIGURE 20-5 ■ Electromyographic recording in essential tremor involving side-to-side movement of the fourth finger. Recordings were made with concentric needle electrodes in muscles that adduct and abduct the finger. (Recording made with John Ravits, MD.)

Mild postural cerebellar tremor is less well defined. The group includes tremors that are transient and more rapid (up to 10 Hz), and that have distal predominance.

Kinetic tremor without postural tremor usually is ascribed to cerebellar dysfunction and is often called cerebellar intention tremor. It may occur also with a postural tremor. The lesions can be in the cerebellum or cerebellar pathways. Kinetic tremor is characterized by rhythmic oscillations about the target of movement; EMG studies show alternating activity in antagonist muscles. It should be differentiated from sequential irregular, inaccurate movements toward the target, which have been named serial dysmetria (Fig. 20-6).[16]

Other Tremors

Wilson disease can present with tremor as its sole manifestation, although other movement disorders and psychiatric disturbances are commonly present as well. The tremor is an action tremor present with posture and kinetic movement. Physiologic analysis shows alternating activity in antagonist muscles at 3 to 5 Hz.

Postural tremor may be seen in the setting of congenital or acquired peripheral neuropathies. The pathophysiology is obscure. The tremor seen with hereditary

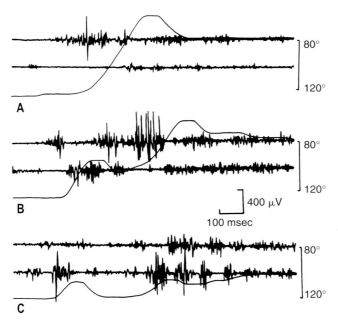

FIGURE 20-6 ■ Attempted voluntary elbow flexion movements of 40 degrees by a patient with alcoholic cerebellar degeneration. In each part a single trial is shown; the first trace is biceps electromyogram (EMG), the second trace is triceps EMG, and the third trace is elbow angle. **A**, Prolonged initial agonist burst. **B**, Serial dysmetria. **C**, Intention tremor. (From Sabra AF, Hallett M: Action tremor with alternating activity in antagonist muscles. Neurology, 34:151, 1984, with permission.)

sensorimotor neuropathy type 1 simply may be essential tremor that is co-inherited.[17] Physiologically, the frequency is in the range of 6 to 8 Hz, and EMG studies show a mixture of synchronous and alternating activity in antagonist muscles. It is likely that, in many circumstances, slowing of nerve conduction in the peripheral loop will give rise to delays that create instability.[18] In other circumstances, studies suggest a coexisting central oscillator.[19]

Palatal tremor, also known as palatal myoclonus, is characterized by rhythmic movements of the palate at approximately 3 Hz. There are two separate disorders: essential palatal tremor, which manifests an ear click; and symptomatic palatal tremor, which is associated with cerebellar disturbances.[20] The palatal movements are caused by activation of the tensor veli palatini muscle in essential palatal tremor and of the levator veli palatini muscle in the symptomatic disorder. In symptomatic palatal tremor, the palatal movements may be accompanied by synchronous movements of adjacent muscles such as the external ocular muscles, tongue, larynx, face, neck, diaphragm, or even limb muscles. Symptomatic palatal tremor is associated with hypertrophy of the inferior olive and many authorities consider it to arise there, but the generator for essential palatal tremor probably differs.

Task-Specific Tremors

Primary writing tremor is task-specific and appears only with handwriting and a few additional skilled tasks. It is not seen with all skilled tasks and is not produced by posture or goal-directed movement in general. The condition probably is underdiagnosed because it is often confused with essential tremor and tremulous writer's cramp. Although the originally described patient had tremor with synchronous activity, subsequent experience suggests that the tremor is more commonly alternating in antagonist muscles with a frequency of 5 to 6 Hz.[21]

Orthostatic tremor is a tremor of the legs that occurs only when standing; it is not present when voluntary movements of the legs are made while lying down, nor is it present with walking.[22] The tremor in leg muscles is at about 16 Hz, is not influenced by peripheral feedback, and is synchronous between homologous leg muscles. The site of the central generator is unknown.

Psychogenic Tremor

Tremor can be a conversion symptom. Such tremors can take many forms, but the most common are action tremors with alternating activity in antagonist muscles.

Often they violate rules of clinical behavior with sudden starts and stops, and disappearance with distraction, but the distinction can be difficult. Psychogenic tremors vary in amplitude more than expected. Clinical neurophysiologic assessment can be very helpful.[23] Accelerometry in most tremors shows a narrow peak frequency that does not change over short periods; in psychogenic tremors the peak may be broad and change frequently. While organic tremors differ in frequency in different limbs, psychogenic tremors are more commonly exactly the same frequency. An important feature useful for physiologic analysis is that the tremor frequency may be entrained or altered by requested tapping at different rates by another body part.

OTHER INVOLUNTARY MOVEMENTS

Three EMG patterns may underlie involuntary movements.[1,24] One pattern, which can be called *tonic*, resembles slow voluntary movements and is characterized by continuous or almost continuous EMG activity lasting for the duration of the movement, from 200 to 1000 msec or longer. Activity can be solely in the agonist muscle, or there can be some co-contraction of the antagonist muscle with the agonist. Another pattern, which can be called *ballistic*, resembles voluntary ballistic movements with a triphasic pattern. There is a burst of activity in the agonist muscle lasting 50 to 100 msec; a burst of activity in the antagonist muscle lasting 50 to 100 msec; and then return of activity in the agonist, often in the form of another burst. The third pattern, which can be called *reflex*, resembles the burst occurring in many reflexes, including H reflexes and stretch reflexes. The EMG burst duration is 10 to 30 msec, and EMG activity in the antagonist muscle is virtually always synchronous.

Myoclonus

Myoclonus is characterized by quick muscle jerks, either irregular or rhythmic.[24,25] There are many types of myoclonus and no common etiologic, physiologic, or therapeutic features that bind them together. Myoclonus can be focal, involving only a few adjacent muscles; generalized, involving many or most of the muscles in the body; or multifocal, involving many muscles but in different jerks. Myoclonus can be spontaneous; activated or accentuated by voluntary movement (action myoclonus); and activated or accentuated by sensory stimulation (reflex myoclonus). Rhythmic (segmental) myoclonus has the appearance of a rest tremor but typically is unaffected by action, stimulation, or even sleep. In this disorder, a segment of the spinal cord (spinal myoclonus) or

brainstem (palatal myoclonus) produces persistent rhythmic repetitive discharges usually unaffected by sleep. A number of contiguous muscles produce synchronous contractions at a rate of 0.5 to 3 Hz. Because of the slow speed of the movements, palatal myoclonus is often called palatal tremor.

By defining epileptic myoclonus as myoclonus that is a fragment of epilepsy, it is possible to divide irregular myoclonus into epileptic and nonepileptic myoclonus.[24,25] The physiologic characteristics of epileptic myoclonus are as follows: (1) EMG burst length of 10 to 50 msec; (2) synchronous antagonist activity; and (3) an electroencephalographic (EEG) correlate. (The technique of EMG–EEG correlation is described later.) The EMG shows a reflex pattern. Nonepileptic myoclonus shows the following: (1) EMG burst lengths of 50 to 300 msec; (2) synchronous or asynchronous antagonist activity; and (3) no EEG correlate (Fig. 20-7). The EMG patterns are either ballistic or tonic.

Examples of epileptic myoclonus are cortical reflex myoclonus, reticular reflex myoclonus, and primary generalized epileptic myoclonus; these are discussed later in relation to EMG–EEG analysis. Examples of nonepileptic myoclonus include dystonic myoclonus; essential myoclonus (e.g., ballistic movement overflow myoclonus); exaggerated startle; physiologic phenomena (e.g., hypnic jerks); and periodic movements of sleep. Frequent

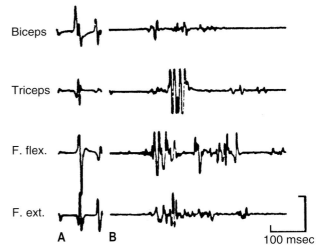

FIGURE 20-7 ■ Comparison of (**A**) "reflex" and (**B**) "ballistic" electromyographic appearance underlying different types of myoclonus. *A* is from a patient with reticular reflex myoclonus. *B* is from a patient with ballistic movement overflow myoclonus. Vertical calibration is 1 mV for *A* and 0.5 mV for *B*. (From Chadwick D, Hallett M, Harris R et al: Clinical, biochemical, and physiological features distinguishing myoclonus responsive to 5-hydroxytryptophan, tryptophan with a monoamine oxidase inhibitor and clonazepam. Brain, 100:455, 1977, with permission.)

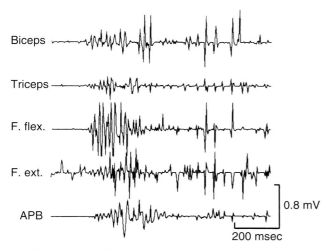

Biceps

Triceps

F. flex.

F. ext.

APB

0.8 mV

200 msec

FIGURE 20-8 ■ Electromyographic recording of action myoclonus. An initial long burst of activity is associated with lifting the arm. Myoclonus is associated with the subsequent brief, synchronous discharges. APB, abductor pollicis brevis. (From Hallett M, Chadwick D, Marsden CD, unpublished observations.)

myoclonus may have the appearance of tremor. In the case of action myoclonus, this may be confusing clinically, but EMG analysis is definitive (Fig. 20-8). Psychogenic myoclonus is a common presentation of psychogenic movement disorders, and the burst pattern is always nonepileptic in type.[23]

Tic

Tics are quick, involuntary, repetitive movements that occur at irregular intervals. The unique feature of a tic is that it is not completely involuntary. Most patients describe a psychic tension that builds up inside them and can be relieved by the tic movement. Hence the tics can be suppressed voluntarily for some time at the expense of increasing psychic tension; patients "let the tic happen" (or perhaps even "make the tic") to relieve the tension. Tic movements, which can be simple or complex, look like quick voluntary movements both clinically and electromyographically.[26] EMG bursts vary from 50 to 200 msec in duration and may have a ballistic or tonic pattern.

Dystonia and Athetosis

The involuntary movements of dystonia and athetosis are similar, and the use of one term rather than the other often seems more a matter of situation and semantics than of physiology.[27] The movements are typically slow but can be quick and may be sustained for a second or longer when the involuntary contraction is at its maximum. Dystonia often contains some sustained postures, while athetosis is slow, continuous movement.

Dystonia often is used to describe proximal twisting movements and athetosis for more distal "flowing" movements. Dystonic and athetotic movements often are characterized by co-contraction of antagonist muscles.[28,29] Although normal voluntary movement commonly is characterized by reciprocal inhibition, there may be some co-contraction. The co-contraction of dystonia and athetosis is excessive, with the appearance of increased tension at the joint. Some dystonic and athetotic movements are fully involuntary, arising at rest independent of will. Other movements arise as excessive, unwanted concomitants to voluntary movements. This phenomenon is called overflow, with the implication that the motor control command is sent to too many muscles with too much intensity. All of this may be caused by a failure of surround inhibition in the motor system.[28,30] EMG studies can document these phenomena. The shortest EMG bursts seen even with dystonic myoclonus are in the range of 100 to 300 msec.

Dyskinesia, Ballism, and Chorea

Dyskinesia describes choreic movements seen in selected circumstances (e.g., a late consequence of neuroleptic drugs or with levodopa toxicity). Ballism describes wild, large-amplitude choreic movements; these usually involve one side of the body and then are called hemiballismus. The most appropriate adjective to describe chorea is "random." Random muscles throughout the body are affected at random times and make movements of random duration. Movements can be brief (e.g., myoclonus) or long (e.g., dystonia). Usually, they are totally beyond voluntary control, but in some mild cases the movements can be suppressed temporarily. EMG patterns are reflex, ballistic, and tonic (Table 20-1, Fig. 20-9).

TABLE 20-1 ■ EMG Appearance in Different Types of Involuntary Movements

| Disorder | EMG Pattern | | | Examples/Comment |
	Reflex	Ballistic	Tonic	
Myoclonus	X			Epileptic myoclonus
		X		Ballistic movement overflow myoclonus
			X	Dystonic myoclonus
Tic		X	X	Not fully involuntary
Dystonia			X	Also athetosis
Chorea	X	X	X	Also dyskinesia, ballism

Modified from Hallett M: Analysis of abnormal voluntary and involuntary movements with surface EMG. p. 907. In Desmedt JE (ed): Motor Control Mechanisms in Health and Disease. Raven, New York, 1983, with permission.

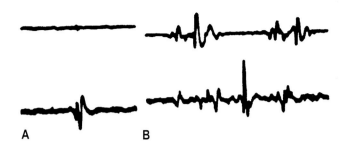

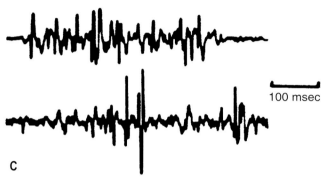

100 msec

FIGURE 20-9 ■ Electromyographic recording of three involuntary movements in a woman with senile chorea. The top trace is from biceps, and the bottom trace is from triceps. **A**, "Reflex" pattern. **B**, "Ballistic" pattern. **C**, "Tonic" pattern. (From Hallett M: Analysis of abnormal voluntary and involuntary movements with surface EMG. p. 907. In Desmedt JE (ed): Motor Control Mechanisms in Health and Disease. Raven, New York, 1983, with permission.)

Asterixis

Asterixis is a brief lapse in tonic innervation.[31] It appears as an involuntary jerk superimposed on a postural or intentional movement. Careful observation often reveals that the jerk is in the direction of gravity, but this may be difficult to detect because a quick compensatory antigravity movement to restore limb position often follows the lapse. The involuntary movement is usually irregular, but when asterixis comes rapidly there may be the appearance of tremor. EMG analysis shows characteristic synchronous pauses in antagonist muscles (Fig. 20-10). Asterixis is also called negative myoclonus.[31,32] When there is an EEG correlate, the physiology is generally similar to epileptic myoclonus, as described earlier.

DERANGEMENTS OF VOLUNTARY MOVEMENT

Clumsiness or slowness of voluntary movements can be analyzed by examining the EMG and kinematic pattern of attempted fast and slow voluntary movements.[6] Earlier in this chapter the normal patterns were described, and it has been shown already how intentional movement brings out intentional tremor or serial dysmetria in patients with cerebellar disorders. Examination of the initial part of attempted rapid movement (i.e., the triphasic ballistic movement pattern) is often illuminating.

Corticospinal Tract Lesions

With corticospinal tract lesions, the first agonist or antagonist EMG bursts (or both) are prolonged. In addition, routine EMG reveals a reduced interference pattern on maximal effort.

Cerebellar Lesions

With cerebellar lesions, the first agonist and/or antagonist EMG bursts are prolonged without a reduced interference pattern. The prolongations can be marked, and there is a good correlation of the acceleration time of the

FIGURE 20-10 ■ Electromyographic (EMG) and accelerometric recording of asterixis. EMG is from flexors and extensors of the wrist, and the accelerometer was on the dorsum of the hand.

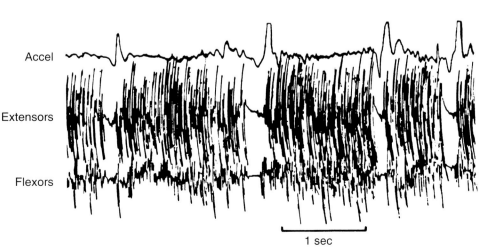

Accel

Extensors

Flexors

1 sec

movement with the duration of the first agonist burst. Unwanted prolongation of acceleration time should predispose to hypermetria. The antagonist burst can be delayed as well.

Parkinsonian Bradykinesia

Parkinsonian bradykinesia is characterized by abnormal patterning, with multiple bursts having the appearance of repetitive cycles of the triphasic pattern to complete the movement (Fig. 20-11). Study of reaction time and movement time is helpful for quantification of Parkinson disease because slowness is such a central aspect of the disease.[33]

Dystonia and Athetosis

With dystonia and athetosis, there is excessive activity (including co-contraction activity) in the antagonist. Excessive activity also overflows into muscles not needed for the action. EMG burst length can be prolonged. In athetosis, particularly, there are a variety of abnormal patterns of antagonist activity that appear to block the movement from occurring.

ELECTROMYOGRAPHIC–ELECTROENCEPHALOGRAPHIC CORRELATION

As noted in the discussion of myoclonus, it can be useful to identify the EEG events occurring at the time of a movement. This can be accomplished for both voluntary and involuntary movements. Events in the ongoing EEG can be correlated with EMG events, but it is more informative to average the EEG with respect to the EMG.[1,24,32] Just as sensory evoked cerebral potentials are time-locked to the stimulus, these movement-related EEG potentials must be time-locked to a phase of the EMG, such as its onset. A great deal of attention is devoted to that part of the potential preceding movement onset because it may relate to generation of the movement; the part of the potential after movement onset includes feedback from the movement itself. The movement potential can be analyzed for the presence of consistent positive and negative waves, and the topography and time relationship of these to the movement can be determined.

A series of waves called the movement-related cortical potentials (MRCPs) are associated with self-paced voluntary movements of normal subjects.[34,35] The most prominent is the Bereitschaftspotential (BP), a widespread

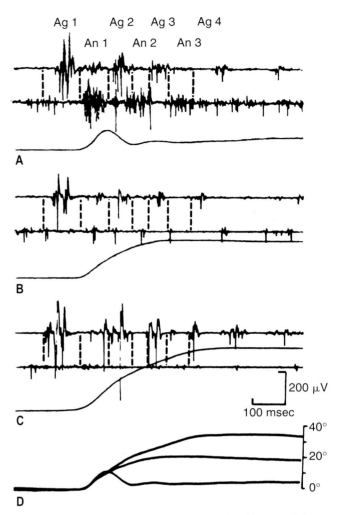

FIGURE 20-11 ■ Ballistic movements of a 68-year-old man with Parkinson disease. **A**, Attempted 10-degree movement. **B**, Attempted 20-degree movement. **C**, Attempted 40-degree movement. In *A*, *B*, and *C* the traces are, from top down, biceps electromyogram (EMG), triceps EMG, and position of the elbow. **D**, The three position traces superimposed. The parts of the figure were aligned so that the movements all began at the same time from the beginning of the traces. The dashed vertical lines are discontinuous straight lines, indicating the correspondence of the timing of EMG bursts in the different movements. The agonist bursts are labeled Ag 1, Ag 2, Ag 3, and Ag 4; the antagonist bursts are An 1, An 2, and An 3. (From Hallett M, Khoshbin S: A physiological mechanism of bradykinesia. Brain, 103:301, 1980, with permission.)

negativity that gradually increases for approximately 1,000 msec before the movement. In the 400 msec before the movement, the negativity increases in slope and can be referred to as the negative slope (NS'). The early and late parts of the BP are referred to most easily as BP1 and BP2.[34] Immediately before the movement, the negativity becomes most marked, first over the motor cortex contralateral to the moving limb and then over the frontal cortex; this is the motor potential (MP).

Stimulation may produce involuntary movements (i.e., reflex myoclonus) and evoke responses in the EEG. In the evoked response, the waves that precede the provoked movement can be analyzed for their relationship to the movement. If the timing and topography of an event in the movement potential before a spontaneous involuntary movement are similar to the timing and topography of an event in the evoked response before the provoked movement, the physiologic mechanism may be similar.

Myoclonus

The use of these techniques can distinguish the three types of epileptic myoclonus described earlier.[24,25,32]

Cortical reflex myoclonus is a fragment of focal or partial epilepsy. Each myoclonic jerk involves only a few adjacent muscles, but larger jerks with involvement of more muscles can be seen. The disorder is commonly multifocal and accentuated by action and sensory stimulation. The genesis of cortical reflex myoclonus is thought to be hyperexcitability of sensorimotor cortex, with each jerk representing the discharge of a small region activated by a paroxysmal depolarization shift (PDS). The EEG recognizes the discharge as a focal negative event preceding spontaneous and reflexly induced myoclonic jerks. The event with reflex jerks is a giant P1–N2 component of the somatosensory evoked potential (Fig. 20-12).

Reticular reflex myoclonus is a fragment of a type of generalized epilepsy. These jerks usually are generalized, with proximal more than distal and flexor more than extensor predominance. Voluntary action and sensory stimulation increase the jerking. The genesis of the myoclonus is thought to be hyperexcitability of a portion of the caudal brainstem reticular formation. A spike can be seen in the EEG often associated with the myoclonic jerk, but because it follows the first EMG manifestation and is not time-locked to the jerk, it does not seem responsible for the jerk. The first activated muscles are those innervated by cranial nerve XI; this strongly suggests a brainstem origin.

Primary generalized epileptic myoclonus is a fragment of primary generalized epilepsy. The most common clinical manifestation is a small, focal jerk that often involves only the fingers and that sometimes has been called minipolymyoclonus. Generalized body jerks can also be seen. This type of myoclonus is thought to arise from the firing of a hyperexcitable cortex driven synchronously by

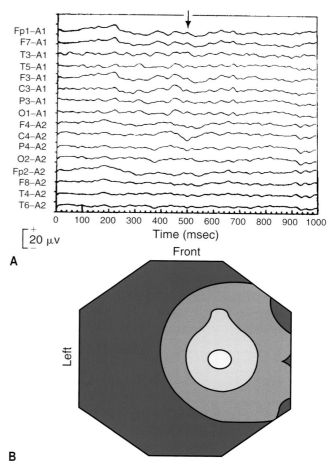

FIGURE 20-12 ■ Electromyographic correlate of myoclonic jerks in a patient with a cortical reflex myoclonus variant in association with Alzheimer disease. **A,** Electroencephalographic (EEG) activity collected before and after myoclonic jerk that occurred in left wrist extensors beginning at 500 msec in the recording. Traces are averages of 32 events. **B,** Topographic display of the EEG data, showing contralateral central negativity (at the time of the arrow in *A*). (From Wilkins DE, Hallett M, Berardelli A et al: Physiologic analysis of the myoclonus of Alzheimer's disease. Neurology, 34:898, 1984, with permission.)

ascending subcortical impulses. The EEG correlate is a slow, bilateral, frontocentrally predominant negativity similar to the wave of a primary generalized paroxysm.

Other Movement Disorders

Movement-related cortical potentials can be used in a number of situations to elucidate the physiology of a disorder. For example, although the tics in Tourette syndrome look like voluntary movements with EMG, there is no BP preceding them (although there may be a small BP2); this suggests a difference between the two types of movement.[26] In patients with psychogenic involuntary movements, a normal-looking BP often precedes the movements.[23] This suggests that the brain is using a mechanism similar to that for self-generated movements.

Studies of MRCPs in Parkinson disease have been controversial. One of the difficulties is that MRCPs change with age and level of dopaminergic medication, and these variables must be controlled carefully. Dopamine, for example, will increase the negativity of the BP, even in normal subjects. Some authors find no abnormality of the BP, whereas others find a deficit in the negativity. A deficit in the negativity may be in the BP1 only.

In dystonia, MRCPs associated with self-paced finger movement in patients with hand dystonia may show deficiency of the BP2 component, but this is not always seen.[36] Symptomatic dystonia has also been investigated. With bilateral lesions, patients showed abnormal BP1 and BP2 bilaterally, whereas with unilateral lesions the problem was worse for the symptomatic hand. These results are more extreme than are those for more mildly affected patients with idiopathic dystonia, and they confirm a reduced excitability of primary sensorimotor cortex.

Although generally subtle abnormalities of the BP occur in Parkinson disease and dystonia, major deficiencies of the negativity occur in patients with cerebellar deficits.[37] This is particularly true of patients with dentate lesions or lesions of the superior cerebellar peduncle. In two patients with cerebellar stroke, it was demonstrated that the MRCP was depressed acutely, but this recovered together with clinical improvement.[38]

ELECTROMYOGRAPHIC RESPONSES TO STIMULATION

Reference has already been made to involuntary movements (e.g., reflex myoclonus) that can be produced by stimulation. Numerous other aspects of movement disorders, including the pathophysiology, can be evaluated with different types of stimulation and recording techniques. Such methods are useful for analyzing the following reflexes, and are particularly valuable in the assessment of tone.

Monosynaptic Reflex

The monosynaptic reflex can be analyzed by the tendon jerk or H reflex. To obtain a meaningful measure of the response, the amplitude of the maximal reflex must be compared with the amplitude of the EMG in maximum voluntary effort or the amplitude of the EMG produced by supramaximal stimulation of the nerve to that muscle (H/M ratio).[1] Unfortunately, there is a large interindividual variability that makes the measurement less useful than it might be. The H/M ratio is enhanced in spasticity but not in rigidity or in dystonia. Furthermore, in spasticity, H reflexes may appear in muscles in which they are not seen ordinarily (e.g., the small hand muscles). The excitability of the H reflex can be assessed by comparing the amplitude of a second H reflex as a function of time with a first H reflex.[39] This relationship, the H-reflex recovery curve, is altered in spasticity and other disorders of movement, but because of lack of specificity it is not used often.

A clinically useful test is vibratory inhibition of the H reflex.[40] In normal subjects, the amplitude of the H reflex is inhibited markedly by vibration of the muscle. Vibration is a strong stimulus for Ia afferents, although other afferents will be activated as well. The inhibition has been attributed largely to presynaptic inhibition from polysynaptic effects of the homonymous Ia afferents, but postactivation depression may also be responsible for some of the effect. H reflexes are tested with and without vibration. Vibration is applied to the tendon of the muscle being studied. The effect can be seen over a wide range of vibrations, but typically a frequency of about 100 Hz is used with an excursion of about 1 mm. The effect can be studied over the range of H-reflex amplitudes. The percentage of inhibition is considered a measure of intensity of presynaptic inhibition. Vibratory inhibition is often reduced dramatically in spasticity. It is also reduced in the stiff-person syndrome and in dystonia, but is normal in parkinsonian rigidity.

Flexor Reflex

Flexor reflexes are spinal polysynaptic reflexes that can be produced by trains of electrical stimuli delivered to cutaneous or mixed nerves.[1] The normal flexor reflex consists of two EMG components. The first component appears at a higher threshold. The latency of the first component ranges from 50 to 60 msec in different individuals, whereas the second component may have a latency of 110 msec to more than 400 msec, depending upon the strength of the stimulus. Increasing the stimulus strength decreases the latency and increases the duration and amplitude of both components. These reflexes are enhanced in spasticity. The involuntary movements in periodic movements in sleep may be released flexor reflexes.[41]

Blink Reflex

In normal subjects, if a second blink reflex is produced at an interval of less than 3 seconds after a first blink reflex, the R2 component of the second blink reflex is reduced in amplitude compared with that of the first blink reflex.[1,42] The amount of inhibition is proportional to the interval between the two stimuli eliciting the blink reflexes. The curve relating the amplitude of the second R2 to the interval between the stimuli is called the blink reflex recovery cycle. Normal values can be determined, and patients with blepharospasm show less inhibition than normal. Abnormalities of blink reflex recovery have been demonstrated also in generalized dystonia, spasmodic torticollis, and spasmodic dysphonia. In the last two conditions, abnormalities can be found even without clinical involvement of the eyelids. The abnormality is not specific because it is also found in Parkinson disease. In Huntington disease there may be more inhibition than normal.

Reciprocal Inhibition

Reciprocal inhibition is the spinal process of inhibition of a motor neuron pool when the antagonist motor neuron pool is activated.[1] This can be studied by assessing the influence on an H reflex of stimulation of a nerve with afferents from muscles antagonist to the muscle where the H reflex is produced. There are several normal periods of inhibition, depending on the interval between the stimulus to the antagonist nerve and that eliciting the H reflex. The period of inhibition best understood is that occurring when the two nerves are stimulated close to the same time. This inhibition is mediated by the Ia inhibitory interneuron. In the arm, reciprocal inhibition has been studied by looking at the effects of radial nerve stimulation upon the H reflex of the flexor carpi radialis. Via various pathways, and therefore at various time intervals after the radial nerve stimulus, the radial afferent traffic can inhibit the motor neuron pool of this muscle. The first period of inhibition is caused by disynaptic Ia inhibition; the second period of inhibition is probably presynaptic inhibition; and little is known about the third period of inhibition. Reciprocal inhibition is reduced in patients with dystonia, including those with generalized dystonia, writer's cramp, spasmodic torticollis, and blepharospasm. It should be noted that reciprocal inhibition can be abnormal even in asymptomatic arms, as is the situation with blepharospasm. Reciprocal inhibition studies can be used as a sensitive method for detecting abnormality in patients with dystonia; however, the method is not specific. Reciprocal inhibition is also reduced abnormally in patients with Parkinson disease.

Stretch Reflexes and Tone Assessment

Tone is defined as the response to passive stretch. Study of EMG responses to controlled stretches can provide physiologic insights and permit quantitative analysis. Devices containing torque motors can deliver controlled stretches. The stretch can be produced by altering the force, or torque, of the motor; or by altering the position of the shaft of the motor. The perturbation can be a single step or more complex, such as a sinusoid. The mechanical response of the limb can also be measured: the positional change if the motor alters force, or the force changes if the motor alters position. Such mechanical measurements can directly mimic and quantify the clinical impression.[1]

An extensive literature has developed about the short- and long-latency EMG responses to controlled stretches and the changes that occur in spasticity and rigidity. The short-latency reflex is the monosynaptic reflex. Reflexes occurring at a longer latency than this are designated "long latency." If a pathway ascends to the brainstem or higher, it could be called "long loop."

In general, when a relaxed muscle is stretched, only a short-latency reflex is produced. When a muscle is stretched while it is active, one or more distinct long-latency reflexes are produced following the short-latency reflex and before the time needed to produce a voluntary response to the stretch (Fig. 20-13). These reflexes are recognized as separate because of brief time gaps between them, giving rise to the appearance of distinct "humps" on a rectified EMG trace. Each component reflex, short or long in latency, has about the same duration, approximately 20 to 40 msec. They appear to be true reflexes in that their appearance and magnitude depend primarily on the amount of background force that the muscle was exerting at the time of the stretch and the mechanical parameters of the stretch; they do not vary much with whatever the subject might want to do after experiencing the muscle stretch. By contrast, the voluntary response that occurs after a reaction time from the stretch stimulus is strongly dependent on the will of the subject.

Studies of stretch reflexes in spasticity show that the short-latency reflex is enhanced and the magnitude of enhancement is correlated with the clinical impression of increased tone, as might have been anticipated. Long-latency reflexes are commonly absent or reduced,

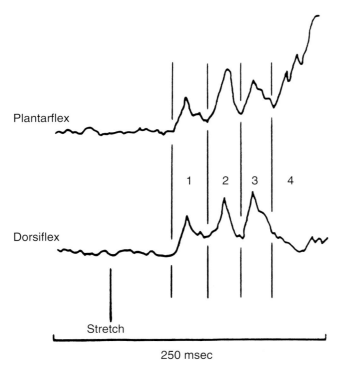

FIGURE 20-13 ■ Averaged and rectified electromyographic responses of triceps surae to dorsiflexion stretch with the subject exerting a background plantarflexion force. The subject was asked to plantarflex (top) or dorsiflex (bottom) the ankle after feeling the perturbation. 1, short-latency reflex; 2 and 3, two long-latency reflexes; 4, voluntary response. (From Berardelli A, Hallett M, Kaufman C et al: Stretch reflexes of triceps surae in normal man. J Neurol Neurosurg Psychiatry, 45:513, 1982, with permission.)

Electrical Stimulation of Mixed and Cutaneous Nerves

Electrical stimulation of a mixed nerve while the limb is at rest will produce only an M wave and an F response in the muscles innervated by that nerve. Electrical stimulation of a cutaneous nerve will not produce any response. If a mixed nerve or a cutaneous nerve is stimulated while the muscles are active, however, additional responses will be produced.[1] With mixed nerve stimulation, there is a short-latency response that seems analogous to the H reflex and one or more long-latency responses. One of these long-latency responses, which has been called LLRII,[43] may have a transcortical pathway similar to some of the long-latency reflexes to stretch. Long-latency responses may be enhanced in Parkinson disease and are reduced in Huntington disease. With cutaneous nerve stimulation, the pattern of response is variable, depending on the particular nerve and muscle. The pattern consists of alternate periods of excitation and inhibition. For example, when recording from the first dorsal interosseous muscle and stimulating the index finger, there will be an excitatory period (E1) followed by alternate inhibition and excitation (I1, E2, and I2). The pathways subserving these responses are not clear, although in some circumstances there appears to be a correspondence between E2 and LLRII of the mixed nerve response. In spasticity and Huntington disease, E2 is decreased markedly, whereas in Parkinson disease, I1 is enhanced.

but they may be present or even enhanced. In some patients they do appear to contribute to increased tone; the clinical correlation is not yet well understood.

Studies of stretch reflexes in rigidity show that the long-latency reflexes are enhanced and that the magnitude of the enhancement is correlated with the clinical impression of increased tone. In rigidity, long-latency reflexes appear even at rest, when normally no long-latency reflexes are seen (Fig. 20-14). The physiology of these long-latency reflexes is not clear, although enhancement of group II-mediated reflexes may play a role. Thus, investigation of stretch reflexes in patients with increased tone would serve to implicate short- or long-latency mechanisms (roughly correlating with spasticity and rigidity) and provide a means of quantification.

In Huntington disease, long-latency reflexes may be diminished markedly in the hand muscles (although not in more proximal muscles). Although the physiologic significance of this alteration is not clear, the result may be useful diagnostically.

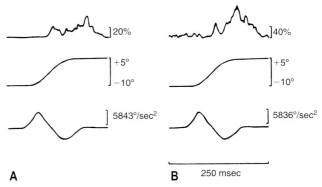

FIGURE 20-14 ■ Averaged and rectified electromyographic responses of triceps surae (top traces) for a patient with Parkinson disease when (**A**) at rest and (**B**) exerting a background plantarflexion force. The middle traces are the ankle angle and the bottom traces are ankle acceleration. Note the unusual morphology of the long-latency stretch reflexes and their presence even at rest. (From Berardelli A, Sabra AF, Hallett M: Physiological mechanisms of rigidity in Parkinson disease. J Neurol Neurosurg Psychiatry, 46:45, 1983, with permission.)

Startle Reflex

The startle reflex is a rapid, generalized motor response to a sudden, surprise stimulus.[44,45] The most extensively studied human startle response is that which occurs to loud noises. It is an oligosynaptic reflex mediated in the brainstem. The startle response is distinctive on EMG testing with surface electrodes. The pattern is bilaterally symmetric with an invariable blink; other craniocervical muscles almost always are activated, but recruitment in the limbs is variable. The onset latency of EMG activity is 30 to 40 msec in orbicularis oculi, 55 to 85 msec in masseter and sternocleidomastoid, 85 to 100 msec in biceps brachii, 100 to 125 msec in hamstrings and quadriceps, and 130 to 140 msec in tibialis anterior. There is synchronous activation of antagonist muscles with an EMG burst duration of 50 to 400 msec. Habituation generally occurs after four or five stimuli. Increased startle responses are excessive or evoked by stimuli that would not be effective in most people. This is identified most easily by loss of habituation. Increased startle reflexes are characteristic of a variety of disorders, including hereditary hyperekplexia.

C Reflexes

With reflex myoclonus, a late response may appear in a relaxed muscle after stretch, mixed nerve stimulation, or cutaneous nerve stimulation. This response, which would not normally be present, may also be seen in muscles outside of the region of the nerve stimulated or even throughout the body. This additional response, sometimes called a C reflex, is a myoclonic movement produced by the stimulation (Fig. 20-15).[24,32] Such responses are manifestations of hyperexcitability of the nervous system and typically reflect exaggerations of one of the normal reflexes described above.

STUDIES WITH TRANSCRANIAL MAGNETIC STIMULATION

Transcranial magnetic stimulation (TMS) is being used actively in research to illuminate the pathophysiology of many different movement disorders. In general, however, these studies have not had a significant impact on clinical practice, where diagnosis and differential diagnosis are the principal aims of electrophysiologic studies. A recent review of the clinical utility of transcranial magnetic stimulation concluded that its only possible clinical utility was in the differential diagnosis of parkinsonian

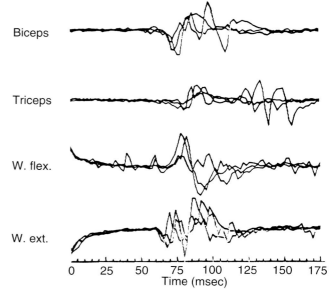

FIGURE 20-15 ■ Electromyographic recording of C reflex in a patient with Alzheimer disease and myoclonus. The three superimposed traces show a consistent synchronous response to ipsilateral median nerve stimulation at time 0. (From Wilkins DE, Hallett M, Berardelli A et al: Physiologic analysis of the myoclonus of Alzheimer's disease. Neurology, 34:898, 1984, with permission.)

syndromes, although more data are needed to support this conclusion.[46]

In Parkinson disease, central motor conduction time is typically normal, but it can be delayed in multiple system atrophy and progressive supranuclear palsy. Abnormalities in all the parkinsonian conditions are found in studies of the silent period and short intracortical inhibition, although data are not complete.[46] The silent period is an absolute or relative silence in tonic EMG activity following stimulation. With low stimulus intensities, it can be seen even without a motor evoked potential (MEP), but typically it follows an MEP. The silent period may depend on mechanisms involving gamma-aminobutyric acid (GABA)$_B$. In Parkinson disease, the silent period lengthens with effective levodopa or surgical therapy. Studies of short intracortical inhibition most commonly examine MEP inhibition by a subthreshold stimulus given 2 to 4 msec before the transcranial magnetic stimulus that evokes the MEP. This inhibition is caused by activation of intracortical GABA$_A$ mechanisms, and it too is generally abnormal in all the parkinsonian conditions. It is called short intracortical inhibition to differentiate it from another period of inhibition with a longer time interval between the conditioning and test stimuli.

In dystonia, a number of abnormalities have been identified, such as diminished short intracortical inhibition and a shortened silent period.[28] Intermediate abnormalities can be found in nonmanifesting carriers of the gene for generalized dystonia.[47] Generally, the findings are not specific, however, and for this reason, the studies cannot be used for diagnostic purposes. A particular problem in this regard is psychogenic dystonia; curiously, most of the abnormalities in inhibition are similar in organic and psychogenic dystonia.[48] Another TMS technique, called paired associative stimulation, can evaluate plasticity of the central nervous system. Patients with organic dystonia show enhanced plasticity, whereas those with psychogenic dystonia are normal on this test.[49] It is possible that in the future such testing may help to distinguish patients with psychogenic dystonia.

The MEP is reduced by stimulation over the cerebellum at an interval of 5 to 7 msec before stimulation over the motor cortex. This effect is reduced in patients with cerebellar damage and can be used as an objective method for defining cerebellar abnormality.[50]

MONITORING DISEASE SEVERITY IN PARKINSON DISEASE

Great progress has been made in the medical and surgical treatment of Parkinson disease. Although there are clinical rating scales, it is worth noting the possible physiologic tests that can produce quantitative measures. Compact devices can be made to measure some or all of the principal signs.[51] The most important defects in patients with Parkinson disease are bradykinesia and akinesia, movement slowness and freezing. Bradykinesia can be measured by assessment of movement time in simple or more complex motor tasks. The more complex the task in terms of simultaneous and sequential elements, the more abnormal will be the behavior. Self-generated movements are more likely to be abnormal than are triggered movements. Such tasks might include the grooved pegboard and gait. The EMG can be monitored during the task, looking for the tremulous nature of the voluntary pattern. Reaction time abnormalities can be assessed and, contrary to the tasks best for movement time, abnormalities are best found in the most simple tasks.[33]

Parkinsonian tremor can be assessed with accelerometry or gyroscopes and the amplitude measured.[52] Since tremor varies considerably over the day, long periods of measurement are likely better than just a brief test.

Rigidity can be measured with a variety of devices that stretch different joints as described earlier. Rigidity can be measured at rest, with reinforcement (i.e., with voluntary movement of the opposite limb), and during movement. Reinforcement brings out abnormalities better than does the simple resting state. There is some controversy as to whether the EMG reflex responses correlate well with rigidity; for this reason, mechanical measurements are better.

REFERENCES

1. Hallett M, Berardelli A, Delwaide P et al: Central EMG and tests of motor control. Report of an IFCN Committee. Electroencephalogr Clin Neurophysiol, 90:404, 1994
2. Hallett M (ed): Movement Disorders. Handbook of Clinical Neurophysiology. Vol 1. Elsevier, Amsterdam, 2003
3. Dohle C, Freund HJ: Kinesiology. p. 191. In Hallett M (ed): Movement Disorders. Handbook of Clinical Neurophysiology. Vol 1. Elsevier, Amsterdam, 2003
4. Elble RJ: Accelerometry. p. 181. In Hallett M (ed): Movement Disorders. Handbook of Clinical Neurophysiology. Vol 1. Elsevier, Amsterdam, 2003
5. Hallett M: Electromyography. p. 7. In Hallett M (ed): Movement Disorders. Handbook of Clinical Neurophysiology. Vol 1. Elsevier, Amsterdam, 2003
6. Berardelli A, Hallett M, Rothwell JC et al: Single-joint rapid arm movements in normal subjects and in patients with motor disorders. Brain, 119:661, 1996
7. Elble RJ: Tremor: clinical features, pathophysiology, and treatment. Neurol Clin, 27:679, 2009
8. Hallett M: Overview of human tremor physiology. Mov Disord, 13(Suppl 3):43, 1998
9. Raethjen J, Deuschl G: Tremor. Curr Opin Neurol, 22:400, 2009
10. Deuschl G, Fietzek U, Klebe S et al: Clinical neurophysiology and pathophysiology of parkinsonian tremor. p. 377. In Hallett M (ed): Movement Disorders. Handbook of Clinical Neurophysiology. Vol 1. Elsevier, Amsterdam, 2003
11. Hallett M, Deuschl G: Are we making progress in the understanding of tremor in Parkinson's disease? Ann Neurol, 68:780, 2010
12. Elble RJ, Deuschl G: An update on essential tremor. Curr Neurol Neurosci Rep, 9:273, 2009
13. Louis ED: Essential tremor: evolving clinicopathological concepts in an era of intensive post-mortem enquiry. Lancet Neurol, 9:613, 2010
14. Deuschl G, Elble RJ: The pathophysiology of essential tremor. Neurology, 54:S14, 2000
15. Paviour DC, Jager HR, Wilkinson L et al: Holmes tremor: application of modern neuroimaging techniques. Mov Disord, 21:2260, 2006
16. Hallett M: Classification and treatment of tremor. JAMA, 266:1115, 1991
17. Cardoso FE, Jankovic J: Hereditary motor-sensory neuropathy and movement disorders. Muscle Nerve, 16:904, 1993
18. Bain PG, Britton TC, Jenkins IH et al: Tremor associated with benign IgM paraproteinaemic neuropathy. Brain, 119:789, 1996

19. Pedersen SF, Pullman SL, Latov N et al: Physiological tremor analysis of patients with anti-myelin-associated glycoprotein associated neuropathy and tremor. Muscle Nerve, 20:38, 1997

20. Deuschl G, Toro C, Valls-Solé J et al: Symptomatic and essential palatal tremor. 1. Clinical, physiological, and MRI analysis. Brain, 117:775, 1994

21. Bain PG, Findley LJ, Britton TC et al: Primary writing tremor. Brain, 118:1461, 1995

22. Piboolnurak P, Yu QP, Pullman SL: Clinical and neurophysiologic spectrum of orthostatic tremor: case series of 26 subjects. Mov Disord, 20:1455, 2005

23. Hallett M: Physiology of psychogenic movement disorders. J Clin Neurosci, 17:959, 2010

24. Hallett M, Shibasaki H: Myoclonus and myoclonic syndromes. p. 2765. In Engel J Jr, Pedley TA (eds): Epilepsy: A Comprehensive Textbook. Vol 3. Lippincott, Williams & Wilkins, Philadelphia, 2008

25. Hallett M: Myoclonus and other involuntary movements. p. 1749. In Brown WF, Bolton CF, Aminoff MJ (eds): Neuromuscular Function and Disease. Vol 2. WB Saunders, Philadelphia, 2002

26. Hallett M: Neurophysiology of tics. Adv Neurol, 85:237, 2000

27. Sanger TD, Chen D, Fehlings DL et al: Definition and classification of hyperkinetic movements in childhood. Mov Disord, 25:1538, 2010

28. Hallett M: Neurophysiology of dystonia: the role of inhibition. Neurobiol Dis, 42:177, 2011

29. Berardelli A, Rothwell JC, Hallett M et al: The pathophysiology of primary dystonia. Brain, 121:1195, 1998

30. Beck S, Richardson SP, Shamim EA et al: Short intracortical and surround inhibition are selectively reduced during movement initiation in focal hand dystonia. J Neurosci, 28:10363, 2008

31. Shibasaki H: Pathophysiology of negative myoclonus and asterixis. Adv Neurol, 67:199, 1995

32. Shibasaki H, Hallett M: Electrophysiological studies of myoclonus. Muscle Nerve, 31:157, 2005

33. Hallett M: Parkinson revisited: pathophysiology of motor signs. Adv Neurol, 91:19, 2003

34. Shibasaki H, Hallett M: What is the Bereitschaftspotential? Clin Neurophysiol, 117:2341, 2006

35. Jahanshahi M, Hallet M (eds): The Bereitschaftspotential: Movement Related Cortical Potentials. Kluver Academic/Plenum, New York, 2003

36. Zeuner KE, Peller M, Knutzen A et al: Slow pre-movement cortical potentials do not reflect individual response to therapy in writer's cramp. Clin Neurophysiol, 120:1213, 2009

37. Ikeda A, Shibasaki H, Nagamine T et al: Dissociation between contingent negative variation and Bereitschaftspotential in a patient with cerebellar efferent lesion. Electroencephalogr Clin Neurophysiol, 90:359, 1994

38. Gerloff C, Altenmuller E, Dichgans J: Disintegration and reorganization of cortical motor processing in two patients with cerebellar stroke. Electroencephalogr Clin Neurophysiol, 98:59, 1996

39. Koelman JH, Willemse RB, Bour LJ et al: Soleus H-reflex tests in dystonia. Mov Disord, 10:44, 1995

40. Bour LJ, Ongerboer de Visser BW, Koelman HTM et al: Soleus H-reflex tests in spasticity and dystonia: a computerized analysis. J Electromyography Kinesiol, 1:9, 1991

41. Bara-Jimenez W, Aksu M, Graham B et al: Periodic limb movements in sleep: state-dependent excitability of the spinal flexor reflex. Neurology, 54:1609, 2000

42. Aramideh M, Ongerboer de Visser BW: Brainstem reflexes: electrodiagnostic techniques, physiology, normative data, and clinical applications. Muscle Nerve, 26:14, 2002

43. Deuschl G: Long-latency reflexes following stretch and nerve stimulation. p. 285. In Hallett M (ed): Movement Disorders. Handbook of Clinical Neurophysiology. Vol 1. Elsevier, Amsterdam, 2003

44. Matsumoto J, Fuhr P, Nigro M et al: Physiological abnormalities in hereditary hyperekplexia. Ann Neurol, 32:41, 1992

45. Matsumoto J, Hallett M: Startle syndromes. p. 418. In Marsden CD, Fahn S (eds): Movement Disorders 3. Butterworth–Heinemann, Oxford, 1994

46. Chen R, Cros D, Curra A et al: The clinical diagnostic utility of transcranial magnetic stimulation: report of an IFCN committee. Clin Neurophysiol, 119:504, 2008

47. Edwards MJ, Huang YZ, Wood NW et al: Different patterns of electrophysiological deficits in manifesting and non-manifesting carriers of the DYT1 gene mutation. Brain, 126:2074, 2003

48. Espay AJ, Morgante F, Purzner J et al: Cortical and spinal abnormalities in psychogenic dystonia. Ann Neurol, 59: 825, 2006

49. Quartarone A, Rizzo V, Terranova C et al: Abnormal sensorimotor plasticity in organic but not in psychogenic dystonia. Brain, 132:2871, 2009

50. Ugawa Y, Terao Y, Hanajima R et al: Magnetic stimulation over the cerebellum in patients with ataxia. Electroencephalogr Clin Neurophysiol, 104:453, 1997

51. Goetz CG, Stebbins GT, Wolff D et al: Testing objective measures of motor impairment in early Parkinson's disease: feasibility study of an at-home testing device. Mov Disord, 24:551, 2009

52. Salarian A, Russmann H, Wider C et al: Quantification of tremor and bradykinesia in Parkinson's disease using a novel ambulatory monitoring system. IEEE Trans Biomed Eng, 54:313, 2007

Evaluation of the Autonomic Nervous System

MICHAEL J. AMINOFF

Autonomic disturbances are a characteristic feature of certain neurologic disorders; may be a cause of death in others; and sometimes complicate general medical disorders, such as diabetes mellitus. For most clinical purposes, autonomic function is evaluated by a number of simple noninvasive tests. These tests have an important role in several clinical contexts. First, they help to confirm a clinical diagnosis of dysautonomia and to exclude other causes of symptoms. Second, they provide an indication of the extent and severity of autonomic involvement and indicate whether the sympathetic and parasympathetic divisions are affected equally or whether one is involved selectively. Third, they may permit the site of the lesion to be localized more precisely, although this sometimes requires more sophisticated or invasive studies. Finally, autonomic function tests may be helpful in the evaluation of small-fiber neuropathies. In this chapter, attention is directed primarily at investigations that can be undertaken conveniently in a clinical neurophysiology laboratory. The enteric component of the autonomic nervous system is also important, but it will not be discussed here because it is usually not the focus of clinical neurophysiologists.

ANATOMY

Details of the anatomy of the autonomic nervous system are provided in standard textbooks; only a short summary of certain aspects of clinical relevance is provided here to facilitate understanding of clinical test procedures and their interpretation.

Afferent Pathways and Central Structures

Autonomic afferent fibers pass along autonomic or somatic peripheral nerves to the central nervous system (CNS), but their precise pathways have not been well defined. Fibers from the retina pass along the optic nerve and tract to the pretectal nucleus and then to pupilloconstrictor neurons in the Edinger–Westphal nucleus. The trigeminal nerve carries afferent fibers from the cornea and the nasal and oropharyngeal mucosa to the trigeminal nuclei and the nucleus tractus solitarius; their activation causes lacrimation and nasal and oral secretions. The glossopharyngeal and vagus nerves carry afferent impulses from baroreceptors in the carotid sinus and aortic arch to the brainstem (Fig. 21-1). Cardiac afferent fibers also pass in the vagus nerve and sympathetic nerves. Afferent impulses travel in the vagus nerve from the tracheobronchial tree and abdominal viscera to the nodose ganglion and nucleus tractus solitarius. Somatic afferent fibers also influence autonomic activity. Sensory neurons projecting to the sympathetic system reside in the dorsal root ganglia and relay information to the dorsal horns of the spinal cord.

A number of regions within the CNS have an important role in modulating autonomic function. These include the frontal and parietal cortical regions, which may influence heart, blood pressure, and respiratory functions. The cingulate cortex is involved in controlling sphincter (bladder and bowel) functions, and bilateral lesions therefore may lead to sphincter disturbances. The temporal lobe and amygdala have autonomic functions, and autonomic features are well-known accompaniments of seizures arising in these regions. The hypothalamus, cerebellum, and various brainstem nuclei also have major roles.[1] Afferent fibers from arterial baroreceptors and chemoreceptors end in the nucleus tractus solitarius in the dorsomedial medulla, and this nucleus also receives input from neocortical, forebrain, diencephalic, and rostral brainstem structures (see Fig. 21-1).

In turn, it projects to the nucleus ambiguus and dorsal nucleus of the vagus and to the lateral reticular formation; it thus influences the cardiovascular and gastrointestinal systems. Various pontine and medullary regions are involved in the regulation of ventilation.

Sympathetic Efferent Pathways

Descending fibers from the brainstem conduct impulses to the preganglionic sympathetic neurons, which are located in the intermediolateral columns of the spinal cord between about T1 and L2. The axons of these neurons pass to the sympathetic trunk in the white rami communicantes (Fig. 21-2). The sympathetic trunk, on each side of the vertebral column, consists of a chain of ganglia connected by longitudinally running fibers. Within the sympathetic trunk, the axons synapse in the paravertebral ganglia with second-order neurons. Some of the preganglionic axons pass up or down in the sympathetic trunk to ganglia at other levels before synapsing. There are 3 paired sympathetic ganglia in the cervical region, 12 in the thoracic region, 4 in the lumbar region, 4 or 5 sacrally, and 1 unpaired ganglion in the coccygeal region. The inferior cervical and first thoracic ganglia may fuse to form the stellate ganglion. Unmyelinated postganglionic fibers pass back to the spinal nerves in

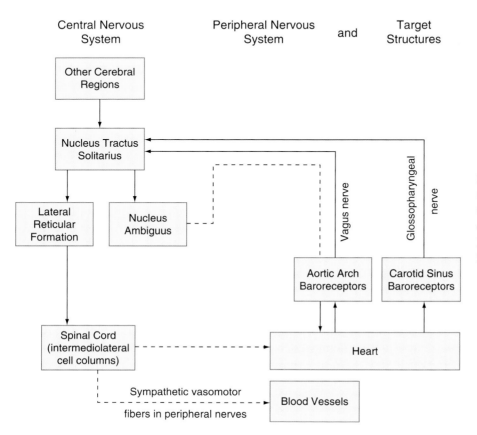

FIGURE 21-1 ■ Diagrammatic representation of the anatomic pathways involved in the baroreceptor reflex regulation of cardiovascular function. (From Aminoff MJ: Electromyography in Clinical Practice. 3rd Ed. Churchill Livingstone, New York, 1998, with permission.)

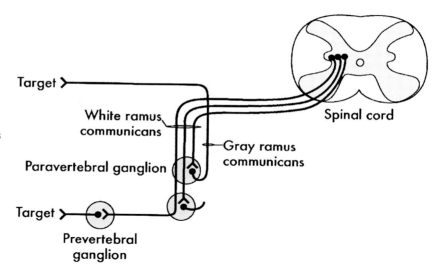

FIGURE 21-2 ▪ Sympathetic efferent pathways from the spinal cord.

the gray rami communicantes or form perivascular plexuses along major arteries as they pass to their final destinations.

Some preganglionic sympathetic fibers pass through the sympathetic ganglia without a synapse to form the splanchnic nerves; these fibers synapse in the prevertebral (preaortic) ganglia (i.e., the celiac, superior mesenteric, and inferior mesenteric ganglia), from which postganglionic fibers pass to the viscera in the hypogastric, splanchnic, and mesenteric plexuses (Table 21-1).

The head and neck are innervated by preganglionic neurons in the T1 and T2 segments through the superior cervical ganglion and the upper four cervical spinal nerves. The upper limb is supplied by preganglionic neurons in the T2 to T8 segments and the stellate ganglion, with varying contributions from the middle cervical and upper thoracic ganglia. The legs are supplied from the T10 to L2 segments through the paravertebral ganglia. Postganglionic sympathetic fibers differ in their properties, depending on their target organ. Thus, cutaneous sympathetic fibers have differing conduction velocities, depending on whether they are vasomotor or sudomotor in function.[2]

Parasympathetic Efferent Pathways

The parasympathetic cranial and sacral outflow is summarized in Table 21-2. The peripheral ganglia are located close to the target organs so that the postganglionic pathways are short.

CLINICAL ASPECTS OF DYSAUTONOMIA

The clinical features of dysautonomia are described in standard textbooks, but a brief summary is provided here as they point to the need for investigation and are

reflected by the manner in which patients are investigated. The most disabling feature is probably an impaired regulation of blood pressure, especially postural hypotension or paroxysmal hypertension. Other cardiovascular abnormalities include syncope, disturbances of cardiac rhythm, and facial flushing. Disturbances of sweating are also common and are manifest by impaired

TABLE 21-1 ▪ The Sympathetic Outflow from the Thoracolumbar Cord

Outflow			Target Structure
SECOND-ORDER NEURON IN PARAVERTEBRAL GANGLIA			
			Eyes
			Salivary glands
			Face
			Head
			Upper limbs
			Heart
			Tracheobronchial tree
			Lungs
			Pulmonary vessels
			Trunk
			Lower limbs
SECOND-ORDER NEURON IN PREVERTEBRAL GANGLIA			
Nerve	*Ganglion*	*Plexus*	
Greater splanchnic	Celiac	Hypogastric	Liver, bile ducts, gallbladder
			Pancreas
			Spleen
			Stomach
			Small intestine
			Proximal colon
Lesser splanchnic	Superior mesenteric	Splanchnic	Small intestine
			Colon
Lumbar splanchnic	Inferior mesenteric	Mesenteric	Distal colon
			Bladder
			Genitalia

TABLE 21-2 ▪ Parasympathetic Efferent System

	Nerve	Peripheral Ganglia	Target Structure
Brainstem outflow	Oculomotor	Ciliary	Eye
	Facial	Pterygopalatine	Palatine glands
		Submandibular	Submaxillary glands
			Sublingual glands
	Glossopharyngeal	Otic	Parotid glands
	Vagus	Ganglia or plexuses related to target organs	Heart
			Airways and lungs
			Abdominal viscera
Sacral outflow (S2–S4)	Pelvic	Pelvic	Distal colon and rectum
			Bladder
			Genitalia

From Aminoff MJ: Electromyography in Clinical Practice. 3rd Ed. Churchill Livingstone, New York, 1998, with permission.

thermoregulatory sweating (anhidrosis or hypohidrosis that may lead to hyperpyrexia if the ambient temperature is high) or hyperhidrosis. Symptoms of gastrointestinal dysfunction include dysphagia from esophageal peristalsis or impaired relaxation of the esophageal sphincter; early satiety, postprandial discomfort, gastric fullness or distension, and vomiting from gastroparesis; and intestinal pseudo-obstruction, constipation, or diarrhea from altered intestinal motility. Urinary frequency, urgency, and incontinence are features of bladder involvement in some patients, whereas hesitancy, retention, or overflow incontinence occurs in other patients, depending on the site of the lesion. Fecal incontinence may occur. Sexual disturbances are common. Erectile dysfunction may have many causes, including an underlying dysautonomia. Ejaculatory failure may also occur. Lesions of the sacral roots or pelvic nerves may be responsible and, in women, may lead to a failure of arousal. The effect of cord lesions depends on their completeness and segmental level. Neuro-ophthalmologic disturbances are other manifestations of a dysautonomia that are well described and beyond the scope of this chapter.

A questionnaire for measuring autonomic symptoms has been developed and validated.[3] It may be useful for assessing autonomic symptoms in clinical trials and epidemiologic studies.

In patients being evaluated for symptoms suggestive of dysautonomia, non-neurologic causes of their complaints require exclusion because they are often reversible. Clinical evaluation is directed with this in mind. The history may suggest an iatrogenic or toxic cause. The neurologic examination may suggest the cause of a dysautonomia. In particular, it may reveal evidence of a polyneuropathy or of a focal CNS lesion, or a combination of signs (parkinsonism with or without upper or lower motor neuron or cerebellar signs) indicative of a degenerative disorder (e.g., multisystem atrophy).

TESTS OF AUTONOMIC FUNCTION

Involvement of the adrenergic system is tested by assessing peripheral vasomotor function and blood-pressure control under various circumstances; sympathetic cholinergic function by measures of thermoregulatory sweating; and parasympathetic impairment primarily by the heart rate responses to various maneuvers.

Cardiovascular Tests

Tests of cardiovascular function are important and provide information about both the parasympathetic and sympathetic divisions of the autonomic nervous system.

HEART RATE VARIATION

In normal resting subjects the heart rate is determined mainly by background vagal activity. The laboratory tests of heart rate variation are therefore mainly tests of parasympathetic function.

Heart Rate Variation with Breathing

An increase in heart rate occurs during inspiration because of decreased cardiac vagal activity; thus, it is blocked by atropine but not by propranolol.[4] The variation in heart rate that occurs depends on the rate and depth of breathing. The test therefore must be standardized if it is to be used for clinical purposes. Normal values are affected by age, which must also be taken into account. The difference between the maximum and minimum heart rate during breathing decreases with increasing age and is diminished or absent in diabetes and other disorders that affect central or peripheral autonomic pathways, as shown in Figure 21-3.

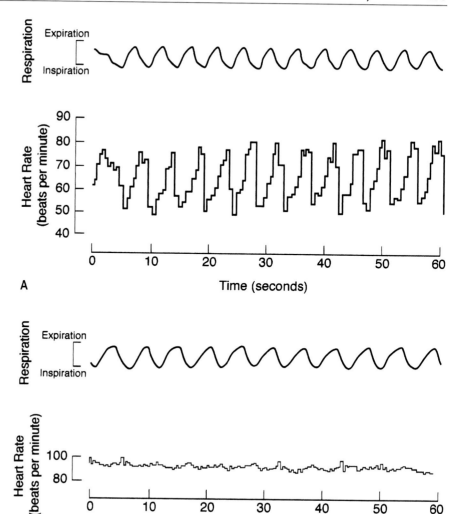

FIGURE 21-3 ▪ **A**, Effect of deep breathing on heart rate in a normal subject, showing a tachycardia during inspiration and a brady-cardia with expiration. **B**, The heart rate response is markedly blunted in patients with dysautonomia, as shown in a patient with multisystem atrophy.

For clinical purposes, the recumbent patient is asked to rest quietly for 5 minutes, and then is asked to take deep breaths at the rate of six per minute, for 1 minute. The timing of the breaths can be directed verbally or by any other convenient means. The heart rate can be measured with a rate monitor or by recording the RR intervals on an electrocardiogram (ECG). The ECG may be displayed on a chart recorder or on standard electro-myographic equipment.

If the heart rate is measured directly, the difference between the highest and lowest rate during the minute of deep breathing is determined. When the ECG is recorded, several different measurements of RR varia-tion may be made.[5,6] The measurements made most commonly are of (1) the difference between the longest and the shortest RR interval during the period of deep breathing; and (2) the expiratory/inspiratory (E/I) ratio, which is the ratio of the mean of the maximum RR intervals in expiration to the mean of the minimum RR intervals in inspiration.

The normal range of heart rate variation is age dependent,[5,7] but normal subjects generally have differ-ences in heart rate exceeding 15 beats per minute. Values of less than 10 beats per minute are abnormal. From a review of the existing literature, Freeman indicated a likely decline in heart rate variability of 3 to 5 beats per minute per decade in normal subjects.[8] The use of a single normal value regardless of age therefore reduces the utility of the test, leading to false-negative results in younger patients and false-positive results in older sub-jects.[8] The E/I ratio decreases with age, but up to the age of 40 years, ratios less than 1.2 may be regarded as abnormal.[7]

Other factors affecting the results in normal subjects include the time of the test (with increased heart rate variability occurring at night), body weight, physical fit-ness, medication, and body position.[8] If possible, anticho-linergic medications (including over-the-counter cold medications) and antidepressants should not be taken for at least 48 hours before testing, and patients should not drink caffeinated or alcoholic beverages or smoke tobacco for 3 hours before testing.[4]

Heart Rate Response to Change in Posture

Immediate Increase in Heart Rate with Standing

Heart rate and blood pressure responses to postural change can be measured conveniently on a tilt-table. The patient lies supine until consistent values are obtained for at least 5 (preferably 10) minutes. The patient then is tilted to be in a 60-degree head-up position and the heart rate and blood pressure are monitored. The normal decline in systolic and diastolic pressures should not exceed 25 and 10 mmHg, respectively. The heart rate normally increases by about 10 to 30 beats per minute, but the response declines with age.[7]

30:15 Ratio

On changing from a recumbent to a standing position, a tachycardia normally occurs and is followed after about 20 seconds by a bradycardia that reaches a relatively stable rate at about the 30th beat after standing (Fig. 21-4). The ratio of the RR intervals that correspond to the 30th and 15th heartbeats is therefore used widely as a measure of parasympathetic function. This 30:15 ratio decreases with age, but in young adults a ratio of less than 1.04 is regarded as abnormal. The ratio of the absolute maximum to minimum RR interval is sometimes preferred. Atropine blocks the heart rate response to standing, indicating that it depends on vagal innervation of the heart. The biphasic response is not present with passive tilting.

Power Spectral Analysis of Heart Rate

Various modifications of heart rate testing have been described but are not in widespread use. Power spectral analysis has been described of the heart rate at rest and after postural change. Two major peaks of interest on the power spectrum occur at rest: a high-frequency peak (greater than 0.15 Hz) representing heart rate changes with respiration (parasympathetic activity), and a low-frequency peak (at 0.05 to 0.15 Hz) that reflects sympathetic and parasympathetic activity.[6,9,10] Another component, at very low frequency (less than 0.05 Hz), also occurs, but its physiologic origin is unclear.[11] A shift in the power spectrum from high to low frequencies occurs with a change in posture to the upright position and may reflect sympathetic activation. Although the results of power spectral analysis may correlate with the results of other tests of autonomic function, the lack of correlation between commonly used indices from power spectral analysis of heart rate variability and cardiac norepinephrine spillover casts doubt on the validity of such analysis to indicate cardiac sympathetic tone.[12]

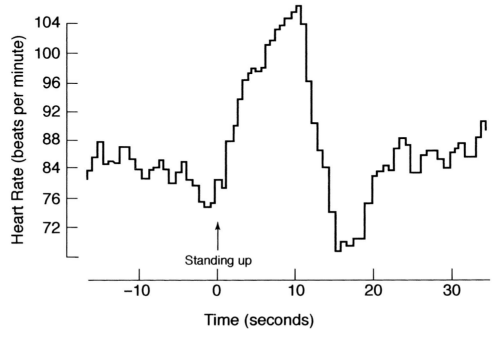

FIGURE 21-4 ■ Heart rate response to standing in a normal subject, showing an initial tachycardia that is maximal at about the 15th beat after standing, and a subsequent bradycardia.

RESPONSE TO THE VALSALVA MANEUVER

The Valsalva maneuver consists of a forced expiration against a closed glottis or mouthpiece with a calibrated air-leak. Characteristic changes in heart rate and blood pressure occur during and after performance of the maneuver and relate to changes in cardiac vagal efferent and sympathetic vasomotor activity as a result of stimulation of carotid sinus and aortic arch baroreceptors and other intrathoracic stretch receptors. For clinical purposes, it may be adequate simply to record the heart rate responses with a heart rate monitor (Fig. 21-5) or an ECG. For more detailed information of the changes in heart rate and blood pressure, however, it is necessary to use a servo-plethysmomanometer device (Finapres) or record from an intra-arterial needle (Fig. 21-6).

The test is performed with the subject in a semirecumbent position with a rubber clip over the nose. The subject is then required to blow into a mouthpiece (with a calibrated air-leak) connected to a mercury manometer and to maintain an expiratory pressure of 40 mmHg for 15 seconds while the heart rate is recorded. The normal response has four stages. Stages 1 and 3 are artifactual and are characterized by an increase (stage 1) or a decline (stage 3) in blood pressure because of the increase or decrease, respectively, in intrathoracic pressure at the beginning and end of the maneuver. In stage 2, the reduction in venous return leads to a progressive decline in systolic, diastolic, and pulse pressure, accompanied by a tachycardia resulting from increased cardiac sympathetic activity. The decline in blood pressure is arrested after about 5 to 8 seconds by a reflex vasoconstriction. With release of the blow at the end of the maneuver,

the artifactual decline in mean blood pressure as a result of the release of intrathoracic pressure (stage 3) is followed by a rebound in blood pressure to above resting levels because of the persisting peripheral vasoconstriction and the increased cardiac output that follows the increased venous return to the heart. This overshoot in the blood pressure, which varies in extent depending upon age, is accompanied by a compensatory, vagally induced bradycardia.

Abnormalities of the Valsalva response in dysautonomic patients may take the form of a loss of the tachycardia in stage 2 or of the bradycardia in stage 4; or a lower heart rate in stage 2 than in stage 4. Other abnormalities include a decline in mean blood pressure in stage 2 to less than 50 percent of the resting mean pressure or loss of the overshoot in systolic pressure in stage 4 (see Fig. 21-6). With isolated impairment of efferent sympathetic vasoconstriction, the blood pressure fails to show an overshoot in stage 4, and consequently there is no compensatory bradycardia despite otherwise intact baroreflex pathways.

When the response to the Valsalva maneuver is studied simply by recording the ECG, the Valsalva ratio is calculated by dividing the longest interbeat interval occurring after the maneuver by the shortest interbeat interval during it. The highest ratio from three successive attempts, each separated by 2 minutes, is recorded. The ratio reflects both parasympathetic (vagal) and sympathetic function. The normal range of values depends on age, the duration of the forced expiration, and the extent to which intrathoracic pressure is increased. A value of 1.1 or less is regarded commonly as abnormal and a

FIGURE 21-5 ▪ Normal heart rate response to the Valsalva maneuver, recorded with a heart rate monitor. A tachycardia occurs during the forced expiration, and a bradycardia occurs on release of the maneuver.

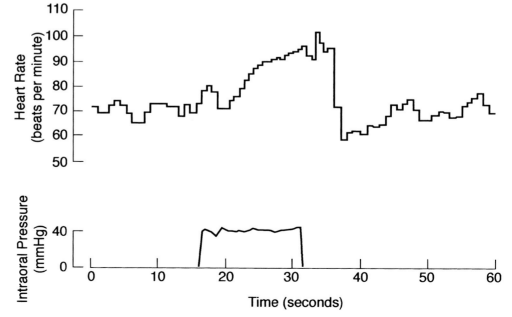

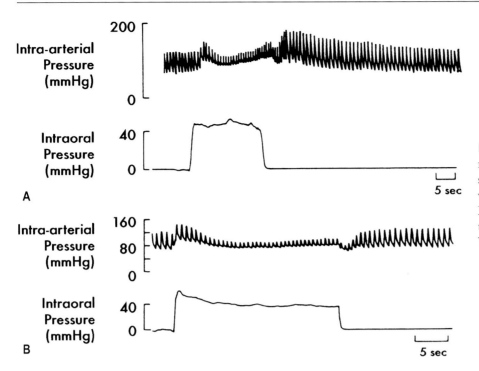

FIGURE 21-6 ■ Valsalva response as recorded intra-arterially. **A**, Normal response. **B**, Abnormal response in a patient with multisystem atrophy. (From Aminoff MJ: Electromyography in Clinical Practice. 3rd Ed. Churchill Livingstone, New York, 1998, with permission.)

value greater than 1.2 as normal, but in normal subjects younger than 40 years the ratio usually exceeds 1.4. Low values sometimes are recorded in patients with heart and lung disease. The Valsalva ratio is sometimes normal when the blood pressure response is abnormal.

BLOOD PRESSURE VARIATION

Change in Posture

The effect of postural change on blood pressure is important. The blood pressure is recorded with the subject supine and at rest for at least 10 minutes. The patient then stands with the arm held horizontally to avoid the hydrostatic effect of the column of blood in the dependent arm leading to a falsely elevated blood pressure. The blood pressure is taken immediately on standing and then at 1-minute intervals for 5 minutes. In normal subjects a slight decline in systolic pressure may occur, and diastolic pressure typically increases slightly. A decline that is greater than 20 mmHg in systolic pressure or 10 mmHg in diastolic pressure within 3 minutes of gaining an upright posture generally is regarded as abnormal.[13]

A tilt-table can also be used to evaluate postural changes in blood pressure, but the response may differ from that obtained by standing because there is less enhancement of the venous return to the heart by contraction of leg and abdominal muscles, and thus greater peripheral pooling of blood. After the patient has been supine for 10 minutes, the table is tilted to an angle of at least 60 degrees, and the patient remains in this upright position for 10 minutes. Blood pressure can be measured with a sphygmomanometer or by continuous recordings from digital arteries using the Finapres device mentioned earlier, which accurately records pressure changes. Prolonged testing (for up to 60 minutes) on a tilt-table at an angle of at least 60 degrees is being used increasingly to evaluate patients with suspected syncope.

The measurement of blood pressure in the sitting and standing positions actually has low diagnostic accuracy, and the more time-consuming method of head-up tilt-testing is preferred.[14] Many studies have shown that blood pressure changes with posture are unrelated to age, but there is no agreement on this point and asymptomatic postural hypotension is common in elderly patients. Postural hypotension occurs in a variety of medical contexts including cardiac disease, endocrine disorders, and hypovolemia, and in patients taking medications such as antihypertensive drugs, dopaminergic medication, and CNS depressants. Thus, detailed investigation may be necessary to clarify the cause of the postural hypotension, including other tests of autonomic function such as the response to the Valsalva maneuver.

Isometric Exercise

Sustained handgrip increases heart rate and blood pressure, partly by central command and partly by changes in contracting muscles that activate fibers subserving the afferent limb of the reflex arc.

The semirecumbent subject is required to maintain a pressure of 30 percent of maximal handgrip pressure for 5 minutes. The change in diastolic blood pressure is defined as the difference between the last value recorded before release of handgrip pressure and the mean resting value over the 3 minutes of recording preceding the isometric exercise.[15] An increase in diastolic pressure of at least 15 mmHg is normal and is not dependent on age. The test is not used widely, however, because the results are not as reproducible as the response to postural change.

CUTANEOUS VASOMOTOR CONTROL

Cutaneous blood flow is altered by stimuli such as a sudden inspiratory gasp, mental stress, startle, or alteration in temperature of another part of the body. Such changes in blood flow can be examined by plethysmography or laser Doppler velocimetry, as illustrated in Figure 21-7. In normal subjects, an inspiratory gasp leads to a digital vasoconstriction through a spinal or brainstem reflex. The response is lost in the presence of a cord lesion or dysfunction of sympathetic efferent fibers to the digit under study, such as in patients with a polyneuropathy or entrapment neuropathy. A cold stimulus to the opposite hand, such as water at 4°C, similarly leads to reflex vasoconstriction. The digital vasoconstriction that occurs in response to mental stress (e.g., performing mental arithmetic despite

distraction, or startle from a sudden loud noise) causes a transient increase in sympathetic vasomotor activity and thus evaluates sympathetic efferent pathways directly. Normal subjects sometimes have no response, however, leading to false-positive results.

TESTS OF BAROREFLEX SENSITIVITY AT REST

The relationship between heart rate and blood pressure can be analyzed on a beat-to-beat basis, quantifying the mathematical relationship between increase in systolic pressure and decline in heart rate, and vice versa. The slope of the regression between spontaneous increments or decrements in blood pressure and alterations in heart rate or RR interval will provide a measure of baroreflex sensitivity. Values in the order of 6 to 8 msec per mmHg have been calculated, and correlate with values obtained by phenylephrine infusion.[16] At present, the method is more of academic interest than practical relevance.

MYOCARDIAL SCINTIGRAPHY

Metaiodobenzylguanidine (MIBG) competes for the same cellular transporter mechanisms as norepinephrine in postganglionic adrenergic neurons. MIBG is actively transported into sympathetic nerve terminals by the norepinephrine transporter and thus accumulates predominantly in

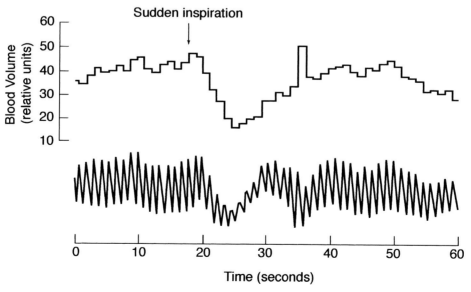

FIGURE 21-7 ■ Effect of a sudden deep inspiration on blood volume of the index finger, recorded photoplethysmographically by an infrared emitter and detector on the pad of the finger. The upper trace shows the amplitude of each pulse in relative units. The lower trace is the sensor output after amplification and reflects absolute blood volume in the finger. Each wave represents a heartbeat, and the amplitude of the waves reflects blood volume in the region of the sensor. The apparent shift of the direct-current signal component results from the long time-constant used to prevent loss of signal information.

organs with high sympathetic activity such as the adrenal gland, liver, spleen, and heart. When labeled with a radioactive tracer, MIBG accumulation can be visualized and measured by scintigraphy. Myocardial MIBG scintigraphy thus can be used to provide a measure of postganglionic sympathetic cardiac innervation. It has been used to evaluate cardiac innervation and has shown that patients with Parkinson disease have lower myocardial MIBG uptake than healthy controls.[17]

Sweat Tests

Disturbances of sweating are common in dysautonomia and can be evaluated by several different approaches. Techniques that have not gained widespread acceptance (e.g., the sweat imprint technique) will not be discussed. The density of nerve fibers innervating sweat glands in skin biopsy specimens can also be determined to provide a structural measure that complements clinical and electrophysiologic measures.[18]

THERMOREGULATORY SWEAT TEST

The thermoregulatory sweat test evaluates central and efferent sympathetic sudomotor function. The patient is warmed with a radiant heat cradle so as to increase the body temperature by 1°C. The skin is covered with a powder that changes color when moist, the most commonly used being alizarin red. This permits the presence and

distribution of sweating to be characterized. Disturbances may reflect preganglionic or postganglionic lesions. A symmetrical distal loss is suggestive of a polyneuropathy. Patchy or segmental anhidrosis may suggest a disorder such as leprosy or Ross (Ross–Adie) syndrome.[19] The procedure is somewhat time consuming and messy, and requires the patient to be unclothed.

SYMPATHETIC SKIN RESPONSE AND RELATED RESPONSES

A simple test of sudomotor function is the so-called galvanic skin response. A reduction in the electrical resistance of the skin occurs in response to a deep inspiration or noxious stimulus. It is related to increased sudomotor activity. This can be detected as a voltage or current change between the region under study and an indifferent area (Fig. 21-8).

The sympathetic skin response (SSR) represents the change in voltage measured at the skin surface following a single electrical or magnetic stimulus. It depends in part on the electrical activity arising from sweat glands and is recorded conveniently and quickly in a clinical neurophysiology laboratory. Pairs of surface electrodes are placed on the hands and feet, with the active electrodes on the palmar or plantar surface and the remote electrodes placed dorsally; limb temperature is maintained at 32 to 34°C. The electrical stimulus has a duration of 0.1 msec and an intensity of 5 to 20 mA, and is delivered randomly to a mixed or cutaneous nerve at the

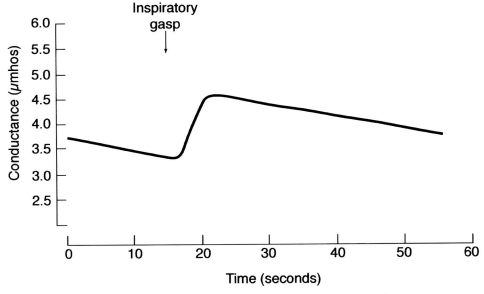

FIGURE 21-8 ■ Galvanic skin response recorded in a normal subject in response to a sudden deep inspiration. There is a change in skin conductance (which is the reciprocal of resistance and is measured in mhos) that is determined by applying a constant voltage across a pair of surface electrodes and measuring the resultant current.

contralateral wrist or ankle. The interstimulus interval should be at least 30 seconds. Magnetic stimuli at the neck have also been used.[20] The response is filtered at a bandpass of 0.1 or 0.5 to 1,000 or 2,000 Hz. A response can be obtained in normal subjects, but at present only its absence and not the absolute values of latency or amplitude are held to be of pathologic significance for clinical purposes. Responses are typically biphasic, with a negative initial potential followed by a positive deflection, the amplitude of which correlates with sweat production.[21] The latency in the upper limb is in the order of 1.5 sec and in the lower limb is about 2 sec. This long latency reflects the slow conduction velocity of postganglionic C fibers (approximately 1 m/sec). Abnormalities in the SSR correlate reasonably well with other sweat tests.[21] Although useful and simple to perform, the SSR is variable, habituates rapidly, and is nonquantitative in nature.[22] The SSR is absent in some patients with axonal neuropathies but generally is preserved in those with demyelinative neuropathies.

SUDOMOTOR AXON REFLEX TESTING

The intradermal injection of acetylcholine (5 to 10 mg) causes local sweating and piloerection if the postganglionic sympathetic fibers are intact. This provides a simple, nonquantitative test of sudomotor and pilomotor functions.

Sweat output in response to an axon reflex can be measured directly and accurately in a specially designed chamber placed on the skin. Iontophoresed acetylcholine activates axon terminals, generating impulses that pass antidromically to a branch point and then are conducted orthodromically down another axon to its terminals, where acetylcholine is released, generating a sweat response. Quantitative sudomotor axon reflex testing (QSART) is a sensitive means of assessing postganglionic sympathetic function and yields reproducible results. It requires sophisticated and expensive equipment, however, so that it is used only in a limited number of centers.

Plasma Catecholamine Levels and Infusions

The resting plasma norepinephrine level has been used to provide an index of sympathetic function. The main utility of this measurement is to indicate whether a sympathetic lesion is preganglionic, postganglionic, or both, because this is of pharmacologic importance. The level is diminished with postganglionic but not with preganglionic lesions. The plasma norepinephrine level normally increases on changing from a supine to standing position, but this increment may be attenuated or absent in patients with either pre- or postganglionic lesions.

The infusion of pressor drugs also helps to localize sympathetic lesions by demonstrating the presence and severity of denervation supersensitivity. Exaggerated pressor responses and a lower response threshold to sympathomimetic drugs (e.g., phenylephrine, norepinephrine, or epinephrine) are characteristic of degeneration of postganglionic sympathetic fibers. The blood pressure and heart rate are recorded with the patient at rest and then after intravenous infusion of the pressor agent at different doses.

With infusion of graded doses of pressor drugs having no direct effect on heart rate, baroreflex sensitivity may be measured by the relationship between changes in heart rate and blood pressure. As mentioned earlier, the baroreflex sensitivity is indicated by the slope of the line obtained by plotting the rate of each heartbeat against the systolic pressure of the preceding beat, and is a measure of vagal activity and baroreflex afferents.

Tests of Pupillary Function

A sympathomimetic agent applied topically leads to dilatation of denervated pupils at concentrations that are ineffective in normal pupils because of denervation sensitivity. For example, 0.1 percent epinephrine, applied to the conjunctival sac, does not affect the normal pupil but leads to dilatation when postganglionic sympathetic fibers are affected. Cocaine hydrochloride (4 percent) instilled into the conjunctival sac normally causes pupillary dilatation, but the response is reduced or absent with lesions of the oculosympathetic pathways. Thus, in Horner syndrome, occurring from an interruption of peripheral sympathetic pathways, the response to cocaine is lost. The responses to 6-hydroxyamphetamine distinguish preganglionic from postganglionic oculosympathetic lesions because pupillary dilatation occurs only when postganglionic sympathetic fibers are intact.

There is usually no response of normal pupils to the instillation of very weak solutions of parasympathomimetic agents (e.g., methacholine 2.5 percent or pilocarpine 0.125 percent), but pupillary constriction occurs when parasympathetic innervation is impaired because of denervation supersensitivity.

Intraneural Recordings

Intraneural recording of postganglionic sympathetic activity in humans has been important in adding to understanding about the operation of the autonomic nervous system in health and disease.[23–25] The topic is considered further in Chapter 14. At present, however, such approaches do not have a major role in diagnosing dysautonomias for clinical purposes and therefore are not considered further.

Other Investigative Techniques

Radiologic studies and urologic procedures such as uroflowmetry and measurement of urethral pressure profiles are not the province of clinical neurophysiologists and are not considered further. Sphincteric electromyography (EMG), pudendal and perineal nerve conduction studies, and evaluation of certain pelvic reflexes have also been used as a means of evaluating autonomic function. Those techniques useful in evaluating sacral function are considered further in Chapter 31.

SELECTION OF TESTS

No full comparative study of autonomic function tests has been reported, but certain general comments can be made. Adequate assessment of autonomic function requires tests of the control of heart rate, blood pressure, and sweating, with evaluation of both sympathetic and parasympathetic pathways.[26] Five simple noninvasive tests of cardiovascular reflexes have been deemed adequate for assessment of diabetic autonomic neuropathy: the heart rate responses to (1) the Valsalva maneuver, (2) standing (30:15 ratio), and (3) deep breathing; and the blood pressure responses to (4) standing and (5) sustained handgrip. Definite autonomic neuropathy is indicated by an abnormality in two or more tests.

An autonomic reflex screen yielding a ten-point composite autonomic scoring scale (CASS) of autonomic function has been described by Low and colleagues at the Mayo Clinic.[27] It involves the QSART and measurement of orthostatic blood pressure and heart rate response to tilt, heart rate response to deep breathing, the Valsalva ratio, and beat-to-beat blood pressure measurements during phases II and IV of the Valsalva maneuver, tilt, and deep breathing. Confounding effects of age and sex are corrected. Thus the presence and severity of postganglionic sudomotor, adrenergic, and cardiovagal function are assessed.

Abnormalities in two or more of a range of tests (i.e., cardiovascular responses to postural change, isometric exercise, deep breathing, and the Valsalva maneuver; thermoregulatory sweat tests; and plasma norepinephrine levels) are generally adequate to confirm the presence of a dysautonomia.

TEST FINDINGS IN SPECIFIC DISORDERS

The pattern of autonomic abnormalities may help to suggest certain disorders, even though both sympathetic and parasympathetic functions eventually come to be affected.

Central Nervous System

Disorders of the CNS associated with autonomic failure include multisystem atrophy (MSA), pure autonomic failure (PAF), and Parkinson disease. Dysautonomic symptoms are common after spinal cord injury.

Multisystem atrophy is a progressive neurodegenerative disorder characterized by autonomic dysfunction; parkinsonism; upper motor neuron deficits; ataxia; and, sometimes, by lower motor neuron signs. Depending on the clinical features, the disorder may be designated as MSA with predominant parkinsonism or predominant ataxia.[28] When dysautonomic symptoms are especially conspicuous, the older term, *Shy–Drager syndrome*, is often used. A review of the autonomic aspects of the disorder has been published in detail elsewhere.[29]

In pure autonomic failure, orthostatic hypotension, commonly associated with bladder dysfunction, impotence, and impaired sweating, is not accompanied by clinical evidence of CNS involvement. In MSA, pathologic changes in the autonomic nervous system involve predominantly the preganglionic neurons, whereas in PAF the sympathetic ganglia and postsynaptic neurons are affected more severely.

In both MSA and PAF, postural hypotension is often dramatic. Impaired thermoregulatory sweating and abnormal heart rate responses to deep breathing, the Valsalva maneuver, and postural change are also found. Resting plasma norepinephrine levels are reduced in PAF but not in MSA; in both disorders there is no increment with head-up tilt, and standing levels are low.[30]

In Parkinson disease, postural hypotension has often been reported and, when present, may be iatrogenic, is often asymptomatic, and may be delayed in its occurrence after postural change.[31] The literature is conflicting, but in the author's experience the cardiovascular reflexes are often preserved.[32] However, several recent studies have suggested that many patients with Parkinson disease have cardiac sympathetic denervation, as shown by scintigraphy, accounting for the postural hypotension.[33,34] In such patients, responses to the Valsalva maneuver are also abnormal. The findings in one large study suggested that pronounced vasomotor and cardiac sympathetic dysfunction was the primary cause of orthostatic hypotension, although impaired baroreceptor reflexes may have a minor contributory role.[35] Abnormalities of the sympathetic skin response[36,37] and of heart rate variation[36] have been found, but some investigators have reported normal heart rate variability.[38] Other dysautonomic symptoms (e.g., disturbances of bladder or gastrointestinal function and excessive salivation) are relatively common.

It may not be possible to distinguish Parkinson disease from MSA when the autonomic nervous system is involved.[39] Even the cardiovascular and plasma norepinephrine responses to adrenergic agonists fail to distinguish reliably between them.[40] The evidence suggests that generalized noradrenergic denervation occurs with similar severity in Parkinson disease accompanied by postural hypotension and in PAF.[41] Interestingly, myocardial sympathetic degeneration correlates with the severity of bradykinesia and rigidity but not with tremor, suggesting that myocardial sympathetic degeneration and hypokinetic-rigid symptoms develop in a closely coupled manner.[42] Deep brain stimulation of the subthalamic nucleus improves postural hypotension in some patients.[43]

Minor abnormalities of autonomic function may occur in patients with progressive supranuclear palsy but are uncommon.[44] Mild dysautonomic findings also may be encountered in Huntington disease, even at a presymptomatic stage of the disease.[32,45–47]

In patients with the rare syndrome of congenital deficiency of dopamine-β-hydroxylase, there is pure sympathetic failure but normal cholinergic function, including sweating. Postural hypotension is an early feature.

Spinal cord injury may have a major impact on autonomic function, causing, for example, neurogenic shock, cardiac dysrhythmias, postural hypotension, autonomic hyperreflexia, abnormalities of temperature regulation and sweating, and disturbances of sphincter and sexual function. Cardiovascular disturbances increase with the level of injury and its severity. Patients with spinal cord injury are at increased risk for heart disease and stroke. Based upon neuroanatomic principles, a framework has been suggested with which to communicate the effects of specific spinal cord injuries on various autonomic functions.[48]

Peripheral Nervous System

Autonomic disturbances are an expected accompaniment of many peripheral neuropathies, even though they have received far less attention than the motor and sensory disturbances that occur. Such a dysautonomia may be an incidental finding that is more of academic interest than clinical relevance, as in certain entrapment neuropathies. It may be a minor feature of neuropathies such as chronic inflammatory demyelinating neuropathy (CIDP) or that associated with acquired immunodeficiency syndrome (AIDS); and a major factor of others, such as the Guillain–Barré syndrome or diabetic neuropathy. The dysautonomia may be the presenting feature of the neuropathy or simply an inconsequential accompaniment, its most disabling (even life-threatening) feature or an asymptomatic manifestation recognized only by laboratory investigations. It may develop acutely, reaching a maximum within 4 weeks, or evolve more insidiously.

Clinically, the dysautonomia may involve sympathetic or parasympathetic fibers, or both (pandysautonomia); similarly, an adrenergic or cholinergic predominance may occur. With generalized sympathetic involvement, postural hypotension and anhidrosis are conspicuous, whereas with parasympathetic involvement there is a fixed heart rate, xerostomia, xerophthalmia, gastrointestinal dysfunction (e.g., colicky abdominal pain, nausea, vomiting, satiety, bloating, gastric fullness, and diarrhea, sometimes alternating with constipation), bladder dysfunction, and—in men—sexual disturbances such as erectile dysfunction. With localized involvement, the site of the pathologic process governs manifestations.

Autonomic testing has an important role in documenting autonomic involvement in patients with peripheral neuropathies, especially when autonomic neuropathy or distal small-fiber sensory polyneuropathy is suspected clinically.[49]

ACUTE PERIPHERAL DYSAUTONOMIAS

Idiopathic Autonomic Neuropathies

Patients present with an acute, monophasic autonomic neuropathy but little, if any, somatic disturbance. There may be evidence of preceding viral infection, or the neuropathy may represent a paraneoplastic disorder. Such associations suggest an underlying immunologic disturbance; this is supported by studies showing high titers of ganglionic acetylcholine receptor antibody in 40 to 50 percent of patients.[50] In patients with a paraneoplastic etiology, other autoantibodies may be found as well or instead, including antineuronal nuclear antibody 1 (ANNA-1 or anti-Hu) or 2 (ANNA-2), Purkinje cell antibody 2 (PCA-2), and collapsin response-mediator protein 5 antibody (CRMP-5). Such antibodies may be important in suggesting the likely site of any underlying primary tumor.

Patients with a pandysautonomia typically complain of dizziness, lightheadedness, visual blurring or fading out, near-syncope, or even loss of consciousness on standing (from postural hypotension); heat intolerance, anhidrosis, or hypohidrosis; and gastrointestinal disturbances. Clinical examination generally confirms the presence of postural hypotension, but repeated examination is sometimes necessary to do so. Other common findings include a fixed heart rate, dry skin, dilated pupils, urinary retention, and paralytic ileus. Autonomic function tests are abnormal and reflect these clinical findings. In addition, thermoregulatory sweat tests or QSART are abnormal, nerve biopsy may show perivascular round cell infiltration, and skin biopsy reveals loss of epidermal C fibers. In patients with high titers of ganglionic acetylcholine receptor antibody, analysis of sudomotor function by thermoregulatory sweat test and QSART suggests postganglionic dysfunction with involvement of both the ganglia and postganglionic nerve fibers; increasing elevation of antibody levels results in increased postganglionic dysfunction.[51] Nerve conduction studies are usually normal, but sometimes mild sensory changes are found. The prognosis is variable, with only about 30 percent making a good recovery, usually within 1 year of onset.[52] Treatment is supportive, but immunomodulating therapy may be worthwhile in those with a progressive or life-threatening disorder. Paraneoplastic dysautonomia may remit with treatment of the underlying malignancy.

Guillain–Barré Syndrome

The somatic features of the Guillain–Barré syndrome are well recognized, but it is the autonomic disturbances that generally are responsible for the fatal outcome that sometimes occurs. Cardiac arrhythmias (most commonly a sinus tachycardia), paroxysmal hypotension or hypertension, and postural hypotension are the most disabling features.[53] Disturbances of bladder or gastrointestinal function also occur. The postural hypotension is multifactorial and may relate to inactivity and bedrest, efferent sympathetic denervation, baroreceptor deafferentation, volume depletion, cardiac abnormalities, or some combination of these and other factors. Autonomic function studies reveal an abnormal Valsalva response, abnormal heart rate responses to induced hypertension or deep breathing, and abnormal sweat tests. The dysautonomia is treated symptomatically and supportively. This may require adrenergic blockade for hypertension or a demand pacemaker for bradyarrhythmias. The dysautonomia typically recovers without long-term sequelae.

The acute dysautonomia of Guillain–Barré syndrome is distinguished by its somatic accompaniments from the acute dysautonomia that sometimes arises as an isolated phenomenon. This latter disorder may be a variant of Guillain–Barré syndrome, but this remains to be established.

Botulism

Botulism, which typically occurs within 36 hours of the ingestion of contaminated food, results from the toxin produced by the type B strain of *Clostridium botulinum*, which impairs acetylcholine release from nerve terminals. It is characterized initially by the development of blurred vision, ptosis, dysphagia, and weakness of the extraocular muscles; and then by facial and more widespread weakness associated with cholinergic failure. Autonomic involvement is signaled by xerophthalmia, xerostomia, anhidrosis, constipation, paralytic ileus, and urinary retention, and studies indicate the presence of abnormal sudomotor function, high resting heart rate, reduced heart rate variation, and significant postural hypotension.[54] The electrophysiologic features resemble those of the Lambert–Eaton syndrome. Single-fiber EMG is abnormal, indicating a disorder of neuromuscular transmission that is presynaptic in nature. In the absence of associated muscle weakness, it is sometimes difficult to distinguish the disorder clinically from acute idiopathic cholinergic autonomic neuropathy.

Other Causes of Acute Dysautonomia

Dysautonomic symptoms may accompany the acute motor neuropathy of porphyria, and are a feature of certain iatrogenic and toxic neuropathies (e.g., related to use of vinca alkaloids[55] or paclitaxel [Taxol][56]; or following exposure to organic solvents or acrylamide). The circumstances in which they develop usually suggest the underlying etiology, and treatment is supportive, combined with avoidance of the offending agent. In most instances, autonomic function studies have not been undertaken and would anyway add little to the evaluation and management of patients.

CHRONIC AUTONOMIC NEUROPATHIES

Autonomic involvement occurs most commonly in axonal (as opposed to demyelinating) neuropathies, and especially in small-fiber neuropathies. Such small-fiber neuropathies are often difficult to recognize clinically or electrophysiologically. Patients typically present with pain, dysesthesias, and allodynia beginning in the feet and then extending proximally in the legs before coming to involve the upper limbs. Evidence of sympathetic involvement is also present. Clinical examination reveals normal power and tendon reflexes, and the only sensory deficit is an impaired appreciation of pinprick and temperature in the legs. Sudomotor abnormalities may be detected by thermoregulatory sweat tests or QSART.[57]

The autonomic nervous system is affected in many peripheral neuropathies, although the clinical manifestations may be mild. Autonomic dysfunction is clinically important in neuropathies associated with diabetes, primary amyloidosis, and familial amyloid polyneuropathy, and in some cases of hereditary sensory neuropathy, particularly the Riley–Day syndrome, as well as in the acute disorders discussed in the preceding section. In most other neuropathies, autonomic dysfunction is usually of only minor clinical importance. In entrapment neuropathies, for example, postganglionic sympathetic fibers mediating the cutaneous vasoconstrictor response to an inspiratory gasp may be involved, indicating that small- and large-diameter fibers are affected, but this is of little diagnostic relevance.

Diabetes

Autonomic neuropathy occurs in about 20 percent of diabetic patients, sometimes as an isolated neurologic finding but more commonly as part of a more widespread neuropathic process. It may present with erectile dysfunction, postural lightheadedness, exercise intolerance, postprandial bloating, early satiety, gastrointestinal motility disturbances, impaired bladder control, and disturbances of sweating. Resting tachycardia may be present. Abnormalities in tests of parasympathetic function (heart rate response to breathing, change of posture, and the Valsalva maneuver) occur early, whereas abnormalities of sympathetic efferent function (blood pressure response to change in posture and isometric exercise) generally develop at a later stage. Reduced cardiovascular autonomic function, as reflected by heart rate variability, is associated with an increased risk of silent myocardial ischemia and death.[58] Abnormalities of sudomotor function are well described. The QSART is commonly abnormal and indicates involvement of distal postganglionic sympathetic fibers. The functional abnormalities in diabetic peripheral neuropathy seem to affect C-fiber subclasses differentially, depending on the type of diabetes, as reflected by studies of axon-reflex responses to injected acetylcholine and the nociceptor (flare) response.[59]

Amyloid Neuropathy

Primary amyloidosis and familial amyloid polyneuropathy of Portuguese type (FAP type 1) are often complicated by autonomic failure resulting from loss of predominantly unmyelinated and small myelinated peripheral fibers and cell loss in the intermediolateral columns of the cord.[60]

Postural hypotension and impotence are common early symptoms; alternating constipation and diarrhea, distal anhidrosis, urinary retention, and cardiac arrhythmias are also common. Tests of sympathetic and parasympathetic function are typically abnormal.[61]

Familial Dysautonomia

Familial dysautonomia (Riley–Day syndrome or hereditary sensory and autonomic neuropathy type III) is manifest in childhood. Autonomic disturbances include impaired lacrimation, hyperhidrosis, postural hypotension, and poor temperature control. Widespread abnormalities of autonomic function may be detected on testing.[62] Neuroimaging reveals abnormalities consistent with concomitant cerebral pathology.[63]

Postural Orthostatic Tachycardia Syndrome

This syndrome is characterized by postural intolerance accompanied by an increase in heart rate of at least 30 beats per minute on standing or tilt-testing. Postural hypotension does not occur. Symptoms relate to cerebral hypoperfusion and sympathetic overactivity. The disorder is often preceded by a viral illness and may relate, at least in part, to some combination of partial peripheral sympathetic denervation, hypovolemia, venous pooling, beta-receptor supersensitivity, psychologic factors, prolonged deconditioning, and impaired neuroregulatory mechanisms.[64] Accompanying features include xerostomia, xerophthalmia, nausea, and postprandial bloating. The response to head-up tilt is characterized by a marked tachycardia within about 2 minutes. The response to the Valsalva maneuver indicates impaired peripheral vasoconstriction, but cardiovagal responses are normal.[62] Thermoregulatory sweat tests commonly reveal distal impairment, and the QSART shows that the lesion is postganglionic.[65,66] Patients sometimes respond to a high-salt diet, copious fluids, postural training, fludrocortisone, midodrine, and low-dose propranolol or cardioselective beta-adrenoceptor blockers.[67]

Other Autonomic Neuropathies

In Adie syndrome (tonic pupils with areflexia), sympathetic failure is sometimes present and segmental anhidrosis (Ross syndrome) may occur. Pathologic studies have indicated reduced cholinergic sweat-gland innervation in areas of hypohidrosis, implying a selective degenerative process of cholinergic sudomotor neurons.[68] A Horner syndrome sometimes is encountered, however, and other dysautonomic symptoms may also be present, suggesting a generalized abnormality of ganglion cells or their projections.[69] Symptoms resulting from vasomotor and respiratory dysfunction may worsen with time.[70]

In patients with *chronic renal failure*, the degree of autonomic dysfunction relates to the impairment of nerve conduction.[71] Parasympathetic cardiovascular abnormalities are more common than sympathetic abnormalities such as postural hypotension and abnormalities of the SSR. The baroreceptor reflexes may also be impaired. Although dysautonomic symptoms are frequent in patients undergoing long-term hemodialysis, abnormalities in tests of autonomic function are less common.[72]

Dysautonomic manifestations, other than impaired sweating distally, are uncommon in *alcoholic peripheral neuropathy*, except when the neuropathy is severe or coexists with Wernicke encephalopathy, which is accompanied by central autonomic dysfunction. However, alcohol-dependent patients admitted to a psychiatric department were found to have a higher incidence than normal subjects of parasympathetic (vagal) disturbances of cardiovascular function as measured by heart rate variability.[73] Cardiovascular autonomic dysfunction may occur in alcoholic and nonalcoholic chronic *liver disease*. In nonalcoholic chronic liver disease, abnormalities in both sympathetic and parasympathetic function tests have been found, with a poor relationship to liver function parameters.[74] Autonomic neuropathy signifies a worse prognosis than otherwise.[75]

In *rheumatoid arthritis*, involvement of postganglionic sympathetic efferent fibers leads to impaired sweating, and vagal involvement leads to abnormalities in the heart rate response to standing, the Valsalva maneuver, and respiration, especially in patients with peripheral neuropathy; pupillary autonomic dysfunction may also occur.[76] Autonomic abnormalities may occur in other connective tissue diseases, including *systemic lupus erythematosus*, *mixed connective tissue disease*, and *Sjögren syndrome*.

Leprosy has been associated with autonomic dysfunction. Patchy anhidrosis is the most common finding, but cardiovascular abnormalities, including postural hypotension, also occur. Abnormalities in cardiovascular parasympathetic tests are more common and occur earlier than cardiovascular sympathetic abnormalities. Nevertheless, abnormalities of cutaneous vasomotor reflexes may be found in patients with leprosy[77] and in the apparently healthy contacts of such patients,[78] and, when combined with electrophysiologic testing of peripheral nerve function, may provide a means of determining the spectrum of involved fibers.[79]

Syncope, impotence, bladder and bowel dysfunction, and anhidrosis are common in patients with *human immunodeficiency virus* infection. Abnormal autonomic function test results become more common and more severe in patients with AIDS; up to 80 percent of patients with AIDS have abnormalities.[80,81]

Diphtheria sometimes causes a demyelinating motor polyneuropathy, and this may be associated with abnormalities in parasympathetic cardiovascular function; sympathetic abnormalities are not found.[82]

During the chronic phase of *Chagas disease*, which is widespread in South America, the gastrointestinal tract and heart may be affected. Clinical manifestations include cardiac arrhythmias, sudden death, and postural hypotension, with abnormal cardiovascular reflexes.[83]

It is generally believed that only minor, infrequent disturbances in autonomic function occur in CIDP but, in one study, a variety of abnormalities, including SSR abnormalities, were found in 50 percent of patients.[84] The abnormalities may involve sympathetic or parasympathetic components; in the former, both vasomotor and sudomotor fibers may be affected.

In patients with *hereditary neuropathies*, pupillary reflexes may be abnormal and sweating is sometimes impaired distally, but cardiovascular reflexes usually are preserved in patients with hereditary motor and sensory neuropathy types I and II.[85] In hereditary sensory and autonomic neuropathies other than Riley–Day syndrome (discussed earlier), anhidrosis is the most common dysautonomic feature.

The dysautonomic manifestations of Fabry disease include hypohidrosis or anhidrosis and gastrointestinal dysfunction with indigestion, nausea, belching, esophageal reflux, abdominal pain, flatus, and diarrhea. Overt symptoms of postural hypotension do not occur. Autonomic tests reveal pupillary abnormalities, abnormal tear and saliva production, widespread anhidrosis, reduced cutaneous flare response to scratch and intradermal histamine, and abnormal colonic motility.[86] Despite the absence of cardiovascular symptoms, testing may reveal reduced changes in heart rate on standing and decreased baroreflex sensitivity.[87] Enzyme replacement therapy may lead to improvement or normalization of sweating, as shown by QSART or thermoregulatory sweat tests,[88] and improved baroreflex function.[87]

REFERENCES

1. Aminoff MJ: Autonomic nervous system. p. 93. In Fogel BS, Schiffer RB, Rao SM (eds): Neuropsychiatry. Williams & Wilkins, Baltimore, 1996
2. Wallin BG, Elam M: Microneurography and autonomic dysfunction. p. 243. In Low PA (ed): Clinical Autonomic Disorders. Little, Brown, Boston, 1993

3. Suarez GA, Opfer-Gehrking TL, Offord KP et al: The Autonomic Symptom Profile: a new instrument to assess autonomic symptoms. Neurology, 52:523, 1999

4. Shields RW, Jr: Heart rate variability with deep breathing as a clinical test of cardiovagal function. Cleve Clin J Med, 76 Suppl 2:S37, 2009

5. Stålberg EV, Nogués MA: Automatic analysis of heart rate variation. I. Method and reference values in healthy controls. Muscle Nerve, 12:993, 1989

6. Linden D, Diehl RR: Comparison of standard autonomic tests and power spectral analysis in normal adults. Muscle Nerve, 19:556, 1996

7. Ingall TJ, McLeod JG, O'Brien PC: The effect of ageing on autonomic nervous system function. Aust N Z J Med, 20: 570, 1990

8. Freeman R: Autonomic testing. p. 483. In Brown WF, Bolton CF, Aminoff MJ (eds): Neuromuscular Function and Disease. WB Saunders, Philadelphia, 2002

9. Freeman R, Cohen RJ, Saul JP: Transfer function analysis of respiratory sinus arrhythmia: a measure of autonomic function in diabetic neuropathy. Muscle Nerve, 18:74, 1995

10. Freeman R, Saul JP, Roberts MS et al: Spectral analysis of heart rate in diabetic autonomic neuropathy. Arch Neurol, 48:185, 1991

11. Hilz MJ: Quantitative autonomic functional testing in clinical trials. p. 1899. In Brown WF, Bolton CF, Aminoff MJ (eds): Neuromuscular Function and Disease. WB Saunders, Philadelphia, 2002

12. Goldstein DS: Neuroscience and heart-brain medicine: the year in review. Cleve Clin J Med, 77: Suppl 3:S34, 2010

13. Lahrmann H, Cortelli P, Hilz M et al: EFNS guidelines on the diagnosis and management of orthostatic hypotension. Eur J Neurol, 13:930, 2006

14. Cooke J, Carew S, O'Connor M et al: Sitting and standing blood pressure measurements are not accurate for the diagnosis of orthostatic hypotension. QJM, 102:335, 2009

15. McLeod JG: Evaluation of the autonomic nervous system. p. 381. In Aminoff MJ (ed): Electrodiagnosis in Clinical Neurology. 4th Ed. Churchill Livingstone, New York, 1999

16. Pitzalis MV, Matropasqua F, Passantino A et al: Comparison between noninvasive indices of baroreceptor sensitivity and the phenylephrine method in post-myocardial infarction patients. Circulation, 97:1362, 1998

17. Rascol O, Schelosky L: ^{123}I-metaiodobenzylguanidine scintigraphy in Parkinson's disease and related disorders. Mov Disord, 24:Suppl 2,S732, 2009

18. Gibbons CH, Illigens BM, Wang N et al: Quantification of sweat gland innervation: a clinical–pathologic correlation. Neurology, 72:1479, 2009

19. Fealey RD: Thermoregulatory sweat test. p. 245. In Low PA (ed): Clinical Autonomic Disorders. 2nd Ed. Lippincott-Raven, Philadelphia, 1997

20. Ellaway PH, Kuppuswamy A, Nicotra A et al: Sweat production and the sympathetic skin response: improving the clinical assessment of autonomic function. Auton Neurosci, 155:109, 2010

21. Maselli RA, Jaspan JB, Soliven BC et al: Comparison of sympathetic skin response with quantitative sudomotor axon reflex test in diabetic neuropathy. Muscle Nerve, 12:420, 1989

22. Toyokura M, Murakami K: Reproducibility of sympathetic skin response. Muscle Nerve, 19:1481, 1996

23. Wallin BG, Elam M: Microneurography and autonomic dysfunction. p. 233. In Low PA (ed): Clinical Autonomic Disorders. 2nd Ed. Lippincott-Raven, Philadelphia, 1997

24. Dotson R, Ochoa J, Marchettini P et al: Sympathetic neural outflow directly recorded in patients with primary autonomic failure: clinical observations, microneurography, and histopathology. Neurology, 40:1079, 1990

25. Wallin BG, Charkoudian N: Sympathetic neural control of integrated cardiovascular function: insights from measurement of human sympathetic nerve activity. Muscle Nerve, 36:595, 2007

26. American Academy of Neurology: Assessment: clinical autonomic testing report of the Therapeutic and Technology Assessment Sub-Committee of the American Academy of Neurology. Neurology, 46:873, 1996

27. Low PA: Composite autonomic scoring scale for laboratory quantification of generalized autonomic failure. Mayo Clin Proc, 68:748, 1993

28. Gilman S, Wenning GK, Low PA et al: Second consensus statement on the diagnosis of multiple system atrophy. Neurology, 71:670, 2008

29. Mathias CJ: Multiple system atrophy and autonomic failure. J Neural Transm Suppl, 70:343, 2006

30. Low PA, Bannister R: Multiple system atrophy and pure autonomic failure. p. 555. In Low PA (ed): Clinical Autonomic Disorders. 2nd Ed. Lippincott-Raven, Philadelphia, 1997

31. Jamnadas-Khoda J, Koshy S, Mathias CJ et al: Are current recommendations to diagnose orthostatic hypotension in Parkinson's disease satisfactory? Mov Disord, 24:1747, 2009

32. Aminoff MJ: Other extrapyramidal disorders. p. 577. In Low PA (ed): Clinical Autonomic Disorders. 2nd Ed. Lippincott-Raven, Philadelphia, 1997

33. Goldstein DS: Dysautonomia in Parkinson's disease: neurocardiological abnormalities. Lancet Neurol, 2:669, 2003

34. Goldstein DS, Holmes CS, Dendi R et al: Orthostatic hypotension from sympathetic denervation in Parkinson's disease. Neurology, 58:1247, 2002

35. Oka H, Yoshioka M, Onouchi K et al: Characteristics of orthostatic hypotension in Parkinson's disease. Brain, 130:2425, 2007

36. Zakrzewska-Pniewska B, Jamrozik Z: Are electrophysiological autonomic tests useful in the assessment of dysautonomia in Parkinson's disease? Parkinsonism Relat Disord, 9:179, 2003

37. Haapaniemi TH, Korpelainen JT, Tolonen U et al: Suppressed sympathetic skin response in Parkinson disease. Clin Auton Res, 10:337, 2000

38. Holmberg B, Kallio M, Johnels B et al: Cardiovascular reflex testing contributes to clinical evaluation and differential diagnosis of parkinsonian syndromes. Mov Disord, 16:217, 2001

39. Riley DE, Chelimsky TC: Autonomic nervous system testing may not distinguish multiple system atrophy from Parkinson's disease. J Neurol Neurosurg Psychiatry, 74:56, 2003

40. Lipp A, Sandroni P, Low PA et al: Systemic postganglionic adrenergic studies do not distinguish Parkinson's disease from multiple system atrophy. J Neurol Sci, 281:15, 2009

41. Sharabi Y, Imrich R, Holmes C et al: Generalized and neurotransmitter-selective noradrenergic denervation in Parkinson's disease with orthostatic hypotension. Mov Disord, 23:1725, 2008

42. Spiegel J, Hellwig D, Farmakis G et al: Myocardial sympathetic degeneration correlates with clinical phenotype of Parkinson's disease. Mov Disord, 22:1004, 2007

43. Stemper B, Beric A, Welsch G et al: Deep brain stimulation improves orthostatic regulation of patients with Parkinson disease. Neurology, 67:1781, 2006

44. Williams DR, Lees AJ: What features improve the accuracy of the clinical diagnosis of progressive supranuclear palsy-parkinsonism (PSP-P)? Mov Disord, 25:357, 2010

45. Chaudhuri KR: Autonomic dysfunction in movement disorders. Curr Opin Neurol, 14:505, 2001

46. Bär KJ, Boettger MK, Andrich J et al: Cardiovagal modulation upon postural change is altered in Huntington's disease. Eur J Neurol, 15:869, 2008

47. Andrich J, Schmitz T, Saft C et al: Autonomic nervous system function in Huntington's disease. J Neurol Neurosurg Psychiatry, 72:726, 2002

48. Alexander MS, Biering-Sorensen F, Bodner D et al: International standards to document remaining autonomic function after spinal cord injury. Spinal Cord, 47:36, 2009

49. England JD, Gronseth GS, Franklin G et al: Practice parameter: the evaluation of distal symmetric polyneuropathy: the role of autonomic testing, nerve biopsy, and skin biopsy (an evidence-based review). Report of the American Academy of Neurology, the American Association of Neuromuscular and Electrodiagnostic Medicine, and the American Academy of Physical Medicine and Rehabilitation. Muscle Nerve, 39:106, 2009

50. Vernino S, Low PA, Fealey RD et al: Autoantibodies to ganglionic acetylcholine receptors in autoimmune autonomic neuropathies. N Engl J Med, 343:847, 2000

51. Kimpinski K, Iodice V, Sandroni P et al: Sudomotor dysfunction in autoimmune autonomic ganglionopathy. Neurology, 73:1501, 2009

52. Suarez GA, Fealey RD, Camilleri M et al: Idiopathic autonomic neuropathy: clinical, neurophysiologic, and follow-up studies on 27 patients. Neurology, 44:1675, 1994

53. Zochodne DW: Autonomic involvement in Guillain–Barré syndrome: a review. Muscle Nerve, 17:1145, 1996

54. Topakian R, Heibl C, Stieglbauer K et al: Quantitative autonomic testing in the management of botulism. J Neurol, 256:803, 2009

55. Tarlaci S: Vincristine-induced fatal neuropathy in non-Hodgkin's lymphoma. Neurotoxicology, 29:748, 2008

56. Jerian SM, Sarosy GA, Link CJ et al: Incapacitating autonomic neuropathy precipitated by taxol. Gynecol Oncol, 51:277, 1993

57. Stewart JD, Low PA, Fealey RD: Distal small fiber neuropathy: results of tests of sweating and autonomic cardiovascular reflexes. Muscle Nerve, 15:661, 1992

58. Vinik AI, Maser RE, Mitchell BD et al: Diabetic autonomic neuropathy. Diabetes Care, 26:1553, 2003

59. Berghoff M, Kilo S, Hilz MJ et al: Differential impairment of the sudomotor and nociceptor axon-reflex in diabetic peripheral neuropathy. Muscle Nerve, 33:494, 2006

60. Ando Y, Suhr OB: Autonomic dysfunction in familial amyloidotic polyneuropathy (FAP). Amyloid, 5:288, 1998

61. Bernardi L, Passino C, Porta C et al: Widespread cardiovascular autonomic dysfunction in primary amyloidosis: does spontaneous hyperventilation have a compensatory role against postural hypotension? Heart, 88:615, 2002

62. Axelrod FB: Familial dysautonomia. Muscle Nerve, 29:352, 2004

63. Axelrod FB, Hilz MJ, Berlin D et al: Neuroimaging supports central pathology in familial dysautonomia. J Neurol, 257:198, 2010

64. Low PA, Sandroni P, Joyner M et al: Postural tachycardia syndrome (POTS). J Cardiovasc Electrophysiol, 20:352, 2009

65. Low PA, Vernino S, Suarez G: Autonomic dysfunction in peripheral nerve disease. Muscle Nerve, 27:646, 2003

66. Peltier AC, Garland E, Raj SR et al: Distal sudomotor findings in postural tachycardia syndrome. Clin Auton Res, 20:93, 2010

67. Raj SR, Black BK, Biaggioni I et al: Propranolol decreases tachycardia and improves symptoms in the postural tachycardia syndrome: less is more. Circulation, 120:725, 2009

68. Sommer C, Lindenlaub T, Zillikens D et al: Selective loss of cholinergic sudomotor fibers causes anhidrosis in Ross syndrome. Ann Neurol, 52:247, 2002

69. Shin RK, Galetta SL, Ting TY et al: Ross syndrome plus: beyond Horner, Holmes–Adie, and harlequin. Neurology, 55:1841, 2000

70. Guaraldi P, Mathias CJ: Progression of cardiovascular autonomic dysfunction in Holmes–Adie syndrome. J Neurol Neurosurg Psychiatry, 82:1046, 2011

71. Wang SJ, Liao KK, Liou HH et al: Sympathetic skin response and R–R interval variation in chronic uremic patients. Muscle Nerve, 17:411, 1995

72. Nowicki M, Zwiech R, Dryja P et al: Autonomic neuropathy in hemodialysis patients: questionnaires versus clinical tests. Clin Exp Nephrol, 13:152, 2009

73. Rechlin T, Orbes I, Weis M et al: Autonomic cardiac abnormalities in alcohol-dependent patients admitted to a psychiatric department. Clin Auton Res, 6:119, 1996

74. Oliver MI, Miralles R, Rubíes-Prat J et al: Autonomic dysfunction in patients with non-alcoholic chronic liver disease. J Hepatol, 26:1242, 1997

75. Hendrickse MT, Thuluvath PJ, Triger DR: Natural history of autonomic neuropathy in chronic liver disease. Lancet, 339:1462, 1992

76. Schwemmer S, Beer P, Schölmerich J et al: Cardiovascular and pupillary autonomic nervous dysfunction in patients with rheumatoid arthritis—a cross-sectional and longitudinal study. Clin Exp Rheumatol, 24:683, 2006

77. Wilder-Smith EP, Wilder-Smith AJ, Nirkko AC: Skin and muscle vasomotor reflexes in detecting autonomic dysfunction in leprosy. Muscle Nerve, 23:1105, 2000

78. Wilder-Smith E, Wilder-Smith A, Egger M: Peripheral autonomic nerve dysfunction in asymptomatic leprosy contacts. J Neurol Sci, 150:33, 1997

79. Abbot NC, Beck JS, Mostofi S et al: Sympathetic vasomotor dysfunction in leprosy patients: comparison with electrophysiological measurement and qualitative sensation testing. Neurosci Lett, 206:57, 1996

80. Ruttimann S, Hilti P, Spinas GA et al: High frequency of human immunodeficiency virus-associated autonomic neuropathy and more severe involvement in advanced stages of human immunodeficiency virus disease. Arch Intern Med, 151:2441, 1991

81. Welby SB, Rogerson SJ, Beeching NJ: Autonomic neuropathy is common in human immunodeficiency virus infection. J Infect, 23:123, 1991

82. Idiaquez J: Autonomic dysfunction in diphtheritic neuropathy. J Neurol Neurosurg Psychiatry, 55:159, 1992

83. Fernandez A, Hontebeyrie M, Said G: Autonomic neuropathy and immunological abnormalities in Chagas' disease. Clin Autonom Res, 2:409, 1992

84. Lyu RK, Tang LM, Wu YR et al: Cardiovascular autonomic function and sympathetic skin response in chronic inflammatory demyelinating polyradiculoneuropathy. Muscle Nerve, 26:669, 2002

85. Ingall TJ, McLeod JG: Autonomic dysfunction in hereditary motor and sensory neuropathy (Charcot–Marie–Tooth disease). Muscle Nerve, 14:1080, 1991

86. Cable WJL, Kolodny EH, Adams RD: Fabry disease: impaired autonomic function. Neurology, 32:498, 1982

87. Hilz MJ, Marthol H, Schwab S et al: Enzyme replacement therapy improves cardiovascular responses to orthostatic challenge in Fabry patients. J Hypertens, 28:1438, 2010

88. Schiffmann R, Floeter MK, Dambrosia JM et al: Enzyme replacement therapy improves peripheral nerve and sweat function in Fabry disease. Muscle Nerve, 28:703, 2003

Evoked Potentials and Related Techniques

Visual Evoked Potentials, Electroretinography, and Other Diagnostic Approaches to the Visual System

ARI J. GREEN

Clinical electrophysiology of the visual system provides an important adjunct to the bedside evaluation of patients with neurologic diseases. It provides the only means available for objective assessment of visual function, especially of the retina and optic nerve, and requires less active participation than subjective evaluations such as perimetry and visual acuity testing. Electrophysiologic techniques can also provide localizing information in the visual pathway and—given the functional organization of the visual system—adjustment of stimulus parameters can be used to define the specific cell type or subpathways affected by an injury. Electrophysiologic techniques play an important role in discriminating diseases of the retina and optic nerve when the distinction cannot be made on standard clinical grounds alone. They also may have use in distinguishing types of injuries of the optic nerve (e.g., glaucomatous, inflammatory, or metabolic), based on assessments tailored to the evaluation of particular functional systems (such as motion or color). The utility of visual electrophysiology is established firmly in the diagnosis and monitoring of patients with ophthalmologic conditions, including neurologic conditions with well-recognized ophthalmologic manifestations such as multiple sclerosis (MS). In addition, clinical research suggests that visual electrophysiology could be used to investigate other neuroinflammatory and neurodegenerative diseases, with the visual system used as a model.

ANATOMY OF THE ANTERIOR VISUAL SYSTEM

The neurosensory retina is one of the three traditional anatomic subdivisions of the central nervous system (the others being brain and spinal cord). The projections of the retina are characterized extremely well and make up a significant volume of the cerebral hemispheres. Of our senses, vision has the greatest amount of cortical surface area dedicated to processing its output and up to 40 percent of the brain has been estimated to be devoted to this effort.

At peak function, the human eye can discriminate up to 10 million shades of color, is sensitive to the flux of a single photon in a darkened room,[1] and can detect flashes of light as brief as 10 to 20 msec. These physiologic features of the human visual system are embedded in the anatomic substrate that makes up the retina, visual pathways, visual cortex, and accessory visual areas. The retina is comprised of 110 million cells divided into at least ten anatomic layers and three primary subsets of neurons. More than 50 different cell types have been described, and ten different neurotransmitters play an important role in retinal physiology.[2–4] Photoreceptors are the primary sensory neurons of the retina and the most abundant of all the retinal cell types (approximately 90 million rods and 5 million cones on average). They are positioned in the deepest layers of the retina (closest to the retinal pigment epithelium, choroid, and sclera), meaning that light has to traverse all the other layers of the retina before interacting with a photoreceptor (Fig. 22-1). Photoreceptors evidence intrinsic photosensitivity and participate in basic phototransduction—

turning light into neuronal signal. Photoreceptors respond to light by converting 11-cis-retinal to 11-trans-retinal, resulting in the hyperpolarization of the neuron and leading to a reduction in release of glutamate from its synaptic terminal.[5]

Photoreceptors are subdivided further into two classes of cells: rods and cones (which are distinguished from one another both by the morphology of their outer segments and by the type of opsin they contain). Rods are highly sensitive to light and evidence peak function in low light conditions. Cones, by contrast, are color sensitive and provide their predominant perceptual input under bright-light (photopic) conditions. In normal individuals there are three cone subtypes (short-, medium-, and long-wavelength), each tuned to a different peak spectral sensitivity within the visible spectrum. Cone and rod distribution is not uniform throughout the retina, as cones are concentrated in the fovea, making up nearly all the photoreceptors in the central 1 degree of the retina,

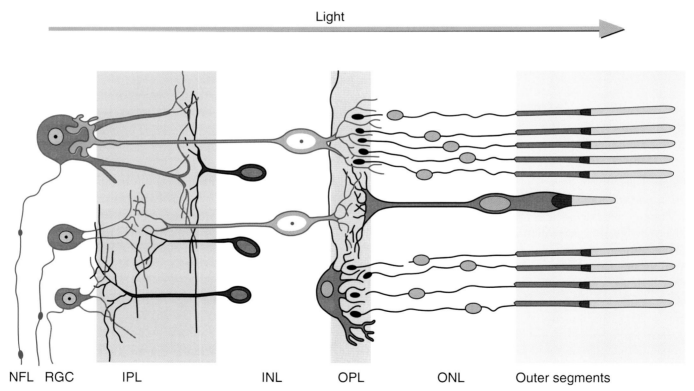

Light

NFL RGC   IPL   INL   OPL   ONL   Outer segments

FIGURE 22-1 ■ Classic schematic representation of human retina by Ramón y Cajal. NFL, nerve fiber layer (axons of retinal ganglion cells that become optic nerve); RGC, retinal ganglion cells; IPL, inner plexiform layer (synapses between dendrites of retinal ganglion cells and both amacrine and bipolar cell axons); INL, inner nuclear layer (somata of amacrine, bipolar, and horizontal cells: note how horizontal cells connect across bipolar cell receptive fields); OPL, outer plexiform layer (synapses between bipolar cell dendrites, horizontal cells, and photoreceptor axons); ONL, outer nuclear layer (somata of photoreceptors); outer segments, light-responsive segment of photoreceptors. The shape of the outer segment is the basis of the name "rods" and "cones." Note that the receptive field (dendritic arbor) for the retinal ganglion cells is generally greater than the receptive field for bipolar cells, which in turn is greater than the receptive field for individual photoreceptors. (Instituto Cajal, Consejo Superior de Investigaciones Científicas, Madrid, circa 1900.)

with a steep decline in density out to about 3 degrees eccentricity, beyond which they are distributed evenly throughout the retina. Rods, by contrast, have a peak density around 6 to 8 degrees from the center of the retina, but also show declining density with greater eccentricity outside of this boundary.[5,6]

The middle layers of the retina consist of interneurons that perform the initial processing and organizing of visual information, including the distribution of visual data into parallel processing streams. Photoreceptors synapse with the cells of the inner nuclear layer (bipolar and horizontal cells) in the outer plexiform layer of the retina. Horizontal cells provide a wide neural network for inter-retinal feedback and processing of visual information (see Fig. 22-1). Their organization is likely the basis for the antagonistic, concentric, center-surround response characteristics of bipolar and retinal ganglion cells.[7] Signals arising from photons striking photoreceptors in the receptive field of a single bipolar cell or retinal ganglion cell converge on two separate pools, some of which enhance neuronal firing and others of which inhibit neuronal responses. These stripes of inhibitory and excitatory input are organized in a target-like pattern and their size is not symmetric across the retina. Neurons with larger receptive fields and thereby larger "centers" and "surrounds" can be found at greater eccentricity from central vision. The center-surround organization of retinal neurons likely plays an important part in the sensitivity of the retina to the pattern-reversal electrophysiologic techniques described later.[8] Furthermore, there are many subtypes of bipolar cells, each of which synapses with either groups of rods or cones exclusively. Bipolar cells can be characterized as **ON** or **OFF** based on how they respond to photoreceptor hyperpolarization and their response to the reduction of glutamate input that results (depolarizing in the case of ON-bipolar cells).[2,4]

Finally, retinal ganglion cells constitute the primary output neurons of the retina. They receive input from the bipolar cells (via amacrine cells) and synapse primarily in the thalamus, as well as in the tectum and hypothalamus. There are approximately 1.2 million retinal ganglion cells in the human retina, 70 percent of which are found in the central 30 degrees of the retina. It is important to note that retinal ganglion cells typically receive input from a large number of bipolar cells (which, in turn, have received input from a number of photoreceptors).[9,10] As a consequence, the receptive field of retinal ganglion cells frequently is substantially larger than the corresponding receptive field of the photoreceptors or bipolar cells that provide its input (see Fig. 22-1). In addition, ganglion (and bipolar cells) do not respond equally to a stimulus at all points in their receptive field because of their center-surround organization.[11]

There are four primary types of retinal ganglion cells. Magnocellular (also known as alpha or Y-type) retinal ganglion cells have a large receptive field and a large axonal diameter (and hence faster conduction of their action potential). They are concentrated outside of the macula and are tuned primarily for detection of contrast and motion. Parvocellular retinal ganglion cells, conversely, have a smaller receptive field, a smaller axonal diameter, and a relatively slower conduction time, and are concentrated in the macula. Many parvocellular retinal ganglion cells are tuned also for the discrimination of color. Koniocellular retinal ganglion cells are the smallest in size and least well characterized.[11,12] Finally, a class of intrinsically photosensitive retinal ganglion cells containing melanopsin are distributed evenly throughout the retina. These melanopsin-containing retinal ganglion cells likely underlie subjective luminance sensitivity, provide some—if not most—of the afferent input for the pupillary response, and help entrain the circadian rhythm.[13] In addition to participating in the continued segregation and analysis of visual data, retinal ganglion cells carry retinal information to the brain for further processing.

After traversing the inner surface of the retina, retinal ganglion cell axons coalesce into the optic nerve, which carries visual information through the orbit and into the brain. The axons are myelinated once they exit the eye posterior to the lamina cribrosa. Visual information from the two eyes arrives together at the optic chiasm before undergoing an anatomic separation that reflects their functional segregation by hemifield. These axons travel via the optic tract to synapse in the thalamus (sensory visual information), hypothalamus (circadian rhythm), and midbrain tectum (luminance sensitivity and pupillary response). Each of the first three subtypes of retinal ganglion cells synapse in different layers of the lateral geniculate nucleus (LGN) of the thalamus, where visual information is processed further before being taken to the visual cortex for additional processing and decoding.[14,15] Only a small number of melanopsin-containing retinal ganglion cells synapse in the intergeniculate leaflet of the LGN; the majority of them synapse in the midbrain and hypothalamus.[16]

The predominant subnucleus of the LGN (the dorsal LGN) receives retinal input segregated by eye and retinal ganglion cell subtype. Inputs from magnocellular retinal ganglion cells and parvocellular retinal ganglion cells are separated into distinct lamellae, while **ON** and **OFF** retinal ganglion cells are also separated in less distinct laminae within these lamellae. The interneurons of the dorsal LGN are also involved in signal processing of visual information. In contrast to retinal ganglion cells, neurons in the LGN are selectively responsive to stimuli with a particular orientation or direction of motion. However, similar to retinal ganglion cells, relay neurons in the dorsal LGN display a center-surround response profile, which means that the LGN enhances the discriminating power of the retinal input and allows for small variations in the visual scene to be highlighted by the visual cortex.[17,18] Dorsal LGN cells send their axons primarily to the primary visual cortex (Brodmann area 17), which surrounds the calcarine fissure in the occipital cortex. This is also referred to as the striate cortex because of the unique Gennari stripe that can be identified on histologic cross-section and which itself provides horizontal interconnections between areas of the primary visual cortex.[15]

Outputs from the dorsal LGN primarily terminate in layer 4 of the striate cortex (one of the so-called granular cortical layers).[19] The striate cortex (also called V1 or primary visual cortex) dedicates 65 percent of its area to the central 15 degrees of the visual field (out of approximately 150 degrees and 120 degrees across the horizontal and vertical meridians, respectively). Primary visual cortex maintains the general retinotopic organization of visual information with visual information from central vision directly including the depths and banks of the calcarine fissure. Cortex dedicated to the peripheral field includes the surrounding cortical areas anteriorly to the parieto-occipital fissure and posteriorly along the surface of the occipital pole.[15,19] In total, striate cortex comprises approximately 4 percent of the whole human cortical surface, and more than half of this is dedicated to macular vision.[15,20] Visual information arising from the portion of the retina subserving central vision is therefore relatively "over-represented," which has important consequences for the visual evoked potential.

Visual information is deciphered and processed further in accessory visual cortex, which includes a wide swath of neighboring cortex in areas that have been distinguished based on functional determinants (V2–V6). These areas do not have the precise anatomic and histologic landmarks of the Gennari stripe and are characterized best via functional characterization in the primate, although lesional studies demonstrate their existence in humans. Outside V1, the stream of visual information changes significantly and no longer is characterized by the serial relay of visual information and stepwise modulation of visual data. Instead, extrastriate visual processing reflects a loose hierarchy with ample feedback and feedforward loops of interconnection. Although the retinotopic organization is maintained in some of these regions, others demonstrate neurons with extremely large receptive fields tuned for particular features of the visual scene, such as faces (including emotional state), animals, or rates of motion. Two classic pathways arising from the visual cortex include the so-called dorsal stream carrying visual information to the parietal lobes for spatial identification ("Where?") and the ventral stream carrying information to the temporal lobes for object identification ("What?"). In addition, much of the primary visual cortex is comprised of layers (besides layer 4C) that receive inhibitory and modulating inputs from extrastriate areas that help to focus visual processing power on features deemed salient.[14,15,19,20]

When considering the implications of the organizational structure of the visual system for clinical electrophysiology, it is important to remember that visual perception is not the consequence of parallel stimulation of afferent neurons, but that each layer of the visual system influences how much of the arriving visual input is transmitted to the next relay. Furthermore, our visual system is designed to discriminate variation in the visual scene, not strictly to quantify the intensity of visual stimuli. This objective is encoded in the architecture and physiology of the system for processing visual information. Understanding this purpose for our visual system is important in understanding how a particular visual stimulus will drive an electrophysiologic response and how injury might impact the response recorded.

CLINICAL ELECTROPHYSIOLOGY OF THE VISUAL SYSTEM

Visual evoked potentials (VEPs) are cortically generated electrical potentials recorded over the scalp in response to a visual stimulus. Electroretinograms (ERGs) are retinally generated potentials recorded from the cornea or periorbital skin. However, the size of the potentials elicited in both the VEP and ERG is small compared with ambient electrical signals that reflect the ongoing activity of brain, heart, and muscle. Therefore, signal-averaging techniques are employed to help resolve both the VEP and the ERG from background electrical potentials related to nonstimulus activity or ambient conditions ("noise"). The amount of signal averaging required is entirely dependent on the signal-to-noise ratio (SNR), but a reasonable rule of thumb for pattern-reversal full-field VEPs is that 50 to 250 averaged samples are required to achieve an adequate SNR.[21,22] Averaging paradigms are determined partially by the stimulus and specific technique being employed, as averaging is not always required for ERG acquired with a contact lens electrode (and less averaging typically is required for the ERG than VEP).[23,24] In general, averaging is achieved by recording the responses to repeated stimulation, and clinical studies require several minutes of recording time. The noise reduction provided by averaging can be calculated by the inverse of the square root of the number of averages and there are therefore diminishing returns afforded by increased averaging.[22]

BASIC ASPECTS OF THE ERG

ERG can be recorded from the corneal surface by a contact lens embedded with a corneal ring electrode and a conjunctival reference, or from periorbital skin by small foil electrodes attached at the lateral canthi. Dermal electrodes significantly improve patient comfort and are recommended particularly for children and infants, but usually require additional signal averaging to optimize SNR.[23]

The standard ERG stimulus is a high-intensity light stimulus such as a strobe light or a Ganzfeld (German for "whole-field") stimulator (a hollow dome to which a patient affixes the gaze to obtain a brief but uniform stimulus to the entire retina). The stimulus used can be modulated to optimize assessment of rod or cone response. Cones have a shorter refractory period and therefore a higher-frequency stimulus can be used (30 Hz) to aid in the assessment of their function. (Rods provide minimal response at a frequency greater than 20 Hz.) It is particularly important to utilize methods to optimize cone responses, as there are over ten times more rods than cones, and the rod response on ERG is an order of magnitude greater than the cone response. Colored filters can also be employed to isolate rod and cone responses further. Rod responses have their peak spectral sensitivity in near blue light (510-nm wavelength) and cones as a group have their peak sensitivity in the yellow range (560 nm). Furthermore, red cones exhibit a response with little to no contamination from rods, given the limited overlap in peak sensitivities. In addition, ambient lighting conditions can be varied to help distinguish rod and cone responses. This is significant because the retinal diseases for which ERG is clinically useful have differential effects on rod and cone populations.[24,25]

The ERG typically is recorded with a patient's pupils dilated after the application of mydriatics. This helps to ensure uniform illumination of the retina and prevent pupillary responses from influencing the character of the ERG tracing. The ERG can also be recorded after light adaptation (photopic) to quench the effects of rods, or dark adaptation (scotopic) to enhance rod contribution. There is a fair amount of variability in the protocols

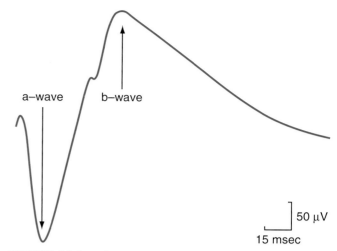

FIGURE 22-2 ■ Schematic representation of dark-adapted electroretinogram at 3.0 candela*seconds/meter^2 (combined cone-rod response). Note the smaller negative a-wave followed by the larger positive-amplitude b-wave.

employed but, as an example, dark adaptation usually requires that the patient sit in a darkened room for 30 minutes prior to recording.[24,25]

Although there are differing conventions among ophthalmologists and neurologists, ERG waveforms frequently are described as negative when the tracing dips below the baseline and positive when they cross above it (Fig. 22-2). ERG typically is analyzed by evaluating the first negative deflection (a-wave) and the subsequent positive deflection (b-wave). In photopic recordings, especially with a bright flash as stimulus, a high-amplitude positive wave may precede the a-wave. The a-wave reflects the depolarization of photoreceptors en masse (rods or cones predominantly depending on stimulus parameters and preconditioning state), and the b-wave reflects the activation of the retinal interneurons from the inner nuclear layer.[24,25] The times to peak of the a- and b-waves are referred to as "implicit time" rather than "latency." In normal individuals the a-wave is observed at around 15 msec and the b-wave at around 30 to 35 msec in photopic ERGs. In photopic recordings the implicit times are usually shorter (faster) but the amplitude of the response is usually lower than in dark-adapted ERGs. Additional c- and d-waves have been described and attributed to retinal pigment epithelium and OFF bipolar cells, respectively,[26,27] but these are not assessed routinely in the clinic.

Pattern-Reversal ERGs

The ERG can also be recorded with an alternating checkerboard or other pattern-reversal stimulus. The pattern-reversal ERG (PERG) is described by the same conventions that govern flash ERG. (Positive deflections are recorded above the baseline, and negative below.) It is characterized by a negative wave at approximately 50 msec (N50) and a positive deflection at around 95 msec (P95). The P95 (also referred to as the PERG b-wave) is thought to reflect activation of the retinal ganglion cells, as some of these cells are tuned to sense spatial contrast, and the implicit time of the PERG implicates neuronal populations downstream from the photoreceptors. In an extremely large retrospective case series, it was reported that subjects with abnormal VEPs and known disease of the anterior visual pathway frequently lost the N95 component of their PERG but almost always showed complete preservation of the P50. However, PERG amplitudes are small and sometimes unreliable and, as a consequence, PERG has found application primarily as a research tool.[24,25,28,29]

FLASH AND PATTERN-REVERSAL VEPs

Prior to 1970, VEPs were only elicited using a diffuse stroboscopic or Ganzfeld flash as the stimulus. Additional stimulus approaches were developed subsequently, including checkerboard pattern-reversal and sinusoidal grating patterns. The flash VEP is much less sensitive than pattern-reversal VEPs for detecting abnormalities such as optic neuritis.[28,30] In addition, flash VEP responses have higher interindividual variation and are more dependent on the patient's state of arousal than pattern-reversal VEP, limiting their routine clinical utility.[30] Their primary clinical use is restricted to patients who are unable to fixate or who are suspected of feigning complete blindness.

Transient and Steady-State VEPs

After stimulation, a transient, cortically generated response is tied to the relevant stimulus (the "transient VEP") and consists of a series of potentials that are alternately positive and negative in polarity. They are labeled on the basis of their polarity and latency. With repeated high-frequency (over 4-Hz) stimulation, however, cortical responses remain constant—or nearly so—with respect to amplitude and phase ("steady-state VEP"). Regan likened transient evoked potentials to providing a "kick" and measuring the response, whereas steady-state responses are similar to "shaking a system gently" and studying the harmonic oscillation that develops.[31] There is some evidence that steady-state and transient VEPs provide complementary data.[30,32–34] The frequency of stimulation in the steady-state VEP can be varied to distinguish responses from the magnocellular (40 to 50 Hz) and parvocellular systems (15 to 20 Hz) in the macaque[31] but this has not been demonstrated to have clinical utility in humans. Interestingly, the observed frequency at which patients with MS appear to have the most profound dysfunction with steady-state VEPs is similar to the frequency at which critical flicker fusion deficits are observed.[30] However, the steady-state VEP is used primarily in evaluating subjects who cannot communicate or otherwise participate in examinations for the assessment of acuity (infants and small children); other applications are restricted largely to the research laboratory at this time.

Interpretation of the Transient Pattern-Reversal VEP

Peak response for the transient full-field pattern-reversal VEP occurs approximately 50 to 250 msec after the stimulus. By convention in clinical neurophysiology (as opposed to ophthalmology) laboratories, the recording arrangements for VEPs are such that electrical potentials that lead to an upward deflection are termed negative, while those with a downward slope are termed positive. There are two primary features to each deflection that can be described: (1) the time elapsed since the stimulus (latency) and (2) the magnitude of deflection from the baseline (amplitude). Normal ranges used for references are dependent on the size, luminance, contrast, and temporal characteristics of the stimulus (see next section). Varying other features of the stimulus, such as the color or shape, have less well-characterized influences on the response but also result in differences.[35–38]

By convention, most recordings are evaluated using the "Queen Square" montage, which includes a midoccipital electrode placed 5 cm above the inion, referenced to a midfrontal electrode placed 12 cm above the nasion (MO–MF). To complete the montage, leads usually are also placed 5 cm to the left (LO) and right (RO) of the MO lead. This placement is obviously very similar to the Fz, Oz, O1, and O2 lead placement from the International 10–20 system and this array can be used as an alternative.

In most individuals, the first response of the full-field pattern-reversal VEP recorded midoccipitally is a negative deflection termed the N75. However, given lack of consistency of both the presence and latency of the N75, by convention full-field VEPs usually are assessed by evaluating the first major positive deflection that occurs at around 100 msec and is therefore designated the P100 component (Fig. 22-3). This positive deflection does not necessarily have the largest amplitude, nor is

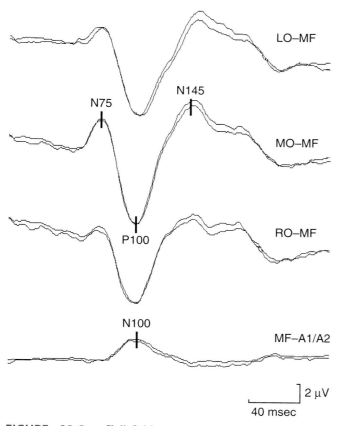

FIGURE 22-3 ■ Full-field pattern-reversal checkerboard visual evoked potential from the right eye of a normal healthy 22-year-old woman (check size 32 minutes of arc). The P100 at the MO–MF channel has a latency of 99 msec.

it always the earliest positive response that is seen, but it is the most reproducible. Following the P100, the next negative deflection is referred to as the N145 (see Fig. 22-3). In patients with hemianopia, stimulation of the affected hemifield leads to absent responses or marked variation in the normal amplitude distribution in the contralateral hemifield (LO–MF or RO–MF), but a good response is seen ipsilateral to the "blind" hemifield (Fig. 22-4, *A* and *B*).[38] However, this method is unreliable compared to dipole source localization, and the ease of obtaining standard automated perimetry has relegated this finding to one of academic interest.

The exact cortical source of the full-field VEP has not been determined unequivocally. It has been suggested that the N75 reflects input from the dorsal LGN to the striate cortex (via the optic radiations), whereas the P100 may reflect a secondary inhibitory response at V1 or excitatory outflow to the accessory visual cortical areas (V2 to V5).[28,38–41] There have been several reports of VEPs persisting even in cases of bilateral destruction of the primary visual cortex, including in 4 of 19 patients with complete cortical blindness.[42]

LATENCY

Latency of the VEP generally is defined as the time from the stimulus to a prespecified feature of the record, typically the peak of the component of interest. Approaches include measurement of latency to the point of the maximal positive (or negative) deflection but this has the drawback that flat or noisy components may be challenging to characterize. An alternative approach is to measure the latency to peak by interpolation—in the case of the P100, a straight line is drawn from the downward slope of the N75 and the upward slope of the N145, and the P100 latency is measured at the point of their intersection. The delineation of abnormal latency for the P100 on full-field VEP is laboratory specific. It is of critical importance that the same methods used for establishment of laboratory references are employed at the time of clinical analysis. Any deviation from a standard approach should be explained clearly in a laboratory report.

Latency delay of the full-field VEP is often interpreted as evidence of demyelinating injury to the visual pathway (Fig. 22-5). Abnormality of latency is defined routinely as a value exceeding the mean by more than 2.5 standard deviations.[28] Assuming a gaussian distribution for the reference population, this means that 99.4 percent of normal individuals should fall within this reference range. Given this stringent requirement for abnormality, it is important to note that some individuals with injury to the visual pathway still may be classified as normal. As a consequence, most investigators also evaluate interocular latency differences to improve sensitivity. The optimal cut-off for interocular latency should be defined within an individual clinical laboratory but standard values range from 6 to 10 msec.[43,44] Consideration must be given to anterior segment (cataract or other ocular media opacities) or outer retinal diseases (such as diabetic eye disease or myopic degeneration) before changes are attributed to optic nerve disease. This is an additional strength to the combined approach, described later.

AMPLITUDE

P100 amplitude is highly variable and, as a consequence, delineation of amplitude abnormality in the full-field VEP is not based on a simple numerical value. There is a high degree of interindividual variability in amplitude on pattern-reversal VEPs in healthy subjects, and the range of observed values is not subject to a gaussian distribution, making it difficult to establish normal values. Furthermore, there may be interocular differences in amplitude of up to 200 percent and repeated VEPs in the same individual may show variability in

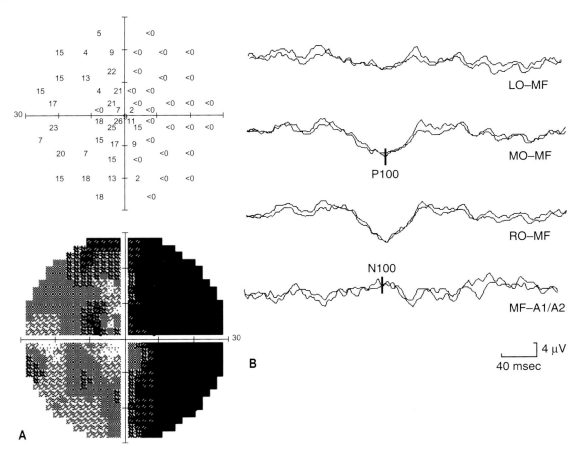

FIGURE 22-4 ■ **A**, Static perimetry (30-2 equivalent from Haag Streit Octopus-900) from a 55-year-old man with a history of demyelinating injury to his left optic radiation (right hemifield defect in addition to reduced thresholds throughout the field). **B**, Full-field visual evoked potential from the same patient showing amplitude loss contralateral to the field loss (LO–MF). Latency is also delayed in the MO–MF recording to 145 msec.

amplitude of a similar extent as well, depending on the subject's state of arousal and other patient- and condition-specific factors.[45,46] Accordingly, caution should be exercised in characterizing a recording as abnormal based on amplitude criteria alone.[47]

Technical Issues for Recording VEPs

As with all clinical electrophysiologic recordings, careful electrode placement with attention to impedance reduction is critical to generating reliable and useful recordings. Because of responses that occur around 60 Hz, bandpass filters at this frequency are not recommended, so ambient electrical noise must be kept to a minimum.[21,28]

LUMINANCE AND CONTRAST

Luminance is defined as the intensity of light from the visible spectrum per unit area traveling in a given direction (usually expressed in candelas/meter^2 [cd/m^2]). Ambient lighting conditions (and preconditioning) can have a significant effect on recordings, and maintenance of luminance conditions is critical for undertaking a reliable study. The luminance of both the stimulus and the ambient conditions should be monitored. The necessary conditions for appropriate ERG recordings are set by the type of study being performed (described earlier). VEPs preferably are recorded under ambient photopic conditions in a standard, normally illuminated room. Patients and normal subjects (laboratory references) should be recorded under the same lighting conditions. The mean luminance at the center of the field is recommended to be at least 50 cd/m^2 but optimally should approximate background luminance. The luminance of the display is also an important factor influencing the VEP, and regular calibration of the system or the use of self-calibrating units is recommended.[28]

Contrast is the luminance difference between two adjacent elements in the visual scene and is defined by the following equation:

$$C = L_{max} - L_{min}/L_{max} + L_{min}$$

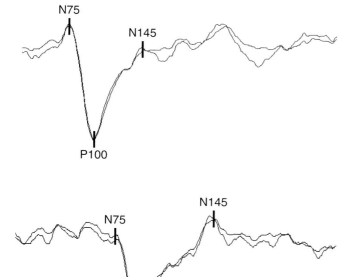

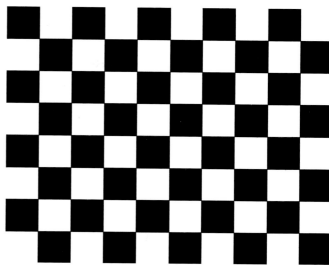

FIGURE 22-6 ▪ Full-field visual evoked potential checkerboard stimulus. Each square alternates in tandem, with half the squares black and half white at any one time point. To maintain fixed luminance across the stimulus, either an even number or large number of odd squares is required.

FIGURE 22-5 ▪ Abnormal full-field visual evoked potential with latency delay in the right eye of a 25-year-old woman with a history of optic neuritis 1 year earlier. The P100 latency was 104 msec with left eye stimulation, and 165 msec with right eye stimulation. Recording is between midoccipital and midfrontal electrodes.

where C indicates contrast level, L_{max} is the brighter luminance element, and L_{min} is the darker luminance element. Contrast is particularly important when considering the electrophysiologic response generated by a pattern-reversal stimulus. Given the sensitivity of the human visual system for detecting differences, pattern-reversal VEP and ERG responses are dependent on contrast. Low-contrast responses have smaller amplitudes and broader peaks than those elicited using patterns with high contrast. Therefore, maintenance of contrast levels in the patterned stimulus used for eliciting VEPs and ERGs is important for ensuring that findings can be compared reliably to laboratory reference ranges, especially at lower contrast levels. In particular, for pattern-reversal VEP, amplitudes decrease with contrast levels below 40 percent.[37]

STIMULUS PARAMETERS

Two types of visual stimulus are used commonly in visual electrophysiology: the unpatterned flash or a strongly patterned stimulus that undergoes reversals of its basic elements (typically black and white). Flash stimuli usually are described in terms of stimulus intensity (luminance) and the frequency at which the stimulus repeats. In addition, for

ERG recordings, the preconditioning environment is important (as described earlier).

There are two predominant patterns that can be employed: alternating bars or checkerboard (Fig. 22-6). Alternating bars (also referred to as gratings) can have sharp boundaries between the stimulus elements (square wave) or the pattern can blend between regions of high and low luminance (sinusoidal pattern). The shape of pattern elements and their size can impact the response waveform significantly and therefore need to be maintained carefully.[48–50] The size of the stimulus at the retina will depend on its size on the monitor and the distance of the subject from the screen. The total stimulus size will determine the area of the visual field subject to stimulation, and check size will impact the neuronal cell population which is generating the response (especially among ganglion and bipolar cells). Based on the nonuniformity in the size of the receptive fields for ganglion cells across the retina, larger check sizes will generate more of their response from the peripheral retina, and vice versa.

Check sizes that are small run the risk of being confounded by refractive errors,[51] whereas large check sizes will only exhibit alternating luminance in a small number of the total ganglion cells in the field (those with a large enough receptive field or those whose center-surround edge lies at the boundary of the check). Recommendations by the International Federation of Clinical Neurophysiology (IFCN) therefore suggest the use of checks that subtend 24 to 32 minutes of visual arc. In spite of this, some research suggests that varying check size can enhance the diagnostic yield of VEP.[52]

Regardless of the stimulus parameter employed, maintaining fixed luminance throughout the pattern-reversal cycle is important. Therefore, the mean field luminance should be identified for the patterns that are utilized in the clinical laboratory. Most clinics utilize predesigned all-in-one visual electrophysiology packages, many of which can be outfitted as an extension of a unit devised for other purposes. The use of these systems has the advantage that certain features of standardization, such as the stimulus display and amplifier settings, are preset to meet recommended guidelines for recordings. However, given the potential impact of other laboratory-specific factors, such as background lighting conditions, ambient electrical noise, and distance between the subject and the stimulus display, care still must be taken to ensure reproducible and reliable recordings.

Most of these systems adhere to international guidelines, simplifying the process of standardization and quality assurance in the clinic.[28] However, such guidelines still recommend that every laboratory establish its own specific reference values. Given the dependence of reliable and informative VEPs on these parameters, the IFCN has established a number of recommendations for the practicing clinical electrophysiologist to optimize standardization. These include a description of the stimulus parameter employed, mean luminance of the field, size of the field, and rate of presentation. Additional patient demographic characteristics (age and sex) and ophthalmologic assessments to be documented include: (1) the patient's visual acuity, (2) the patient's ability to fixate, (3) the patient's pupillary size at the time of recording, and (4) a description of known visual field defects or known optical aberrations (such as cataracts or other impaired ocular media) that could influence the patient's ability to visualize the stimulus fully.[28] Adherence to these recommendations helps to ensure that results are interpreted reliably.

STIMULUS OPTIONS

It has been suggested that, rather than requiring pattern reversal of the stimulus at each sector, displaying the pattern when shown from a neutral gray background (called pattern-pulse) can improve the accuracy of the multifocal technique (discussed later) by reducing false-positive results. In addition, this technique has been employed with larger sectors for multifocal recordings—nicknamed sparse multifocal VEP—allowing for more rapid

recording times.[53] Adjustments in contrast level and stimulus color have also been suggested to improve VEP sensitivity, but have yet to be developed for widespread use.[54]

TIME BASE OF RECORDINGS

The relevant epoch (time base) and required filters for recording are determined by the nature of the stimulus employed. For standard full-field VEPs, recording should be made for at least 250 msec after each stimulus. Given that multifocal VEPs are performed with continuous recording, the epoch can be modified during analysis. However, a standard time window of 200 to 250 msec usually is employed and will avoid second-order responses.

COMPARISON OF FULL-FIELD AND MULTIFOCAL TRANSIENT VEPs

Traditional VEPs are recorded in response to a stimulus that varies consistently across a large portion of the visual field (see Fig. 22-6). In contrast, the multifocal VEP technique divides the visual field into a fixed number of sectors, each of which follows its own sequence of stimulus changes. Each sector can have one of two states, which—as with the full-field VEP—are inverted checkerboards (Fig. 22-7). Rather than recording each sector seque-ntially, which would be prohibitively time consuming, in the multifocal approach a stimulation method is employed that allows for simultaneous recording and rapid analysis of the summed response to derive the contribution from each individual sector. In order to achieve this, there are two basic requirements: (1) the stimulation sequence for

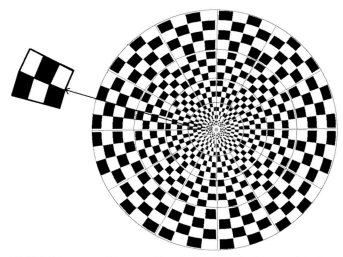

FIGURE 22-7 ■ The multifocal visual evoked potential stimulus, with 120 sectors. Inset of a single sector from the central field second ring (arrow).

each sector must be independent of the sequence for any other sector; and (2) the stimulus state of each sector during any given epoch is independent of its state during any other epoch. Each sector follows the same underlying sequence, but starts and finishes at a different point in the series.[55,56]

The multifocal VEP is recorded using the same electrodes, filters, and amplifier settings as the conventional full-field VEP. The waveforms are generally analogous to those seen in full-field VEP, although there is usually a phase reversal at the horizontal meridian (Fig. 22-8) caused by the involution of the calcarine fissure. However, the standard occipitofrontal VEP montage relatively oversamples the inferior visual field (by use of the midfrontal reference) and therefore sampling of the entire field is optimized by the use of occipital recording electrodes and an occipital reference. Two different montages have been employed to perform multifocal VEP recordings. Standard recording arrangements include four leads: one at the inion, another 2 cm above the inion, and the last two 3 cm to the right and left of the line bisecting these first two electrodes.[57,58] An alternative montage with electrodes placed 2 cm above and 2 cm below the inion ("bipolar occipital-straddle placement") likely results in improved SNR in potentials from the superior visual field[59,60] but may lead to greater contamination with muscle artifact from the neck and shoulders.

Initially, it was hoped that the multifocal VEP could provide an objective means of performing the standard visual field with less participation from subjects. However, intersubject variability caused by differences in the position of the calcarine fissure with respect to external landmarks and variability in the pattern of sulcal arrangement and cortical folding have made it difficult to define absolute normal standard values. To overcome the issues generated by intersubject variability in the multifocal VEP, it has become conventional to compare interocular differences in the multifocal VEP to assess for lateralizing deficits (Fig. 22-9).[61,62] This allows for the detection of deficits that would be missed on standard VEPs[62] or identification of normal areas in a subject who otherwise would be thought to be abnormal across the field (Fig. 22-10).

The macula constitutes approximately 1 percent of the surface area of the retina (10 to 15 mm^2 out of 1,000 mm^2). However, at the cortical level, nearly two-thirds of striate cortex subserves macular vision. Given this tremendous relative cortical "over-representation" of the macula, multifocal VEP sectors are scaled for cortical magnification with smaller check sizes centrally and larger ones peripherally.[63] This scaling of the sectors also necessitates that the multifocal VEP stimulus be concentric rings rather than a rectangular display (see Fig. 22-7). The sensitivity of pattern-reversal VEPs suffers from the limitations imposed by macular over-representation

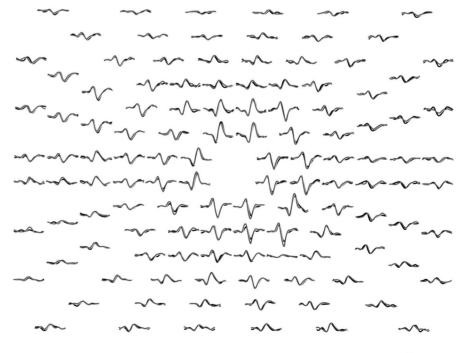

FIGURE 22-8 ■ Normal multifocal visual evoked potential from a 35-year-old healthy man. Right eye represented with black tracings and left eye represented with blue tracings. Notice the symmetry of the waveforms between the two eyes. Also note the phase reversal across the horizontal meridian caused by the calcarine fissure.

]500 nV
200 msec

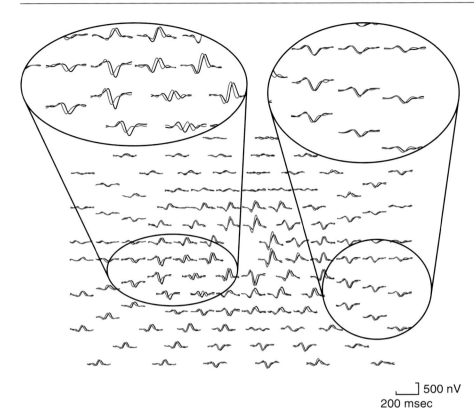

FIGURE 22-9 ■ Abnormal multifocal visual evoked potential with focal areas of latency delay seen in the nasal (left) hemifield of the right eye relative to the left eye (central three rings; left inset) and matched latency (right inset). Right eye represented with black tracings and left eye represented with blue tracings.

⌐____⌐ 500 nV
200 msec

(see Fig. 22-10). As indicated by the optic neuritis treatment trial, patients with optic neuritis can suffer injury to any of the topographic areas of the visual field, and by extension, to any of the fiber tracts in the anterior visual pathway.[64] Given the small central checks in multifocal VEP, it is particularly sensitive to refractive error and other optical aberrations.[65] As a result, clinicians must either correct for these deficits at the time of recording or consider them when analyzing a study.

In addition, while concentrating on a stimulus may or may not be important for the reliability of recordings, steady fixation is essential, as derivations of the local response are dependent on the maintained location of each sector in visual space. Therefore, it is unreliable to record from patients with fixation deficits such as primary position nystagmus. Fixation is monitored routinely during multifocal VEP recordings by a pupil camera mounted on the stimulator.

Using source localization procedures and a broader array of electrodes than is used in routine clinical practice, it has been argued the multifocal VEP is derived primarily from primary visual cortex, as compared to the full-field pattern-reversal VEP which has significant contributions from extrastriate cortex.[66] This argument may be undercut by the observation that summed multifocal VEP latencies across the field are longer when compared to full-field VEP latencies across the field.[67] This difference in latency may be explained in part by the increased representation of the peripheral field—which may have slightly longer latencies—in the multifocal VEP. Regardless, given the differences in stimulus, electrode placement, and cortical source localizations, the full-field VEP cannot be considered as the simple summation of multifocal VEPs across the field.[55,57]

The multifocal VEP can be used to monitor for progression within an individual patient. In both normal subjects and patients, the multifocal VEP demonstrates equivalent or superior test repeatability when compared to standard automated perimetry.[68,69] The relatively restricted dynamic range in the superior field with some electrode montages may limit detection of an abnormality in this area.

MULTIFOCAL ERG

In a manner akin to that described above, methodologies can be modified to record ERG responses from local retina areas, as well as the summed response. Using the same pseudorandom sequence, local flashes (rather than small alternating checkerboards) can be used. Unlike the required modification to the recording montage for multifocal VEPs, the same electrode placement is used for

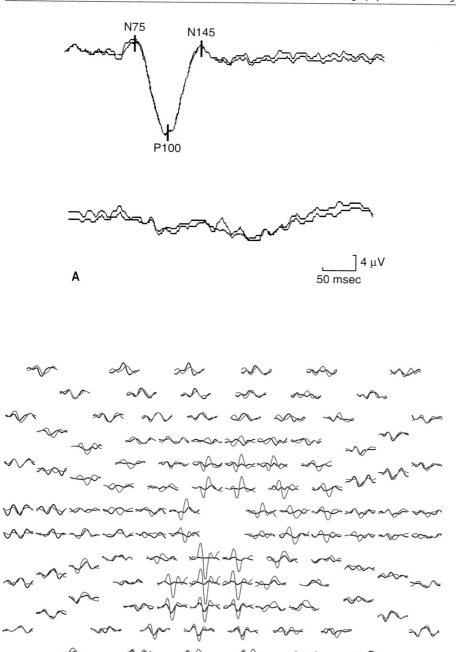

A

]4 µV
50 msec

B

]500 nV
200 msec

FIGURE 22-10 ▪ **A**, Full-field visual evoked potential (VEP) of a 23-year-old woman with a history of optic neuritis, showing normal but delayed (131 msec) responses to stimulation of the left eye (top) and poorly formed, if any, response from the right eye (bottom). Responses are recorded between the midoccipital and midfrontal electrodes to 32-min checks. **B**, Multifocal VEP of the same subject, showing amplitude decrement centrally to right eye stimulation (black tracings) with preserved symmetric responses peripherally. This also demonstrates the macular over-representation of the full-field VEP, as the response is dominated by the central sectors.

multifocal ERG and standard flash ERG. Multifocal ERG amplitudes can be compared across the field, similar to a visual field (Fig. 22-11). The multifocal ERG has less interindividual variability than multifocal VEPs. It is important to note that a dark-adapted state cannot be maintained with the multifocal ERG and therefore this test primarily assesses cone response.[25] In contrast to the standard generation of a multifocal VEP, which is derived from the first slice of the second-order kernel, multifocal ERG is derived from the first-order kernel. This also makes understanding its derivation more straightforward than multifocal VEP.[61]

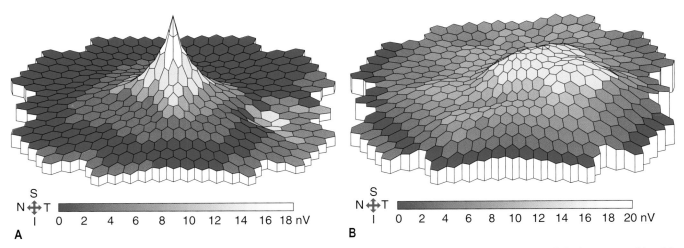

FIGURE 22-11 ■ **A**, Topographic representation of amplitudes from multifocal electroretinography (ERG) in a normal healthy 33-year-old man. **B**, Topographic representation of amplitudes from multifocal ERG in a 38-year-old woman with cone-predominant retinal dystrophy. Note the loss of the sharp central peak and relatively preserved amplitudes in the periphery.

PATIENT FACTORS INFLUENCING RECORDINGS

Head Size and Gender

A number of studies indicate that average P100 latencies are shorter (and amplitudes greater) for women than men. As early as the 1970s, it was suggested that brain volume and pathway length may explain these differences[21,70] However, gender differences may be secondary to differences in head size rather than reflecting a sex-specific effect.[71] Our own experience suggests that this relationship is observed in subjects with multiple sclerosis but no optic neuritis (Fig. 22-12). In spite of this, most laboratories have not used head size to correct for normal referenced latency values.

Age

VEP amplitudes peak in late adolescence and exhibit a modest decline in early adulthood. However, after that point, consistent amplitude is maintained over many years. Latency increases with age, especially for small check sizes and lower total luminance settings. This has been attributed to age-related declines in average pupil size,[72] but contradictory data suggest that other factors

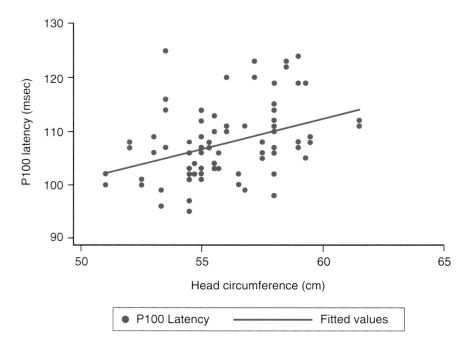

FIGURE 22-12 ■ Data correlating full-field P100 latency to head size in 40 subjects (77 eyes) with multiple sclerosis and no optic neuritis. R = approximately 0.4. (© Ari Green, 2011.)

may underlie this change.[73,74] Our own data suggest that, irrespective of pupil size, multifocal VEP latency increases with age, particularly in men. SNR does not vary with age from the third to tenth decade of life.[75]

Pupil Size

It has been theorized that, because of changes in levels of retinal illumination, large pupils can shorten VEP latency. Pupillary dilatation does not lead to a significant latency shortening of the full-field flash VEP,[76] but it does affect latency of the full-field pattern-reversal VEP.[72] Pupil size has also been shown to affect latency but not amplitude of multifocal VEPs,[77] but both amplitude and latency of the multifocal ERG.[78] It is standard practice for pattern-reversal VEPs to be recorded with normal pupils, whereas ERGs are recorded with pupils pharmacologically dilated.

Temperature

Body temperature has been shown not to influence full-field VEP latencies, except in patients with demyelinating injury in whom the occurrence of temperature-dependent clinical symptoms is well known.[21]

Effects of Anterior Segment Disease

Steady-state VEPs can be used to predict postoperative visual function in patients with a dense cataract.[79] This suggests that the impact of cataract on VEP characteristics is unlikely to be profound. However, it is well known that unilateral central cataracts can lead to interocular latency differences in full-field transient VEPs, and opacity of the ocular media is known to impact both ERG and VEP outcomes.[80] Similar findings have been reported with multifocal VEPs and multifocal ERGs.[63] As a consequence, awareness of large uncorrected refractive errors or anterior segment disease—especially when unilateral—is required when analyzing study results.

CLINICAL APPLICATIONS OF TRANSIENT FULL-FIELD AND MULTIFOCAL VEPs

Multiple Sclerosis and Optic Neuritis

Given the reduced requirement for patient participation in VEP recordings, VEPs sometimes are employed to help in discriminating organic from psychosomatic visual complaints. However, subtle visual impairment may not be detectable with standard VEPs. In addition, there is controversy over whether patients can influence their VEP results by daydreaming or meditation.[81] Technologists need to monitor patient attention and visual fixation, as failure to maintain gaze can influence the VEP findings, especially with multifocal recordings.

VEPs can be used to confirm a diagnosis of acute optic neuritis. The amplitude of the full-field pattern-reversal VEP usually is attenuated and, if present, the response is usually delayed significantly. If vision is worse than 20/80, the waveform is frequently absent. In cases of optic neuritis in which the diagnosis is in question, VEPs can be invaluable (Fig. 22-13). However, the VEP results need to be evaluated in the context of ophthalmologic assessment, as latency delay can be caused by outer retinal or anterior segment disease. With visual recovery, the amplitude returns but prolonged latency with a mean delay of around 35 msec is seen in about 90 percent of patients.[30]

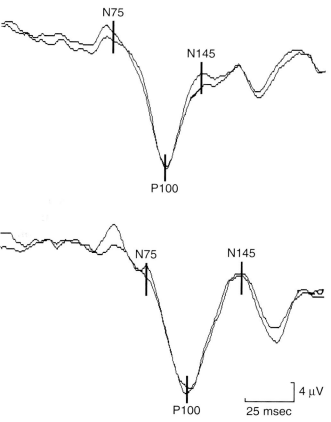

FIGURE 22-13 ■ Full-field visual evoked potential recorded between the midoccipital and midfrontal regions in a 49-year-old woman with complaints of mild eye pain who had slight disc swelling on examination. There was no prior history of optic neuritis. The P100 latency was 99 msec to left eye stimulation (top) and 112 msec to right eye stimulation (bottom). Interocular difference of more than 8 msec is considered evidence of right eye abnormality in our laboratory.

In the period following an acute optic neuritis, VEP latency delays become progressively less pronounced in the involved eye over the following 1 to 2 years. This relative improvement in latency delay is most dramatic in the first 3 to 6 months and is believed to be secondary to remyelination or ion channel reorganization on the denuded axon. Interestingly, in the unaffected fellow eyes of subjects, increasing latency times are observed, especially in individuals who go on to develop MS.[30] Persistent latency delay or amplitude decrement on multifocal VEP after an episode of optic neuritis has been associated with a greater risk of progression to MS.[82,83]

A general review of the literature demonstrates that nearly all subjects with clinically confirmed MS and a history of optic neuritis will have latency delay on pattern-reversal VEP (either in absolute or interocular terms). Older studies reported latency delay among subjects with "clinically definite" MS and no optic neuritis at high rates as well (60 to 95 percent), although, among subjects undergoing diagnostic work-up for MS, these rates were lower (35 to 80 percent, varying with the probability that MS was indeed the diagnosis) and dependent on stimulus method employed (including check size). The author's own experience suggests that rates of latency delay may be even lower when using the VEP to identify patients at the earliest stages of disease.

In older patients, in whom the diagnosis of nonarteritic ischemic optic neuropathy is under consideration, amplitude recovery is less common and latency frequently is delayed by less than 10 msec and almost never by more than 40 msec.[84–88] Therefore, in unusual cases, the VEP can help play a role in distinguishing ischemic from inflammatory demyelinating optic neuropathies. In patients with significant and persistent degradation in visual acuity after an ischemic optic neuropathy (worse than 20/80), the full-field VEP generally is lost completely and not simply delayed.[85,86,88]

Using stimulus patterns of various sizes, it has been reported that a small number of subjects have latency delay in their wider field (approximately 20 degrees from point of fixation), while "central field" full-field VEPs with smaller stimulus and check sizes (central 4 degrees) are normal.[30] This suggests that the location of deficits can influence the sensitivity of the full-field VEP. In a group of patients with recent demyelinating optic neuritis, multifocal VEPs have been shown to be more sensitive for detecting latency delays in the affected eye (89 percent versus 73 percent). This difference may be the consequence of greater detection of latency delays outside of central vision with multifocal VEPs.[89] Optic disc drusen have been reported to impact latency responses on multifocal but not full-field VEPs.[90] This suggests that multifocal VEPs are more sensitive to local injury than full-field VEPs. Our own experience supports this observation, as small, localized, central or peripheral areas of latency delay are missed or difficult to confirm on full-field VEPs. In addition, widened P100 waveforms ("temporal dispersion"), which have been the subject of long-standing controversy in the analysis of full-field VEP recordings, sometimes can be seen to reflect localized defects identifiable on the multifocal VEP (Fig. 22-14).

VEPs and ERGs, especially elicited by the multifocal technique, can improve the sensitivity of subjective visual assessments such as perimetry. Traquair famously described the visual field as representing "an island of vision surrounded by a sea of blindness."[91] Standard automated perimetry is employed routinely to perform standardized, consistent assessments of visual function beyond central vision. It has become the standard measure of disease progression in disorders such as glaucoma and has an important role in measuring visual dysfunction in MS.[64] In patients with visual complaints but normal perimetry, electrophysiologic recordings can be useful in establishing the presence of dysfunction or disease (Fig. 22-15).[54]

Other factors may also influence the difference in sensitivity between the techniques. As mentioned earlier, the full-field VEP is not just the simple sum of the waveforms from the multifocal VEP, given the differences in stimulus parameters and recording paradigms. In patients with optic neuritis, there is a modest but not perfect correlation between full-field VEPs and multifocal VEPs in both latency and amplitude.[89] Patients with an abnormal latency on full-field VEP but unusual waveform morphology sometimes can be found to have entirely normal VEPs using the multifocal technique (Fig. 22-16).

Peripheral Demyelinating Diseases

In addition to demyelinating diseases of the central nervous system (CNS), chronic demyelinating diseases of the peripheral nervous system have been associated with VEP abnormalities. In chronic inflammatory demyelinating polyneuropathy, a number of studies have reported rates of CNS demyelination that vary from 47 to 75 percent.[92,93] These subjects do not always have evidence of additional CNS involvement on magnetic resonance imaging.

Neurodegenerative Diseases

Patients with Alzheimer disease have been reported to complain of visual disturbances without abnormalities that can be identified on standard ophthalmologic

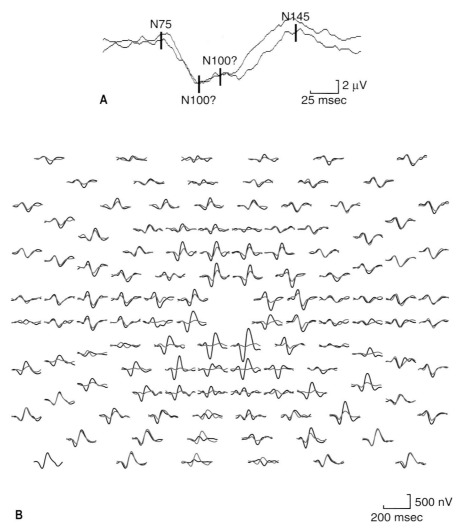

FIGURE 22-14 ▪ **A**, Full-field visual evoked potential (VEP) recorded between the midoccipital and midfrontal regions in a 53-year-old woman, with temporal dispersion of the response that is challenging to interpret. **B**, Multifocal VEP confirms abnormality by demonstrating central amplitude decrement in the left eye (blue tracings).

assessment.[94–96] A small but consistent literature suggests that retinal ganglion cell loss can be detected at autopsy in patients with Alzheimer disease[97–101] and that these patients lose axons of retinal ganglion cells during the course of their disease.[100,102,103] Although small studies have reached varying conclusions, the majority of investigations have reported changes on PERG and full-field VEP in patients with Alzheimer disease.[96,103,104] Although statistically significant differences have been reported when comparing groups, these differences are not sufficient to use current electrophysiologic techniques for the diagnosis or monitoring of patients with Alzheimer disease. These findings are consistent with

retinal imaging data demonstrating that patients with this disease have thinner retinal nerve fiber layer on optical coherence tomography[97,100–102] and retinal pathology data that document a reduction in retinal ganglion cells at the end of life.[98,99]

Patients with Parkinson disease have been reported to have prolonged latency on full-field VEP, and reduced amplitudes on both scotopic and photopic pattern ERGs, as well as normalization after administration of dopaminergic medications.[105] Similarly, when patients are administered dopamine antagonist medications, they have been reported to demonstrate similar prolongation of VEP latency and reduced ERG amplitudes.[106,107]

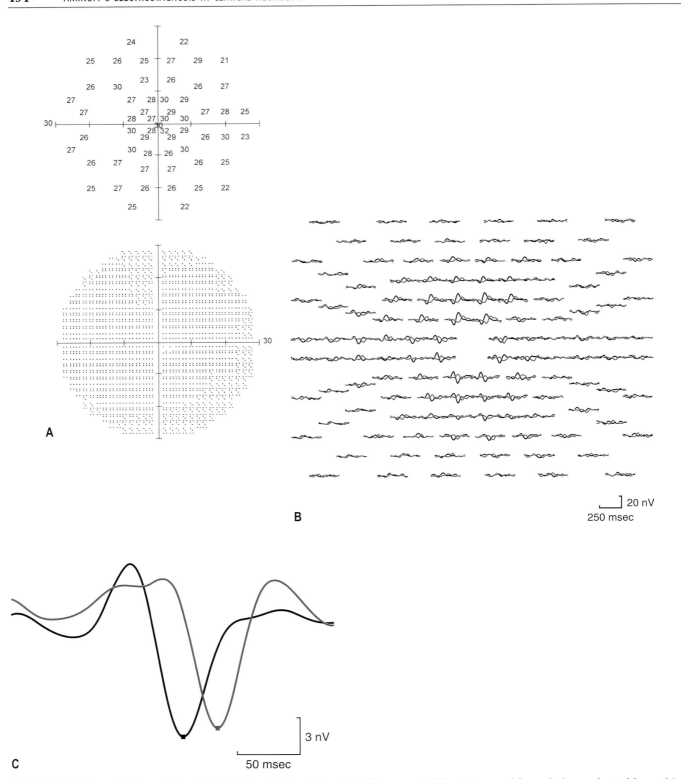

FIGURE 22-15 ▪ **A**, Normal visual field (30-2 equivalent Haag Streit Octopus-900) in a 55-year-old man being evaluated for multiple sclerosis with a history of possible optic neuritis in his left eye. **B**, Abnormal multifocal visual evoked potential (VEP) showing diffuse latency delay in the left eye (blue) on the same patient, helping to confirm prior demyelinating injury. **C**, Summed response of multifocal VEP showing a 35 msec difference between the right and left eyes (126 msec and 161 msec, respectively).

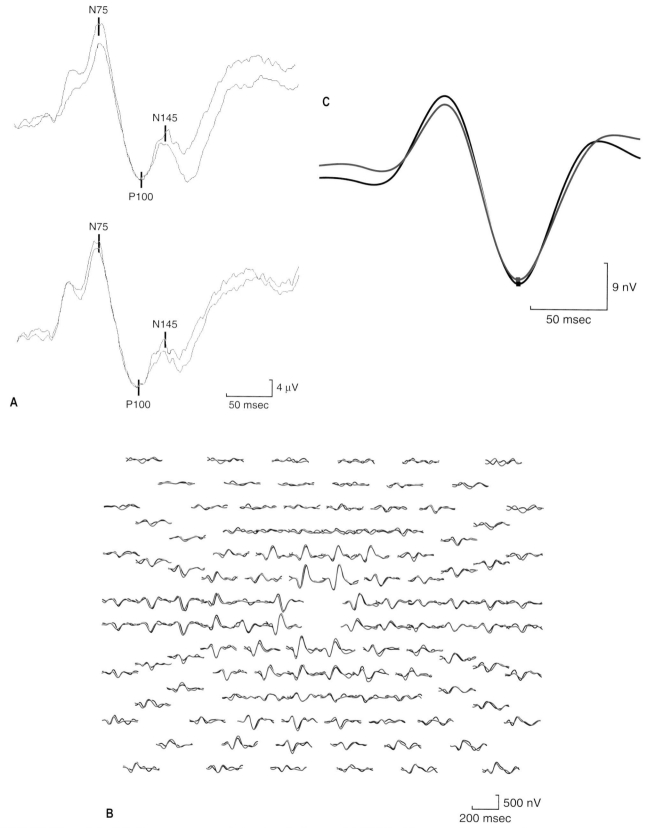

FIGURE 22-16 ■ **A**, Full-field pattern-reversal visual evoked potential (VEP) with unusual waveform from a 26-year-old woman with a history of transverse myelitis. Responses were recorded between the midoccipital and midfrontal electrodes. The P100 latencies were 178 msec and 179 msec to stimulation of left and right eyes, respectively, raising concern about disseminated disease despite a normal brain magnetic resonance image. **B**, Normal multifocal VEP on the same patient. **C**, Summed responses of multifocal VEP on the same patient showing normal morphology, as well as significantly shorter and normal latencies of 125 msec from each eye.

CLINICAL APPROACH TO ERG FOR NEUROLOGISTS

The full-field ERG plays an important role in the diagnosis of a number of conditions encountered by neurologists, including retinal dystrophies, vitamin A deficiency, paraneoplastic conditions (cancer-associated retinopathy; melanoma-associated retinopathy), X-linked retinoschisis (retinal separation), and retinal ischemia (especially old retinal artery occlusions). It is also useful in diagnosing and monitoring retinal inflammatory disorders (e.g., bird shot chorioretinopathy) and medication-induced injury (e.g., hydroxychloroquine toxicity). In retinal dystrophies, the ERG is frequently abnormal even before the patient has any significant visual impairment. In many of these conditions, both the a- and b-waves are attenuated significantly or are absent.[25,108] Retinal dystrophies are encountered most frequently by neurologists when part of a syndrome such as Kearns–Sayre syndrome or the neuropathy, ataxia, and retinitis pigmentosa (NARP) syndrome. Outer retinal degeneration is also significant enough to attenuate the ERG in many disorders involving peroxisomal dysfunction (Zellweger syndrome, Refsum disease, and adrenoleukodystrophy). These conditions are discovered most often in infancy or childhood.[25,108]

In some conditions there is a selective reduction in b-wave amplitude. In these situations, the b-wave is smaller rather than larger than the a-wave, and therefore the recording does not return to baseline after the b-wave. This pattern of abnormality implies that the injury involves the inner nuclear layer with relative preservation of photoreceptor function. It is seen most frequently in cases of old retinal ischemia, retinoschisis, and paraneoplastic conditions. In central retinal artery occlusions, ERG is most useful when the injury is only partial, and it may also provide objective assessment of severity. In this setting, the a-wave amplitude may be reduced as well. In contrast, with central retinal vein occlusions the effect is most pronounced on the b-wave alone.[25,108] Selective b-wave attenuation is usually most evident on the scotopic flash ERG. Finally, the ERG is essential to the diagnosis of paraneoplastic retinal disorders, as structural abnormalities occur late in these disorders and a high index of suspicion is required before ordering the confirmatory serologic tests.[109,110]

ERG can also be useful in (1) subjects with an abnormal VEP but unusual features suggesting primary retinal rather than neurologic dysfunction, and (2) patients with unexplained visual loss in whom examination and retinal imaging cannot distinguish optic nerve from retinal injury.[25,108] It has been suggested that, for diagnostic use, the multifocal VEP should be done in conjunction with a multifocal ERG to determine whether observed localized defects are from optic nerve or retina.[25,58] In our experience, this should also include retinal imaging, which can aid further in properly defining anatomic localization (discussed in the next section).

OTHER INVESTIGATIVE TECHNIQUES

In the modern neuro-ophthalmology clinic, many techniques can be employed to assist the evaluation of patients. As with all clinical diagnostic measures, electrophysiologic studies sometimes fail to detect relevant disease or, conversely, suggest abnormality in a subject who is otherwise normal. VEP abnormalities have been reported in a variety of outer retinal diseases,[111–113] and it has been suggested that unexpected VEP results are best interpreted in combination with the ERG. As a consequence, electrophysiologic studies cannot replace standard clinical examination techniques such as funduscopy, indirect ophthalmoscopy and visual acuity assessments. Furthermore, judicious use of ancillary techniques such as retinal imaging, automated perimetry, and detailed assessments of visual function (color vision performance, low contrast acuity) can help to extend the diagnostic reliability of electrophysiologic investigations. In particular, a combined approach can be valuable to help delineate the potential cause of visual dysfunction in individuals with unusual clinical features.

Optical coherence tomography (OCT) is an important method for the assessment of the structural integrity and health of the visual system. Using an infrared light source in the range of approximately 840 nm, it can be used to image the retina and obtain both cross-sectional and volumetric images of retinal structures. It can serve as an important tool to complement and inform the interpretation of electrophysiologic recordings. OCT can be employed to augment the standard ophthalmologic examination and to quantify retinal structures that otherwise are assessed qualitatively. Recent advances permit image resolution in the axial plane in the order of 2 µm, and extremely high reproducibility makes longitudinal assessments feasible and informative.

In the assessment of patients with possible MS and optic neuritis, for example, OCT can play an adjunctive role in determining whether a borderline VEP abnormality actually reflects disease. During an episode of acute retrobulbar neuritis, patients will often have mild swelling of the nerve fiber layer, beyond the resolution of most trained clinicians (Fig. 22-17). This is especially

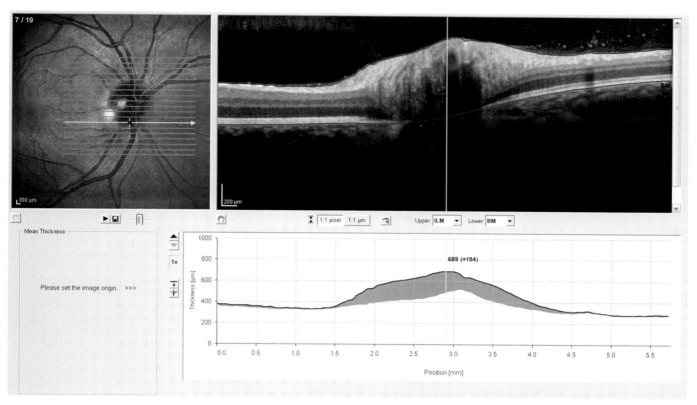

FIGURE 22-17 ■ Optical coherence tomography B-scan through the disc (right) and infrared fundus photo (left) of a 49-year-old woman with eye pain and mild delay of the visual evoked potential (VEP) as indicated by an increased interocular latency difference (the same patient as in Fig. 22-13). Disc swelling evidence of papillitis and VEP prolongation suggests that this is not disc edema but swelling due to anterior inflammatory injury. Note the swelling and the layers of the retina that can be identified.

true in cases where the demyelinating lesion is in the anterior portion of the nerve (typically, anterior to the orbital canal). Conversely, in patients with swelling of the retinal nerve fiber layer on OCT, VEP can help to establish whether the injury is likely to be demyelinating or related to increased intracranial pressure (Fig. 22-18). However, both compressive and infiltrative optic neuropathies can cause swelling and delayed VEP latency. It has also been reported previously that VEP prolongation can be observed in patients with central serous retinopathy,[112] a self-limited condition in which the neurosensory retina suffers a flat serous detachment from the posterior pole and then usually spontaneously re-anneals over weeks to months. Given its clinical characteristics, including the presence of subacute visual blurring in a young patient (albeit without pain), central serous retinopathy can be mistaken for optic neuritis. OCT, ophthalmologic examination, or both can be used to diagnose the retinopathy unequivocally (Fig. 22-19).

In patients with MS, either with or without a history of optic neuritis, nerve fiber layer thinning is observed and usually predominates in the fibers of the papillomacular bundle—that is, the temporal quadrant (Fig. 22-20). This can aid in the interpretation of a borderline VEP finding.

In general, electrophysiologic studies of the visual system can play an important role in the diagnosis and management of patients with a variety of neurologic and ophthalmologic conditions. Their use, in conjunction with other methods for assessing and monitoring visual function and ophthalmologic health, can aid in improving diagnostic accuracy and may come to play an important role in disease prognostication.

ACKNOWLEDGMENTS

The author thanks Chris Songster, Ami Cuneo, and Rachel Nolan for help with the illustrations.

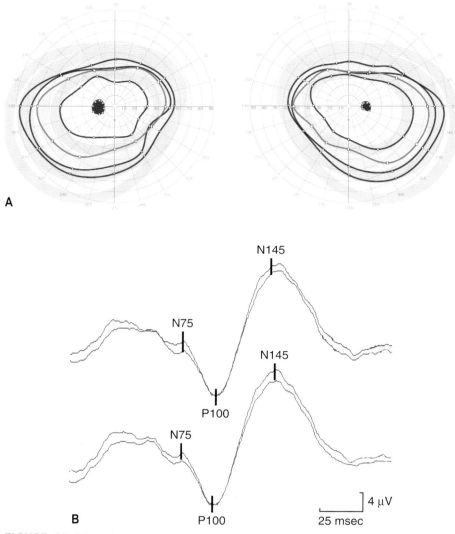

FIGURE 22-18 ■ **A**, Automated kinetic perimetry obtained with a Haag-Streit Octopus-900 in a 33-year-old man with disc swelling or papillitis. Note the enlarged blind spot in the left eye (shaded). Also note relative constriction of isopters in the left eye. **B**, Full-field pattern-reversal visual evoked potential from left (top) and right eye (bottom) shows normal symmetric P100 latency (112 msec) and amplitude bilaterally. This demonstrates that the swelling is likely papilledema rather than papillitis or infiltration.

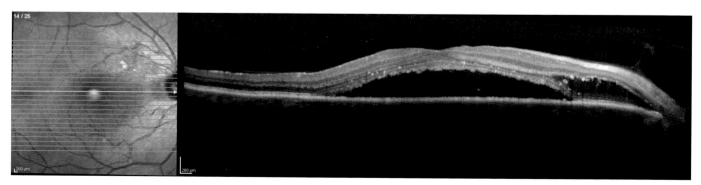

FIGURE 22-19 ■ Retinal photo (left) and optical coherence tomography (OCT) B-scan through the macula (right) of the right eye in a patient with multiple sclerosis and painless visual blurring, confirming a diagnosis of central serous retinopathy rather than optic neuritis. Note the dark fluid-filled space beneath the retina in the OCT. Central serous retinopathy can be worsened by administration of steroids. (© Ari Green, 2011.)

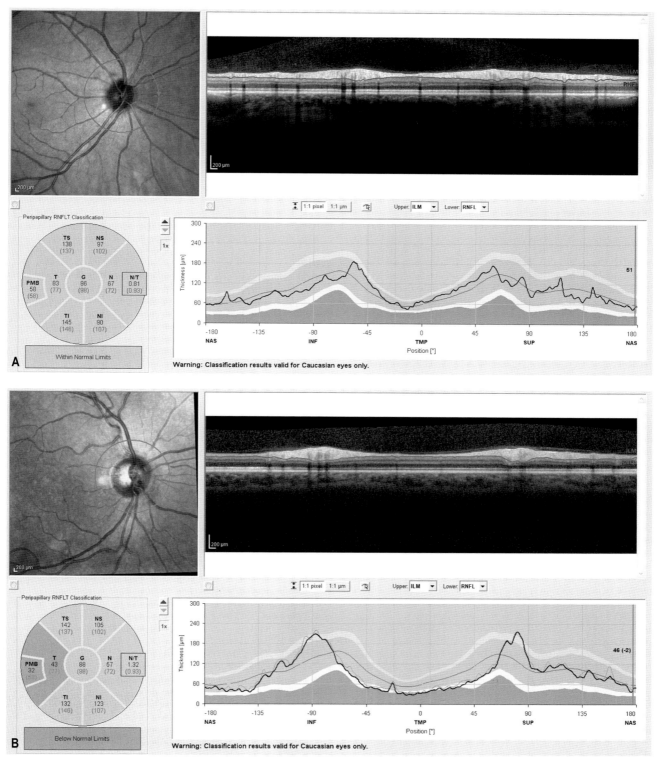

FIGURE 22-20 ▪ **A**, Circular circumpapillary optical coherence tomography (OCT) B-scan in a normal healthy subject showing normal nerve fiber layer thickness. Numbers in the clock face represent nerve fiber layer thickness in micrometers. **B**, Circular circumpapillary OCT B-scan in a 32-year-old woman with multiple sclerosis showing characteristic loss of nerve fiber in the temporal quadrant of the OCT.

REFERENCES

1. Rieke F, Baylor DA: Single-photon detection by rod cells of the retina. Rev Mod Physics, 70:1027, 1998
2. Cook T: Cell diversity in the retina: more than meets the eye. Bioessays, 25:921, 2003
3. Stryer L: The molecules of visual excitation. Scientific Amer, 257:42, 1987
4. Vaney DI: Retinal neurons: cell types and coupled networks. Prog Brain Res, 136:239, 2002
5. Masland RH: The fundamental plan of the retina. Nat Neurosci, 4:877, 2001
6. Curcio CA, Sloan KR: Packing geometry of human cone photoreceptors: variation with eccentricity and evidence for local anisotropy. Vis Neurosci, 9:169, 1992
7. Packer OS, Dacey DM: Receptive field structure of H1 horizontal cells in macaque monkey retina. J Vis Sci, 2:272, 2002
8. Derrington AM, Lennie P, Wright MJ: The mechanism of peripherally evoked responses in retinal ganglion cells. J Physiol, 289:299, 1979
9. Wassle H, Boycott BB: Functional architecture of the mammalian retina. Physiol Rev, 71:447, 1991
10. McGuire BA, Stevens JK, Sterling P: Microcircuitry of beta ganglion cells in cat retina. J Neurosci, 6:907, 1986
11. Curcio CA, Allen KA: Topography of ganglion cells in the human retina. J Comp Neurol, 300:5, 1990
12. Rockhill RL, Daly FJ, MacNeil MA et al: The diversity of ganglion cells in a mammalian retina. J Neurosci, 22:3831, 2002
13. Do MT, Yau KW: Intrinsically photosensitive retinal ganglion cells. Physiol Rev, 90:1547, 2010
14. Kupper C: The projection of the macula in the lateral geniculate nucleus of man. Am J Ophthalmol, 54:597, 1962
15. Celesia GG, Demarco PJ: Anatomy and physiology of the visual system. J Clin Neurophys Sci, 11:482, 1994
16. Gooley JJ, Lu J, Fischer D et al: A broad role for melanopsin in nonvisual photoreception. J Neurosci, 23:7093, 2003
17. Singer W: Control of thalamic transmission by corticofugal and ascending reticular pathways in the visual system. Physiol Rev, 57:386, 1977
18. Kaplan E, Purpura K, Shapley R: Contrast affects the transmission of visual information through the mammalian lateral geniculate nucleus. J Physiol, 391:267, 1987
19. Callaway EM: Local circuits in the primary visual cortex of the macaque monkey. Annu Rev Neurosci, 21:47, 1998
20. Horton JC, Hoyt WF: The representation of the visual field in human striate cortex. A revision of the classic Holmes map. Arch Ophthalmol, 109:816, 1991
21. Kriss A: Recording technique. p. 1. In Halliday AM (ed): Evoked Potentials in Clinical Testing. Churchill Livingstone, New York, 1993
22. Hassan U, Anwar MS: Reducing noise by repetition: introduction to signal averaging. Eur J Physics, 31:453, 2010
23. Hidajat RR, McLay JL, Elder MJ et al: A comparison of two patient-friendly ERG electrodes. Australas Phys Eng Sci Med, 26:30, 2003
24. Marmor MF, Fulton AB, Holder GE et al: International Society for Clinical Electrophysiology of Vision: ISCEV Standard for full-field clinical electroretinography (2008 update). Doc Ophthalmol, 118:69, 2009
25. Lam BL: Electrophysiology of Vision. Clinical Testing and Applications. Taylor & Francis, Boca Raton, FL, 2005
26. Samuels IS, Sturgill GM, Grossman GH et al: Light-evoked responses of the retinal pigment epithelium: changes accompanying photoreceptor loss in the mouse. J Neurophysiol, 104:391, 2010
27. Moschos M, Brouzas D: C wave of electroretinogram and visual evoked response in optic neuritis due to demyelinating diseases. Ophthalmologica, 204:149, 1992
28. Celesia GG, Brigell MG: Recommended standards for pattern electroretinograms and visual evoked potentials. International Federation of Clinical Physiology. Electroencephalogr Clin Neurophysiol Suppl, 52:45, 1999
29. Kaufman D, Celesia GG: Simultaneous recording of pattern electroretinogram and visual evoked responses in neuro-ophthalmologic disorders. Neurology, 35:644, 1985
30. Halliday AM: The visual evoked potential in the investigation of diseases of the optic nerve. p. 195. In Halliday AM (ed): Evoked Potentials in Clinical Testing. Churchill Livingstone, New York, 1993
31. Regan D, Lee BB: A comparison of the human 40Hz response with the properties of macaque ganglion cells. Vis Neurosci, 10:439, 1993
32. Milner BA, Regan D, Heron HR: Differential diagnosis of multiple sclerosis by visual evoked potential recording. Brain, 97:755, 1974
33. Vialatte FB, Maurice M, Dauwels J et al: Steady-state visually evoked potentials: focus on essential paradigms and future perspectives. Prog Neurobiol, 90:418, 2010
34. Kirkham TH, Coupland SG: Abnormal electroretinograms and visual evoked potentials in chronic papilledema using time-difference analysis. Can J Neurol Sci, 8:243, 1981
35. Pompe MT, Kranjc BS, Brecelj J: Visual evoked potentials to red-green stimulation in schoolchildren. Vis Neurosci, 23:447, 2006
36. Rudvin I: Visual evoked potentials for reversals of red-green gratings with different chromatic contrasts: asymmetries with respect to isoluminance. Vis Neurosci, 22:749, 2005
37. Spekreijse H, van der Twell LH, Zuidema T: Contrast evoked responses in man. Vision Res, 13:1577, 1973
38. Kuroiwa Y, Celesia GG: Visual evoked potentials with hemifield pattern stimulation. Their use in the diagnosis of retrochiasmatic lesions. Arch Neurol, 38:86, 1981
39. Schroeder CE, Tenke CE, Givre SJ et al: Striate cortical contribution to the surface-recorded pattern-reversal VEP in the alert monkey. Vision Res, 31:31, 1991

40. Givre SJ, Schroeder CE, Arezzo JC: Contribution of extrastriate area V4 to the surface-recorded flash VEP in the awake macaque. Vision Res, 34:415, 1994

41. Kraut MA, Arezzo JC, Vaughan HG, Jr: Inhibitory processes in the flash evoked potential of the monkey. Electroencephalogr Clin Neurophysiol, 76:440, 1990

42. Aldrich MS, Alessi AG, Beck RW et al: Cortical blindness: etiology, diagnosis, and prognosis. Ann Neurol, 21:149, 1987

43. Kupersmith MJ, Nelson JI, Seiple WH et al: The 20/20 eye in multiple sclerosis. Neurology, 33:1015, 1983

44. Robinson K, Rudge P, Small DG et al: A survey of the pattern reversal visual evoked response (PRVER) in 1428 consecutive patients referred to a clinical neurophysiology department. J Neurol Sci, 64:225, 1984

45. Joost W, Bach M, Schulte-Maunting J: Influence of mood on visually evoked potentials: a prospective longitudinal study. Int J Psychophysiol, 12:147, 1992

46. Oken BS, Chiappa KH, Gill E: Normal temporal variability of the P100. Electroencephalogr Clin Neurophysiol, 68:153, 1987

47. Bemelmans NA, Tilanus MA, Cuypers MH et al: Pattern-reversal visual evoked potentials in patients with epiretinal membrane. Am J Ophthalmol, 123:97, 1997

48. Ristanovic D, Hajdukovic R: Effects of spatially structured stimulus fields on pattern reversal VEPs. Electroencephalogr Clin Neurophysiol, 51:599, 1981

49. Sokol S, Jones K, Nadler D: Comparison of the spatial response properties of the human retina and cortex as measured by simultaneously recorded pattern ERGs and VEPs. Vision Res, 23:723, 1983

50. Kurita-Tashima S, Tobimatsu S, Nakayama-Hiromatsu M et al: Effect of check size on the pattern reversal VEP. Electroencephalogr Clin Neurophysiol, 80:161, 1991

51. Sokol S, Moskowitz A: Effects of retinal blur on the peak latency of the pattern evoked potential. Vision Res, 19:747, 1979

52. Neima D, Regan D: Pattern visual evoked potentials and spatial vision in retrobulbar neuritis and MS. Arch Neurol, 41:198, 1984

53. Fortune B, Hood DC: Conventional pattern-reversal VEPs are not equivalent to summed multifocal VEPs. Invest Ophthalmol Vis Sci, 44:1364, 2003

54. Hoffman MB: Investigating visual function with multifocal VEP. p. 139. In Lorenz B, Borruat FX (eds): Essentials in Ophthalmology: Pediatric Ophthalmology, Neuro-Ophthalmology, Genetics. Springer, New York, 2008

55. Baseler HA, Sutter EE, Klein SA et al: The topography of visual evoked response properties across the visual field. Electroencephalogr Clin Neurophysiol, 90:65, 1994

56. Hood DC, Greenstein VC: Multifocal VEP and ganglion cell damage: applications and limitations for the study of glaucoma. Prog Retin Eye Res, 22:201, 2003

57. Klistorner AI, Graham SL, Grigg JR et al: Multifocal topographic visual evoked potential: improving objective detection of local visual field defects. Invest Ophthalmol Vis Sci, 39:937, 1998

58. Klistorner AI, Graham SL, Grigg JR et al: Electrode position and the multi-focal visual-evoked potential: role in objective visual field assessment. Aust N Z J Ophthalmol Suppl:1, S91, 1998

59. Hood DC, Zhang X, Rodarte C et al: Determining abnormal interocular latencies of multifocal visual evoked potentials. Doc Ophthalmol, 109:177, 2004

60. Shimada Y, Horiguchi M, Nakamura A: Spatial and temporal properties of interocular timing differences in multifocal visual evoked potentials. Vision Res, 45:365, 2005

61. Slotnick SD, Klein SA, Carney T et al: Electrophysiological estimate of human cortical magnification. Clin Neurophysiol, 112:1349, 2001

62. Beck RW, Cleary PA, Trobe JD et al: The effect of corticosteroids for acute optic neuritis on the subsequent development of multiple sclerosis. The Optic Neuritis Study Group. N Engl J Med, 329:1764, 1993

63. Winn BJ, Shin E, Odel JG et al: Interpreting the multifocal visual evoked potential: the effects of refractive errors, cataracts, and fixation errors. Br J Ophthalmol, 89:340, 2005

64. Slotnick SD, Klein SA, Carney T et al: Using multi-stimulus VEP source localization to obtain a retinotopic map of human primary visual cortex. Clin Neurophysiol, 110:1793, 1999

65. Klistorner A, Fraser C, Garrick R et al: Correlation between full-field and multifocal VEPs in optic neuritis. Doc Ophthalmol, 116:19, 2008

66. Fortune B, Demirel S, Zhang X et al: Repeatability of normal multifocal VEP: implications for detecting progression. J Glaucoma, 15:131, 2006

67. Fortune B, Demirel S, Zhang X et al: Comparing multifocal VEP and standard automated perimetry in high-risk ocular hypertension and early glaucoma. Invest Ophthalmol Vis Sci, 48:1173, 2007

68. Guthkelch AN, Bursick D, Sclabassi RJ: The relationship of the latency of the visual P100 wave to gender and head size. Electroencephalogr Clin Neurophysiol, 68:219, 1987

69. Gregori B, Pro S, Bombelli F et al: VEP latency: sex and head size. Clin Neurophysiol, 117:1154, 2006

70. Wright CE, Williams DE, Drasdo N: The influence of age on the electroretinogram and visual evoked potential. Doc Ophthalmol, 59:365, 1985

71. Celesia G, Kaufman D, Cone S: Effects of age and sex on pattern electroretinograms and visual evoked potentials. Electroencephalogr Clin Neurophysiol, 68:161, 1987

72. Sokol S, Moscowitz A, Towle V: Age-related changes in the latency of the visual evoked potential: influence of check size. Electroencephalogr Clin Neurophysiol, 51:559, 1981

73. Fortune B, Zhang X, Hood DC et al: Normative ranges and specificity of the multifocal VEP. Doc Ophthalmol, 109:87, 2004

74. Skalka H, Holman J: Effect of pupillary dilatation in flash VER testing. Doc Ophthalmol, 63:321, 1986

75. Martins A, Balachandran C, Klistorner AI et al: Effect of pupil size on multifocal pattern visual evoked potentials. Clin Experiment Ophthalmol, 31:354, 2003

76. Gonzalez P, Parks S, Dolan F et al: The effects of pupil size on the multifocal electroretinogram. Doc Ophthalmol, 109:67, 2004

77. Mori H, Momose K, Nemoto N et al: Application of visual evoked potentials for preoperative estimation of visual function in eyes with dense cataract. Graefes Arch Clin Exp Ophthalmol, 239:915, 2001

78. Galloway NR: Electrophysiological testing of eyes with opaque media. Eye, 2:615, 1988

79. Ruseckaite R, Maddess T, Danta G et al: Sparse multifocal stimuli for the detection of multiple sclerosis. Ann Neurol, 57:904, 2005

80. Arvind H, Graham S, Leaney J et al: Identifying preperimetric functional loss in glaucoma: a blue-on-yellow multifocal visual evoked potentials study. Ophthalmology, 116:1134, 2009

81. Bumgartner J, Epstein CM: Voluntary alteration of visual evoked potentials. Ann Neurol, 12:12, 1982

82. Fraser C, Klistorner A, Graham S et al: Multifocal visual evoked potential latency analysis: predicting progression to multiple sclerosis. Arch Neurol, 63:847, 2006

83. Klistorner A, Graham S, Fraser C et al: Electrophysiological evidence for heterogeneity of lesions in optic neuritis. Invest Ophthalmol Vis Sci, 48:4549, 2007

84. Holder GE: Electrophysiological assessment of optic nerve disease. Eye, 18:1133, 2004

85. Janaky M, Fulup Z, Paiffy A et al: Electrophysiological findings in patients with nonarteritic ischemic optic neuropathy. Clin Neurophysiol, 117:1158, 2006

86. Mukartihal GB, Radhakrishan S, Ramasubba Reddy et al: Statistical analysis of visual evoked potentials in optic neuritis and ischemic optic neuropathy subjects. Conf Proc IEEE Eng Med Biol Soc, 2:1193, 2005

87. Parisi V, Gallinaro G, Ziccardi L: Electrophysiological assessment of visual function in patients with nonarteritic ischaemic optic neuropathy. Eur J Neurol, 15:839, 2008

88. Wilson WB: Visual evoked response differentiation of ischaemic optic neuritis from the optic neuritis of multiple sclerosis. Am J Ophthalmol, 86:520, 1978

89. Klistorner A, Fraser C, Garrick R et al: Correlation between full-field and multifocal VEPs in optic neuritis. Doc Ophthalmol, 116:19, 2008

90. Grippo TM, Ezon I, Kanadani FN et al: The effects of optic disc drusen on the latency of the pattern-reversal checkerboard and multifocal visual evoked potentials. Invest Ophthalmol Vis Sci, 50:4199, 2009

91. Scott GI: Traquair's Clinical Perimetry. 7th Ed. Henry Kimpton, London, 1957

92. Stojkovic T, de Seze J, Hurtevent JF et al: Visual evoked potentials study in chronic idiopathic inflammatory demyelinating polyneuropathy. Clin Neurophysiol, 111: 2285, 2000

93. Uncini A, Gallucci M, Lugaresi A et al: CNS involvement in chronic inflammatory demyelinating polyneuropathy: an electrophysiological and MRI study. Electromyogr Clin Neurophysiol, 31:365, 1991

94. Cronin-Golomb A, Corkin S, Rizzo JF et al: Visual dysfunction in Alzheimer's disease: relation to normal aging. Ann Neurol, 29:41, 1991

95. Jackson GR, Owsley C: Visual dysfunction, neurodegenerative diseases, and aging. Neurol Clin, 21:709, 2003

96. Katz B, Rimmer S: Ophthalmologic manifestations of Alzheimer's disease. Surv Ophthalmol, 34:31, 1989

97. Berisha F, Feke GT, Trempe CL et al: Retinal abnormalities in early Alzheimer's disease. Invest Ophthalmol Vis Sci, 48:2285, 2007

98. Blanks JC, Torigoe Y, Hinton DR et al: Retinal pathology in Alzheimer's disease. I. Ganglion cell loss in foveal/parafoveal retina. Neurobiol Aging, 17:377, 1996

99. Blanks JC, Schmidt SY, Torigoe Y et al: Retinal pathology in Alzheimer's disease. II. Regional neuron loss and glial changes in GCL. Neurobiol Aging, 17:385, 1996

100. Danesh-Meyer HV, Birch H, Ku JY et al: Reduction of optic nerve fibers in patients with Alzheimer disease identified by laser imaging. Neurology, 67:1852, 2006

101. Guo L, Duggan J, Cordeiro MF: Alzheimer's disease and retinal neurodegeneration. Curr Alzheimer Res, 7:3, 2010

102. Lu Y, Li Z, Zhang X, Ming B et al: Retinal nerve fiber layer structure abnormalities in early Alzheimer's disease: evidence in optical coherence tomography Neurosci Lett, 480:69, 2010

103. Paquet C, Boissonnot M, Roger F et al: Abnormal retinal thickness in patients with mild cognitive impairment and Alzheimer's disease. Neurosci Lett, 420:97, 2007

104. Krasodomska K, Lubienski W, Potemkowski A et al: Pattern electroretinogram (PERG) and pattern visual evoked potential (PVEP) in the early stages of Alzheimer's disease. Doc Ophthalmol, 121:111, 2010

105. Archibald NK, Clarke MP, Mosimann UP et al: The retina in Parkinson's disease. Brain, 132:1128, 2009

106. Bartel P, Blom M, Robinson E et al: Effects of chlorpromazine on pattern and flash ERGs and VEPs compared to oxazepam and to placebo in normal subjects. Electroencephalogr Clin Neurophysiol, 77:330, 1990

107. Stanzione P, Fattapposta F, Tagliati M et al: Dopaminergic pharmacological manipulations in normal humans confirm the specificity of the visual (PERG-VEP) and cognitive (P300) electrophysiologic alterations in Parkinson's disease. Electroencephalogr Clin Neurophysiol, 41:216, 1990

108. Gouras, P: Electroretinography. p. 427. In Aminoff MJ (ed): Electrodiagnosis in Clinical Neurology. 5th Ed. Elsevier Churchill Livingstone, Philadelphia, 2005

109. Thirkill CE: Cancer associated retinopathy. Neuro-ophthalmology, 13:297, 1994

110. Berson EL, Lessell S: Paraneoplastic night blindness with malignant melanoma. Am J Ophthalmol, 106:307, 1988

111. Janaky M, Palffy A, Horvath G et al: Pattern reversal electroretinograms and visual evoked potentials in retinitis pigmentosa. Doc Ophthalmol, 177:27, 2008

112. Lennerstrand G: Delayed visual cortical potentials in retinal disease. Acta Ophthalmol, 60:497, 1982

113. Weinstein GW, Odom JV, Cavendar S: Visually evoked potentials and electroretinography in neurologic evaluation. Neurol Clin, 9:225, 1991

Visual Evoked Potentials in Infants and Children

EILEEN E. BIRCH and VIDHYA SUBRAMANIAN

Visual evoked potentials (VEPs) are massed electrical signals generated by occipital cortical areas 17, 18, and 19 in response to visual stimulation. VEPs differ from the electroencephalogram (EEG) in that the EEG represents ongoing activity of wide areas of the cortex, whereas the VEP is a specific occipital lobe response triggered by a visual stimulus, primarily dependent on the functional integrity of vision in the central visual field. Thus, VEPs can be used to assess the integrity or maturational state of the visual pathway in infants and preverbal children.

The basic methodology for recording VEPs is straightforward and is described in the Visual Evoked Potentials Standard developed by the International Society for Clinical Electrophysiology in Vision (ISCEV).[1] An active electrode is placed on the scalp over the visual cortex (Oz), along with a reference electrode at Fz and a ground electrode at Cz or on the ear lobe. Signals are led from the electrodes through a preamplifier, which is located near the infant to boost signal amplitude prior to further contamination by outside noise sources. The preamplifier also typically acts as a bandpass filter. From the preamplifier the signal is led into a computer capable of averaging VEPs. The main purpose of filtering and signal averaging is to improve the signal-to-noise ratio. The VEP is contaminated by EEG, as well as by outside noise sources. However, since the VEP in response to a given

pattern is fairly constant in amplitude and latency (or phase) while the EEG occurs randomly with respect to the visual stimulus, stimulus averaging will decrease the unwanted contamination by EEG and other noise sources in proportion to the square root of the number of VEPs averaged.

Most commercial equipment for recording the VEP is not designed specifically for use with infants and young children and therefore requires several modifications for use in this patient population. Since it is important that the infant be visually alert and attentive to patterned stimuli, it is helpful to have some small toys that can be dangled in front of the video display when collecting pattern VEPs. The majority of the VEP response is generated by the cortical projection of the macular area (central 6 to 8 degrees of the visual field[2,3]); therefore, the toys must be very small or open in the center so as not to block the stimulus from reaching the macula. An observer must watch the infant and signal to the averaging equipment when the infant is looking at the pattern and when the infant is looking elsewhere. Both hand-held buttons and foot pedals can be constructed for this purpose. Sudden head and body movements, including yawns, crying, or vigorous sucking, can produce large-amplitude broad-band electrical artifacts. Accordingly, the averaging or analysis equipment must contain hardware or software to reject these artifacts because averaging alone is not sufficient to eliminate their contribution to the recorded response. Alternatively, trials containing artifacts can be deleted manually from the signal average.

Minimum standards for reporting VEPs have been published.[1] At least two averages should be obtained, to demonstrate reproducibility of waveforms. Traces of VEP recordings should have a clear indication of polarity, time in milliseconds, and amplitude in microvolts. The ISCEV recommends that VEP traces be presented as positive upwards, although in many clinical neurophysiology laboratories the traces are presented with a downward deflection representing positivity at the active electrode. Normative values and normal tolerance limits for amplitude and latency should be reported along with the results. Since VEP latency, amplitude, and waveform change with age, comparison to same-age normative values is useful in clinical practice.

VEPs are elicited by a temporal change in visual stimulation. Three types of visual stimuli commonly are used to elicit VEPs: luminance (light) flashes, pattern onset/offset, and pattern contrast reversal. Each of these stimuli may be presented as single events or in a repetitive manner. When the light flashes, pattern onset/offset, or contrast reversal occurs infrequently (i.e., at 1 Hz or less), the entire VEP waveform can be seen; this is called a *transient* response. Peak-to-peak amplitudes and latencies of several major peaks can be measured (Fig. 23-1). When the light flashes or pattern reversals are repeated frequently at regular intervals (at rates of 6 Hz or higher), a simpler periodic waveform is seen; this is called a *steady-state* response. Response amplitude and phase are measured.

TRANSIENT LUMINANCE (FLASH) VEPs

Transient luminance VEPs are obtained in response to a strobe light or flashing light-emitting diode (LED) display or goggles. The flash should subtend at least 20 degrees and should have a stimulus strength of 2.7 to 3.3 cd/m^2.[1] The flash rate should be 1.0 Hz $\pm$ 10 percent.[1] The transient luminance flash VEP is a complex waveform with multiple negative and positive changes in voltage. Various approaches have been taken to naming the peaks and troughs in this response, which has led to some difficulty in interpreting differences among studies. Recently, recommendations for standardized reporting of VEP data have been made by the ISCEV.[1] As shown in Figure 23-1, peaks are designated as positive and negative in numerical sequence (P1, P2, P3 and N1, N2, N3). The most commonly reported amplitude is the N2-P2 peak-to-peak amplitude.

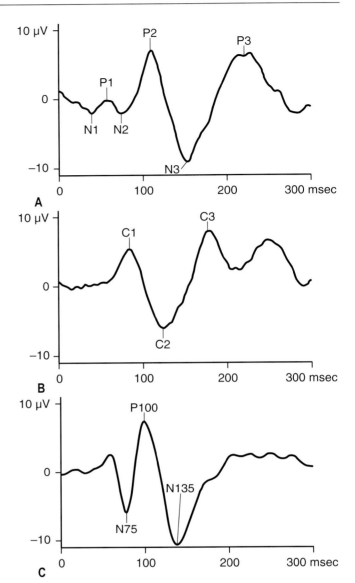

FIGURE 23-1 ▪ Normal transient flash (**A**), transient pattern onset/offset (**B**), and transient pattern-reversal (**C**) visual evoked potentials. The system of naming of positive and negative peaks proposed by the International Society for Clinical Electrophysiology of Vision[1] is indicated.

Using both source localization techniques in humans and intracortical recording in primates, several recent studies suggest that the transient luminance flash VEP primarily reflects the activity of striate and extrastriate cortex.[4–6] In addition, some wavelets in the VEP appear to be subcortical in origin.[5–7] These subcortical wavelets are not major components of the flash VEPs obtained from patients with healthy striate and extrastriate cortical areas. However, flash VEPs have been recorded in newborns who lack functional striate and extrastriate cortex.[8,9] These VEPs may have reflected subcortical function that was more apparent in the VEP when the cortical components of the response were missing. Thus, the presence of a flash VEP response cannot be taken as unequivocal evidence of cortical function.

PATTERN ONSET/OFFSET VEPs

Pattern onset/offset VEPs are obtained in response to a pattern abruptly exchanged with a diffuse background. The pattern should subtend at least 15 degrees and the pattern and diffuse fields should be well matched in mean luminance.[1] Pattern onset duration should be 200 msec separated by 400 msec of diffuse background.[1] In most cases, a minimum of two pattern-element sizes should be included, 1 degree and 15 minutes,[1] but normal newborns may not respond to the 15-minute pattern-element size. Pattern VEPs primarily reflect activity of the striate and extrastriate cortex.[10-13] The pattern onset/offset VEP contains three peaks in adults: a positive peak followed by a negative peak and a second positive peak. As shown in Figure 23-1, ISCEV proposes that these components be termed C1, C2, and C3. Amplitude is measured from the preceding negative peak. Pattern onset/offset VEPs are useful for evaluating infants and children with nystagmus, as they are less sensitive than pattern-reversal VEPs to confounding by involuntary eye movements and poor fixation stability.

PATTERN-REVERSAL VEPs

Pattern-reversal VEPs are elicited by abrupt contrast reversal. The pattern should subtend at least 15 degrees and, typically, a minimum of two pattern-element sizes are included, 1 degree and 15 minutes.[1] Pattern reversal at 1 Hz (2 reversals per sec) yields transient VEPs, whereas higher reversal rates (e.g., 6 to 10 Hz) yield steady-state VEPs. In adults, the transient pattern-reversal VEP typically contains a small negative peak followed by a large positive peak and a second negative peak. As shown in Figure 23-1, ISCEV proposes that these components be termed N75, P100, and N135 to indicate their polarity and their approximate latency (in milliseconds) in normal adults. The most commonly reported amplitude is the N75-P100 peak-to-peak amplitude. The steady-state pattern-reversal VEP has a relatively simple, almost sinusoidal waveform; amplitude and phase of the response typically are reported. Since the mean luminance of the pattern remains constant throughout the contrast reversals, pattern-reversal VEPs reflect pattern sensitivity rather than light sensitivity.

Using intracerebral recording in awake humans, Ducati and co-workers found that P100 appears to be generated by the pyramidal cells in layer IV of area 17.[6] However, imaging studies in humans point to the source of the early phase of the P100 peak as being in dorsal extrastriate cortex of the middle occipital gyrus, whereas the late phase of P100 appears to be generated by the ventral extrastriate cortex of the fusiform gyrus.[13] There have been no reports of pattern-reversal VEPs being recorded in newborns who lack functional striate and extrastriate cortex. Thus, the presence of a pattern-reversal VEP response may be a good indicator of the integrity of cortical function.

NORMAL MATURATION OF VEPs

Visual responses have been documented in preterm infants as young as 24 weeks gestational age (GA), but these responses are rudimentary. Infants tested at 22 to 23 weeks GA had very poor or absent VEPs.[14] Considerable visual development occurs during the third trimester of gestation and the first post-term year. While, on funduscopic examination, the fovea appears mature soon after term birth, detailed anatomic studies have shown that neither the migration of cone photoreceptors toward the foveal pit nor the movement of ganglion cells away from the foveal pit is complete during the first months of life.[15] Moreover, the fine anatomic structure of the foveal cone photoreceptors, which subserve fine detail vision, is not mature until at least 4 years of age.[15] Myelination of the optic nerve and tract is incomplete at term birth and continues to increase for 2 years postnatally.[16] Although the number of cells in the primary visual cortex appears to be complete at birth, considerable increases in cell size, synaptic structure, and dendritic density take place during the first 6 to 8 months of life.[17,18] One approach to monitoring the progress of anatomic maturation has been to evaluate developmental changes in the VEPs of healthy alert infants. These data also provide a baseline for assessment of the degree of visual impairment in pediatric patients.

Flash VEP amplitudes may be influenced by arousal state, but latency is less affected.[19,20] The mean latency of N3 across various arousal states (awake, drowsy, active sleep, and quiet sleep) was within 15 msec in preterm infants at 30 to 37 weeks GA, but sleep significantly reduced N3 amplitude.[21] Similarly, the mean latencies of P1 for the alert state and the sleep state were within 15 msec at 40 weeks GA.[22] Pattern VEPs are affected by arousal state; good-quality pattern VEP recordings require an alert, attentive infant whose eyes are focused on the pattern.

Amplitude and Latency of Transient Luminance (Flash) VEPs

In preterm infants less than 30 weeks GA, a single long-latency (about 300 msec) negative peak is the most prominent component of the flash VEP (Fig. 23-2).[14,22,23] This peak has been identified by some authors as N1, since it is the earliest negative peak observed in young infants. However, other authors have suggested that this peak corresponds to the N3 component of the mature waveform and that the N1 and N2 peaks are "missing."[14] Some difficulty in establishing correspondence between peaks in infant and adult waveforms occurs because the early negative peak in young infants is often bifid, with two subpeaks that may or may not be symmetric in amplitude.[14,21,23,24]

In Figure 23-2, flash VEP latency from various studies is plotted to show the maturation of the early negative peak, which appears to correspond to the adult's N3 (adult latency, 150 msec). Tsuneishi and colleagues assessed changes in the early negative peak longitudinally and found that latency decreased at a rate of 4.6 msec per week between 30 and 40 weeks GA.[20,24] Pike and colleagues report a similar rate of 5.5 msec per week between 28 and 42 weeks GA.[25] There is some evidence that the change in latency does not occur smoothly but, instead, occurs in "spurts" of at least 6 msec,[20,24] possibly reflecting the myelination process in the visual pathway.

At term (40 weeks GA), earlier negative components are present in the waveform which shorten in latency with age; these appear to correspond to N2 (adult latency, 75 msec) and N1 (adult latency, 40 msec). As seen in Figure 23-2, Pike and associates report that the earliest negative components can be obtained from infants as young as 34 weeks GA,[25] while all other studies indicate that these components arise at term (40 weeks GA). Yet, even in that study, only at term age did all infants simultaneously have both an early N0 and N1. One possible explanation for this finding is that Pike and colleagues[25] included only infants who later had normal neurologic examinations over the first 2 years of life.

The youngest infants reported to show an early positive peak with a latency of approximately 200 msec were between 30 and 35 weeks GA.[26] This positive peak likely corresponds to the P2 peak in the adult waveform (latency, 100 msec). P2 is consistently present in all normal neonates from 37 weeks GA on, and is present in 90 percent of neurologically normal infants by 35 to 36 weeks GA.[27] When present, the latency of the positive component decreases from about 220 msec at 34 weeks GA to 150 to 190 msec at term and to 100 msec by 8 to12 weeks post-term age (48 to 52 weeks GA) (Fig. 23-3).[20,23,28] The P2 peak is clearly identifiable in the VEPs of healthy infants by 6 weeks post-term (46 weeks GA), and its amplitude exceeds that of N3 by 8 weeks post-term (48 weeks GA).[28,29]

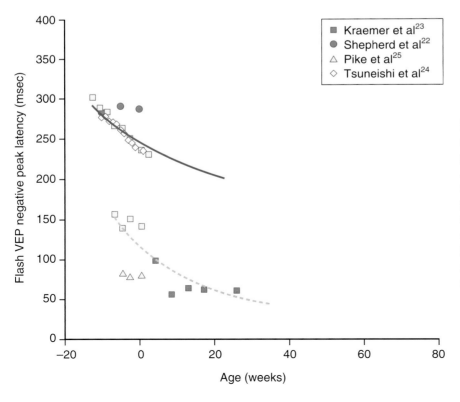

FIGURE 23-2 ■ Latency of the major negative components of the flash visual evoked potential in preterm and term infants.[22–25] Age at 0 weeks corresponds to 40 weeks gestational age (term). Two exponential decay fits are plotted; the solid line summarizes the maturational trend for N3 latency. Note that the initial negative peak was bifid in many infants and the latency of each component is reported separately. The dashed line summarizes the maturational trend for N1 latency.

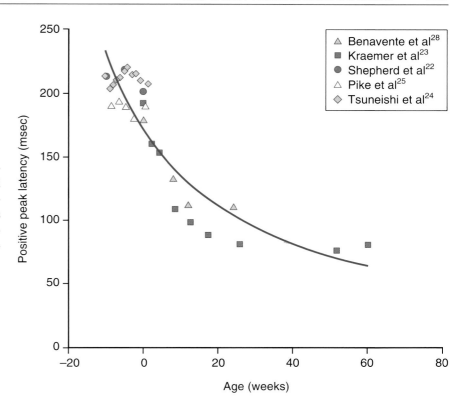

FIGURE 23-3 ▪ Latency of the major positive component of the transient flash visual evoked potential in preterm and term infants.[22–25,28] Age at 0 weeks corresponds to 40 weeks gestational age (term). An exponential decay fit summarizes the mean maturational trend.

A rapid increase in the amplitudes of most of the flash VEP peaks occurs during early childhood, with the largest amplitudes present at about 6 years of age. Amplitudes of the various peaks reach adult levels by about 16 years of age. The maturational changes in amplitude, however, are age trends that are present despite very large individual differences in amplitude within any given age group. This variability limits the utility of flash VEP amplitude in detecting developmental visual abnormalities. Clinical evaluation has focused largely on the latency of the negative component and appearance of the first positive peak (which corresponds to P2 in adults). Prolonged latency of the initial negative peak (more than 370 msec) and the absence of the positive peak at 40 weeks GA or older have been linked to poor outcomes in preterm infants.[22]

Steady-state flash VEPs have been used to investigate the maturation of temporal resolution during infancy.[30] The data suggest three phases in maturation. During the first month of life (40 to 44 weeks GA) temporal resolution shows little maturation, improving from 15 Hz to 19 Hz. During the next 5 months, temporal resolution matures rapidly to 45 Hz, and then undergoes further maturation, slowly approaching the adult level (55 Hz) by 9 months of age. In addition, the optimal stimulus frequency—that is, the frequency that elicited the largest amplitude response—increases with age during the first 2 years of life.[31]

Amplitude and Latency of Pattern VEPs

The presence, amplitude, and latency of pattern VEPs change with maturation and age.[32–42] With large pattern-element sizes, transient pattern-reversal VEPs can be recorded from preterm infants as early as 30 weeks GA. At this age the pattern-reversal VEP to a large-element checkerboard (each check subtending about 2 degrees of visual angle) has a simple waveform consisting of a single positive peak with a latency of approximately 330 msec. As shown in Figure 23-4, latency for large-element patterns decreases to about 250 msec by 40 weeks GA (term), 150 msec by 10 weeks post-term (50 weeks GA), and 110 msec by 25 weeks post-term (65 weeks GA).[32,36–40] For small pattern-element sizes (less than 15 minutes), transient pattern-reversal VEPs may not be recordable up to 50 to 54 weeks GA.[35,38]

Beyond 4 weeks post-term (44 weeks GA), the VEP waveform changes from a simple one to a more complex waveform with multiple peaks, and peak latency grows progressively shorter (Fig. 23-5).[33] Latency is dependent on pattern-element size, with latency to large-element patterns decreasing rapidly over the first months of life and latency to small-element patterns decreasing more gradually (see Figs. 23-4 and 23-5).[32–40] Similar changes in latency have been reported for transient pattern onset/offset VEPs.[36]

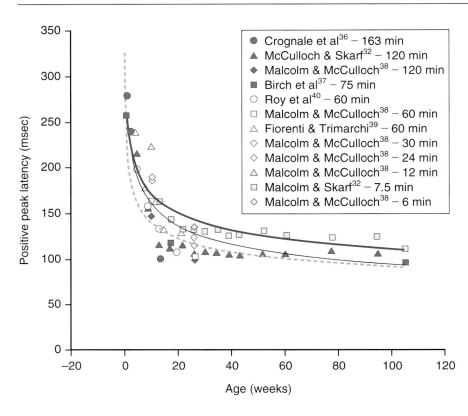

FIGURE 23-4 ■ Latency of the major positive component of the transient pattern-reversal visual evoked potential in preterm and term infants.[32,36–40] Age at 0 weeks corresponds to 40 weeks gestational age (term). Studies are presented in the inset box along with the pattern-element size used (in minutes of arc): large (dark blue symbols and dotted line), medium (open symbols and thin black line), and small (light blue symbols and heavy line) checks. All studies used checkerboard patterns except that of Fiorentini and Trimarchi,[39] which used black and white stripes. The lines are exponential decay fits to the data.

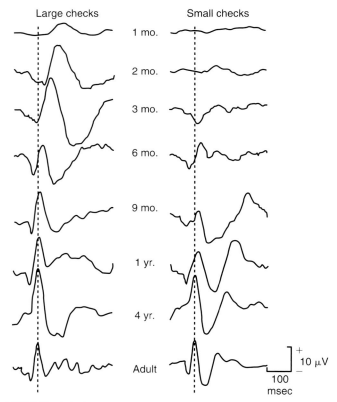

FIGURE 23-5 ■ Pattern-reversal transient visual evoked potentials obtained from visually normal infants, children, and an adult in response to large (60-minute arc) and small (15-minute arc) checks. (From Moskowitz A, Sokol S: Developmental changes in the human visual system as reflected by the latency of the pattern reversal VEP. Electroencephalogr Clin Neurophysiol, 56:1, 1983, with permission.)

Steady-state pattern VEPs can be recorded from preterm infants as early as 35 weeks GA when large pattern-element sizes and relatively slow pattern alternation rates are used.[41] As infants mature, responses can be recorded to progressively smaller pattern-element sizes and progressively faster pattern-alternation rates.[41,42]

Visual Acuity Development

The pattern VEP has been used to estimate visual acuity in infants for the past 35 years.[43] Just as a standard eye chart for measuring visual acuity contains letters ranging from very large to quite small, a pattern VEP acuity test includes a group of checkerboard or striped grating patterns with elements that range from coarse to fine. In both cases, the goal is to determine the finest pattern that the patient's visual system can resolve. When the VEP is used, visual acuity is estimated most often by examining the relationship between amplitude and pattern-element size. Ideally, many pattern-element sizes would be evaluated to pinpoint the exact size at which a response can no longer be recorded. With the limited attention span of infants and young children, typically a limited set of four to six patterns is presented. Particularly in clinical settings where there is often little prior information on which to base a choice of the optimal pattern-element sizes, logarithmic spacing between pattern-element sizes in the test series is used (so that, for example, each pattern size is one-half that of the previous pattern in the series). Logarithmic spacing of a wide range of pattern-element sizes despite a small number of steps maximizes the possibility that acuity can be estimated from the data obtained. Linear regression of amplitude on pattern-element size is used to extrapolate the pattern-element size that corresponds to 0.0-μV amplitude in order to provide the visual acuity estimate.

Many pediatric laboratories and clinics have adopted the *sweep VEP* for acuity testing in recent years.[44] Sweep VEP protocols present pattern-element sizes to the infant in rapid succession during a 10-second sweep. Using Fourier analytic techniques to extract the VEP responses to each of the brief stimuli (specifically, the amplitude and phase of the harmonics of the stimulation rate), sufficient information can be obtained from the VEP records to estimate visual acuity from only a few brief test trials. This technique has three significant advantages. First, test time is reduced. Second, the infant's behavioral state changes little during the brief recording session. Third, since many more pattern-element sizes are included in the test protocol, linear spacing in the series can be used and a more accurate estimate of acuity can be obtained (Fig. 23-6).

Two classic studies of the maturation of visual acuity during infancy using transient pattern VEPs were conducted during the mid 1970s by Sokol[34] and by Marg and associates.[45] From an initial visual acuity of 1.30 logMAR (20/400 Snellen equivalent) at 4 weeks of age, visual acuity rapidly matured to nearly adult levels (0.2 to 0.0 logMAR; 20/30 to 20/20 Snellen equivalent) by 6 to 7 months of age. MAR represents the minimum angle of resolution. Although some controversy remains, it appears that visual acuity matures according to age corrected for preterm birth (GA) rather than age from birth (Fig. 23-7).

Over the past 10 years, we have gathered a substantial normative data set for monocular and binocular sweep VEP acuity maturation during the first 2 years of life.[43] Overall, sweep VEP acuity improves from about 0.75 logMAR (20/105 Snellen equivalent) at 6 weeks of age to about 0.37 logMAR (20/45) at 26 weeks of age and 0.25 logMAR (20/35) by 55 weeks of age (see Fig. 23-7). The acuity improvements parallel postnatal anatomic maturation, including the migration of cone photoreceptors toward the foveal pit, changes in the fine anatomic structure of the foveal cone photoreceptors,[15,46] myelination of the optic nerve and tract,[16] increases in cortical cell size, synaptic structure and dendritic density,[17,18] and elimination of supernumerary synapses in visual cortex.[17] Visual acuity measured by pattern onset/offset VEP matures more rapidly than acuity measured by pattern-reversal VEP, which may be the result of different aspects of pattern vision maturing at different rates.

After 15 weeks of age, mean binocular sweep VEP acuity is better than mean monocular sweep VEP acuity by

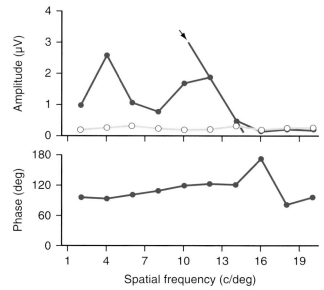

FIGURE 23-6 ▪ In the sweep visual evoked potential protocol, the amplitude versus linear pattern-element size function may have a nonmonotonic shape with multiple peaks. Linear regression of amplitude on log pattern-element size and extrapolation to 0 μV is performed on the final descending limb of the function. Sample data from a 10-month-old healthy infant are shown. Filled circles show the amplitude and phase of the visual response to each pattern-element size (spatial frequency). Open circles show the amplitude of noise during the same recording period. The diagonal line (arrow) illustrates the linear regression; acuity is estimated to be 14.5 c/deg, which corresponds to a Snellen equivalent of approximately 20/40.

about 0.03 logMAR (equivalent to about a half-line on an eye chart). The variability of binocular sweep VEP acuity within an age group (e.g., 17-week-old infants), defined as 95 percent of the normal distribution, is about ±0.23 logMAR around the mean. Variability is slightly greater for monocular sweep VEP acuity at ±0.29 logMAR.

Within the normative sample, mean interocular acuity differences are small in each age group, averaging less than 0.1 logMAR (equivalent to about 1 line on an eye chart). However, the range of interocular differences comprising 95 percent of the normal distribution varies with age. At 6 weeks, 95 percent of interocular differences fall within ±0.29 logMAR (equivalent to about 3 lines on an eye chart) while, by 46 weeks post-term age (86 weeks GA), 95 percent of interocular differences fall within ±0.18 logMAR (equivalent to about 2 lines on an eye chart).

Normative longitudinal measurements of sweep VEP acuity over the first 18 months of life have also been reported for preterm and full-term infants.[43,47] These data have direct clinical utility in that they provide a method for determining whether a change in an individual's acuity over time represents a significant change.

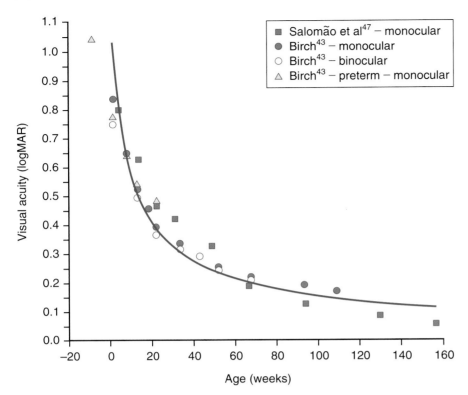

FIGURE 23-7 ▪ Monocular (filled symbols) and binocular (open symbols) sweep visual evoked potential acuity as a function of age in weeks.[43,47] Age at 0 weeks corresponds to 40 weeks gestational age (term). Preterm monocular acuity (blue triangles) development matches term infant acuity development when age is adjusted for preterm birth. The line is an exponential decay fit to the data.

In other words, such data provide a baseline for the evaluation of progression, recovery, or response to treatment in individual patients. The rate of sweep VEP acuity development (slope) ranged from −0.34 to −0.89 logMAR/log weeks in a normative sample of 53 healthy term infants tested on five occasions during the first 18 months of life. The rate of acuity development during infancy may be more predictive of long-term visual acuity outcome than the infant's acuity determined from a single acuity test.[48]

CLINICAL USE OF THE VEP IN INFANTS AND CHILDREN

Technical Issues

In the projection from the retina to the occipital cortex, the central 10 degrees of the visual field are predominant, with the peripheral visual field more sparsely represented. The electrical signals recorded from the scalp over the occipital lobe even more strongly reflect this central visual field area because the central projection is on the exposed surface of the occipital cortex, whereas the peripheral projection lies deep within the calcarine fissure. This situation enhances the sensitivity of VEP protocols to disruption of central vision, which subserves the ability to fixate and to perform the many finely

detailed visual tasks that make up daily life, such as reading or face recognition. However, a child with poor central vision or noncentral fixation may fail to produce a reliable VEP response despite substantial residual visual function.

Several patient characteristics limit the ability to obtain VEPs. In general, patients must be alert and quiet, able to look at the center of the stimulus, and able to focus on the stimulus. Sleepy or sedated patients, as well as patients under anesthesia, produce poor or variable VEP results at best and paradoxical and misleading VEP results at worst. Head and body movements, including yawning, crying, and vigorous sucking, can lead to muscle artifacts in the VEP records, which are sometimes so large that the VEP signal cannot be recognized. Patients who are unable to maintain gaze at the center of the stimulus have variable or absent VEP responses, even when significant visual function is present. Nystagmus is a particular problem because central fixation is impaired and the involuntary eye movements themselves may generate electrical artifacts. Failure to accommodate to bring pattern stimuli into focus on the retina or uncorrected refractive error substantially reduces the amplitudes of pattern VEP responses and may lead to nondetectable VEPs in children who see quite well when the stimuli are in proper focus.

Patients with neurologic diseases present some additional problems for VEP testing. Accurate electrode placement, which is accomplished by careful measurement relative to skull landmarks, may not be possible in patients with abnormal brain anatomy. Artificial alterations in brain anatomy, such as the placement of shunts, may interfere with the ability to record a signal at some sites on the scalp.

Disorders of the Optic Nerve, Chiasm, and Tract

Optic nerve hypoplasia is an ocular malformation diagnosed clinically on the basis of an abnormally small optic nerve head, optic nerve pallor, the "double-ring sign," and tortuous retinal vessels. Functional vision outcome varies widely in this group and outcome is not always associated clearly with the appearance of the optic nerve head. Long-term visual outcome of infants with bilateral optic nerve hypoplasia is correlated with the signal-to-noise ratio of the pattern-onset VEP[49] and amplitude of the flash VEP.[50]

Colobomas of the optic nerve are a rare malformation in which the optic disc is excavated. Like optic nerve hypoplasia, visual function outcomes with coloboma are highly variable. Transient pattern-reversal VEPs appear to be more suitable for analyzing vision in these patients than flash VEPs in predicting functional vision, although flash VEPs are also altered in cases of serious malformation.[51]

The carrier state of Leber hereditary optic neuropathy, a maternally inherited disease associated with mitochondrial point mutations that leads to profound visual impairment, may be detectable via transient pattern VEPs.[52] Prolonged P100 and N135 latencies for 15-minute checks and N135 latencies for 60-minute checks have been reported in asymptomatic carriers. In affected children, VEPs become abnormal immediately after the onset of acute visual loss, and may even be abnormal before symptoms appear in some patients.[53]

Although the current recommendation for screening and monitoring of optic pathway gliomas in children with neurofibromatosis type 1 is an annual ophthalmologic examination, such an examination of young children may be difficult or the findings equivocal. Magnetic resonance imaging (MRI) is very sensitive, but cost and risks to the child preclude its routine use. VEPs have been proposed as a possible alternative or aid in identifying which patients need MRI examinations, and have been reported to have high sensitivity (more than 90 percent) and good specificity (60 to 83 percent).[54–56] Longitudinal changes in flash VEP may be predictive of MRI-assessed changes in optic glioma size and extension.[57]

Pattern-reversal VEPs are abnormal during the acute phase of optic neuritis in children, with a well-preserved waveform but delayed P100.[58] P100 delays may be a sensitive indicator of ethambutol toxicity in children, consistent with the elevated risk for optic neuritis associated with treatment for tuberculosis.[59] With recovery, VEP latency returns to within the normal range in approximately 33 percent of cases, and shows improvement in the remainder.[58] Optic neuritis and the accompanying VEP latency abnormality are most often unilateral in children; bilateral VEP abnormality is associated with an elevated risk for the subsequent diagnosis of multiple sclerosis.[60]

Cortical Visual Impairment

Cortical visual impairment, often referred to as "cortical blindness" before residual visual function was established in many patients, is characterized by severe visual impairment, normal pupillary responses, normal fundus, and no nystagmus. It rarely occurs in isolation; almost all patients have developmental delays and neurologic abnormalities. In early VEP studies of cortical visual impairment, VEPs ranged from normal to nondetectable, which suggested that VEP testing was of little use in evaluating this group of children. These wide-ranging results were probably due to differences in stimulation and recording protocols, in eligibility criteria for the patient cohort, and in timing of the test relative to the onset of visual loss. More recent studies document that virtually all children with carefully defined cortical visual impairment have either abnormal flash or pattern VEPs, or both, and that topographic recording can increase further the sensitivity of VEP protocols in this context.[61,62] VEP acuity is correlated with the Huo scale (a clinical scale of visual function) in children with moderate to severe cortical visual impairment.[63]

About two-thirds of infants with cortical visual impairment show improvements in visual acuity with increasing age. The catch-up phase can be short and highly accelerated in some infants, but for other infants improvement can be protracted.[64,65] It should be noted that there are also reports of abnormal VEPs in children who subsequently recover vision,[66] of behaviorally blind children with normal VEPs who later show recovery,[67,68] and of patients with normal VEPs who remain blind due to damage at higher levels of the visual system beyond area 17.[69,70] VEP testing may also be useful in distinguishing gaze disturbances that limit the infant's ability to fix and follow a visual stimulus, such as oculomotor apraxia, from cortical visual impairment.[65]

In delayed visual maturation, transient flash VEPs are reduced in amplitude and delayed in timing.[69–71] As these findings are also characteristic of infants with permanent cortical visual impairment, it is not possible to use the flash VEP to distinguish infants who will recover from those who will have long-term visual impairment. Delayed myelination of the optic nerves may underlie the flash VEP abnormalities.[72] Pattern VEPs are normal in cases of delayed visual maturation and may provide an avenue for establishing prognosis.[73] Caution is needed when interpreting normal pattern VEPs as good prognostic indicators in a child who appears blind, however, because there are rare reports of children with normal pattern VEPs who are blind due to dysfunction of visual areas beyond area 17.[74]

Flash VEPs are prognostic in cases of acute-onset cortical blindness following surgery, trauma, infectious disease, or hypoxia.[75–77] Within this carefully defined subset of patients with cortical visual impairment, tested immediately after the onset of visual impairment, over 90 percent with normal transient flash VEPs recovered normal visual function. Among those with abnormal or absent transient flash VEPs, over 90 percent had long-term visual impairment or blindness. Thus, flash VEPs have substantial prognostic value when recorded immediately after acute onset of cortical visual loss in pediatric patients.

Perinatal Asphyxia and High-Risk Neonates

Serial measurements of transient flash VEPs during the first week of life may have prognostic value in cases of perinatal asphyxia. McCulloch and colleagues reported that neonates with normal flash VEPs or only transient abnormalities during the first week of life had no long-term visual dysfunction.[78] Among neonates who had no recordable flash VEP response during the first week of life, only one achieved normal vision, while three were blind and two had significant visual impairment. Among children with cerebral visual impairment and a history of neonatal hypoxic-ischemic encephalopathy, VEPs can be used to document visual acuity and to track the slow visual improvement that may occur over 2 to 4 years postnatally.[79]

Flash VEPs have been used to assess the degree of visual impairment in high-risk neonates. Abnormalities in flash VEPs have been demonstrated in infants with grade III intraventricular hemorrhage, but not in infants with milder hemorrhage; the abnormal responses may reflect subcortical rather than cortical visual dysfunction.[27] Abnormal flash VEPs are common in infants with periventricular low-density masses[19]; absence of one or more components of the flash VEP or increased latency of the components has been found in all infants with periventricular leukomalacia. Normal flash VEPs were found in 88 percent of very-low-birthweight infants with normal computed tomographic scans.[19] Flash VEP latency in infants is correlated with their performance on visual-cognitive tasks in the Bayley Scales of Infant Development-II at age 2 years.[80] A recent study by O'Connor and colleagues reported that sweep VEP acuity at 7 to 12 months, but not at 1 to 6 months, was predictive of acuity outcome at age 4 to 8 years in a cohort of children with birthweights of less than 2,000 grams.[81]

Antiepileptic Medications

VEPs are used widely for the evaluation of sensory pathways in epileptic patients receiving different antiepileptic drugs.[82–84] It has been suggested that some antiepileptic drugs can affect VEPs significantly,[85,86] although other authors did not find any difference in evoked potentials between epileptic patients and controls. The controversy may arise from the study of very different cohorts, with some authors examining patients who have just started therapy but the large majority examining adult patients who have received polytherapy for a long time.

Infants with infantile spasms treated with vigabatrin may suffer visual loss due to retinal toxicity. When specialized VEP methodology was used for the assessment of contrast sensitivity and visual fields in preverbal children, treated children were found to show reduced peak contrast sensitivity[87] and visual field defects.[88] Sweep VEP visual acuity may be reduced in infants on vigabatrin therapy, and reduced visual acuity is correlated with retinal toxicity as identified by reduced electroretinogram amplitude.[89]

Cerebral White Matter Disorders

Cerebral white matter disorders include demyelination, hypomyelination, and dysmyelination of white matter from neurodegenerative, metabolic, inflammatory, or developmental defects. Flash VEP abnormalities, such as increased latencies or generally altered waveforms, are present in many but not all children with cerebral white matter disorders.[90] Very few patients with progressive disease have shown a normal flash VEP at any time during development. In general, increased latency correlates with progressive disease, and highly abnormal or nonrecordable flash VEPs are associated with severe disability and poor prognosis.[90] Most infants (more than 75 percent) who develop periventricular leukomalacia have abnormal flash VEPs during the first 2 weeks of life[91] and sweep VEP visual acuity usually is affected severely.[92]

Boys with adrenoleukodystrophy show prolonged flash VEP latency when posterior white matter lesions are present, but asymptomatic boys do not; instead, they exhibit higher than normal flash VEP amplitudes.[93,94] Despite extensive involvement of the central nervous system in mucopolyaccharidosis III, however, nearly all affected children have normal flash VEPs.[95]

Phenylketonuria

Most studies of children and adolescents with phenylketonuria report increased latency of the P100 wave.[96–99] There are some reports of associations between prolonged P100 latency and recent exposure to high phenylalanine levels, the mean phenylalanine level during the first decade of life, the level of phenylalanine measured on the day of the VEP recording, and the age at discontinuation of dietary therapy for phenylketonuria. However, others have found no association with clinical or metabolic measures. Correlations between prolonged latency and severity of cerebral white matter abnormalities on MRI are also controversial.

Prenatal Substance Exposure

Alterations in the flash or pattern VEPs of children prenatally exposed to moderate levels of alcohol, marijuana, tobacco, or other illicit drugs have been noted.[100] Most striking is a delay in P1 latency during the first weeks following birth. Infants exposed to hydroxychloroquine prenatally exhibit delayed pattern VEPs at 3 to 7 months of age,[101] and those exposed to methadone have atypical, immature, or nondetectable flash VEPs during the first week of life.[102]

Methylmercury can produce widespread adverse effects on the development and functioning of the human central nervous system, especially in some fishing communities where infants are exposed prenatally or during early childhood. Prolonged P100 latency has been reported[103] and neuropathologic studies confirm lesions in the visual cortex.[104,105] VEP abnormalities have also been associated with prenatal exposure to organic solvents[106] and with chronic exposure to toxic molds[107] and lead.[108]

Visual Loss of Unknown Etiology and Malingering

VEPs can be a useful adjunct in evaluating children with visual loss of unknown etiology, particularly in distinguishing visual impairment from malingering in children who have a normal ophthalmologic examination. Children who are familiar with eye charts are unfamiliar with striped patterns on video displays and often provide evidence of normal visual acuity in a VEP protocol. Abnormal VEP responses are not necessarily indicative of visual impairment since patients can willfully degrade VEP responses by defocusing the patterns.

REFERENCES

1. Odom J, Bach M, Brigell M et al: ISCEV standard for clinical visual evoked potentials (2009). Doc Ophthalmol, 120:111, 2009
2. Sakaue H, Katsumi O, Mehta M et al: Simultaneous pattern reversal ERG and VER recordings. Effect of stimulus field and central scotoma. Invest Ophthalmol Vis Sci, 31:506, 1990
3. Rabin J, Swittkes E, Crognale M: Visual evoked potentials in three-dimensional color space: correlates of spatiochromatic processing. Vision Res, 34:2657, 1994
4. van der Marel E, Dagnelie G, Spekreijse H: Subdurally recorded pattern and luminance EPs in the alert rhesus monkey. Electroencephalogr Clin Neurophysiol, 57:354, 1984
5. Kraut M, Arezzo J, Vaughan HG, Jr: Intracortical generators of the flash VEP in monkeys. Electroencephalogr Clin Neurophysiol, 62:300, 1985
6. Ducati A, Fava E, Motti E: Neuronal generators of the visual evoked potentials: intracerebral recording in awake humans. Electroencephalogr Clin Neurophysiol, 71:89, 1988
7. Schanel-Klitsch E, Siegfried J: Developmental differences in visual evoked potential slow waves and high frequency wavelets across the lifespan: effects of luminance variation of flash and background. p. 198. In Barber C, Blum T (eds): Evoked Potentials III. Butterworth, Boston, 1987
8. Snyder R: Subcortical visual function in the newborn. Pediat Neurol, 6:333, 1990
9. Dubowitz LMS, Vries LD, Mushin J et al: Visual function in the newborn infant: is it cortically mediated? Lancet, 1(8490):1139, 1986
10. Spekreijse H, Dagnelie G, Maier J et al: Flicker and movement constituents of the pattern reversal response. Vision Res, 25:1297, 1985
11. Dagnelie G, de Vries M, Maier J et al: Pattern reversal stimuli: motion or contrast? Doc Ophthalmol, 31:343, 1986
12. Schroeder C, Tenke C, Givre S et al: Striate cortical contribution to the surface-recorded pattern-reversal VEP in the alert monkey. Vision Res, 31:1143, 1991
13. Di Russo F, Martinez A, Sereno M et al: Cortical sources of the early components of the visual evoked potential. Hum Brain Map, 15:95, 2001
14. Taylor MJ, Menzies R, MacMillan LJ et al: VEPs in normal full-term and premature neonates: longitudinal versus cross-sectional data. Electroencephalogr Clin Neurophysiol, 68:20, 1987
15. Hendrickson A: Morphological development of the primate retina. p. 287. In Simons K (ed): Early Visual Development: Normal and Abnormal. Oxford University Press, New York, 1993

16. Magoon EH, Robb RM: Development of myelin in human optic nerve and tract. A light and electron microscope study. Arch Ophthalmol, 99:655, 1981

17. Huttenlocher PR, De Courten C: The development of synapses in striate cortex of man. Hum Neurobiol, 6:1, 1987

18. Garey L: Structural development of the visual system of man. Hum Neurobiol, 3:75, 1984

19. Kurtzberg D, Vaughan H: Electrophysiologic assessment of auditory and visual function in the newborn. Clin Perinatol, 12:277, 1985

20. Tsuneishi S, Casaer P, Fock J et al: Establishment of normal values for flash visual evoked potentials (VEPs) in preterm infants: a longitudinal study with special reference to two components of the N1 wave. Electroencephalogr Clin Neurophysiol, 96:291, 1995

21. Whyte H, Pearce J, Taylor M: Changes in the VEP in preterm neonates with arousal states, as assessed by EEG monitoring. Electroencephalogr Clin Neurophysiol, 68: 223, 1987

22. Shepherd A, Saunders K, McCulloch D et al: Prognostic value of flash visual evoked potentials in preterm infants. Dev Med Child Neurol, 41:9, 1999

23. Kraemer M, Abrahamsson M, Sjostrom A: The neonatal development of the light flash visual evoked potential. Doc Ophthalmol, 99:21, 1999

24. Tsuneishi S, Casaer P: Stepwise decrease in VEP latencies and the process of myelination in the human visual pathway. Brain Dev, 19:547, 1997

25. Pike A, Marlow N, Reber C: Maturation of flash visual evoked potentials in preterm infants. Early Hum Dev, 54:215, 1999

26. Ellingson R: Cortical electrical responses to visual stimulation in the human infant. Electroencephalogr Clin Neurophysiol, 12:663, 1960

27. Placzek M, Mushin J, Dubowitz LMS: Maturation of the visual evoked response and its correlation with visual acuity development in preterm infants. Dev Med Child Neurol, 27:448, 1985

28. Benavente I, Tamargo P, Tajada N et al: Flash visually evoked potentials in the newborn and their maturation during the first six months of life. Doc Ophthalmol, 110:255, 2005

29. Ellingson RG, Lathrop GH, Danahy T et al: Variability of visual evoked potentials in human infants and adults. Electroencephalogr Clin Neurophysiol, 34: 113, 1973

30. Apkarian P: Temporal frequency responsivity shows multiple maturational phases: state-dependent visual evoked potential luminance flicker fusion from birth to 9 months. Vis Neurosci, 10:1007, 1993

31. Pieh C, McCulloch DL, Shahani U et al: Maturation of steady-state flicker VEP in infants. Doc Ophthalmol, 118:109, 2009

32. McCulloch D, Skarf B: Development of the human visual system: monocular and binocular pattern VEP latency. Invest Ophthalmol Vis Sci, 32:2372, 1991

33. Moskowitz A, Sokol S: Developmental changes in the human visual system as reflected by the latency of the pattern reversal VEP. Electroencephalogr Clin Neurophysiol, 56:1, 1983

34. Sokol S: Measurement of infant visual acuity from pattern reversal evoked potentials. Vision Res, 18:33, 1978

35. McCulloch D, Orbach H, Skarf B: Maturation of the pattern-reversal VEP in human infants: a theoretical framework. Vision Res, 39:3673, 1999

36. Crognale M, Kelly J, Chang B et al: Development of pattern visual evoked potentials: longitudinal measurements in human infants. Optom Vis Sci, 74:808, 1997

37. Birch EE, Birch DG, Petrig B et al: Retinal and cortical function of very low birthweight infants at 36 and 57 weeks post-conception. Clin Vision Sci, 5:363, 1990

38. Malcolm C, McCulloch D: Pattern-reversal visual evoked potentials in infants: gender differences during early visual maturation. Dev Med Child Neurol, 44:345, 2002

39. Fiorentini A, Trimarchi C: Development of temporal properties of pattern electroretinogram and visual evoked potentials in infants. Vision Res, 32:1609, 1992

40. Roy MS, Barsoum-Homsy M, Orquin J et al: Maturation of binocular pattern visual evoked potentials in normal full-term and preterm infants from 1 to 6 months of age. Pediatr Res, 37:140, 1995

41. Birch EE, Birch DG, Hoffman DR et al: Dietary essential fatty acid supply and visual acuity development. Invest Ophthalmol Vis Sci, 33:3242, 1992

42. Porciatti V: Temporal and spatial properties of the pattern-reversal VEPs in infants below 2 months of age. Hum Neurobiol, 3:97, 1984

43. Birch E: Assessing infant acuity, fusion, and stereopsis with visual evoked potentials. p. 353. In Heckenlively J (ed): Principles and Practice of Clinical Electrophysiology. Mosby Year Book, St. Louis, 2006

44. Norcia A, Tyler C: Spatial frequency sweep VEP: visual acuity during the first year of life. Vision Res, 25:1399, 1985

45. Marg E, Freeman D, Peltzman P et al: Visual acuity development in human infants: evoked potential measurements. Invest Ophthalmol Vis Sci, 15:150, 1976

46. Hendrickson AE: Primate foveal development: a microcosm of current questions in neurobiology. Invest Ophthalmol Vis Sci, 35:3129, 1994

47. Salomão SR, Ejzenbaum F, Berezovsky A et al: Age norms for monocular grating acuity measured by sweep-VEP in the first three years of age. Arq Bras Oftalmol, 71:475, 2008

48. Jeffrey B, Weems J, Salomão S et al: Prediction of visual acuity outcome following perinatal cortical insult. Paper presented at the annual meeting of the American Association for Pediatric Ophthalmology and Strabismus, San Diego, 2001

49. Weiss A, Kelly J: Acuity, ophthalmoscopy, and visually evoked potentials in the prediction of visual outcome in infants with bilateral optic nerve hypoplasia. J AAPOS, 7:108, 2003

50. McCulloch DL, Garcia-Filion P, Fink C et al: Clinical electrophysiology and visual outcome in optic nerve hypoplasia (ONH). Br J Ophthalmol, 94:1017, 2010

51. Tormene A, Riva C: Electroretinogram and visual-evoked potentials in children with optic nerve coloboma. Doc Ophthalmol, 96:347, 1999

52. Salomão S: Pattern-reversal visually evoked potential (VEP) in asymptomatic carriers from an extensive Brazilian pedigree with 11778 Leber's hereditary optic neuropathy (LHON). Invest Ophthalmol Vis Sci, 44:E-Abstract 936, 2003

53. Hung H, Kao L, Huang C: Clinical features of Leber's hereditary optic neuropathy with the 11778 mitochondrial DNA mutation in Taiwanese patients. Chang Gung Med, 26:41, 2003

54. Ng Y, North K: Visual evoked potentials in the assessment of optic gliomas. Pediatr Neurol, 24:44, 2002

55. North K, Cochineas C, Tang E et al: Optic gliomas in neurofibromatosis type 1: role of visual evoked potentials. Pediatr Neurol, 10:117, 1994

56. Wolsey DH, Larson SA, Creel D et al: Can screening for optic nerve gliomas in patients with neurofibromatosis type I be performed with visual-evoked potential testing? J AAPOS, 10:307, 2006

57. Falsini B, Ziccardi L, Lazzareschi I et al: Longitudinal assessment of childhood optic gliomas: relationship between flicker visual evoked potentials and magnetic resonance imaging findings. J Neurooncol, 88:87, 2008

58. Suppiej A, Gaspa G, Cappellari A et al: The role of visual evoked potentials in the differential diagnosis of functional visual loss and optic neuritis in children. J Child Neurol, 26:58, 2011

59. Menon V, Jain D, Saxena R et al: Prospective evaluation of visual function for early detection of ethambutol toxicity. Br J Ophthalmol, 93:1251, 2009

60. Wilejto M, Shroff M, Buncic JR et al: The clinical features, MRI findings, and outcome of optic neuritis in children. Neurology, 67:258, 2006

61. Whiting S, Jan J, Wong P: Permanent visual cortical impairment in children. Dev Med Child Neurol, 27:730, 1985

62. Frank Y, Kurtzberg D, Kreuzer J et al: Flash and pattern-reversal visual evoked potential abnormalities in infants and children with cortical blindness. Dev Med Child Neurol, 34:305, 1992

63. Good W: Development of a quantitative method to measure vision in children with chronic cortical visual impairment. Trans Am Ophthalmol Soc, 99:253, 2001

64. Clarke M, Mitchell K, Gibson M: The prognostic value of flash visual evoked potentials in the assessment of non-ocular visual impairment in infancy. Eye, 11:398, 1997

65. Weiss A, Kelly J, Phillipis O: The infant who is visually unresponsive on a cortical basis. Ophthalmology, 108: 2076, 2001

66. Kupersmith M, Nelson J: Preserved visual evoked potential in infant cortical blindness. Neuro-ophthalmology, 6:85, 1986

67. Sokol S, Hedges T, Moskowitz A: Pattern VEPs and preferential looking acuity in infantile traumatic blindness. Clin Vision Sci, 2:59, 1987

68. Regan D, Regal D, Tibbles J: Evoked potentials during recovery from blindness recorded serially from an infant and his normally sighted twin. Electroencephalogr Clin Neurophysiol, 54:465, 1982

69. Harel S, Holtzman M, Feinsod M: Delayed visual maturation. Trans Am Ophthalmol Soc, 104:653, 1983

70. Mellor D, Fielder A: Dissociated visual development: electrodiagnostic studies in infants that are slow to see. Dev Med Child Neurol, 22:327, 1980

71. Fielder AR, Russell-Eggitt IR, Dodd KL et al: Delayed visual maturation. Trans Ophthalmol Soc, 104: 653, 1985

72. Baker RS, Schmeisser ET, Epstein AD: Visual system electrodiagnosis in neurologic disease of childhood. Pediatr Neurol, 12:99, 1995

73. Lambert S, Kriss A, Taylor D: Delayed visual maturation: a longitudinal clinical and electrophysiological assessment. Ophthalmology, 96:524, 1989

74. Bodis-Wollner I, Atkin A, Raab E et al: Visual association cortex and vision in man: pattern-evoked occipital potentials in a blind boy. Science, 198:638, 1977

75. Taylor M, McCulloch D: Prognostic value of VEPs in young children with acute onset of cortical blindness. Pediat Neurol, 7:111, 1991

76. Barnet A, Manson J, Wilner E: Acute cerebral blindness in childhood: six cases studied clinically and electrophysiologically. Neurol, 20:1147, 1970

77. Kupersmith M, Nelson J, Carr R: The visual evoked potential as a prognosticator in childhood cortical blindness. Ann Neurol, 14:146, 1983

78. McCulloch D, Taylor M, Whyte H: Visual evoked potentials and visual prognosis following perinatal asphyxia. Arch Ophthalmol, 109:229, 1991

79. Lim M, Soul JS, Hansen RM et al: Development of visual acuity in children with cerebral visual impairment. Arch Ophthalmol, 123:1215, 2005

80. Feng JJ, Wang TX, Yang CH et al: Flash visual evoked potentials of infants with different birth weights. World J Pediatr, 6:163, 2010

81. O'Connor A, Birch E, Leffler J et al: Visual evoked potential (VEP) and preferential-looking (PL) grating acuity as predictors of long-term visual impairment in low birth weight children. Invest Ophthalmol Vis Sci, 44:E-Abstract 2712, 2003

82. Harding G, Herrick C, Jeavons P: A controlled study of the effect of sodium valproate on photosensitive epilepsy and its prognosis. Epilepsia, 19:555, 1987

83. Cosi V, Callieco R, Galimberti C: Effect of vigabatrin on evoked potentials recordings in patients with epilepsy. Br J Clin Pharmacol, 27:61, 1989

84. Drake M, Pakalnis A, Padamadan H et al: Effect of antiepileptic drug monotherapy and polypharmacy on visual and auditory evoked potentials. Electromyogr Clin Neurophyiol, 29:55, 1989

85. Martinovic Z, Ristanovic D, Dokic-Ristanovic D et al: Pattern reversal evoked potentials recorded in children with generalized epilepsy. Clin Electroencephalogr, 21: 233, 1990

86. Cosi V, Callieco R, Galimberti C: Effect of vigabatrin on visual, brainstem auditory, and somatosensory evoked potentials in epileptic patients. Eur Neurol, 28:42, 1988

87. Mirabella G, Morong S, Buncic JR et al: Contrast sensitivity is reduced in children with infantile spasms. Invest Ophthalmol Vis Sci, 48:3610, 2007

88. Harding G, Robertson K, Spencer E et al: Vigabatrin: its effect on the electrophysiology of vision. Doc Ophthalmol, 104:213, 2002

89. Durbin S, Mirabella G, Buncic JR et al: Reduced grating acuity associated with retinal toxicity in children with infantile spasms on vigabatrin therapy. Invest Ophthalmol Vis Sci, 50:4011, 2009

90. Kristjansdottir R, Sjostrom A, Uverbrant P: Ophthalmological abnormalities in children with cerebral white matter disorders. Eur J Pediatr Neurol, 6:25, 2002

91. Tinelli F, Pei F, Guzzetta A et al: The assessment of visual acuity in children with periventricular damage. Vision Res, 48:1233, 2008

92. Kidokoro H, Okumura A, Kato T et al: Electroencephalogram and flash visual evoked potentials for detecting periventricular leukomalacia. Neuropediatrics, 39:226, 2008

93. Furushima W, Inagaki M, Gunji A et al: Evaluation of preclinical onset in patients with the childhood form of cerebral adrenoleukodystrophy. No To Hattatsu, 40:301, 2008

94. Furushima W, Inagaki M, Gunji A et al: Early signs of visual perception and evoked potentials in radiologically asymptomatic boys with X-linked adrenoleukodystrophy. J Child Neurol, 24:927, 2009

95. Husain AM, Escolar ML, Kurtzberg J: Neurophysiologic assessment of mucopolysaccharidosis III. Clin Neurophysiol, 117:2059, 2006

96. Jones S, Turano G, Kriss A et al: Visual evoked potentials in phenylketonuria: association with brain MRI, dietary state, and IQ. J Neurol Neurosurg Psychiatry, 59:260, 1995

97. Leuzzi V, Cardona F, Antonozzi I et al: Visual, auditory, and somatosensorial evoked potentials in early and late treated adolescents with phenylketonuria. J Clin Neurophysiol, 11:602, 1994

98. Giovannini M, Valsasina R, Villani R: Pattern reversal visual evoked potentials in phenylketonuria. J Inher Metab Dis, 11:416, 1986

99. Korinthenberg R, Ullrich K, Fullenkemper F: Evoked potentials and electroencephalography in adolescents with phenylketonuria. Neuropediatrics, 19:175, 1988

100. Scher M, Richardson G, Robles N et al: Effects of prenatal substance exposure: altered maturation of visual evoked potentials. Pediatr Neurol, 18:236, 1998

101. Renault F, Flores-Guervera R, Renaud C et al: Visual neurophysiological dysfunction in infants exposed to hydroxychloroquine in utero. Acta Paediatr, 98:1500, 2009

102. McGlone L, Mactier H, Hamilton R et al: Visual evoked potentials in infants exposed to methadone in utero. Arch Dis Child, 93:784, 2008

103. Murata K, Weihe P, Renzoni A et al: Delayed evoked potentials in children exposed to methylmercury from seafood. Neurotoxicol Teratol, 21:343, 1999

104. Choi B: The effects of methylmercury on the developing brain. Prog Neurobiol, 32:447, 1989

105. Tokuomi H, Uchino M, Imamura S et al: Minimata disease (organic mercury poisoning): neuroradiologic and electrophysiologic studies. Neurology, 32:1369, 1982

106. Till C, Rovet J, Koren G et al: Assessment of visual functions following prenatal exposure to organic solvents. Neurotoxicology, 24:725, 2003

107. Anyanwu E, Campbell A, Vojdani A: Neurophysiological effects of chronic indoor environmental toxic mold exposure on children. Sci World J, 3:281, 2003

108. Altmann L, Sveinsson K, Kramer U et al: Visual functions in 6-year-old children in relation to lead and mercury levels. Neurotoxicol Teratol, 20:9, 1998

Brainstem Auditory Evoked Potentials: Methodology, Interpretation, and Clinical Application

ALAN D. LEGATT

Following a transient acoustic stimulus, such as a click or a brief tone pip, the ear and parts of the nervous system generate a series of electrical signals with latencies ranging from milliseconds to hundreds of milliseconds. These auditory evoked potentials (AEPs) are conducted through the body tissues and can be recorded from electrodes placed on the skin to evaluate noninvasively the function of the ear and portions of the nervous system activated by the acoustic stimulation. These short-latency or brainstem auditory evoked potentials (BAEPs) have proven to be valuable tools for hearing assessment, diagnosis of neurologic disorders, and intraoperative monitoring.

OVERVIEW OF AUDITORY EVOKED POTENTIALS

AEPs have been divided into short-latency components, with latencies of under 10 msec in adults; long-latency AEPs, with latencies exceeding 50 msec; and middle-latency AEPs, with intermediate latencies (Fig. 24-1). The earliest components derive from electrical processes within the inner ear and action potentials in the auditory nerve. AEP components generated within the brainstem may reflect both action potentials and postsynaptic potentials. Auditory-evoked neural activity becomes

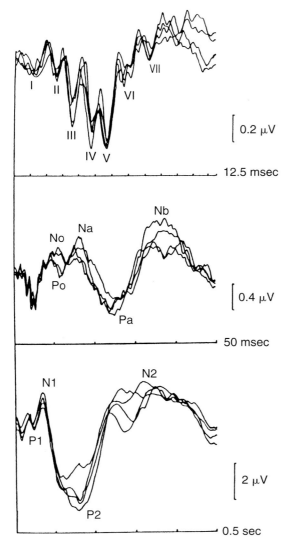

FIGURE 24-1 ■ Short-latency (top), middle-latency (middle), and long-latency (bottom) auditory evoked potentials (AEPs) elicited by monaural click stimuli and recorded in a vertex-mastoid channel with vertex positivity plotted as a downward deflection. Note the differing epoch durations of the three AEPs. (From Picton TW, Hillyard SA, Krausz HI et al: Human auditory evoked potentials. I. Evaluation of components. Electroencephalogr Clin Neurophysiol, 36:179, 1974, with permission.)

affected increasingly by temporal dispersion as the post-stimulus latency increases and as the contribution of short-duration electrical phenomena (e.g., action potentials) is eliminated. Thus, AEP components that are longer in latency are also wider, and the middle- and long-latency AEP components are generated predominantly by postsynaptic potentials within areas of cerebral cortex that are activated by the acoustic stimulus. AEP components are also affected increasingly by the state of the subject and by anesthesia as their latency increases.

Long-latency AEPs are affected profoundly by the degree to which the subject is attending to the stimuli and

analyzing stimulus features (Fig. 24-2). They have therefore been used as probes of cognitive processes, but their variability, as well as uncertainty about the precise identity of their cortical generators, limits their utility for neurologic diagnosis. Middle-latency AEPs are small; are subject to contamination by myogenic signals; and are rather variable from subject to subject, which also limits their clinical application. Both middle- and long-latency AEPs are affected prominently by surgical anesthesia.

Short-latency AEPs have achieved the greatest clinical utility because they are relatively easy to record and their waveforms and latencies are highly consistent across normal subjects. They are unaffected by the subject's degree of attention to the stimuli and are almost identical in the waking and sleeping states,[1] aside from minor differences related to changes in body temperature.[2] Sedation also

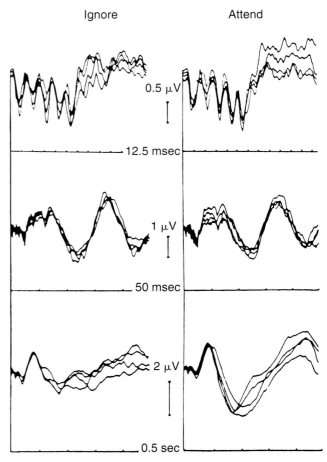

FIGURE 24-2 ■ Effect of attention on auditory evoked potentials. Trains of clicks that were occasionally lower in intensity were presented, and the subject was asked either to ignore the clicks (left) or to attend to them and count the number of softer ones (right). Recording conditions were otherwise the same as Figure 24-1. (From Picton TW, Hillyard SA: Human auditory evoked potentials. II: Effects of attention. Electroencephalogr Clin Neurophysiol, 36:191, 1974, with permission.)

produces only minor changes in BAEPs, and has been employed during BAEP recordings. However, the use of sedation for evoked potential recordings has been reduced markedly owing to concerns about monitoring and the care of patients during conscious sedation.[3] Because a typical surgical level of anesthesia produces only minor alterations in BAEPs (Fig. 24-3),[4,5] they can be used for intraoperative monitoring of the ears and the auditory pathways.

The earliest electrical signals produced by the auditory system in response to a transient stimulus, constituting the electrocochleogram (ECochG), initially were recorded by electrodes placed directly in the middle ear.[6] Extratympanic recordings of the ECochG yielded smaller signals that required signal averaging to achieve an adequate signal-to-noise ratio.[7] Signal averaging also permitted recording of small time-locked signals originating from other locations. Additional deflections with latencies of several milliseconds after auditory stimulation were recorded first in humans during signal-averaged ECochG studies by Sohmer and Feinmesser.[8] Jewett and co-workers identified the short-latency scalp-recorded AEPs as far-field potentials volume-conducted from the brainstem, described the components and their properties, and established the Roman numeral labeling of the peaks that is used in most laboratories (Fig. 24-4).[9,10] A far-field potential is a potential (voltage) recorded at a sufficiently large distance from its source that small movements of the recording electrode have no significant effect on the waveform.

Although short-latency AEPs commonly are called brainstem auditory evoked potentials, this term is not completely accurate because the roster of generators clearly includes the distal (with respect to the brainstem) cochlear nerve and may also include the thalamocortical auditory radiations, neither of which is within the brainstem. Nonetheless, the designation BAEP is used in this

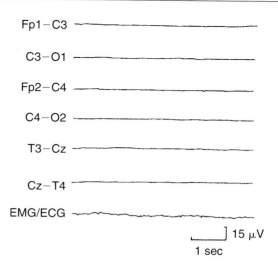
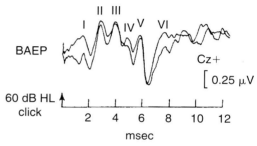

FIGURE 24-3 ▪ Brainstem auditory evoked potentials recorded during surgery in a patient anesthetized with isoflurane at a concentration sufficient to render the electroencephalogram isoelectric. Although the amplitudes of waves IV, V, VI, and VII were reduced by anesthesia, the latencies of waves I through V were not significantly different from those recorded in this patient in the unanesthetized state. (From Stockard JJ, Pope-Stockard JE, Sharbrough FW: Brainstem auditory evoked potentials in neurology: methodology, interpretation, and clinical application. p. 514. In Aminoff MJ [ed]: Electrodiagnosis in Clinical Neurology. 3rd Ed. Churchill Livingstone, New York, 1992, with permission.)

FIGURE 24-4 ▪ Normal brainstem auditory evoked potential recorded between the vertex (Cz) and the right ear lobe (A2) following right ear stimulation in a 23-year-old woman. Two averages of 2,000 sweeps each are superimposed. Vertex-positive peaks, shown here as upward deflections, are labeled with Roman numerals according to the convention of Jewett and Williston.[10] Downgoing peaks after waves I and V are labeled IN and VN, respectively. An electrical stimulus artifact appears at the beginning of the tracings.

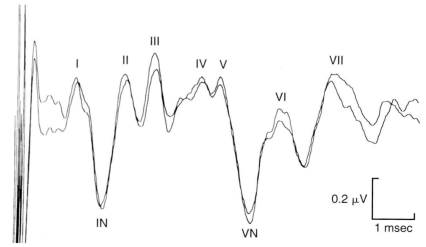

chapter because it is the most widely used and understood term. Other synonyms or related designations include auditory brainstem response, far-field electrocochleography, and brainstem audiometry.

STANDARD BAEP RECORDING TECHNIQUES

This section describes the standard techniques used to record BAEPs in adult subjects. BAEP recording techniques for infants and children are described in Chapter 25, and intraoperative BAEP monitoring is discussed in Chapter 30. The American Clinical Neurophysiology Society has published guidelines for clinical BAEP recordings.[11,12]

Stimulation

BAEPs are elicited most commonly by brief acoustic click stimuli that are produced by delivering monophasic square pulses of 100-μsec duration to headphones or other electromechanical transducers at a rate of about 10 Hz. A rate of exactly 10 Hz or another submultiple of the power line frequency should be avoided; otherwise, the inevitable line frequency artifact will be time-locked to the stimuli and will not be removed by the averaging process. Audiometric headphones having a relatively flat frequency response are desirable so that "broad-band" clicks, whose energy is spread over a wide frequency range, will be produced.

The stimulus intensity should be loud enough to elicit a clear BAEP waveform without causing discomfort or ear damage; 60 to 65 dB HL is a typical level. If hearing loss is present, stimulus intensity may be adjusted accordingly so that stimulation is at 60 to 65 dB SL. (It should be noted that dB HL is decibels relative to the threshold of a normal population, dB SL is decibels relative to the threshold of the ear being tested, and dB nHL is decibels relative to the threshold of the specific control population used to establish a laboratory's normative database.) Reduced stimulus intensities are also useful during BAEP recordings, as discussed later in this chapter. The subjective click threshold should be measured in all subjects in whom this is possible, to recognize hearing loss and to determine the stimulus level corresponding to 0 dB SL.

Stimuli are delivered monaurally, so that a normal BAEP to stimulation of one ear does not obscure the presence of an abnormal response to stimulation of the other ear. An acoustic stimulus delivered to one ear via headphones can reach the other ear via air and bone conduction with a volume attenuation of 40 to 70 dB and generate an evoked potential by stimulation of the contralateral ear (Fig. 24-5).[13,14] To prevent this contralateral stimulation from occurring and possibly being misinterpreted as a BAEP arising from stimulation of the ipsilateral ear, the contralateral ear is masked with continuous white noise at an intensity 30 to 40 dB below that of the BAEP stimulus. Acoustic crosstalk also occurs with ear-insert transducers, though the signal reaching the opposite ear is attenuated to an even greater extent, typically 70 to 100 dB.[14]

If the electrical square pulse causes the diaphragm of the acoustic transducer to move toward the patient's ear, a propagating wave of increased air pressure, termed

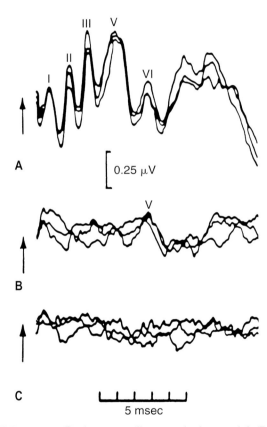

FIGURE 24-5 ■ Brainstem auditory evoked potentials (BAEPs) to monaural stimulation from a patient with one nonfunctioning ear. **A**, Stimulation of the unaffected ear elicits a normal BAEP. **B**, When contralateral noise masking is not used, stimulation of the nonfunctioning ear produces a delayed wave V because of air and bone conduction of the stimulus to the other ear. **C**, When masking noise is delivered to the unaffected ear, stimulation of the nonfunctioning ear does not elicit any reproducible BAEPs. (Modified from Chiappa K, Gladstone KJ, Young RR: Brain stem auditory evoked responses. Studies of waveform variations in 50 normal human subjects. Arch Neurol, 36:81, 1979, with permission.)

a *compression click* (also called a *condensation click*) is produced. Reversing the polarity of the electrical square pulse that activates the transducer produces a *rarefaction click*. BAEPs to rarefaction and compression clicks may differ (most prominently in patients with a cochlear high-frequency hearing loss),[15] and averaging the responses to the two click polarities together may produce a composite waveform with less diagnostic utility. Therefore, a single stimulus polarity should be used unless alternating polarities are necessary for canceling the electrical stimulus artifact or cochlear microphonic. Rarefaction clicks are generally preferable because they tend to yield BAEPs with better definition of the components; this may be because the initial cochlear movements produced by rarefaction clicks are in a direction that depolarizes the hair cells. In evaluating a patient's BAEPs, the normative data used should have been acquired with the same stimulus polarity used to test the patient.

Recording

Recording electrodes typically are placed at the vertex (location Cz of the International 10–20 System) and at both ear lobes. (The ear lobes ipsilateral and contralateral to the stimulated ear are labeled Ai and Ac, respectively.) Electrodes at the mastoids (labeled Mi and Mc) may be substituted for the ear-lobe placements, although wave I tends to be smaller. Such placement, in combination with increased pickup of muscle noise, yields a poorer signal-to-noise ratio for wave I with mastoid leads than with ear-lobe leads. The ground electrode is often placed on the forehead, but its precise location is not critical. Metal cup or pellet electrodes may be used; needle electrodes should be avoided. Electrode impedance should be less than 5 kohm. Optimally, the same type of electrode should be used at all recording positions, and electrode impedance should be as consistent as possible across all recording electrodes, because mismatched electrode impedances can increase the amount of noise in the BAEP data.[16]

BAEPs should be recorded between Cz and either Ai or Mi. A minimum of a two recording-channel system, with Cz–Ac or Cz–Mc in the second channel, has been recommended because this channel may aid in the identification of waves IV and V, which may be fused in the channel 1 waveform.[12] An Ac–Ai or Mc–Mi channel may assist in the identification of wave I, and can be substituted in channel 2 when necessary, or can be recorded as a standard part of all tests if more than two recording channels are available.

The raw analog data are amplified by high input-impedance differential amplifiers with a common mode rejection ratio of at least 80 dB (10,000 : 1).[11] A typical analog filter bandpass is 100 Hz or 150 Hz to 3,000 Hz (−3 dB points). The analog gain depends on the input window of the analog-to-digital converter; a value of approximately 100,000 is typical.

Data typically are digitized over an epoch duration or analysis time of approximately 10 msec. (The analysis time in some recording systems is actually 10.24 msec.) However, a longer analysis time of 15 msec may be required for recording pathologically delayed BAEPs, BAEPs to lowered stimulus intensities (as when recording a latency–intensity study), BAEPs in children, and BAEPs during intraoperative monitoring. The Nyquist criterion requires analog-to-digital conversion with a sampling rate of at least 6,000 Hz (2 × 3,000 Hz) in each channel to avoid aliasing, but higher sampling rates are required for accurate reproduction of the BAEP waveform and precise measurement of peak latencies. The analog-to-digital conversion should use at least 256 points per epoch; sampling of a 10.24-msec epoch at 256 time points corresponds to a sampling interval of 0.4 msec and a sampling rate of 25,000 Hz.

Far-field BAEPs are too small to be visible in unaveraged raw data, and so signal averaging is required. The improvement in the signal-to-noise ratio is proportional to the square root of the number of data epochs included in the average. Automatic artifact rejection is used to exclude sweeps with high-amplitude noise from the average. The number of epochs per trial is typically 2,000, although a larger number may be required if the signal-to-noise ratio is poor (usually reflecting a low-amplitude BAEP or noisy raw data). At least two separate averages should be recorded and superimposed to assess reproducibility of the BAEP waveforms. Latency replication to within 1 percent of the sweep time and amplitude replication to within 15 percent of the peak-to-peak amplitude have been recommended as standards for adequate reproducibility.[11]

Waveform Identification and Measurement

When recording far-field potentials such as the BAEPs, the two electrodes connected to the inputs of a differential amplifier cannot be considered active and reference electrodes. The voltage distributions of the BAEPs extend over most, if not all, of the head, and no cephalic electrode can be considered to be truly inactive for all components. For example, wave V in the Cz–Ai BAEP waveform largely reflects positivity at the vertex, whereas wave I is derived from a negativity around the stimulated ear that is picked up by the Ai electrode. Thus, both input electrodes must be specified when describing a BAEP waveform.

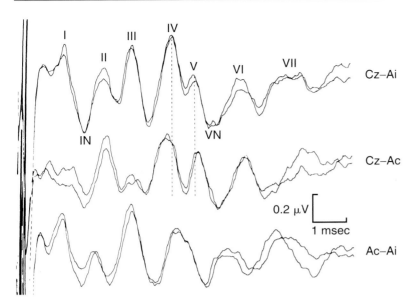

FIGURE 24-6 ■ Brainstem auditory evoked potentials recorded simultaneously from three different recording electrode linkages following monaural stimulation. The vertical dashed lines indicate the peak latencies of waves IV and V in the Cz–Ai waveforms. Note the decreased wave IV latency and the increased wave V latency in the Cz–Ac waveforms.

The Cz–Ai BAEP typically is displayed so that positivity at the vertex relative to the stimulated ear is displayed as an upward deflection, and the upward-pointing peaks are labeled with Roman numerals according to the convention established by Jewett and Williston[10] (see Fig. 24-4; Fig. 24-6). The downward-pointing peaks are labeled with the suffix N according to the peak that they follow; for example, downward peak IN follows upward wave I. The downward deflection following wave V, which has also been labeled the slow negativity (SN), is typically wider than the positive components and the earlier negative peaks.

Recognition and identification of the components in BAEP waveforms obtained with standard recording techniques will now be described. Modifications in the recording paradigm that can be used to enhance specific BAEP components are discussed later in this chapter.

The BAEP waveform typically begins with an electrical stimulus artifact that is synchronous with stimulus production at the transducer. Wave I is the first major upgoing peak of the Cz–Ai BAEP. It appears as an upgoing peak of similar amplitude in the Ac–Ai waveform and is markedly attenuated or absent in the Cz–Ac waveform (see Fig. 24-6). The cochlear microphonic may be visible as a separate peak preceding wave I, especially if the stimulus artifact is small. Its scalp distribution is similar to that of wave I. They may be distinguished by reversing the stimulus polarity, which will reverse the polarity of the cochlear microphonic; wave I may show a latency shift, but will not reverse polarity.

A bifid wave I is occasionally present and represents contributions to wave I from different portions of the cochlea. The earlier of the two peaks, which reflects activation of the base of the cochlea, corresponds to the single wave I that is typically present in the Cz–Ai waveform. Reversal of stimulus polarity can be used to distinguish a bifid wave I from a cochlear microphonic followed by (a single) wave I.

In contrast to wave I, wave IN is present at substantial amplitude in the Cz–Ac channel (see Fig. 24-6). This downgoing deflection is usually the earliest BAEP component in that waveform.

Wave II is typically the first major upward deflection in the Cz–Ac waveform because wave I is markedly attenuated or absent there. When present, wave II is usually of similar amplitude in the Cz–Ai and Cz–Ac channels (see Fig. 24-6). However, wave II may be small and difficult to identify in some normal subjects.

A substantial wave III is usually present in both the Cz–Ai and Ac–Ai channels. Wave III in the Cz–Ac waveform is usually substantially smaller than that in the Cz–Ai waveform (see Fig. 24-6). This difference helps to distinguish it from wave II, whose amplitude is little changed by the change in the ear electrode. The peak latency of wave III decreases slightly, whereas that of wave II increases slightly when the inverting amplifier input is changed from Ai to Ac; thus, the Cz–Ai waveform tends to give better separation of waves II and III than does the Cz–Ac waveform. A bifid wave III occasionally is observed as a normal variant (Fig. 24-7); the wave III latency in such waveforms can be scored as midway between the peak latencies of the two subcomponents. Rarely, wave III may be poorly formed or absent in a patient with a clear wave V and a normal I–V interpeak interval; this finding is best interpreted as a normal variant waveform.

Waves IV and V are often fused into a IV/V complex whose morphology varies from one subject to another, and may differ between the two ears in the same person

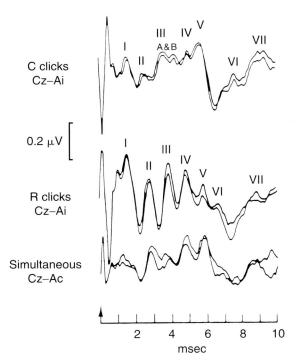

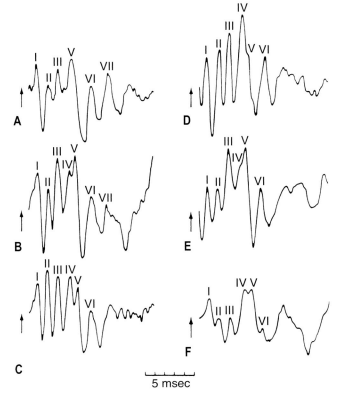

FIGURE 24-7 ▪ Brainstem auditory evoked potentials recorded from a normal subject following stimulation with compression (C) and rarefaction (R) clicks. Prominent differences in wave shape are evident between the two stimulus polarities. The latency of wave VI and the relative amplitudes of waves IV and V are affected markedly by the click polarity. The lowest point in the waveform after wave V precedes wave VI with compression clicks and follows wave VI with rarefaction clicks. A bifid wave III is present in the Cz–Ai waveform elicited by compression clicks. (By permission of the Mayo Foundation.)

FIGURE 24-8 ▪ Various IV/V complex morphologies in Cz–Ai waveforms recorded in normal subjects. (From Chiappa K, Gladstone KJ, Young RR: Brain stem auditory evoked responses. Studies of waveform variations in 50 normal human subjects. Arch Neurol, 36:81, 1979, with permission.)

(Fig. 24-8). The IV/V complex is often the most prominent component in the BAEP waveform. It usually is followed by a large negative deflection that lasts several milliseconds and brings the waveform to a point below the prestimulus baseline. Occasionally, the most negative point in the waveform follows wave VI (see Fig. 24-7), which could lead to misinterpretation of wave VI as an abnormally delayed wave V. The identity of wave V can be clarified by changes in recording montage or click polarity (see Figs. 24-6 and 24-7) or by reducing the stimulus intensity and/or increasing the stimulus rate to attenuate wave VI relative to wave V. In distinguishing between a totally fused IV/V complex and a single wave IV or V, Epstein notes that the former has a "base" that is greater than 1.5 msec in duration, whereas the width of a single wave is less than 1.5 msec.[17]

When waves IV and V overlap in the Cz–Ai waveform, the wave V latency measurement used for BAEP interpretation should be taken from the second subcomponent of the IV/V complex, even if this is not the highest peak (in contrast to the amplitude measurement used to calculate the IV/V:I amplitude ratio, which is taken from the highest point in the complex). Measurement of the peak latency of wave V may be inaccurate if V appears only as an inflection on the falling edge of wave IV (see Fig. 24-8) and it may be impossible if they are fused smoothly. Two approaches may be used in such cases. The first involves measurement of wave V latency in a Cz–Ac recording channel. The overlapping peaks are separated more clearly there because the latency of wave IV is typically earlier, and that of wave V is later, than in the Cz–Ai waveform (see Fig. 24-6). However, because of these latency shifts, wave V latency values measured in a Cz–Ac waveform should be compared with normative data in which the latency of wave V was also measured in a Cz–Ac recording. The other approach is to reduce the stimulus intensity to attenuate wave IV relative to wave V and permit accurate measurement of the peak latency of wave V. That latency value cannot be compared with normative data obtained at a higher stimulus intensity, but the I–V interpeak interval can be evaluated because it is affected minimally by changes in stimulus intensity.

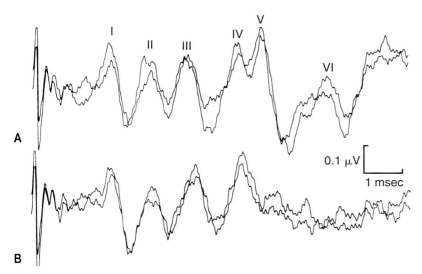

FIGURE 24-9 ■ Brainstem auditory evoked potentials (BAEPS) to left ear stimulation recorded (Cz–Ai) during surgery for a basilar artery aneurysm. The aneurysm ruptured and the basilar artery was clipped transiently to control the bleeding. The patient suffered a brainstem infarct. **A,** Clear waves I through VI were present in these BAEPs recorded just before the aneurysm ruptured. **B,** BAEPs recorded after the clip was removed show a loss of waves V and VI. Waves I through IV were unaffected. (Modified from Legatt AD, Arezzo JC, Vaughan HG, Jr: The anatomic and physiologic bases of brain stem auditory evoked potentials. Neurol Clin, 6:681, 1988, with permission.)

It is important to distinguish wave V from wave IV. If wave V were delayed abnormally, but an earlier and larger wave IV (which dominated the IV/V complex) were mistaken for wave V, the BAEP abnormality might be missed. If the latency of an apparent wave V is abnormally short, efforts should be made to determine whether this peak is, in fact, a dominant wave IV. Lesions that affect wave V almost always also affect wave IV, but rarely wave IV may be unaltered (Fig. 24-9).

Clinical interpretation of BAEPs is based predominantly on the latencies of waves I, III, and V. Once these peaks have been identified and their latencies measured, the I–III, III–V, and I–V interpeak intervals are calculated. The latency of wave I has also been labeled the peripheral transmission time (PTT) and the I–V interpeak interval has been called the central transmission time (CTT). Differences of component latencies and interpeak intervals between stimulation of the right and left ears are also calculated.

The amplitudes of wave I and the IV/V complex are measured, each with respect to the most negative point that follows it in the waveform (I to IN and IV/V to VN), and their ratio is calculated. An excessively small IV/V:I amplitude ratio can identify as abnormal some BAEP waveforms in which all component latencies and interpeak intervals are normal (Fig. 24-10). It sometimes has been called the V:I amplitude ratio. However, most studies establishing the value of this quantity measured the amplitude from the highest peak of the IV/V complex to VN, not from the wave V peak to VN. Measuring the latter may give an abnormally small ratio in normal waveforms in which the peak of wave IV is much higher than that of wave V.

Patient Relaxation and Sedation

The amplifier bandpass used for BAEP recordings filters out all of the delta, theta, alpha, and beta bands of the electroencephalogram (EEG), and the biologically derived noise in the recordings is derived predominantly from muscle activity. Therefore, patient relaxation

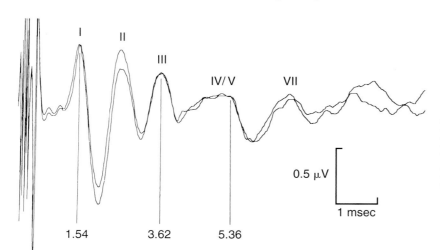

FIGURE 24-10 ■ Brainstem auditory evoked potential (Cz–Ai) in a 27-year-old woman with probable multiple sclerosis. The IV/V:I amplitude ratio is 0.28; all absolute latencies and interpeak intervals are normal. The stimulus intensity was 65 dB nHL.

during the recording session is essential to obtain "clean" waveforms with a good signal-to-noise ratio. Patients usually are tested while lying comfortably so that their neck musculature is relaxed. Patients should be requested to let their mouth hang open if the muscles of mastication are tensed. They are encouraged to sleep during testing because this aids relaxation and will not alter the BAEPs.

If the patient cannot relax sufficiently, sedation can be induced with agents such as chloral hydrate, a short-acting barbiturate, or a benzodiazepine; these have little or no effect on BAEPs in the usual sedative doses.

MODIFICATIONS TO BAEP RECORDING TECHNIQUES

Reducing the Stimulus Artifact

The transient electrical current in the transducer that generates the acoustic stimulus produces a transient electromagnetic field, which in turn induces a voltage in the patient and in the recording leads. This voltage creates an electrical stimulus artifact that, if large and prolonged, may overlap with wave I and impair the identification and measurement of that component. Using shielded headphones and headphones with piezoelectric transducers instead of voice coil transducers can reduce this artifact.[18] Transducers that are connected to an ear insert by flexible plastic tubing several centimeters in length may also be used to mitigate this problem. The BAEPs, including wave I, are delayed by the time required for the acoustic stimulus to propagate through the plastic tube, but the electrical stimulus artifact remains simultaneous with transducer activation; the increased temporal separation between them permits greater decay of the electrical artifact before wave I. The greater distance between the transducer and the earlobe or mastoid recording site also serves to reduce the amplitude of the electrical stimulus artifact. The delay introduced by the plastic tube must be considered when one interprets BAEP latencies; passage through the tube may also change the acoustic properties of the stimulus. Ideally, the normative data used for BAEP interpretation should have been acquired with the same techniques that are used to test the patients. When ear inserts are used, they may be covered with metal foil to serve as near-field recording electrodes for wave I, thereby yielding a larger wave I.

Responses to compression and rarefaction clicks may be averaged together to reduce the electrical stimulus artifact by cancellation. Most evoked potential recording systems have an option for alternating the click polarity during stimulus delivery. This option should be avoided if possible during diagnostic testing because the BAEPs elicited by the two click polarities may differ.[15] Stimulus artifact is usually more of a problem in the operating room environment, and alternating click polarity is often necessary during intraoperative BAEP monitoring. In this setting, the BAEPs are being compared with signals recorded earlier in the same patient with the identical stimulus paradigm, so the admixture of responses to the two stimulus polarities is less of a problem.

Improving the Resolution of Specific Components

Wave I may be small and difficult to record in some patients, especially if hearing loss is present. Several techniques can be used to obtain a clearer wave I. Because wave I is a near-field potential, relatively small movements of the Ai/Mi recording electrode can have a substantial effect on its amplitude. Thus, alternative electrode positions around the stimulated ear can be used. An electrode within the external auditory canal yields an even larger wave I, and may take the form of a metal foil covering on an ear insert or a spring-leaf electrode that makes contact with the wall of the canal.

Although wave I appears predominantly because of the presence of a near-field negativity at the Ai electrode, the horizontal orientation of its dipole projects a small positivity to the contralateral ear. Accordingly, an Ac–Ai recording channel can yield a somewhat larger and clearer wave I than that in the standard Cz–Ai recording.

Modifications in stimulus parameters are also useful in obtaining a clearer wave I. Alternating stimulus polarity can be useful by attenuating a large stimulus artifact that is obscuring wave I or by helping to differentiate wave I from the cochlear microphonic. A reduction in the stimulus repetition rate may yield a clearer wave I. Increasing the stimulus intensity is particularly helpful in improving the clarity of wave I and may be used if that peak is not clearly identifiable at standard intensities in the presence of hearing loss. One caveat is that in patients with a high-frequency hearing loss of cochlear origin, this maneuver yields interpeak intervals that are shorter than those of normal subjects. This difference in interpeak intervals probably reflects contributions to wave I from different portions of the cochlea. At normal intensities, the earliest peak, which reflects activation of the base of the cochlea, predominates. At higher intensities, a somewhat longer-latency component becomes increasingly prominent. If the earlier component is missing because of high-frequency hearing loss, and if stimulus intensity is increased, the wave I that appears may predominantly reflect the longer-latency contribution; the I–III and I–V interpeak intervals are thus shorter than those that would have been measured from the usual wave I. Measurement of the PTT from this longer-latency subcomponent would decrease the sensitivity of the test for recognition of prolonged I–III or I–V interpeak intervals.

Wave V is often fused with wave IV into a IV/V complex in the Cz–Ai BAEP waveform. A Cz–Ac recording channel helps to identify wave V by increasing the separation between the peaks of these two components; the latency of wave IV is shorter and that of wave V is longer than in the Cz–Ai recording (see Fig. 24-6). Because of this latency shift, the latency of wave V in a patient's Cz–Ac waveform should be compared with normal values derived from Cz–Ac recordings in control subjects.

Modifications of the stimulus parameters can also be used to identify wave V if it is unclear when standard recording techniques are used. Wave V is the BAEP component most resistant to the effects of decreasing stimulus intensity (Fig. 24-11) or increasing stimulus rate. If either of these stimulus modifications is performed progressively until only one component remains, that peak can be identified as wave V and then traced back through the series of waveforms to identify wave V in

the BAEP recorded with the standard stimulus. Occasionally, wave V may be present following stimulation with one click polarity but not the other (Fig. 24-12). Therefore, recording a BAEP with the opposite stimulus polarity may be useful if wave V is not identifiable with the standard laboratory protocol.

Stimulation at Several Intensities

In a patient with a conductive hearing loss, the stimulus intensity reaching the cochlea is less than that delivered to the external ear, and an abnormal BAEP with a delayed or absent wave I may result. If the stimulus intensity is increased to compensate for the conductive hearing loss, and no coexisting sensorineural hearing loss is present, a normal BAEP will be recorded. In contrast, BAEPs that are delayed as a result of abnormally slowed neural conduction do not normalize when the stimulus intensity is increased (Fig. 24-13). Thus, increasing the stimulus intensity can help to differentiate peripheral from neural abnormalities, especially when wave I is not clear. The degree of hearing loss can be estimated by the elevation of the subjective auditory click threshold; increasing the stimulus intensity to compensate for this elevation is thus equivalent to stimulating at a specific intensity above that threshold

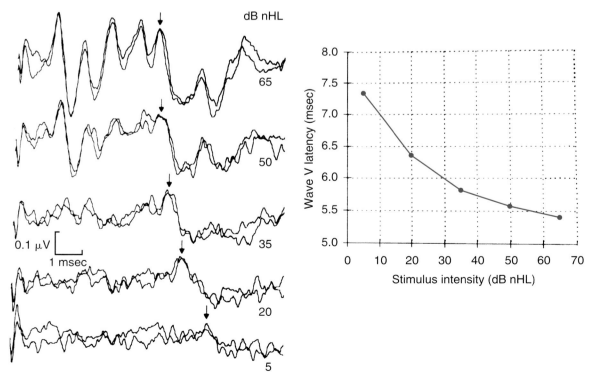

FIGURE 24-11 ■ Brainstem auditory evoked potentials (BAEPs) recorded at progressively lower stimulus intensities are shown on the left. Wave V latencies (arrows) are measured and then plotted as a function of stimulus intensity to give the latency–intensity curve on the right. This 35-year-old woman with dizziness and tinnitus had normal BAEPs and normal magnetic resonance imaging findings.

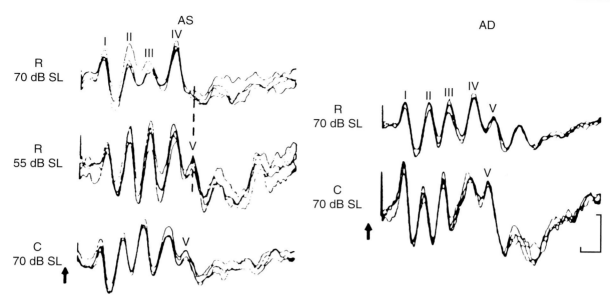

FIGURE 24-12 ▪ Brainstem auditory evoked potentials elicited by rarefaction (R) and compression (C) clicks of several different intensities. Wave V is absent following left ear (AS) stimulation with 70 dB SL rarefaction clicks but appears when the stimulus intensity is decreased to 55 dB SL or when stimulus polarity is reversed. A clear wave V is present following right ear (AD) stimulation with 70 dB SL clicks of either polarity. The calibration bars are 0.25 μV and 1.0 msec. (From Emerson RG, Brooks EB, Parker SW et al: Effects of click polarity on brainstem auditory evoked potentials in normal subjects and patients: unexpected sensitivity of wave V. Ann N Y Acad Sci, 388:710, 1982, with permission.)

(e.g., at 60 to 65 dB SL rather than at 60 to 65 dB HL). The normative data to which such recordings are compared should also have been recorded at a specific intensity in dB SL, rather than dB HL.

If each ear is stimulated at several different intensities, and the latency of wave V is graphed as a function of stimulus intensity, a latency–intensity curve is produced (see Fig. 24-11). Examination of latency–intensity curves may help to classify a patient's hearing loss.[19] A shift of the curve to a higher intensity level without a change in its shape suggests conductive hearing loss, whereas a change in the shape of the curve with an increased slope suggests sensorineural hearing loss. Latency–intensity curves may also reveal abnormalities that are not demonstrated by BAEP recordings at the standard, relatively high stimulus intensity typically used in BAEP studies performed for neurologic diagnosis.[20]

Rapid Stimulation

A stimulus rate of approximately 10 Hz is used for routine clinical testing; this is because some of the BAEP components become attenuated and less clearly defined and the interpeak intervals lengthen as the rate is increased substantially above this. Measurement of the BAEP threshold is based solely on the presence or absence of wave V because it is the last BAEP component to disappear as the stimulus intensity is reduced. Because wave V is relatively resistant to the effects of rapid stimulation, recordings

made solely for threshold measurement can be accomplished more rapidly by increasing the stimulus rate to 50 to 70 Hz. However, rapid stimulation can make BAEPs undetectable, especially in premature infants. Thus, infants who appear to have a hearing loss on BAEP screening using rapid stimulation should be retested using a slower stimulation rate.[21]

When stimuli are delivered at a rate of about 10 Hz, the neural elements generating the BAEPs have approximately 100 msec to recover after responding to one stimulus before they must respond to the next. It has been speculated that, in some pathologic states, action potential propagation or synaptic transmission occurs normally with recovery times of this magnitude but is delayed when recovery times are shorter. If this were the case, more rapid stimulation would demonstrate BAEP abnormalities in some patients with normal BAEPs to the standard stimuli, thus increasing the sensitivity of the test. Rapid stimulation has been reported to increase the test sensitivity of BAEPs in patients with neurologic abnormalities in some, but not all, studies.

Alternative Auditory Stimuli

The standard BAEP stimulus is a "broad-band" click produced when an electrical square pulse is delivered to the headphone or other electromechanical transducer. It is generated predominantly by the region of the cochlea responding to 2,000- to 4,000-Hz sounds, although wave

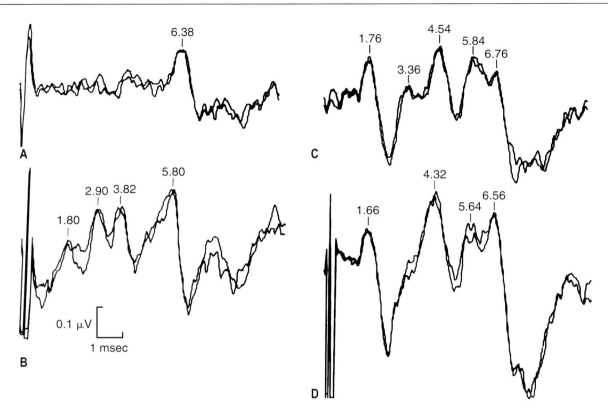

FIGURE 24-13 ■ Brainstem auditory evoked potentials (BAEPs) elicited by two different stimulus intensities in two patients and recorded in Cz–Ai montage. **A**, Left ear stimulation at 70 dB nHL elicits an abnormally delayed wave V in a 36-year-old woman with a peripheral hearing loss in the left ear. Wave I is not visible. **B**, When the stimulus intensity is increased to 85 dB nHL, wave I becomes identifiable and the latency of wave V is decreased markedly. Interpeak intervals are normal. **C**, Left ear stimulation at 65 dB nHL in a 14-year-old boy with a fourth ventricular tumor elicits clear BAEPs with a normal wave I latency and an abnormally delayed wave V. The I–III and I–V interpeak intervals both are prolonged abnormally. **D**, An increase in the stimulus intensity to 85 dB nHL causes a slight decrease in all component latencies. Wave V remains abnormally delayed, and the I–III and I–V interpeak intervals remain abnormally prolonged.

V may also receive contributions from lower-frequency regions of the cochlea. BAEPs have also been recorded following stimulation with brief tone pips, in an effort to probe specific parts of the cochlea. This method can be used to determine thresholds at different frequencies for BAEP audiometry. Tone pips most often are generated with stimuli consisting of brief bursts of sine waves. The burst cannot be stopped and started abruptly because an audible "click" containing many frequencies would be produced. Instead, the sine wave stimulus is amplitude-modulated with a rise-time, plateau, and fall-time to reduce (although not eliminate) the energy content of the stimulus at other frequencies. A filtered click, which is obtained by passing a broad-band click through a bandpass filter, has also been used as a frequency-specific stimulus.

Another technique that can be used to obtain frequency-specific information from BAEPs is acoustic masking. In one approach, the broad-band clicks used to elicit the BAEPs are superimposed on white noise that has been highpass-filtered by using different cut-off

frequencies in different runs. Each BAEP waveform is generated predominantly by the unmasked region of the cochlea and represents a response to frequencies lower than the cut-off frequency used during that run. Subtraction of one such response from another yields a "derived" response that estimates the response to the frequency band between the cut-off frequencies of the two runs (Fig. 24-14). The subtraction process yields waveforms with relatively poor signal-to-noise ratios, however.[22]

Frequency-specific stimuli and frequency-specific masking can be combined by embedding tone pips in continuous notched noise. The latter is white noise that has been notch-filtered to remove the basic frequency of the tone pip. Shaping a pure tone into a pip with an onset and an offset introduces power at other frequencies into its frequency spectrum, which would impair the frequency specificity of the test, but the notched noise masks the responses to frequencies other than the basic frequency of the tone pip. BAEP audiograms produced with such stimuli are similar to behavioral audiograms in the same

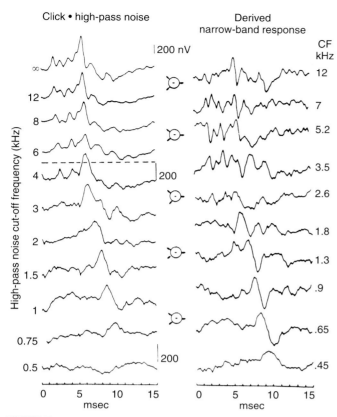

Click • high-pass noise   Derived
                                narrow-band response

FIGURE 24-14 ■ Derivation of frequency-specific brainstem auditory evoked potentials (BAEPs) with high-pass noise masking. Alternating-polarity, 170-μsec-duration clicks at an intensity of 60 dB SL were delivered at a rate of 13 Hz. The noise, which was delivered to the same ear, was highpass-filtered with cascaded filters to produce a filter function with a slope of 96 dB per octave. The BAEPs elicited by the clicks in the presence of the masking noise are shown in the left column; the number at the left of each waveform indicates the cut-off frequency of the noise filter. The uppermost waveform (marked "∞") is the conventional BAEP, without masking noise. The derived responses, obtained by calculating the differences between pairs of adjacent BAEPs from the left column, are shown in the right column. CF, central frequency assigned to each derived waveform, based on the characteristics of the noise filter. (From Don M, Eggermont JJ: Analysis of the click-evoked brainstem potentials in man using high-pass noise masking. J Acoust Soc Am, 63:1084, 1978, with permission.)

subject.[22] Wave V is broader in the frequency-specific BAEPs elicited by the lower frequencies; when these are recorded, reducing the low-cut (high-pass) analog filter in the evoked potential averager to 30 Hz may yield a clearer wave V and more reliable results.[19]

Stimulation with relatively prolonged, low-frequency tone bursts (e.g., 200- to 500-Hz tone bursts lasting 10 to 15 msec each) produces an evoked potential that contains oscillatory components at the frequency of the tone (Fig. 24-15). The frequency-following response and the BAEPs do not appear to have the same neural

generators.[23] Whereas the BAEPs reflect activity originating in the base of the cochlea, the frequency-following response predominantly reflects activity originating in lower-frequency regions of the cochlea. However, the clinical utility of frequency-following responses for assessing hearing in the lower frequencies has been limited by the technical difficulties associated with recording them and by their relatively high thresholds.

BAEPs may also be elicited by bone-conducted stimuli.[24,25] This is most useful in assessing patients who may have conductive hearing losses, such as neonates in whom BAEPs performed with air-conducted stimuli are suggestive of a hearing loss.

BAEPs to Electrical Stimuli

BAEPs can also be recorded following electrical stimulation of eighth nerve fibers through the electrodes of a cochlear prosthesis. This can be used to assess the proximity of these electrodes to the spiral ganglion during implantation and the adequacy of eighth nerve stimulation during programming of the processor,[26,27] though recording of the evoked eighth nerve compound action potential through a different set of electrodes may prove to be a more useful tool for the latter application.[28] Recording of BAEPs to electrical stimulation at the promontorium has proven to be a poor predictor of the

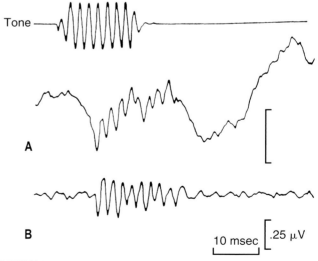

FIGURE 24-15 ■ Averaged frequency-following response to a 500-Hz tone burst, recorded between the vertex and linked ears with amplifier filter bandpass of (**A**) 8 Hz to 10,000 Hz and (**B**) 200 Hz to 1,000 Hz. The acoustic stimulus, recorded by a microphone at the subject's earpiece, is shown at the top. Note the latency shifts between the onset and the offset of the stimulus and the response. (From Marsh JT, Brown WS, Smith JC: Far-field recorded frequency-following responses: correlates of low pitch auditory perception in humans. Electroencephalogr Clin Neurophysiol, 38:113, 1975, with permission.)

success of cochlear implantation in children.[29] However, recording of BAEPs to electrical stimulation via an intracochlear electrode has been shown to correlate well with auditory outcomes, and may prove to be useful in guiding therapy in young children with questionable auditory nerve integrity.[30]

Magnetic Recording of BAEPs

Since the BAEP generators are far from the surface of the head, it is difficult to record the magnetic fields corresponding to the BAEPs, and such recordings are not practical for clinical use. However, prolonged averaging with a large number of epochs per average can yield magnetic signals within the latency range of the BAEPs.[31] Studies of these signals may produce evidence about the generators of the BAEPs. The most consistent peaks of the magnetic BAEPs correspond in latency to waves IN and V of the electrical BAEPs that are elicited by the same acoustic stimulus.[31]

EFFECTS OF VARYING STIMULUS PARAMETERS

Stimulus Polarity

Responses to rarefaction and compression clicks delivered to the same ear may differ (see Fig. 24-7). Component latencies following rarefaction clicks are usually, although not always, shorter than those following compression clicks. The BAEP latency differences between the two stimulus polarities tend to be greatest in patients with cochlear high-frequency hearing loss. BAEP peaks tend to be clearer with rarefaction clicks because of fusion of adjacent components when compression clicks are used, although again there are exceptions. The presence of wave V following one click polarity, but not the opposite, has been reported as an uncommon finding in patients referred for BAEP studies (see Fig. 24-12); the significance of this finding is unclear.

Stimulus Intensity

As the stimulus intensity is decreased, the latencies of all BAEP components increase (see Fig. 24-11). The increase is caused predominantly by a latency shift of wave I; the interpeak intervals are relatively constant until the stimulus intensity nears threshold. Component amplitudes decrease as the stimulus intensity is lowered, but with different patterns. Wave I shows the most rapid attenuation as the stimulus intensity is lowered, and it usually is lost before waves III and V. Wave V is attenuated

to a lesser degree at lower stimulus intensities and is the last peak to disappear; its disappearance defines the BAEP threshold. At lower intensities, the IV/V:I amplitude ratio is increased because of the greater degree of attenuation of wave I.

Stimulus Rate

Increasing the stimulus rate increases both the absolute latencies of the BAEP components and the interpeak intervals. As the stimulus rate is increased above approximately 10 per sec, component amplitudes decrease and the peaks tend to become less well defined. Wave V is most resistant to these effects. Thus, a stimulation rate of approximately 10 Hz is preferable for routine clinical testing, but more rapid rates may be used to facilitate recordings to measure the wave V threshold.

GENERATORS AND SCALP TOPOGRAPHIES OF BAEPs

In their first detailed description of BAEPs, Jewett and Williston hypothesized that most of the BAEP components represented composites of contributions of multiple generators.[10] This premise is supported by the bifid wave III seen in some normal BAEPs (see Fig. 24-7), which contains two subcomponents that overlap in most subjects. The effects of variations in stimulus parameters on the topography of wave II suggest that this component arises from more than one generator.[32] Shifts in the latencies of many BAEP peaks across various scalp recording locations (see Fig. 24-6) indicate that these peaks represent summations of overlapping components. Intraoperative recordings in humans[33] and detailed intracranial mapping studies in animals[34,35] have also demonstrated multiple generators for many BAEP components.

The complexity of the generators of human BAEPs (Fig. 24-16) derives in part from the pattern of connections within the auditory pathways, with ascending fibers both synapsing in and bypassing various relay nuclei. It also reflects the presence of two bursts of activity in the auditory nerve, seen as the N1 and N2 action potentials of the ECochG, which can drive the more rostral pathways. Because of both of these factors, several different structures within the infratentorial auditory pathways may be active and may generate field potentials simultaneously.

Although most early reports of generators based on clinicopathologic correlations stated that their conclusions and summary figures were probably simplifications, many subsequent authors and investigators have assumed a

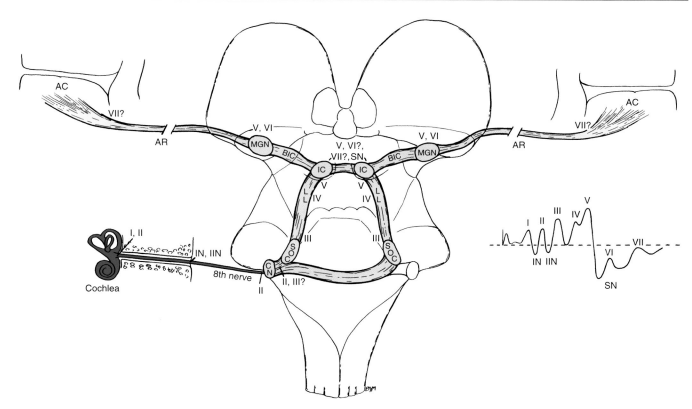

FIGURE 24-16 ■ Diagram showing the probable generators of the human brainstem auditory evoked potentials. SN, slow negativity after wave V; AC, auditory cortex; AR, auditory radiations; BIC, brachium of the inferior colliculus; CN, cochlear nucleus; IC, inferior colliculus; LL, lateral lemniscus; MGN, medial geniculate nucleus; SOC, superior olivary complex. (From Legatt AD, Arezzo JC, Vaughan HG, Jr: The anatomic and physiologic bases of brain stem auditory evoked potentials. Neurol Clin, 6:681, 1988, with permission.)

one-peak to one-generator correspondence. Inasmuch as human intracranial and clinical data tend to identify only the major generator of each wave, it is important to realize that other generators may provide significant contributions that may be unmasked if the major contribution is lost. If these contributions were construed as the contribution of the major generator, the clinical interpretation of these BAEPs could be erroneous.

Wave I

Wave I arises from the first volley of action potentials in the auditory nerve at the most distal (i.e., closest to the cochlea) portion of the nerve. It represents the same electrical phenomenon as the N1 component of the eighth nerve compound action potential in the ECochG, as confirmed by simultaneous BAEP and ECochG recordings.[36] There may also be a small contribution from the cochlear summating potential that precedes and overlaps with the N1 in ECochG recordings from the human external auditory meatus.[37]

The origin of wave I in the most distal portion of the auditory nerve is demonstrated by its presence in some patients who fulfill clinical and electroencephalographic criteria for brain death (Figs. 24-17 and 24-18) and by its occasional persistence after section of the auditory nerve during acoustic neuroma surgery (Fig. 24-19). The lateral location of the generator accounts for its surface distribution, a circumscribed negativity around the stimulated ear. Wave I therefore appears in Cz–Ai and Ac–Ai recordings but is minimal or absent in Cz–Ac recordings. The magnetic BAEP does not contain a clear peak at the latency of wave I.[31] This may reflect the trajectory of the distal eighth nerve and the fact that the magnetoencephalogram is relatively insensitive to radial currents.

Wave IN

Propagating action potentials can produce far-field potentials at points where the impedance of the tissue surrounding the nerve changes.[38,39] The afferent volley in the auditory nerve generates wave IN as it passes the internal auditory meatus and moves from a nerve encased in bone to one surrounded by cerebrospinal fluid. Human intracranial recordings at the internal

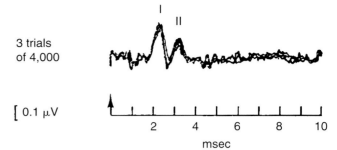

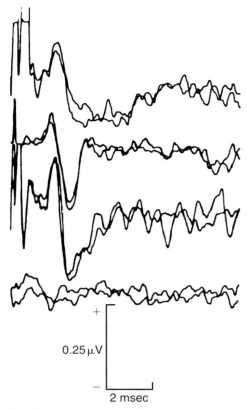

FIGURE 24-17 ■ Brainstem auditory evoked potentials from four patients fulfilling clinical and electroencephalographic criteria for brain death. Wave I is present in the upper three waveforms, and an even larger wave IN is present in the middle two. (Modified from Starr A: Auditory brain-stem responses in brain death. Brain, 99:543, 1976, with permission.)

auditory meatus contain a large peak synchronous with IN (Fig. 24-20),[33] and experimental inactivation of the intracranial eighth nerve reduces or eliminates wave IN but spares wave I in animals.[40] The first prominent peak in the magnetic BAEP corresponds in timing to wave IN, and the localization of its equivalent current dipole is

FIGURE 24-18 ■ Brainstem auditory evoked potentials in a 52-year-old woman with complete brain death, including necrosis of the cochlear nuclei, verified at postmortem examination. Waves I and II are both present. Simultaneous electrocochleography suggested that the latter originated in the N2 component of the eighth nerve action potential. (By permission of the Mayo Foundation.)

consistent with the eighth nerve at the internal auditory meatus.[31] Because IN originates in a cranial nerve, it may persist and may be even larger than wave I in brain-dead patients (see Fig. 24-17) and in patients in whom an acoustic neuroma has eliminated all centrally generated BAEP components (Fig. 24-21).

Just as the upward-pointing wave I corresponds to a negativity around the stimulated ear, the downward-pointing wave IN is synchronous with a positivity at the mastoid and in the ECochG.[41] However, the field of IN also includes a far-field negativity around the vertex. Thus, in contrast to wave I, wave IN is prominent in Cz–Ac BAEP waveforms (see Fig. 24-6).

Wave II

Sounds at the intensity levels used for BAEP recordings elicit two volleys of activity within the auditory nerve, corresponding to the N1 and N2 components of the

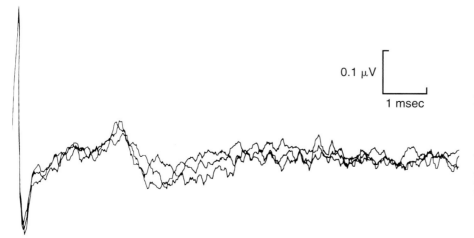

FIGURE 24-19 ■ Intraoperative brainstem auditory evoked potential (Cz–Ai recording) to left ear stimulation showing persistence of wave I after sacrifice of the intracranial eighth nerve during resection of a left-sided acoustic neuroma. (Modifed from Legatt AD, Arezzo JC, Vaughan HG, Jr: The anatomic and physiologic bases of brain stem auditory evoked potentials. Neurol Clin, 6:681, 1988, with permission.)

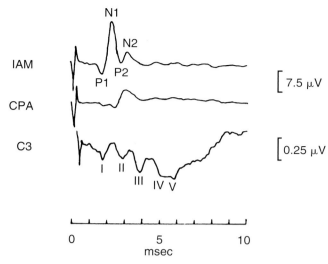

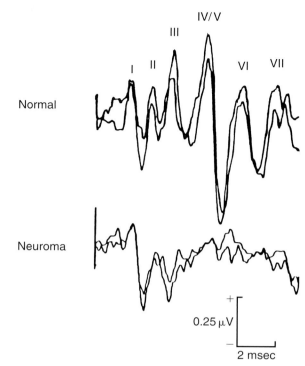

FIGURE 24-20 ■ Brainstem auditory evoked potentials (BAEPs) recorded directly from the human eighth nerve at the internal auditory meatus (top) and at the cerebellopontine angle (middle), as well as far-field scalp BAEPs (bottom). The onset and peak of P1 are coincident with those of the scalp-recorded wave I, whereas N1 corresponds to component IN. Negativity with respect to the scalp muscle reference is displayed as an upward deflection in this figure. (From Hashimoto I, Ishiyama Y, Yoshimoto T et al: Brain-stem auditory evoked potentials recorded directly from human brain-stem and thalamus. Brain, 104:841, 1981, with permission.)

FIGURE 24-21 ■ Presence of waves I, IN, II, and IIN but absence of all subsequent waves in a patient with an acoustic neuroma. A normal Cz–Ai brainstem auditory evoked potential is shown for comparison. (Modified from Starr A, Hamilton AE: Correlation between confirmed sites of neurological lesions and abnormalities of far-field auditory brainstem responses. Electroencephalogr Clin Neurophysiol, 41:595, 1976, with permission.)

eighth nerve action potential in the ECochG. When the N2 component begins in the distal auditory nerve, the activity of the first volley has propagated to the proximal auditory nerve or cochlear nucleus, and both contribute to the generation of wave II.

The contribution from N2 in the distal auditory nerve is confirmed by simultaneous BAEP and ECochG recordings[36] and by recordings from the intracranial eighth nerve (see Fig. 24-20).[33] It arises from the same location and is generated in the same way as wave I, and has a similar topography.[42] The N2 contribution accounts for the presence of wave II in patients with acoustic neuromas that have destroyed the proximal eighth nerve and eliminated all later BAEP components (see Fig. 24-21),[43] in a patient with a lower brainstem lesion that compromised the proximal eighth nerve as far as the internal meatus (wave IN was eliminated),[44] and in some brain-dead patients (see Fig. 24-18).[43] The wave II in Figure 24-22, recorded in a patient with an acoustic neuroma that markedly delayed wave V, can also be attributed to the distal eighth nerve. Waves I and II were delayed equally, a reflection of peripheral auditory dysfunction. Wave V was delayed to a much greater extent, the difference representing slowed conduction through the eighth

nerve. Because wave II did not show this additional delay, it must have originated distal to the tumor.

The origin of the more rostrally generated part of wave II is controversial. It is the earliest component affected by pontomedullary cerebrovascular accidents involving the cochlear nucleus.[45] This finding has been interpreted as implying a generator within the brainstem, specifically the cochlear nucleus or its outflow. Dissection within the pons can eliminate the far-field wave II in the Cz–Ac channel, whereas the near-field wave II recorded at the ipsilateral ear persists, indicating that the former is generated within the brainstem.[46] Intracranial recordings over the pons and from within the ventricular system have also been interpreted as indicating a generator within the brainstem (Fig. 24-23).[33] However, when the propagating N1 volley is recorded at multiple sites along the intracranial eighth nerve, the peak latency of the compound action potential at the brainstem end of the nerve approximates that of wave II, thus suggesting a contribution from the proximal eighth nerve (see Fig. 24-20).[33,47] Møller and Jannetta estimated auditory nerve conduction times

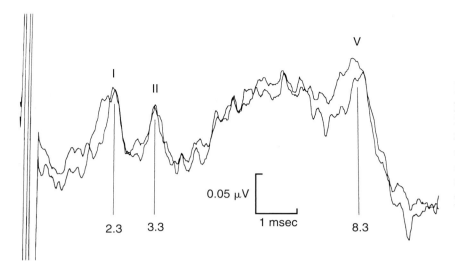

FIGURE 24-22 ■ Brainstem auditory evoked potentials (Cz–Ai) to right ear stimulation in a 36-year-old man with a right-sided acoustic neuroma. The stimulus intensity has been increased to 85 dB nHL. The absolute latencies of waves I and II are abnormally delayed, and the I–V interpeak interval is abnormally prolonged.

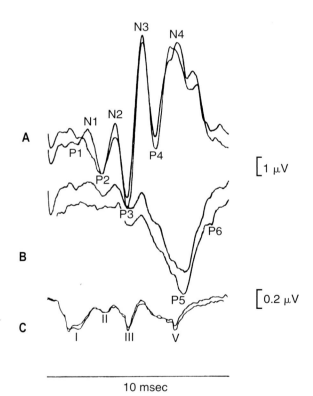

FIGURE 24-23 ■ Human brainstem auditory evoked potentials (BAEPs) to binaural stimulation recorded during surgery from the midline dorsal pons (**A**) at the level of the facial colliculi and (**B**) the midline dorsal mesencephalon at the level of the inferior colliculi, as well as (**C**) the far-field BAEP. Negativity with respect to the scalp muscle reference is displayed as an upward deflection in this figure. (From Hashimoto I, Ishiyama Y, Yoshimoto T et al: Brain-stem auditory evoked potentials recorded directly from human brain-stem and thalamus. Brain, 104:841, 1981, with permission.)

and believed that timing considerations ruled out a contribution of postsynaptic cochlear nucleus activity to wave II.[47]

These data can be reconciled,[48] and it is likely that activity within the proximal end of the auditory nerve and postsynaptic activity within the cochlear nucleus both contribute to wave II. Because the auditory nerve terminals are within the substance of the cochlear nucleus, the distinction between a proximal auditory nerve generator and a cochlear nucleus generator does not have a major impact on the anatomic localization of the cause of a wave II abnormality. The brainstem generator is usually predominant and produces a scalp topography with maximal amplitude over the dorsal part of the head and a clear wave II in the Cz–Ac waveform. The presence of an additional generator in the distal auditory nerve is clinically important, however, because it may produce a wave II in a patient whose entire brain, including the brainstem, is not functioning (see Fig. 24-18). If wave II were regarded as originating entirely within the brainstem, its presence would be interpreted as incompatible with a diagnosis of brain death.

Wave IIN

As it passes the internal auditory meatus, the N2 volley of the eighth nerve compound action potential can generate a downgoing peak, wave IIN, in the BAEP waveform in the same manner as the N1 volley gives rise to wave IN. Human intracranial recordings at the internal auditory meatus have demonstrated compound action potential peaks corresponding to both IN and IIN.[33] Like IN, wave

IIN may be recorded from patients in whom an acoustic neuroma has eliminated all centrally generated BAEP components (see Fig. 24-21).

Wave III

Wave III also probably represents a composite of contributions from multiple generators. It occasionally has a bifid waveform (see Fig. 24-7), and may be more abnormal either ipsilateral or contralateral to the major pathology in patients with asymmetric lesions. Human lesion data localize the major generators of wave III to the caudal pontine tegmentum. Most patients with lesions in this region that involve the superior olivary complex have a normal wave II but abnormal wave III. Wave III is present and is usually normal in patients with lesions confined to the middle or upper pons or mesencephalon.[49] Intracranial recordings are also consistent with a pontine generator (see Fig. 24-23).[33] Latency shifts as a function of rostrocaudal position[33,50] suggest a contribution from activity ascending in the lateral lemniscus as well.

Although wave III may receive a contribution from cochlear nucleus activity driven by the N2 volley of the eighth nerve compound action potential, the available data suggest that it is generated predominantly in the superior olivary complexes or their outflow within the lateral lemniscus. The scalp distribution of wave III includes both an amplitude maximum over the dorsal portion of the scalp and a substantial horizontally oriented component; thus, wave III is prominent in Cz–Ai, Cz–Ac, and Ac–Ai BAEP waveforms.

Wave IV

Wave IV is affected by tumors or cerebrovascular accidents of the midpons or rostral pons. Its generators are close to or overlapping with, but not identical to, those of wave V; waves IV and V are usually either both affected or both unaffected by brainstem lesions, but they may be affected differentially by multilevel demyelination, a brainstem infarct (see Fig. 24-9),[48] or a small brainstem hemorrhage in the lateral lemniscus.[51] Intracranial recordings demonstrate a large positivity coincident with wave IV over the dorsal pons (see Fig. 24-23).[33] Latency shifts observed at serial intracranial recording positions are consistent with propagating action potentials within the ascending brainstem auditory pathways. Also, wave IV may persist in the presence of a lesion of the inferior colliculus that eliminates wave V (Fig. 24-24).[52] Thus, wave IV appears to reflect activity predominantly in ascending auditory fibers within the

dorsal and rostral pons, caudal to the inferior colliculus. Although the nucleus of the lateral lemniscus has been implicated as a BAEP generator in animal studies, human data are insufficient to confirm its contribution to wave IV.

Wave V

Waves IV and V are the earliest components that are absent and usually are the earliest that are abnormal in patients with lesions of the midpons, rostral pons, or mesencephalon.[49,51,53–55] Occasionally, waves II and III are delayed in latency with rostral brainstem tumors (Fig. 24-25); this delay may be caused by pressure on more caudal structures or it may reflect effects on descending pathways.[56] In intracranial recordings, the positive peak corresponding to wave V is largest near the inferior colliculus contralateral to the stimulated ear (Fig. 24-26).[50,57] The equivalent current dipole for the wave V peak in the magnetic BAEP is also contralateral to the stimulated ear, though the dipole locates posterior and lateral to the lateral lemniscus and the inferior colliclus.[31] Wave V inverts to a negativity over the dorsal pons, in contrast to earlier waves, which do not display an inversion between the pons and the mesencephalon (see Fig. 24-23). Ipsilateral near-field responses recorded near the inferior colliculus are smaller and do not match the latency of wave V as well. These data are consistent with generation of wave V at the level of the mesencephalon, either from the inferior colliculus itself or, as some authors have suggested,[58,59] from the fibers in the rostral portion of the lateral lemniscus as they terminate in the inferior colliculus. Normal BAEPs with a clear wave V have been reported following damage in the region of the inferior colliculus caused by brainstem stroke,[59,60] head trauma,[61] and injury during resection of pineal region tumors,[62,63] but it is not clear that the colliculi were destroyed totally in these cases. In contrast, Hirsch and associates reported a case in which a highly focal lesion involving the inferior colliculus eliminated wave V of the BAEP (see Fig. 24-24).[52]

Intracranial data also suggest that the mesencephalon contralateral to the stimulated ear is the major generator of wave V. Clinically, however, unilateral abnormalities of wave V are associated most often with ipsilateral pathology, although there are exceptions.[51,54,64] On the scalp, the amplitude of wave V is maximal in the midline, and a large wave V is present in both the Cz–Ai and the Cz–Ac waveforms.

The monkey homolog of the human wave V, which likewise predominantly reflects activity in the mesencephalon

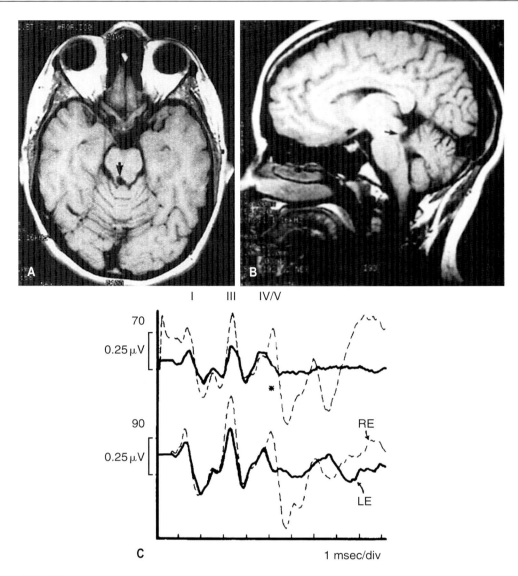

FIGURE 24-24 ▪ **A**, Axial and **B**, sagittal MRI in a patient who developed left-sided hearing impairment following gamma-knife treatment for a midbrain arteriovenous malformation that had bled. The treatment caused a lesion in the right inferior colliculus (black arrows). **C**, Brainstem auditory evoked potentials (BAEPs) recorded in this patient at two different stimulus intensities (70 and 90 dB). BAEPs to left ear (LE) stimulation are shown as solid lines, whereas those to right ear (RE) stimulation are shown as dashed lines. Wave IV is present for both stimulus lateralities, but wave V and following downgoing peak, VN, are absent following left ear stimulation. (Modified from Hirsch BE, Durrant JD, Yetiser S et al: Localizing retrocochlear hearing loss. Am J Otol, 17:537, 1996, with permission.)

(contralateral more than ipsilateral),[35] also contains contributions from other structures, including the medial geniculate nucleus, auditory radiations, and lateral lemniscus within the pons. The lemniscal contribution reflects the multiple bursts of activity that are present at all levels of the auditory system. Because wave V may be eliminated by mesencephalic lesions,[52] the lemniscal contribution is most likely not of clinical significance in humans.

Depth recordings within the human medial geniculate nucleus suggest that activity in this structure contributes to wave V (Fig. 24-27),[33,65] but this contribution does not affect the clinical interpretation of BAEPs. The normal wave V recorded in patients with rostral midbrain or supratentorial lesions is generated predominantly in the mesencephalon, just as it is in normal individuals; absence of the geniculate contribution is not apparent. Conversely, a lesion that eliminates the mesencephalic

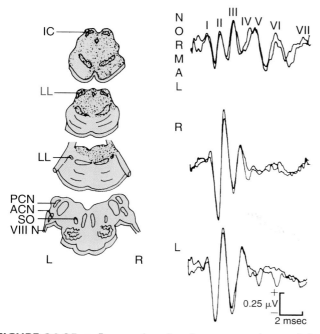

FIGURE 24-25 ■ In a patient in whom a germinoma (stipples) destroyed most of the mesencephalon and pons, including the right but not the left lateral lemniscus, waves I through III were present following stimulation of either the right (R) or the left (L) ear, but later brainstem auditory evoked potential (BAEP) components were absent. The latencies of waves II and III were abnormally delayed, but the wave I latencies were normal. A normal Cz–Ai BAEP is shown at the top for comparison. IC, inferior colliculus; LL, lateral lemniscus; PCN, posterior cochlear nucleus; ACN, anterior cochlear nucleus; SO, superior olivary nucleus. (From Starr A, Hamilton AE: Correlation between confirmed sites of neurological lesions and abnormalities of far-field auditory brainstem responses. Electroencephalogr Clin Neurophysiol, 41:595, 1976, with permission.)

generators of wave V will remove the auditory input to the medial geniculate nucleus and eliminate its contribution to the BAEP waveform as well.

Wave VI

Abnormalities of wave VI, with normal waves I through V, have been described in patients with tumors of the rostral midbrain and caudal thalamus at the level of the medical geniculate nucleus and the brachium of the inferior colliculus. Depth recordings within the human medial geniculate demonstrate large near-field peaks coincident with wave VI; both positive (see Fig. 24-27[33,66]) and negative[65] peaks have been recorded. The polarity differences most likely reflect differences in the position of the electrode relative to the

equivalent dipole of the wave VI generator within the geniculate. The scalp topography of wave VI also provides evidence for generation of wave V within the medial geniculate nuclei or their outflow tracts.[48]

The monkey homolog of the human wave VI also contains a contribution from the inferior colliculus,[35] a reflection of the multiple bursts of activity within the auditory system. A large wave VI peak is visible in recordings from electrodes placed directly on the human inferior colliculus when the large slow-wave components in them are removed by filtering (see Fig. 24-26).[57] Thus, the inferior colliculus may contribute to the human wave VI.

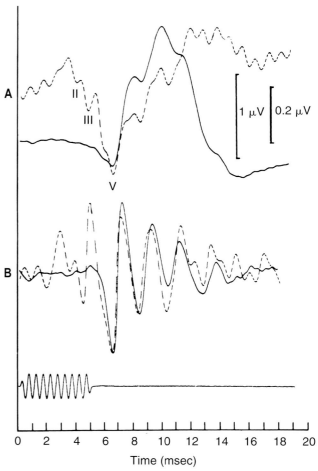

FIGURE 24-26 ■ Brainstem auditory evoked potentials (BAEPs) recorded during surgery from the human inferior colliculus (solid lines) compared with the far-field BAEP (dashed lines). **A**, Low-pass filtered waveforms. **B**, Digitally filtered waveforms. Negativity with respect to the reference is displayed as an upward deflection in this figure. Calibration bars: 1 μV for inferior colliculus recordings and 0.2 μV for far-field BAEP. (From Møller AR, Jannetta PJ: Interpretation of brainstem auditory evoked potentials: results from intracranial recordings in humans. Scand Audiol, 12:125, 1983, with permission.)

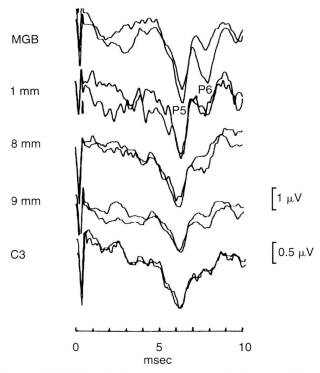

FIGURE 24-27 ■ Brainstem auditory evoked potentials recorded by a thalamic depth electrode passed near or through the medial geniculate in a human patient. The two large positive peaks can be traced to the scalp (bottom waveform). Binaural stimulation was used. Negativity with respect to the scalp muscle reference is displayed as an upward deflection in this figure. (From Hashimoto I, Ishiyama Y, Yoshimoto T et al: Brain-stem auditory evoked potentials recorded directly from human brain-stem and thalamus. Brain, 104:841, 1981, with permission.)

This mesencephalic contribution could generate a wave VI in a patient with bilateral geniculate damage. Conversely, wave VI is absent in Cz–Ai and Cz–Ac recordings in some normal individuals. Thus, neither the presence of a normal wave VI nor the complete absence of this component provides clinically useful information about the status of the medial geniculate nuclei. BAEPs cannot be used to assess the status of the auditory pathways rostral to the mesencephalon.

Wave VII

Wave VII is so often absent in conventionally recorded normal BAEPs that its absence in pathologic states cannot be used to ascertain its generators. The scalp topography of wave VII supports its generation near the auditory cortex, predominantly contralaterally.

Intracranial recordings demonstrate a large near-field peak at latency of wave VII or its simian homolog in the region of inferior colliculus in both humans (see Fig. 24-26[57]) and monkeys,[35] again most likely originating in the repeated bursts of activity that occur in this structure following a single auditory stimulus.

As was the case with wave VI, the common absence of wave VII in normal individuals and the possibility of a mesencephalic contribution (which could produce a wave VII in the face of more rostral damage) mean that assessment of wave VII does not provide clinically useful information about the status of the auditory pathways.

Wave VN

The large downward deflection following wave V has a slower time course than do the preceding upward-pointing peaks; this, most likely, predominantly reflects postsynaptic potentials within brainstem auditory nuclei, primarily the inferior colliculus.[48]

CLINICAL INTERPRETATION OF BAEPs

Waves II, IV, VI, and VII are sometimes not identifiable in normal individuals, and their peak latencies display more interindividual variability than do the peak latencies of waves I, III, and V. Amplitude measurements of the individual components are also highly variable across subjects, but the ratio between the amplitude of the IV/V complex and that of wave I has proved to be a clinically useful measure. Therefore, clinical interpretation of a patient's BAEPs is based predominantly on the presence or absence of waves I, III, and V, and on measurements of the wave I latency (PTT), the I–V interpeak interval (CTT), the I–III and III–V interpeak intervals, the right-left differences of these values, and the IV/V:I amplitude ratios. Measurement of right-left differences increases test sensitivity because the intersubject variability of these measures is less than that of the absolute component latencies and interpeak intervals from which they were derived (Fig. 24-28).

Normative Data

The control data used to derive normal values should have been acquired under the same conditions used to test the patient, including the polarity, rate, and intensity of the stimulus and the filter settings used for data recording, because alteration in any of these parameters can change the latencies or amplitudes of BAEP components.

As is the case with all evoked potentials, calculation of normal ranges must take into account the distribution of

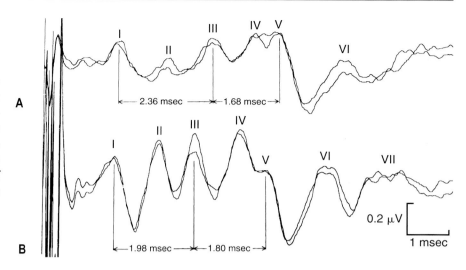

FIGURE 24-28 ■ Brainstem auditory evoked potentials (Cz–Ai) to (**A**) left ear and (**B**) right ear stimulation in a 23-year-old man with a left-sided acoustic neuroma. The I–III, III–V, and I–V interpeak intervals are within normal limits bilaterally, but the right-left differences of the I–III and I–V interpeak intervals are abnormally large.

values in the control population.[11,67,68] A value that is not distributed normally can be transformed into a normal or gaussian distribution to calculate the mean and standard deviation, or a nonparametric statistical measure such as percentiles can be used. The limits of the normal range are typically set at 2.5 or 3 standard deviations from the mean of normally distributed data. A BAEP may be classified as abnormal if any of several measurements is abnormal. The performance of multiple tests increases the possibility of a false-positive result,[69] so the more conservative limit (3 standard deviations) is preferable for evaluation of each measured value.

Because the I–V and III–V interpeak intervals are, on average, shorter in women than in men,[70,71] some laboratories establish separate normal values for the two genders.

Delay Versus Absence of Components

Evoked potentials represent the summated activity of large populations of neurons firing in synchrony; the electrical signal produced by a single cell is too small to be seen at the scalp. If the timing of neuronal activity is delayed uniformly across the cell population, a delayed evoked potential component will result. If the delay is nonuniform and the electrical signals are desynchronized (a process called *temporal dispersion*), the summation may not produce a recognizable evoked potential component. Because the same pathophysiologic process (i.e., delay in neural activity) can cause either delay or absence of a BAEP peak, both of these findings should be interpreted similarly. They both indicate dysfunction, but not necessarily complete loss of activity, in a part of the infratentorial auditory pathways.

Significance of Specific BAEP Abnormalities

ABNORMALITIES OF WAVE I

Because wave I originates in the distal portion of the auditory nerve, abnormalities (delay or absence) of wave I usually reflect peripheral auditory dysfunction, either conductive or cochlear, or pathology involving the most distal portion of the eighth nerve. An audiogram is useful to identify and quantify the degree of hearing loss; a BAEP waveform with a poorly formed or absent wave I but a clear wave V may reflect high-frequency hearing loss.

If all BAEP components are absent with the standard stimulus, an attempt should be made to elicit them by using a longer analysis time (typically 15 msec) and a higher stimulus intensity. The increased stimulus artifact caused by the latter may necessitate the use of alternating stimulus polarity. Because peripheral auditory dysfunction is sufficient to cause complete absence of BAEPs, a waveform in which no BAEP components are identifiable provides no information about the status of the brainstem auditory pathways.

Cochlear dysfunction may reflect intracranial pathology because the cochlea receives its blood supply from the intracranial circulation via the internal auditory artery. This vessel, which is usually a branch of the anterior inferior cerebellar artery, passes through the internal auditory canal alongside the eighth nerve. Cochlear ischemia or infarction may result from compression of the internal auditory artery within the canal or from occlusion of its parent vessel.[20,72,73] Thus, wave I may be delayed or absent in patients with basilar artery thrombosis or other posterior circulation vascular disease,[60,73–75] acoustic nerve tumors (see Fig. 24-22; Fig. 24-29), or brain death (see Fig. 24-17[76]) caused by interference with the blood supply of the cochlea.

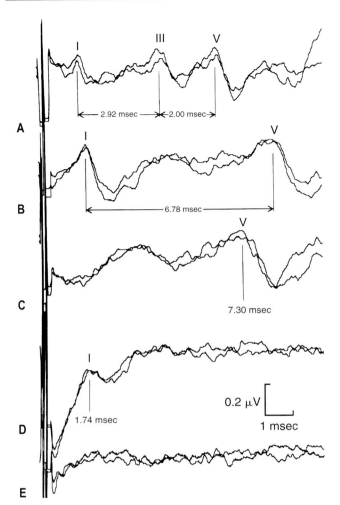

FIGURE 24-29 ■ Brainstem auditory evoked potentials recorded (Cz–Ai) in five patients (**A** to **E**) with acoustic neuromas following stimulation ipsilateral to the tumor. The stimulus intensity was increased to 85 dB nHL in all cases.

With mild cochlear ischemia, BAEPs may be normal to standard, high-intensity stimuli but become abnormally delayed or absent as the stimulus intensity is lowered. Examination of latency–intensity curves may increase the sensitivity of BAEPs for detecting small acoustic neuromas.[20] The latency–intensity curve may normalize following resection of a small acoustic neuroma (Fig. 24-30), thereby demonstrating the reversibility of the cochlear ischemia.

ABNORMALITIES OF THE I–III INTERPEAK INTERVAL

Prolongation of the I–III interpeak interval, either absolute (in comparison to normal limits) or relative (excessive right-left difference) in the presence of a prolonged CTT (I–V interpeak interval), reflects an abnormality within the neural auditory pathways between the distal eighth nerve on the stimulated side and the lower pons. Absence of waves III and V carries the same significance.

However, the rare absence of wave III in the presence of a clear wave V with a normal I–V interpeak interval should not be interpreted as an abnormality.

Interpretation of a prolonged I–III or III–V interpeak interval when the I–V interpeak interval is normal is less clear. Owing to the complexity of the brainstem auditory pathways, the neural activity that generates wave V may not arise from propagation of the same neural activity that generates wave III; the III–V interpeak interval therefore would not actually measure propagation of neural signals between the two sets of anatomic generators. Thus, it is prudent to refrain from interpreting a prolonged III–V interpeak interval as an abnormality in the presence of a normal CTT. In contrast, the I–III interpeak interval does reflect propagation of neural signals from the generator of wave I to the generator(s) of wave III because all auditory afferent activity must pass through the distal eighth nerve on its way to the brainstem. Thus, it is logical to interpret a prolonged I–III interpeak interval as an abnormality, whether or not the corresponding CTT is also prolonged.

Abnormality of the I–III interpeak interval is the characteristic BAEP finding in eighth nerve lesions such as acoustic neuromas (see Fig. 24-29), although there may be a simultaneous peripheral abnormality if the internal auditory artery has been compromised. Abnormal I–III interpeak intervals can also result from other processes such as demyelinating disease, brainstem tumors, or vascular lesions of the brainstem. In a patient with unilateral auditory nerve pathology, prolongation of the I–III interpeak interval will be found on stimulation of the ear on the side of the lesion. In patients with unilateral brainstem lesions and unilateral I–III abnormalities (i.e., abnormal BAEPs to stimulation of one ear and normal BAEPs to stimulation of the other), the ear in which stimulation produces the abnormal BAEP waveform is most often ipsilateral to the lesion, but there are rare exceptions.

ABNORMALITIES OF THE III–V INTERPEAK INTERVAL

Prolongation of both the I–V and III–V interpeak intervals, or complete absence of the IV/V complex in the presence of a wave III, reflects an abnormality within the neural auditory pathways between the lower pons and the mesencephalon. As explained earlier, prolongation of the III–V interpeak interval is best not interpreted as an abnormality if the I–V interpeak interval is normal.

Abnormalities in the III–V interpeak interval are seen in a variety of disease processes involving the brainstem, including demyelination, tumor, and vascular disease. If the disease process also involves the lower pons or eighth nerve, both the I–III and the III–V interpeak

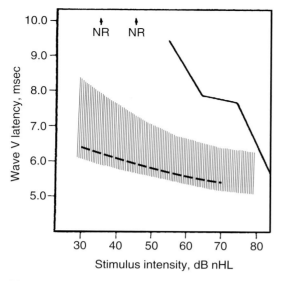 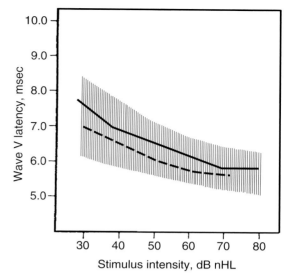

FIGURE 24-30 ▪ Left: Latency–intensity curves to left ear (solid line) and right ear (*dashed line*) stimulation recorded before surgery in a 52-year-old woman with a left-sided intracanalicular acoustic neuroma. The wave V latency to 70-dB SL (85-dB nHL) stimulation of the left ear was normal, but as the stimulus intensity was decreased, the latency–intensity curve went outside the normal range (*shaded*) and then the brainstem auditory evoked potentials (BAEPs) disappeared (NR, no response). The tumor was resected completely with intra-operative monitoring of BAEPs and facial nerve function. Right: After the resection, the patient's latency–intensity curves were normal bilaterally. Her audiogram was normal and her speech discrimination score in the left ear was 100 percent. (From Legatt AD, Pedley TA, Emerson RG et al: Normal brain-stem auditory evoked potentials with abnormal latency–intensity studies in patients with acoustic neuromas. Arch Neurol, 45:1326, 1988, with permission.)

intervals may be prolonged within the same waveform (Fig. 24-31). In patients with unilateral brainstem lesions and unilateral III–V interpeak interval abnormalities, the ear in which stimulation produces the abnormal BAEP waveform is most often, although not always, ipsilateral to the lesion.[53,64]

ABNORMALITIES OF THE *IV/V:I* AMPLITUDE RATIO

An abnormally small IV/V:I amplitude ratio (see Fig. 24-10) reflects dysfunction within the auditory pathways between the distal eighth nerve and the mesencephalon. Because

waves I and V are affected differentially by stimulus intensity, the amplitude ratio should be measured at the same intensity used to establish the normative data. Decreasing the stimulus intensity will attenuate wave I more than wave V, and thus inflate the ratio and perhaps cause the abnormality to be missed. Conversely, increasing the stimulus intensity beyond the normal level could increase wave I and give a false-positive result.

Suboptimal placement of the Ai recording electrode may decrease the amplitude of wave I because that component is recorded as a near-field negativity around the

FIGURE 24-31 ▪ Brainstem auditory evoked potentials (BAEPs) (Cz–Ai) to stimulation of each ear in a 35-year-old woman with multiple sclerosis. **A**, BAEPs to left ear stimulation are normal. **B**, The I–III and III–V interpeak intervals are both abnormally prolonged following right ear stimulation.

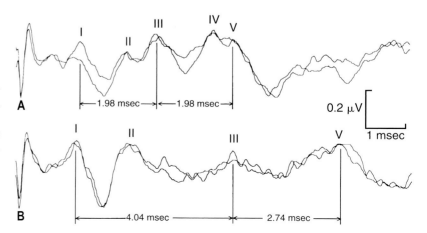

stimulated ear. Such placement may increase the IV/V:I amplitude ratio artifactually and perhaps cause an abnormality to be missed. Fortunately, electrode-position shifts are unlikely to cause a false-positive result; because the IV/V complex is recorded predominantly as a far-field potential, small displacements of the Cz recording electrode will not attenuate the IV/V complex substantially.

Portion of the Auditory System Assessed by BAEPs

All primary afferent auditory neurons synapse in the cochlear nucleus, but the ascending auditory pathways after that structure are extremely complex. The cochlear nucleus projects to several different brainstem nuclei both ipsilaterally and contralaterally, and projections from subsequent auditory nuclei (e.g., the superior olivary complex) also both synapse in and bypass more rostral nuclei. These various projections do not all serve the same function, and it appears that they do not all contribute equally to the BAEPs.

FUNCTIONAL SUBSETS

Because the BAEP peaks are narrow, the neuronal populations that generate them must be synchronized extremely well. Some neurons within the brainstem auditory system have morphologic and physiologic features that minimize temporal dispersion.[77] Neurons with such characteristics are required for sound localization. An anatomically distinguishable neuronal subsystem for sound localization is present within the brainstem, and it appears that these are the neurons that generate the BAEPs. In human patients, BAEP abnormalities are highly correlated with difficulty in correctly lateralizing click pairs with interaural time delays.[78] In contrast, pure tone audiometry and speech discrimination may be normal in patients with grossly abnormal BAEPs.[79,80] Also, normal BAEPs may be present in patients with infratentorial lesions causing profound impairment of speech perception,[62,63] though this finding conceivably could reflect interruption of the auditory pathways rostral to the inferior colliculi. Dipole analysis of BAEPs provides another indication of their relationship to the sound localization system; some components show changes that depend on the position of the sound source.[81]

CROSSED AND UNCROSSED PATHWAYS

Ascending projections from the cochlear nucleus are bilateral but are more extensive contralaterally than ipsilaterally. Despite this anatomic asymmetry, the BAEPs appear to reflect predominantly activity in the ipsilateral ascending pathways because unilateral brainstem lesions that produce unilateral abnormalities involving either the I–III or the III–V interpeak interval usually do so on stimulation of the ear ipsilateral to the lesion.

ROSTROCAUDAL EXTENT

Although some of the BAEP components may receive contributions from the medial geniculate nucleus and auditory radiations, BAEPs as currently performed do not provide reliable, clinically useful assessment of these structures. BAEPs can be used only to assess the status of the ear, auditory nerve, and brainstem auditory pathways up through the level of the mesencephalon.

ROLE OF DESCENDING PATHWAYS

Waves I and II may be quite large in patients with rostral brainstem pathology that causes abnormalities of wave V (see Figs. 24-10 and 24-25). This increase in waves I and II probably reflects loss of activity in descending inhibitory pathways originating in or traversing the region of the inferior colliculus.[56] Growth of wave I concurrent with loss of wave V has been observed in serial BAEP studies of preterminal patients in whom brain death subsequently developed.[82,83] In a patient with an extra-axial tumor compressing the brainstem, removal of the tumor with decompression of the brainstem led to an increase in the amplitude of wave V and a decrease in the amplitude of wave I.[84]

In a patient with a mesencephalic lesion and an attenuated IV/V complex, enlargement of wave I because of disinhibition will decrease the IV/V:I amplitude ratio even further. This mechanism therefore acts to enhance the sensitivity of the IV/V:I amplitude ratio in the detection of brainstem damage.

Relationship Between BAEPs and Hearing

CATEGORIZATION OF ABNORMALITIES

BAEP abnormalities can be divided into a "central" pattern, in which the CTT (I–V interpeak interval) is prolonged; and a "peripheral" pattern, in which wave I is delayed. A single waveform may contain both abnormalities (see Fig. 24-22). Clinically, hearing losses are divided into conductive and sensorineural categories. These categories do not correspond to the BAEP categories, however; the relationship among them and the anatomic location of the abnormality are shown in Table 24-1.

TABLE 24-1 ■ **Classification of Hearing Loss**

Clinical Classification	Location of Pathology	BAEP Classification
Conductive hearing loss	— External or middle ear	} Peripheral hearing loss
Sensorineural hearing loss {	Inner ear (cochlea)	
	Eighth nerve or brainstem (retrocochlear)	— "Central" hearing loss

Although much of the I–III interpeak interval represents the conduction time of the afferent volley along the auditory nerve, abnormalities of the I–III interpeak interval are common in patients with multiple sclerosis (MS). This observation is not surprising in light of the histologic structure of the auditory nerve. Most of the other cranial nerves (except I and II, which are actually central nervous system tracts) are histologically peripheral nerves; their myelin is produced by Schwann cells, except for a short segment at the nerve root. In contrast, eighth nerve fibers are ensheathed along most of their lengths by central-type myelin, produced by oligodendrocytes; the transition to peripheral-type myelin produced by Schwann cells occurs near the distal end of the nerve. Therefore, in MS the eighth nerve is vulnerable to demyelination along most of its length, and magnetic resonance imaging has demonstrated involvement of the eighth nerve in MS.[85,86] Although it might at first glance seem inappropriate to include the conduction time along the eighth cranial nerve in the "central" conduction time (I–V interpeak interval), it is actually reasonable to do so because most of that conduction is through fibers with central-type myelin.

PERIPHERAL HEARING LOSS

The BAEP waveform to a broad-band click predominantly reflects activity originating in the base of the cochlea. It is mediated by neurons with characteristic frequencies in the 2,000- to 4,000-Hz range. Thus, significant high-frequency hearing losses in this frequency band typically produce BAEP abnormalities, whereas BAEPs are relatively insensitive to isolated low-frequency hearing losses. As described earlier, frequency-specific stimulus and acoustic masking paradigms can increase the accuracy with which BAEP recordings detect and quantify hearing loss in several frequency ranges.

In patients with peripheral auditory dysfunction, high stimulus intensities can correct, partially or completely, BAEP abnormalities that become obvious at lower stimulus intensities (see Figs. 24-13 and 24-30). Thus, BAEP studies that are used to screen for hearing loss should be performed with multiple stimulus intensities, and latency–intensity curves should be constructed. BAEP

studies intended to diagnose conduction abnormalities within the neural auditory pathways can be performed with a single, relatively high (e.g., 60 to 65 dB nHL) stimulus intensity.

CENTRAL AUDITORY PATHWAY ABNORMALITIES

Because BAEPs reflect activity in only a subset of the auditory pathways, dysfunction in another portion of the auditory system can affect hearing without altering the BAEPs. For example, patients with bilateral temporal lobe infarctions involving the auditory cortex may be deaf and yet have completely normal BAEPs.[87,88]

Conversely, BAEPs may be abnormal in patients with brainstem disease who have normal hearing. Unilateral brainstem lesions only rarely cause hearing loss because the ascending projections from each ear are bilateral. In addition, lesions (whether unilateral or bilateral) that affect the short-latency, highly synchronized subsystem involved in sound localization may spare other portions of the brainstem auditory pathways that are sufficient to maintain normal perception. Even if the disease process affects the brainstem auditory pathways globally, abnormal BAEPs do not necessarily imply hearing loss. If BAEPs are present but delayed, the information that a suprathreshold auditory stimulus has occurred still reaches higher auditory centers; it just does so a few milliseconds later. Thus, the audiogram may be normal. As previously discussed, the absence of a component may reflect temporal dispersion rather than conduction block, so hearing may even be present when there is no identifiable wave V.[89]

The possibility of normal hearing in the presence of abnormal BAEPs enhances their clinical utility. It is precisely because they can detect subtle neuronal dysfunction that is not clinically apparent on the neurologic and audiologic examination that BAEPs (and visual and somatosensory evoked potentials as well) are a valuable addendum to the clinical evaluation of patients with suspected neurologic disease.

In patients with auditory symptoms that are suspected of being functional, an abnormal BAEP study demonstrates the existence of pathology within the auditory system. However, a normal study does not prove that the symptoms are psychogenic. The lesion in such a patient may have spared the short-latency, highly synchronized brainstem subsystem that generates the BAEPs but damaged other parts of the auditory system enough to produce symptoms. Malingerers cannot volitionally make their BAEPs abnormal (with components delayed or absent), but if they maintain a degree of tension in their cranial and neck muscles, the EMG activity picked up by the recording electrodes may be sufficient to prevent recording of an interpretable BAEP study.[90]

BAEP in Specific Neurologic Conditions

The final section of this chapter describes BAEP findings in the neurologic conditions for which diagnostic BAEP recordings are performed most commonly in adults. Screening for hearing impairment and evaluation for possible neurodegenerative disorders are important additional indications for BAEP testing in the pediatric population (discussed in Chapter 25).

ACOUSTIC NEUROMA

Many different BAEP patterns are seen in patients with acoustic neuromas (see Fig. 24-29). In several large published series,[91,92] abnormal BAEPs to standard high-intensity stimuli were found in more than 95 percent of patients with acoustic neuromas. The probability of abnormal BAEPs is less in patients with small (less than 1 cm) tumors, though some investigators have reported sensitivities greater than 90 percent.[93,94] In patients with small, intracanalicular tumors in whom BAEPs to standard high-intensity stimuli are normal, latency–intensity studies may reveal abnormal cochlear function resulting from compression of the internal auditory artery (see Fig. 24-30).[20] Acoustic neuromas typically originate from the distal vestibular nerve at the vestibular ganglion, and the auditory portion of the nerve may be unaffected early in the course of the disease.

As an acoustic neuroma enlarges, it begins to compress the auditory nerve. Such compression produces prolongation of the I–III interpeak interval (see Figs. 24-28 and 24-29, *A*) and eventually complete eradication of wave III and subsequent BAEP components (see Fig. 24-29, *D*). In some cases, wave V becomes delayed but persists, whereas wave III (see Fig. 24-29, *B*) or waves I and III

(see Fig. 24-29, *C*) are lost. Wave II may be relatively spared, a reflection of the contribution to that component originating in the distal eighth nerve (see Fig. 24-22).

Simultaneous with I–III interpeak interval abnormalities, wave I may become delayed as the degree of cochlear ischemia increases (see Fig. 24-22). Infarction of the cochlea may cause elimination of all BAEPs (see Fig. 24-29), a common finding with large tumors in patients who have major hearing loss or who are completely deaf. As acoustic neuromas expand within the posterior fossa, they begin to compress the brainstem. Prolongation of the III–V interpeak interval in response to stimulation of the ear contralateral to the tumor (Fig. 24-32) is indicative of brainstem compression by a large tumor.

The pattern of BAEP abnormality on the side of the tumor can be used to predict the likelihood of hearing preservation during surgical resection of the tumor.[95]

OTHER POSTERIOR FOSSA TUMORS

BAEPs are almost always abnormal in brainstem gliomas and other intrinsic brainstem tumors. Exceptions are tumors that are located entirely within the medulla, neither directly involving the auditory pathways nor affecting them by compression or deformation. Abnormalities in the I–III or III–V interpeak interval, or a combination of both, may be present, depending on the location of the tumor and the extent to which it affects surrounding brainstem tissue. Serial recordings may show deterioration of the BAEPs because of tumor growth. When a brainstem tumor shrinks in response to treatment, the BAEPs may demonstrate an improvement in conduction within the brainstem auditory pathways.[96]

Extra-axial posterior fossa tumors can also produce BAEP abnormalities because of brainstem compression; the pattern of the abnormality depends on the location

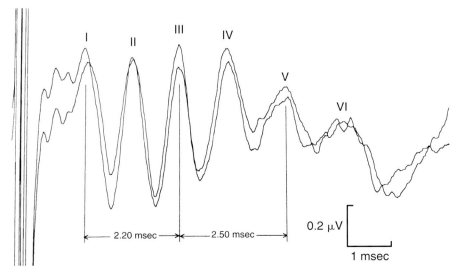

FIGURE 24-32 ■ Brainstem auditory evoked potentials (Cz–Ai) to stimulation of the ear contralateral to a large cerebellopontine angle tumor that was compressing the brainstem. The I–V and III–V interpeak intervals are both abnormally prolonged. This tumor was a meningioma, but a large acoustic neuroma could produce the same changes by the same mechanism.

of the tumor and on which structures are being compressed. Although the earliest BAEP changes seen with acoustic neuromas (which usually arise distally within the internal auditory canal) are typically I–III interpeak interval abnormalities and wave I abnormalities to stimulation ipsilateral to the tumor, posterior fossa tumors arising in other locations may first produce abnormalities in the III–V interpeak interval because of brainstem compression without evidence of eighth nerve compromise. BAEPs may show improvement following decompression of the brainstem because of tumor resection or tumor shrinkage in response to treatment.

CEREBROVASCULAR DISEASE

The effect of a brainstem stroke on BAEPs depends on the location and type of the stroke and on the extent of involvement of the auditory pathways, and may be quite limited (see Fig. 24-9). BAEPs are usually normal in patients with medullary infarcts[60,97] or lesions confined to the basis pontis, cerebral peduncles, and cerebellar hemispheres[60]; however, they may be affected if edema or ischemia compromises brainstem function outside the area of infarction. Shimbo and co-workers studied BAEPs in 55 patients with posterior circulation strokes and found that they were abnormal in all patients with lesions of the pontine tegmentum or the cerebellar peduncles.[60] BAEPs may have prognostic significance; the presence of BAEP abnormalities is associated with an adverse clinical outcome.[60]

Abnormalities in the I–III or III–V interpeak interval, or a combination of both, may be seen in patients with brainstem strokes. Posterior circulation vascular disease can also interfere with the blood supply to the cochlea by the internal auditory artery. If a cochlear stroke accompanies the brainstem stroke, all BAEP components will be absent following stimulation of that ear.

BAEP abnormalities are found in most patients with vertebrobasilar transient ischemic attacks if they are recorded acutely.[98] These findings tend to resolve over time,[98,99] and the yield of abnormalities was lower in studies in which the BAEPs were recorded more than a week after the last transient ischemic attack.[100] Persistent BAEP changes may represent small infarcts that are clinically silent.

DEMYELINATING DISEASE

One of the major clinical applications of evoked potential testing has been in patients suspected of having a demyelinating disease such as MS. The diagnosis of definite MS requires a demonstration that multiple sites within the nervous system are involved. Evoked potentials can detect conduction slowing and temporal dispersion caused by subclinical demyelination and thus help to demonstrate the involvement of areas besides those accounting for the patient's clinical signs.

Following an episode of demyelination, signs and symptoms may clear because of remyelination or the establishment of nonsaltatory conduction, but the conduction velocity usually does not return to baseline. Nonsaltatory conduction in a completely demyelinated fiber is slow. In remyelination, the new myelin is usually thinner than the original and the internodes are shorter; both of these anatomic changes contribute to a slowed conduction velocity. Thus, evoked potentials can demonstrate a residual abnormality related to a prior symptom that has cleared and confirm that it is related to demyelination.

The reported sensitivity of BAEPs in patients with MS varies widely among published studies. The discrepancies are in part caused by differences in the criteria used to determine abnormality of BAEPs, as well as differences in the patient populations being studied (e.g., definite rather than probable MS). As an example of the latter, in one study of 202 patients with the disease,[101] abnormal BAEPs were found in approximately 20 percent of the patients with possible or probable MS and in 47 percent of the patients with clinically definite MS. The abnormality rate was even higher (57 percent) in a subgroup of patients with definite MS and symptoms or signs of a brainstem lesion.

In a meta-analysis by Chiappa covering 1,000 patients with MS (in various categories) reported in the literature,[102] abnormal BAEPs were found in 46 percent. When subdivided by categories of disease, the rate of abnormal BAEPs was 67 percent in patients with definite MS, 41 percent in probable MS, and 30 percent in possible MS.

BAEPs may display various patterns of abnormality in MS, depending on the areas that are involved by the disease process. Abnormalities in the I–III or III–V interpeak interval, or a combination of both, may be seen. Another pattern seen in MS is an abnormally small IV/V:I amplitude ratio in the presence of normal component latencies and interpeak intervals (see Fig. 24-10).

As noted earlier, MS may affect the eighth nerve itself. Involvement of the eighth nerve would be expected to cause a I–III interpeak interval abnormality of the BAEPs. However, prolongations of the PTT (wave I latency) have also been noted in patients with MS.[103] Multiple audiologic tests failed to reveal an otologic cause for the BAEP abnormalities in these patients, and the latency prolongations increased or decreased

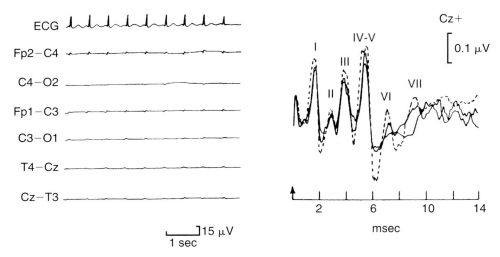

FIGURE 24-33 ■ Electroencephalogram (EEG) and brainstem auditory evoked potentials (BAEPs) from a 35-year-old woman who was comatose following a mixed drug overdose with central nervous system depressant drugs and a respiratory arrest. The clinical examination was consistent with brain death, and the EEG showed periods of complete suppression of electrical cerebral activity (left) lasting up to 18 minutes. The patient subsequently made a full neurologic recovery, and her EEG became normal. BAEPs recorded during a 13-minute EEG suppression while she was comatose (solid lines) and after she had recovered (dotted line) were both normal. (From Stockard JJ, Sharbrough FW: Unique contributions of short-latency auditory and somatosensory evoked potentials to neurologic diagnosis. p. 231. In Desmedt JE [ed]: Clinical Uses of Cerebral, Brainstem and Spinal Somatosensory Evoked Potentials. Karger, Basel, 1980, with permission.)

coincident with exacerbation or remission of the patients' clinical symptoms. Thus, it seems most likely that demyelinating disease itself can cause wave I abnormalities, and it should be considered as a possible cause of a PTT prolongation found in a patient being evaluated for possible MS.

COMA AND BRAIN DEATH

Coma can be caused by bilateral cerebral hemispheric dysfunction, brainstem dysfunction, or metabolic abnormalities that cause diffuse brain dysfunction. The BAEP findings depend on the cause of the coma and, for structural lesions, on the location of the pathology. BAEPs are typically normal in patients with coma caused entirely by supratentorial disease, although they may deteriorate subsequently because of transtentorial herniation.[82,83] Abnormal BAEPs in patients with supratentorial infarctions or hemorrhages are correlated with poor clinical outcomes.[104,105] Patients who are comatose because of brainstem lesions will have BAEP abnormalities and clinical findings that depend on the location of the pathology. The finding of normal-appearing BAEPs in a patient whose examination shows widespread brainstem dysfunction should prompt suspicion of a metabolic etiology such as a drug overdose; BAEPs are highly resistant to central nervous system depressant drugs and may be nearly normal in patients who clinically have no brainstem function (Fig. 24-33).

There have been many published reports of BAEPs in coma. Most of the patients studied were comatose following head trauma, although brainstem strokes were also included in some series. In several studies, BAEPs were shown to have prognostic value: patients in whom they were normal or who showed relatively mild latency or amplitude abnormalities were more likely to survive with good functional outcomes than were those in whom BAEPs were grossly abnormal or absent.[106–108] However, BAEPs were not thought to provide useful prognostic information in other reports,[109,110] predominantly because many patients with normal or nearly normal BAEPs died or had persistent severe neurologic impairment. This is not surprising; the unfavorable outcomes in these patients may have reflected brain damage outside the region of the brainstem generating the BAEPs. All of the studies showed that patients with markedly abnormal BAEPs are likely to have poor neurologic outcomes. These outcomes are attributable to the brainstem damage demonstrated by the BAEPs.

Several technical considerations should be kept in mind when performing and interpreting BAEP studies in comatose patients. Endotracheal tubes and positive-pressure ventilation interfere with eustachian tube function, and in patients who are chronically intubated, a middle ear effusion or pressure change may develop and cause conductive hearing loss, which appears as a wave I abnormality in the BAEP recording.

Body temperature should be noted when testing comatose patients because hypothermia causes alteration of the BAEPs; both interpeak latencies and the PTT will show reversible increases as the patient's temperature declines.[111,112] Hypothermia commonly is encountered (and may be profound) during intraoperative monitoring.

Some comatose patients are treated with barbiturate anesthesia. BAEPs can persist with only minor changes despite high doses of barbiturates in both human patients and animals. High doses of intravenous lidocaine can transiently abolish BAEPs, however.[113]

The locked-in syndrome typically results from infarction or demyelination affecting the motor tracts in the ventral pons. Patients with the locked-in syndrome are by definition not in coma because they are aware and can respond with eye movements, but a comatose state may be diagnosed unless the clinician is aware of the possibility of the syndrome and checks for it. BAEPs may be either normal[114–116] or abnormal[114,117] in patients with the locked-in syndrome, depending on the extent to which the lesion extends outside the ventral pons and involves the auditory pathways.

Typically, the BAEP recording in brain death contains no identifiable components, consists of wave I alone, or contains only a wave I followed by a wave IN (see Fig. 24-17). Reversal of stimulus polarity may be necessary to distinguish an apparent persistent wave I from the cochlear microphonic. Rarely, waves II and IIN may also be present and reflect the contribution to these components from the auditory nerve (see Fig. 24-18).[43] The presence of wave III is not compatible with total cessation of function of the entire brainstem because this component is generated within the lower pons, with a possible contribution from the cochlear nucleus. Rarely, persistence of wave III, and possibly of wave V as well, demonstrate persistent function of some brainstem structures in comatose patients meeting all clinical and EEG criteria for brain death, though none of the patients in whom this has been reported has survived.[76]

The absence of wave I in a comatose patient reflects ear or eighth nerve damage. Loss of the eighth nerve compound action potential eliminates input to the brainstem auditory pathways. Thus, a waveform in which no BAEP components are identifiable does not provide an assessment of the brainstem auditory pathways. Although consistent with brain death, it cannot be used as evidence that the brainstem is nonfunctional.

REFERENCES

1. Campbell KB, Bell I, Bastien C: Evoked potential measures of information processing during natural sleep. p. 89. In Broughton RJ, Ogilvie RD (eds): Sleep, Arousal, and Performance. Birkhauser, Boston, 1992
2. Litscher G: Continuous brainstem auditory evoked potential monitoring during nocturnal sleep. Int J Neurosci, 82:135, 1995
3. American Academy of Pediatrics Committee on Drugs: Guidelines for monitoring and management of pediatric patients during and after sedation for diagnostic and therapeutic procedures. Pediatrics, 89:1110, 1992
4. Banoub M, Tetzlaff JE, Schubert A: Pharmacologic and physiologic influences affecting sensory evoked potentials: implications for perioperative monitoring. Anesthesiology, 99:716, 2003
5. Legatt AD: Mechanisms of intraoperative brainstem auditory evoked potential changes. J Clin Neurophysiol, 19:396, 2002
6. Ruben RJ, Bordley JE, Lieberman AT: Cochlear potentials in man. Laryngoscope, 71:1141, 1961
7. Yoshie N, Ohashi T, Suzuki T: Non-surgical recording of auditory nerve action potentials in man. Laryngoscope, 77:76, 1967
8. Sohmer H, Feinmesser M: Cochlear action potentials recorded from the external ear in man. Ann Otol Rhinol Laryngol, 76:427, 1967
9. Jewett DL, Romano MN, Williston JS: Human auditory evoked potentials: possible brain stem components detected at the scalp. Science, 167:1517, 1970
10. Jewett DL, Williston JS: Auditory-evoked far fields averaged from the scalp of humans. Brain, 94:681, 1971
11. American Clinical Neurophysiology Society: Guideline 9A: Guidelines on evoked potentials. J Clin Neurophysiol, 23:125, 2006
12. American Clinical Neurophysiology Society: Guideline 9C: Guidelines on short-latency auditory evoked potentials. J Clin Neurophysiol, 23:157, 2006
13. Chiappa KH: Brain stem auditory evoked potentials: methodology. p. 157. In Chiappa KH (ed): Evoked Potentials in Clinical Medicine. 3rd Ed. Raven, New York, 1997
14. Roeser RJ, Clark JL: Clinical masking. p. 253. In Roeser RJ, Valente M, Hosford-Dunn H (eds): Audiology: Diagnosis. Thieme, New York, 2000
15. Schwartz DM, Morris MD, Spydell JD et al: Influence of click polarity on the brainstem auditory evoked response (BAER) revisited. Electroencephalogr Clin Neurophysiol, 77:445, 1990
16. Legatt AD: Impairment of common-mode rejection by mismatched electrode impedances: quantitative analysis. Am J EEG Technol, 35:296, 1995
17. Epstein CM: The use of brain stem auditory evoked potentials in the evaluation of the central nervous system. Neurol Clin, 6:771, 1988
18. Hughes JR, Fino J: Usefulness of piezoelectric earphones in recording the brain stem auditory evoked potentials: a new early deflection. Electroencephalogr Clin Neurophysiol, 48:357, 1980

19. Arnold SA: The auditory brain stem response. p. 451. In Roeser RJ, Valente M, Hosford-Dunn H (eds): Audiology: Diagnosis. Thieme, New York, 2000

20. Legatt AD, Pedley TA, Emerson RG et al: Normal brainstem auditory evoked potentials with abnormal latency–intensity studies in patients with acoustic neuromas. Arch Neurol, 45:1326, 1988

21. Klein AJ, Alvarez ED, Cowburn CA: The effects of stimulus rate on detectability of the auditory brain stem response in infants. Ear Hearing, 13:401, 1992

22. Stapells DR, Picton TW, Durieux-Smith A et al: Thresholds for short-latency auditory-evoked potentials to tones in notched noise in normal-hearing and hearing-impaired subjects. Audiology, 29:262, 1990

23. Hoormann J, Falkenstein M, Hohnsbein J et al: The human frequency-following response (FFR): normal variability and relation to the click-evoked brainstem response. Hearing Res, 59:179, 1992

24. Cone-Wesson B, Ramirez GM: Hearing sensitivity in newborns estimated from ABRs to bone-conducted sounds. J Am Acad Audiol, 8:299, 1997

25. Yang EY, Stuart A, Mencher GT et al: Auditory brain stem responses to air- and bone-conducted clicks in the audiological assessment of at-risk infants. Ear Hearing, 14:175, 1993

26. Wackym PA, Firszt JB, Gaggl W et al: Electrophysiologic effects of placing cochlear implant electrodes in a perimodiolar position in young children. Laryngoscope, 114:71, 2004

27. Waring MD: Intraoperative electrophysiologic monitoring to assist placement of auditory brainstem implant. Ann Otol Rhinol Laryngol, 106:Suppl 166, 33, 1995

28. Brown CJ: Clinical uses of electrically evoked auditory nerve and brainstem responses. Curr Opin Otolaryngol Head Neck Surg, 11:383, 2003

29. Nikolopoulos TP, Mason SM, Gibbin KP et al: The prognostic value of promontory electric auditory brain stem response in pediatric cochlear implantation. Ear Hearing, 21:236, 2000

30. Song MH, Bae MR, Kim HN et al: Value of intracochlear electrically evoked auditory brainstem response after cochlear implantation in patients with narrow internal auditory canal. Laryngoscope, 120:1625, 2010

31. Parkkonen L, Fujiki N, Mäkelä JP: Sources of auditory brainstem responses revisited: contribution by magnetoencephalography. Hum Brain Mapping, 30:1772, 2009

32. Ananthanarayan AK, Durrant JD: On the origin of wave II of the auditory brain stem evoked response. Ear Hearing, 12:174, 1991

33. Hashimoto I, Ishiyama Y, Yoshimoto T et al: Brain-stem auditory evoked potentials recorded directly from human brain stem and thalamus. Brain, 104:841, 1981

34. Achor LJ, Starr A: Auditory brain stem responses in the cat. I. Intracranial and extracranial recordings. Electroencephalogr Clin Neurophysiol, 48:154, 1980

35. Legatt AD, Arezzo JC, Vaughan HG, Jr: Short-latency auditory evoked potentials in the monkey. II. Intracranial generators. Electroencephalogr Clin Neurophysiol, 64:53, 1986

36. Gersdorff MCH: Simultaneous recordings of human auditory potentials: transtympanic electrocochleography (ECoG) and brainstem-evoked responses (BER). Arch Otorhinolaryngol, 234:15, 1982

37. Chatrian GE, Wirch AL, Edwards KH et al: Cochlear summating potential recorded from the external auditory meatus of normal humans. Amplitude-intensity functions and relationships to auditory nerve compound action potential. Electroencephalogr Clin Neurophysiol, 59:396, 1984

38. Chimento TC, Williston JS, Jewett DL et al: The 3-channel Lissajous' trajectory of the auditory brain-stem response. VIII. Isolated frog sciatic nerve in a volume conductor. Electroencephalogr Clin Neurophysiol, 68:380, 1987

39. Kimura J, Kimura A, Ishida T et al: What determines the latency and amplitude of stationary peaks in far-field recordings? Ann Neurol, 19:479, 1986

40. Legouix JP, Pierson A: Investigations on the sources of whole-nerve action potentials recorded from various places in the guinea pig cochlea. J Acoust Soc Am, 56:1222, 1974

41. Portmann M, Cazals Y, Negrevergne M et al: Transtympanic and surface recordings in the diagnosis of retrocochlear disorders. Acta Otolaryngol, 89:362, 1980

42. Scherg M, Von Cramon D: A new interpretation of the generators of BAEP waves I–V: results of a spatio-temporal dipole model. Electroencephalogr Clin Neurophysiol, 62:290, 1985

43. Stockard JJ, Pope-Stockard JE, Sharbrough FW: Brainstem auditory evoked potentials in neurology: methodology, interpretation, and clinical application. p. 503. In Aminoff MJ (ed): Electrodiagnosis in Clinical Neurology. 3rd Ed. Churchill Livingstone, New York, 1992

44. Curio G, Oppel F, Scherg M: Peripheral origin of BAEP wave II in a case with unilateral pontine pathology: a comparison of intracranial and scalp recordings. Electroencephalogr Clin Neurophysiol, 66:29, 1987

45. Hopf HC: Die Generatoren der AEP-Wellen-II-III. Flogerungen aus Befunden bei definierten Hirnstammprozessen. Akt Neurol, 12:58, 1985

46. Legatt AD, Gordon DS, Flamm ES: BAEP changes during surgery for an intra-pontine cavernous hemangioma: evidence that wave II is composite. Muscle Nerve, 28:S81, 2003

47. Møller AR, Jannetta PJ: Compound action potentials recorded intracranially from the auditory nerve in man. Exp Neurol, 74:862, 1981

48. Legatt AD, Arezzo JC, Vaughan HG, Jr: The anatomic and physiologic bases of brain stem auditory evoked potentials. Neurol Clin, 6:681, 1988

49. Cohen M, Luxon L, Rudge P: Auditory deficits and hearing loss associated with focal brainstem haemorrhage. Scand Audiol, 25:133, 1996

50. Curio G, Oppel F: Intraparenchymatous ponto-mesencephalic field distribution of brain-stem auditory evoked potentials in man. Electroencephalogr Clin Neurophysiol, 69:259, 1988

51. Cho TH, Fischer C, Nighoghossian N et al: Auditory and electrophysiological patterns of a unilateral lesion of the lateral lemniscus. Audiol Neurootol, 10:153, 2005

52. Hirsch BE, Durrant JD, Yetiser S et al: Localizing retrocochlear hearing loss. Am J Otol, 17:537, 1996

53. Scaioli V, Savoiardo M, Bussone G et al: Brain-stem auditory evoked potentials (BAEPs) and magnetic resonance imaging (MRI) in a case of facial myokymia. Electroencephalogr Clin Neurophysiol, 71:153, 1988

54. Fischer C, Bognar L, Turjman F et al: Auditory evoked potentials in a patient with a unilateral lesion of the inferior colliculus and medial geniculate body. Electroencephalogr Clin Neurophysiol, 96:261, 1995

55. Chu N-S: Brainstem auditory evoked potentials: correlation between CT midbrain-pontine lesion sites and abolition of wave V or the IV–V complex. J Neurol Sci, 91:165, 1989

56. Musiek FE: Neuroanatomy, neurophysiology, and central auditory assessment. Part III: Corpus callosum and efferent pathways. Ear Hearing, 7:349, 1986

57. Møller AR, Jannetta PJ: Evoked potentials from the inferior colliculus in man. Electroencephalogr Clin Neurophysiol, 53:612, 1982

58. Møller AR, Jannetta PJ: Interpretation of brainstem auditory evoked potentials: results from intracranial recordings in humans. Scand Audiol, 12:125, 1983

59. Kimiskidis VK, Lalaki P, Papagiannopoulos S et al: Sensorineural hearing loss and word deafness caused by a mesencephalic lesion: clinicoelectrophysiologic correlations. Otol Neurotol, 25:178, 2004

60. Shimbo Y, Sakata M, Hayano M et al: Topographical relationships between the brainstem auditory and somatosensory evoked potentials and the location of lesions in posterior fossa stroke. Neurol Med Chir, 43:282, 2003

61. Hu C-J, Chan K-Y, Lin T-J et al: Traumatic brainstem deafness with normal brainstem auditory evoked potentials. Neurology, 48:1448, 1997

62. Masuda S, Takeuchi K, Tsuruoka H et al: Word deafness after resection of a pineal body tumor in the presence of normal wave latencies of the auditory brain stem response. Ann Otol Rhinol Laryngol, 109:1107, 2000

63. Meyer B, Kral T, Zentner J: Pure word deafness after resection of a tectal plate glioma with preservation of wave V of brain stem auditory evoked potentials. J Neurol Neurosurg Psychiatry, 61:423, 1996

64. Zanette G, Carteri A, Cusumano S: Reappearance of brain-stem auditory evoked potentials after surgical treatment of a brain-stem hemorrhage: contributions to the question of wave generation. Electroencephalogr Clin Neurophysiol, 77:140, 1990

65. Velasco M, Velasco F, Almanza X et al: Subcortical correlates of the auditory brain stem potentials in man: bipolar EEG and multiple unit activity and electrical stimulation. Electroencephalogr Clin Neurophysiol, 53:133, 1982

66. Hashimoto I: Auditory evoked potentials from the human midbrain: slow brain stem responses. Electroencephalogr Clin Neurophysiol, 53:652, 1982

67. Oken BS: Statistics for evoked potentials. p. 565. In Chiappa KH (ed): Evoked Potentials in Clinical Medicine. 3rd Ed. Raven, New York, 1997

68. Sand T: Statistical properties of ABR amplitudes and latencies. Implications for computation of reference limits and relation to click phase. Scand Audiol, 19:131, 1990

69. van Dijk JG, Jennekens-Schinkel A, Caekebeke JFV et al: What is the validity of an "abnormal" evoked or event-related potential in MS? Auditory and visual evoked and event-related potentials in multiple sclerosis patients and normal subjects. J Neurol Sci, 109:11, 1992

70. Chan YW, Woo EK, Hammond SR et al: The interaction between sex and click polarity in brain-stem auditory potentials evoked from control subjects of Oriental and Caucasian origin. Electroencephalogr Clin Neurophysiol, 71:77, 1988

71. Lopez-Escamez JA, Salguero G, Salinero J: Age and sex differences in latencies of waves I, III and V in auditory brainstem response of normal hearing subjects. Acta Otorhinolaryngol Belg, 53:109, 1999

72. Eggermont JJ, Don M: Mechanisms of central conduction time prolongation in brainstem auditory evoked potentials. Arch Neurol, 43:116, 1986

73. Ferbert A, Buchner H, Bruckmann H et al: Evoked potentials in basilar artery thrombosis: correlation with clinical and angiographic findings. Electroencephalogr Clin Neurophysiol, 69:136, 1988

74. Rao TH, Libman RB: When is isolated vertigo a harbinger of stroke? Ear Nose Throat J, 74:33, 1995

75. Yamasoba T, Kikuchi S, Higo R: Deafness associated with vertebrobasilar insufficiency. J Neurol Sci, 187:69, 2001

76. Facco E, Munari M, Gallo F et al: Role of short latency evoked potentials in the diagnosis of brain death. Clin Neurophysiol, 113:1855, 2002

77. Trussell LO: Synaptic mechanisms for coding timing in auditory neurons. Annu Rev Physiol, 61:477, 1999

78. Levine RA, Gardner JC, Fullerton BC et al: Effects of multiple sclerosis brainstem lesions on sound lateralization and brainstem auditory evoked potentials. Hearing Res, 68:73, 1993

79. Kaga K, Shindo M, Tanaka Y: Auditory brain stem responses and nonsense monosyllable perception test findings for patients with auditory nerve and brain stem lesions. Laryngoscope, 96:1272, 1986

80. Pillion JP, Moser HW, Raymond GV: Auditory function in adrenomyeloneuropathy. J Neurol Sci, 269:24, 2008

81. Polyakov A, Pratt H: Electrophysiologic correlates of direction and elevation cues for sound localization in the human brainstem. Int J Audiol, 42:140, 2003

82. Garcia-Larrea L, Bertrand O, Artru F et al: Brain-stem monitoring. II. Preterminal BAEP changes observed until brain death in deeply comatose patients. Electroencephalogr Clin Neurophysiol, 68:446, 1987

83. Hall JW III, Mackey-Hargadine JR, Kim EE: Auditory brain-stem response in determination of brain death. Arch Otolaryngol, 111:613, 1985

84. Musiek FE, Weider DJ, Mueller RJ: Reversible audiological results in a patient with an extra-axial brainstem tumor. Ear Hearing, 4:169, 1983

85. Yamasoba T, Sakai K, Sakurai M: Role of acute cochlear neuritis in sudden hearing loss in multiple sclerosis. J Neurol Sci, 146:179, 1997

86. Bergamaschi R, Romani A, Zappoli F et al: MRI and brainstem auditory evoked potential evidence of eighth cranial nerve involvement in multiple sclerosis. Neurology, 48:270, 1997

87. Ho KJ, Kileny P, Paccioretti D et al: Neurologic, audiologic, and electrophysiologic sequelae of bilateral temporal lobe lesions. Arch Neurol, 44:982, 1987

88. Bahls FH, Chatrian GE, Mesher RA et al: A case of persistent cortical deafness: clinical, neurophysiologic, and neuropathologic observations. Neurology, 38:1490, 1988

89. Kraus N, Özdamar Ö, Stein L et al: Absent auditory brain stem response: peripheral hearing loss or brain stem dysfunction? Laryngoscope, 94:400, 1984

90. Legatt AD: Evoked potentials in the assessment of patients with suspected psychogenic sensory symptoms. p. 209. In Hallett M, Lang A, Jankovic J et al (eds): Psychogenic Movement Disorders and Other Conversion Disorders. Cambridge University Press, Cambridge, 2011

91. Barrs DM, Brackmann DE, Olson JE et al: Changing concepts of acoustic neuroma diagnosis. Arch Otolaryngol, 111:17, 1985

92. Zappia JJ, O'Connor CA, Wiet RJ et al: Rethinking the use of auditory brainstem response in acoustic neuroma screening. Laryngoscope, 107:1388, 1997

93. El-Kashlan HK, Eisenmann D, Kileny PR: Auditory brain stem response in small acoustic neuromas. Ear Hearing, 21:257, 2000

94. Dornhoffer JL, Helms J, Hoehmann DH: Presentation and diagnosis of small acoustic tumors. Otolaryngol Head Neck Surg, 111:232, 1994

95. Matthies C, Samii M: Management of vestibular schwannomas (acoustic neuromas): the value of neurophysiology for evaluation and prediction of auditory function in 420 cases. Neurosurgery, 40:919, 1997

96. Weston PF, Manson JI, Abbott KJ: Auditory brainstem-evoked response in childhood brainstem glioma. Childs Nerv Syst, 2:301, 1986

97. Itoh A, Kim YS, Yoshioka K et al: Clinical study of vestibular-evoked myogenic potentials and auditory brainstem responses in patients with brainstem lesions. Acta Otolaryngol Suppl, 545:116, 2001

98. Factor SA, Dentinger MP: Early brain-stem auditory evoked responses in vertebrobasilar transient ischemic attacks. Arch Neurol, 44:544, 1987

99. Rossi L, Amantini A, Bindi A et al: Electrophysiological investigations of the brainstem in the vertebrobasilar reversible attacks. Eur Neurol, 22:371, 1983

100. Benna P, Bianco C, Costa P et al: Visual evoked potentials and brainstem auditory evoked potentials in migraine and transient ischemic attacks. Cephalalgia, 5:Suppl 2, 53, 1985

101. Chiappa KH, Harrison JL, Brooks EB et al: Brainstem auditory evoked responses in 200 patients with multiple sclerosis. Ann Neurol, 7:135, 1980

102. Chiappa KH: Use of evoked potentials for diagnosis of multiple sclerosis. Neurol Clin, 6:861, 1988

103. Rimpel J, Geyer D, Hopf HC: Changes in the blink responses to combined trigeminal, acoustic and visual repetitive stimulation, studied in the human subject. Electroencephalogr Clin Neurophysiol, 54:552, 1982

104. Haupt WF, Birkmann C, Halber M: Serial evoked potentials and outcome in cerebrovascular critical care patients. J Clin Neurophysiol, 17:326, 2000

105. Burghaus L, Liu WC, Dohmen C et al: Evoked potentials in acute ischemic stroke within the first 24 h: possible predictor of a malignant course. Neurocrit Care, 9:13, 2008

106. Ottaviani F, Almadori G, Calderazzo AB et al: Auditory brain-stem (ABRs) and middle latency auditory responses (MLRs) in the prognosis of severely head-injured patients. Electroencephalogr Clin Neurophysiol, 65:196, 1986

107. Facco E, Martini A, Zuccarello M et al: Is the auditory brain-stem response (ABR) effective in the assessment of post-traumatic coma? Electroencephalogr Clin Neurophysiol, 62:332, 1985

108. Krieger D, Adams H-P, Rieke K et al: Prospective evaluation of the prognostic significance of evoked potentials in acute basilar occlusion. Crit Care Med, 21:1169, 1993

109. Cant BR, Hume AL, Judson JA et al: The assessment of severe head injury by short-latency somatosensory and brainstem auditory evoked potentials. Electroencephalogr Clin Neurophysiol, 65:188, 1986

110. Anderson DC, Bundli S, Rockswold GL: Multimodality EPs in closed head trauma. Arch Neurol, 41:369, 1984

111. Markand ON, Lee BI, Warren C et al: Effects of hypothermia on brainstem auditory evoked potentials in humans. Ann Neurol, 22:507, 1987

112. Rodriguez RA, Edmonds HL Jr, Auden SM et al: Auditory brainstem evoked responses and temperature monitoring during pediatric cardiopulmonary bypass. Can J Anaesth, 46:832, 1999

113. García-Larrea L, Artu F, Bertrand O et al: Transient drug-induced abolition of BAEPs in coma. Neurology, 38:1487, 1988

114. Bassetti C, Mathis J, Hess CW: Multimodal electrophysiological studies including motor evoked potentials in patients with locked-in syndrome: report of six patients. J Neurol Neurosurg Psychiatry, 57:1403, 1994

115. Landi A, Fornezza U, De Luca G et al: Brain stem and motor evoked responses in "locked-in" syndrome. J Neurosurg Sci, 38:123, 1994

116. Budak F, Ilhan A, Ozmenoglu M et al: Locked-in syndrome: a case report. Clin Electroencephalogr, 25:40, 1994

117. Seales DM, Torkelson RD, Shuman RM et al: Abnormal brainstem auditory evoked potentials and neuropathology in "locked-in" syndrome. Neurology, 31:893, 1981

Brainstem Auditory Evoked Potentials in Infants and Children

TERENCE W. PICTON, MARGOT J. TAYLOR, and ANDRÉE DURIEUX-SMITH

Brainstem auditory evoked potentials (BAEPs) are used in pediatrics to detect and measure hearing loss in children who cannot be tested behaviorally and to evaluate the auditory brainstem pathways in children who may have neurologic problems. Recording pediatric BAEPs requires close cooperation between audiologists and neurologists because it is impossible to interpret these responses correctly without paying careful attention to both the ear and the brain.

SPECIAL TECHNICAL CONSIDERATIONS IN CHILDHOOD

Sleep

BAEPs in children are smaller than in adults, and the background electrical noise from the electroencephalogram (EEG) and scalp muscles is often higher. Whenever possible, infants and young children should be tested while asleep because sleep reduces both EEG and muscle artifact. Newborn infants quickly fall asleep after feeding. Most older infants will sleep through a 1-hour recording session if they are awakened early on the day of the test. After the electrodes are applied, the infant is left with the mother in a darkened, sound-attenuated room to

feed and fall asleep. Children older than 18 months of age usually will be quiet for the procedure, provided that it is introduced to them slowly and gently. If necessary, sleep may be assisted by oral diazepam (0.2 to 0.3 mg/kg) or chloral hydrate (30 to 50 mg/kg), but only if adequate facilities for resuscitation are immediately available. General anesthesia is occasionally necessary in extremely disturbed children and those with severe involuntary movement disorders. Most anesthetics cause small dose-related changes in the latency and amplitude of the responses but do not affect the detection of the different waves or the assessment of thresholds.

Stimuli

BAEPs commonly are evoked by clicks. Each recording should be made with clicks of only one polarity. In patients with high-frequency hearing loss, latency differences between the responses to condensation and rarefaction clicks may distort the responses when using clicks with alternating polarity. Recording separate responses to condensation and rarefaction clicks allows brainstem responses to be distinguished from stimulus artifacts and cochlear microphonics.[1]

For most purposes, responses are recorded using monaural stimuli. If binaural stimuli are used, the examiner should be aware that the binaural response approximates the sum of the responses from each ear. A unilateral hearing loss thus may not be noticed. If the threshold for one ear differs by more than 40 dB from the other ear, contralateral masking to prevent cross-hearing is necessary. Some systems automatically present masking in the contralateral ear.

The intensity of the click is calibrated relative to normal hearing thresholds (nHL) for adults. The acoustic intensity of 0 dB nHL is approximately 30 dB peak-to-peak equivalent sound pressure level (peSPL).[2,3] The earphones should be placed or held so that they do not slip off the ear or occlude the ear canal. Some BAEP systems use an earphone with a light circumaural seal and a transparent cover that allows the examiner to observe the ear canal. Insert earphones are perhaps the best way of attenuating the stimulus artifact and preventing collapse of the ear canal.

The stimuli are presented at rates between 10 and 100 Hz. Wave I is best recorded at rates between 10 and 20 Hz. Wave V is recorded most efficiently at 50 to 100 Hz because its amplitude is relatively insensitive to increasing rates. Maximum length sequences provide an effective way of presenting stimuli at rates greater than 100 Hz without running into problems of overlap.[4,5]

Clicks contain energy at all audiometric frequencies, and simple click-evoked BAEPs cannot assess auditory thresholds at different frequencies. Thresholds for the click-evoked BAEP are related most closely to behavioral thresholds between 2,000 and 4,000 Hz. However, children with high-frequency hearing losses and normal hearing at 1,000 Hz can still show BAEPs (albeit delayed) down to nearly normal thresholds. Furthermore, although absent click-evoked potentials usually indicate severe high-frequency loss, they provide very little information about the extent of low-frequency hearing. Procedures for assessing frequency-specific thresholds use two main techniques: (1) limiting the responsiveness of the auditory system by masking; and (2) concentrating the acoustic energy in the stimuli by using tones.

The derived-response technique records the responses to clicks in high-pass masking noise. Different high-pass cut-off frequencies are used for the masking noise, and sequential subtraction of the recordings yields the derived responses to the frequencies between the filter settings. This technique has been used to evaluate the hearing of infants and the development of the cochlea.[6]

Brief tones are another way of evaluating frequency-specific thresholds. The most commonly used tones have linear rise and fall times of 2 cycles each and a plateau of 1 cycle.[7] Brief tones have significant energy in frequencies other than their nominal frequency, and BAEPs to brief tones may be evoked by this spectral splatter. Notched noise or broad-band masking may be used to limit responsiveness to the frequencies of the tone.[8] Determining the thresholds for BAEPs evoked by tones may provide important information about hearing in infancy and childhood.[9,10]

Continuous tones with sinusoidal amplitude modulation have energy limited to the carrier frequency and two side bands separated from the carrier by the frequency of modulation. These frequency-specific stimuli can evoke steady-state responses at the frequency of the modulation.[11] In adults and older children, prominent steady-state responses can be recorded at frequencies near 40 Hz. Unfortunately, these responses are attenuated by sleep and are difficult to record in infants and young children. Responses at frequencies of 70 to 100 Hz are probably the steady-state version of the transient BAEP and can be recorded reliably in sleeping infants.[12–14]

BAEP thresholds to bone-conducted stimuli are important when assessing middle ear function. The bone vibrator should be positioned over the temporal bone posterior and superior to the ear and held in place by an elastic headband or the examiner's hand.[15,16] The skull bones of infants are not meshed tightly together, and bone-conducted stimuli are not distributed equally through the skull. BAEPs recorded between the vertex and the ipsilateral mastoid in infants are larger and have slightly lower thresholds than those recorded between the vertex and the contralateral mastoid. This asymmetry may aid in the evaluation of whether inner-ear function differs between the ears in infants with bilateral conductive hearing loss. Steady-state responses recorded using bone-conducted stimuli show a similar asymmetry.[17]

Recording

BAEPs are recorded between surface electrodes placed on the vertex and the ipsilateral mastoid or ear lobe. If the scalp electrode is located on the forehead, wave V will be smaller but still recognizable. In young infants the vertex electrode is best located in the midline anterior to the fontanelle. In newborn infants, the electrodes should be attached to the scalp with nonirritating tape and saline jelly. In older children, an adhesive paste or collodion and gauze may be used. Collodion should not be used in neonates because of skin sensitivity.

The authors recommend recording simultaneously from two channels: (1) vertex to ipsilateral mastoid;

and (2) vertex to contralateral mastoid. It is then unnecessary to switch electrodes when the baby rolls over during sleep and the examiner decides to stimulate the upper ear rather than risk wakefulness by rolling the baby back. A mastoid-to-mastoid recording, which can sometimes make wave I easier to recognize, can be obtained by subtracting one vertex recording from the other.

Because the infant's response is slower than that of the adult, the recording sweep should be longer (15 or 20 msec) and the low-frequency cut-off of the filters should be lower (20 to 30 Hz) than in adults.[18] This adjustment is particularly important when responses to low-intensity stimuli are being examined. Settings similar to those for adults (10-msec sweeps and 100- to 3,000-Hz filter bandpass) are used in much of the literature and are acceptable for older children. Normative data for latencies and amplitudes are specific to the filter settings.

DEVELOPMENTAL CHANGES

Normal Neonates

The BAEP of infants probably is best introduced through the response of the normal newborn (Fig. 25-1). In general, the neonatal BAEP is about one-half the size of the adult BAEP. Wave V is particularly small, and the average V/I amplitude ratio in the normal newborn is about 1.5, whereas in adults it is over 2. These numbers are based on a low-frequency cut-off of 20 or 30 Hz; raising this setting will decrease the V/I ratio. The V/I ratio may decrease with increasing stimulus intensity because wave I increases more than wave V. The general morphology of the response differs in several other ways: in the neonate, wave I is often double-peaked, a prominent negative wave follows wave I, and the negative wave after wave III is small.

As in adults, the peak latencies of the infant's response increase with decreasing intensity, and the I–V latency increases with increasing rates of stimulation. A rarefaction click usually evokes an earlier wave I than a condensation click. Because wave I of newborns may be double-peaked, latency values involving this wave will differ with the rules used for its measurement. Benchmark latencies for the BAEP in full-term neonates are a I–V latency of 5 msec and a wave V latency of 7 msec at 70 dB nHL.[19]

The scalp distribution of the neonatal BAEP is very different from that of the adult response.[20] This difference may be related to the different orientations of the neonatal auditory pathways or to incomplete myelination in

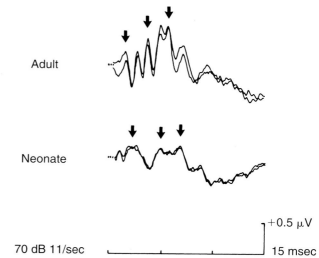

FIGURE 25-1 ■ Typical brainstem auditory evoked potentials from a normal adult and a normal neonate (40 weeks gestational age). In the adult the responses were recorded between electrodes on the vertex and the ipsilateral mastoid. In the newborn infant the responses were recorded between an electrode just anterior to the anterior fontanelle and an electrode on the ipsilateral mastoid. The polarity convention of this and all subsequent figures is that positivity at the scalp relative to the mastoid is represented by an upward deflection. For both subjects the stimulus was a 70-dB nHL rarefaction click presented at a rate of 11 per second. Each tracing represents the average of 2,000 individual responses. The stimulus artifacts recorded in the first 0.5 msec of the sweep have been removed from the recordings. The arrows indicate waves I, III, and V for both the adult and the neonatal response.

parts of the pathway. In the neonate, wave I is often larger on a mastoid-to-mastoid recording than on a vertex-to-mastoid recording. The dipoles underlying waves III and V are also oriented more laterally. On a recording between the vertex and the contralateral mastoid, waves III and V are small and appear to have opposite polarity to those recorded on the ipsilateral montage (Fig. 25-2). The small size of the contralateral recording in the neonate makes the response very difficult to recognize at low intensities, and when assessing thresholds care must be taken to ensure that the electrode montage is correct. The scalp distribution of the BAEP becomes similar to that of the adult BAEP by the end of the first year of life.[21]

The BAEP can be recorded in normal newborn infants with stimulus intensities as low as 30 dB nHL, provided that the infant is asleep, sufficient averaging is performed, and the acoustic noise in the environment is low. If the recording parameters are optimized, responses can be recorded with stimuli as low as 10 dB nHL. Figure 25-3 shows BAEPs recorded near threshold in a normal newborn infant.

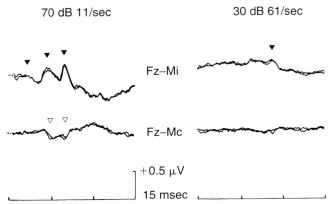

FIGURE 25-2 ■ Ipsilateral and contralateral recording montages in the neonatal brainstem auditory evoked potential (BAEP). These responses were recorded from a newborn infant at 38 weeks gestational age. On the left are responses to 70-dB nHL clicks presented at a rate of 11 Hz, and on the right are responses to 30-dB nHL clicks presented at a rate of 61 Hz. The upper tracings represent recordings between the forehead and the mastoid ipsilateral to stimulation, whereas the lower tracings represent recordings between the forehead and the mastoid contralateral to stimulation. In the BAEP recorded at high intensity with the ipsilateral montage, waves I, III, and V are clearly visible (filled triangles). On the contralateral montage, waves III and V are much smaller in amplitude and have an opposite polarity (open triangles). At the lower intensity, wave V is recognizable on the ipsilateral montage (filled triangle), but there is no clear response on the contralateral montage.

Premature Infants

BAEPs can be recorded in premature infants as early as a gestational age of 26 weeks.[22] In these infants they are evoked only by stimuli presented at high intensity and slow rates. The amplitude of the response, particularly wave V, is smaller than that in full-term neonates. The latencies of all the components of the response decrease with increasing conceptional age. Wave V shows a greater change with age than does wave I, and thus the I–V interpeak latency also decreases with age. From 36 to 40 weeks gestational age the latency of wave I decreases by about 0.1 msec, whereas the latency of wave V decreases by 0.4 msec. The increase in latency and decrease in amplitude of wave V that occur with increasing stimulus rate are more marked in premature infants than in full-term infants.[23] Figure 25-4 shows the BAEPs from a normal premature infant and a term infant.

The BAEPs of a premature infant and a full-term infant who have reached the same conceptional age are similar in morphology and interpeak latencies. However, the absolute latencies of specific peaks in the BAEP of premature infants are longer by about 0.3 msec, and this difference persists over the first 2 years of life.[24] This might be partly related to the greater incidence of otitis media in babies born prematurely. In premature infants

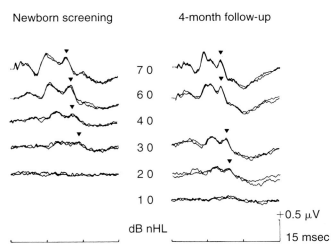

FIGURE 25-3 ■ Threshold studies during infancy. On the left are shown the responses recorded in a newborn infant at a gestational age of 37 weeks. On the right are shown follow-up results taken 4 months later. Responses were evoked by rarefaction clicks presented at a rate of 61 Hz. For the neonatal recordings, wave V is clearly recognizable (triangle) down to 30 dB nHL. Four months later, the responses can be recognized down to 20 dB nHL.

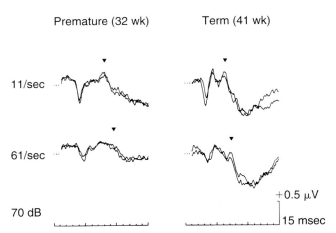

FIGURE 25-4 ■ Brainstem auditory evoked potentials (BAEPs) in premature infants. On the left are shown BAEPs recorded from a premature infant (gestational age 32 weeks), and on the right are shown responses from a term infant (gestational age 41 weeks). The upper tracings represent the responses to 70-dB nHL clicks presented at a rate of 11 Hz, and the lower tracings represent responses recorded at a stimulus rate of 61 Hz. The response of the premature infant is smaller and later than the response of the term infant, and increasing the stimulus rate to 61 Hz causes a greater change in the latency and amplitude of wave V (triangles).

who are small for gestational age, wave V is shorter in latency than in normal premature infants, but the latency does not change as much with increasing age.[25]

Postnatal Maturation

BAEPs recorded from infants within the first few hours after birth differ significantly from those recorded a day after birth.[26] Wave I is delayed just after birth by about 0.8 msec, probably because of residual fluid in the middle ear. However, there is also a significant difference in the I–V interval of 0.2 msec, which indicates some central changes over the first day of life.

In normal children the BAEP to monaural stimulation matures to the adult pattern by the age of about 3 years.[27–29] After this age, the child's BAEP has latencies that are similar to those of the adult, although some subtle differences remain. Table 25-1 presents normative developmental data from the authors' laboratories in Ottawa and Toronto.

The different components of the BAEP mature differently. Wave I latency reaches adult values by 2 months. Waves III and V show a rapid decrease in latency over the first several months and then a slower decrease to reach adult normal values at the end of the third year. The amplitude of wave V shows a marked increase after 6 months but does not reach adult values until about 5 years. The developmental changes in the latencies of the BAEP can be interpreted in terms of the differential maturation of axonal conduction time and synaptic transmission, and by the changes in the length of the auditory pathways.[30,31]

The threshold for detecting the BAEP decreases by about 10 dB in the first 3 months of life and by a further 5 dB by the end of the first year. These changes probably are related to several factors, including the resolution of neonatal conductive hearing loss and maturation of the cochlea and brainstem. Figure 25-3 illustrates this improvement in threshold.

Gender causes significant differences in BAEPs, but there is some controversy in the literature about when these differences become significant. Some studies of neonates have found a significantly shorter latency of wave V in female babies, whereas other studies have found no differences. More consistent latency differences between males and females show up somewhere between a few months of age and puberty.[32,33] The major differences involve the I–III and I–V interpeak latencies. The amplitude of wave V is larger in girls, with this difference becoming apparent by 3 years of age. These latency and amplitude differences probably are caused by gender-related differences in the length of the basilar membrane.[34]

EVALUATION OF HEARING

Hearing Impairment in Infancy

Between 1 and 3 per 1,000 children are born with a sensorineural hearing loss that requires treatment.[35] The cost of hearing impairment to the individual and to society is a result of the decreased communication ability of the hearing-impaired individual. Even mild hearing loss can impede the normal development of speech and language. Conductive hearing losses can be treated medically or surgically; sensorineural hearing losses can be treated with hearing aids, cochlear implants, and communication development training (e.g., "aural habilitation"). A major determinant of how well a hearing-impaired individual ultimately communicates is the age at which the impairment is detected and treatment instituted. It is therefore essential to identify and assess hearing-impaired infants as soon as possible.[36–38]

	Latency (msec)				Amplitude (μV)	
Age	I	III	V	I–V	V	V/I
Premature (36-wk gestational age)	2.1 (0.3)	5.0 (0.4)	7.4 (0.4)	5.3 (0.3)	0.4	1.5
Full-term neonate	2.0 (0.3)	4.8 (0.3)	7.0 (0.3)	5.0 (0.3)	0.5	1.6
6 wk	1.8 (0.2)	4.4 (0.3)	6.6 (0.3)	4.9 (0.3)	0.5	1.6
3 mo	1.7 (0.2)	4.3 (0.3)	6.4 (0.3)	4.7 (0.3)	0.6	1.6
6 mo	1.7 (0.2)	4.1 (0.3)	6.2 (0.3)	4.6 (0.3)	0.6	1.8
12 mo	1.7 (0.2)	4.0 (0.3)	6.0 (0.3)	4.3 (0.2)	0.6	2.0
2 yr	1.7 (0.2)	3.8 (0.2)	5.7 (0.2)	4.0 (0.2)	0.6	2.2

TABLE 25-1 ■ Normative Values for Pediatric BAEPS*

*These values are for BAEPs elicited by 70-dB nHL rarefaction clicks presented at a rate of 11 Hz. Standard deviations are given in parentheses for latencies but not for amplitudes because the latter are not distributed normally.

TABLE 25-2 ■ Risk Factors for Hearing Loss in Neonates

1. Family history of hereditary childhood hearing loss
2. Congenital perinatal infection (e.g., cytomegalovirus, rubella, herpes, toxoplasmosis, syphilis)
3. Anatomic malformations involving the head or neck
4. Birth weight < 1,500 g
5. Hyperbilirubinemia at levels requiring exchange transfusion
6. Ototoxic medications
7. Bacterial meningitis
8. Apgar scores of 0–4 at 1 min or 0–6 at 5 min
9. Mechanical ventilation for longer than 5 days
10. Stigmata of syndromes known to include sensorineural hearing loss (e.g., Waardenburg or Usher syndrome)

There are clearly defined risk factors for hearing loss in the newborn period (Table 25-2).[35] Most of the risk factors for hearing loss (except family history) are present in infants treated in a neonatal intensive care unit (NICU), and many children with significant hearing loss are admitted to an NICU. One early approach to the detection of hearing impairment was therefore to record BAEPs in babies at risk for hearing impairment and babies being discharged from an NICU.[39]

Unfortunately, about 40 percent of infants with significant hearing loss do not show any risk factors.[35] A consensus panel of the National Institutes of Health in the United States therefore recommended universal screening of all newborn infants for hearing impairment.[40] Behavioral testing is not an effective approach to the evaluation of hearing in the first few months of life. Some babies have reflex responses to sound, but sleepy or sick babies may not. Furthermore, because behavioral responses are elicited mainly by loud sounds, hearing losses of mild or moderate degree may not show any abnormality on behavioral testing. BAEPs and otoacoustic emissions are objective techniques for evaluating auditory function in infants. Two main approaches are now used for newborn hearing screening.[41] One approach is to screen all infants with otoacoustic emissions and then to use BAEPs to assess infants who lack otoacoustic emissions. Another approach is to use automated techniques for recording BAEPs to low-intensity sounds in the initial screening test.

Otoacoustic emissions are sounds that originate in the cochlea and can be recorded in the external ear canal using a sensitive microphone. They can be evoked either by presenting a brief stimulus (click or tone) and recording the acoustic energy in the external ear canal over the subsequent 20 msec, or by presenting two tones of different frequency and recording the acoustic energy at the distortion products of these frequencies. Because they take less time than BAEPs, automated procedures using otoacoustic emissions are used widely to identify children who need to be evaluated further for possible hearing impairment.[42,43] As otoacoustic emissions depend on the normal activity of hair cells, they are not recorded when cochlear hearing loss exceeds about 40 dB. If emissions are present, cochlear function is sufficiently normal that treatment is probably not indicated. If they are absent, hearing loss is present, but the severity of this loss is not known. Infants who fail this test therefore should be assessed with BAEPs to confirm a persistent hearing loss and to assess its severity. Screening with otoacoustic emissions will miss infants with auditory neuropathy, who usually have normal cochlear function. BAEP screening therefore is recommended in the NICU, where there is a greater incidence of auditory neuropathy than in well-baby nurseries.[44]

Although most significant childhood hearing losses are present at birth, a hearing impairment can develop during the first few years of life.[41] Any parental concern about the hearing of a child should lead to an audiologic evaluation. Infants with certain congenital disorders such as rubella or cytomegalovirus infection may show a deterioration in hearing after birth. All children exposed to postnatal risk factors (e.g., meningitis, encephalitis, skull fracture, and ototoxic medication) should have their hearing tested. It is also important to monitor the auditory status of infants who have risk factors for chronic middle ear effusions (e.g., prematurity, Down syndrome, cleft palate, unilateral atresia of the external auditory canal, or other craniofacial malformations). All children with delayed intellectual development should also be tested, because hearing loss could explain or exacerbate their cognitive problems.

Newborn Hearing Assessment with BAEPs

The click-evoked BAEPs provide a quick assessment of the general hearing threshold and evaluate the neurologic integrity of the brainstem auditory pathways. This evaluation can be used as an initial hearing test (especially for infants in an NICU), as a follow-up test after screening with otoacoustic emissions, and as the initial step in a full objective audiometric evaluation.

Hearing is assessed by using 30-dB nHL monaural clicks presented at a rate of 61 Hz; 4,000 responses are averaged. If replicated responses are not recognizable, the testing is continued at higher intensities until an auditory threshold is obtained. Replicate BAEPs are also obtained for each ear by using 70-dB nHL clicks presented monaurally at a rate of 11 Hz. These responses allow assessment of neurologic function as well as hearing. Any infant not showing responses at 30 dB is retested at the age of 3 to 5 months. By that time, normal thresholds have developed in many of these infants, perhaps because a perinatal conductive loss has resolved. The authors initially hesitated between using 30 and 40 dB nHL as the screening level. Screening at 40 dB greatly reduces the number of follow-up tests and should not miss an infant with a sensorineural hearing loss requiring amplification. However, approximately 40 percent of the babies with a 40-dB threshold in the newborn period showed persistent conductive losses on follow-up. Because we considered it important to monitor these infants, we decided to screen at 30 dB nHL. Screening at 3 months is more accurate than screening in the neonatal period because transient neonatal conductive losses have resolved. Nevertheless, it is important to assess infants while they are in the hospital in case they do not return for follow-up. Figure 25-5 shows the BAEPs

obtained on screening and at follow-up for an infant with bilateral sensorineural hearing loss.

A large study has evaluated a similar protocol in over 7,000 infants.[45] This study used accurate ways to calibrate ear-canal sound levels and precise measures of the signal-to-noise ratio to determine when a response was present. More than 99 percent of newborn infants could be tested, and more than 90 percent of these passed the test (at 30 dB nHL). The rest were followed up with more extensive audiometric testing, leading to the identification of sensorineural hearing loss in about 2 percent of the tested population.[46]

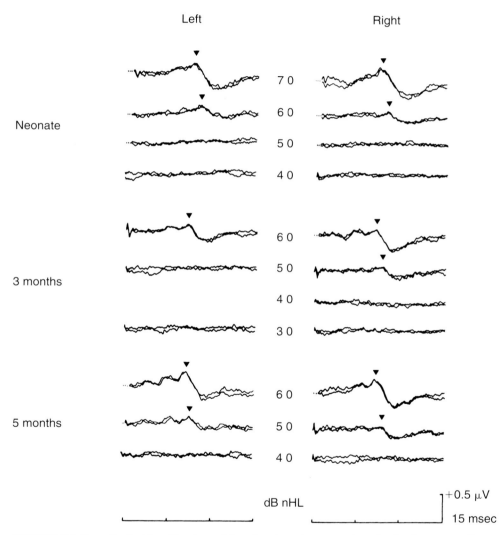

FIGURE 25-5 ▪ Early identification of hearing impairment using the brainstem auditory evoked potential. This child was born after 38 weeks gestation with a birthweight of 3,210 g. The postnatal course was complicated by perinatal asphyxia and seizures. The initial screening test done on discharge from the neonatal intensive care unit is shown in the upper part of the figure. Responses to clicks at 61 Hz were recognizable only down to 60 dB nHL (triangles), which indicates bilateral moderate hearing impairment. Follow-up studies shown in the middle and lower part of the figure confirmed this impairment with thresholds between 50 and 60 dB nHL. After the second follow-up test, the child was fitted with a hearing aid on the right ear and enrolled in the aural habilitation program. By the age of 2 years the child was able to comprehend well and to speak two-word phrases with good voice quality and intonation.

BAEP thresholds in the neonatal period closely predict the high-frequency thresholds of the behavioral audiogram obtained when the child is old enough to provide accurate behavioral thresholds. One study defined significant hearing loss on follow-up as a sensorineural loss with thresholds above 40 dB nHL and found that abnormal BAEP results (neonatal BAEP thresholds above 40 dB nHL) correctly detected 98 percent of the hearing-impaired babies (sensitivity), with only 4 percent false-positive results (96 percent specificity).[47] Another defined the target population as those requiring hearing aids and found a sensitivity of 86 percent and specificity of 100 percent.[48]

Between 10 and 30 percent of babies in an NICU have a transient conductive hearing loss that resolves within the first few months of life.[48,49] Furthermore, conductive hearing losses may occur by the time of follow-up in a baby who was normal in the neonatal period. Infants who have conductive losses in the neonatal period are more likely to have repeat otitis later than are those with normal neonatal hearing.

Some infants may show transient abnormalities of the BAEP in the newborn period with normal recordings several months later.[50] When the otoacoustic emissions are normal, these findings suggest a transient auditory neuropathy.[51]

Some children with normal thresholds for clicks in the newborn period show significant hearing loss at follow-up.[48] Passing a neonatal screening test is no guarantee that the child's hearing is normal or that it will continue to be normal. In some infants, sensorineural hearing loss may develop after birth. However, most of the hearing-impaired children who showed normal click-evoked

BAEPs in infancy have an audiometric pattern with normal thresholds somewhere between 1 and 4 kHz and significant hearing losses at other frequencies (Fig. 25-6). Normal neonatal BAEPs occurred because the broadband click elicited a response from the frequency region with normal thresholds.

Auditory steady-state responses may also be used to screen for hearing loss in newborn infants.[38,52] Either clicks or modulated noise may be used to evoke responses that can be recorded accurately and quickly in the frequency domain.

Evoked Potential Audiometry

The click-evoked BAEP gives a general indication of hearing but does not provide the frequency-specific thresholds of an "audiogram." This information is essential to fitting hearing aids. By 6 months of age a normal child will turn to look for a faint sound, and this response can be reinforced by such stimuli as an animated toy on the correctly localized speaker. This approach can provide an accurate assessment of hearing in most children from 6 months to 2 years. As the child gets older, increasingly refined tests become available. Objective testing is necessary in all children before the age of 6 months and in those older children who cannot give reliable thresholds with behavioral testing (e.g., those with cognitive disturbances, emotional disturbance, or multiple handicaps).

The main goal of evoked potential audiometry is to determine thresholds at frequencies between 500 and 4,000 Hz in each ear. Evoked potential audiometry in infants and children usually begins with click stimuli. Thresholds for the BAEP (wave V) are estimated to within

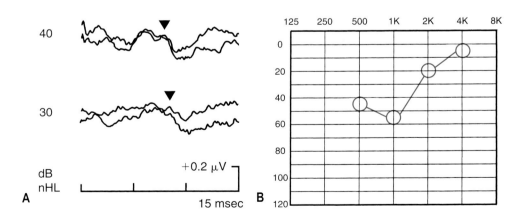

FIGURE 25-6 ■ Follow-up audiograms in infants screened for hearing loss in the neonatal period. This child was born at term and was admitted to the neonatal intensive care unit because of perinatal asphyxia. The brainstem auditory evoked potentials in infancy showed normal thresholds. **A**, Responses to 40- and 30-dB nHL clicks presented at a rate of 61 Hz to the right ear. Wave V is recognizable (triangle) at both intensities. **B**, Audiogram obtained at age 3 years. Although the thresholds at 2,000 and 4,000 Hz are within normal limits, the hearing at 500 and 1,000 Hz is significantly impaired. Both ears showed a similar hearing impairment, and the child was fitted with hearing aids after the audiogram.

10 dB using rapid stimulus rates (50 to 80 Hz). Under reasonable recording conditions (i.e., a quiet child in a quiet room), the BAEP in a child older than 6 months of age should be detected to within 20 dB of the normal adult behavioral threshold for the click. The threshold for the click-evoked BAEP does not give any information about the response to specific frequencies but can provide a general estimate of hearing, particularly at high frequencies. The next step estimates thresholds at different frequencies by using techniques such as derived responses, tone pips in noise, or steady-state responses.

The most widely studied technique for estimating the audiogram in infants and young children involves recording the BAEPs to brief tones.[9,53] A meta-analysis of many such studies indicates that thresholds are estimated between 10 and 20 dB above behavioral thresholds for frequencies between 500 and 4,000 Hz.[54] The variability of the threshold estimation is such that any individual threshold will be within 10 to 20 dB of this mean difference between the physiologic and behavioral thresholds. The basic protocol presents brief tones with alternating onset polarity at a rate of 40 to 50 per second. BAEPs are recorded with a low-frequency cut-off no greater than 30 Hz to obtain two replicate averages of 2,000 trials each. Ipsilateral notch-noise masking will make the thresholds frequency specific. If notch-noise masking is not used, the estimated thresholds may be inaccurate if the slope between adjacent frequencies on the audiogram is steep. Bone conduction thresholds for clicks or tones should be obtained if air conduction thresholds are elevated. Alternating polarity is essential to attenuate the stimulus artifact when recording bone conduction responses.

Auditory steady-state responses can also be used to estimate the audiogram in infants.[12–14] Because multiple responses can be obtained simultaneously, the time taken to estimate the audiogram is significantly less than that required when using BAEPs to brief tones.

BAEP Evaluation of Specific Hearing Disorders

Bacterial meningitis is the most common cause of acquired sensorineural hearing loss in childhood. All children with meningitis should be assessed audiometrically before leaving the hospital. Because the incidence of this disease is high in the first year of life, the BAEP is often a necessary part of this assessment. The BAEP is probably more accurate than behavioral testing, particularly if the hearing impairment is transient, unilateral, or mild. The incidence of hearing loss in children recovering from meningitis is between 25 and 60 percent when BAEP testing is performed.[55–57] The hearing loss is conductive

in about one-quarter, cochlear in one-half, and retrocochlear in the remaining one-quarter of the children.

The BAEP is essential in the evaluation of infants born with atresia of the external auditory meatus (Fig. 25-7). In a child with unilateral atresia, the status of the normal ear can be assessed easily by BAEPs. During the first few years of life, the BAEP may also be helpful if middle ear disease is suspected in the good ear. In a child with bilateral atresia, the BAEP can demonstrate function of the inner ear (see Fig. 25-7) and may suggest (if the scalp topography of the response is asymmetric) that only one inner ear is functioning.

Otitis media and middle ear effusions are very common in the first 3 years of life. It is important to monitor the hearing of children who experience recurrent middle ear disease. Because of the age of the children, monitoring will often require objective tests of auditory function, such as those provided by the BAEP. The conductive hearing losses associated with otitis media show up in the BAEP as elevated thresholds and a delay in all of the waves. The degree of delay can provide an estimate of the amount of hearing loss, although variability in the response may obscure small changes in threshold. BAEPs are very helpful in monitoring infants with cleft palate, who are susceptible to recurrent middle ear effusions.[58]

Ototoxic medications are often used in infancy and childhood, particularly in intensive care nurseries. Because infants and young children are unable to complain of auditory deterioration during the course of treatment, the BAEP may provide an objective means of monitoring

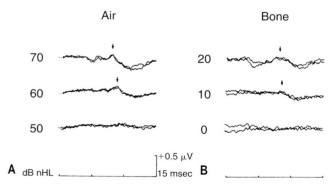

FIGURE 25-7 ■ Congenital atresia of the external auditory meatus. This child was born at term with no abnormality other than bilateral absence of the pinna and external auditory canal. She was referred for testing at the age of 4 months. **A**, Responses to air-conducted rarefaction clicks presented at a rate of 61 Hz to the left ear. The arrows indicate wave V. The responses to right ear stimulation showed a similar elevated threshold at 60 dB nHL. **B**, Responses to an alternating click presented through a bone conduction transducer placed on the forehead. Responses are clearly visible down to 10 dB nHL. This pattern indicates that at least one cochlea is functioning well.

hearing and detecting neurotoxicity, particularly if the treatment is prolonged.[59-61]

Treatment of Sensorineural Hearing Loss

Once sensorineural hearing loss is detected, it is essential to provide the patient with amplification. Fitting hearing aids normally requires frequency-specific and ear-specific estimates of hearing thresholds, acoustic measurements of infants' external ear (real-ear to coupler differences), and the gain characteristics of the aid. The amplification and compression of the aid are adjusted so that the frequencies and intensities of the normal speech spectrum become audible. A final confirmation of a satisfactory hearing aid is the subject's ability to discriminate speech with the aid. The most important use of the BAEPs or auditory steady-state responses in the fitting of hearing aids is to provide an accurate audiogram when this cannot be obtained behaviorally. Other possible uses of physiologic testing are to determine maximum levels of amplification and to demonstrate the discriminability of the aided sounds. As they can be evoked by amplitude-modulated tones, which are frequency specific and stable over time, auditory steady-state responses are unlikely to be distorted by amplification in either a sound-field speaker or a hearing aid. These responses may be used to assess aided thresholds (Fig. 25-8).[62] A more important use of the auditory steady-state

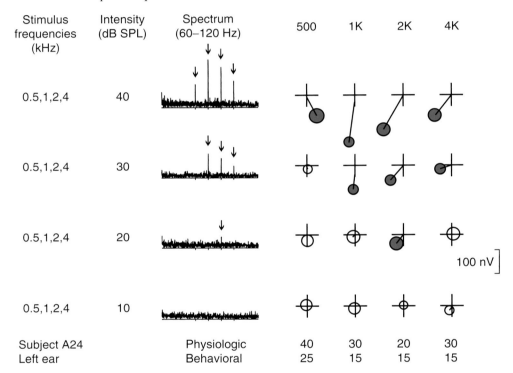

FIGURE 25-8 ■ Auditory steady-state responses in the evaluation of aided thresholds. For these recordings four amplitude-modulated tones were presented simultaneously to the subject through a sound-field speaker. The carrier frequencies of the tones were 500, 1,000, 2,000, and 4,000 Hz. Each carrier frequency had its own signature modulation frequency: 81, 89, 97, and 105 Hz for the 500-, 1,000-, 2,000-, and 4,000-Hz carrier frequencies, respectively. The subject was a 12-year-old child with a bilateral sensorineural hearing impairment. The test was performed with a hearing aid in the left ear. The potentials evoked by the amplitude-modulated tones were converted into the frequency domain to provide measurements of amplitude at different frequencies. The middle column shows the amplitude spectrum from 60 to 120 Hz. The locations of the four modulating frequencies are noted on the baseline of the spectra. At the right are shown the responses at each of the modulating frequencies (measuring the responses to each of the tones), plotted with polar coordinates to show both amplitude and phase. The circles represent the confidence limits for the response. If the origin of the polar plot is not included within the circle (shaded), the response is significantly different from zero. In this child the physiologic responses are recognizable to within 15 dB of the thresholds that were measured with behavioral techniques. This approach therefore may provide a means of objectively evaluating aided thresholds in younger children who, unlike this child, are unable to provide behavioral responses.

responses would be to demonstrate the ability of the brain to discriminate changes in the frequency and intensity of amplified sounds.

Cochlear implants can provide stimulation of auditory nerve fibers in children who are so severely hearing impaired that they get little or no benefit from hearing aids. It is customary to record the BAEPs in response to very loud clicks in children being considered for cochlear implants to determine any residual cochlear function. Some of these children show a vertex negative wave at about 3 msec that probably represents activation of vestibular nerve or nucleus rather than any residual function in the hair cells and auditory nerve fibers.[63] Figure 25-9 shows a waveform that may represent this type of response. Electrically elicited BAEPs provide essential information for preoperative evaluation of surviving neural elements in the auditory pathways and for intraoperative assessment of the implant's function.[64,65] After the operation, BAEPs may be used to check the continuing function of the implanted device, to adjust the intensity levels in the external processor, and to monitor the development of the auditory pathways. The waveform of the electrically evoked response is similar to that of the acoustically evoked BAEP. The latencies of the waves are shorter, and wave I usually is obscured by stimulus artifact. Wave V latency is usually about 4.0 msec and changes by only about 0.5 msec from high to low intensity.

Neurology of Hearing

The BAEP does not really assess "hearing." Children with disorders of auditory perception may have normal BAEPs. In these children, normal BAEP thresholds indicate that they probably will not benefit from amplification. Some of these children may have abnormalities of the later auditory evoked potentials. Patients with abnormal BAEPs because of neurologic dysfunction probably do not have normal hearing. However, they may have much more hearing than is apparent from the BAEP findings. For example, demyelination in the auditory pathways may desynchronize neuronal discharges and render it impossible to record a BAEP. Such pathology may interfere with auditory perception that requires accurate timing without significantly affecting the hearing of pure tones or speech. Most infants with neurologically abnormal BAEPs will still show normal BAEP thresholds. However, BAEPs recorded for evaluating auditory thresholds in patients with known neurologic disorders must be interpreted cautiously. Particular attention must be paid to the latency and threshold of wave I, and electrocochleography using electrodes in the external or middle ear may aid in the assessment of inner ear function. In all children treated for hearing loss without good behavioral testing, close cooperation is important between the audiologist and the therapist treating the child and the family. The child should perform better with the hearing aid than without.

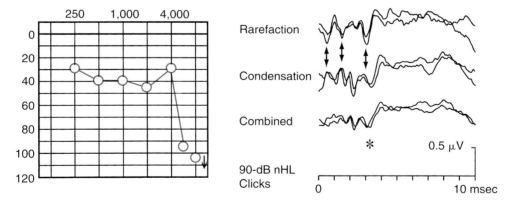

FIGURE 25-9 ■ Absent brainstem auditory evoked potentials (BAEPs) in a patient with only mild hearing loss. This figure represents the audiogram and the BAEPs of a 17-year-old girl with a history of jaundice at birth and difficulty with speech perception. Results are shown for the left ear. On the left of the figure, the pure-tone audiogram shows mild hearing loss, except for frequencies greater than 4,000 Hz. On the right of the figure are shown the BAEPs in response to 90-dB nHL clicks. These BAEPs show small waveforms out to about 4 msec that reverse in polarity when the stimulus is changed from a condensation to a rarefaction click (two-headed arrows). These mainly represent cochlear microphonics and not neural potentials. When the condensation and rarefaction responses are combined, a vertex negative wave (asterisk) can be noted at a peak latency of approximately 3 msec. This may represent a response of the vestibular rather than the cochlear system.

Auditory Neuropathy

The relationship between hearing and BAEPs (and between audiology and neurology) is particularly important in patients with a disorder that has come to be known as auditory neuropathy.[66-69] This disorder is characterized by abnormal function in the auditory pathways beginning in the auditory nerve, despite normal function in the external hair cells of the cochlea. The auditory nerve problems are demonstrated by absent or severely abnormal BAEPs, beginning at wave I; the relative preservation of hair cell function is demonstrated by otoacoustic emissions or cochlear microphonics. Patients typically have only a mild or moderate elevation of pure-tone thresholds but a significantly reduced ability to discriminate speech. Other abnormalities are a lack of middle ear muscle reflexes and no evidence of contralateral suppression of the otoacoustic emissions.[70] When recording BAEPs it is important to record separate responses to rarefaction and condensation clicks because the cochlear microphonics may be quite prominent and may mimic abnormal BAEPs (see Fig. 25-9).[1] The disorder might be caused by an abnormality of the inner hair cells, of the afferent auditory nerve fibers, or of the synapse between them.[69] The disorder may be idiopathic or occur in association with certain definite pathologies such as hyperbilirubinemia[71,72] and hereditary sensorimotor neuropathies.[69] A report of a temperature-dependent form suggests that demyelination may play a role.[73] In certain cases, as the disorder progresses, the otoacoustic emissions disappear, perhaps owing to withdrawal of cochleotrophic factors.[74] The diagnosis becomes much less certain if the emissions are absent. The fact that auditory neuropathy occurs in newborn infants suggests that newborn hearing screening should involve both otoacoustic emissions and BAEPs. Otoacoustic emissions alone would miss newborns with auditory neuropathy, whereas BAEPs alone would indicate a hearing loss but would not recognize its special character. Auditory neuropathy is difficult to treat because amplification may not improve speech perception. Low-gain frequency-modulated systems may improve the acoustic signal-to-noise ratio, and speech perception may be supported with lip reading or other communication aids. Cochlear implants may help in some patients.[75,76]

NEUROLOGIC APPLICATIONS

The BAEP is very useful in investigating neurologic disorders that may damage the brainstem auditory pathway. The BAEP is usually abnormal with brainstem tumors, is almost always abnormal with leukodystrophies, and is often abnormal with degenerative diseases that affect white matter. It is a valuable part of the neurologic workup in children with degenerative processes, encephalopathy, ataxia, or coma. In patients in whom the extent of brain damage has not been determined fully, the BAEP can demonstrate whether the brainstem has been affected significantly. However, the BAEP and the auditory pathways that generate this response are resistant to many neurologic insults and can be normal in a child who is far from normal neurologically. Furthermore, although an abnormal BAEP may demonstrate and localize dysfunction in the auditory pathway, it cannot define the etiology of this dysfunction.

When the BAEP is recorded for neurologic purposes, it is essential not to consider the results in isolation. The BAEP evaluates only the auditory pathways of the brainstem. Diagnosis and prognosis in pediatric neurology require information about the whole nervous system. Multimodality evoked potential studies are very helpful in distinguishing different disorders by the different patterns of abnormality.[77,78] By surveying the extent of brain damage, they can also contribute to a more accurate prognosis.

Repeated testing is often helpful. Comparison of the results may assist in prognosis. Furthermore, if the BAEP is abnormal, monitoring the BAEP may aid in following treatment. BAEPs in children with acquired immunodeficiency syndrome (AIDS) provide an example. Some delays in I–V latency occur, particularly at rapid rates of stimulation,[79] and abnormalities may be improved by treatment.[80]

In many pediatric disease processes, abnormalities of the BAEP become apparent only when comparisons are made between groups of affected and normal subjects. Such comparisons may indicate that the disease affects the brainstem auditory pathways, but they do not aid in the diagnosis of individual patients, many of whom have normal BAEPs.

For neurologic assessment, identification of wave I is essential inasmuch as the absence or delay of subsequent waves identifies dysfunction within the brainstem auditory pathways. A low rate of stimulation (10 to 20 Hz) and a relatively high intensity (70 to 90 dB nHL) should be used. BAEPs to stimulation of the left and right ears should be recorded separately and, as with all evoked potential testing, replication is essential. If wave I is abnormal or absent, it is necessary to evaluate hearing thresholds either behaviorally or by using wave V of the BAEP.

Tumors

The BAEP is generally abnormal in patients with tumors of the posterior fossa, which are far more common in children than in adults. Abnormalities of the response can demonstrate a brainstem lesion and assist in its localization. Although magnetic resonance imaging (MRI) is the most helpful diagnostic procedure in children with suspected tumors of the posterior fossa, the BAEP is useful as an inexpensive test when the index of suspicion is relatively low, as a means of confirming a small tumor or of determining the significance of a questionable radiographic abnormality, and as an effective way of monitoring progression during treatment.

BAEP abnormalities beginning after wave I and before wave III indicate a lesion of the pons or auditory nerve (Fig. 25-10). The lateralization of such a lesion usually can be determined by noting from which ear the more abnormal response is obtained. The BAEP is a sensitive means for the early detection of acoustic neuromas.[81] These tumors are rare in childhood and usually occur bilaterally in association with neurofibromatosis type 2. Genetic studies, MRI, and BAEP recordings are important means of detecting and monitoring children with this disorder.[82]

Abnormalities of the BAEP beginning after wave III indicate lesions of the upper pons or midbrain (see Fig. 25-10). An increased I–V latency without a clear wave III indicates some dysfunction of the auditory nerve or brainstem but is not more specific in localizing the lesion.

Brainstem gliomas are particularly likely to produce abnormal BAEPs. In the authors' experience, the BAEPs have been abnormal in 26 children with tumors involving the pons or midbrain. Furthermore, in only 2 of these patients have the BAEPs not predicted correctly the side predominantly involved. Both children had large mass effects in the brainstem, and the BAEPs may well have reflected functional rather than structural effects of the lesion. In three children with thalamic tumors, a small or delayed wave V was found, probably reflecting pressure on the midbrain. Far-field somatosensory evoked potentials (SEPs) were more useful in assessing these tumors. In children with cerebellar tumors, the BAEP is usually abnormal, depending on whether the auditory pathway is affected by tumor extension or mass effect. The BAEP may be helpful in monitoring brainstem function during operations on posterior fossa tumors and in assessing the effects of surgical resection, radiation, and chemotherapy. Figure 25-11 shows the BAEP studies of a child before and after resection of a cerebellar cyst.

Neurofibromatosis type 1 (von Recklinghausen disease) is an inherited disorder that affects the cell growth of neural tissue and can lead to tumor formation. Evoked potentials can help to detect abnormalities and monitor progression of the disease. The authors have found that 11 of 25 children with neurofibromatosis type 1 had an abnormally delayed I–III or I–V interpeak interval (Fig. 25-12). One child had an auditory nerve tumor, another had a brainstem glioma, and the others are being monitored. This incidence of abnormal BAEPs is similar to that reported by other investigators.[83,84] The yield of abnormalities is even greater with multimodality evoked potentials or MRI. Evoked potentials are clearly useful for detecting cerebral abnormalities in children with neurofibromatosis, but the significance of these abnormalities is uncertain. Some abnormalities may represent tumor formation, but others probably indicate nonneoplastic local areas of brain dysplasia. More long-term follow-up will determine the value of monitoring patients with neurofibromatosis.

Developmental Disorders

Hydrocephalus typically is associated with severe BAEP abnormalities, although normal BAEPs occasionally may occur. The most common abnormality is a decrease in the amplitude of the later components, with a significantly reduced V/I amplitude ratio or an absent wave V.[85] The relationship of the BAEP abnormality to the hydrocephalus is unclear. Abnormal recordings may be related partially to the ventricular dilatation because the BAEP can improve when the child is treated successfully with a shunt. They may also be caused by developmental abnormalities of the brainstem that occur in association with hydrocephalus.

The Arnold–Chiari malformation is present in most patients with myelomeningocele, but it may occur occasionally without either myelomeningocele or any associated hydrocephalus. It can cause symptoms related to medullary compression, the most important being swallowing difficulties and apneic episodes. Brainstem decompensation sometimes can lead to respiratory failure and death. Several studies have investigated whether BAEPs in children with the Arnold–Chiari malformation can predict the emergence of these clinical symptoms and the need for brainstem decompression. In children with myelomeningocele, the longest central conduction times occur in those with hydrocephalus and neurologic symptoms.[86] Brainstem decompression may lead to resolution of the medullary symptoms and improvement in the BAEP. However, one study found abnormal BAEPs in 72 percent of 18 children older than 5 years of age with myelomeningocele and hydrocephalus, none of whom had clinical symptoms.[87] MRI is probably the most helpful test in determining brainstem compression, but the BAEP may be helpful in evaluating the general neurologic prognosis.

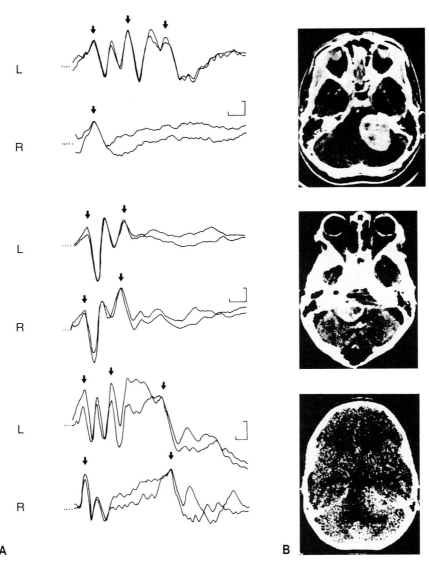

A

B

FIGURE 25-10 ■ Brainstem auditory evoked potentials (BAEPs) in the evaluation of children with tumors of the posterior fossa. **A**, Responses to 70-dB nHL click stimuli presented at a rate of 11 Hz. Responses to left (L) and to right (R) ear stimuli were recorded with electrodes on the vertex and ipsilateral mastoid or ear lobe. Waves I, III, and V are identified with arrows. The calibration lines represent 0.5 μV and 2 msec. The third set of tracings was recorded with a sweep of 15 msec rather than 10 msec. **B**, Computed tomographic (CT) scans from these children. All scans were obtained with contrast enhancement. The scans are printed such that the left side of the patient is on the left of the scan. The patient whose tracings are shown at the top of the figure was a 16-year-old girl with right-sided hearing loss and headaches. Her audiogram showed a severe right-sided hearing loss for pure tones with no detectable speech discrimination. Only the first component of the response was recognized in the BAEP to right ear stimulation. The CT scan showed a right acoustic neuroma. The tracings in the middle part of the figure were obtained from an 8-year-old girl with ataxia and slurred speech. On examination she showed bilateral sixth nerve palsies and a left seventh nerve palsy. The BAEPs in response to left ear stimulation showed no components after wave III. In response to right ear stimulation, there were questionable waves IV and V of small amplitude. The CT scan showed an enhancing tumor in the left pons. The patient underwent shunting but did poorly and died 6 months later. Pathology revealed a malignant astrocytoma. The bottom tracings are from a patient examined for ataxia and vomiting. The BAEPs show a severely delayed I–V interval (7.9 msec) for right ear stimulation, with no clear wave III. The response to left ear stimulation showed normal components I, II, and III and a delayed wave V. The CT scan showed a contrast-enhancing mass in the right pontine region pushing the fourth ventricle backward and to the left. An exploratory operation revealed an unresectable astrocytoma.

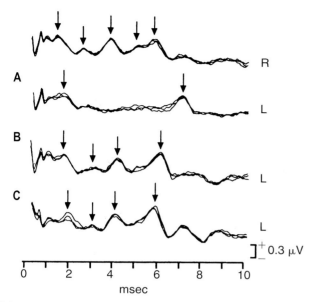

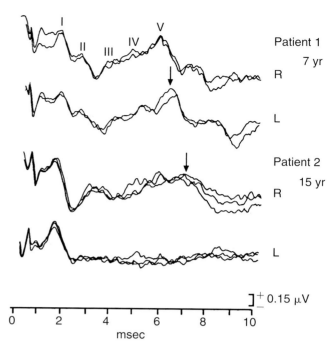

FIGURE 25-11 ■ Monitoring tumor progression with brainstem auditory evoked potentials (BAEPs). These recordings were obtained in a girl aged 7 years who presented with behavior problems and seizures following a skull fracture 3 years earlier. Her BAEP was abnormal. **A,** With left-ear (L) stimulation with 80-dB nHL clicks presented at 11 Hz, wave III was not recognizable and wave V was delayed significantly; the response to stimulation of the right ear (R) was normal. Radiologic studies showed a cystic tumor of the left cerebellum, which was removed 1 month later. Subsequent recordings after 2 months (**B**) and 3 years (**C**) showed improvement of the BAEP to normal. Arrows indicate the various components of the response.

The authors studied BAEPs after myelomeningocele repair in 47 neonates between 1 day and 3 months of age to determine whether the BAEP had prognostic value regarding the child's neurologic outcome.[88] In this series, 69 percent had abnormal BAEPs; some had small waves IV and V, whereas others had a normal wave I and poorly defined and delayed later components (Fig. 25-13). BAEPs were abnormal in all infants with symptomatic Arnold–Chiari malformation and in 47 percent of nonsymptomatic patients. More interestingly, 87 percent of the infants with abnormal BAEPs had central neurologic abnormalities on follow-up at 2 years of age, whereas 81 percent of the infants with normal BAEPs had normal cerebral function on follow-up. Thus, the BAEP was highly predictive of neurologic outcome. BAEPs are also useful during surgical decompression of Arnold–Chiari malformations, to help determine the extent of decompression needed and to reduce the risk of neurologic injury.[89]

Hydranencephalic infants have normal BAEPs, although later auditory responses, visual evoked potentials (VEPs), and cortical SEPs are absent.[90,91]

FIGURE 25-12 ■ The brainstem auditory evoked potentials (BAEPs) from two patients with neurofibromatosis. The top pair of traces, from a 7-year-old, show normal responses to 70-dB nHL clicks at 11 Hz for the right ear (R), but delayed III–V and I–V latencies for the left (L) (2.4 and 4.7 msec, respectively). Magnetic resonance imaging revealed only a small focal nodule deep in the right cerebellum. Neurofibromatosis type 1 was diagnosed in this patient at age 4 years, and she had a positive family history and café-au-lait spots. Apart from some developmental delay, her neurologic examination is normal. The second pair of traces is from a 15-year-old boy with neurofibromatosis type 2. Computed tomography showed bilateral acoustic neuromas (L greater than R), a cystic lesion in the upper cervical cord, and a lesion in the left jugular foramen. The BAEPs were recorded in response to 80-dB nHL click stimuli at 11 Hz before surgical excision of the left acoustic neuroma. Only wave I is present on the left; on the right, the peaks after wave I are poorly delineated and delayed (I–V interpeak latency of 5.3 msec).

Myelin Disorders

Disorders affecting the myelin sheath initially delay the later components of the BAEP. As the disorder progresses, these later components decrease in amplitude and finally disappear until only wave I is present. Because these findings are probably the result of desynchronization rather than disruption of transmission in the auditory pathway, they usually occur before definite auditory symptoms.

Combined use of the EEG and the BAEP in children with progressive neurologic disorders may help to differentiate between gray and white matter diseases. Gray matter diseases cause paroxysmal EEG abnormalities

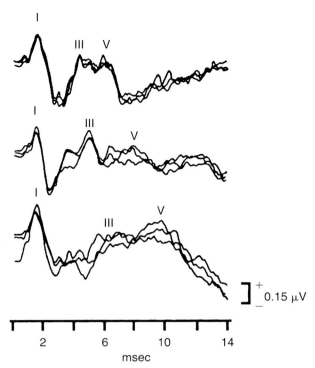

FIGURE 25-13 ■ Brainstem auditory evoked potentials (BAEPs) in infants with myelomeningocele and hydrocephalus. These recordings were taken from three different infants after repair of the myelomeningocele and before any shunting. The first infant had normal BAEPs. An associated Arnold–Chiari malformation was present, but there was no definite hydrocephalus and no shunt was placed. The second infant shows a small delayed wave V. The third infant shows delayed and poorly formed waves III and V. Both the second and the third infants had severe hydrocephalus and underwent shunting at 2 weeks of age. All recordings were in response to 90-dB nHL monaural clicks at 11 Hz. The responses were similar for stimulation of either the left or the right ear. For clarity, the figure shows only one of the responses for each infant.

and tend not to affect the BAEP. White matter diseases cause diffuse EEG slowing and abnormal BAEPs. The BAEP can demonstrate the demyelinating nature of the disease process very early in its course and may be helpful in differentiating among the leukodystrophies. The BAEPs are so consistently abnormal in the various leukodystrophies that another diagnosis should be considered if the BAEP is normal. Figure 25-14 shows typical BAEPs recorded in children with different leukodystrophies.

In the infantile leukodystrophies (e.g., Krabbe disease or Pelizaeus–Merzbacher disease), the BAEPs are very abnormal, with only the early waves being recognizable.[92–95] We have not seen normal BAEPs in any children with these disorders, even though the disease has been diagnosed clinically in children as young as

1 month of age. The BAEPs may aid in the differential diagnosis inasmuch as such marked BAEP abnormalities are not seen in other disorders with similar clinical features.

In older children with demyelinating disorders, abnormalities of the BAEP are less severe. In metachromatic and adrenal leukodystrophies, the initial abnormality is an increase in interpeak latencies, particularly between waves I and III. The abnormalities increase with clinical severity. Even in patients who are still neurologically normal, the BAEPs are abnormal and useful as an early diagnostic test for leukodystrophy.[96,97] Carriers of the sex-linked gene for adrenoleukodystrophy also have abnormal BAEPs.[98]

Multimodal evoked potential studies have long been used to evaluate adult demyelinating disorders such as multiple sclerosis. Although rarer in children, multiple sclerosis is often a difficult diagnostic dilemma because of the fluctuating symptoms and because children are often unreliable observers. As with adults, MRI and multimodal evoked potential studies are important.[99] In a series of 24 children with multiple sclerosis, we found abnormal BAEPs in 4. Although they were not abnormal in isolation, BAEPs helped to demonstrate multiple lesions.

Metabolic and Degenerative Disorders

The BAEP is abnormal in many metabolic disorders. Those that affect the BAEP probably cause significant disruption of cerebral myelin. Inherited metabolic disorders associated with abnormal BAEPs are maple syrup urine disease, pyruvate decarboxylase deficiency, and phenylketonuria. Four of five children with nonketotic hyperglycinemia have had prolonged I–V intervals.[100] BAEPs are normal in children with abetalipoproteinemia, although the VEPs and SEPs are often abnormal.[101,102] We have also found abnormal BAEPs in patients with Leber disease, propionic acidemia, and Kearn–Sayre syndrome; in five of six patients with cerebrohepatorenal (Zellweger) syndrome; and in one of three patients with Menkes kinky hair disease.

Leigh syndrome, or subacute necrotizing encephalomyelopathy, results from a number of metabolic abnormalities in pyruvate metabolism. Within this broad grouping are patients with deficiencies of pyruvate dehydrogenase, cytochrome oxidase, complex 1, and complex 5, as well as other mitochondrial disorders. The BAEPs in these patients are often abnormal, but the abnormalities vary with the metabolic disorder and with the age of the patient.[103] Typical BAEPs in the various disorders associated with this syndrome are shown in Figure 25-15.

The BAEPs are also abnormal in several degenerative brain disorders that do not specifically affect the white

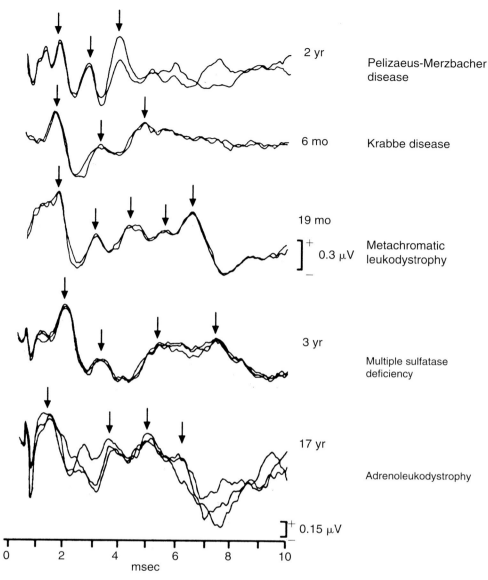

FIGURE 25-14 ▪ Brainstem auditory evoked potentials (BAEPs) recorded in patients with various leukodystrophies. Individual components are indicated by arrows. The top traces are from a 2-year-old with Pelizaeus–Merzbacher disease. Only waves I to III are present, at normal latencies. The second traces are from a 6-month-old with Krabbe disease. The BAEP shows only waves I to III, with a delayed I-III interpeak latency of 3.2 msec. The third traces are from a patient who was asymptomatic but who had metachromatic leukodystrophy confirmed by absent arylsulfatase A activity in enzymatic assays in fibroblasts; the child was investigated because of a symptomatic sibling. The I–III and I–V interpeak latencies are prolonged (2.7 and 4.8 msec, respectively). The fourth trace is from a 3-year-old with multiple sulfatase deficiency. Her BAEPs show prolonged absolute and interpeak latencies (I–III and I–V are 3.3 and 5.4 msec, respectively). The final trace is from a boy with adrenoleukodystrophy. The BAEPs show poorly defined waves, with delayed III–V and I–V intervals (2.5 and 4.8 msec, respectively) and a low-amplitude wave V. All responses were to monaural 80-dB nHL clicks presented at 11 per second. For clarity, only the response from one ear is shown. The upper calibration refers to the top three tracings and the lower to the bottom two tracings.

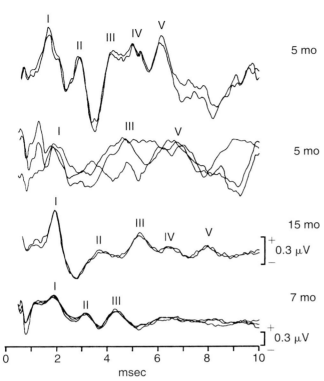

FIGURE 25-15 ■ Brainstem auditory evoked potentials (BAEPs) in Leigh syndrome. This figure presents recordings from four patients with autopsy-proven Leigh syndrome in whom the underlying metabolic defects were known. The top traces are from a patient with complex 1 deficiency, who typically has normal BAEPs. The second set of traces, from a patient with pyruvate dehydrogenase deficiency, shows poorly defined BAEPs with interpeak latencies just at the upper limits of normal for his age. The third traces are from a patient with complex 4 or cytochrome oxidase deficiency with delayed interpeak latencies and low-amplitude waves IV and V. The bottom traces are from a patient with complex 5 deficiency, it shows normal waves I to III, but absent later waves. The upper vertical calibration refers to the upper three responses, which were evoked by 70-dB nHL clicks presented at 11 Hz. The lower calibration refers to the bottom response, which was elicited by 80-dB nHL clicks. For clarity, only the response from one ear is shown in each case.

matter (e.g., Gaucher disease[104] and Niemann–Pick disease[105]). The BAEPs are often abnormal when Wilson disease affects the nervous system.[106] We have recorded normal BAEPs in children in whom this disorder has been diagnosed and treated early. BAEP abnormalities may nevertheless occur in children with Wilson disease without clear neurologic symptoms. In these degenerative disorders, the BAEP abnormalities reflect whether the disease involves the brainstem auditory pathways.

Hurler syndrome (mucopolysaccharidosis I) is a progressive lysosomal storage disease transmitted as an autosomal-recessive trait. The clinical manifestations result from an accumulation of mucopolysaccharides in various tissues. Coarse facies, dwarfism, cognitive disturbances, hepatosplenomegaly, and joint contractures typically develop in these children. Both conductive and sensorineural hearing loss occur. A therapy for this syndrome is bone marrow transplantation. The authors have studied seven of these children (aged 11 months to 3 years); all have had abnormal BAEPs before transplantation. These abnormalities ranged from increased interpeak latencies (indicating brainstem dysfunction) to increased absolute latencies (probably caused by conductive hearing loss) to an absence of waves (which could indicate both hearing loss and brainstem dysfunction). These findings are illustrated in Figure 25-16. Five of these children were evaluated after bone marrow transplantation. In one patient, the BAEPs recorded 1 year after transplantation showed residual mild hearing loss in one ear. In all the other patients, normal BAEPs were seen on postoperative follow-up studies, although this normalization occurred over a 1- to 4-year period. The BAEPs may well be an effective means of monitoring recovery in these children.

The abnormal BAEPs in Friedreich ataxia (Fig. 25-17) can help to exclude other hereditary ataxias in which the BAEPs are normal. In agreement with these BAEP findings, neuropathologic studies have shown cell loss and gliosis in the brainstem of patients with Friedreich ataxia but not in ataxia telangiectasia. The BAEPs in Friedreich ataxia exhibit a characteristic rostrocaudal loss of waves beginning very early in the course of the disease.[107–109] This typical BAEP abnormality can be very helpful because young children with ataxia do not always have the differentiating signs (e.g., telangiectasia or cardiomyopathy) that allow easy discrimination among ataxias in older children and adults. The BAEPs reflect both the rate of progression and the severity of Friedreich ataxia.[109]

Certain disorders such as kernicterus have a specific predilection for the auditory pathways.[72] In acute bilirubin encephalopathy, BAEPs are absent or severely abnormal. BAEP abnormalities vary with the "bilirubin toxicity," an index that takes into account serum bilirubin, albumin binding, and pH.[110] The BAEP is particularly important in evaluating the preterm infant with possible kernicterus, as it may be more sensitive than MRI in these patients.[111] The BAEP is a good means of detecting and monitoring the hearing loss that is so often a part of chronic bilirubin encephalopathy. This hearing loss is usually an auditory neuropathy, with preserved otoacoustic emissions.

In general, BAEP abnormalities increase with progression of the degenerative diseases. Repeated tests therefore

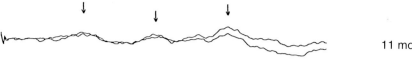

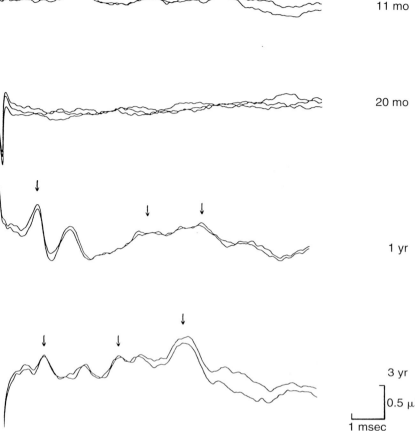

FIGURE 25-16 ■ Brainstem auditory evoked potentials (BAEPs) from three different children with Hurler syndrome. The responses were elicited by 70-dB nHL clicks presented at 11 Hz. The top three recordings were obtained before bone marrow transplantation. The recordings illustrate the types of BAEP abnormalities found in these children. The top trace shows delayed waves beginning at wave I, probably caused by conductive hearing loss (seen in two cases). The second trace shows a complete absence of waves that could represent both hearing loss and brainstem dysfunction (seen in two cases). The third trace shows a prolonged interpeak latency indicating brainstem dysfunction (seen in three cases). The fourth trace shows a normal BAEP following bone marrow transplantation in the same child as in the top trace.

can help to quantify the rate of progression, a measurement that is often difficult in young children. BAEP interpeak latencies can improve during the treatment of certain metabolic disorders. For example, BAEPs improve in infants with hyperbilirubinemia after exchange transfusions[112] or phototherapy.[113,114] BAEPs have also been used to monitor the neurologic status of children with metabolic disorders who are treated with peritoneal dialysis and dietary restrictions (Fig. 25-18).

Malnutrition sufficient to cause marasmus or kwashiorkor causes abnormalities of the BAEP, particularly increasing the I–V interpeak latency.[115] Long-term effects and the relation of BAEP abnormalities to treatment and to other evidence of neurologic abnormality remain to be determined.

Neurotoxic Disorders

BAEPs can help to demonstrate the neurologic effects of environmental toxins such as lead and mercury.[116,117] The effects are usually small and are demonstrated mainly by group comparisons with normal children and by correlations with serum levels of the toxin. Although they cannot demonstrate abnormalities clearly in individual children, they can demonstrate the deleterious neurologic effects of a population's exposure to the toxins.

Prenatal exposure to toxins can cause abnormalities of the infant BAEP. Fetal alcohol syndrome may affect the auditory system in many ways.[118,119] The most common abnormality is a peripheral conductive hearing loss, related to abnormal development of the external and middle ear and to chronic otitis. The BAEPs are delayed in these patients. In addition, there may be central effects in the brainstem auditory pathways (causing increased interpeak latencies in the BAEP) or in the responses of the auditory cortex. Prenatal cocaine exposure can also cause delayed latencies of the BAEP[120] but the effects of cocaine may be more manifest in cortical evoked potentials.[121] Interestingly, maternal smoking causes a significant decrease in BAEP latencies, perhaps related to the effects of nicotine on synaptic processing.[122]

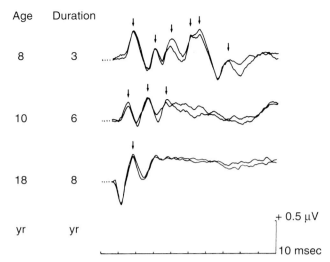

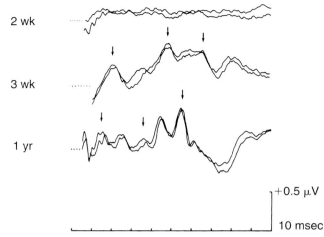

FIGURE 25-17 ■ Friedreich ataxia. The brainstem auditory evoked potentials (BAEPs) to 80-dB nHL clicks presented at the rate of 11 Hz are shown for three different patients. For simplicity, only responses obtained from one ear are shown in each case. The first tracing is from an 8-year-old child with a mild ataxia for 3 years, areflexia, posterior column signs, and extensor plantar reflexes. The second tracing is from a 10-year-old patient who had been ataxic for 6 years and who also had cord signs and cardiomyopathy. The third tracing is from a patient aged 18 years who had been ataxic for 8 years. This patient had severe ataxia, spinal cord signs, cardiomyopathy, dysarthria, and peripheral neuropathy. The BAEPs show a progressive attenuation of the later components of the response with increasing duration and severity of the disease process. The arrows indicate the identified waves. The first tracing shows normal waves I to VI, the second tracing shows only waves I to III, the third tracing shows no recognizable components after wave I.

Anoxia

The BAEPs recorded in infants and children with anoxic brain damage are often abnormal. Prolonged anoxia caused by congenital cardiac disease results in increased I–V interpeak latencies.[123] BAEPs are perhaps more clinically helpful in evaluating the effects of a specific anoxic episode or period to determine the extent of the anoxic damage and the prognosis for recovery.[124–128] The most common abnormalities are attenuation and delay of the later components of the response (Fig. 25-19). The significance of the abnormality depends on the age of the child, the persistence of the abnormality over repeated testing, and the clinical findings.

In infants and young children, the abnormal BAEPs that follow an anoxic episode are prognostically less significant than in older children or adults. Severely abnormal BAEPs have been recorded in asphyxiated premature infants who develop normally despite

FIGURE 25-18 ■ Monitoring the treatment of a metabolic disorder. This child was seen at 2 weeks of age with seizures progressing to coma. The tracing at the top of the figure represents the brainstem auditory evoked potentials (BAEPs) to 80-dB nHL stimuli presented to the right ear at a rate of 11 Hz. There were no recognizable components. At that time, the serum ammonia level was markedly elevated. A diagnosis of proprionic acidemia was made, and the patient was treated with peritoneal dialysis and dietary restrictions. The second tracing, done 1 week later, showed recognizable waves I, III, and V (arrows) at normal latencies for her age. Since then, the patient has continued with a diet low in methionine, isoleucine, valine, and threonine. At the age of 1 year, the BAEPs have shown the normal maturational decrease in latency.

persistence of the BAEP abnormality.[50] In older children, the central nervous system is less resilient than it is in neonates, and abnormal BAEPs following an anoxic episode are more likely to indicate irreversible damage. The BAEP may then be helpful in predicting long-term neurologic sequelae after hypoxia. An abnormally small V/I amplitude ratio indicates a poor prognosis. In asphyxiated children who were not born prematurely, an abnormally small wave V in the presence of normal or only mildly attenuated waves I and III is associated with severe neurologic abnormalities on follow-up examination.[124] Such a pattern likely is caused by anoxic damage in the midbrain. When measurements of the V/I ratio are made, care must be taken not to attenuate wave V by using clicks with too high an intensity or amplifiers with too high a low-frequency cut-off.

Abnormal BAEPs recorded on only one occasion are not very helpful in predicting the long-term neurologic sequelae of anoxia at any age. Although normal responses are usually positive prognostic signs, and absent responses are usually negative signs, BAEPs that are absent or abnormally delayed must be repeated until they stabilize. The resilience of the child's brain is such that

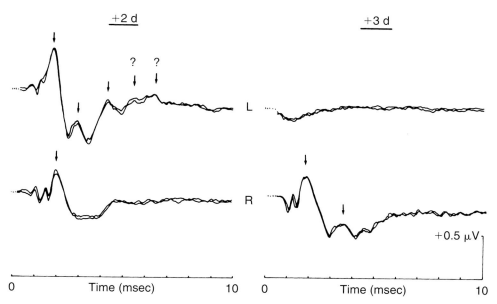

FIGURE 25-19 ■ Effects of anoxia on the brainstem auditory evoked potential (BAEP). These tracings were obtained from a 2-year-old who had a cardiac arrest after asphyxia caused by acute epiglottitis. The initial EEG showed a burst-suppression pattern. On the second day of hospitalization, the EEG showed electrocerebral inactivity. The BAEPs at that time (2 d) showed a normal wave I with severely attenuated or absent later components. The responses to left (L) ear stimulation with 90-dB nHL clicks are shown at the top, and the responses to right (R) ear stimulation are shown at the bottom. On the third day (3 d), the BAEP to left ear stimulation showed an absence of all waves. The EEG continued to show electrocerebral inactivity. There were no spontaneous respirations, and the patient died on the fourth day of hospitalization.

absent BAEPs can return to normal within a few weeks.[129] The BAEPs may also deteriorate in the first day or two after an anoxic episode. Improvement or deterioration of the BAEP may occur before or in parallel with clinical changes. When BAEPs remain persistently abnormal or absent after an anoxic episode, infants do not do well. The BAEP examines function only in the auditory pathways and cannot evaluate anoxic damage in other areas of the brain. The prognosis after asphyxia depends on the results of many clinical and laboratory tests, of which the BAEP is only one. Later auditory evoked potentials and responses in other sensory modalities may provide important additional information about the extent of neurologic damage.

The effects of anoxia on the BAEP may be more evident when stimuli are presented at rapid rates. The neurologic effects of perinatal anoxia may be detected and followed using BAEPs that are recorded using maximum length sequences that allow stimuli to be presented at rates of several hundred per second.[130,131] These studies have found abnormally decreased amplitudes and prolonged latencies in newborns after perinatal asphyxia. These abnormalities corrrelated with

neurodevelopmental deficits on follow-up examinations. Infants with anoxia due to chronic lung disease also show abnormalities of the BAEP but these affect the more central (III–V) rather than the peripheral (I–II) latencies.[126]

Because anoxia can damage the cochlea as well as the brain, it is important to assess the BAEP at threshold as well as at high intensity. In the authors' experience, anoxia can cause a profound cochlear hearing loss or a moderate loss with recruitment. In the latter cases, responses at high intensity may be normal.

BAEPs in infants who have apneic episodes and are at risk for sudden infant death are usually normal.[132,133] Abnormalities reported in earlier studies were small and were probably the result of apneic episodes rather than a sign of a brainstem cause for them.[133] The authors have found the BAEP to be so consistently normal in these children that its use is not recommended in screening infants who may be at risk for sudden infant death. During a routine follow-up examination of infants who had been treated in the NICU, we recorded completely normal BAEPs in a baby who died without obvious cause on the night after the recording.

Head Injury, Coma, and Brain Death

BAEPs in children with head injuries provide information similar to those recorded in adults.[134–136] In general, absent or abnormal BAEPs in a comatose child indicate a poor prognosis. This is particularly true if the BAEPs are persistently abnormal and no peripheral hearing loss is present. A normal BAEP is not necessarily a good prognostic sign because the cerebral cortex can be damaged extensively without affecting the BAEP. The authors have often seen normal BAEPs in comatose children who died within a day. SEPs have been found to be more useful as a general prognostic indicator.[137,138] Localization of the brain damage in head-injured children is determined better from the combined recording of evoked potentials to auditory, somatosensory, and visual stimuli than from BAEPs alone.

Peripheral hearing loss is not uncommon after head injury. Unilateral absence of BAEPs suggests the possibility of a transverse fracture of the temporal bone with damage to the cochlea or auditory nerve. Endotracheal intubation can result in middle ear effusions, which will delay all components of the BAEP. In these children, high-intensity clicks are often necessary to elicit a recognizable wave I.

The BAEPs may be a helpful adjunct in the clinical diagnosis of brain death. BAEPs in 51 pediatric patients with clinically established brain death (following head injury and other causes) showed a recognizable wave I was present in about a third of the patients (an incidence higher than in adults) but no waves III or V.[139] The BAEPs were more compatible with the clinical diagnosis of brain death than the EEG, which often showed residual activity.

Cognitive Disorders

Several studies have found abnormal BAEPs in patients with autism spectrum disorder.[140–142] The findings have included abnormally delayed interpeak latencies and raised thresholds. The abnormalities are not pathognomonic for autism because a group of autistic patients without cognitive disturbances or epilepsy showed completely normal BAEPs.[143] The auditory abnormalities that they represent are probably part of a diffuse or multifocal brain dysfunction and are not related directly to the autistic behavior. Nevertheless, distorted auditory input certainly could exacerbate the underlying disorder and further impede normal development.

Rett syndrome is a disorder in girls characterized by cognitive disturbances, autistic behavior, ataxia, and stereotyped hand movements. The EEG is quite abnormal, with multifocal spike discharges and slowing. BAEPs sometimes show a specific delay in the III–V interval.[144] However, the authors have found BAEPs to be normal in 15 of 16 cases of Rett syndrome (the only abnormal case having a delayed III–V interpeak interval), which is consistent with other reports.[145]

BAEPs with abnormal waveforms and raised thresholds have also been found in intellectually challenged children.[146,147] Patients with Down syndrome show an interesting decrease in interpeak latencies that is not related to head size or hearing loss. Although some early studies reported smaller BAEP waves in undifferentiated cognitive disturbances, such has not been our experience.

Neurologic damage in infancy can go undetected because the infant has not yet developed to a stage where the damaged tissue is used. BAEPs may be helpful in documenting brain damage in the perinatal period.[148,149] An extensive study of the development of the BAEP in infancy differentiated a group of infants at risk for central nervous system damage from a group of healthy infants on the basis of the amplitudes of waves III and V.[149] The at-risk infants failed to show the normal maturational increase in amplitude of these waves. Unfortunately, because of the large intersubject variability in amplitude measurements, it is impossible to make any definite comments about individual babies. Furthermore, it is as yet uncertain whether the BAEP abnormalities are related to the actual neurologic and intellectual outcome of the high-risk infants. Because the BAEPs were evoked by binaural stimuli, their small amplitude in some children may have related to unilateral conductive hearing loss.

A common reason for BAEP referral in childhood is a delay in the development of speech and language. After cognitive disturbances, a hearing impairment is the most common cause of delayed speech and language. Many cognitively impaired children have a hearing impairment in addition to their neurologic disorder. Children with delayed speech and language who have normal intelligence and no peripheral hearing loss may have a central auditory dysfunction. Some of these children have abnormalities of the BAEP.[150,151] More extensive studies of auditory evoked potentials at all latencies[152] and of the auditory steady-state responses may help to classify these abnormalities of auditory perception.

A new approach to auditory processing disorders records the brainstem evoked potentials to speech stimuli instead of clicks. The responses to a brief consonant-vowel stimulus such as "da" show a combination of transient responses (to the onset and offset of the stimulus) and a frequency-following response to the vowel. These responses can show abnormalities in children with communication disorders that are not evident in the BAEPs to simple clicks.[153–156]

CONCLUDING COMMENTS

The BAEP can provide important information about a child's cochlear and brainstem function. The results of BAEP testing must be interpreted cautiously. It is particularly difficult to evaluate hearing when neurologic abnormalities are present and to evaluate brainstem function when peripheral hearing is impaired. Furthermore, the BAEP must never be considered in isolation. It can indicate dysfunction but cannot determine the specific etiology of this dysfunction. Its great advantages are that it does not require the cooperation of the child and that it provides replicable measurements of latency, amplitude, and threshold. BAEPs are therefore an essential part of the audiologic test battery and a helpful adjunct to the neurologic examination.

ACKNOWLEDGMENTS

We appreciate the financial support of the Canadian Institutes of Health Research, the National Health Research and Development Program, the Ontario Deafness Research Foundation, the Research Foundation of the Hospital for Sick Children, and the Research Institute of the Children's Hospital of Eastern Ontario. Richard Mowrey, Chris Edwards, Linda Moran, Janice Pearce, Lynn MacMillan, Nancy Keenan, Patricia Van Roon, and Sandra Champagne helped with the recordings.

REFERENCES

1. Berlin CI, Bordelon J, St John P et al: Reversing click polarity may uncover auditory neuropathy in infants. Ear Hear, 19:37, 1998
2. Stapells DR, Picton TW, Smith AD: Normal hearing thresholds for clicks. J Acoust Soc Am, 72:74, 1982
3. Richter U, Fedtke T: Reference zero for the calibration of audiometric equipment using 'clicks' as test signals. Int J Audiol, 44:478, 2005
4. Lasky RE, Perlman J, Hecox K: Maximum length sequence auditory evoked brainstem responses in human newborns and adults. J Am Acad Audiol, 3:383, 1992
5. Jiang ZD, Brosi DM, Wilkinson AR: Brainstem auditory evoked response recorded using maximum length sequences in term neonates. Biol Neonate, 76:193, 1999
6. Ponton CW, Eggermont JJ, Coupland SG et al: Frequency specific maturation of the eighth nerve and brainstem auditory pathway: evidence from derived ABRs. J Acoust Soc Am, 91:1576, 1992
7. Fedtke T, Richter U: Reference zero for the calibration of air-conduction audiometric equipment using 'tone bursts' as test signals. Int J Audiol, 46:1, 2007
8. Stapells DR, Gravel JS, Martin BA: Thresholds for auditory brainstem responses to tones in notched noise from infants and young children with normal hearing and sensorineural hearing loss. Ear Hear, 16:361, 1995
9. Sininger YS, Abdala C, Cone-Wesson B: Auditory threshold sensitivity of the human neonate as measured by auditory brainstem response. Hear Res, 104:27, 1997
10. Ribeiro FM, Carvallo RM: Tone-evoked ABR in full-term and preterm neonates with normal hearing. Int J Audiol, 47:21, 2008
11. Picton TW: Auditory steady-state and following responses: dancing to the rhythms. p. 285. In Picton TW (ed): Human Auditory Evoked Potentials. Plural, San Diego, 2010
12. Lins OG, Picton TW, Boucher B et al: Frequency-specific audiometry using steady-state responses. Ear Hear, 17:81, 1996
13. Van Maanen A, Stapells DR: Multiple-ASSR thresholds in infants and young children with hearing loss. J Am Acad Audiol, 21:535, 2010
14. Van Maanen A, Stapells DR: Normal multiple auditory steady-state response thresholds to air-conducted stimuli in infants. J Am Acad Audiol, 20:196, 2009
15. Foxe JJ, Stapells DR: Normal infant and adult auditory brainstem responses to bone-conducted tones. Audiology, 23:95, 1993
16. Small SA, Stapells DR: Multiple auditory steady-state response thresholds to bone-conduction stimuli in young infants with normal hearing. Ear Hear, 27:219, 2006
17. Small SA, Stapells DR: Normal ipsilateral/contralateral asymmetries in infant multiple auditory steady-state responses to air- and bone-conduction stimuli. Ear Hear, 29:185, 2008
18. Picton TW, Durieux-Smith A, Moran LM: Recording auditory brainstem responses from infants. Int J Pediatr Otolaryngol, 28:93, 1994
19. Durieux-Smith A, Edwards CG, Picton TW et al: Auditory brainstem responses to clicks in neonates. J Otolaryngol, 14:Suppl 14, 12, 1985
20. Edwards CG, Durieux-Smith A, Picton TW: Neonatal auditory brainstem responses from ipsilateral and contralateral recording montages. Ear Hear, 6:175, 1985
21. Stapells DR, Mosseri M: Maturation of the contralaterally recorded auditory brainstem response. Ear Hear, 12:167, 1991
22. Cox LC, Martin RJ, Carlo WA et al: Early ABRs in infants undergoing assisted ventilation. J Am Acad Audiol, 4:13, 1993
23. Lasky RE: A developmental study on the effect of stimulus rate on the auditory evoked brain-stem response. Electroencephalogr Clin Neurophysiol, 59:411, 1984
24. Eggermont JJ, Salamy A: Maturational time course for the ABR in preterm and full term infants. Hear Res, 33:35, 1988
25. Eldredge L, Salamy A: Functional auditory development in preterm and full term infants. Early Hum Dev, 45:215, 1996
26. Adelman C, Levi H, Linder N et al: Neonatal auditory brain-stem response threshold and latency: 1 hour to 5 months. Electroencephalogr Clin Neurophysiol, 77:77, 1990

27. Gorga MP, Kaminski JR, Beauchaine KL et al: Auditory brainstem responses from children 3 months to 3 years of age: normal patterns of response. J Speech Hear Res, 32:281, 1989

28. Jiang ZD, Zheng MS, Sun DK et al: Brain stem auditory evoked responses from birth to adulthood: normative data of latency and interval. Hear Res, 54:67, 1991

29. Jiang ZD, Zhang L, Wu YY et al: Brain stem auditory evoked responses from birth to adulthood: development of wave amplitude. Hear Res, 68:35, 1993

30. Ponton CW, Moore JK, Eggermont JJ: Auditory brain stem response generation by parallel pathways: differential maturation of axonal conduction time and synaptic transmission. Ear Hear, 17:402, 1996

31. Moore JK, Ponton CW, Eggermont JJ et al: Perinatal maturation of the auditory brain stem response: changes in path length and conduction velocity. Ear Hear, 17:411, 1996

32. O'Donovan CA: Latency of brainstem response in children. Br J Audiol, 14:23, 1980

33. Thivierge J, Côté R: Brainstem auditory evoked response: normative values in children. Electroencephalogr Clin Neurophysiol, 77:309, 1990

34. Don M, Ponton CW, Eggermont JJ et al: Gender differences in cochlear response time: an explanation for gender amplitude differences in the unmasked auditory brain-stem response. J Acoust Soc Am, 94:2135, 1993

35. Fortnum H: Epidemiology of permanent childhood hearing impairment: implications for neonatal hearing screening. Audiol Med, 1:155, 2003

36. Durieux-Smith A, Fitzpatrick E, Whittingham J: Universal newborn hearing screening: a question of evidence. Int J Audiol, 47:1, 2008

37. Nelson HD, Bougatsos C, Nygren P: Universal newborn hearing screening: systematic review to update the 2001 US Preventive Services Task Force Recommendation. Pediatrics, 122(1):e266, 2008

38. Picton TW: Infant hearing assessment: opening ears. p. 449. In Picton TW (ed): Human Auditory Evoked Potentials. Plural, San Diego, 2010

39. Galambos R, Wilson MJ, Silva DP: Identifying hearing loss in the intensive care nursery: a 20-year summary. J Am Acad Audiol, 5:151, 1994

40. National Institutes of Health: Early identification of hearing impairment in infants and young children. NIH Consensus Statement, 11:1, 1993

41. Joint Committee on Infant Hearing: Year 2000 position statement: principles and guidelines for early hearing detection and intervention programs. Pediatrics, 106:798, 2000

42. Norton SJ, Gorga MP, Widen JE et al: Identification of neonatal hearing impairment: transient evoked otoacoustic emissions during the perinatal period. Ear Hear, 21:425, 2000

43. Gorga MP, Norton SJ, Sininger YS et al: Identification of neonatal hearing impairment: distortion product otoacoustic emissions during the perinatal period. Ear Hear, 21:400, 2000

44. Joint Committee on Infant Hearing: Year 2007 position statement: principles and guidelines for early hearing detection and intervention programs. Pediatrics, 120:898, 2007

45. Sininger YS, Cone-Wesson B, Folsom RC et al: Identification of neonatal hearing impairment: auditory brain stem responses in the perinatal period. Ear Hear, 21:383, 2000

46. Norton SJ, Gorga MP, Widen JE et al: Identification of neonatal hearing impairment: summary and recommendations. Ear Hear, 21:529, 2000

47. Hyde ML, Riko K, Malizia K: Audiometric accuracy of the click ABR in infants at risk for hearing loss. J Am Acad Audiol, 1:59, 1990

48. Durieux-Smith A, Picton TW, Bernard PH et al: Prognostic validity of brainstem electric response audiometry (BERA) in infants of a neonatal intensive care unit (NICU). Audiology, 30:249, 1991

49. Stockard JE, Curran JS: Transient elevation of threshold of the neonatal auditory brainstem response. Ear Hear, 11:21, 1990

50. Stockard JE, Stockard JJ, Kleinberg F et al: Prognostic value of brainstem auditory evoked potentials in neonates. Arch Neurol, 40:360, 1983

51. Psarommatis I, Riga M, Douros K et al: Transient infantile auditory neuropathy and its clinical implications. Int J Pediat Otorhinol, 70:1629, 2006

52. Sturzebecher E, Cebulla M, Neumann K: Click-evoked ABR at high stimulus repetition rates for neonatal hearing screening. Int J Audiol, 42:59, 2003

53. Stapells DR: Frequency-specific evoked potential audiometry in infants. p. 13. In Seewald RC (ed): A Sound Foundation through Early Amplification 1998. Proceedings of the First International Conference. Phonak AG, Basel, 2000

54. Stapells DR: Threshold estimation by the tone-evoked auditory brainstem response: a literature meta-analysis. J Speech Lang Path Audiol, 24:74, 2000

55. Ozdamar O, Kraus N, Stein L: Auditory brainstem responses in infants recovering from bacterial meningitis: audiologic evaluation. Arch Otolaryngol, 109:13, 1983

56. Ozdamar O, Kraus N: Auditory brainstem responses in infants recovering from bacterial meningitis: neurological evaluation. Arch Neurol, 40:499, 1983

57. Bao X, Wong V: Brainstem auditory-evoked potential evaluation in children with meningitis. Pediatr Neurol, 19:109, 1998

58. Moran LM, Durieux-Smith A, Malizia K: Brainstem electric response audiometry (BERA) in the evaluation of hearing loss in infants with cleft palate. J Speech Lang Pathol Audiol, 13:43, 1989

59. Chayasirisobhon S, Yu L, Griggs L et al: Recording of brainstem evoked potentials and their association with gentamicin in neonates. Pediatr Neurol, 14:277, 1996

60. Berg AL, Spitzer JB, Garvin JH: Ototoxic impact of cisplatin in pediatric oncology patients. Laryngoscope, 109:1806, 1999

61. Poblano A, Belmont A, Sosa J et al: Amikacin alters auditory brainstem conduction time in newborns. J Perinat Med, 31:237, 2003

62. Picton TW, Durieux-Smith A, Champagne SC et al: Objective evaluation of aided thresholds using auditory steady-state responses. J Am Acad Audiol, 9:315, 1998

63. Mason S, Garnham C, Hudson B: Electric response audiometry in young children before cochlear implantation: a short latency component. Ear Hear, 17:537, 1996

64. Gordon KA, Papsin BC, Harrison RV: Activity-dependent developmental plasticity of the auditory brain stem in children who use cochlear implants. Ear Hear, 24:485, 2003

65. Picton TW: Cochlear implants: body electric. p. 569. In Picton TW (ed): Human Auditory Evoked Potentials. Plural, San Diego, 2010

66. Starr A, Picton TW, Sininger YS et al: Auditory neuropathy. Brain, 119:741, 1996

67. Rance G, Beer DE, Cone-Wesson B et al: Clinical findings for a group of infants and young children with auditory neuropathy. Ear Hear, 20:238, 1999

68. Sininger Y, Starr A (eds): Auditory Neuropathy. Singular, San Diego, 2001

69. Picton TW: Auditory neuropathy: when time is broke. p. 535. In Picton TW (ed): Human Auditory Evoked Potentials. Plural, San Diego, 2010

70. Berlin C, Hood LJ, Cecola RP et al: Does type I afferent neuron dysfunction reveal itself through lack of efferent suppression? Hear Res, 65:40, 1993

71. Stein L, Tremblay K, Pasternak J et al: Brainstem abnormalities in neonates with normal otoacoustic emissions. Semin Hear, 17:197, 1996

72. Shapiro SM: Bilirubin toxicity in the developing nervous system. Pediatr Neurol, 29:410, 2003

73. Starr A, Sininger Y, Winter M et al: Transient deafness due to temperature-sensitive auditory neuropathy. Ear Hear, 19:169, 1998

74. Deltenre P, Mansbach AL, Bozet C et al: Auditory neuropathy with preserved cochlear microphonic potentials and secondary loss of otoacoustic emissions. Audiology, 38:187, 1999

75. Shallop JK, Peterson A, Facer GW et al: Cochlear implants in five cases of auditory neuropathy: postoperative findings and progress. Laryngoscope, 111:555, 2001

76. Mason JC, De Michele A, Stevens C et al: Cochlear implantation in patients with auditory neuropathy of varied etiologies. Laryngoscope, 113:45, 2003

77. Taylor MJ: Evoked potentials in paediatrics. p. 489. In Halliday AM (ed): Evoked Potentials in Clinical Testing. 2nd Ed. Churchill Livingstone, Edinburgh, 1993

78. Taylor MJ, Saliba E, Laugier J: Use of evoked potentials in preterm neonates. Arch Dis Child (Fetal Neonatal Ed), 74: F70, 1996

79. Frank Y, Vishnubhakat SM, Pahwa S: Brainstem auditory evoked responses in infants and children with AIDS. Pediatr Neurol, 8:262, 1992

80. Brivio L, Tornaghi R, Musetti L et al: Improvement of auditory brainstem responses after treatment with zidovudine in a child with AIDS. Pediatr Neurol, 7:53, 1990

81. Pikus AT: Pediatric audiologic profile in type 1 and type 2 neurofibromatosis. J Am Acad Audiol, 6:54, 1995

82. Evans DG, Newton V, Neary W et al: Use of MRI and audiological tests in presymptomatic diagnosis of type 2 neurofibromatosis (NF2). J Med Genet, 37:944, 2000

83. Pensak ML, Keith RW, Digman PS et al: Neuroaudiologic abnormalities in patients with type 1 neurofibromatosis. Laryngoscope, 99:702, 1989

84. Duffner PK, Cohen ME, Seidel FG et al: The significance of MRI abnormalities in children with neurofibromatosis. Neurology, 39:373, 1989

85. Edwards CG, Durieux-Smith A, Picton TW: Auditory brainstem response audiometry in neonatal hydrocephalus. J Otolaryngol, 14:Suppl 14, 40, 1985

86. Lütschg J, Meyer E, Jeanneret-Iseli C: Brainstem auditory evoked potentials in meningomyelocele. Neuropediatrics, 16:202, 1985

87. Docherty TB, Herbaut AG, Sedgwick EM: Brainstem auditory evoked potential abnormalities in myelomeningocoele in the older child. J Neurol Neurosurg Psychiatry, 50:13, 1987

88. Taylor MJ, Boor R, Keenan NK et al: Brainstem auditory and visual evoked potentials in infants with myelomeningocele. Brain Dev, 18:99, 1996

89. Anderson RC, Dowling KC, Feldstein NA et al: Chiari I malformation: potential role for intraoperative electrophysiologic monitoring. J Clin Neurophysiol, 20:65, 2003

90. Lott IT, McPherson DL, Starr A: Cerebral cortical contributions to sensory evoked potentials: hydranencephaly. Electroencephalogr Clin Neurophysiol, 64:218, 1986

91. Kaga K, Yasui T, Yuge T: Auditory behaviors and auditory brainstem responses of infants with hypogenesis of cerebral hemispheres. Acta Otolaryngol, 122:16, 2002

92. Garg BP, Markand ON, DeMyer WE: Usefulness of BAEP studies in the early diagnosis of Pelizaeus–Merzbacher disease. Neurology, 33:955, 1983

93. Yamanouchi H, Kaga M, Iwasaki Y et al: Auditory evoked responses in Krabbe disease. Pediatr Neurol, 9:387, 1993

94. Nezu A: Neurophysiological study in Pelizaeus–Merzbacher disease. Brain Dev, 17:175, 1995

95. Wang PJ, Young C, Liu HM et al: Neurophysiologic studies and MRI in Pelizaeus–Merzbacher disease: comparison of classic and connatal forms. Pediatr Neurol, 12:47, 1995

96. Kaga K, Tokoro Y, Tanaka Y et al: The progress of adrenoleukodystrophy as revealed by auditory evoked responses and brain stem histology. Arch Otorhinolaryngol, 228:17, 1980

97. De Meirleir LJ, Taylor MJ, Logan WJ: Multimodal evoked potential studies in leukodystrophies of children. Can J Neurol Sci, 15:26, 1988

98. Schmidt S, Traber F, Block W: Phenotype assignment in symptomatic female carriers of X-linked adrenoleukodystrophy. J Neurol, 248:36, 2001

99. Guilhoto LM, Osorio CA, Machado LR et al: Pediatric multiple sclerosis: report of 14 cases. Brain Dev, 17:9, 1995

100. Markand ON, Garg BP, Brandt IK: Nonketotic hyperglycinemia: electroencephalographic and evoked potential abnormalities. Neurology, 32:151, 1982

101. Brin MF, Pedley TA, Lovelace RE et al: Electrophysiologic features of abetalipoproteinemia. Neurology, 36:669, 1986

102. Fagan ER, Taylor MJ: Longitudinal multimodal evoked potential studies in abetalipoproteinemia. Can J Neurol Sci, 14:617, 1987

103. Taylor MJ, Robinson BH: Evoked potentials in children with oxidative metabolic defects leading to Leigh's syndrome. Pediatr Neurol, 8:25, 1992

104. Lacey DJ, Terplan K: Correlating auditory evoked and brainstem histologic abnormalities in infantile Gaucher's disease. Neurology, 34:539, 1984

105. Aisen M, Rapoport S, Solomon G: Brainstem auditory evoked potentials in two siblings with Niemann–Pick disease. Brain Dev, 7:431, 1985

106. Hsu YS, Chang YC, Lee WT et al: The diagnostic value of sensory evoked potentials in pediatric Wilson disease. Pediatr Neurol, 29:42, 2003

107. Taylor MJ, McMenamin JB, Andermann E et al: Electrophysiological investigation of the auditory system in Friedreich's ataxia. Can J Neurol Sci, 9:131, 1982

108. Cassandro E, Mosca F, Sequino L et al: Otoneurological findings in Friedreich's ataxia and other inherited neuropathies. Audiology, 25:84, 1986

109. Taylor MJ, Chan-Lui WY, Logan WJ: Longitudinal evoked potential studies in hereditary ataxias. Can J Neurol Sci, 12:100, 1985

110. Esbjörmer E, Larsson P, Leissner P et al: The serum reserve albumin concentration or monoacetyldiaminodiphenyl sulphone and auditory evoked responses during neonatal hyperbilirubinaemia. Acta Paediatr Scand, 80:406, 1991

111. Okumura A, Kidokoro H, Shoji H et al: Kernicterus in preterm infants. Pediatrics, 123:e1052, 2009

112. Chin KC, Taylor MJ, Perlman M: Improvement in auditory and visual evoked potentials in jaundiced preterm infants after exchange transfusion. Arch Dis Child, 60:714, 1985

113. Hung KL: Auditory brainstem responses in patients with neonatal hyperbilirubinemia and bilirubin encephalopathy. Brain Dev, 11:297, 1989

114. Tan KL, Skurr BA, Yip YY: Phototherapy and the brainstem auditory evoked response in neonatal hyperbilirubinemia. J Pediatr, 120:306, 1992

115. Durmaz S, Karagol U, Deda G et al: Brainstem auditory and visual evoked potentials in children with protein-energy malnutrition. Pediatr Int, 41:615, 1999

116. Rothenberg SJ, Poblano A, Schnaas L: Brainstem auditory evoked response at five years and prenatal and postnatal blood lead. Neurotoxicol Teratol, 22:503, 2000

117. Counter SA: Neurophysiological anomalies in brainstem responses of mercury-exposed children of Andean gold miners. J Occup Environ Med, 45:87, 2003

118. Rössig C, Wässer S, Oppermann P: Audiologic manifestations in fetal alcohol syndrome assessed by brainstem auditory-evoked potentials. Neuropediatrics, 25:245, 1994

119. Church MW, Eldis F, Blakley BW et al: Hearing, language, speech, vestibular, and dentofacial disorders in fetal alcohol syndrome. Alcohol Clin Exp Res, 21:227, 1997

120. Tan-Laxa MA, Sison-Switala C, Rintelman W et al: Abnormal auditory brainstem response among infants with prenatal cocaine exposure. Pediatrics, 113:357, 2004

121. Cone-Wesson B: Prenatal alcohol and cocaine exposure: influences on cognition, speech, language, and hearing. J Commun Disord, 38:279, 2005

122. Kable JA, Coles CD, Lynch ME et al: The impact of maternal smoking on fast auditory brainstem responses. Neurotoxicol Teratol, 31:216, 2009

123. Sunaga Y, Sone K, Nagashima K et al: Auditory brainstem responses in congenital heart disease. Pediatr Neurol, 8:437, 1992

124. Hecox KE, Cone B: Prognostic importance of brainstem auditory evoked responses after asphyxia. Neurology, 31:1429, 1981

125. Jiang ZD, Liu XY, Shi BP et al: Brainstem auditory outcomes and correlation with neurodevelopment after perinatal asphyxia. Pediatr Neurol, 39:189, 2008

126. Jiang ZD, Brosi DM, Wilkinson AR: Differences in impaired brainstem conduction between neonatal chronic lung disease and perinatal asphyxia. Clin Neurophysiol, 121:725, 2010

127. Fisher B, Peterson B, Hicks G: Use of brainstem auditory-evoked response testing to assess neurologic outcome following near drowning in children. Crit Care Med, 20:578, 1992

128. Kaga K, Ichimura K, Kitazumi E et al: Auditory brainstem responses in infants and children with anoxic brain damage due to near-suffocation or near-drowning. Int J Pediatr Otorhinolaryngol, 36:231, 1996

129. Taylor MJ, Houston BD, Lowry NJ: Recovery of auditory brainstem responses in severe hypoxic-ischemic insult. N Engl J Med, 309:1169, 1983

130. Jiang ZD, Brosi DM, Shao XM et al: Maximum length sequence brainstem auditory evoked responses in term neonates who have perinatal hypoxia-ischemia. Pediatr Res, 48:639, 2000

131. Jiang ZD, Brosi DM, Wang J et al: Time course of brainstem pathophysiology during first month in term infants after perinatal asphyxia, revealed by MLS BAER latencies and intervals. Pediatr Res, 54:680, 2003

132. Kileny P, Finer N, Sussman P et al: Auditory brainstem responses in sudden infant death syndrome: comparison of siblings, "near-miss", and normal infants. J Pediatr, 101:225, 1982

133. Stockard JJ: Brainstem auditory evoked potentials in adult and infant sleep apnea syndromes, including sudden infant death syndrome and near-miss for sudden infant death. Ann N Y Acad Sci, 388:443, 1982

134. De Meirleir LJ, Taylor MJ: Evoked potentials in comatose children: auditory brainstem responses. Pediatr Neurol, 2:31, 1986

135. Bosch Blancafort J, Olesti Marco M, Poch Puig JM et al: Predictive value of brain-stem auditory evoked potentials in children with post-traumatic coma produced by diffuse brain injury. Childs Nerv Syst, 11:400, 1995

136. Butinar D, Gostisa A: Brainstem auditory evoked potentials and somatosensory evoked potentials in prediction of post-traumatic coma in children. Eur J Physiol, 431:Suppl 2, R289, 1996

137. De Meirleir LJ, Taylor MJ: Prognostic utility of SEPs in comatose children. Pediatr Neurol, 3:78, 1987

138. Becca J, Cox PN, Taylor MJ et al: Somatosensory evoked potentials for prediction of outcome in acute severe brain injury. J Pediatr, 126:44, 1995

139. Ruiz-Lopez MJ, Martinez de Azagra A, Serrano A et al: Brain death and evoked potentials in pediatric patients. Crit Care Med, 27:412, 1999

140. Taylor MJ, Rosenblatt B, Linschoten L: Auditory brainstem response abnormalities in autistic children. Can J Neurol Sci, 9:429, 1982

141. Maziade M, Merette C, Cayer M et al: Prolongation of brainstem auditory-evoked responses in autistic probands and their unaffected relatives. Arch Gen Psychiatry, 57:1077, 2000

142. Rosenhall U, Nordin V, Brantberg K et al: Autism and auditory brain stem responses. Ear Hear, 24:206, 2003

143. Courchesne E, Courchesne RY, Hicks G et al: Functioning of the brainstem auditory pathway in non-retarded autistic individuals. Electroencephalogr Clin Neurophysiol, 61:491, 1985

144. Pelson RO, Budden SS: Auditory brainstem response findings in Rett syndrome. Brain Dev, 9:514, 1987

145. Verma NP, Nigro MA, Hart ZH: Rett syndrome a gray matter disease? Electrophysiologic evidence. Electroencephalogr Clin Neurophysiol, 67:327, 1987

146. Squires N, Ollo C, Jordan R: Auditory brainstem responses in the mentally retarded: audiometric correlates. Ear Hear, 7:83, 1986

147. Jiang ZD, Wu YY, Liu XY: Early development of brainstem auditory evoked potentials in Down's syndrome. Early Hum Dev, 23:41, 1990

148. Kitamoto I, Kukita J, Kurukawa T et al: Transient neurologic abnormalities and BAEPs in high-risk infants. Pediatr Neurol, 6:319, 1990

149. Salamy A, Mendelson T, Tooley WH et al: Differential development of brainstem potentials in healthy and high-risk infants. Science, 210:553, 1980

150. Maison S, Duclaux R, Ferber-Viart C et al: Clinical interest of brainstem auditory evoked potentials in 72 children with inadequate language development. Int J Neurosci, 88:261, 1996

151. Blegvad B, Hvidegaard T: Hereditary dysfunction of the brainstem auditory pathways as the major cause of speech retardation. Scand Audiol, 12:179, 1983

152. Mason SM, Mellor DH: Brain-stem, middle latency and late cortical evoked potentials in children with speech and language disorders. Electroencephalogr Clin Neurophysiol, 59:297, 1984

153. Johnson K, Nicol T, Zecker et al: Auditory brainstem correlates of perceptual timing deficits. J Cogn Neurosci, 19:376, 2007

154. Russo NM, Bradlow AR, Skoe E et al: Deficient brainstem encoding of pitch in children with autism spectrum disorders. Clin Neurophysiol, 119:1720, 2008

155. Banai K, Hornickel JM, Skoe E et al: Reading and subcortical auditory function. Cereb Cortex, 19:2699, 2009

156. Skoe E, Kraus N: Auditory brainstem response to complex sounds: a tutorial. Ear Hear, 31:302, 2010

Somatosensory Evoked Potentials

MICHAEL J. AMINOFF and ANDREW EISEN

The development of sophisticated imaging techniques has had a great impact on the role of somatosensory evoked potentials (SEPs) in the clinical setting. Their role in the evaluation of most neurologic diseases is limited; nevertheless, as described in this chapter, SEPs are valuable as a diagnostic and prognostic test in several clinical situations. Their role in the operating room and intensive care unit has expanded, and interest remains high in SEPs as a research tool for unraveling fundamental aspects of central sensory physiology.[1]

Stimulation of a mixed nerve is used most commonly to evoke the SEP. This type of stimulus activates predominantly—if not entirely—the large-diameter, fast-conducting group Ia muscle and group II cutaneous afferent fibers. The number of axons that are activated synchronously is large, so the response is relatively large and easy to record. The SEP amplitude is almost maximal when the peripheral nerve action potential is only 50 percent of its maximum. This translates into a stimulus intensity of about twice sensory threshold, which is well tolerated by patients.[2] Selective intrafascicular nerve stimulation has provided evidence for a direct muscle afferent fiber (Ia) projection to the human somatosensory cortex. However, when a mixed nerve is stimulated, both group Ia muscle afferents and cutaneous group II afferents contribute to the resulting SEP, and this method detects selective impairment of sensory modalities poorly. Results can be normal even when selective sensory deficits are considerable. Discrimination can be improved by using a variety of mechanical or thermal stimuli.[3] These techniques selectively activate specific sensory end-organs. Unfortunately, because of the rather small number of axons stimulated and the wide range of their conduction velocities, the SEPs elicited are usually small in amplitude and desynchronized. Many hundreds of responses need to be averaged, and even then the onset latency may be difficult to identify. These issues have limited the clinical utility of SEPs elicited by mechanical and thermal stimulation.[4,5]

Selective ablation of the dorsal columns in animals greatly attenuates or abolishes the SEP, thus indicating that within the spinal cord the SEP is mediated predominantly via the dorsal columns. Therefore, diseases of the dorsal columns, with associated impairment of vibration and position sensation, invariably are associated with abnormalities of the SEP.[6] Conversely, spinal cord lesions that do not interrupt the dorsal columns are often associated with a relatively normal SEP after mixed nerve stimulation.[7] Tourniquet-induced ischemia in humans has been shown to abolish short-latency before long-latency SEP components, which suggests that the short-latency components are mediated by different centrally conducting afferent tracts.

Although, in general, the SEP is best recorded over the somatosensory cortex, topographic mapping indicates that several of its components are distributed widely over the scalp, and some are recorded maximally outside the somatosensory cortex.[8–10] The SEP monitors more than just the somatosensory pathways. For example, abnormalities occur commonly in certain primary diseases of the motor system (e.g., amyotrophic lateral sclerosis) and should not cause concern.[11]

STIMULATION TECHNIQUES

Mixed Nerve Stimulation

Electrical stimulation of a mixed nerve initiates a relatively synchronous volley that elicits a sizeable SEP. It therefore has become the standard for clinical use.[12] The stimulus intensity required to elicit an SEP of maximum amplitude should be one that induces a mixed nerve action potential just exceeding 50 percent of its maximum amplitude. This will elicit a slight twitch of the muscle, indicating that motor as well as sensory axons are activated. Stimulation of Ia afferents is not uncomfortable, even at repetition rates of 5 Hz. Their threshold for activation is lower than that of motor axons (as indicated by the intensity required to induce an H reflex). If the stimulus intensity is too high, occlusion of the rapidly converging afferent impulses may occur, depending on the limb that is stimulated. A short-duration (200 to 300 μsec) stimulus is popular, but stimuli of longer duration (1,000 μsec) and appropriately lower intensity are more likely to activate preferentially the group Ia and II afferents. A repetition rate of 3 Hz is convenient and without discomfort, and faster rates are usually tolerable. Repetition rates of up to 15 Hz do not alter the SEP. Sometimes electrocardiographic artifacts are troublesome, a point particularly relevant when trying to obtain noncephalic, referential recordings of SEPs elicited by stimulation of nerves in the lower limbs. This problem usually can be solved by using the electrocardiogram to trigger the stimulus.

Cutaneous Nerve Stimulation

Use of cutaneous nerve stimulation has particular application to peripheral nerve diseases and should be considered in several circumstances:

1. To assess the integrity of specific cutaneous nerves that are not studied readily by conventional sensory nerve conduction techniques (e.g., the lateral femoral cutaneous, saphenous, and antebrachial cutaneous nerves). Sensory nerve action potentials can be difficult to record from these nerves, whereas the corresponding SEP is usually of sufficient size to measure with ease.[13,14]
2. To measure peripheral sensory conduction when not otherwise possible because the sensory nerve action potential is small or absent. In hereditary sensory motor neuropathy types I, II, and III, sensory nerve action potentials are often absent; but the SEP, although dispersed, can be elicited from stimulation of two or more sites along a cutaneous nerve, and thereby allows one to deduce a conduction velocity.
3. To evaluate isolated root function. When compared with mixed nerve stimulation, the segmental specificity of cutaneous stimulation is increased, even though most cutaneous nerves are derived from at least two sensory segments.
4. To assess dubious patchy numbness for medicolegal reasons by stimulating homologous areas of affected and normal skin supplied through cutaneous terminals.

Dermatomal Stimulation

Dermatomal stimulation is even more segmentally specific than is cutaneous nerve stimulation, which invariably activates two or more dermatomes. However, the ascending volley is sometimes very desynchronized, making the SEP difficult to interpret. The technique has been used most often to assess function of the lumbosacral roots. For L5, the medial side of the first metatarsophalangeal joint or the dorsal surface of the foot between the first and second toes is stimulated. For S1, the lateral side of the fifth metatarsophalangeal joint is stimulated. Care must be taken to avoid stimulus spread to neighboring dermatomes, underlying muscle (which induces activity of Ia afferents), and digital cutaneous nerves. Such stimulus specificity can be achieved if the stimulus is kept at 2.5 times the sensory threshold, which gives about 80 percent of the maximum amplitude. Normative data for the L5 and S1 dermatomes are well established.

Laser Stimulation

Because of the high specificity of radiant heat for nociceptor activation, laser-evoked brain potentials (LEPs) are a suitable tool for testing small-fiber and spinothalamic tract function. The CO_2 laser pulse is absorbed completely within the epidermis and activates a very limited number of superficial afferents, mostly A-delta fibers, belonging predominantly to the pain system.[15]

A pathway from cortical layer 6 to the thalamus directly excites relay cells and indirectly inhibits them via the thalamic reticular nucleus. Laser-scanning photostimulation, which specifically activates cell bodies or dendrites, has been used to understand the circuit organization of this cortical feedback stimulating the primary somatosensory cortex.[16] LEP components have been recorded by intracranial electrodes and these mirrored the ones picked up from the Cz lead, thus suggesting that they probably are generated by the opposite pole of the same cortical sources producing the scalp responses. In the intracranial traces, there was no evidence of earlier potentials possibly generated within the thalamus or of subcortical far-field responses. This means that the nociceptive signal amplification occurring within the cerebral cortex is necessary to produce identifiable LEP components.[17]

Based on studies in normal subjects, as well as in patients with sensory loss, the ascending signals following CO_2 laser stimulation are conducted through A-delta fibers and the spinothalamic tract.[18,19] The peripheral and spinal cord components of the LEP are not detectable, whereas a cortical potential can be recorded with a wide distribution on the scalp and with a maximal amplitude at the vertex. Using a modified technique, conduction velocity has been determined in C-fibers (2 m/sec) as well as in A-delta fibers (10 m/sec) of the spinothalamic tract.[20]

LEPs have been demonstrated to complement quantitative sensory testing in assessing the relationship between skin nerve denervation and regeneration.[21] They have also been used to document posterior root impairment objectively in patients with acute monosegmental radiculopathy.[22] Such studies open the perspective of electrophysiologically differentiating the presence or absence of posterior root pathology in patients with similar clinical symptoms but possibly different prognoses.[22]

LEPs have been evaluated during sleep.[23] In the awake subject, nonpainful stimulation evokes early- and middle-latency components (N20, P30, and N60), and painful stimulation additionally evokes later pain-specific components (N130 and P240) at the Cz electrode. During sleep, N20 and P30 do not change in amplitude, N60 shows a slight but significant amplitude reduction, and N130 and P240 decrease markedly or disappear entirely.[23]

Contact Heat Stimulation

A specially designed, commercially available, contact heat stimulator can be used to deliver recurrent heat stimuli at a specified temperature to the skin while the cerebral responses, mediated primarily by A-delta fibers, are recorded over the scalp. The thermode has a circular contact area of 572.5 mm^2 with stimulators in two layers working together; two thermocouples embedded within its outer coating measure the skin temperature. The thermode allows for very rapid heating and cooling of the skin. SEPs elicited by contact heat stimulators have been used to assess the function of A-delta fibers in patients with neuropathy.[24] The response latencies of such SEPs are longer than those elicited by laser stimulation, perhaps because of the longer duration of the stimuli and the time required to conduct the heat through the skin to stimulate nociceptors.[25] The approach is easier to use in the clinic than laser stimulation, does not require eye protection, and has a lesser risk of inducing burns or erythema.[26]

RECORDING AND FILTERING OF SEPs

Surface or needle electrodes can be used for recording SEPs. Scalp needle electrodes are inserted easily into the scalp but are not popular because of their higher impedance, the discomfort caused during insertion, and concern about infection. Now that disposable needles are widely available, they are preferred when needle electrodes are to be used. Recording montages are either "cephalic bipolar," in which both electrodes are placed on the head; or "referential," with the reference electrode placed at a noncephalic site. A cephalic bipolar montage has the advantage of being relatively free from noise and is preferred for routine clinical use; however, small-amplitude, far-field potentials, which reflect activity within subcortical structures, are largely canceled. The Cz′–Fz derivation generally is used for recording the cortical component of tibial SEPs, but considerable intersubject and intrasubject variation exists in the cortical distribution of tibial SEP components. In particular, P37 in the Cz′–Fz recording may be very small, even in normal subjects, and a Cz′–Cc derivation as the single cortical bipolar recording arrangement may be better suited for routine clinical examinations.[27] Far-field potentials can be recorded only with noncephalic references (e.g., with the reference electrode placed on the opposite mastoid, shoulder, arm, hand, or knee; linked mastoids or ear lobes may also be used).

Multichannel recording using both cephalic and noncephalic montages is advantageous; however, the number of channels (recording derivations) used should be dictated by the specific reason for performing the SEP study. For example, in field distribution and brain-mapping studies, 16 or more channels may be important, whereas one channel is sufficient when the SEP is being used to assess peripheral nerve disease.

The near-field potentials recorded with a bipolar cephalic derivation are characteristically of negative polarity and of relatively large amplitude. The amplitude of near-field potentials falls rapidly as the electrode is moved away from the generator source. Some small-amplitude far-field potentials may also be recorded with bipolar cephalic derivations, but this is too variable for clinical purposes, and referential recording is required to identify far-field potentials with confidence. These potentials are characteristically of small amplitude, and are recorded with equal ease and amplitude over a wide area of the scalp. They are usually positive and monophasic at the active electrode, reflecting a moving front approaching the recording electrode, but under some circumstances they may be biphasic and of either polarity.

Different recording montages are used in different laboratories, depending on the purpose of the study, and recommendations by various professional organizations also differ in their details. For general clinical purposes, a common but minimal montage for recording median or other upper-limb SEPs is between the ipsilateral and contralateral Erb's point (channel 1); the fifth cervical spine and contralateral Erb's point (channel 2); midway between the ipsilateral C3/4 and P3/4 (CP placement; also known as C3′ or C4′, located 2 cm behind the C3 or C4 placements) and the contralateral Erb's point (channel 3); and contralateral and ipsilateral CP placements (channel 4). For the tibial SEP, recordings may be made between the distal and proximal regions of the popliteal fossa (channel 1); the L1 and L3 spine (channel 2); Cz or CPz (Cz′) and Fz or Fpz (channel 3); and the ipsilateral CP placement and Fpz (channel 4).

Small-amplitude components of the SEP are composed of both high and low frequencies, and filtering can be problematic. Too wide a bandpass results in a "noisy" SEP, whereas a restrictive bandpass attenuates either the high- or low-frequency components, depending on the settings chosen. There is no "correct" filter setting; the choice is best related to the particular task at hand. For general purposes, a relatively broad bandpass (10 to 2,500 Hz) is suitable, but even the same bandpass has differing effects, depending on the amplifiers used. It is reasonable to experiment with different filter settings for a given recording device. Restrictive filtering of between 150 and 300 to 3,000 Hz enhances high-frequency, small-amplitude, near- and far-field components, but does so at the expense of the low-frequency components.

Restrictive analog filtering induces a phase shift of components, which invariably causes distortion of these components and may create artifactual components. Digital filtering, available on some equipment, is designed for zero phase shift and does not distort components. Digital filtering does not create new peaks, but it greatly enhances those normally present (Fig. 26-1). This

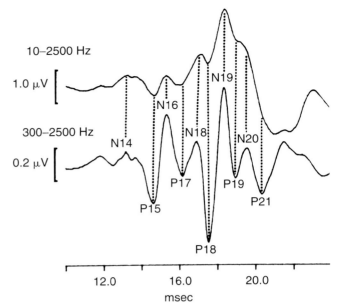

FIGURE 26-1 ■ Effect of restrictive digital filtering designed for zero phase shift on the median nerve somatosensory evoked potential recorded between the contralateral C3 or C4 electrode and a reference at Fpz. The top trace shows the response (average of 1,024 trials) obtained by using an analog bandpass of 10 to 2,500 Hz. The lower trace shows the response when it was digitally filtered (300 to 2,500 Hz). No new waves have been "created," but all components are recognized more easily. There has been no phase shift. (From Eisen A, Roberts K, Low M et al: Questions regarding the sequential neural generator theory of the somatosensory evoked potential raised by digital filtering. Electroencephalogr Clin Neurophysiol, 59:388, 1984, with permission.)

characteristic is of particular importance for recording SEPs evoked by leg stimulation because it makes the small-amplitude components more easily identifiable (Fig. 26-2). Human median nerve SEPs exhibit a brief oscillatory burst of low amplitude (less than 500 nV) and high frequency (about 600 Hz), which can be isolated by digital filtering. These oscillations are superimposed on the primary cortical response N20, but the N20 component and the high-frequency oscillations are dissociated functionally and represent independent SEP components. The N20 response is generated mainly by excitatory postsynaptic potentials in pyramidal cells of Brodman area 3b, whereas the high-frequency oscillations seem to be generated intracortically by postsynaptic inhibitory interneurons.[28,29]

MEASUREMENT OF THE SEP

Several characteristics of the SEP can be measured, including onset latency, peak latency, interpeak latency, amplitude (including the presence or absence of

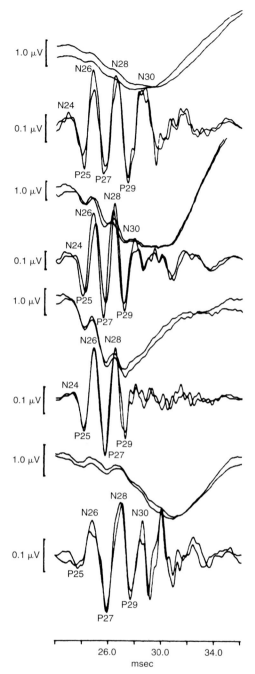

FIGURE 26-2 ■ Somatosensory evoked potentials (SEPs) evoked by fibular (peroneal) nerve stimulation in four normal subjects and recorded between Cz and the C3 or C4 electrode contralateral to the side of stimulation. The top pair of each set of traces is a routine analog recording with a bandpass of 2 to 2,500 Hz; the bottom pair of each set is the same SEP after digital filtering at 300 to 2,500 Hz. N26 and N28 are considered the median N18 and N20 equivalents but are seldom recognized in routine recordings. (From Eisen A, Roberts K, Low M et al: Questions regarding the sequential neural generator theory of the somatosensory evoked potential raised by digital filtering. Electroencephalogr Clin Neurophysiol, 59:388, 1984, with permission.)

components), morphology, and dispersion of the SEP. Side-to-side comparisons may be useful. Latency is the easiest SEP feature to measure and standardize, but it gives rather limited information. Other characteristics (e.g., morphology or dispersion) are more variable and difficult to interpret.

Latency varies with limb length, whereas interpeak transit (conduction) times are reliable parameters that are independent of limb length and are usually independent of peripheral nerve disease. Central afferent pathways do not mature at the same rate as peripheral pathways, and adult values for conduction velocity are not attained until 7 or 8 years of age. Aging is associated with prolongation of SEP latencies. This prolongation is not simply a reflection of slowed peripheral conduction because central conduction times are also slowed significantly. Latency or interpeak conduction times are considered abnormal when they are more than 3 standard deviations above the normal mean. They are measured easily but may be normal in the face of obvious clinical impairment. It is important to be aware that SEP components may come to be so attenuated that they cannot be recognized, particularly in the case of SEPs evoked by stimulation of leg nerves. Care is required to distinguish between a delayed SEP and an absent component; when a component is absent, the subsequent component may be mistaken for the missing potential and the latency of the SEP erroneously considered to be delayed.

There is an asymmetry of the median-derived SEP in relation to handedness. This occurs only at the cortical level. However, both functional and morphologic cortical asymmetry of somatosensory representation appears to vary independently of motor and language functions.[30] Other factors that modify the SEP include acute and regular exercise, which shortens SEP latency and decreases its amplitude,[31] and attention. There are differences between elderly and young subjects in the brain mechanisms underlying selective attention. The median SEP amplitude increases during a selective attention condition in young subjects but not in the elderly, who are unable to divert their attention from the electrical stimuli being delivered to the median nerve. These observations agree with recent hypotheses that suggest a decrease of the inhibitory control of attention mechanisms during aging.[32]

Absence of components normally present is regarded as abnormal. The absolute amplitude of SEP components is quite variable, but an interside difference exceeding 50 percent is regarded as abnormal by many clinical neurophysiologists.[33] A difference of this extent may be indicative either of central conduction block or of considerable neuronal/axonal loss. However, complex facilitatory and occlusive synaptic interactions can result in "central gain" within the nervous system and may prevent amplitude reduction in the SEP and thereby mask axonal or neuronal loss. Amplitude reduction of the SEPs also occurs during voluntary movement, a phenomenon commonly known as "gating." This presumably prevents irrelevant afferent inputs during movement from reaching consciousness. The gating effect takes place at the cortical level; subcortical SEP components remain unchanged during movement.[34-36] Gating of SEPs is selective to muscles utilized for specific tasks and may persist after repetitive movements, leading to an altered pattern and level of cortical processing. It has been proposed that this results in plastic changes in the cortex that may be relevant to the development of overuse syndromes.[37] SEP amplitude increases in the elderly, and "giant" potentials typify hereditary myoclonic epilepsy.[38]

The morphology (shape) and dispersion of the SEP are difficult features to quantitate, but both may be abnormal before or in the absence of latency prolongation or amplitude reduction. Computer-assisted methods for quantifying both dispersion and morphology of the SEP have been described, but the methodology is not suitable for routine clinical use.

NEURAL GENERATORS OF THE SEP

The different SEP components are designated by their polarity and latency. Polarity at the active electrode is indicated as either positive (P) or negative (N). Debate continues regarding the origin of some SEP components, and no agreement has been reached regarding the numerical latency value ascribed to each component.[39] The origin of specific, early-latency SEP components elicited by median and tibial nerve stimulation and recorded over the scalp is shown in Table 26-1, which summarizes the most widely held views at this time.

It is accepted generally that the different components of the SEP predominantly reflect sequential activation of neural generators excited by the ascending volley. This concept is appealing because it provides a rational base for interpreting an absent or abnormal component in relation to a specific anatomic lesion. However, factors other than neural generators (i.e., synapses in relay nuclei) are important in the origin of some SEP components, particularly the small far-field potentials recorded with noncephalic references. In particular, stationary far-field peaks (e.g., P9, P11, P13, and P14 evoked by median nerve stimulation) reflect propagated volleys of action potentials traveling in axons and can be recorded as the traveling volley approaches but before it actually reaches the active recording electrode. As shown in

TABLE 26-1 ■ Origin of Far-Field and Near-Field Somatosensory Potential Components

Component	Generator	Comments
MEDIAN NERVE		
Far-field potentials		
P9	Just distal to the brachial plexus	Sometimes bilobed P9a and P9b (depending on arm position)
P11	Posterior root entry (presynaptic)	
P13/P14	Medial lemniscus (postsynaptic)	P13 may reflect synaptic activity of posterior horn interneurons
N18	Between the upper pons and midbrain	N18 remains intact after thalamic lesions
Near-field potentials		
N20	Area 3b in the posterior bank of the rolandic fissure	Diagnostically the most useful peak to measure
P22	Motor area 4	Increases with age
P27	Parietal cortex	
N30	Supplementary motor area	Decreases with age
TIBIAL NERVE		
Far-field potentials		
P18	Sacral plexus	Analogous to median P9
P31	Gracile nucleus	Analogous to median P14
N34	Brainstem	Analogous to median N18
Near-field potential		
P37/N37	Primary somatosensory cortex	Analogous to median N20 Multiple cortical generators are involved

From Aminoff MJ, Eisen AA: Somatosensory evoked potentials. Muscle Nerve, 21:277, 1998, with permission of the American Association of Neuromuscular and Electrodiagnostic Medicine.

Figure 26-3, this property results from physical changes in the surrounding volume conductor, including the resistance or impedance of the volume conductor, sites of axonal branching, and anatomic orientation of the traveling impulse.

Neurosurgical interventions allow for intracerebral near-field recordings of SEPs from the deep lemniscal and thalamocortical system. Such studies of subcortically recorded SEPs have helped to establish concepts on the generators of the components that correspond to the scalp responses peaking in the first 15 msec after median nerve stimulation. These reflect successive activation of the lemniscal system at the spinal entry zone of the peripheral nerve, the posterior column, the cuneate nucleus, and the medial lemniscus.[40]

Of the far-field potentials in the median and tibial SEPs, it seems likely that relay nuclei are responsible only for the generation of P13 and P31, respectively[41]; the other potentials probably reflect electrophysical change

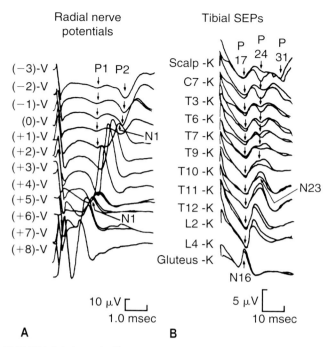

Radial nerve
potentials

Tibial SEPs

A

B

10 µV
1.0 msec

5 µV
10 msec

FIGURE 26-3 ▪ **A**, Somatosensory evoked potentials (SEPs) recorded antidromically from the superficial radial nerve with a referential recording technique. The active electrode was placed at different points at 1.5-cm increments along the course of the nerve over the dorsum of the hand and second digit. The 0 level represented the base of the digit, with the other recording sites indicated by a number from the 0 level, a minus sign being assigned for more distal placements. The reference electrode was placed around the fifth digit (V). P1 and P2 are stationary positive peaks. P1 becomes apparent when the active electrode is at the junction between the arm and the wrist, and P2 does so when this electrode is at the junction between the wrist and the finger. **B**, Tibial SEPs recorded referentially with active electrodes over the scalp, along the spine, and near the gluteal fold, and reference electrodes at the knee (K) after the tibial nerve was stimulated at the ankle. Stationary positive peaks (P17 and P24) are present; they occurred at the junction between the leg and the thigh (pelvic girdle, sacral plexus) and the peripheral and central nervous system (conus medullaris, posterior columns), respectively. At the junctional zones is an electrophysical change in the surrounding volume conductor, in part or in whole responsible for the stationary far-field potentials. (From Kimura J, Mitsudome A, Yamada T et al: Stationary peaks from a moving source in far-field recording. Electroencephalogr Clin Neurophysiol, 58:351, 1984, with permission.)

in the surrounding volume conductor.[42,43] The near-field components N20 and N37 are generated neurally but probably reflect multiple and even independent thalamocortical projections.

The clinical usefulness of middle-latency SEPs (P40, N60) is still controversial because these components show considerable interindividual variability even in healthy subjects. Nevertheless, middle-latency SEPs following stimulation of the median nerve are considered a sensitive measure of cortical function, and several studies have reported their reliability for objective assessment and quantification of cerebral dysfunction and prognostic evaluation in patients with a variety of diseases.[44] Amplitude and latency of middle-latency SEPs increase gradually with age in normal subjects.[44]

Long-latency components are distributed bilaterally, with the greatest amplitude being at the vertex. They relate to nonspecific thalamocortical projection systems involved in habituation, adaptation, and arousal. These components are of large amplitude (between 10 and 40 µV), so as few as 50 averaged epochs are required to obtain a measurable response. Unfortunately, their recovery time takes several seconds, which necessitates a stimulus repetition rate that is lower than once every 5 seconds to avoid significant attenuation of the response. Recovery function of given SEP components is not determined simply by the number of synapses interposed between the stimulus site and the generator source of the response in the central nervous system (CNS). There appears to be a structural or functional process of low-cut filtering in the primary sensory cortex.[45]

Spinal SEPs

Spinal SEPs can be recorded over the cervical and thoracolumbar regions. They are considerably smaller in amplitude than SEPs recorded over the scalp, which limits their clinical usefulness. However, the difference in latency between the scalp and cervical or lumbar SEPs is a measure of central sensory conduction, which remains a major clinical application of spinal SEPs. When a combined vertical and horizontal array of electrodes is placed over the neck, and a noncephalic reference is used, the cervical SEP elicited by median nerve stimulation consists of three distinct components (Fig. 26-4): (1) the proximal plexus volley (PPV); (2) the posterior (dorsal) column volley (DCV); and (3) a cervical component (CERV N13/P13) that possibly is generated at the level of the posterior gray matter of the cervical cord. These occur with onset latencies of approximately 10, 12, and 13 msec, respectively. With a cephalic reference, these components become fused, although some or all of the subcomponents may be appreciated as small deflections superimposed on the main negativity. The latency difference between the peak of the main negativity of the spine-recorded response, usually measuring between 12 and 14 msec, and the N20 cortical SEP component gives a "central conduction time" between the lower part of the brainstem and the primary sensory cortex that measures about 5.5 msec.

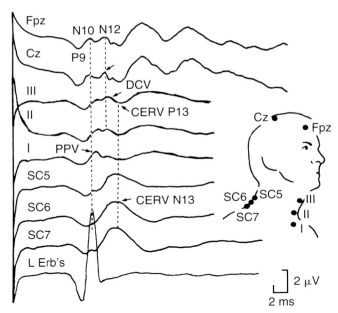

FIGURE 26-4 ■ Left median somatosensory evoked potential (SEP) recorded from different electrode locations with a contralateral elbow reference. The cervical SEP has three components. PPV (the proximal plexus volley) is recorded at the scalp as a far-field negativity (N10); DCV (the posterior or dorsal column volley) is also recorded at the scalp as a far-field negativity (N12); and CERV N13/P13 is recorded at the scalp as a far-field positivity P13 (not labeled). Corresponding components can be recognized for the thoracolumbar spinal SEP. (Modified from Emerson RG, Seyal M, Pedley TA: Somatosensory evoked potentials following median nerve stimulation. 1. The cervical components. Brain, 107:169, 1984, with permission.)

Thoracolumbar spinal SEPs are even smaller than cervical spinal SEPs and can be difficult to elicit in obese subjects. Nevertheless, by using a knee or iliac crest reference, an SEP elicited by tibial nerve stimulation at the ankle can be recorded over the thoracolumbar spine and, like the cervical SEP, has several subcomponents. An initial traveling wave, N18, can be recorded over the lower lumbar spine and is akin to the cervical PPV evoked by median nerve stimulation; it indicates that the volley has passed through the sacral plexus. It can be seen in scalp-recorded far-field potentials as a small positivity designated P18. A second component, N22, is recorded with maximal amplitude over the lower thoracic spine (T10 to L1). It is a stationary peak and its latency remains constant even when the recording electrodes are moved several segments rostrally or caudally. It is probably akin to the median-evoked DCV and represents postsynaptic activity in the lumbar gray matter generated in response to input from axon collaterals. The third component is a negative traveling wave, N24, with a latency that shortens from the caudal to the rostral thoracic cord; it

is most evident over the lower thoracic cord, however, and reflects a propagated volley in the posterior columns that is equivalent to the DCV potential recorded over the neck with median nerve stimulation.

SEPs IN DISORDERS OF THE PERIPHERAL NERVOUS SYSTEM

The main clinical reason to record SEPs is to identify and localize a lesion involving the somatosensory pathways. The presence of an SEP abnormality, however, may provide no further information than could have been obtained by clinical examination, and normal findings do not exclude the possibility of organic disease as a cause of the symptoms. Furthermore, the presence of an SEP abnormality does not indicate the nature of the disease process. Nevertheless, the recording of SEPs may provide information of diagnostic relevance, may help characterize disease processes, and may determine the extent of pathologic involvement.

Disorders of the Peripheral Nerves

In general, SEPs have a definite role in the investigation of the peripheral nervous system when conventional techniques (see Chapter 13) cannot be used because the site of pathology is so proximal or because the nature of the lesion is such that responses cannot otherwise be recorded.

SEPs have been used to determine sensory conduction velocity in distal segments of a nerve and can provide results comparable to those obtained by peripheral nerve conduction studies if the stimulus is applied in turn to two or more sites along the course of the nerve. In several early studies, for example, scalp-recorded SEPs were found to be absent or delayed in patients with a variety of polyneuropathies and mononeuropathies. Such a sophisticated approach is unnecessary if similar information can be obtained by routine conduction studies, but it may be an important means of identifying extensive or localized lesions of peripheral nerves and of determining sensory conduction velocity when sensory nerve action potentials cannot be recorded peripherally by conventional techniques. In such circumstances, afferent conduction velocity, as determined by the SEPs, is slowed, usually in proportion to the degree of slowing in motor conduction velocity, but occasionally is within the normal range. The absence of peripheral responses presumably results from dispersal of impulse traffic by the underlying pathology, and the preservation of cortically generated SEPs probably reflects central amplification by a reorganization and synchronization of afferent volleys at different synaptic levels. Central amplification of a preserved but attenuated response derived from a few normally conducting axons is probably also responsible for the apparently normal afferent conduction velocity found occasionally. Accordingly, the very factor that permits afferent conduction velocity to be determined by the SEP technique when it otherwise cannot be measured sometimes may result in misleadingly normal values.

In patients in whom a diagnosis of a demyelinating sensorimotor polyneuropathy cannot be confirmed by conventional motor and sensory nerve conduction studies— either because they are normal or because distal sensory studies are normal but motor studies are abnormal— SEP studies may reveal proximal involvement of sensory nerves, thereby suggesting the correct diagnosis.[46,47] SEP studies may also be helpful in showing proximal sensory nerve dysfunction in patients with a pure sensory ataxia.[46] Such proximal involvement typically is not found in diabetic polyneuropathy and other length-dependent neuropathies.[47]

In Guillain–Barré syndrome, conduction is normal in distal segments of the nerves in up to 20 percent of patients at an early stage of the disorder. Conduction slowing in the proximal segments of peripheral nerves has been demonstrated with SEPs (e.g., by an increase in the interpeak interval between the responses recorded over Erb's point and the cervical spine or by the finding of a small dispersed cervical response) in a number of patients with Guillain–Barré syndrome. In general, however, the median-derived SEPs are less sensitive than F-waves for detecting proximal pathology in patients with this syndrome.[48] Accordingly, in patients with suspected Guillain–Barré syndrome, SEP studies probably are best reserved for occasions when peripheral nerve conduction and F-wave studies are normal.

The SEP findings have been used with those of other electrodiagnostic tests to support the belief that a continuity exists between Bickerstaff brainstem encephalitis and Miller Fisher syndrome. In one instance, for example, an absent median-derived N20 (despite normal peripheral function), together with a diffusely slowed electroencephalogram (EEG) and absent R2 of the blink reflex, suggested central involvement, whereas facial conduction studies and F-wave and H-reflex studies suggested peripheral pathology.[49]

Skin denervation often is associated with reduced thermal sensitivity, and this has led to studies of contact heat evoked potentials in patients with neuropathy. A specially designed, commercially available contact heat stimulator delivers recurrent heat stimuli at a specified temperature to the skin while the cerebral responses, mediated by A-delta or C fibers, are recorded over the scalp. In patients with pathologic evidence of skin denervation, the amplitude of the SEPs is reduced and correlates with the degree of denervation. Latencies are prolonged.[24] The technique thus provides a means of evaluating small-fiber function in patients with peripheral neuropathy. It also shows promise for distinguishing neuropathy from other chronic pain states, and sometimes shows abnormalities in symptomatic patients without significant loss of intraepidermal fibers or abnormality of quantitative sensory testing.[26]

Another approach to assessing small-fiber function is with pain-related SEPs elicited by painful electrical stimuli. A concentric planar electrode has been devised that delivers stimuli limited to the superficial layers of the dermis and that therefore depolarizes mainly superficial nociceptive A-delta fibers. In a study of HIV-associated sensory neuropathy, all 19 had abnormal pain-related SEPs, with the latency and amplitude of the responses correlating with the intraepidermal nerve-fiber density, whereas standard nerve conduction studies were abnormal in only 8 instances.[50]

Focal nerve lesions may be detected and evaluated by SEP studies. Thus, common entrapment syndromes (e.g., median nerve compression in the carpal tunnel[51]) have been diagnosed by this means, although such an approach is usually unnecessary. However, the technique may be used to monitor recovery in patients after complete section of a peripheral nerve because a response may be recorded from the scalp at a time when a potential cannot be recorded from the nerve itself. SEPs have been used to evaluate focal lesions involving the proximal segments of sensory nerves, which may not be accessible for conventional nerve conduction studies. Such an application complements the use of F waves to evaluate conduction through proximal motor fibers. The approach may be useful, for example, in documenting abnormalities in patients with such disorders as meralgia paresthetica.[52,53]

Finally, SEPs may be useful in the evaluation of patients with distal axonopathies (e.g., those related to toxin exposure) inasmuch as these conditions may involve the terminal portions of central as well as peripheral axons. Indeed, in patients with cisplatin neuropathy, CNS involvement—as evidenced by slowing of central conduction of the tibial-derived SEP—occurred with doses of cisplatin that caused peripheral nerve changes, suggesting that loss of large fibers in the posterior columns was secondary to degeneration of posterior root ganglion cells.[54] In the authors' experience, however, SEPs are always normal in patients with symptoms possibly related to occupational toxic exposure when peripheral nerve conduction studies are normal.

Plexus Lesions

In patients with injuries to the brachial plexus, the location of the lesion influences the outcome; root avulsion carries a poor prognosis, whereas a postganglionic lesion may require surgical treatment and may be followed by recovery. Conventional nerve conduction studies can help in determining the probable site of injury. Patients with preganglionic lesions have preserved sensory nerve action potentials despite clinical sensory loss. However, the recording of SEPs over the scalp and spine following the stimulation of arm nerves has been held to enhance the accuracy of electrophysiologic assessment because any attenuation of N13 relates to the total proportion of damaged fibers, whereas attenuation of N9 reflects the proportion damaged postganglionically. Unfortunately, such a theoretical approach has not been of practical use in a clinical context and has now been abandoned.

A preganglionic lesion may be partially or completely obscured electrophysiologically by coexisting postganglionic damage to the same fibers; this is a major limitation of electrophysiologic techniques for evaluating plexus lesions. In occasional patients, however, the findings are of help in localizing the lesion, as when peripheral sensory nerve action potentials are attenuated (but present) but SEPs are absent over the spine and scalp, a situation suggesting that multiple root avulsions have occurred in addition to more peripheral lesions. Nevertheless, in most instances, the information derived from SEP studies concerning the site and extent of plexus injury can be obtained more quickly and conveniently by needle electromyography (EMG).

The recording of SEPs may be useful in certain other contexts. The operative appearance of the brachial plexus may be misleading because nerve fascicles may appear intact even though anatomic disruption has occurred. In this regard, intraoperative stimulation of specific roots while responses are recorded from the contralateral portion of the scalp may help in establishing their functional continuity with the cord. More useful in this context is the epidural recording of evoked spinal cord potentials.[55] Intraoperative SEP recording can be especially helpful when ruptured nerves are to be treated by grafting. The presence of a cortical response to stimulation of the proximal stump makes a second, more rostral lesion unlikely, whereas the lack of a response usually is associated with a poor outcome.

Thoracic Outlet Syndrome

Characteristic electrophysiologic changes may occur in patients with cervical ribs or bands that are causing neurogenic thoracic outlet syndrome. Typical findings include a small or absent ulnar sensory nerve action potential; chronic partial denervation in the small muscles of the hand, especially in the muscles of the thenar eminence; and prolongation of the F-wave latencies from these muscles. In many patients with suspected thoracic outlet syndrome, however, clinical examination is normal, and needle EMG and nerve conduction studies reveal no abnormalities. The designation *non-neurogenic syndrome* is used in such circumstances.

In patients with suspected thoracic outlet syndrome, the ulnar-derived SEP is abnormal in many—but not necessarily all—patients with objective neurologic signs. It typically has a poorly formed potential at Erb's point, with or without abnormalities of the responses over the spine or scalp, such as an attenuated N13 response or a prolonged N9–N13 interpeak interval. Occasionally, needle EMG is abnormal but the SEP is normal, or vice versa. Thus, the recording of SEPs is of limited diagnostic importance in patients with the neurogenic variety of thoracic outlet syndrome.

In patients with the non-neurogenic syndrome, the SEPs elicited by median, ulnar, or superficial radial nerve stimulation are usually normal in the authors' experience and that of others.[56] Reports of abnormalities in this syndrome are usually difficult to interpret because of the nature of the claimed abnormalities or because the clinical and electrophysiologic findings were not provided in sufficient detail to allow for independent evaluation.

Cervical Spondylotic Radiculopathy or Myelopathy

Short-latency SEPs have been used to evaluate patients with cervical spondylosis, but the findings do not distinguish spondylosis from other cervical lesions. Most of the published studies concern SEPs elicited by stimulation of the median or ulnar nerve trunks. Patients with pain and paresthesias but without neurologic signs often have normal responses, whereas those with a more severe spondylotic radiculopathy causing objective neurologic signs may have abnormal SEPs, with delayed or lost components, regardless of whether a myelopathy is also present. Some authors emphasize that amplitude rather than latency of the responses reflects nerve lesions caused by spondylotic deformities. In general, however, the nature of the surface-recorded SEP abnormality does not help in indicating either the severity of the neurologic disorder or the long-term prognosis, and in some patients with a spondylotic myelopathy, the SEP findings may be entirely normal. Thus, the SEPs elicited by stimulation of nerve trunks in the arms are no better than careful clinical examination in determining the severity and prognosis of cervical spondylosis. They are of no help in the selection of patients for surgery, and such a decision should be made on clinical grounds.

It is possible that axons arising in the lumbosacral region are more likely to be affected by cervical compression than are fibers from the arms. Whether the recording of sural-derived SEPs in patients without clinical evidence of myelopathy will help in determining which patients with cervical spondylosis are at risk for the development of a cord deficit clinically is not known.

Lumbosacral Radiculopathy

It is hard to account for reports that fibular- or tibial-derived SEPs are abnormal in a high percentage of patients with lumbosacral radiculopathy because stimulation of a nerve derived from several segments would not be expected to lead to an SEP abnormality in patients with an isolated root lesion. Fibers traversing the unaffected roots would presumably generate a normal response, and this accords with the authors' experience.

Cutaneous nerves can be stimulated at selected sites so that segmental specificity is better than with stimulation of mixed nerve trunks. For example, the musculocutaneous nerve can be stimulated in the forearm for testing C5, median nerve fibers in the thumb to test C6, median nerve fibers along the adjoining surfaces of the second and third fingers for C7, and the ulnar nerve in the little finger to test C8. For evaluating lumbosacral roots, the saphenous nerve can be stimulated at the knee and ankle for L3 and L4, respectively; the superficial fibular (peroneal) nerve at the ankle to test L5; and the sural nerve at the ankle for S1. In our experience, however, only about 50 to 60 percent of patients with lumbosacral radiculopathies confirmed by imaging studies have abnormal scalp-recorded SEPs derived from such stimulation. Abnormalities usually involve parameters that vary considerably in normal subjects or that are hard to quantify (e.g., amplitude reduction and abnormal morphology), thereby limiting the clinical relevance of the technique; prolongation in latency is found only occasionally. Although some have claimed a higher yield for the technique in detecting radicular involvement, the sensitivity and specificity are insufficient to make it clinically useful.[57,58]

SEPs have been recorded in response to dermatomal stimulation in the L5 or S1 territory. The typical response recorded at the vertex (referenced to the midfrontal region or the contralateral C3'/C4' position) consists of a positive–negative-positive complex, the initial positivity having a latency of about 50 msec (Fig. 26-5). Early reports claimed a high yield of abnormalities in patients with surgically verified L5 or S1 root entrapment from a herniated disc, but it is unclear how criteria of abnormality were selected. In our experience, dermatomal SEPs enable an isolated radicular lesion to be localized correctly in only about 25 percent of patients. A latency abnormality is relatively uncommon, the usual finding being loss or marked attenuation of the response (see Fig. 26-5). In general, needle EMG is the single most useful electrophysiologic approach for evaluating root lesions, but dermatomal SEPs sometimes provided complementary information by revealing unsuspected root dysfunction.[58] Dumitru and Dreyfuss similarly found the utility of dermatomal SEPs was limited in patients with suspected unilateral L5 or S1 root lesions because they do not have both high specificity and high sensitivity.[57]

There are several reasons that dermatomal or cutaneous nerve stimulation does not lead to a higher yield of abnormal SEPs in patients with isolated root lesions. First, the cutaneous nerves are not entirely specific segmentally, and there is overlap in dermatomal territories. Second, conduction slowing in the small segment that is compressed will be masked by the normal conduction that occurs in the greater part of the pathway under study. This masking effect will be reduced if the responses recorded over the spine rather than scalp are utilized to determine normality or abnormality. Third, even if conduction block occurs in some fibers, it will be masked by the preserved conduction in others and will not be recognized because of the marked interside variation in amplitude that occurs in normal subjects.

A new approach to the electrophysiologic diagnosis of radiculopathy has been with dermatomal LEPs,[59] but the data are insufficient to reach any conclusions at the present time.

In patients with polyradiculopathies such as occur in lumbar spinal stenosis, some authors have suggested that dermatomal SEP studies may be of value in defining the extent of root involvement,[60,61] but detailed studies are required to establish this.

SEPs IN DISORDERS OF THE CENTRAL NERVOUS SYSTEM

SEP findings may help in the detection and localization of lesions of the central somatosensory pathways but are never pathognomonic of specific diseases. The role of SEPs in clinical evaluation of the CNS is best discussed under several different headings.

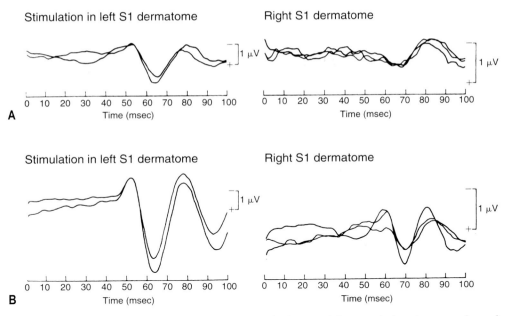

FIGURE 26-5 ▪ Dermatomal somatosensory evoked potentials recorded at the contralateral C3' or C4' electrodes, with reference to Cz, on stimulation in the S1 dermatome on either side in two patients. (The C3' and C4' locations are 2 cm behind the C3 and C4 placements in the international 10–20 system.) Two or three trials, each the average of 512 responses, have been superimposed. An upward deflection indicates relative negativity at C3' or C4' (or positivity at Cz). The responses to stimulation of the left S1 dermatome are normal. **A**, Loss of the first upward deflection of the response to right-sided stimulation. **B**, Prolonged response latency to stimulation in the right S1 dermatome. These findings are suggestive of a right S1 radiculopathy in each case, but the former is encountered more commonly than the latter. (Modified from Aminoff MJ, Goodin DS, Barbaro NM et al: Dermatomal somatosensory evoked potentials in unilateral lumbosacral radiculopathy. Ann Neurol, 17:171, 1985, with permission.)

Detection of Lesions in Somatosensory Pathways

MULTIPLE SCLEROSIS

SEP and other evoked potential studies were often performed in the past to evaluate patients with suspected multiple sclerosis (MS) but their role in this context has been supplanted largely by neuroimaging studies. Nevertheless, their utility in MS still merits some comment. The presence of SEP abnormalities may reveal subclinical lesions involving the central somatosensory pathways and thus may help establish that multiple lesions are present in patients with clinical evidence of only one lesion that spares these pathways. Furthermore, an SEP abnormality may indicate that vague sensory complaints have an organic basis when this is otherwise uncertain because the findings on clinical sensory examination are equivocal.

The likelihood of finding an SEP abnormality is greater in patients in whom the diagnosis of MS is definite than in patients in whom it is only a possibility; in other words, it increases as diagnostic certainty increases. Abnormalities

are not always found, even among patients with definite MS, in whom the incidence of abnormalities is about 80 percent, regardless of whether any clinical sensory disturbance is present. However, it is in the nosologic category of possible MS that ancillary studies are needed to help establish the diagnosis, and the incidence of subclinical SEP abnormalities is then only about 25 to 35 percent. The highest yield is from SEPs elicited by stimulation of a nerve in the legs rather than a nerve in the arms.

The likelihood of finding an SEP abnormality increases if a clinical sensory disturbance is present in the stimulated limb; in such circumstances, SEPs provide little further information than could have been obtained by physical examination. SEP abnormalities are even more common if pyramidal signs are present in the stimulated limb or in the legs, presumably because of the close anatomic relationship of the corticospinal and ascending sensory pathways in the spinal cord. Thus, in patients with a pyramidal deficit, an SEP abnormality does not necessarily indicate the presence of a separate pathologic lesion but merely may reflect an extensive lesion affecting both motor and sensory pathways.

The relative usefulness of the different evoked potential techniques in detecting subclinical involvement of different afferent systems in patients with suspected MS has been examined. The highest diagnostic yield is with SEPs, whereas brainstem auditory evoked potentials (BAEPs) are the least useful. Whether such differences relate to the length and extent of the tracts being tested or to differential susceptibility to pathologic involvement is unclear.

Abnormalities may take several forms, including delay or absence of components of the response or an altered morphology (Figs. 26-6 and 26-7). A commonly encountered abnormality in the response to median nerve stimulation consists of loss, attenuation, or increased

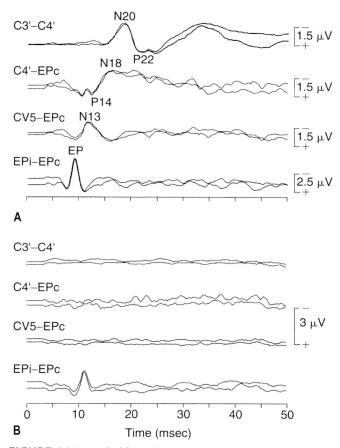

FIGURE 26-6 ■ **A**, Normal somatosensory evoked potential (SEP) elicited by stimulation of the right median nerve at the wrist. Responses were recorded over the brachial plexus at ipsilateral Erb's point (EPi), over the fifth cervical spine (CV5), and over the ipsilateral scalp (C4′) with contralateral Erb's point (EPc) used as a reference, as well as over the contralateral scalp (C3′) referenced to the ipsilateral scalp (C4′). An N9 potential is seen over Erb's point, an N13 over the cervical spine, subcortical far-field P14 and N18 potentials over the ipsilateral scalp area, and an N20 over the contralateral "hand" area (C3′) of the scalp. **B**, Abnormal SEP to right median nerve stimulation in a patient with definite multiple sclerosis. A normal response was recorded at Erb's point, but no clear response is seen over the neck or scalp.

dispersion of the cervical (N13) component with preservation of the cortically generated components. Central conduction time can be calculated from the interpeak latency of various components of the SEP if it is assumed that only a single afferent projection system is involved in the generation of these components. There may be a significant side-to-side difference in conduction time in patients with MS, sometimes as the sole abnormality.

Because so much of the literature has emphasized the role of evoked potential techniques in the evaluation of patients with suspected MS, it sometimes is assumed that multimodality evoked potential abnormalities or subclinical SEP abnormalities are diagnostic. Such is not the case. Multimodality abnormalities may also be found, for example, in patients infected with human immunodeficiency virus (HIV) and in other disorders such as vitamin B_{12} and vitamin E deficiency states[62] and the hereditary spinocerebellar degenerations.[63] SEP abnormalities may also be found in some varieties of hereditary spastic paraplegia.[64,65] The electrophysiologic findings are therefore not diagnostic in themselves and must be interpreted in the clinical context in which they are obtained.

Some clinicians have suggested that evoked potential techniques may be useful for monitoring disease progression and evaluating experimental therapeutic agents for MS. However, there is sometimes a marked disparity between the clinical and electrophysiologic changes, as well as excessive variability between test sessions of the response to stimulation of a clinically involved afferent pathway, even when the clinical deficit is stable. Changes in previously abnormal evoked potentials do not necessarily reflect the site of new lesions, and electrophysiologic changes accompanying clinical exacerbations sometimes occur in pathways not affected clinically by the relapse.

Various new techniques have been utilized to enhance the yield of SEPs in patients with suspected multiple sclerosis, including the recording of LEPs to evaluate function of the spinothalamic tracts[66] and of the high-frequency (600-Hz) oscillations superimposed on the N20 component of the median-derived SEP, which are generated in the thalamocortical projection neurons and at the primary somatosensory cortex.[67] Such approaches may provide further insight into the pathophysiology of MS and the cause of neurologic deficits, but are of little diagnostic utility.

In summary, SEPs may provide information of diagnostic relevance in patients with MS by helping to establish the presence of multiple lesions when they are not evident clinically. Such a multiplicity of lesions does not in itself establish the diagnosis, however, and must be integrated with other clinical and laboratory findings

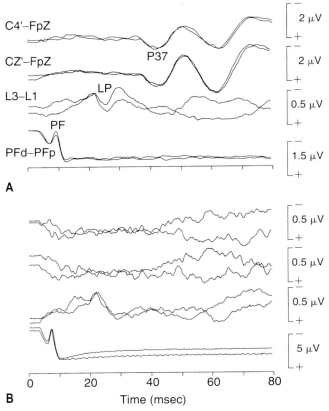

FIGURE 26-7 ▪ **A**, Normal response recorded over the popliteal fossa, the scalp, and the spine with stimulation of the right tibial nerve at the ankle. A well-marked potential is recorded over the nerve at the popliteal fossa between the distal and the proximal electrodes (PFd and PFp), and a lumbar potential (LP) is recorded between the third and the first lumbar vertebrae (L3–L1). A positivity is seen at Cz′ and the contralateral scalp area (C4′) with reference to Fpz. **B**, Somatosensory evoked potential to right tibial nerve stimulation in a patient with definite multiple sclerosis. An initial potential is recorded over the nerve in the popliteal fossa and over the lumbar spine, but no response can be identified over the scalp.

because disseminated lesions may occur in other neurologic disorders. SEPs have a limited role in monitoring the course of MS or in evaluating its response to treatment. The SEP findings may also help to predict which patients presenting with a first-episode acute myelitis are likely to go on and develop MS.[68]

OTHER NEUROLOGIC DISORDERS

SEPs may be abnormal in disorders of the CNS other than MS, depending on the site of pathologic involvement. In patients with impaired pain and temperature appreciation but no other sensory loss, SEPs elicited by stimulation of nerve trunks in the affected limbs are similar to those obtained from clinically uninvolved limbs and are normal.

Spinal Cord Dysfunction

Patients with spinal cord tumors (Fig. 26-8) or *vascular malformations*[69] may have abnormal SEPs when the lesion involves the afferent pathways being stimulated. Serial SEP studies have been used to detect retethering of the spinal cord in patients who have undergone repair of spinal dysraphic lesions. The SEP findings, however, do not necessarily correlate with clinical status and are of little utility.[70]

An upper cervical myelopathy caused by a small foramen magnum may occur in *achondroplasia*. SEPs—in particular, analysis of their subcortical components—are useful in the detection of early or subclinical cervical myelopathy and allow early neurosurgical decompression to prevent permanent damage.[71] Compressive myelopathy at the craniocervical junction may also complicate *mucopolysaccharidoses*, and SEPs have been used to detect such involvement, sometimes at a subclinical stage.[72]

In *Friedreich ataxia*, the median-derived SEP commonly shows marked attenuation of the Erb's point potential, with little, if any, delay in this or the major cervical component. The cortical response may be normal but is often dispersed, broadened, or delayed, which suggests that central conduction is slowed.

Patients with *hereditary spastic paraplegia* or *hereditary cerebellar ataxia* may also have abnormal SEPs, with loss of spinal or cortical components or marked cortical delay.[63-65] The SEP may be abnormal when there is no clinical sensory loss. These patients, as well as those with Friedreich ataxia, may also have abnormality of the evoked potentials elicited by visual or auditory stimulation. Patients with *olivopontocerebellar atrophy* may have normal SEPs or attenuated or absent responses.[73]

SEPs may be abnormal in patients who are *HIV seropositive*, with a prolonged central conduction time suggesting pathology involving the posterior columns of the spinal cord. In one study, for example, median- and tibial-derived SEPs were recorded in 15 HIV-seropositive patients without acquired immunodeficiency syndrome (AIDS) and in 23 patients with AIDS. The AIDS patients had delayed latencies of the cortical responses to tibial nerve stimulation that were attributed to slowed spinal conduction. In the non-AIDS patients, spinal latency and conduction time from the gluteal crest to T12 generally increased over a 2-year period.[74] Others have reported that SEPs are helpful in aiding the diagnosis of AIDS-associated myelopathy, especially when a

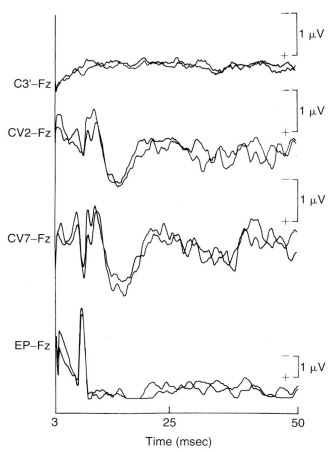

FIGURE 26-8 ■ Somatosensory evoked potential following stimulation of the right median nerve at the wrist in a 15-year-old boy with a structural lesion at the level of the foramen magnum. There is a reproducible Erb's point potential, and responses can also be recorded over the cervical spine, but no response can be elicited over the scalp. (From Aminoff MJ: The use of somatosensory evoked potentials in the evaluation of the central nervous system. Neurol Clin, 6:809, 1988, with permission.)

peripheral neuropathy coexists; abnormalities of tibial central conduction time correlated with the clinical diagnosis of myelopathy, and analysis of peripheral and central latencies permitted neuropathy and myelopathy to be distinguished in individual cases.[75] Whether SEP studies will have a useful role in predicting which patients with HIV infection are likely to develop a clinical myelopathy, or whether they will provide information of prognostic relevance is unknown.

The recording of lower limb SEPs may be useful in the evaluation of patients with *human T-cell lymphotropic virus type I–associated myelopathy* (tropical spastic paraparesis). Subclinical lesions of afferent pathways may be detected, and central sensory conduction time correlates with disability.[76]

Brainstem Lesions

SEPs are normal in patients with Wallenberg syndrome but are usually abnormal when lesions involve the medial lemniscus. Thus, they may be abnormal in patients with *"locked-in" syndrome* because of pontine infarction, although the findings vary considerably in different patients and are therefore of little clinical utility.[77]

Thalamic Lesions

The SEP findings in patients with thalamic infarcts or neoplasms depend on the extent of these lesions. Generally, they parallel the clinical findings (i.e., they are abnormal when significant clinical deficits are present), although such is not always the case. Laterally placed lesions tend to affect the tibial SEP, and more mesially situated lesions tend to affect the median SEP. This tendency agrees with clinical observations that lateral lesions generally cause more severe involvement of the lower extremity than of the upper, whereas the opposite is true for mesial lesions. With subcortical infarcts, the short-latency SEP is relatively preserved in comparison to the midlatency and long-latency components. With regard to tumors involving the thalamus, the SEP sometimes is relatively preserved with slowly growing noninfiltrating extrinsic tumors, whereas extrinsic mass lesions compressing the thalamus acutely influence the SEPs more markedly, sometimes leading to loss of both median- and tibial-derived SEPs. Patients with intrinsic thalamic tumors and a clinical sensory deficit usually have very abnormal SEPs.

Hemispheric Lesions

In patients with sensory loss from parietal lesions caused by vascular pathology, SEPs to median nerve stimulation are often abolished over the affected hemisphere. SEPs are typically normal in patients with no sensory deficit and virtually abolished in patients with moderate or severe cortical sensory loss. In a few patients, however, a discrepancy exists between the clinical and SEP findings, the SEPs being normal despite cortical sensory deficits, or being absent despite preserved sensation.

In patients with a single circumscribed hemispheric lesion involving the parietal lobe, abnormalities of some but not other SEP components have been described, but these are of academic rather than of clinical or diagnostic relevance in this era of advanced imaging techniques and merit no discussion here.

Although it has been suggested that the SEP findings may be of prognostic relevance in the evaluation of patients who have had a stroke,[78] neither SEPs nor motor evoked potentials are widely used for this purpose and seem little better than a detailed neurologic examination in predicting outcome.

Prognostic Guide

COMA AND BRAIN DEATH

There seems little doubt that median-derived SEPs provide useful prognostic information in comatose patients. Among patients with bilateral loss of the N20–P22 response, the likely outcome is death or a persistently vegetative state, with no meaningful recovery of cognition. With unilateral loss of the N20–P22 response, a functional level is regained in some instances but a major residual neurologic deficit is likely. Many but not all patients with bilaterally preserved N20–P22 responses have a good outcome and regain useful function. The value of recording SEPs in comatose patients with suspected brain death also seems clear. In response to median nerve stimulation, N13–N14 components may be recorded over the neck, indicating that the stimulus-generated signal reached the cord-medulla, but later components should not be present.[79]

In a review of 44 published studies regarding the use of SEPs to predict outcome after severe brain injury, Carter and Butt found positive likelihood ratio, positive predictive value, and sensitivity were 4.04, 71.2 percent, and 59 percent, respectively, for normal SEPs predicting a favorable outcome; and 11.41, 98.5 percent, and 46.2 percent, respectively, for bilaterally absent SEPs predicting an unfavorable outcome (i.e., severe disability, vegetative state, or death).[80] Of 777 patients, only 12 with bilaterally absent responses had favorable outcomes. This false-positive rate declined to less than 0.5 percent for bilaterally absent SEPs when patients with focal lesions, subdural or extradural fluid collections, and decompressive craniotomy in the preceding 48 hours were excluded. Early recovery after injury can be detected by SEPs, despite sedative medication.[81] Initial SEPs relate to outcome, but the findings may change so that normal responses become abnormal, or vice versa. Thus, the SEP findings recorded at any one time may not be sufficiently reliable to provide a satisfactory prognostic guide in individual cases. The recording of both SEPs and cognitive event-related potentials may increase utility further.[82]

SEPs have also been used to evaluate patients in anoxic-ischemic coma. The prognosis can often be determined by careful clinical examination, but the SEP findings may be important in supplementing the clinical findings.[83] In a study of 60 patients who were comatose following cardiac arrest, a bad outcome was best predicted by combining the clinical findings with the SEP results. Thus, a Glasgow coma score of less than 8 on clinical examination at 48 hours, combined with loss or abnormality of the early cortical components of the median SEP, is highly predictive of a bad outcome.[84] Some clinical features may be modified by induced hypothermia, making the SEP and EEG findings especially important in this context.[83]

A systematic review of the literature, published in 1998, found that bilateral absence of early cortical SEPs within the first week was highly specific (100 percent) for a poor outcome (i.e., death or persistent vegetative state) in patients in anoxic-ischemic coma. Because SEPs are less susceptible to metabolic changes and drugs than is the clinical state or the EEG, the authors concluded that they were the most useful method for predicting poor outcome.[85] Indeed, their absence for more than 72 hours signals a poor prognosis, regardless of whether patients are sedated or made hypothermic.[86] A more recent meta-analysis confirms the value of SEPs in predicting outcome of hypoxic coma, especially within the first 24 hours, when it is superior to clinical markers such as the absence of a motor response.[87] A study by Robinson and colleagues found that adults in coma from hypoxic-ischemic encephalopathy who had absent SEPs had less than a 1 percent chance of recovering consciousness.[88] However, rare cases have been reported in which recovery of consciousness and cognitive function occurred despite bilaterally absent N20 responses after cardiac arrest treated by hypothermia.[89] Further comment on brain death is made in Chapter 35.

SPINAL INJURIES

Numerous studies have documented the SEP changes that occur with spinal injury. Responses to stimulation of a nerve below the level of the lesion may be normal, delayed, attenuated, or lost. The changes depend in part on the severity of the cord lesion and on when the examination is performed in relation to the injury.

When it first became possible to record SEPs in a clinical context, it was hoped that the presence or absence of a response over the scalp to stimulation of a nerve below the level of the lesion would provide a reliable guide to the completeness of cord injuries. Unfortunately, however, it is often not possible to record any cortical response during the acute stage in patients with clinically incomplete traumatic cord lesions. Thus, the technique, as used at present, may not permit early recognition of the totality of the lesion reliably, although preserved responses or their early return after injury indicates an incomplete lesion and therefore implies a good prognosis.

Again, intraoperative or postoperative improvement in SEPs following surgical decompression in patients with cord injuries may be followed by clinical improvement. Certainly, the normalization of a previously abnormal or absent response may precede clinical change in such circumstances and implies a better prognosis than otherwise.

Although it has been suggested that serial studies may be helpful for monitoring progess after spinal surgery, it is not clear whether this confers any practical advantage over clinical examination. Unless it does, there seems to be little need to apply complex technology to monitoring change in clinical or functional status, especially in patients for whom no further therapeutic maneuvers can be offered.

SEPs have been used intraoperatively to monitor cord function. Intraoperative recording of SEPs has been used most often to monitor patients undergoing corrective surgery for scoliosis in the hope of detecting evidence of any cord damage at an early stage, when it might be reversible. Numerous studies have been published in this regard, but the low surgical morbidity had made it difficult to determine whether the monitoring procedure actually reduced the incidence of major neurologic complications. The study by Nuwer and co-workers, however, does suggest that monitoring is important in this regard.[90] Postoperative clinical deficits may occur despite preservation of the SEPs during intraoperative monitoring. Such false-negative results may occur for several reasons. First, the operative procedure may lead to a lesion that does not involve the somatosensory pathways being monitored. Second, if the pathways being monitored are already abnormal and a pre-existing electrophysiologic and neurologic deficit is present, further use of SEPs to monitor the affected pathway may not be possible. Third, perioperative complications may develop after discontinuation of the monitoring procedure. Fourth, interpretation of the SEPs may be confounded by technical factors or by the effect of hypotension or general anesthetics on the response. Further discussion of this aspect is provided in Chapter 30, but the stimulation of motor pathways in conjunction with the recording of SEPs may enhance the value of electrophysiologic monitoring of cord function intraoperatively.

Other Applications

SEP abnormalities have been described in a number of other disorders, but the findings are more of academic interest than of practical clinical relevance. They have been noted, for example, following upper- or lower-limb stimulation in patients with *amyotrophic lateral sclerosis*,[91,92]

as might have been expected from previous clinical and pathologic reports of sensory involvement. Abnormalities may involve not only the N20 peak of the median SEP but also certain longer-latency components. Laser-evoked SEPs have been studied because of the pain experienced by some patients with amyotrophic lateral sclerosis. The latencies and amplitudes of certain components were increased but no correlation was found between the electrophysiologic changes, pain intensity and clinical features.[93] Patients with *bulbospinal neuronopathy* may have abnormal SEPs elicited from the arms and legs[94]; those with juvenile *focal spinal muscular atrophy* of the upper limb (Hirayamo syndrome) may have abnormal upper-limb SEPs, with attenuated Erb's point and N13 responses but normal N20 responses and peak latencies.[95]

Median-derived SEPs may be abnormal in *dystrophia myotonica*, the findings suggesting peripheral or central conduction delays, or both, but there is no apparent relationship between the individual SEP findings and severity of the clinical disorder.[96] Evidence of altered cortical excitability has been observed when SEPs are elicited by paired stimuli of the median nerve,[97] but this is more of theoretical interest than practical relevance.

In *Wilson disease*, multimodality evoked potential studies may be abnormal, with subclinical dysfunction occurring in the major sensory pathways in accord with the neuropathologic and neuroradiologic evidence of widespread degeneration of the brain. In *Huntington disease*, central somatosensory conduction time is normal, but the amplitude of the early cortical components may be reduced with little or no change in latency; this may correlate with the CAG trinucleotide repeat length.[98] SEP attenuation may also parallel the course of the disease.[99] Such findings are of no clinical relevance at the present time.

In patients with congenital indifference to pain and no clinical evidence of any other disorder of the nervous system, SEPs are normal. Some patients with sensory symptoms have no consistent objective clinical signs, and the possibility is raised that the symptoms do not have an organic basis. In this context, an abnormal SEP implies an organic cause of the symptoms. Normal SEPs and peripheral sensory nerve conduction studies support any clinical suspicions that the symptoms are not organic in origin but do not in themselves establish this point with certainty. Indeed, SEPs may be normal in patients with pure sensory stroke caused by, for example, lacunar infarcts.

In patients with intractable neuropathic pain, spinal cord stimulation is sometimes therapeutically helpful, and the results of a recent study suggest that preoperative

SEPs may have a role in predicting outcome and thus in selecting patients for treatment by this means. In particular, a significantly abnormal central conduction time was associated with a lack of therapeutic response, whereas 75 percent of those with normal preoperative SEPs responded well.[100] Clearly, such an approach merits further appraisal.

REFERENCES

1. Amantini A, Amadori A, Fossi S: Evoked potentials in the ICU. Eur J Anaesthesiol Suppl, 42:196, 2008

2. Cruccu G, Aminoff MJ, Curio G et al: Recommendations for the clinical use of somatosensory-evoked potentials. Clin Neurophysiol, 119:1705, 2008

3. Spiegel J, Hansen C, Baumgartner U et al: Sensitivity of laser-evoked potentials versus somatosensory evoked potentials in patients with multiple sclerosis. Clin Neurophysiol, 114:992, 2003

4. Ohara S, Crone NE, Weiss N et al: Cutaneous painful laser stimuli evoke responses recorded directly from primary somatosensory cortex in awake humans. J Neurophysiol, 91:2734, 2004

5. Arendt-Nielsen L, Chen AC: Lasers and other thermal stimulators for activation of skin nociceptors in humans. Neurophysiol Clin, 33:259, 2003

6. Sonoo M: Anatomic origin and clinical application of the widespread N18 potential in median nerve somatosensory evoked potentials. J Clin Neurophysiol, 17:258, 2000

7. Aminoff MJ, Eisen AA: AAEM minimonograph 19: Somatosensory evoked potentials. Muscle Nerve, 21:277, 1998

8. Yamada T, Matsubara M, Shiraishi G et al: Topographic analyses of somatosensory evoked potentials following stimulation of tibial, sural and lateral femoral cutaneous nerves. Electroencephalogr Clin Neurophysiol, 100:33, 1996

9. Durak K, Chen AC, Arendt-Nielsen L: 3D topographic study of the diode laser evoked potentials (LEPs) to painful stimulation of the trigeminal sensory area. Brain Topogr, 16:133, 2004

10. Valeriani M, Restuccia D, Barba C et al: Central scalp projection of the N30 SEP source activity after median nerve stimulation. Muscle Nerve, 23:353, 2000

11. Hamada M, Hanajima R, Terao Y et al: Median nerve somatosensory evoked potentials and their high-frequency oscillations in amyotrophic lateral sclerosis. Clin Neurophysiol, 118:877, 2007

12. Nuwer MR, Aminoff M, Desmedt J et al: IFCN recommended standards for short latency somatosensory evoked potentials. Report of an IFCN committee. Electroencephalogr Clin Neurophysiol, 91:6, 1994

13. Seror P: Lateral femoral cutaneous nerve conduction v somatosensory evoked potentials for electrodiagnosis of meralgia paresthetica. Am J Phys Med Rehabil, 78:313, 1999

14. Rabie M, Drory VE: A test for the evaluation of the lateral cutaneous branch of the iliohypogastric nerve using somatosensory evoked potentials. J Neurol Sci, 238:59, 2005

15. Spiegel J, Hansen C, Treede RD: Laser-evoked potentials after painful hand and foot stimulation in humans: evidence for generation of the middle-latency component in the secondary somatosensory cortex. Neurosci Lett, 216:179, 1996

16. Lam YW, Sherman SM: Functional organization of the somatosensory cortical layer 6 feedback to the thalamus. Cereb Cortex, 20:13, 2010

17. Valeriani M, Truini A, Le Pera D et al: Laser evoked potential recording from intracerebral deep electrodes. Clin Neurophysiol, 120:790, 2009

18. Cruccu G, Iannetti GD, Agostino R et al: Conduction velocity of the human spinothalamic tract as assessed by laser evoked potentials. Neuroreport, 11:3029, 2000

19. Rossi P, Serrao M, Amabile G et al: A simple method for estimating conduction velocity of the spinothalamic tract in healthy humans. Clin Neurophysiol, 111:1907, 2000

20. Qiu Y, Innui K, Wang X et al: Conduction velocity of the spinothalamic tract in humans as assessed by CO_2 laser stimulation of C-fibers. Neurosci Lett, 311:181, 2001

21. Rage M, Van Acker N, Facer P et al: The time course of CO_2 laser-evoked responses and of skin nerve fibre markers after topical capsaicin in human volunteers. Clin Neurophysiol, 121:1256, 2010

22. Quante M, Hauck M, Gromoll M et al: Dermatomal laser-evoked potentials: a diagnostic approach to the dorsal root. Norm data in healthy volunteers and changes in patients with radiculopathy. Eur Spine J, 16:943, 2007

23. Wang X, Inui K, Qiu Y et al: Effects of sleep on pain-related somatosensory evoked potentials in humans. Neurosci Res, 45:53, 2003

24. Chao CC, Hsieh SC, Tseng MT et al: Patterns of contact heat evoked potentials (CHEP) in neuropathy with skin denervation: correlation of CHEP amplitude with intraepidermal nerve fiber density. Clin Neurophysiol, 119:653, 2008

25. Iannetti GD, Zambreanu L, Tracey I: Similar nociceptive afferents mediate psychophysical and electrophysiological responses to heat stimulation of glabrous and hairy skin in humans. J Physiol, 577:235, 2006

26. Atherton DD, Facer P, Roberts KM et al: Use of the novel Contact Heat Evoked Potential Stimulator (CHEPS) for the assessment of small fibre neuropathy: correlations with skin flare responses and intra-epidermal nerve fibre counts. BMC Neurol, 7:21, 2007

27. Miura T, Sonoo M, Shimizu T: Establishment of standard values for the latency, interval and amplitude parameters of tibial nerve somatosensory evoked potentials (SEPs). Clin Neurophysiol, 114:1367, 2003

28. Gobbele R, Waberski TD, Thyerlei D et al: Functional dissociation of a subcortical and cortical component of high-frequency oscillations in human somatosensory evoked potentials by motor interference. Neurosci Lett, 350:97, 2003

29. Urasaki E, Genmoto T, Akamatsu N et al: The effects of stimulus rates on high frequency oscillations of median nerve somatosensory-evoked potentials: direct recording study from the human cerebral cortex. Clin Neurophysiol, 113:1794, 2002

30. Jung P, Baumgartner U, Bauermann T et al: Asymmetry in the human primary somatosensory cortex and handedness. Neuroimage, 19:913, 2003

31. Bulut S, Ozmerdivenli R, Bayer H: Effects of exercise on somatosensory-evoked potentials. Int J Neurosci, 113:315, 2003

32. Valeriani M, Ranghi F, Giaquinto S: The effects of aging on selective attention to touch: a reduced inhibitory control in elderly subjects? Int J Psychophysiol, 49:75, 2003

33. Miura T, Sonoo M, Shimizu T: Establishment of standard values for the latency, interval and amplitude parameters of tibial nerve somatosensory evoked potentials (SEPs). Clin Neurophysiol, 114:1367, 2003

34. Insola A, Le Pera D, Restuccia D et al: Reduction in amplitude of the subcortical low- and high-frequency somatosensory evoked potentials during voluntary movement: an intracerebral recording study. Clin Neurophysiol, 115:104, 2004

35. Kanovsky P, Bares M, Rektor I: The selective gating of the N30 cortical component of the somatosensory evoked potentials of median nerve is different in the mesial and dorsolateral frontal cortex: evidence from intracerebral recordings. Clin Neurophysiol, 114:981, 2003

36. Klostermann F, Gobbele R, Buchner H et al: Differential gating of slow postsynaptic and high-frequency spike-like components in human somatosensory evoked potentials under isometric motor interference. Brain Res, 922:95, 2001

37. Murphy BA, Taylor HH, Wilson SA et al: Rapid reversible changes to multiple levels of the human somatosensory system following the cessation of repetitive contractions: a somatosensory evoked potential study. Clin Neurophysiol, 114:1531, 2003

38. Valeriani M, Restuccia D, Di Lazzaro V et al: The pathophysiology of giant SEPs in cortical myoclonus: a scalp topography and dipolar source modelling study. Electroencephalogr Clin Neurophysiol, 104:122, 1997

39. Sonoo M: Generators of subcortical components of SEPs and their clinical applications. Suppl Clin Neurophysiol, 59:113, 2006

40. Mauguière F, Allison T, Babiloni C et al: Somatosensory evoked potentials. Electroencephalogr Clin Neurophysiol Suppl, 52:79, 1999

41. Valeriani M, Restuccia D, Di Lazzaro V et al: Dipolar generators of the early scalp somatosensory evoked potentials to tibial nerve stimulation in human subjects. Neurosci Lett, 238:49, 1997

42. Sonoo M, Kobayashi M, Genba-Shimizu K et al: Detailed analysis of the latencies of median nerve SEP components: 1. Selection of the best standard parameters and the establishment of the normal value. Electroencephalogr Clin Neurophysiol, 100:319, 1996

43. Sonoo M, Genba-Shimizu K, Mannen T et al: Detailed analysis of the latencies of median nerve somatosensory evoked potential components: 2. Analysis of subcomponents of the P13/14 and N20 potentials. Electroencephalogr Clin Neurophysiol, 104:296, 1997

44. Zumsteg D, Wieser HG: Effects of aging and sex on middle-latency somatosensory evoked potentials: normative data. Clin Neurophysiol, 113:681, 2002

45. Hoshiyama M, Kakigi R: New concept for the recovery function of short-latency somatosensory evoked cortical potentials following median nerve stimulation. Clin Neurophysiol, 113:535, 2002

46. Yiannikas C, Vucic S: Utility of somatosensory evoked potentials in chronic acquired demyelinating neuropathy. Muscle Nerve, 38:1447, 2008

47. Tsukamoto H, Sonoo M, Shimizu T: Segmental evaluation of the peripheral nerve using tibial nerve SEPs for the diagnosis of CIDP. Clin Neurophysiol, 121:77, 2010

48. Olney RK, Aminoff MJ: Electrodiagnostic features of the Guillain–Barré syndrome: the relative sensitivity of different techniques. Neurology, 40:471, 1990

49. Ogawara K, Kuwabara S, Yuki N: Fisher syndrome or Bickerstaff brainstem encephalitis? Anti-GQ1b IgG antibody syndrome involving both the peripheral and central nervous systems. Muscle Nerve, 26:845, 2002

50. Obermann M, Katsarava Z, Esser S et al: Correlation of epidermal nerve fiber density with pain-related evoked potentials in HIV neuropathy. Pain, 138:79, 2008

51. Ilkhani M, Jahanbakhsh SM, Eghtesadi-Araghi P et al: Accuracy of somatosensory evoked potentials in diagnosis of mild idiopathic carpal tunnel syndrome. Clin Neurol Neurosurg, 108:40, 2005

52. Seror P: Somatosensory evoked potentials for the electrodiagnosis of meralgia paresthetica. Muscle Nerve, 29:309, 2004

53. Cordato DJ, Yiannikas C, Stroud J et al: Evoked potentials elicited by stimulation of the lateral and anterior femoral cutaneous nerves in meralgia paresthetica. Muscle Nerve, 29:139, 2004

54. Krarup-Hansen A, Helweg-Larsen S, Schmalbruch H et al: Neuronal involvement in cisplatin neuropathy: prospective clinical and neurophysiological studies. Brain, 130:1076, 2007

55. Murase T, Kawai H, Masatomi T et al: Evoked spinal cord potentials for diagnosis during brachial plexus surgery. J Bone Joint Surg Br, 75:775, 1993

56. Komanetsky RM, Novak CB, Mackinnon SE et al: Somatosensory evoked potentials fail to diagnose thoracic outlet syndrome. J Hand Surg (Am), 21:662, 1996

57. Dumitru D, Dreyfuss P: Dermatomal/segmental somatosensory evoked potential evaluation of L5/S1 unilateral/unilevel radiculopathies. Muscle Nerve, 19:442, 1996

58. Lomen-Hoerth C, Aminoff MJ: Clinical neurophysiologic studies: which test is useful and when? Neurol Clin, 17:65, 1999

59. Quante M, Lorenz J, Hauck M: Laser-evoked potentials: prognostic relevance of pain pathway defects in patients with acute radiculopathy. Eur Spine J, 19:270, 2010

60. Fisher MA: Electrophysiology of radiculopathies. Clin Neurophysiol, 113:317, 2002

61. Kraft GH: Dermatomal somatosensory-evoked potentials in the evaluation of lumbosacral spinal stenosis. Phys Med Rehabil Clin North Am, 14:71, 2003

62. Misra UK, Kalita J, Das A: Vitamin B12 deficiency neurological syndromes: a clinical, MRI and electrodiagnostic study. Electromyogr Clin Neurophysiol, 43:57, 2003

63. Velázquez Pérez L, Sánchez Cruz G, Canales Ochoa N et al: Electrophysiological features in patients and presymptomatic relatives with spinocerebellar ataxia type 2. J Neurol Sci, 263:158, 2007

64. Sartucci F, Tovani S, Murri L et al: Motor and somatosensory evoked potentials in autosomal dominant hereditary spastic paraparesis (ADHSP) linked to chromosome 2p, SPG4. Brain Res Bull, 74:243, 2007

65. Bruyn RP, van Dijk JG, Scheltens P et al: Clinically silent dysfunction of dorsal columns and dorsal spinocerebellar tracts in hereditary spastic paraparesis. J Neurol Sci, 125:206, 1994

66. Spiegel J, Hansen C, Baumgartner U et al: Sensitivity of laser-evoked potentials versus somatosensory evoked potentials in patients with multiple sclerosis. Clin Neurophysiol, 114:992, 2003

67. Gobbele R, Waberski TD, Dieckhofer A et al: Patterns of disturbed impulse propagation in multiple sclerosis identified by low and high frequency somatosensory evoked potential components. J Clin Neurophysiol, 20:283, 2003

68. Gajofatto A, Monaco S, Fiorini M et al: Assessment of outcome predictors in first-episode acute myelitis: a retrospective study of 53 cases. Arch Neurol, 67:724, 2010

69. Linden D, Berlit P: Spinal arteriovenous malformations: clinical and neurophysiological findings. J Neurol, 243:9, 1996

70. Li V, Albright AL, Sclabassi R et al: The role of somatosensory evoked potentials in the evaluation of spinal cord retethering. Pediatr Neurosurg, 24:126, 1996

71. Boor R, Fricke G, Brühl K et al: Abnormal subcortical somatosensory evoked potentials indicate high cervical myelopathy in achondroplasia. Eur J Pediatr, 158:662, 1999

72. Boor R, Miebach E, Brühl K et al: Abnormal somatosensory evoked potentials indicate compressive cervical myelopathy in mucopolysaccharidoses. Neuropediatrics, 31:122, 2000

73. Okajima Y, Chino N, Saitoh E et al: Two types of abnormal somatosensory evoked potentials in chronic cerebellar ataxias. Am J Phys Med Rehabil, 70:96, 1991

74. Smith T, Jakobsen J, Trojaborg W: Somatosensory evoked potentials during human immunodeficiency virus (HIV) infection. Electroencephalogr Clin Neurophysiol, 75:S142, 1990

75. Tagliati M, Di Rocco A, Danisi F et al: The role of somatosensory evoked potentials in the diagnosis of AIDS-associated myelopathy. Neurology, 54:1477, 2000

76. Moritoyo H, Arimura K, Arimura Y et al: Study of lower limb somatosensory evoked potentials in 96 cases of HTLV-I-associated myelopathy/tropical spastic paraparesis. J Neurol Sci, 138:78, 1996

77. Gutling E, Isenmann S, Wichmann W: Electrophysiology in the locked-in-syndrome. Neurology, 46:1092, 1996

78. Lee SY, Lim JY, Kang EK et al: Prediction of good functional recovery after stroke based on combined motor and somatosensory evoked potential findings. J Rehabil Med, 42:16, 2010

79. Facco E, Munari M, Gallo F et al: Role of short latency potentials in the diagnosis of brain death. Clin Neurophysiol, 113:1855, 2002

80. Carter BG, Butt W: Review of the use of somatosensory evoked potentials in the prediction of outcome after severe brain injury. Crit Care Med, 29:178, 2001

81. Claassen J, Hansen HC: Early recovery after closed traumatic head injury: somatosensory evoked potentials and clinical findings. Crit Care Med, 29:494, 2001

82. Lew HL, Dikmen S, Slimp J et al: Use of somatosensory-evoked potentials and cognitive event-related potentials in predicting outcomes of patients with severe traumatic brain injury. Am J Phys Med Rehabil, 82:53, 2003

83. Rossetti AO, Oddo M, Logroscino G et al: Prognostication after cardiac arrest and hypothermia: a prospective study. Ann Neurol, 67:301, 2010

84. Bassetti C, Bomio F, Mathis J et al: Early prognosis in coma after cardiac arrest: a prospective clinical, electrophysiological, and biochemical study of 60 patients. J Neurol Neurosurg Psychiatry, 61:610, 1996

85. Zandbergen EG, de Haan RJ, Stoutenbeek CP et al: Systematic review of early prediction of poor outcome in anoxic-ischaemic coma. Lancet, 352:1808, 1998

86. Samaniego EA, Mlynash M, Caulfield AF et al: Sedation confounds outcome prediction in cardiac arrest survivors treated with hypothermia. Neurocrit Care, 15:113, 2011

87. Lee YC, Phan TG, Jolley DJ et al: Accuracy of clinical signs, SEP, and EEG in predicting outcome of hypoxic coma: a meta-analysis. Neurology, 74:572, 2010

88. Robinson LR, Micklesen PJ, Tirschwell DL et al: Predictive value of somatosensory evoked potentials for awakening from coma. Crit Care Med, 31:960, 2003

89. Leithner C, Ploner CJ, Hasper D et al: Does hypothermia influence the predictive value of bilateral absent N20 after cardiac arrest? Neurology, 74:965, 2010

90. Nuwer MR, Dawson EG, Carlson LG et al: Somatosensory evoked potentials spinal cord monitoring reduces neurologic deficits after scoliosis surgery: results of a large multicenter survey. Electroencephalogr Clin Neurophysiol, 96:6, 1995

91. Daube JR: Electrodiagnostic studies in amyotrophic lateral sclerosis and other motor neuron disorders. Muscle Nerve, 23:1488, 2000

92. Gregory R, Mills K, Donaghy M: Progressive sensory nerve dysfunction in amyotrophic lateral sclerosis: a prospective clinical and neurophysiological study. J Neurol, 240:309, 1993

93. Simone IL, Tortelli R, Samarelli V et al: Laser evoked potentials in amyotrophic lateral sclerosis. J Neurol Sci, 288:106, 2010

94. Polo A, Teatini F, D'Anna S et al: Sensory involvement in X-linked spino-bulbar muscular atrophy (Kennedy's syndrome): an electrophysiological study. J Neurol, 243:388, 1996

95. Polo A, Curro'Dossi M, Fiaschi A et al: Peripheral and segmental spinal abnormalities of median and ulnar somatosensory evoked potentials in Hirayama's disease. J Neurol Neurosurg Psychiatry, 74:627, 2003

96. Fierro B, Daniele O, Aloisio A et al: Neurophysiological and radiological findings in myotonic dystrophy patients. Eur J Neurol, 5:89, 1998

97. Mochizuki H, Hanajima R, Kowa H et al: Somatosensory evoked potential recovery in myotonic dystrophy. Clin Neurophysiol, 112:793, 2001

98. Beniczky S, Keri S, Antal A et al: Somatosensory evoked potentials correlate with genetics in Huntington's disease. Neuroreport, 13:2295, 2002

99. Lefaucheur JP, Ménard-Lefaucheur I, Maison P et al: Electrophysiological deterioration over time in patients with Huntington's disease. Mov Disord, 21:1350, 2006

100. Sindou MP, Mertens P, Bendavid U et al: Predictive value of somatosensory evoked potentials for long-lasting pain relief after spinal cord stimulation: practical use for patient selection. Neurosurgery, 52:1374, 2003

Somatosensory Evoked Potentials in Infants and Children

MICHAEL J. AMINOFF

Examination of the sensory pathways is particularly difficult in infants and young children, and the recording of somatosensory evoked potentials (SEPs) is therefore important as a means of providing objective information about the functional integrity of the somatosensory pathways.[1–3] As in adults, SEPs are helpful in diagnosing certain disorders, localizing lesions, following the response to therapies, and monitoring the integrity of the sensory pathways during procedures that may put them at especial risk. In the pediatric population, they can also provide information on the development and maturity of the sensory pathways.

Cortical SEPs can be recorded from at least the 27th week of estimated gestational age (i.e., the age in weeks of the infant at birth as calculated from the mother's last menstrual period; EGA).[4] Although the responses at this time may be difficult to record, are sometimes absent, show marked individual variation, and may differ from those recorded later in life, they show that the somatosensory pathways can conduct impulses from the periphery to the cerebral cortex. In fact, Taylor and colleagues were able to record SEPs in all of 22 preterm infants ranging between 27 and 32 weeks EGA. The waveform consisted of triphasic positive and negative components with latencies that decreased rapidly over the preterm period. There appeared to be no differences in the maturational changes as a function of gestational age at birth.

The generators of the various components of the SEPs elicited by stimulations of limb nerves were discussed in Chapter 26, to which the reader is referred. Guidelines for recording SEPs are available.[5]

The various components of SEPs are labeled by their polarity and expected latency. Given the differences in length and maturity of the nervous system that exist between adults and children, the latencies of the individual components—and thus their designations—also differ. Table 27-1 shows selected componenets of the median- and tibial-derived SEPs, with their usual latencies for adults and young children.

METHODOLOGY

Techniques for recording median SEPs in infants and children are well described. A stimulus rate of 4.1 Hz, stimulus intensity just above motor threshold, and sweep time of 50 or 100 msec are used widely. In normal infants, a bandpass of 10 or 30 to 3,000 Hz, with 100 k gain, commonly is preferred because it allows better differentiation of the early positive and negative cerebral components in the recordings.[6] A bandpass of 5 to 1,500 Hz is helpful in some cases, however, to facilitate recording of late slow waves which may be the first indication of the presence of cortical potentials.[6] For recording the median SEP, a common montage is between the ipsilateral and contralateral Erb's point (channel 1);

TABLE 27-1 ■ **Selected Components of the Median and Tibial Somatosensory Evoked Potential in Children and Adults**

	Origin	Adults	Children	
			Term infants*	1–8 yrs
Median SEPs	Brachial plexus	N9/P9	–	N7/P7
	Medial lemniscus	P13–P14	P10	P9–10
	Cortical area 3b	N20	N27–30	N16
	Cortical motor area 4	P22	P36–39	P20
Tibial SEPs	Sacral plexus	P18	–	P11
	Lumbar potential	N22	N8	N14
	Gracile nucleus	P31	–	P21
	Somatosensory cortex	P37	Variable (P33)	P28

*The most pronounced maturational changes occur in the first 6 weeks of life. Methodological differences make it difficult to compare values obtained by different authors for infants. The values shown here, derived from the literature, are provided simply as a guide.

the fifth cervical spine and contralateral Erb's point (channel 2); midway between the ipsilateral C3/4 and P3/4 (CP placement; also known as C3′ or C4′, located behind the C3 or C4 placements in the international 10–20 system), and the contralateral Erb's point (channel 3); and contralateral and ipsilateral CP placements (channel 4). In infants, recordings are sometimes made at a site 1 cm above the axilla rather than at the ipsilateral Erb's point to obtain more reliable recording of the Erb's point potential.[7] Figure 27-1 shows median SEPs in a child of 7 years and another aged 23 months.

For the tibial nerve, recordings are made from over the popliteal fossa (channel 1) and the L1 spine (channel 2) referenced to the sixth thoracic spine, and over the C7 spine (channel 3) and CPz (channel 4) referenced to Fz. Methods are similar to those used in adults. An example of a tibial SEP recorded in an 8-year-old boy is provided in Figure 27-2. Normative data corrected for height are helpful for evaluating latency values. The scalp-recorded tibial SEP is not seen in infants younger than 31 weeks conceptual age (CA; i.e., EGA plus the legal age), and its presence in older infants is variable[8]; not all components are recorded, even at term.[9]

Recordings ideally should be made with the patient awake, as cortical components are affected by sleep, but this is not always possible. Sedation should be avoided if possible in infants younger than 3 months of

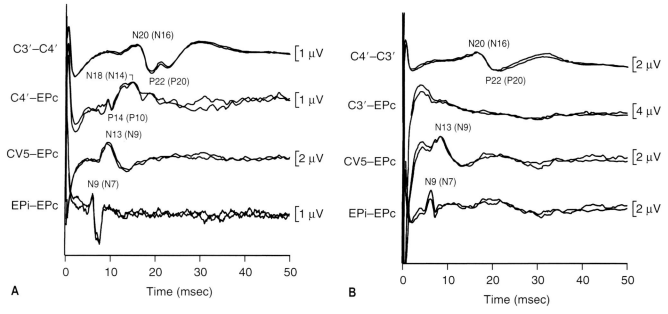

FIGURE 27-1 ■ **A**, Somatosensory evoked potential (SEP) elicited by stimulation of the right median nerve at the wrist in a 7-year-old boy. Responses were recorded over the brachial plexus at ipsilateral Erb's point (EPi), over the fifth cervical spine (CV5), and over the ipsilateral scalp in the centroparietal region (C4′) with contralateral Erb's point (EPc) used as a reference, as well as over the contralateral centroparietal scalp (C3′) referenced to the ipsilateral scalp (C4′). Negativity at the active electrode is indicated by an upward deflection. Components are labeled by their designation in adults, with the designation in children shown in parentheses. An N9 (N7) potential is seen over Erb's point, an N13 (N9) over the cervical spine, subcortical far-field P14 (P13) and N18 (N14) potentials over the ipsilateral scalp area, and an N20 (N16) over the contralateral "hand" area (C4′) of the scalp. The responses are normal, and the N20 (N16) latency is 16.2 msec. **B**, SEP to stimulation of the left median nerve in a 23-month-old girl. Recording derivation as marked. The N20 (N16) in this child is 16.6 msec. The similarity of the recordings in *A* and *B* is readily apparent, and both are similar to the recordings in adults (see Chapter 26), except for the latency differences.

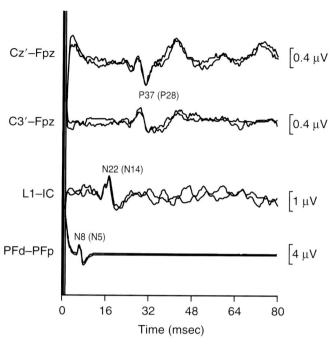

FIGURE 27-2 ■ Normal response recorded over the popliteal fossa, the spine, and the scalp with stimulation of the left tibial nerve at the ankle in an 8-year-old boy (4 feet 4 inches in height), with a history of high arches and abnormal cutaneous sensation in the legs. A well-marked potential is recorded over the nerve at the popliteal fossa between the distal and the proximal electrodes (PFd and PFp), and a lumbar potential (N14; the N22 equivalent) is recorded over the first lumbar vertebra with the reference at the iliac crest (L1–IC). A positivity (P37 equivalent) is seen at Cz′ and the contralateral scalp area (C3′) with reference to Fpz and has a latency of 30 msec.

age,[3] but may be necessary in older infants and children. Sedation or anesthesia may attenuate the cortical SEP components and affect component latencies.

EFFECTS OF MATURATION AND RELATED FACTORS

Maturation of Structures in the Nervous System

It is difficult to determine the effects of maturation on the somatosensory system because a number of different factors are involved including—but not limited to—change in the length of the sensory pathway and the myelination of different parts of the sensory pathway at different times.

As the human infant develops, nerve fibers myelinate and the diameter and length of peripheral nerves increase.[10,11] In newborns, the conduction velocity of peripheral nerves increases linearly with CA from approximately 20 m/sec at 33 weeks CA to 33 m/sec at 44 weeks

CA.[12] The conduction velocity of peripheral nerves continues to increase with age during early childhood,[13] with maximal values attained at 18 to 27 postnatal months for the sural nerve.[14]

Maturation of the spinal cord occurs later than that of peripheral nerves. At 26 weeks CA, the spinal canal finishes at the level of the fourth lumbar vertebra, whereas by term it is at about the second lumbar vertebra. As summarized by Gilmore, myelin first appears in the fasciculus cuneatus at 14 weeks CA and in the fasciculus gracilis at 22 to 24 weeks CA in humans.[12] With maturation, fiber diameter and conduction velocity increase, exceeding the effects of elongation of the spinal cord in early infancy.[8] Cracco and co-workers used surface distance measurements to calculate conduction velocities over different segments of the spinal cord in infants and children. Conduction velocity was faster in rostral than in more caudal segments or peripheral nerve, and increased progressively with age. It came to be within the adult range in peripheral nerve by 3 years of age, and in the spinal cord by 5 years.[15] In children, the increase in conduction velocity seems to parallel the increase in length of the cord.[2]

The more rostral parts of the somatosensory system myelinate over a wide range of times, probably accounting, at least in part, for the different times at which scalp-recorded potentials or their various components appear in preterm newborns. In the medial lemniscus, myelination begins at approximately 23 to 25 weeks CA in a caudal-rostral order, being completed probably at about 12 months post-term.[16] The thalamus is known to have no or little myelin at approximately 32 weeks CA, but myelination occurs over the ensuing weeks so that by term, the thalamus usually is myelinated.[17] The somesthetic radiations are not myelinated completely until approximately 12 to 18 months post-term.[16]

In infants, the absence of SEP components may simply reflect the fact that maturation has not proceeded sufficiently for development of either the relevant neural generators or the pathways conducting the potentials of interest. With regard to the median SEP, the cortical potential was recorded consistently after 6 post-term weeks in one study,[7] and after 8 weeks in another.[18] If infants without cerebral potentials at birth are retested at 2 to 3 months, most (80 percent) will have cerebral potentials.[19] Maturational changes occur throughout infancy but are fastest during the first 3 weeks of life.[6] In the preterm and term periods, maturation is reflected mainly as shortening of the latencies and increase in the amplitude of especially the early responses of the SEP.[20]

Fifty-two sets of cortical SEPs were recorded from 23 normal children between the ages of 1 day and 13 weeks with median nerve stimulation by George and Taylor, who found that a component corresponding to the adult P22 became the major component by 2 to 3 weeks of age.[6] Gibson and associates studied the median SEPs in 40 healthy term infants.[21] Identifiable potentials were recorded over the cervical spine in all of them and from the scalp in at least some runs in most (39) infants. The cervical response showed little variation and consisted of a clear negative wave with up to three peaks, the largest having a mean latency of 10.2 ± 0.7 msec, followed by a positive deflection. The cortical response was variable in form and latency between infants and in the same infant at different times. Its morphology could be symmetric, asymmetric, plateau- or M-shaped, of increasing complexity. In some instances the response was absent or ambiguous but usually could be resolved by altering the stimulus frequency or intensity. In the whole group, the mean latency for the potential corresponding to the N20 component was 30.0 ± 6.8 msec, and for the central conduction time was 19.8 ± 6.5 msec. Differences between the different cortical waveforms suggested that the M-shaped form was the most mature response.

With regard to the tibial SEP, there is also some variability in the findings. In 26 babies, aged between 1 day and 3 months, Georgesco and co-workers found no reproducible tibial SEPs over the scalp in 6 instances but, in the other 20 infants, an electropositive component (corresponding to the P37) was found that showed no correlation in its scalp distribution or latency with the baby's size, age, or physiologic state, or the intensity of stimulation.[22] In another study, cortical and spinal SEPs were recorded after median and tibial nerve stimulation in healthy newborns. Spinal SEPs were obtained and recorded readily in all but one neonate after stimulation of both nerves. Cortical SEPs were recorded more frequently after median nerve (87 percent) than tibial nerve stimulation (73 percent) but the shape of cortical SEPs obtained after tibial stimulation was less variable.[23]

In a study of spinal, subcortical, and short-latency cortical SEPs following median or tibial nerve stimulation in 100 sedated or nonsedated children aged between 4 weeks and 13 years, the morphology of the responses was similar to adults, but the initial cortical components of the median SEP showed maturational changes in both interpeak latencies and morphology.[24] The negative peak latencies recorded over Erb's point (N9 equivalent) and the second cervical vertebra (N13 equivalent) following median nerve stimulation, and over the lumbothoracic junction following tibial nerve stimulation were related directly to patient age and limb length. There was no correlation between age and the latencies of either the initial negativity or positivity of the cortical

SEPs after median and tibial nerve stimulation, respectively. Central somatosensory conduction time declined slowly during the first decade and reached adult values after 8 years of age.[24]

The presence, morphology, and latency of the SEP, especially of the cortical component, may reflect the wide time-range over which myelin appears at different sites in the developing central nervous system (CNS).

Age and Height Effects on SEP Latencies

Changes in the length of the pathways mediating the SEPs—as well as maturational changes—influence SEP latency. The latency of the N20 (N16 in the child) component of the median SEP decreases for the first 4 or 5 years of life and then starts to increase with increase in body and arm length.[25,26] The latencies of the Erb's point potential and N13 (N9 in the child) are similar in newborns and older infants,[7] probably remaining stable or decreasing slightly until 4 to 5 years.[26] They then start to increase, reaching adult values in the teenage years.[15]

The central conduction time, calculated from the median SEP as the difference in latency between N20 (N16 in children) and N13 is correlated inversely with age, diminishing as the infant grows. It declined slowly during the first decade, reaching adult values after 8 years of age in one study.[24]

In the SEP elicited by fibular (peroneal) nerve stimulation, the conduction velocity along the peripheral nerve reaches the adult range by 3 years of age, whereas that recorded between the lumbar and cervical spinal cord does not do so until the fifth year.[15]

As regards the tibial SEP, a study of preterm infants revealed that the latencies of the potentials recorded over the lumbar and cervical spine following bilateral simultaneous stimulation decrease with increasing CA, probably because conduction velocities are increasing faster (with myelination) than the length of the conducting pathway.[8] By contrast, latency of the popliteal fossa potential is constant and unrelated to age or length, presumably because leg length[11] and conduction velocity[13] increase at similar rates. The latency of the scalp-recorded equivalent of the P37 in adults (P55) shows marked variation, is independent of most factors, and probably reflects variable rates of cerebral myelination and neuronogenesis, varying states of alertness, and possibly subclinical encephalopathies.[8] In children aged between 1 and 8 years, latencies of the early components of the tibial SEP increase with increasing age or height, whereas that of the scalp-recorded P28 potential (the P37 of adults) correlates only modestly with height and reflects asynchronous maturation of elongating polysynaptic pathways.[2]

Effects of Sleep

Tactile stimulation of the fingertips elicits responses over the scalp that are similar in waveform and latency to the responses evoked by electrical stimulation in term neonates.[27] An initial negative potential (N1) with a latency of 31 to 34 msec is followed by one or two positive deflections, P1 and P2, within about 300 msec from the stimulation. Pihko and associates found that N1 was present clearly only in active sleep and only in a few subjects; both positive potentials were depressed in active sleep.[27]

The effect of sleep on the short-latency median SEP is variable in infants and children. The findings in wakefulness and rapid eye movement (REM) sleep are similar. Hashimoto and associates examined electrically elicited median SEPs in 83 children aged between 1 month and 16 years.[25] Components comparable to the adult N20 remained stable during sleep, whereas P22 demonstrated an increase in peak latency during slow-wave sleep but not during REM sleep. In another study on the effect of sleep on the median SEP in 20 healthy children aged 20 days to 3 years, non-REM sleep influenced the latency and the duration of SEPs, especially in children younger than 1 year.[28] In adults, non-REM sleep may prolong SEP latencies.[29,30]

The effect of sleep on the cortical components of the tibial SEP of infants and children is even more marked and complicated.[12] In some preterm infants, natural sleep actually enhances the appearance of the later cortical potentials.

CLINICAL APPLICATIONS

Prognosis in Coma

Clinical assessments using the Glasgow Coma Scale may be limited for technical reasons, as when it is not possible to examine motor function because of the effects of muscle relaxants or sedatives. Having the means of assessing the integrity of the patient's nervous system electrophysiologically as well as clinically is therefore important in guiding prognostication.

The value of the median-derived SEP for prognosis has been examined in comatose infants and children. Absence of cortical components of the median SEP with preservation of the brainstem auditory evoked potential (BAEP) correlated with loss of cortical function and preservation of brainstem function in five children with hypoxic insults, as might have been anticipated.[31] In children with brainstem pathology, however, the recording of both BAEPs and median SEPs may provide more information than does either test alone,[32] but does not

necessarily provide a better prognostic guide.[33] SEPs are more useful than visual evoked potentials (VEPs) in evaluating prognosis.[34]

De Meirleir and Taylor reported the SEP findings in children who were comatose from a variety of causes.[33] Those with bilaterally absent cortical SEPs died or were left with a severe spastic quadriplegia; those with unilaterally abnormal cortical SEPs developed a residual hemiparesis; and those with normal or only mildly abnormal SEPs that normalized within a few days had normal outcomes.

Goodwin and associates also found that SEPs and BAEPs are useful in predicting outcome in comatose children.[35] They studied 41 children with a variety of disorders admitted to a pediatric intensive care unit with a Glasgow Coma Scale score of less than 8. Survivor outcome was determined at discharge and 1 to 3 years later. There were no false pessimistic predictions (i.e., predictions of a bad outcome when a good outcome actually occurred), and two false optimistic predictions in this series. A comprehensive literature review of coma outcome prediction, using multimodality evoked potential recordings, revealed 20 series with 982 additional patients in whom the predictive errors of false pessimism and false optimism could be determined. Five cases of false pessimism (which declined to three if neonates were excluded) and 99 cases of false optimism were identified in the 982 additional patients.[35]

Beca and co-workers have studied this issue and compared the SEP as a predictor of outcome in acute, severely brain-injured infants and children with prediction using the motor component of the Glasgow Coma Scale. They found that a normal SEP had a positive predictive value (PPV) for favorable outcome (using the Glasgow Outcome Scale) of 93 percent. Absent SEPs were predictive (92 percent) of an unfavorable outcome (either severe disability, survival in a persistent vegetative state, or death).[36] Although an absent motor response to a painful stimulus also had a PPV of 100 percent for an unfavorable outcome, in 23 percent of patients the response could not be evaluated because of the effects of muscle relaxants or sedatives.

In a prospective cohort of 57 consecutive children who were mechanically ventilated for hypoxic-ischemic encephalopathy in a tertiary pediatric intensive care unit, 42 had impaired consciousness or remained in coma after 24 hours. Among this group, an initial cardiopulmonary resuscitation duration longer than 10 minutes and a Glasgow Coma Scale score of less than 5 at 24 hours after admission were associated with an unfavorable outcome (PPV, 91 and 100 percent). A discontinuous electroencephalogram (EEG) and the presence of epileptiform discharges were associated with an unfavorable outcome (PPV, 100 percent for the two criteria). The bilateral absence of the N20 wave on short-latency SEPs had a PPV for unfavorable outcome of 100 percent. Clinical assessment combined with EEG and SEPs thus allows an early prediction of the prognosis of children.[37]

Clinical assessment may be as predictive or have a higher PPV for outcome than electrophysiologic studies, but is often hampered by sedation or paralysis in patients in the intensive care unit. SEPs and other evoked potential studies thus remain a valuable tool for those caring for comatose children.

REYE SYNDROME

In children with Reye syndrome, longitudinal SEPs may be helpful in prognostication. Patient survival in one study was correlated with early recovery of initially absent short-latency (less than 50 msec) cortical components of the median SEP; lack of their recovery was associated with death.[38] Progressive recovery of SEP components later than 100 msec was associated with satisfactory clinical recovery; when these components failed to recover, patients were left with a residual neuropsychologic deficit.

Assessment of Term and Preterm Newborns

The importance of early afferent activity for normal brain development is widely known and indicates the importance of assessing brain responses to afferent stimuli in patients in the neonatal intensive care unit. Evoked potentials are useful clinically in preterm neonates because the neurologic evaluation of these infants is often unreliable.[39] Prediction of outcome for graduates of neonatal intensive care units is helpful in identifying patients requiring early interventions and in guiding how families are counseled.

SEPs, alone or in combination with other electrophysiologic studies, can be helpful for determining prognosis in high-risk newborns.[40-44] In one study, almost one-third of newborns at high risk for neurologic or developmental sequelae had abnormal SEPs with delayed or absent scalp-recorded potentials or a prolonged central conduction time.[42] Patients were tested again at 2 and 6 months of age, and then neurodevelopmental outcome was determined at 1 year. SEP abnormalities that persisted or worsened correlated with severe neurologic impairment, whereas an abnormal SEP that improved or normalized in infancy was associated with only mild to moderate neurologic sequelae.[43] In a subsequent

prospective study of the long-term predictive value of SEPs, BAEPs, and the Einstein Neonatal Neurobehavioral Assessment Scale, 78 high-risk newborns and 28 healthy controls were assessed by these means in the newborn period.[45] At 8 to 9 years of age, 42 subjects and 13 controls were re-evaluated for developmental progress using a range of psychologic, sensorimotor, and neurologic measures. The SEP was most accurate at predicting outcome at school age, with high specificity (83 to 100 percent) across all domains tested and good sensitivity (80 to 100 percent) for intellectual performance and sensorimotor abilities. The BAEP was limited by false negatives, and the neurobehavioral assessment by many false positives. Thus, associations between neonatal SEPs and developmental sequelae remain significant at school age.[45]

Taylor and her co-investigators examined median SEPs and VEPs in asphyxiated term infants who were followed for 18 to 24 months. Electrophysiologic studies were performed in the first 3 days of life, during the first week, and at follow-up visits. The SEPs had high sensitivity (96 percent) and negative predictive power (97 percent); normal SEPs virtually guaranteed normal outcome. VEPs had both a specificity and positive predictive power of 100 percent; abnormal VEPs guaranteed abnormal outcome. Both together had a higher predictive power than either alone.[46] Others have reported similar findings at both intermediate[47,48] and long-term follow-up.[49]

Median SEPs provide reliable data that can help to predict neurologic outcome in preterm infants at risk of periventricular leukomalacia, and the tibial SEP may be even better but is more difficult to obtain.[39]

PREDICTING CEREBRAL PALSY

The above studies bear on the issue of predicting severe motor impairment at an early stage. Infants with prolonged or absent cortical SEPs all demonstrated fixed handicaps after the first year of life, indicating that the SEP is a valuable early indicator of severe motor impairment, although there was a rather high false-negative rate, probably because only the afferent pathway was tested electrophysiologically.[41] In another study, cortical SEPs were always present in the perinatal period in those surviving without major neurologic disability, while they were absent bilaterally in all but one patient with a subsequent diagnosis of cerebral palsy.[50]

In a more detailed study, it was found that SEPs recorded early in the course of the life of a preterm infant predict long-term neurodevelopmental outcome.[51] Thus, unilateral, median SEPs were recorded twice in the first 3 weeks of life in a group of preterm infants. Bilateral SEP abnormalities were associated with the presence of periventricular leukomalacia on head ultrasound and were predictive of later cerebral palsy. False-positive results were frequent. A normal SEP, even when there was periventricular echogenicity on head ultrasound, was associated with a normal outcome in all but one instance. The SEPs were less accurate than the findings of periventricular leukomalacia on ultrasound in the prediction of later cerebral palsy. SEPs done in the first 3 weeks of life therefore may provide additional prognostic information, particularly when the test is normal. Abnormal SEPs in this period must be interpreted cautiously.[51]

Neurodegenerative Disorders

Abnormal spinal and cortical SEP components have been reported in a variety of neurodegenerative disorders. Severe abnormalities have been described in children with polioencephalopathies (primarily disorders affecting gray matter) and leukodystrophies. In children with leukodystrophy (metachromatic leukodystrophy, Pelizaeus–Merzbacher disease (Figs. 27-3 and 27-4), Krabbe disease, adrenoleukodystrophy, Alexander disease, Canavan disease, and multiple sulphatase deficiency), the SEPs were abnormal in all instances. Cortical SEPs were absent in 16 and abnormal in 5 who were

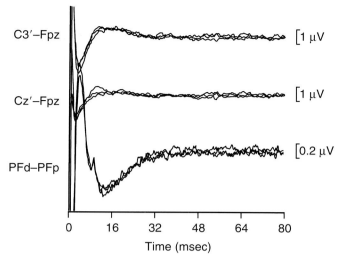

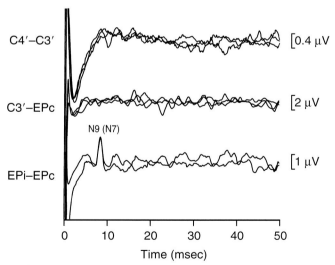

FIGURE 27-3 ▪ Median somatosensory evoked potential recorded in a boy aged 5 years 8 months, with Pelizaeus–Merzbacher disease. Responses were recorded over Erb's point and the scalp as shown; spinal responses were not recorded as, because of laryngo-tracheomalacia, the boy had a tracheostomy and required cervical support. An upward deflection indicates negativity at the active electrode. A peripheral potential is present at Erb's point (N9 equivalent) but central responses are absent.

FIGURE 27-4 ▪ Tibial somatosensory evoked potential recorded in the same patient as in Figure 27-3. Recording montage as shown. An upward deflection indicates negativity at the active electrode. A peripheral response is recorded over the popliteal fossa but there is no response over the scalp.

in the earlier stages of their disease. Cervical SEPs were within normal limits, except for the patients with Krabbe disease and metachromatic leukodystrophy, who showed peripheral slowing.[52]

SEPs are valuable in differentiating adrenomyeloneuropathy from adrenoleukodystrophy.[53] Central conduction time is prolonged in both disorders, but in the former the Erb's point potential is also delayed, indicating slowing in conduction velocity of the peripheral nerve.[53] In a study of 6 patients with adrenomyeloneuropathy showing only mild signs of CNS involvement, median SEPs showed delayed or absent scalp P14 far-field potential in all patients and abnormal spinal N13 in 2. Tibial SEPs showed abnormalities of the subcortical P30 response in all 4 patients in whom scalp-to-ear recording was employed. These findings suggest that neurologic dysfunction is localized in the spinal cord in early stages of the disease, where it is difficult to assess with magnetic resonance imaging (MRI). However, SEPs, which show a typical pattern of abnormality, may be helpful in revealing signs of long-tract involvement and in monitoring treatment.[54]

Rossini and co-workers examined SEPs in patients with several other neurodegenerative disorders.[55,56] Patients with Friedreich ataxia, olivopontocerebellar atrophy, hereditary motor and sensory neuropathy type II (HMSN II), and ataxia-telangiectasia had impaired central conduction and normal or slightly prolonged latencies of peripheral components of the median SEP. In patients with Friedreich ataxia and HMSN II, the peripheral nerve potentials were attenuated.

Lower-extremity SEPs in patients with Friedreich ataxia were characterized by near-normal latencies of peripheral components with impaired central conduction. Similar findings have been reported by others.[57] In olivopontocerebellar atrophy, median SEPs were usually normal but all lower-extremity SEPs were abnormal. Patients with HMSN II usually had normal median SEPs but increased central conduction time in lower-extremity SEPs. In HMSN I, the Erb's point potential was delayed and more rostral potentials were absent.[55] SEPs were normal in patients with familial spastic paraplegia in this study,[55] but others have reported attenuation of the tibial SEPs without latency alterations.[58]

In metabolic disorders such as aminoacidopathies, neuronal storage diseases, and organic acidemias, SEPs may show mild prolongation of central conduction time. Approximately one-third of patients with organic acidemias have abnormal SEPs.[59] Profound delays have been seen in Leigh disease[60] and can be used with other electrophysiologic tests to follow the disease[61]; marked delays are found also in Krabbe disease, as mentioned earlier Patients with classic galactosemia may have abnormal SEPs, especially with tibial nerve stimulation.[62] SEP abnormalities have also been found in patients with Hallervorden–Spatz disease.[63] In neuronal ceroid lipofuscinosis, prolonged central conduction times and high-amplitude cortical components of the SEP have been described. The amplitudes sometimes exceed 40 μV, but this finding is not pathognomonic because it occasionally occurs in other conditions.[64]

Demyelinating diseases such as multiple sclerosis are uncommon but increasingly recognized during childhood. SEPs may be useful in the evaluation of suspected cases, as discussed in Chapter 26.

Structural and Compressive Lesions

Structural and compressive lesions may affect the SEP, depending on their site. Compressive lesions of the cervical spine (e.g., foramen magnum stenosis) commonly are associated with abnormal SEPs. Intrinsic cervical cord lesions (e.g., gliomas and Arnold–Chiari malformations) are associated with SEP abnormalities that correlate with the severity of clinical involvement. In a study of 52 patients aged between 8 months and 20 years (median 7.3 years) with an Arnold–Chiari malformation, for example, abnormal SEPs were found mainly in symptomatic patients, especially in those more than 4 years old, and presumably reflected dysfunction of the brainstem or the upper cervical cord.[65] In another study of infants with myelomeningocele and Arnold–Chiari malformation, the cortical component of the median SEP

(equivalent to the adult N20) was absent or had low amplitude and prolonged latency in all 6 patients with, and in 4 without, clinical signs of brainstem dysfunction, suggesting that they may be a helpful measure of brainstem function in infants with this malformation.[66]

Patients with extrinsic lesions (e.g., spinal stenosis and foramen magnum stenosis secondary to achondroplasia) have also been studied. Nelson and co-workers studied the median and tibial SEPs of 23 achondroplastic patients with and without symptoms of cord involvement.[67] All symptomatic patients and 7 of 16 asymptomatic patients had at least one abnormal SEP, suggesting that SEPs might provide an early indication of cord involvement so that decompressive surgery can be undertaken before neurologic compromise is serious.

In another study to detect myelopathy in patients with achondroplasia, Li and associates recorded median and tibial SEPs in 77 patients aged between 4 months and almost 18 years (mean 2.7 years) using conventional techniques but also noncephalic and mastoid reference electrodes to record the subcortical waveforms generated near the craniocervical junction.[68] The findings were related to the MRI results. Thirty-four patients had abnormal MRI findings including spinal cord compression (28 patients) or myelomalacia (24 instances) at or below the craniocervical junction. The median SEPs had a sensitivity of 74 percent and specificity of 98 percent, including all abnormal upper cervical cord MRI findings; the sensitivity and specificity were 79 and 92 percent, respectively, for cervical cord compression. For the tibial SEPs, sensitivity and specificity were 52 and 93 percent for all abnormal MRI findings, and 59 and 92 percent, respectively, for cervical cord compression. The subcortical SEPs were more sensitive than the conventional recordings. Median SEPs in particular, and especially the subcortical recordings, are thus useful for the detection of cervical myelopathy in children with achondroplasia.

Compressive myelopathy at the craniocervical junction may complicate mucopolysaccharidoses. To detect cervical myelopathy, the median and posterior tibial nerve SEPs, including the subcortical components generated near the craniocervical junction, were recorded in 15 patients aged between 2.4 and 33.4 years (median 8.8 years) with various mucopolysaccharidoses.[69] MRI studies in 13 subjects revealed spinal cord compression at the cranio-cervical junction in 10 patients; 5 patients had an increased signal intensity on the T2-weighted initial MRI indicating high cervical myelomalacia and 4 patients had clinical signs of cervical myelopathy. There was no relationship between the SEPs and spinal cord compression. Abnormal SEPs were found in the patients with myelomalacia on MRI (100 percent sensitivity and specificity) and in the patients with clinical signs of myelopathy (100 percent sensitivity and 91 percent specificity). Abnormal SEPs indicated subclinical cervical myelopathy in 3 subjects. Although cervical cord compression may be present before clinical or electrophysiologic evidence of myelopathy, SEP analysis may help to detect functional impairment of the cervical cord in mucopolysaccharidoses.

Structural cord lesions below the cervical level are often associated with abnormalities in tibial SEPs.[70,71] Recording the spinal components of lower-limb SEPs may be useful in evaluating patients with myelodysplasia and occult spinal dysraphism.[72] The large spinal potential normally recorded over the lower thoracic spine is displaced caudally. In patients with myelographically and operatively confirmed tethering dysraphic lesions, the tibial SEPs were predictive of the level or laterality of the lesion.[73] Similarly, ranking the severity of neurologic impairment and the extent of dysraphism at surgery, as well as the extent of SEP abnormality, revealed a significant association between clinical severity and SEP abnormalities.[73] If the traction is relieved, the SEP may improve.[73] Early detection of clinically significant spinal cord retethering is important for maintaining neurologic function in patients with repaired spinal dysraphic lesions, but serial SEPs do not correlate well with clinical status and are not a useful modality for monitoring patients at risk for retethering.[74]

Structural brainstem lesions commonly are associated with SEP abnormalities, but—depending on the lesion—BAEPs may be more helpful. With the advent of high-resolution neuroimaging, the role of evoked potentials in this context is limited.

Peripheral Lesions

Peripheral nerve, plexus, and root lesions can also be assessed with SEPs in the same manner as described for adults in Chapter 26. With root avulsion, the dorsal root ganglia are intact, so that an Erb's point potential is present but more rostral components are abnormal. With a plexus lesion, the Erb's point potential and more rostral components may be absent depending on the extent of the lesion. The findings in Guillain–Barré syndrome were considered in Chapter 26; in general, F-wave studies are more useful than SEPs for detecting proximal pathology when conventional nerve conduction studies are normal.

Cracco and colleagues recorded spinal SEPs to stimulation of the fibular (peroneal) nerves in the popliteal fossa from 46 insulin-dependent neurologically normal patients with juvenile diabetes.[75] Compared to age-matched control subjects, mean values for overall spinal conduction velocity (L3 to C7 spines) and conduction velocity over rostral spinal cord (T6 to C7 spines) and from the fibular (peroneal) nerve to cauda equina (stimulus site to L3 spine) were significantly lower in the diabetic group. Peripheral nerve conduction velocity alone was slow in 5 patients, and spinal conduction velocity was slow in 8; in 2, both peripheral and spinal velocities were slow. This study suggests that, in addition to impairment of peripheral nerve function, patients with juvenile diabetes without clinical evidence of neurologic involvement can have a defect in spinal afferent transmission.

SEP Monitoring

Intraoperative monitoring is important to reduce the risks of surgical procedures that pose a particular hazard to neurologic structures, and it is discussed in detail in Chapter 30. Surgical repair of congenital cardiovascular disorders that might compromise the spinal cord is a circumstance in which intraoperative SEP monitoring is used in young children and merits brief comment here. Faberowski and associates reported a series of 84 children who underwent aortic coarctation repair.[76] SEP changes occurred in 40 percent of the cases and were often immediately responsive to changes in surgical or anesthetic management; in more than 26 percent of the procedures, interventions (e.g., repositioning the aortic cross-clamp, increasing the blood pressure, or aborting the surgery) were required, based on the SEP changes. No patient sustained a neurologic deficit.

CONCLUDING COMMENTS

SEPs provide a means of reliably assessing the functional integrity of the somatosensory systems in infants and children. Although the effects of maturation and growth complicate interpretation, SEPs may provide clinically useful information for diagnostic or prognostic purposes, or for characterizing more fully the extent of pathologic involvement of various disorders and the response to therapeutic maneuvers.

REFERENCES

1. Cracco JB, Cracco RQ: Spinal, brainstem, and cerebral SEP in the pediatric age group. p. 21. In Cracco RQ, Bodis-Wollner I (eds): Evoked Potentials. Alan R Liss, New York, 1986
2. Gilmore RL, Bass NH, Wright EA et al: Development assessment of spinal cord and cortical evoked potentials after tibial nerve stimulation: effects of age and stature on

normative data during childhood. Electroencephalogr Clin Neurophysiol, 62:241, 1985

3. Gilmore R: Somatosensory evoked potential testing in infants and children. J Clin Neurophysiol, 9:324, 1992

4. Taylor MJ, Boor R, Ekert PG: Preterm maturation of the somatosensory evoked potential. Electroencephalogr Clin Neurophysiol, 100:448, 1996

5. Cruccu G, Aminoff MJ, Curio G et al: Recommendations for the clinical use of somatosensory-evoked potentials. Clin Neurophysiol, 119:1705, 2008

6. George SR, Taylor MJ: Somatosensory evoked potentials in neonates and infants: developmental and normative data. Electroencephalogr Clin Neurophysiol, 80:94, 1991

7. Cracco J, Udani V, Cracco RQ: MN-SSEPs in infants. Electroencephalogr Clin Neurophysiol, 69:79P, 1988

8. Gilmore R, Brock J, Hermansen MC et al: Development of lumbar spinal cord and cortical evoked potentials after tibial nerve stimulation in the pre-term newborns: effects of gestational age and other factors. Electroencephalogr Clin Neurophysiol, 68:28, 1987

9. Gallai V: Maturation of SEPs in pre-term and full-term neonates. p. 95. In Gallai V (ed): Maturation of the CNS and Evoked Potentials. Elsevier, Amsterdam, 1986

10. Ouvrier RA, McLeod JG, Conchin T: Morphometric studies of sural nerve in childhood. Muscle Nerve, 10:47, 1987

11. Merlob P, Sivan Y, Reisner SH: Lower limb standards in newborns. Am J Dis Child, 138:140, 1984

12. Gilmore RL: Somatosensory evoked potentials in infants and children. p. 577. In Aminoff MJ (ed): Electrodiagnosis in Clinical Neurology. 5th Ed. Elsevier Churchill Livingstone, New York, 2005

13. Wagner AL, Buchthal F: Motor and sensory conduction in infancy and childhood: reappraisal. Dev Med Child Neurol, 14:189, 1972

14. Buchthal F, Rosenfalck A, Behse F: Sensory potentials of normal and diseased nerves. p. 442. In Dyck PJ, Thomas PK, Lambert EH (eds): Peripheral Neuropathy. WB Saunders, Philadelphia, 1975

15. Cracco JB, Cracco RQ, Stolove R: Spinal evoked potentials in man: a maturational study. Electroencephalogr Clin Neurophysiol, 46:58, 1979

16. Yakovlev P, Lecours A: The myelogenetic cycles of regional maturation of the brain. p. 3. In Minkowski A (ed): Regional Development of the Brain in Early Life. FA Davis, Philadelphia, 1967

17. Rorke LB, Riggs HE: Myelination of the Brain in the Newborn. p. 15. JB Lippincott, Philadelphia, 1969

18. Willis J, Seales D, Frazier E: Short latency somatosensory evoked potentials in infants. Electroencephalogr Clin Neurophysiol, 59:366, 1984

19. Laureau E, Majnemer A, Rosenblatt B et al: A longitudinal study of short latency somatosensory evoked responses in healthy newborns and infants. Electroencephalogr Clin Neurophysiol, 71:100, 1988

20. Vanhatalo S, Lauronen L: Neonatal SEP—back to bedside with basic science. Semin Fetal Neonatal Med, 11:464, 2006

21. Gibson NA, Brezinova V, Levene MI: Somatosensory evoked potentials in the term newborn. Electroencephalogr Clin Neurophysiol, 84:26, 1992

22. Georgesco M, Radiere M, Seror P et al: Les potentiels cérébraux somesthésiques évoqués à partir du membre inférieur chez le nouveau-né et le nourrisson. Rev Electroencephalogr Neurophysiol Clin, 12:123, 1982

23. Laureau E, Marlot D: Somatosensory evoked potentials after median and tibial nerve stimulation in healthy newborns. Electroencephalogr Clin Neurophysiol, 76:453, 1990

24. Whittle IR, Johnston IH, Besser M: Short latency somatosensory-evoked potentials in children—Part 1. Normative data. Surg Neurol, 27:9, 1987

25. Hashimoto T, Tayama M, Hiura K et al: Short latency somatosensory evoked potential in children. Brain Dev, 5:390, 1983

26. Doria-Lamba L, Montaldi L, Grosso P et al: Short latency evoked somatosensory potentials after stimulation of the median nerve in children: normative data. J Clin Neurophysiol, 26:176, 2009

27. Pihko E, Lauronen L, Wikström H et al: Somatosensory evoked potentials and magnetic fields elicited by tactile stimulation of the hand during active and quiet sleep in newborns. Clin Neurophysiol, 115:448, 2004

28. Fotiou F, Sitzoglou KH, Tsitsopoulos P et al: Effect of N-REM sleep on the cortical SEPs in early life. Electromyogr Clin Neurophysiol, 29:87, 1989

29. Nakano S, Tsuji S, Matsunaga K et al: Effect of sleep stage on somatosensory evoked potentials by median nerve stimulation. Electroencephalogr Clin Neurophysiol, 96:385, 1995

30. Addy RO, Dinner DS, Lüders H et al: The effects of sleep on median nerve short latency somatosensory evoked potentials. Electroencephalogr Clin Neurophysiol, 74:105, 1989

31. Frank LM, Furgiuele TL, Etheridge JE: Prediction of chronic vegetative state in children using evoked potentials. Neurology, 35:931, 1985

32. Lutschg J, Pfenninger J, Ludin HP et al: Brain-stem auditory evoked potentials and early somatosensory evoked potentials in neurointensively treated comatose children. Am J Dis Child, 137:421, 1983

33. De Meirleir LJ, Taylor MJ: The prognostic utility of SEPs in comatose children. Pediatr Neurol, 3:78, 1987

34. Taylor MJ, Farrell EJ: Comparison of the prognostic utility of VEPs and SEPs in comatose children. Pediatr Neurol, 5:145, 1989

35. Goodwin SR, Friedman WA, Bellefleur M: Is it time to use evoked potentials to predict outcome in comatose children and adults? Crit Care Med, 19:518, 1991

36. Beca J, Cox PN, Taylor MJ et al: Somatosensory evoked potentials for prediction of outcome in acute severe brain injury. J Pediatr, 126:44, 1995

37. Mandel R, Martinot A, Delepoulle F et al: Prediction of outcome after hypoxic-ischemic encephalopathy: a prospective clinical and electrophysiologic study. J Pediatr, 141:45, 2002

38. Goff WR, Shaywitz BA, Goff GD et al: Somatic evoked potential evaluation of cerebral status in Reye syndrome. Electroencephalogr Clin Neurophysiol, 55:388, 1983

39. Taylor MJ, Saliba E, Laugier J: Use of evoked potentials in preterm neonates. Arch Dis Child, 74:F70, 1996

40. Lutschg J, Hanggeli C, Huber P: The evolution of cerebral hemispheric lesions due to pre- or perinatal asphyxia (clinical and neuroradiological correlation). Helv Paediatr Acta, 38:245, 1983

41. Gorke W: Somatosensory evoked cortical potentials indicating impaired motor development in infancy. Dev Med Child Neurol, 28:633, 1986

42. Majnemer A, Rosenblatt B, Riley P et al: Somatosensory evoked response abnormalities in high-risk newborns. Pediatr Neurol, 3:350, 1987

43. Majnemer A, Rosenblatt B, Riley PS: Prognostic significance of multimodality evoked response testing in high-risk newborns. Pediatr Neurol, 6:367, 1990

44. Majnemer A, Rosenblatt B: Prediction of outcome at school entry in neonatal intensive care unit survivors, with use of clinical and electrophysiologic techniques. J Pediatr, 127:823, 1995

45. Majnemer A, Rosenblatt B: Prediction of outcome at school age in neonatal intensive care unit graduates using neonatal neurologic tools. J Child Neurol, 15:645, 2000

46. Taylor MJ, Murphy WJ, Whyte HE: Prognostic reliability of somatosensory and visual evoked potentials of asphyxiated term infants. Dev Med Child Neurol, 34:507, 1992

47. de Vries LS, Pierrat V, Eken P et al: Prognostic value of early somatosensory evoked potentials for adverse outcome in full-term infants with birth asphyxia. Brain Dev, 13:320, 1991

48. Harbord MG, Weston PF: Somatosensory evoked potentials predict neurologic outcome in full-term neonates with asphyxia. J Paediatr Child Health, 31:148, 1995

49. White CP, Cooke RW: Somatosensory evoked potentials following posterior tibial nerve stimulation predict later motor outcome. Dev Med Child Neurol, 36:34, 1994

50. Suppiej A, Cappellari A, Franzoi M et al: Bilateral loss of cortical somatosensory evoked potential at birth predicts cerebral palsy in term and near-term newborns. Early Hum Dev, 86:93, 2010

51. Ekert PG, Taylor MJ, Keenan NK et al: Early somatosensory evoked potentials in preterm infants: their prognostic utility. Biol Neonate, 71:83, 1997

52. De Meirleir LJ, Taylor MJ, Logan WJ: Multimodal evoked potential studies in leukodystrophies of children. Can J Neurol Sci, 15:26, 1988

53. Tobimatsu S, Fukui R, Kato M et al: Multimodality evoked potentials in patients and carriers with adrenoleukodystrophy and adrenomyeloneuropathy. Electroencephalogr Clin Neurophysiol, 62:18, 1985

54. Restuccia D, Di Lazzaro V, Valeriani M et al: Abnormalities of somatosensory and motor evoked potentials in adrenomyeloneuropathy: comparison with magnetic resonance imaging and clinical findings. Muscle Nerve, 20:1249, 1997

55. Rossini PM, Zarola F, Di Capua M et al: Somatosensory evoked potentials in neurodegenerative system disorders. p. 125. In Gallai V (ed): Maturation of the CNS and Evoked Potentials. Elsevier, Amsterdam, 1986

56. Rossini PM, Cracco JB: Somatosensory and brainstem auditory evoked potentials in neurodegenerative system disorders. Eur Neurol, 26:176, 1987

57. Taylor MJ, Chan-Lui WY, Logan WJ: Longitudinal evoked potential studies in hereditary ataxias. Can J Neurol Sci, 12:100, 1985

58. Imai T, Minami R, Kameda K et al: Attenuated SEPs with no latency shifts in a family with hereditary spastic paraplegia. Pediatr Neurol, 6:13, 1990

59. Stigsby B, Yarworth SM, Rahbeeni Z et al: Neurophysiologic correlates of organic acidemias: a survey of 107 patients. Brain Dev, 16:Suppl, 125, 1994

60. Taylor MJ, Robinson BH: Evoked potentials in children with oxidative metabolic defects leading to Leigh syndrome. Pediatr Neurol, 8:25, 1992

61. Araki S, Hayashi M, Yasaka A et al: Electrophysiological brainstem dysfunction in a child with Leigh disease. Pediatr Neurol, 16:329, 1997

62. Kaufman FR, Horton EJ, Gott P et al: Abnormal somatosensory evoked potentials in patients with classic galactosemia: correlation with neurologic outcome. J Child Neurol, 10:32, 1995

63. Mutoh K, Okuno T, Ito M et al: Somatosensory evoked potentials in Hallervorden–Spatz-neuroaxonal-dystrophy complex with dorsal column involvement. Clin Electroencephalogr, 21:58, 1990

64. Schmitt B, Thun-Hohenstein L, Molinari L et al: Somatosensory evoked potentials with high cortical amplitudes: clinical data in 31 children. Neuropediatrics, 25:78, 1994

65. Boor R, Schwarz M, Goebel B et al: Somatosensory evoked potentials in Arnold–Chiari malformation. Brain Dev, 26:99, 2004

66. Barnet AB, Weiss IP, Shaer C: Evoked potentials in infant brainstem syndrome associated with Arnold–Chiari malformation. Dev Med Child Neurol, 35:42, 1993

67. Nelson FW, Goldie WD, Hecht JT et al: Short-latency somatosensory evoked potentials in the management of patients with achondroplasia. Neurology, 34:1053, 1984

68. Li L, Müller-Forell W, Oberman B et al: Subcortical somatosensory evoked potentials after median nerve and posterior tibial nerve stimulation in high cervical cord compression of achondroplasia. Brain Dev, 30:499, 2008

69. Boor R, Miebach E, Brühl K et al: Abnormal somatosensory evoked potentials indicate compressive cervical myelopathy in mucopolysaccharidoses. Neuropediatrics, 31:122, 2000

70. Perot PL, Vera CL: Scalp-recorded somatosensory evoked potentials to stimulation of nerves in the lower extremity and evaluation of patients with spinal cord trauma. Ann N Y Acad Sci, 388:359, 1982

71. Mutoh K, Ito M, Okuno T et al: Nontraumatic spinal intramedullary hemorrhage in an infant. Pediatr Neurol, 5:53, 1989

72. Cracco JB, Cracco RQ: Spinal somatosensory evoked potentials: maturational and clinical studies. Ann N Y Acad Sci, 388:527, 1982

73. Roy MW, Gilmore R, Walsh JW: Somatosensory evoked potentials in tethered cord syndrome. Electroencephalogr Clin Neurophysiol, 64:42P, 1986

74. Li V, Albright AL, Sclabassi R et al: The role of somatosensory evoked potentials in the evaluation of spinal cord retethering. Pediatr Neurosurg, 24:126, 1996

75. Cracco J, Castells S, Mark E: Spinal somatosensory evoked potentials in juvenile diabetes. Ann Neurol, 15:55, 1984

76. Faberowski LW, Black S, Trankina MF et al: Somatosensory-evoked potentials during aortic coarctation repair. Cardiothorac Vasc Anesth, 13:538, 1999

Diagnostic and Therapeutic Role of Magnetic Stimulation in Neurology

ROBERT CHEN and NICOLAE PETRESCU

Until about 25 years ago, direct noninvasive investigation of conduction in central motor pathways was not possible. Transcranial magnetic stimulation (TMS) was first described by Barker and co-workers in 1985 as a noninvasive and painless way to stimulate the human brain.[1] Since then, refinements in technique have allowed the technique to be introduced into clinical practice for both diagnostic and therapeutic purposes, and developed as a research tool.

DEVELOPMENT AND TECHNICAL CONSIDERATIONS

A conducting coil is placed tangential to the scalp and a brief, high-current pulse is passed through the coil. Depending on the machine, the current may have a monophasic or biphasic waveform (Fig. 28-1). A rapidly changing magnetic field is produced around the coil, with lines of flux passing perpendicularly to its plane. The magnetic field can reach up to 3 Tesla and lasts approximately 100 μsec. The changing magnetic field

generates an electrical field perpendicular to the magnetic field. In a homogeneous medium, the spatial change in the electric field causes current to flow in loops parallel to the plane of the coil, which is usually tangential to the surface of the scalp. The induced electric field causes ions to flow in the brain, depolarizing or hyperpolarizing neurons. Experimental evidence indicates that stimulation occurs at a lower threshold where axons terminate or bend sharply.[2] Accordingly, stimulation should occur where the electric field is strongest and at points of change in the structure of an axon.

Magnetic coils may take various shapes. Although circular coils are powerful, coils with a figure-of-eight shape are more focal, producing maximal current at the intersection of the circular components. They generate magnetic fields that stimulate outer layers of the cortex.[3] The Hesed coil (H-coil) is yet another configuration, its complex windings allowing for a slower fall-off of magnetic field intensity with depth.[4] The H-coil effects reach deeper than circular or figure-of-eight coils.

The physiologic responses to TMS are best described for the motor cortex. TMS of the motor cortex of

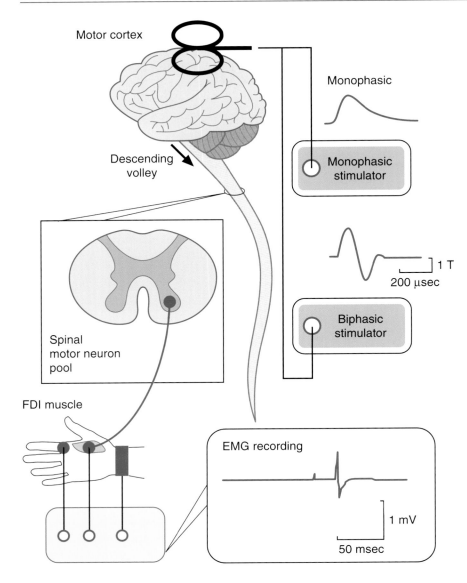

FIGURE 28-1 ▪ Schematic representation of the pathways involved in transcranial magnetic stimulation of the motor cortex. Transcranial magnetic stimulation (TMS) may be applied by monophasic or biphasic stimulators. A focal figure-of-eight coil is being used to stimulate the motor cortical representation of the first dorsal interosseous (FDI) muscle. The spinal motor neuron pool is activated by the descending volleys induced by TMS. The signal arrives at the muscle, where a motor evoked potential can be recorded with surface electromyography (EMG) from the FDI muscle. (Adapted from Ni Z, Chen R: Electrophysiological and pharmacological mechanisms of TMS and rTMS. p. 11. In Mally J (ed): The Repetitive Transcranial Magnetic Stimulation in the Treatment and Rehabilitation of Central Nervous Diseases. Eurobridge, Budapest, 2009, with permission.)

sufficient intensity activates the descending corticospinal fibers (see Fig. 28-1). A single TMS pulse results in multiple volleys in the corticospinal tract. They activate spinal motor neurons that send volleys in the peripheral nerve to cause a muscle twitch, and the stimulation is recorded as a motor evoked potential (MEP) (see Fig. 28-1). A stronger pulse results in wider and deeper areas of activation in the motor cortex.

TMS Parameters

Different TMS measures are used to evaluate cortical excitability and corticospinal transmission, and they are useful in understanding changes in brain physiology in health and disease. The more common measures are discussed here. The motor threshold refers to the lowest TMS intensity capable of eliciting small MEPs, which are usually defined as more than 50 μV in peak-to-peak amplitude for resting muscles or more than 200 μV in active muscles in at least 5 of 10 trials.[5] Although it is largely independent (in adults) of age, gender, and hemisphere, the motor threshold provides information about the excitability of a central core of neurons in the motor cortex, being lower in the cortical representation of intrinsic hand muscles than of lower limb and trunk muscles.[6] This likely reflects differences in the strength of corticospinal projection and neuronal membrane excitability because it increases with drugs that block voltage-gated sodium channels.[7,8] The recruitment curve, also known as stimulus–response curve, refers to the increase in MEP amplitude (Fig. 28-2) with increasing TMS intensity. Compared to motor threshold, this measure assesses neurons that are intrinsically less excitable or spatially further from the center of activation.

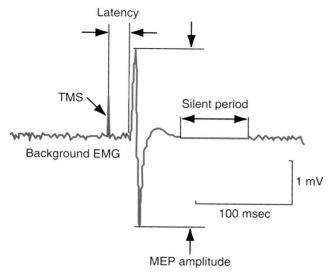

FIGURE 28-2 ▪ Motor evoked potential (MEP) measurements. When transcranial magnetic stimulation (TMS) is delivered during voluntary muscle contraction, an MEP, followed by a silent period, can be recorded. MEP latency is the time from TMS delivery to the onset of MEP, while MEP amplitude usually is measured as the peak-to-peak value but can also be measured as the MEP area. The silent period can be measured from the delivery of TMS, the beginning of the MEP, or the end of MEP to the first recovery of background electromyographic (EMG) activity. (Adapted from Ni Z, Chen R: Electrophysiological and pharmacological mechanisms of TMS and rTMS. p. 13. In Mally J (ed): The Repetitive Transcranial Magnetic Stimulation in the Treatment and Rehabilitation of Central Nervous Diseases. Eurobridge , Budapest, 2009, with permission.)

The slope of the recruitment curve is increased by drugs that increase adrenergic transmission (e.g., dextroamphetamine) and is decreased by sodium and calcium channel blockers (e.g., lamotrigine) and by drugs that enhance the effects of gamma-aminobutyric acid (GABA; e.g., lorazepam).[9] The size of the MEP varies considerably from one stimulus to the next and among individuals.[10]

MEP latency is the time between the delivery of the TMS pulse and the resulting response, and it reflects the conduction time from the cortex to the target muscle (see Fig. 28-2). The conduction time from motor cortex to the motor neuron pool in the spinal cord or brainstem, known as the central motor conduction time (CMCT), can be obtained by subtracting the peripheral conduction time from the MEP latency. A common way[11] to measure CMCT is the F-wave method using the formula

$$\frac{(\text{F-wave latency} + \text{M-wave latency} - 1)}{2}$$

The M wave is the direct muscle response to motor nerve stimulation and the F wave is the muscle response

produced by activation of the alpha motor neuron by the antidromic volley. Electrical or magnetic stimulation of the spine may also be used to establish the peripheral conduction time, especially in proximal muscles where the F-wave method cannot be applied. CMCT usually is measured with the target muscle active, thereby giving the shortest latency from the cortex to the muscle.

Another way to study corticospinal conduction is with the triple-stimulation technique.[10] This is a collision method that synchronizes the response of the motor neurons driven to discharge by the transcranial stimulus, thereby avoiding phase cancellation that accompanies the desynchronization of the biphasic motor unit potentials (Fig. 28-3). Three stimuli are given in sequence and with appropriate delays. The first stimulus is TMS, followed by two supramaximal stimuli given to the nerve supplying the target muscle, first distally then proximally. Thus, only the action potentials elicited initially by TMS descend on the axons of the peripheral nerve and do so in a synchronized manner. Comprehensive descriptions of the technique are available in several publications.[12] It allows precise quantification of central conduction failures caused by reduced excitability or loss of cortical motor neurons and can allow assessment of conduction to muscles other than hand muscles.[12] It is considered two to three times more sensitive than standard TMS procedures to detect corticospinal conduction deficits in patients with central nervous system disorders and is specially suited for the detection and quantification of small changes of central motor conduction.

Stimulating the corticospinal tract at the level of the foramen magnum activates the corticospinal tract at the pyramidal decussation.[13] It produces a single descending volley rather than the multiple volleys from TMS of the motor cortex, and can be used with CMCT to localize a corticospinal tract lesion above or below the foramen magnum.[13]

In addition to testing the corticospinal tract, TMS may be used to investigate the facilitatory and inhibitory mechanisms in the motor cortex. Short-interval intracortical inhibition and intracortical facilitation (ICF) are obtained with paired-pulse studies and reflect interneuron influences in the cortex.[14] In these studies, a conditioning stimulus strong enough to activate cortical neurons but below the threshold for producing descending influence on the spinal cord is applied. A second, suprathreshold test stimulus follows. Intracortical effects produced by the conditioning stimulus modulate the MEP amplitude of the subsequent test stimulus. At interstimulus intervals (ISI) of less than 5 msec, inhibition is produced; facilitation is produced at ISIs of 8 to 30 msec. Short-interval intracortical inhibition likely is mediated largely by $GABA_A$ receptors and can be used to assess

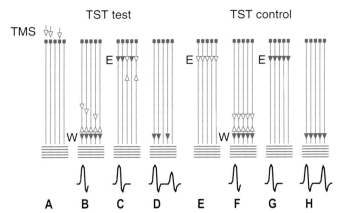

FIGURE 28-3 ■ Principle of the triple-stimulation technique (TST). The motor tract is simplified to five spinal motor neurons and the horizontal lines represent the muscle fibers of the five motor units. Black arrows depict the action potentials that evoke a response (i.e., a trace deflection) and open arrows those that collide. TST test is shown in panels *A* to *D*. **A**, A submaximal transcranial magnetic stimulation (TMS) excites three spinal motor neurons (1, 2, and 4) out of five (large open arrows). **B**, TMS-induced action potentials descend in the axons of these three spinal motor neurons. The three action potentials in axons 1, 2, and 4 are desynchronized. After a delay, a supramaximal stimulus is applied to the peripheral nerve close to the target muscle (W, wrist). The orthodromic wave gives rise to a first negative deflection of the electromyographic trace. The antidromic action potentials collide with the descending action potentials on motor axons 1, 2, and 4. **C**, The action potentials on axons 3 and 5 continue to ascend. After a second delay, a supramaximal stimulus is applied to the proximal nerve, close to the spinal motor neuron (Erb's point, E). In axons 3 and 5, the descending action potentials collide with the ascending action potentials. **D**, A synchronized response from the three motor neurons that initially were excited by TMS is recorded as the second deflection of the TST test trace. TST control is shown in panels *E* to *H*. **E**, A supramaximal stimulus is applied at Erb's point. **F**, After a delay, a supramaximal stimulus applied at the wrist is recorded as the first deflection of the TST control trace. **G**, After another delay, a second supramaximal stimulus is applied at Erb's point. **H**, A synchronized response from the five motor axons is recorded as the second deflection of the TST control trace. The test response is quantified as the ratio of second deflection of the TST test (in *D*) to TST control (in *H*). (Adapted from Chen R, Cros D, Curra A et al: The clinical diagnostic utility of transcranial magnetic stimulation: report of an IFCN committee. Clin Neurophysiol, 119:504, 2008, with permission.)

changes in cortical excitability.[15] ICF may be mediated partly by glutamate.[16]

Long-interval intracortical inhibition is another measure of intracortical inhibition elicited by suprathreshold conditioning and test stimuli at ISIs of 50 to 200 msec.[17]

It likely shares mechanisms with the suppression of voluntary muscle contraction induced by a single suprathreshold TMS pulse known as the silent period.[17] The silent period is a pause in ongoing voluntary EMG activity produced by TMS as a result of spinal cord refractoriness and cortical inhibition (see Fig. 28-2). This type of inhibition appears to be mediated by $GABA_B$ receptors and is modulated by sleep deprivation, muscle fatigue, and repetitive TMS (rTMS).[18,19]

Interhemispheric or transcallosal inhibition induced by motor cortex stimulation can be assessed by the ipsilateral silent period, which refers to interruption of ongoing EMG activities in ipsilateral muscles.[20] Since the ipsilateral silent period is absent or delayed in patients with congenital, acquired, or surgical lesions of the corpus callosum,[20] it is likely due to transcallosal inhibition. Interhemispheric callosal connections can also be studied by a paired-pulse paradigm, with conditioning stimuli over one hemisphere and test stimuli over the opposite hemisphere.[21] Interhemispheric inhibition is produced at ISIs of 8 to 50 msec.[22] Cerebellar TMS suppresses the contralateral motor cortex at ISIs of 5 to 8 msec.[23] The effect was absent in patients with degeneration of the cerebellar cortex or lesions in the cerebellothalamocortical pathway.[24]

Short- and long-latency afferent inhibition refers to effects on cortical excitability produced at latencies of about 20 msec and 200 msec, respectively, after somatosensory stimulation of the hand.[25] Selective blockage by scopolamine suggests that muscarinic cholinergic transmission is involved in mediating short-latency afferent inhibition.

Stimulation Protocols

TMS may be applied as single-pulse TMS, paired-pulse TMS, or repetitively (rTMS). Physiologic effects of rTMS depend on a number of factors such as coil geometry, stimulation site, intensity, frequency, duration of stimulation, and the number of stimulation sessions. rTMS can produce powerful effects that outlast the period of stimulation, producing cortical inhibition with stimulation at low frequencies (1 Hz or lower),[26] and cortical excitation with stimulation at high frequencies (5 Hz or higher).[27] New rTMS approaches include high-frequency bursts of stimuli at theta frequencies (5 Hz), termed theta burst stimulation (TBS).[28] The temporal pattern of the bursts determines whether the protocols are facilitatory (intermittent TBS; iTBS) or inhibitory (continuous TBS; cTBS).[28] Another type of TMS, quadripulse stimulation, consists of four monophasic pulses of the same intensity separated by 1.5 msec, repeatedly given at 0.2 Hz. Quadripulse stimulation induces long-lasting, locally restricted facilitation of motor cortical excitability for up to 75 minutes without affecting the motor thresholds. It thus holds promise for inducing plastic changes in the brain. Since conventional rTMS methods are not able to activate deep brain regions effectively, combining rTMS with the H-coil may help to stimulate deeper brain structures.

Safety Considerations

Overall, single- or paired-pulse TMS is considered safe. The magnetic field generated by TMS may interact with selected metals in cranial implants. The contraindications for single- and paired-pulse TMS are similar to those of magnetic resonance imaging (MRI) and mainly involve the presence of intracranial ferromagnetic material such as aneurysm clips. Some titanium implants are not magnetic and may prove safe for TMS exposure. Removal of glasses, watches, jewelry, and other magnetically reactive accessories is advised. Cardiac pacemakers are considered safe, according to the most recent safety guideline.[29] In patients with implanted electrodes for deep brain stimulation, single- and paired-pulse TMS has been applied safely when the TMS coil is not in close proximity to the implanted pulse generator.[29] Epilepsy may be considered a relative contraindication; the risk of inducing a seizure with single- or paired-pulse TMS is low.[30]

For rTMS, seizure is the most serious acute adverse event, although the overall risk is still low. Since seizures generally are associated with prolonged trains of high-frequency rTMS at high intensities, safety guidelines to limit rTMS stimulation parameters have been published to minimize this risk.[30] Since their publication, the occurrences of seizures with rTMS are related mostly to rTMS parameters exceeding the guidelines, patients treated with drugs that potentially lower seizure threshold, or patients with neurologic disorders known to increase the risk for seizure.[29] Electrode heating or burns when rTMS is administered in patients with scalp electroencephalographic (EEG) electrodes have been reported.[31] The use of low-conductivity plastic and radial notching of electrodes can reduce heating.

Rapid mechanical deformation of the TMS stimulating coil when it is energized produces an intense, broad-band acoustic artifact that may exceed 140 dB of sound pressure level,[32] carrying a potential for hearing damage. The majority of studies in which hearing protection was used report no change in hearing after TMS; hearing protection with ear plugs is recommended.[29] The most common side-effect of TMS is pain.

The intensity of pain experienced varies depending on individual susceptibility, scalp location, coil design, intensity, and frequency of stimulation. Patients and subjects should be warned that TMS, especially rTMS, may not be pleasant and may cause pain; the pain has not been reported to persist for more than a few days.[33]

CLINICAL UTILITY IN NEUROLOGIC DISEASES

TMS can play a significant role as a diagnostic tool. Several TMS measures are promising in the evaluation of myelopathy, amyotrophic lateral sclerosis (ALS), and multiple sclerosis (MS), and others have potential utility in various contexts.[34] The use of TMS has also been explored for intraoperative monitoring (see Chapter 30).

Plasticity, which can be defined as any experience-dependent enduring change in neuronal or network properties, either morphologic or functional,[35] is one of the bases for employing TMS as a therapeutic tool. It is an exciting avenue to explore, as TMS is believed to induce lasting changes in cortical excitability and thus enable functionally significant changes in patients with a large variety of neurologic and psychiatric conditions. The variability in neurophysiologic and behavioral responses to such brain stimulation techniques is high and may limit the therapeutic usefulness of the technique. Factors such as priming, prior voluntary motor activity, parallel voluntary motor activity, age, attention, sex, and pharmacologic influences are thought to contribute to the variability in response, and understanding these determinants is crucial in optimizing therapeutic applications.[36]

Myelopathy

Compressive myelopathy is a good indication for central motor conduction studies. A large study found that upper- and lower-limb CMCT correlated with the severity of cord compression on MRI in patients with myelopathy.[37] In addition, the specificity of using TMS in differentiating between the presence and absence of MRI cord abnormality was 84.8 percent and the sensitivity was 100 percent. TMS may also detect incipient cord compression prior to the development of clinical or radiologic signs. In patients with cervical spondylosis but no clear clinical evidence of a myelopathy, CMCT was abnormal.[38] CMCT findings also correlated with clinical findings better than MRI and localized the affected cervical spinal segments more precisely.[39] Finally, TMS may be used to differentiate myelopathy with radiculopathy from ALS, both of which may have upper and lower motor neuron involvement. Abnormal CMCT to

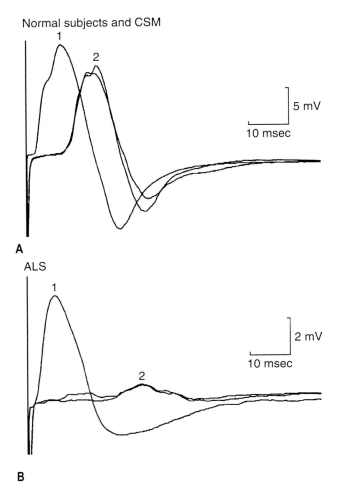

Normal subjects and CSM

A

ALS

B

FIGURE 28-4 ▪ Trapezius muscle recordings as observed in **A**, normal subjects and patients with cervical spondylotic myelopathy (CSM), and **B**, amyotrophic lateral sclerosis (ALS) patients. (1) CMAPs obtained by electrical stimulation of the accessory nerve at the neck. (2) Trapezius motor evoked potentials obtained by transcranial magnetic stimulation (two curves superimposed). (Adapted from Truffert A, Rosler KM, Magistris MR: Amyotrophic lateral sclerosis versus cervical spondylotic myelopathy: a study using transcranial magnetic stimulation with recordings from the trapezius and limb muscles. Clin Neurophysiol, 111:1031, 2000, with permission.)

muscles innervated by nerves emerging above the foramen magnum, such as the trapezius[40] (Fig. 28-4) or the tongue, would be more indicative of ALS than myelopathy.

Amyotrophic Lateral Sclerosis

DIAGNOSTIC UTILITY OF TMS

Several groups have used TMS to investigate patients with motor neuron disease for subclinical upper motor neuron (UMN) dysfunction. An abnormal CMCT,

mostly prolonged, representing subclinical UMN involvement was reported to occur in most ALS patients examined.[41] Prolonged MEP latencies were noted in several ALS patients as well.[42] The sensitivity of TMS for UMN dysfunction in motor neuron disease may improve with the choice of target muscle, as it increased when conduction to orofacial muscles was combined with more conventional muscle recordings,[43] or with use of the triple-stimulation technique.[44,45] To improve specificity, MEPs from the trapezius muscles can be recorded to distinguish from the possible pathophysiologic effects of cervical spondylosis (see Fig. 28-4).[40] In addition, preferential cortical control of the thenar eminence muscles compared to the hypothenar muscles in ALS patients can improve specificity.[46] Changes in motor threshold did not reveal consistent results.[41] In patients with clinically definite ALS, the sensitivity of TMS approached 100 percent in one study.[42] The sensitivity of combining abnormal CMCT and MEP amplitude was only about 50 percent in ALS patients without definite UMN signs.[47] Addition of parameters such as motor threshold and the silent period may yield a higher degree of sensitivity in patients with motor neuron disease and only probable UMN signs (ALS-PUMNS).[48,49] A combination of TMS parameters that include CMCT, triple-stimulation technique, motor threshold, silent period, and short-interval intracortical inhibition is useful in the diagnosis of ALS.[34]

THERAPEUTIC ROLE OF TMS

In a double-blind, placebo-controlled study, bilateral continuous theta-burst stimulation (cTBS) delivered over the primary motor cortex 5 days per week over 6 months reduced the deterioration rate in patients with ALS.[50] Similar results were reported after several cycles of 1-Hz rTMS over the primary motor cortex in ALS.[51] However, a more recent, larger, double-blind, placebo-controlled trial with 5 days of cTBS per week over 12 months found no beneficial effects on the progression of ALS.[52] These results do not exclude the potential efficacy of different protocols of motor cortex stimulation, particularly during the early stages of the disease, as these studies were undertaken in ALS patients with advanced disease.

Stroke and Rehabilitation

DIAGNOSTIC AND PROGNOSTIC ROLE OF TMS

In the acute stage of stroke, the presence of an MEP in the paralyzed limb is a good prognostic sign.[53] Conversely, the absence of the MEP in this situation can be a poor prognostic sign.[54] The presence of ipsilateral

MEPs in the paretic limb from stimulation of the unaffected hemisphere usually is associated with poor recovery.[55] In a chronically paretic limb, MEP presence predicted meaningful gains in stroke patients receiving motor rehabilitation.[56]

TMS cortical motor maps can be used to demonstrate spatial cortical reorganization after stroke rehabilitation. Both mediolateral and anteroposterior shifts in motor cortex representation of the affected limbs correlate with the motor outcome following neurorehabilitation.[57] In addition, improvement in motor performance after constraint-induced movement therapy correlates with enlargement in TMS motor cortical map[58] and with changes in cortical excitability in the lesioned hemisphere.[59]

THERAPEUTIC ROLE OF TMS

The basis for using TMS in stroke rehabilitation is its potential to modulate cortical excitability and plasticity through both high-frequency rTMS (increasing cortical excitability) and low-frequency rTMS (decreasing cortical excitability). In a randomized, sham-controlled study, 3-Hz rTMS to the lesioned motor cortex daily for 10 days in patients with acute ischemic stroke improved disability scores.[60] This effect persisted for at least 10 days after stimulation. In a study involving chronic hemiparetic stroke patients, 10-Hz rTMS enhanced corticomotor excitability and motor performance accuracy on a sequential finger motor task using the paretic hand.[61] Stronger and asymmetric transcallosal inhibition after stroke may lead to reduced activity in the affected hemisphere concomitant with increased activity of the unaffected hemisphere.[62] The magnitude of this inhibition correlated negatively with hand function.[63] Thus, another therapeutic approach is to decrease excitability on the contralesional side. One study found that 1-Hz rTMS reduced the amplitude of MEPs in the contralesional hand, decreased the duration of interhemispheric inhibition, and induced an improvement in pinch acceleration of the affected hand.[64] rTMS likely reduced activity in the inhibitory projections from contralesional to ipsilesional motor cortex, releasing the injured motor cortex and improving its function. Similar positive results were noted in a cross-over, sham-controlled study of ten stroke patients.[65] In a randomized, sham-controlled study in children with subcortical stroke, 1-Hz rTMS for 8 days to the contralesional motor cortex improved function of the affected hand.[66]

Although the majority of studies have focused on chronic stroke, inhibitory rTMS over M1 of the unaffected hemisphere may also be effective in acute stroke patients (less than 6 months after stroke). In one case, inhibitory (1-Hz) rTMS over M1 of the unaffected (contralesional) hemisphere applied repetitively over 5 to 8 days revealed beneficial effects on motor function of the affected hand that lasted for at least 1 week.[67] In patients with strokes 1 to 4 months prior to the intervention, one session of inhibitory rTMS over the contralesional M1 was associated with behavioral improvement of the affected hand immediately after the intervention.[68] A placebo-controlled, double-blinded crossover trial of rTMS in patients who suffered a recent stroke (less than 14 days prior to the intervention) demonstrated significant improvement in dexterity in the paretic hand after a single session of 1-Hz rTMS over the contralesional hemisphere.[69] These findings suggest that therapeutic rTMS could become part of a neurorehabilitative therapy. At present, both inhibitory and facilitatory brain-stimulation techniques have been applied to patients suffering from mild to moderate impairments of hand function after stroke. It is not known if these techniques can improve more severe motor deficits. Despite the overall small number of patients investigated, consistent findings across independent groups suggest that inhibition of contralesional M1 and increasing cortical excitability of ipsilesional M1 may help improve recovery of function of the affected hand after stroke.

A limited number of trials have used facilitatory rTMS to improve language functions in chronic aphasia. Martin and colleagues studied patients with nonfluent aphasia from a stroke that had occurred 6 or more months earlier; 1-Hz rTMS for 2 weeks, applied to the right pars triangularis, a subregion of Broca's area, improved naming at 2 and 8 months of follow-up.[70]

Cognitive Disorders

DIAGNOSTIC AND PATHOPHYSIOLOGIC ASPECTS

Likely related to the cholinergic deficits, TMS studies show that short-latency afferent inhibition is decreased in about 70 percent of patients with Alzheimer disease,[71] but is normal in frontotemporal dementia[72] and mild cognitive impairment (MCI).[73] Abnormality of such inhibition has also been reported in dementia with Lewy bodies,[74] a form of dementia that responds to cholinergic medications. In Alzheimer disease, the increase in short-latency afferent inhibition after a single dose of rivastigmine correlated with favorable changes in cognitive function after treatment for 1 year.[71] This parameter may thus provide diagnostic, therapeutic, and prognostic guidance as a pathophysiologic biomarker for managing dementia patients.

Use of rTMS to Improve Cognitive Deficits

Cognitive deficits are common consequences of traumatic brain injury, stroke, and neurodegenerative disorders. Brain stimulation may provide exciting opportunities for cognitive neurorehabilitation. Improvement in picture naming was observed after bilateral rTMS of the dorsolateral prefrontal cortex in patients with Alzheimer disease.[75] Interestingly, action naming was improved but there was no effect on object naming. In another study, the same group evaluated the effect of rTMS in patients with Alzheimer disease with different degrees of cognitive decline and found improved naming accuracy for both classes of stimuli (actions and objects) in the moderate-to-severe group.[76] The amelioration was short-lived, lasting only for minutes, and although the effect size on action naming was quite robust, the reasons for the discrepancy in action and object naming remain unclear. Because of the short-lived effect, the method may not be suitable as a neurorehabilitation intervention, but is a promising method of patient selection for possible routes of neurorehabilitation. Based on preliminary, small studies, it has been suggested that application of low-frequency rTMS over the right homolog of Broca's area may result in an improved ability to name pictures.[77]

TMS has been used in patients with extinction. Single- and paired-pulse parietal TMS in patients with right brain damage reduced the amount of extinction.[78] High-frequency rTMS over the unaffected parietal cortex in patients with neglect reduced contralateral neglect, but the improvement was short-lived.[79] Patients with unilateral visual neglect have experienced a significant improvement in visuospatial performance that persisted for 15 days after low-frequency rTMS stimulation of the unlesioned cortex.[80] Overall, these results suggest that the hemispheric imbalance due to unilateral brain damage can be diminished by inhibitory stimulation of the unaffected hemisphere, thereby downregulating attentional imbalance in patients with hemispatial neglect. Despite the positive results, these studies should be considered preliminary because they are small, open-labeled, and lacking controls or sham stimulation.

In a randomized, double-blind, sham-controlled study in normal elderly subjects, high-frequency rTMS trains over the prefrontal cortex bilaterally produced improvement in recognition accuracy in an associative memory task.[81] Patients with cerebrovascular disease and mild executive dysfunction had improved executive functioning after high-frequency rTMS of the left prefrontal cortex.[82]

Clinical trials investigating the effects of TMS on cognition have also been carried out in patients with depression as a primary condition or associated with Parkinson disease or stroke. A trend has been found toward cognitive improvement in patients with post-stroke depression when stimulated over the left prefrontal cortex.[83] Overall, high-frequency rTMS (10 to 20 Hz) seems most likely to cause significant cognitive improvement when applied over the left dorsolateral prefrontal cortex, in a range of 10 to 15 successive sessions. Many studies, however, have failed to demonstrate significant cognitive effects but show trends toward selective cognitive improvements. Based on the currently available evidence, the use of TMS to improve cognitive function is unclear and requires further investigation.

Epilepsy

Diagnostic and Pathophysiologic Aspects

Enhanced cortical excitability may be the pathophysiologic substrate of epilepsies and underlie the tendency to develop seizures. By assessing cortical excitability, TMS can give information regarding mechanisms for the genesis of epileptic seizures. Motor threshold is decreased in untreated patients with idiopathic generalized epilepsy.[84] Different classes of antiepileptic drugs have different effects on various cortical circuits activated by TMS. For example, vigabatrin and gabapentin increase intracortical inhibition while carbamazepine, lamotrigine, and phenytoin, which block sodium and calcium channels, elevate the motor threshold.[85] Potentially, TMS can be used to quantify physiologic effects of antiepileptics or implanted brain stimulators in patients with epilepsy.[86]

Therapeutic Role of TMS

Diminished cortical excitability produced by rTMS has been studied as an adjunctive therapy for epilepsy. In the first open-label study, Tergau and colleagues explored the impact of low-frequency rTMS (0.3 Hz) applied for 5 consecutive days on seizure frequency in patients with focal, pharmacoresistant epilepsy.[87] The reduction in the number of epileptic seizures was still prominent 4 weeks after the intervention. Several open-label studies showed a reduction of focal seizure frequency by rTMS with stimulation frequencies of 1 Hz or lower.[88,89] Of three randomized, double-blinded, sham-controlled studies investigating the benefits of rTMS in epilepsy, only one showed a significant reduction of seizure frequency and interictal discharges.[90] In another study, a trend for a reduction of epileptic seizures was found,[91] and in the third study, only significantly reduced epileptiform discharges were documented.[92] Overall, the results suggest a variable efficacy of rTMS in reducing epileptic discharges and in improving the clinical state.

The treatment protocols differed in terms of focality of stimulation, location of stimulation (the epileptogenic zone or the vertex), stimulation intensity, and stimulus frequency, as well as etiology of epilepsy and antiepileptic medications used. No clear picture emerges in terms of which stimulation protocol might be optimal and which patients benefit most from stimulation. Moreover, most studies included pharmacoresistant patients, which may underestimate efficacy. Protocol-optimizing studies and therapeutic studies conducted in a sham-controlled, randomized, double-blinded fashion are required.

Movement Disorders

DIAGNOSTIC STUDIES IN PARKINSONIAN DISORDERS

In Parkinson disease, abnormal cortical excitability has been found with TMS. Most studies found no change in motor threshold or CMCT. However, the silent period is shortened and can be normalized with dopaminergic medication.[93,94] Short-interval intracortical inhibition[95] and presynaptic inhibition,[96] as well as afferent inhibition,[25] are impaired in Parkinson disease.

CMCT is normal in Parkinson disease and corticobasal degeneration, but can be prolonged in patients with multiple system atrophy and progressive supranuclear palsy.[97,98] Therefore, TMS may have a role in demonstrating CMCT abnormalities in patients with parkinsonism-plus syndromes in whom pyramidal signs are equivocal. In patients with parkinsonism, the ipsilateral silent period was abnormal in patients with corticobasal degeneration and progressive supranuclear palsy, and the finding correlated with atrophy of the corpus callosum on MRI, but it was intact in all patients with Parkinson disease and multiple system atrophy.[99,100] Therefore, measurements of the ipsilateral silent period may be useful clinically to differentiate parkinsonian syndromes.

THERAPEUTIC ROLE OF rTMS IN PARKINSON DISEASE

Early studies suggested an improvement in pointing performance and on the Unified Parkinson Disease Rating Scale (UPDRS) after rTMS to the motor cortex.[101] Subthreshold rTMS applied to the motor cortex at both 0.5 Hz and 10 Hz improved motor performance.[102] However, such changes lasted only for minutes. A long-lasting effect of rTMS may be obtained with repeated application over a period of days. In a randomized study, patients receiving 5-Hz rTMS to the motor cortex experienced improvements in the UPDRS motor scores, walking speed, and a self-assessment scale that persisted for over 1 month.[103] In a double-blind, placebo-controlled study, rTMS over 4 weeks using four cortical targets (left and right motor and dorsolateral prefrontal cortex) in each session showed a therapeutic effect that lasted for at least 1 month after treatment ended.[104]

Among such studies, the rTMS parameters such as site of stimulation, stimulation frequencies, and treatment duration varied widely. The most common sites studied are the motor cortex and the dorsolateral prefrontal cortex, which correspond to cortical targets of motor and prefrontal basal ganglia–thalamic loops.[105] Recent systematic reviews of the randomized controlled trials of rTMS in Parkinson disease found that high-frequency rTMS led to a significant improvement in UPDRS scores (Fig. 28-5).[106,107] However, because of the small number of patients in each study and the variability in the patients studied and the rTMS protocols used, the results should be interpreted with caution.[106] Future studies are needed to clarify the optimal stimulation parameters and a large, randomized, blinded, placebo-controlled trial is needed to further define its role in the treatment of Parkinson disease.

Low-frequency rTMS (less than 1 Hz) studies, by contrast, showed no significant reduction in motor UPDRS

FIGURE 28-5 ▪ Individual and pooled effect size for motor part of Unified Parkinson Disease Rating Scale (UPDRS) in patients with Parkinson disease treated with high-frequency repetitive transcranial magnetic stimulation (rTMS). The size of the squares increases with increasing sample size. There was an overall benefit with reduction of UPDRS scores with high-frequency rTMS. (Adapted from Elahi B, Elahi B, Chen R: Effect of transcranial magnetic stimulation on Parkinson motor function—systematic review of controlled clinical trials. Mov Disord, 24:357, 2009, with permission.)

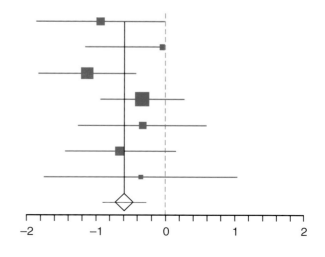

but may be a potential treatment for levodopa-induced dyskinesias.[106] A single session of rTMS at 1 Hz to the supplementary motor area bilaterally lowered the severity of dyskinesias for 30 minutes after stimulation.[108] Repeated administration of 1-Hz rTMS of the motor cortex[109,110] and cTBS to the cerebellum[111] have shown promise also as potential treatment for levodopa-induced dyskinesias.

DYSTONIA

Primary dystonia occurs in the absence of other neurologic abnormalities, generalized dystonia can involve the whole body, and focal dystonia involves abnormal muscle contractions restricted to one part of the body. Physiologic studies in dystonia reveal a decrease in short and long intracortical inhibition.[112,113]

Low-frequency rTMS has been used to induce an increase in inhibition and thus treat dystonia. Normalization of intracortical inhibition was noted with 1-Hz rTMS of the motor cortex,[114] and 1-Hz rTMS of the premotor cortex ameliorated the deficit in reciprocal inhibition in dystonia.[115] Two controlled studies found improvement in handwriting in writer's cramp with low-frequency rTMS over the motor or premotor cortex.[114,116] A recent randomized control study found promising results with low-frequency rTMS over the anterior cingulate cortex in benign essential blepharospasm.[117] Therefore, preliminary studies have suggested that low-frequency rTMS may be a promising method to treat dystonia.

Cerebellar Disorders

Inhibition of the motor cortex from cerebellar stimulation is reduced in patients with cerebellar ataxia,[24,118] whereas normal suppression of the motor cortex is elicited in patients with noncerebellar ataxia. Increase in short-interval intracortical inhibition and reduction of intracortical facilitation is also observed in patients with cerebellar stroke in the superior or the inferior cerebellar artery territories.[119] These results are consistent with the effects of cerebellar stimulation on short- and long-interval intracortical inhibition in normal subjects.[120] Several studies reported increased short-interval intracortical inhibition and reduced intracortical facilitation in cerebellar ataxia.[121,122] Interestingly, different genetic defects may result in different patterns of TMS abnormalities. For example, reduced intracortical facilitation in inherited spinocerebellar ataxia (SCA) may be more specific for SCA2 and SCA3.[123] Similarly, CMCT may be prolonged in patients with Friedreich ataxia[124] and SCA types 1,

2,[125] and 6.[126] Although there is preliminary evidence for abnormal TMS parameters in cerebellar dysfunction, currently there is limited clinical applicability of the technique.

Multiple Sclerosis

PATHOPHYSIOLOGIC AND DIAGNOSTIC ROLE

Demyelinating injury to the corticospinal tract can be measured by CMCT delays. The first notable use of CMCT in demyelinating injury was in MS. Several studies showed a high yield of abnormalities, even in patients without clinical evidence of corticospinal tract involvement, but the probability of an abnormality varies with the choice of tested muscles.[127,128] The sensitivity of detecting corticospinal involvement improves if lower-limb muscles are assessed.[127,129] When combined with other tests, such as sensory evoked potentials and MRI, TMS studies still showed added value.[128]

Most studies indicate a significant correlation between CMCT abnormalities and clinical motor signs or motor disability.[130,131] In fact, a multimodal evoked potential score including CMCT measurements and changes was found to predict the Expanded Disability Status Scale (EDSS) of patients with clinically definite MS 6 to 24 months later.[132,133] A strong correlation was found between EDSS scores and a composite TMS index (CMCT plus ipsilateral silent period duration) in a large series of patients.[134] Prolongation of CMCT is more pronounced in progressive than relapsing-remitting MS.[130,135] CMCT and the triple-stimulation technique are considered to have demonstrated utility in the diagnosis of MS.[34]

THERAPEUTIC ROLE OF TMS

In MS, spasticity likely is caused by hyperexcitability of the stretch reflex arc secondary to lesions of the corticospinal tract. In a double-blind, placebo-controlled study, twice daily sessions of high-frequency rTMS (25 Hz) for 7 consecutive days in MS patients significantly improved self-scoring of ease of everyday activities and clinical spasticity scores, while the stretch reflex threshold increased.[136] In a subsequent study, high-frequency rTMS (25 Hz) over the leg motor area of MS patients with lower-limb spasticity induced a decrease of the soleus muscle H-reflex amplitude.[137] There is thus some preliminary evidence that rTMS can benefit MS patients with spasticity, but further rigorous studies are required to determine optimal protocols, efficacy, and duration of effects.

Migraine

Migraine can be a disabling illness that presents with episodic attacks. The migraine aura is thought to have cortical spreading depression (CSD) as a physiologic substrate, most commonly in the occipital cortex, leading to a visual aura. TMS studies have reported a reduction in phosphene threshold in migraineurs and a threshold increase with prophylactic migraine medications.[138]

A pilot study that randomized migraineurs to either high- or low-intensity paired-pulse TMS over the area of perceived pain during a migraine found a 75 percent decrease in pain intensity from baseline measures. In addition, all patients with aura achieved pain relief with TMS.[139] This study was followed by a multicentered, sham-controlled trial which showed that two TMS pulses applied to the occiput as soon as possible after the beginning of an aura produced significantly higher pain-free rates in the treatment group 2 hours after intervention.[140] For migraine prophylaxis, a small pilot study that used high-frequency rTMS over the left dorsolateral prefrontal cortex showed a significant reduction in migraine.[141] A 5-day course of low-frequency (1 Hz) rTMS over the vertex was associated with decreased frequency of migraine attacks compared to baseline but was not effective when compared with placebo.[142] The efficacy of TMS in the acute treatment of migraine without aura has not been studied rigorously. For rTMS, adequately blinded and powered studies for migraine prevention have not been reported. Further research is warranted.

Chronic Pain

TMS may have a role in the management of chronic pain. The commonest stimulation site is the motor cortex. Although single-pulse TMS could provide some pain relief,[143] the effects were too transient to be an effective treatment. By contrast, rTMS provides longer-lasting pain relief and is most effective when stimulation is more focal, applied at a high rate (greater than 5 Hz), of long duration (at least 1,000 pulses), and applied over repeated sessions.[144] A meta-analysis showed rTMS of the motor cortex is effective in reducing pain and may be more effective in treating centrally than peripherally originated neuropathic pain (Fig. 28-6).[145] Regions other than the motor cortex have been targeted with rTMS and led to amelioration of specific types of pain. For example, 1-Hz rTMS over the right somatosensory cortex improved visceral pain in five patients with chronic pancreatitis.[146] Several studies found rTMS to be predictive

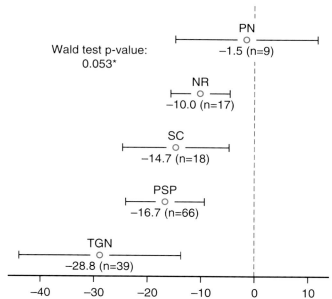

FIGURE 28-6 ■ Diagnosis and treatment effect of repetitive transcranial magnetic stimulation in neuropathic pain. Mean changes (95 percent confidence interval) in percentage of pain based on visual analog scale (VAS) are shown. P value is from the Wald test for the interaction effect of diagnosis and treatment on the percentage change in VAS score. NR, nerve root; PN, peripheral nerve; PSP, post-stroke supraspinal related pain; SC, spinal cord; TGN, trigeminal nerve or ganglion. (Adapted from Leung A, Donohue M, Ronghui X et al: rTMS for suppressing neuropathic pain: a meta-analysis. J Pain, 10:1205, 2009, with permission.)

of the outcome of subsequent chronic epidural stimulation; a positive response to rTMS (pain score decrease of more than 30 to 40 percent) was highly associated with a good outcome at long-term follow-up.[147] To summarize, rTMS can provide significant analgesic effects, but their short duration is a limitation at this time for its application in routine therapeutic practice. Adequately powered studies investigating the long-lasting effects of rTMS would be an appropriate next step in investigating clinical potential in chronic pain management.

Facial Nerve Disorders

In all cases of Bell palsy, there is a greatly diminished (or absent) response to canalicular stimulation from the time of symptom onset to several months later, even when clinical function of the nerve and the response to cortical stimulation are preserved or restored.[148] Figure 28-7 describes the principles of canalicular stimulation with TMS.[34] Focal hypoexcitability of the facial nerve to TMS may thus exist independently of the state of clinical function of the nerve. A bilaterally abnormal response is

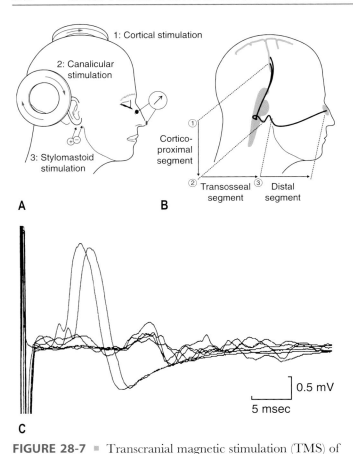

FIGURE 28-7 ■ Transcranial magnetic stimulation (TMS) of the facial nerve and facial representation of the motor cortex. **A**, Placement of the stimulating coil and recording electrodes. (1) Stimulation of the facial representation of the motor cortex is performed over the opposite hemisphere. (2) For canalicular stimulation of the facial nerve, the magnetic coil is placed over the parieto-occipital region (bottom of the coil being over the mastoid). (3) Stylomastoid electrical stimulation is performed in the region of the stylomastoid foramen. Recording may be made from any facial muscle. Recording here is from the nasalis muscle, with the inactive electrode placed on the tip of the nose to reduce volume-conducted activity from other facial muscles. **B**, Three segments of the pathway, as delineated by the stimulation sites. **C**, Examples of normal responses to TMS in facial muscles and superimposed recordings from the nasalis muscle. The first deflection is the response to stylomastoid electrical stimulation. The second deflection is the TMS response evoked by "canalicular" stimulation, of similar size and configuration as the response to stylomastoid electrical stimulation. The third response (superimposition of five successive trials) is the TMS response to cortical stimulation performed during slight voluntary contraction of the nasalis muscle. Latencies are measured to take-off of the negative deflection. Amplitudes are measured from baseline to the negative peak of the compound motor action potential and motor evoked potential. Note that in this normal subject the responses are reproducible but rather small (their average amplitude being 17 percent of the response to stylomastoid stimulation). (Adapted from Chen R, Cros D, Curra A et al: The clinical diagnostic utility of transcranial magnetic stimulation: report of an IFCN committee. Clin Neurophysiol, 119:504, 2008, with permission.)

strongly suggestive of certain etiologies, in particular polyradiculoneuropathy in disorders such as Lyme disease, sarcoidosis, Guillain–Barré syndrome, and human immunodeficiency virus infection.[149] An increase in the transosseal conduction time, as well as a simultaneous slowing of conduction on the distal segment with desynchronization of the response, is characteristic of demyelinating neuropathies such as in Guillain–Barré syndrome, even without accompanying facial weakness.[149] The addition of TMS to conventional electrical stimulation of the facial nerve may help to localize the dysfunction of the nerve along its course and may contribute to identifying the etiology of peripheral facial nerve palsies. Moreover, since it can detect changes in excitability and conduction deficits that do not depend on Wallerian degeneration, TMS can be used immediately after the occurrence of facial nerve palsy.

Tinnitus

An increasing number of rTMS studies on tinnitus have been published and reviews are available.[150] It is likely that tinnitus suppression by rTMS depends on a complex interplay between patient characteristics and stimulation parameters. Most studies applied low-frequency rTMS repeatedly over 5 to 10 days and beneficial clinical effects were observed in about 50 percent of treated subjects.[151,152] Although stimulation parameters varied, the stimulation targets were fairly uniform, mostly temporal or temporoparietal cortex, either on the left side independently of tinnitus laterality or based on individual functional imaging results.[153] By using rTMS in combination with electrophysiologic and neuroimaging methods, further studies should aim to identify optimal cortical stimulation targets and parameters.

The potential of rTMS as a prognostic instrument has been investigated. Patients responding positively to high-frequency rTMS were good surgical candidates for permanent electrical stimulation of the auditory cortex.[154] Thus, high-frequency rTMS may be used as a screening method for implantation of cortical electrodes.

Psychiatric Disorders

The most extensive therapeutic use of rTMS is for depression. In 2008, the United States Food and Drug Administration (FDA) approved rTMS for treatment of medication-resistant depression and regulatory approval for this indication is available in several other countries, including Israel and Canada. It has also been studied in patients with schizophrenia, mania, bipolar disease, and obsessive-compulsive disorder. However, the use of TMS in psychiatry is beyond the scope of this chapter and will not be considered further.

CONCLUDING COMMENTS

TMS has undergone significant developments in recent years. While in the therapeutic realm rTMS most notably has been approved as a clinical tool for treatment-resistant depression, rTMS also holds promise for therapeutic use in neurologic disorders through its ability to modulate excitatory and inhibitory mechanisms in disease. Functional recovery after stroke, cognitive rehabilitation, cortical excitation modulation in epilepsy, movement disorder management, migraine, and pain relief, as well as psychiatric disorders such as schizophrenia and mania, are among the settings and conditions likely to have TMS join their arsenal of management options in the future. The diagnostic and evaluation capabilities of TMS are reflected in the technique's ability to detect physiologic abnormalities. MEP changes are sensitive but not specific in a variety of neurologic disorders, but other parameters such as CMCT and the silent period can help to differentiate movement disorders with parkinsonism and combine with other TMS measures to offer diagnostic clues, not only for demyelinating and UMN diseases, but also for myelopathy and cerebellar disorders. Undoubtedly, TMS will continue to develop into a means to investigate and manage neurologic conditions. Recently developed TMS methodologies, combining TMS with other neurophysiologic investigations such as MRI and EEG, and rigorous trials establishing the effectiveness of TMS as a diagnostic and therapeutic tool in neurologic and psychiatric disorders are promising new directions.

REFERENCES

1. Barker AT, Jalinous R, Freeston IL: Non-invasive stimulation of the human motor cortex. Lancet, II:1106, 1985
2. Amassian VE, Eberle L, Maccabee PJ et al: Modelling magnetic coil excitation of human cerebral cortex with a peripheral nerve immersed in a brain-shaped volume conductor: the significance of fiber bending in excitation. Electroencephalogr Clin Neurophysiol, 85:291, 1992
3. Davey K, Epstein CM, George MS et al: Modeling the effects of electrical conductivity of the head on the induced electric field in the brain during magnetic stimulation. Clin Neurophysiol, 114:2204, 2003
4. Zangen A, Roth Y, Voller B et al: Transcranial magnetic stimulation of deep brain regions: evidence for efficacy of the H-coil. Clin Neurophysiol, 116:775, 2005
5. Rossini PM, Barker AT, Berardelli A et al: Non-invasive electrical and magnetic stimulation of the brain, spinal cord and roots: basic principles and procedures for routine clinical application. Report of an IFCN committe. Electroencephalogr Clin Neurophysiol, 91:79, 1994
6. Chen R, Tam A, Bütefisch C et al: Intracortical inhibition and facilitation in different representations of the human motor cortex. J Neurophysiol, 80:2870, 1998
7. Ziemann U, Lönnecker S, Steinhoff BJ et al: Effects of anti-epileptic drugs on motor cortex excitability in humans: a transcranial magnetic stimulation study. Ann Neurol, 40:367, 1996
8. Chen R, Samii A, Caños M et al: Effects of phenytoin on cortical excitability in humans. Neurology, 49:881, 1997
9. Boroojerdi B, Battaglia F, Muellbacher W et al: Mechanisms influencing stimulus-response properties of the human corticospinal system. Clin Neurophysiol, 112:931, 2001
10. Magistris MR, Rosler KM, Truffert A et al: Transcranial stimulation excites virtually all motor neurons supplying the target muscle. A demonstration and a method improving the study of motor evoked potentials. Brain, 121:437, 1998
11. Mills KR: Magnetic Stimulation of the Human Nervous System. Oxford University Press, Oxford, 1999
12. Magistris MR, Rosler KM: The triple stimulation technique to study corticospinal conduction. Suppl Clin Neurophysiol, 56:24, 2003
13. Ugawa Y, Uesaka Y, Terao Y et al: Clinical utility of magnetic corticospinal tract stimulation at the foramen magnum level. Electroencephalogr Clin Neurophysiol, 101: 247, 1996
14. Kujirai T, Caramia MD, Rothwell JC et al: Corticocortical inhibition in human motor cortex. J Physiol, 471: 501, 1993
15. Ziemann U: TMS and drugs. Clin Neurophysiol, 115:1717, 2004
16. Ziemann U, Chen R, Cohen LG et al: Dextromethorphan decreases the excitability of the human motor cortex. Neurology, 51:1320, 1998
17. Wassermann EM, Samii A, Mercuri B et al: Responses to paired transcranial magnetic stimuli in resting, active, and recently activated muscle. Exp Brain Res, 109:158, 1996
18. Scalise A, Desiato MT, Gigli GL et al: Increasing cortical excitability: a possible explanation for the proconvulsant role of sleep deprivation. Sleep, 29:1595, 2006
19. Taylor JL, Gandevia SC: Transcranial magnetic stimulation and human muscle fatigue. Muscle Nerve, 24:18, 2001
20. Meyer BU, Roricht S, Grafin von Einsiedel H et al: Inhibitory and excitatory interhemispheric transfers between motor cortical areas in normal humans and patients with abnormalities of the corpus callosum. Brain, 118: 429, 1995
21. Ferbert A, Priori A, Rothwell JC et al: Interhemispheric inhibition of the human motor cortex. J Physiol, 453:525, 1992
22. Ni Z, Gunraj C, Nelson AJ et al: Two phases of interhemispheric inhibition between motor related cortical areas and the primary motor cortex in human. Cereb Cortex, 19:1654, 2009
23. Ugawa Y, Uesaka Y, Terao Y et al: Magnetic stimulation over the cerebellum in humans. Ann Neurol, 37:703, 1995
24. Ugawa Y, Terao Y, Hanajima R et al: Magnetic stimulation over the cerebellum in patients with ataxia. Electroencephalogr Clin Neurophysiol, 104:453, 1997
25. Sailer A, Molnar GF, Paradiso G et al: Short and long latency afferent inhibition in Parkinson's disease. Brain, 126:1883, 2003

26. Chen R, Classen J, Gerloff C et al: Depression of motor cortex excitability by low-frequency transcranial magnetic stimulation. Neurology, 48:1389, 1997

27. Pascual-Leone A, Valls-Solé J, Wassermann EM et al: Responses to rapid-rate transcranial magnetic stimulation of the human motor cortex. Brain, 117:847, 1994

28. Huang YZ, Edwards MJ, Rounis E et al: Theta burst stimulation of the human motor cortex. Neuron, 45:201, 2005

29. Rossi S, Hallett M, Rossini PM et al: Safety, ethical considerations, and application guidelines for the use of transcranial magnetic stimulation in clinical practice and research. Clin Neurophysiol, 120:2008, 2009

30. Wassermann EM: Risk and safety in repetitive transcranial magnetic stimulation: report and suggested guidelines from the International Workshop on the Safety of Repetitive Transcranial Magnetic Stimulation, June 5–7, 1996. Electroencephalogr Clin Neurophysiol, 108:1, 1998

31. Roth BJ, Pascual-Leone A, Cohen LG et al: The heating of metal electrodes during rapid-rate magnetic stimulation: a possible safety hazard. Electroencephalogr Clin Neurophysiol, 85:116, 1992

32. Counter SA, Borg E: Analysis of the coil generated impulse noise in extracranial magnetic stimulation. Electroencephalogr Clin Neurophysiol, 85:280, 1992

33. Janicak PG, O'Reardon JP, Sampson SM et al: Transcranial magnetic stimulation in the treatment of major depressive disorder: a comprehensive summary of safety experience from acute exposure, extended exposure, and during reintroduction treatment. J Clin Psychiatry, 69:222, 2008

34. Chen R, Cros D, Curra A et al: The clinical diagnostic utility of transcranial magnetic stimulation: Report of an IFCN committee. Clin Neurophysiol, 119:504, 2008

35. Donoghue JP, Hess G, Sanes JN: Substrates and mechanisms for learning in motor cortex. p. 363. In Bloedel J, Ebner T, Wise SP (eds): Acquisition of Motor Behavior in Vertebrates. MIT Press, Cambridge, 1996

36. Ridding MC, Ziemann U: Determinants of the induction of cortical plasticity by non-invasive brain stimulation in healthy subjects. J Physiol, 588:2291, 2010

37. Lo YL, Chan LL, Lim W et al: Systematic correlation of transcranial magnetic stimulation and magnetic resonance imaging in cervical spondylotic myelopathy. Spine, 29:1137, 2004

38. Travlos A, Pant B, Eisen A: Transcranial magnetic stimulation for detection of preclinical cervical spondylotic myelopathy. Arch Phys Med Rehabil, 73:442, 1992

39. Chan KM, Nasathurai S, Chavin JM et al: The usefulness of central motor conduction studies in the localization of cord involvement in cervical spondylytic myelopathy. Muscle Nerve, 21:1220, 1998

40. Truffert A, Rosler KM, Magistris MR: Amyotrophic lateral sclerosis versus cervical spondylotic myelopathy: a study using transcranial magnetic stimulation with recordings from the trapezius and limb muscles. Clin Neurophysiol, 111:1031, 2000

41. Schriefer TN, Hess CW, Mills KR et al: Central motor conduction studies in motor neurone disease using magnetic brain stimulation. Electroencephalogr Clin Neurophysiol, 74:431, 1989

42. Eisen A, Shytbel W, Murphy K et al: Cortical magnetic stimulation in amyotrophic lateral sclerosis. Muscle Nerve, 13:146, 1990

43. Urban PP, Wicht S, Hopf HC: Sensitivity of transcranial magnetic stimulation of cortico-bulbar vs. cortico-spinal tract involvement in amyotrophic lateral sclerosis (ALS). J Neurol, 248:850, 2001

44. Komissarow L, Rollnik JD, Bogdanova D et al: Triple stimulation technique (TST) in amyotrophic lateral sclerosis. Clin Neurophysiol, 115:356, 2004

45. Rosler KM, Magistris MR: Triple stimulation technique (TST) in amyotrophic lateral sclerosis. Clin Neurophysiol, 115:1715, 2004

46. Weber M, Eisen A, Stewart H et al: The split hand in ALS has a cortical basis. J Neurol Sci, 180:66, 2000

47. Claus D, Brunholzl C, Kerling FP et al: Transcranial magnetic stimulation as a diagnostic and prognostic test in amyotrophic lateral sclerosis. J Neurol Sci, 129: Suppl, 30, 1995

48. Schulte-Mattler WJ, Muller T, Zierz S: Transcranial magnetic stimulation compared with upper motor neuron signs in patients with amyotrophic lateral sclerosis. J Neurol Sci, 170:51, 1999

49. Triggs WJ, Menkes D, Onorato J et al: Transcranial magnetic stimulation identifies upper motor neuron involvement in motor neuron disease. Neurology, 53:605, 1999

50. Di Lazzaro V, Dileone M, Pilato F et al: Repetitive transcranial magnetic stimulation of the motor cortex for hemichorea. J Neurol Neurosurg Psychiatry, 77:1095, 2006

51. Di Lazzaro V, Oliviero A, Saturno E et al: Motor cortex stimulation for amyotrophic lateral sclerosis. Time for a therapeutic trial? Clin Neurophysiol, 115:2004

52. Di Lazzaro V, Pilato F, Profice P et al: Motor cortex stimulation for ALS: a double blind placebo-controlled study. Neurosci Lett, 464:18, 2009

53. Heald A, Bates D, Cartlidge NE et al: Longitudinal study of central motor conduction time following stroke. 2. Central motor conduction measured within 72 h after stroke as a predictor of functional outcome at 12 months. Brain, 116:1371, 1993

54. Trompetto C, Assini A, Buccolieri A et al: Motor recovery following stroke: a transcranial magnetic stimulation study. Clin Neurophysiol, 111:1860, 2000

55. Gerloff C, Bushara K, Sailer A et al: Multimodal imaging of brain reorganization in motor areas of the contralesional hemisphere of well recovered patients after capsular stroke. Brain, 129:791, 2006

56. Stinear CM, Barber PA, Smale PR et al: Functional potential in chronic stroke patients depends on corticospinal tract integrity. Brain, 130:170, 2007

57. Thickbroom GW, Byrnes ML, Archer SA et al: Motor outcome after subcortical stroke correlates with the degree of cortical reorganization. Clin Neurophysiol, 115:2144, 2004

58. Liepert J, Bauder H, Wolfgang HR et al: Treatment-induced cortical reorganization after stroke in humans. Stroke, 31:1210, 2000

59. Liepert J: Motor cortex excitability in stroke before and after constraint-induced movement therapy. Cogn Behav Neurol, 19:41, 2006

60. Khedr EM, Ahmed MA, Fathy N et al: Therapeutic trial of repetitive transcranial magnetic stimulation after acute ischemic stroke. Neurology, 65:466, 2005

61. Kim YH, You SH, Ko MH et al: Repetitive transcranial magnetic stimulation-induced corticomotor excitability and associated motor skill acquisition in chronic stroke. Stroke, 37:1471, 2006

62. Boroojerdi B, Diefenbach K, Ferbert A: Transcallosal inhibition in cortical and subcortical cerebral vascular lesions. J Neurol Sci, 144:160, 1996

63. Murase N, Duque J, Mazzocchio R et al: Influence of interhemispheric interactions on motor function in chronic stroke. Ann Neurol, 55:400, 2004

64. Takeuchi N, Chuma T, Matsuo Y et al: Repetitive transcranial magnetic stimulation of contralesional primary motor cortex improves hand function after stroke. Stroke, 36:2681, 2005

65. Mansur CG, Fregni F, Boggio PS et al: A sham stimulation-controlled trial of rTMS of the unaffected hemisphere in stroke patients. Neurology, 64:1802, 2005

66. Kirton A, Chen R, Friefeld S et al: Contralesional repetitive transcranial magnetic stimulation for chronic hemiparesis in subcortical paediatric stroke: a randomised trial. Lancet Neurol, 7:507, 2008

67. Fregni F, Boggio PS, Valle AC et al: A sham-controlled trial of a 5-day course of repetitive transcranial magnetic stimulation of the unaffected hemisphere in stroke patients. Stroke, 37:2115, 2006

68. Nowak DA, Grefkes C, Dafotakis M et al: Effects of low-frequency repetitive transcranial magnetic stimulation of the contralesional primary motor cortex on movement kinematics and neural activity in subcortical stroke. Arch Neurol, 65:741, 2008

69. Liepert J, Zittel S, Weiller C: Improvement of dexterity by single session low-frequency repetitive transcranial magnetic stimulation over the contralesional motor cortex in acute stroke: a double-blind placebo-controlled crossover trial. Restor Neurol Neurosci, 25:461, 2007

70. Martin PI, Naeser MA, Ho M et al: Research with transcranial magnetic stimulation in the treatment of aphasia. Curr Neurol Neurosci Rep, 9:451, 2009

71. Di Lazzaro V, Oliviero A, Pilato F et al: Neurophysiological predictors of long term response to AChE inhibitors in AD patients. J Neurol Neurosurg Psychiatry, 76:1064, 2005

72. Pierantozzi M, Panella M, Palmieri MG et al: Different TMS patterns of intracortical inhibition in early onset Alzheimer dementia and frontotemporal dementia. Clin Neurophysiol, 115:2410, 2004

73. Sakuma K, Murakami T, Nakashima K: Short latency afferent inhibition is not impaired in mild cognitive impairment. Clin Neurophysiol, 118:1460, 2007

74. Di Lazzaro V, Pilato F, Dileone M et al: Functional evaluation of cerebral cortex in dementia with Lewy bodies. Neuroimage, 37:422, 2007

75. Cotelli M, Manenti R, Cappa SF et al: Effect of transcranial magnetic stimulation on action naming in patients with Alzheimer disease. Arch Neurol, 63:1602, 2006

76. Cotelli M, Manenti R, Cappa SF et al: Transcranial magnetic stimulation improves naming in Alzheimer disease patients at different stages of cognitive decline. Eur J Neurol, 15:1286, 2008

77. Naeser MA, Martin PI, Nicholas M et al: Improved picture naming in chronic aphasia after TMS to part of right Broca's area: an open-protocol study. Brain Lang, 93:95, 2005

78. Oliveri M, Rossini PM, Filippi MM et al: Time-dependent activation of parieto-frontal networks for directing attention to tactile space. A study with paired transcranial magnetic stimulation pulses in right-brain-damaged patients with extinction. Brain, 123:1939, 2000

79. Oliveri M, Bisiach E, Brighina F et al: rTMS of the unaffected hemisphere transiently reduces contralesional visuospatial hemineglect. Neurology, 57:1338, 2001

80. Brighina F, Bisiach E, Oliveri M et al: 1 Hz repetitive transcranial magnetic stimulation of the unaffected hemisphere ameliorates contralesional visuospatial neglect in humans. Neurosci Lett, 336:131, 2003

81. Sole-Padulles C, Bartres-Faz D, Junque C et al: Repetitive transcranial magnetic stimulation effects on brain function and cognition among elders with memory dysfunction. A randomized sham-controlled study. Cereb Cortex, 16:1487, 2006

82. Rektorova I, Megova S, Bares M et al: Cognitive functioning after repetitive transcranial magnetic stimulation in patients with cerebrovascular disease without dementia: a pilot study of seven patients. J Neurol Sci, 229–230:157, 2005

83. Jorge RE, Robinson RG, Tateno A et al: Repetitive transcranial magnetic stimulation as treatment of poststroke depression: a preliminary study. Biol Psychiatry, 55:398, 2004

84. Reutens DC, Berkovic SF, Macdonell RAL et al: Magnetic stimulation of the brain in generalized epilepsy: Reversal of cortical hyperexcitability by anticonvulsants. Ann Neurol, 34:351, 1993

85. Ziemann U, Iliac TV, Pauli C et al: Learning modifies subsequent induction of long-term potentiation-like and long-term depression-like plasticity in human motor cortex. J Neurosci, 24:1666, 2004

86. Molnar GF, Sailer A, Gunraj CA et al: Changes in motor cortex excitability with stimulation of anterior thalamus in epilepsy. Neurology, 66:566, 2006

87. Tergau F, Naumann U, Paulus W et al: Low-frequency repetitive transcranial magnetic stimulation improves intractable epilepsy. Lancet, 353:2209, 1999

88. Rotenberg A, Bae EH, Takeoka M et al: Repetitive transcranial magnetic stimulation in the treatment of epilepsia partialis continua. Epilepsy Behav, 14:253, 2009

89. Joo EY, Han SJ, Chung SH et al: Antiepileptic effects of low-frequency repetitive transcranial magnetic stimulation by different stimulation durations and locations. Clin Neurophysiol, 118:702, 2007

90. Fregni F, Otachi PT, Do VA et al: A randomized clinical trial of repetitive transcranial magnetic stimulation in patients with refractory epilepsy. Ann Neurol, 60:447, 2006

91. Theodore WH, Hunter K, Chen R et al: Transcranial magnetic stimulation for the treatment of seizures: a controlled study. Neurology, 59:560, 2002

92. Cantello R, Rossi S, Varrasi C et al: Slow repetitive TMS for drug-resistant epilepsy: clinical and EEG findings of a placebo-controlled trial. Epilepsia, 48:366, 2007

93. Cantello R, Gianelli M, Bettucci D et al: Parkinson's disease rigidity: magnetic motor evoked potentials in a small hand muscle. Neurology, 91:1449, 1991

94. Priori A, Berardelli A, Inghilleri M et al: Motor cortical inhibition and the dopaminergic system. Pharmacological changes in the silent period after transcranial magnetic brain stimulation in normal subjects, patients with Parkinson's disease and drug-induced parkinsonism. Brain, 117:317, 1994

95. Ridding MC, Inzelberg R, Rothwell JC: Changes in excitability of motor cortical circuitry in patients with Parkinson's disease. Ann Neurol, 37:181, 1995

96. Chu J, Wagle-Shukla A, Gunraj C et al: Impaired presynaptic inhibition in the motor cortex in Parkinson disease. Neurology, 72:842, 2009

97. Abbruzzese G, Tabaton M, Morena M et al: Motor and sensory evoked potentials in progressive supranuclear palsy. Mov Disord, 6:49, 1991

98. Abbruzzese G, Marchese R, Trompetto C: Sensory and motor evoked potentials in multiple system atrophy: a comparative study with Parkinson's disease. Mov Disord, 12:315, 1997

99. Trompetto C, Buccolieri A, Marchese R et al: Impairment of transcallosal inhibition in patients with corticobasal degeneration. Clin Neurophysiol, 114:2181, 2003

100. Wolters A, Classen J, Kunesch E et al: Measurements of transcallosally mediated cortical inhibition for differentiating parkinsonian syndromes. Mov Disord, 19:518, 2004

101. Siebner HR, Rossmeier C, Mentschel C et al: Short-term motor improvement after sub-threshold 5-Hz repetitive transcranial magnetic stimulation of the primary motor hand area in Parkinson's disease. J Neurol Sci, 178:91, 2000

102. Lefaucheur JP, Drouot X, Von Raison F et al: Improvement of motor performance and modulation of cortical excitability by repetitive transcranial magnetic stimulation of the motor cortex in Parkinson's disease. Clin Neurophysiol, 115:2530, 2004

103. Khedr EM, Farweez HM, Islam H: Therapeutic effect of repetitive transcranial magnetic stimulation on motor function in Parkinson's disease patients. Eur J Neurol, 10:567, 2003

104. Lomarev MP, Kanchana S, Bara-Jimenez W et al: Placebo-controlled study of rTMS for the treatment of Parkinson's disease. Mov Disord, 21:325, 2006

105. Wu AD, Fregni F, Simon DK et al: Noninvasive brain stimulation for Parkinson's disease and dystonia. Neurotherapeutics, 5:345, 2008

106. Elahi B, Elahi B, Chen R: Effect of transcranial magnetic stimulation on Parkinson motor function–systematic review of controlled clinical trials. Mov Disord, 24:357, 2009

107. Fregni F, Simon DK, Wu A et al: Non-invasive brain stimulation for Parkinson's disease: a systematic review and meta-analysis of the literature. J Neurol Neurosurg Psychiatry, 76:1614, 2005

108. Brusa L, Versace V, Koch G et al: Low frequency rTMS of the SMA transiently ameliorates peak-dose LID in Parkinson's disease. Clin Neurophysiol, 117:1917, 2006

109. Wagle-Shukla A, Angel MJ, Zadikoff C et al: Low-frequency repetitive transcranial magnetic stimulation for treatment of levodopa-induced dyskinesias. Neurology, 68:704, 2007

110. Filipovic SR, Rothwell JC, van de Warrenburg BP et al: Repetitive transcranial magnetic stimulation for levodopa-induced dyskinesias in Parkinson's disease. Mov Disord, 24:246, 2009

111. Koch G, Brusa L, Carrillo F et al: Cerebellar magnetic stimulation decreases levodopa-induced dyskinesias in Parkinson disease. Neurology, 73:113, 2009

112. Ridding MC, Sheean G, Rothwell JC et al: Changes in the balance between motor cortical excitation and inhibition in focal, task specific dystonia. J Neurol Neurosurg Psychiatry, 39:493, 1995

113. Chen R, Wassermann EM, Cańos M et al: Impaired inhibition in writer's cramp during voluntary muscle activation. Neurology, 49:1054, 1997

114. Siebner HR, Tormos JM, Ceballos-Baumann AO et al: Low frequency repetitive transcranial magnetic stimulation of the motor cortex in writer's cramp. Neurology, 52:529, 1999

115. Huang YZ, Edwards MJ, Bhatia KP et al: One-Hz repetitive transcranial magnetic stimulation of the premotor cortex alters reciprocal inhibition in DYT1 dystonia. Mov Disord, 19:54, 2004

116. Murase N, Rothwell JC, Kaji R et al: Subthreshold low-frequency repetitive transcranial magnetic stimulation over the premotor cortex modulates writer's cramp. Brain, 128:104, 2005

117. Kranz G, Shamim EA, Lin PT et al: Transcranial magnetic brain stimulation modulates blepharospasm: a randomized controlled study. Neurology, 75:1465, 2010

118. Di Lazzaro V, Molinari M, Restuccia D et al: Cerebro-cerebellar interactions in man: neurophysiological studies in patients with focal cerebellar lesions. Electroencephalogr Clin Neurophysiol, 93:27, 1994

119. Liepert J, Kucinski T, Tuscher O et al: Motor cortex excitability after cerebellar infarction. Stroke, 35:2484, 2004

120. Daskalakis ZJ, Paradiso GO, Christensen BK et al: Exploring the connectivity between the cerebellum and motor cortex in humans. J Physiol, 557:689, 2004

121. Restivo DA, Lanza S, Saponara R et al: Changes of cortical excitability of human motor cortex in spinocerebellar ataxia type 2. A study with paired transcranial magnetic stimulation. J Neurol Sci, 198:87, 2002

122. Tamburin S, Fiaschi A, Andreoli A et al: Stimulus-response properties of motor system in patients with cerebellar ataxia. Clin Neurophysiol, 115:348, 2004

123. Schwenkreis P, Tegenthoff M, Witscher K et al: Motor cortex activation by transcranial magnetic stimulation in ataxia patients depends on the genetic defect. Brain, 125:301, 2002

124. Cruz-Martinez A, Palau F: Central motor conduction time by magnetic stimulation of the cortex and peripheral nerve conduction follow-up studies in Friedreich's ataxia. Electroencephalogr Clin Neurophysiol, 105:458, 1997

125. Restivo DA, Giuffrida S, Rapisarda G et al: Central motor conduction to lower limb after transcranial magnetic stimulation in spinocerebellar ataxia type 2 (SCA2). Clin Neurophysiol, 111:630, 2000

126. Lee YC, Chen JT, Liao KK et al: Prolonged cortical relay time of long latency reflex and central motor conduction in patients with spinocerebellar ataxia type 6. Clin Neurophysiol, 114:458, 2003

127. Mayr N, Baumgartner C, Zeitlhofer J et al: The sensitivity of transcranial cortical magnetic stimulation in detecting pyramidal tract lesions in clinically definite multiple sclerosis. Neurology, 41:566, 1991

128. Beer S, Rosler KM, Hess CW: Diagnostic value of paraclinical tests in multiple sclerosis: relative sensitivities and specificities for reclassification according to the Poser committee criteria. J Neurol Neurosurg Psychiatry, 59:152, 1995

129. Jones SM, Streletz LJ, Raab VE et al: Lower extremity motor evoked potentials in multiple sclerosis. Arch Neurol, 48:944, 1991

130. Kidd D, Thompson PD, Day BL et al: Central motor conduction time in progressive multiple sclerosis - Correlations with MRI and disease activity. Brain, 121:1109, 1998

131. Magistris MR, Rosler KM, Truffert A et al: A clinical study of motor evoked potentials using a triple stimulation technique. Brain, 122:265, 1999

132. Leocani L, Rovaris M, Boneschi FM et al: Multimodal evoked potentials to assess the evolution of multiple sclerosis: a longitudinal study. J Neurol Neurosurg Psychiatry, 77:1030, 2006

133. Feuillet L, Pelletier J, Suchet L et al: Prospective clinical and electrophysiological follow-up on a multiple sclerosis population treated with interferon beta-1 a: a pilot study. Mult Scler, 13:348, 2007

134. Schmierer K, Irlbacher K, Grosse P et al: Correlates of disability in multiple sclerosis detected by transcranial magnetic stimulation. Neurology, 59:1218, 2002

135. Humm AM, Magistris MR, Truffert A et al: Central motor conduction differs between acute relapsing-remitting and chronic progressive multiple sclerosis. Clin Neurophysiol, 114:2196, 2003

136. Nielsen JF, Sinkjaer T, Jakobsen J: Treatment of spasticity with repetitive magnetic stimulation; a double-blind placebo-controlled study. Mult Scler, 2:227, 1996

137. Nielsen JF, Sinkjaer T: Long-lasting depression of soleus motoneurons excitability following repetitive magnetic stimuli of the spinal cord in multiple sclerosis patients. Mult Scler, 3:18, 1997

138. Gunaydin S, Soysal A, Atay T et al: Motor and occipital cortex excitability in migraine patients. Can J Neurol Sci, 33:63, 2006

139. Clarke BM, Upton AR, Kamath MV et al: Transcranial magnetic stimulation for migraine: clinical effects. J Headache Pain, 7:341, 2006

140. Lipton RB, Dodick DW, Silberstein SD et al: Single-pulse transcranial magnetic stimulation for acute treatment of migraine with aura: a randomised, double-blind, parallel-group, sham-controlled trial. Lancet Neurol, 9:373, 2010

141. Brighina F, Piazza A, Vitello G et al: rTMS of the prefrontal cortex in the treatment of chronic migraine: a pilot study. J Neurol Sci, 227:67, 2004

142. Teepker M, Hotzel J, Timmesfeld N et al: Low-frequency rTMS of the vertex in the prophylactic treatment of migraine. Cephalalgia, 30:137, 2010

143. Migita K, Uozumi T, Arita K et al: Transcranial magnetic coil stimulation of motor cortex in patients with central pain. Neurosurgery, 36:1037, 1995

144. Cruccu G, Aziz TZ, Garcia-Larrea L et al: EFNS guidelines on neurostimulation therapy for neuropathic pain. Eur J Neurol, 14:952, 2007

145. Leung A, Donohue M, Xu R et al: rTMS for suppressing neuropathic pain: a meta-analysis. J Pain, 10:1205, 2009

146. Fregni F, DaSilva D, Potvin K et al: Treatment of chronic visceral pain with brain stimulation. Ann Neurol, 58:971, 2005

147. Canavero S, Bonicalzi V, Dotta M et al: Low-rate repetitive TMS allays central pain. Neurol Res, 25:151, 2003

148. Schrader M, Schrader V: Reliability of magnetic stimulation in the diagnosis of peripheral facial paralysis of idiopathic origin. Rev Laryngol Otol Rhinol (Bord), 116: 123, 1995

149. Rosler KM, Magistris MR, Glocker FX et al: Electrophysiological characteristics of lesions in facial palsies of different etiologies. A study using electrical and magnetic stimulation techniques. Electroencephalogr Clin Neurophysiol, 97:355, 1995

150. Londero A, Langguth B, De Ridder D et al: Repetitive transcranial magnetic stimulation (rTMS): a new therapeutic approach in subjective tinnitus? Neurophysiol Clin, 36:145, 2006

151. Khedr EM, Rothwell JC, Ahmed MA et al: Effect of daily repetitive transcranial magnetic stimulation for treatment of tinnitus: comparison of different stimulus frequencies. J Neurol Neurosurg Psychiatry, 79:212, 2008

152. Rossi S, De Capua A, Ulivelli M et al: Effects of repetitive transcranial magnetic stimulation on chronic tinnitus: a randomised, crossover, double blind, placebo controlled study. J Neurol Neurosurg Psychiatry, 78:857, 2007

153. Langguth B, Zowe M, Landgrebe M et al: Transcranial magnetic stimulation for the treatment of tinnitus: a new coil positioning method and first results. Brain Topogr, 18:241, 2006

154. De Ridder D, Verstraeten E, Van der KK et al: Transcranial magnetic stimulation for tinnitus: influence of tinnitus duration on stimulation parameter choice and maximal tinnitus suppression. Otol Neurotol, 26:616, 2005

Event-Related Potentials

DOUGLAS S. GOODIN

Averaged evoked potentials have been used widely to record the changes in electrical potential that occur within the nervous system in response to an external stimulus.[1] For clinical purposes, the short-latency brainstem auditory evoked potential (BAEP), somatosensory evoked potential (SEP), and visual evoked potential (VEP) are recorded. In general, these evoked potentials represent an obligate neuronal response to a given stimulus, and both their amplitude and latency depend on the physical characteristics of the eliciting stimulus (see Chapters 22 to 27). Such "exogenous" or "stimulus-related" potentials (SRPs) are independent of whether the subject is attentive to or interested in the stimulus. Indeed, BAEPs, SEPs, and flash VEPs can be recorded even when the subject is asleep.

There is, however, another distinct class of evoked potential: the "endogenous" or "event-related" potentials (ERPs) that can be recorded in response to an external stimulus or event.[2–4] These potential changes, unlike the SRPs just described, occur only when the subject is selectively attentive to the stimulus and are elicited only in circumstances in which the subject is required to distinguish one stimulus (the target) from a group of other stimuli (the nontargets). They depend primarily on the setting in which the target stimulus occurs and are relatively independent of the physical characteristics of that stimulus.[2–4] Thus, ERPs seem to be related to some aspect of the cognitive events associated with the distinction of target from nontarget stimuli. Attempts have even been made to relate ERPs to presumed stages of information processing (e.g., sensory discrimination or response selection) that must be completed successfully before a person can respond selectively to a target stimulus.[5–14] The precise relationship between any such stages and the individual components of the ERP is, however, uncertain. Indeed, it seems most likely that the ERP reflects activity in distributed parallel networks that are responsible for the discriminative behavior.[5,7,15]

Because of this relationship between ERPs and cognitive behavior, considerable interest has developed in the possible clinical use of these potentials in the evaluation of patients who suffer from disorders of cognition. This interest has focused principally on disorders that affect brain function diffusely (e.g., Alzheimer disease, frontotemporal dementia, schizophrenia, or metabolic encephalopathies).

DESCRIPTION OF EVENT-RELATED (ENDOGENOUS) POTENTIALS

Several components of the ERP have been identified; these include Nd[4]; the processing negativity (PN[4]); the mismatch negativity (MMN[4]); P165[5]; N2[12]; P3a[4,16,17]; P3 (or P3b[4,16,17]); N400[18]; and the error negativity (ERN or N_e).[19,20] With the exception of P3 (which is also referred to as the P300 component because of its polarity and latency), these components have not been found consistently in different recording situations. Much of this apparent inconsistency probably relates to two factors. First, these other ERP components are of relatively small amplitude compared with the P3 component and thus are more difficult to separate from background noise when only a few trials are averaged. Second, most of these components occur at relatively short latencies and overlap considerably with the simultaneously occurring SRPs. As a consequence, special procedures such as the subtraction of one waveform from another[4,5,7] are often required for demonstrating them (Fig. 29-1). Most clinical studies therefore have been concerned primarily with the more easily identified N1 and P2 components in response to the frequent tone and the P3 component in response to the rare tone (see Fig. 29-1). For this reason, attention is confined to a discussion of these components of the ERP in the remainder of this chapter.

The simplest experimental design that is used to elicit the P3 response is the so-called oddball paradigm.[2-4] In this design, the subject is presented with a sequence of two distinguishable stimuli, one of which occurs frequently (the frequent stimulus) and the other infrequently (the rare stimulus). The subject is required to count mentally or otherwise respond to one of the two stimuli. Cerebral responses to the rare and frequent stimuli are recorded and averaged separately.

The response to the frequent stimulus consists of a series of waves (the stimulus-related components) that relates, for the most part, to the sensory modality stimulated. For example, to an auditory stimulus this response has been divided into three sequential time periods: (1) early-latency, (2) mid-latency, and (3) long-latency responses (Fig. 29-2). The early-latency (less than 10 msec) response (BAEP) reflects activity in the peripheral and brainstem auditory structures (see Chapter 24). The mid-latency (10 to 50 msec) response is thought to reflect a combination of muscle reflex activity and neural activity that may arise in the thalamocortical radiations, primary auditory cortex, and early association cortex. The neural generators of the long-latency (greater than 50 msec) response are uncertain, although probably the ERP reflects overlapping neural activity from multiple neocortical and limbic regions.[15] This response consists of a large negative (N1)–positive (P2) complex referred to as the "vertex potential" because it has the largest amplitude at the vertex.[4] At least part of this vertex potential seems to reflect activity in neural areas that can be activated by more than one sensory modality. Thus, a similar negative–positive complex is elicited by auditory, visual, and somatosensory stimuli (Fig. 29-3). This response is nevertheless an obligate response of

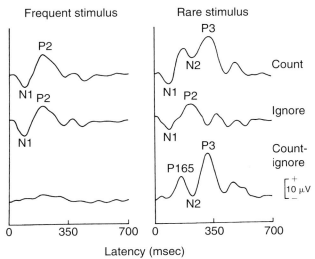

FIGURE 29-1 ■ Long-latency evoked potentials recorded from an electrode at the vertex (Cz) and referred to linked mastoids. The waveforms on the left show the response to a frequent (1,000-Hz) tone that occurred on 85 percent of the trials. The average of 340 trials is shown. The waveforms on the right show the response to a rare (2,000-Hz) tone that occurred on 15 percent of the trials. The average of 60 responses is shown. The sequence of rare and frequent tones (50-msec duration, 60 dB HL, 1.5-second interstimulus interval) was pseudorandom, with the constraint that no two rare tones occurred consecutively. The top row of waveforms represents the response to the rare and frequent stimuli when the subject is required to count the rare tones as they occur. With the frequent stimulus, a negative (N1)–positive (P2) vertex potential is seen. With the rare stimulus, a negative (N1)–positive (apparent P2)–negative (N2)–positive (P3) complex representing, in part, the event-related response is seen. The middle row of waveforms represents the response to the same stimuli when the subject ignores the tone sequence and reads a magazine during the test procedure. The response to both stimuli consists of only the stimulus-related vertex potential. The bottom row of waveforms was obtained by subtraction of the "ignore" waveform from the "count" waveform for the rare and frequent tones, respectively. For the frequent tone, this difference waveform is a flat line because in both conditions only a stimulus-related response is obtained. For the rare tone, the stimulus-related response has been similarly subtracted out and the event-related response (P165, N2, P3) can be seen clearly. (Modified from Goodin DS, Squires KC, Henderson BH et al: An early event-related cortical potential. Psychophysiology, 15:360, 1978, with permission.)

the nervous system to the stimulus and is largely independent of the subject's attention or level of arousal.[4,21] It is, therefore, like the early-latency and mid-latency components, a stimulus-related response.

In contrast, the long-latency response to the rare auditory stimulus is considerably different and consists of a

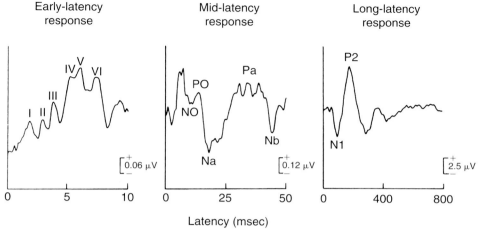

Early-latency response

Mid-latency response

Long-latency response

FIGURE 29-2 ■ Evoked potentials recorded from the vertex (Cz) in response to an auditory stimulus during three sequential time periods show the early-latency (brainstem auditory evoked potential), mid-latency, and long-latency responses.

Latency (msec)

negative (N1)–positive (apparent P2)–negative (N2)–positive (P3) complex (see Fig. 29-1). The first positive wave is termed *apparent* P2 because it represents the sum of the stimulus-related P2 and the event-related P165. This response is quite consistent, in both amplitude and latency, in the same subject performing the same task[14,22–24] even when measured on several different occasions over a period of months (Fig. 29-4). The P3 component of this response has a latency-to-peak of approximately 300 to 400 msec following onset of the rare stimulus; it is of positive polarity and is of maximal amplitude in the midline over the central and parietal regions of the scalp. An evoked potential component with a similar scalp distribution can be recorded to stimuli in any of the sensory modalities (see Fig. 29-3) and can even be recorded (without associated SRPs) when an anticipated stimulus is omitted unexpectedly.[5] The neural generators of this P3 response are not known definitively,

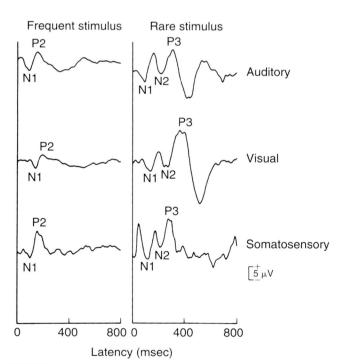

FIGURE 29-3 ■ Long-latency potentials elicited by auditory (top row), visual (middle row), and somatosensory (bottom row) stimuli. The responses to rare and frequent stimuli in each modality are shown. In each case, the frequent stimulus elicited a negative (N1)–positive (P2) response, and the rare stimulus elicited, in addition, an event-related response.

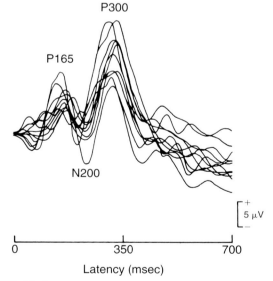

FIGURE 29-4 ■ Event-related potentials recorded from the vertex in response to a rare tone on several occasions over a 2-month period in the same subject. Each trace represents the difference waveform obtained by subtracting the rare-tone "ignore" waveform from the rare-tone "count" waveform (see Fig. 29-1). The event-related response is quite stable in both amplitude and latency over time. (Modified from Goodin DS, Squires KC, Henderson BH et al: An early event-related cortical potential. Psychophysiology, 15:360, 1978, with permission.)

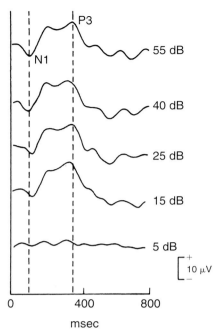

FIGURE 29-5 ■ Event-related potentials recorded from the vertex of a 30-year-old subject in response to rare auditory stimuli of different stimulus intensities (measured in dB HL). A reduction in stimulus intensity did not influence the amplitude or latency of the P3 response (despite an increase in the latency of the stimulus-related N1 component) until a stimulus of 5 dB HL was used, at which point the stimuli were barely perceptible to the subject.

although converging evidence has suggested a temporo-parietal source.[15,25–30]

Several variables alter the amplitude and latency of the SRPs without appreciably affecting the ERPs, and vice versa. For instance, a change in the intensity of stimulation has relatively little effect on the P3 component (Fig. 29-5) but has a major influence on the associated SRPs (see Chapters 22 to 27). Conversely, the P3 is influenced by changes in the ease with which targets can be distinguished from nontargets (Fig. 29-6), by alterations in the ratio of target to nontarget stimuli (Fig. 29-7), or by shifts in the attention of the subject (see Fig. 29-1), whereas SRPs are not.[4,5,7,17,31–33]

RECORDING ARRANGEMENTS

To record ERPs it is necessary to be able to deliver both frequent and rare stimuli and to average separately the cerebral response to each. Any sensory modality can be used, although in clinical practice an auditory stimulus is most common. The stimuli are generally two or three differently pitched tones (see Fig. 29-1) delivered binaurally with a relatively long interstimulus interval

(i.e., greater than 1 second) because of the long refractory period of the vertex potential.

The amplitude of the P3 response is quite large (i.e., 50 to 100 times the amplitude of the BAEP), and therefore an average of the cerebral response to a relatively low number of rare tones is generally sufficient to improve the signal-to-noise ratio to the point that the P3 response can be easily seen (Fig. 29-8). Indeed, the P3 amplitude is often so large that the P3 response can be identified in single trials (see Fig. 29-8). The probability of rare tone occurrence generally is set between 10 and 30 percent, so that approximately 50 responses to the rare tone can be averaged in 10 minutes of recording time. This arrangement seems to be a good balance between the

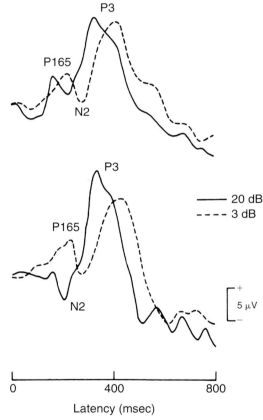

FIGURE 29-6 ■ Event-related potentials (ERPs) (plotted as difference waveforms: see Fig. 29-1) obtained from two subjects at two different levels of task difficulty. In the easy condition (solid lines) the subjects were required to distinguish two tones that differed in intensity by 20 dB, whereas in the difficult condition (dashed lines) the two tones differed in intensity by only 3 dB. The peak latencies of the different components of the ERP are longer in response to the difficult task than to the easy one. (Modified from Goodin DS, Squires KC, Starr A: Variations in early and late event-related components of the auditory evoked potential with task difficulty. Electroencephalogr Clin Neurophysiol, 55:680, 1983, with permission.)

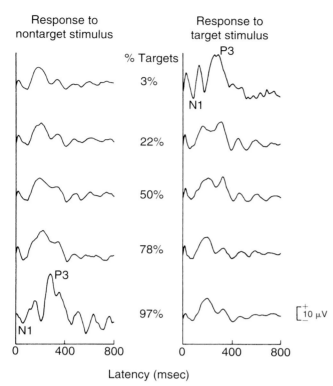

Response to nontarget stimulus Response to target stimulus

% Targets

3%

22%

50%

78%

97%

Latency (msec)

FIGURE 29-7 ▪ Long-latency evoked potentials recorded from the vertex in response to target and nontarget stimuli (tones) when the probability of target stimulus occurrence is altered. With increasing probability that a target stimulus will occur, there is a progressive decrement in the P3 response evoked by target stimuli and a progressive increment in that elicited by nontarget stimuli.

enhancement of P3 amplitude that occurs at smaller ratios of target to nontarget stimuli, the increased response noise associated with fewer trials in the rare tone average, and the difficulty of keeping the subject's attention for longer recording times.

Optimally, multiple recording channels (a minimum of four) are used. Responses are recorded from Fz, Cz, and Pz electrode placements on the scalp referenced to an indifferent (although not necessarily inactive) scalp location such as the mastoids or ear lobe. Eye movements may contaminate the ERP recordings; therefore, at least one channel usually is devoted to monitoring them. Depending on the recording apparatus used, it may be possible to reject automatically trials containing eye movement or to remove digitally eye blink artifacts from the responses and thereby produce less noisy recordings.

The electrical power in these long-latency responses essentially is confined to frequencies under 10 Hz so that the high-frequency cut-off of the filters used (down 3 dB at the cut-off frequencies; roll-off of 12 dB per octave) can be set low enough (e.g., at 40 to 50 Hz) to eliminate any 60-Hz activity that otherwise might degrade the

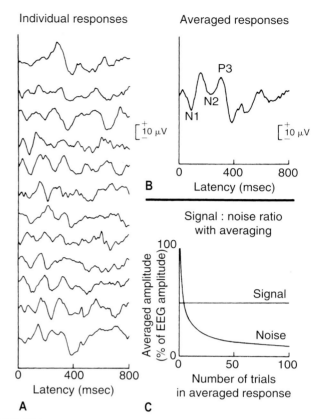

Individual responses   Averaged responses

Latency (msec)

A   **C**

Signal : noise ratio with averaging

Number of trials in averaged response

FIGURE 29-8 ▪ **A,** Long-latency evoked potentials recorded from the vertex of a subject on 12 single trials. In each trial a negative–positive–negative–positive complex can be identified, although it is somewhat variable in both amplitude and latency, presumably partly because of superimposed noise. **B,** Average of these 12 trials. The negative (N1)–positive (apparent P2)–negative (N2)–positive (P3) response can be seen. **C,** Plot showing the improvement in the signal-to-noise ratio that occurs with averaging. The noise is reduced in the average by the square root of the number of trials, whereas the time-locked signal remains constant. The P3 component generally has an amplitude of between 10 and 30 μV. The background electroencephalogram is often approximately 50 μV; thus the initial signal-to-noise ratio in the recording of event-related potentials may be as high as 0.5 : 1. Under such circumstances, even the averaged response to only a few trials is adequate to define the signal.

waveforms. The best low-frequency cut-off is somewhat controversial,[34,35] although it probably should not exceed 1 Hz because much of the power in these recordings is in the 1- to 4-Hz frequency band, and a marked distortion in P3 amplitude begins to occur at this point. In addition, as will occur with any analog lowpass filter, responses will be shifted to earlier latencies at even very low filter settings, so it is important to record both normal control subjects and clinical patients at the same bandpass.[34,35]

NON-NEUROLOGIC FACTORS INFLUENCING THE P3 COMPONENT

Several non-neurologic factors may affect the ERP; it is essential that these factors be taken into account if ERPs are to be recorded in a clinical setting.

Age

Advancing age, during both maturation and senescence, has an important influence on several of the long-latency evoked potential components (Fig. 29-9 and Table 29-1). The data on maturation are limited, but they suggest that

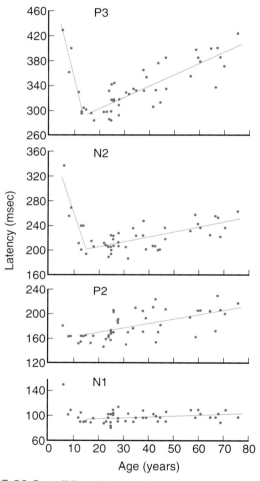

FIGURE 29-9 ■ Effect of age on the components of the long-latency evoked potential. The solid lines represent the regression lines from data obtained from 50 normal subjects. Beginning at about age 15 years, each component increases in latency with age. The rate of this change, however, becomes progressively faster for components with greater initial peak latencies. During maturation (age 6 to 15 years), the effect of age is reversed, at least for the event-related components. (Modified from Goodin DS, Squires KC, Henderson HB et al: Age-related variations in evoked potentials to auditory stimuli in normal human subjects. Electroencephalogr Clin Neurophysiol, 44:447, 1978, with permission.)

the stimulus-related N1 and P2 components have reached their adult latencies at least by the age of 5 or 6 years and perhaps well before.[36-39] The event-related N2 and P3 components, in contrast, are markedly prolonged in young children and progressively decrease in latency with increasing age until reaching adult values in the teenage years or early twenties.[36-39] This apparently differential effect of maturation on the stimulus-related and event-related components may be related to the temporal evolution of cognitive development in children.[36-39]

Beginning in about the midteens, a linear increase occurs in the latency of both the stimulus-related (P2) and the event-related (N2 and P3) components with advancing age (see Fig. 29-9 and Table 29-1). Several studies have corroborated these general findings (Table 29-2), although the rate of these changes has varied somewhat between reports.[22,36,39-49] Although occasional reports have suggested that the age-related change in the latency of the P3 component is curvilinear,[43] most authors have found the P3 latency–age function to be linear.[16,36,40-42,44,45] For example, in a meta-analysis of the existing literature on this issue as of 1996, Polich concluded that the weight of the evidence supported a linear, and not a curvilinear, relationship between the latency of P3 and age.[42] This has continued to be the experience of others.[44,45,47-50] As a result of these discrepancies, it is unclear whether, or in what circumstances, nonlinear factors are important determinants of the P3 latency–age function. For example, even in the study of Anderer and associates,[43] the significance of such curvilinear effects may have been exaggerated by the fact that the four oldest subjects (greater than 80 years) had quite deviant P3 latencies. It would be of interest to know what effect the exclusion of these four subjects from the analysis may have on the significance of the curvilinear nature of the age–latency function. In addition, the results of one study,[49] in which a high level of cognitive function was strictly controlled, indicated that there were no significant age-related changes in either P3 latency or amplitude. Although this study has been criticized,[50] the findings are provocative and clearly worth replication. Regardless, however, even based on this study, when using a specific testing procedure on individuals of uncertain status, a comparison with age-adjusted controls from an unaffected population is appropriate.

This age-related increase in latency occurs at a faster rate for components of longer initial peak latency,[36,40,41,43] which suggests that a relatively uniform slowing of neural transmission occurs with advancing age.[36] The intersubject variability in P3 latency is generally small in relation to the actual peak latency, and most authors report standard errors around the regression line of between 20 and 30 msec (see Table 29-2).

TABLE 29-1 ■ **Age-Related Variations in the Amplitudes and Latencies of Auditory Evoked Potential Components for Normal Subjects Aged 15 to 76 Years**

	Slope	Correlation Coefficient	Standard Error about Regression Line	Value at Age 15 Yr	Significance
STIMULUS-RELATED COMPONENTS					
N1 latency	0.1 msec/yr	0.228	8 msec	94 msec	NS
P2 latency	0.7 msec/yr	0.560	19 msec	168 msec	P < .001
N1–P2 amplitude	−0.2 μV/yr	−0.420	5.56 μV	15.6 μV	P < .01
EVENT-RELATED COMPONENTS					
N2 latency	0.8 msec/yr	0.691	15 msec	199 msec	P < .001
P3 latency	1.6 msec/yr	0.810	21 msec	310 msec	P < .001
N2–P3 amplitude	−0.2 μV/yr	−0.313	7.9 μV	17.7 μV	P < .05

NS, not significant.

From Goodin DS, Squires KC, Henderson BH et al: Age-related variations in evoked potentials to auditory stimuli in normal human subjects. Electroencephalogr Clin Neurophysiol, 44:447, 1978, with permission.

With increasing age, the amplitudes of both the stimulus-related and the event-related components of the long-latency evoked potential also decrease (see Table 29-1). The intersubject variability in amplitude is, however, extremely large, so a single standard error around the normal regression line is equivalent to approximately 60 to 80 percent of the expected P3 amplitude at 60 years of age (see Table 29-2). Such marked variability limits the usefulness of amplitude measurements in a clinical setting.

Sex

Gender is known to have effects on several of the stimulus-related components used clinically (see Chapters 22 to 27). By contrast, this factor does not seem to have any effect on latency of the event-related components,[48,51,52] although the amplitude of P3 may be larger in female subjects.[48]

Drugs

An understanding of the changes in the ERP produced by drugs (in particular, antipsychotics and antidepressants) is extremely important. Certainly, drugs taken in dosages sufficient to produce a metabolic encephalopathy can affect the ERP,[36] but the effect of these particular drugs taken in therapeutic dosages seems to be minimal.[53–55] Thus, an evidence-based review concluded that, while an amplitude reduction was possibly helpful diagnostically, medication status was not a factor.[53]

TABLE 29-2 ■ **Age-Related Changes in the P3 Component of the Event-Related Potential: Comparison of Findings in Different Studies**

	Latency			Amplitude		
	Slope (msec/yr)	Intercept (msec)	SE (msec)	Slope (μV/yr)	Intercept (μV)	SE (μV)
Goodin et al*	+1.64	285	21	−0.18	17.6	5.56
Picton et al*†	+1.71	294	25	−0.15	16.6	4.0
Brown et al*	+1.12	272	‡	−0.15	‡	‡
Pfefferbaum et al*	+0.94	‡	51	−0.13	‡	‡
Emmerson et al*	+1.46	‡	‡	‡	‡	‡
Gordon et al*	+0.91	‡	31	‡	‡	‡
Enoki et al[40]	+1.43	297	21	‡	‡	‡
Iragui et al[41]	+0.88	294	44	−0.10	14.4	5.1
Polich[42]	+0.92	304	32	‡	‡	‡
Anderer et al[43]	+0.92	333	33	−0.15	22.4	5.4
Alain and Woods[44]	+1.4	‡	‡	−0.25	‡	‡
Walhovd and Fjell[45]	+1.65	278	‡	−0.17	19.3	‡
Schiff et al[48]	+1.7	270	30	−0.04	19.3	2.1

*Cited in Goodin.[36]

†Data reported for auditory stimulation with an interstimulus interval of 3.3 seconds and a 30 percent probability of rare tone occurrence.

‡Not reported.

Similarly, Ford and co-workers studied 21 unmedicated schizophrenic patients.[55] The subjects were tested after receiving placebo for 1 week and again after treatment with antipsychotic medication for 4 weeks. Despite significant clinical improvement while taking medication, the amplitude and latency of the N1, N2, and P3 components of the response were unchanged. Consequently, it seems that these medications have relatively minor effects on ERPs in therapeutic dosages.

Several researchers have looked at the effect of other medications on the ERP. Particular interest has been directed at drugs that influence the cholinergic system, and several authors have reported a significant increase in the amplitude and shortening in the latency of the P3 response in patients with Alzheimer disease treated with cholinergic medication.[56–59] Moreover, an opposite effect has been observed with the use of anticholinergic medications or with thiamine.[36,60,61] These changes cannot, however, be interpreted as a specific effect on the generators of the P3 response because P3 amplitude changes may result from a general change in the attention or arousal of the subject, and latency shifts may result from delays at earlier stages of processing.

The effects of anticonvulsant medications on the ERP are less clear-cut. Meador and colleagues studied, in a double-blind crossover trial, the effects of different anticonvulsants on the P3 response in patients with epilepsy.[62] They found no difference in P3 latency or amplitude between patients taking carbamazepine, phenobarbital, or phenytoin in therapeutic doses. Chen and co-workers studied the P3 response in 73 children with newly diagnosed epilepsy, both before and after 6 and 12 months of treatment with antiepileptic medication.[63] They reported that P3 latency was unchanged in the patients receiving valproic acid and carbamazepine but was increased in patients receiving phenobarbital. By contrast, Panagopoulos and colleagues reported that treatment with valproic acid, but not carbamazepine, resulted in prolongation of P3 latency.[64] The reason for such discrepant findings is unclear but may relate, in part, to the fact that different blood levels of the anticonvulsants, particularly in toxic ranges, may affect P3 latency.[65]

Sleep Deprivation

Sleep deprivation has been reported to cause both an increase in the latency and a decrease in the amplitude of the P3 response, perhaps reflecting a decrease in the subject's level of vigilance in the sleep-deprived state.[66]

Fitness

Fitness, as determined by increased oxygen utilization during maximal exercise, has been reported to reduce P3 latency in older subjects.[67–69] In one report, however, the significance of the change was only marginal ($P < .05$), and the finding that increased fitness in younger subjects tended to increase P3 latency makes the conclusion questionable.[67] More importantly, in a recent study comparing ERPs in fit subjects with those in sedentary subjects, no difference was found in P3 latency or amplitude between groups.[68,69] Interestingly, however, following exercise, the P3 amplitude increased and its latency decreased significantly in both groups.[68]

Other Factors

It has been suggested that certain other variables (e.g., the recency of food consumption, body temperature, time of day, season, and position in the menstrual cycle) may affect the P3 response.[70,71] These reports still need to be confirmed, but even if the findings are corroborated, the small magnitude of the reported changes makes it unlikely that these variables will markedly influence the interpretation of clinical studies.

CLINICAL APPLICATIONS

Dementia

Dementia refers to an abnormal deterioration in intellect affecting several areas of cognitive function (e.g., abstraction, orientation, judgment, and memory). As such, it is a symptom of many diseases and is not a diagnosis in itself. By far the most common cause of this symptom, particularly in the elderly, is senile dementia of the Alzheimer type (SDAT), which accounts for more than 50 percent of demented patients in most series. Even though SDAT is a progressive and, at present, untreatable disorder, it is nonetheless important to investigate all patients thoroughly to exclude other, treatable causes. For the most part, a few simple radiologic and laboratory studies are sufficient to exclude treatable causes. However, one sizable category of patients with an apparent deterioration in intellect cannot be distinguished from patients with SDAT by these means, and yet these patients have a treatable disease: pseudodementia caused by depression or other psychiatric illness.

It is in this context, then, that the clinical use of ERPs has attracted widest attention. Because ERPs are sensitive to task variables that relate to cognitive behavior, it seemed likely that they might be altered in patients with disorders of cognition such as dementia. Indeed, several groups have studied the P3 component in demented patients and reported that it is of prolonged latency and reduced amplitude in this group (Fig. 29-10 and Table 29-3).[36,72-85] For example, in one study of 58 demented patients, the P3 latency was more than 2 standard errors above the normal age–latency regression line in 74 percent of patients (Fig. 29-11).[36] Moreover, with the exception of a single patient who had a profound postencephalitic anterograde amnestic syndrome without other cognitive difficulties, all diagnostic categories of dementia showed similar prolongations in P3 latency (Table 29-4). The P3 amplitude was also reduced significantly in the group of demented patients but, because of its large normal variability, amplitude could not be used to distinguish individual patients from normal control subjects.[36] By contrast, only 3.5 percent of the 84 nondemented patients with diverse neurologic and psychiatric disorders had P3 latency prolongations of such magnitude (see Fig. 29-11). These findings, again, were similar in all diagnostic categories, including depressive illness (see Table 29-4).

The published studies generally have corroborated these findings: that P3 latency is significantly prolonged and P3 amplitude is significantly reduced in demented subjects compared with those measures in normal control subjects.[36,72-85] Moreover, most studies have not shown a significant delay in the P3 latency of patients diagnosed with depression. However, such a conclusion

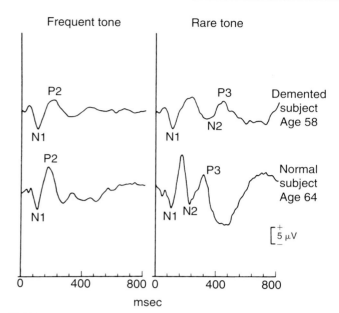

FIGURE 29-10 ■ Long-latency evoked potentials recorded from the vertex in two subjects of similar age, one of whom was demented. The top row shows the response recorded from the demented subject. The bottom row shows the response recorded from the normal subject. The waveforms on the left are the responses to the frequent tone and those on the right are to the rare tone. The latency and amplitude of the N1 and P2 components are similar in the two subjects, but the later event-related components are small and delayed in the response from the demented subject. (From Goodin DS: Electrophysiologic evaluation of dementia. Neurol Clin, 3:633, 1985, with permission.)

TABLE 29-3 ■ P3 Latency in Neurologic and Psychiatric Disease: Percentage Abnormality*			
	Demented Patients	**Psychiatric Patients**	**Nondemented Patients**
Squires et al†	74% (58)	3% (33)‡	4% (51)‡
Brown et al†	61% (18)	0% (7)§	
Pfefferbaum et al†	30% (37)	19% (54)‖	
Leppler and Greenberg†	73% (15)		0% (5)
Gordon et al†	80% (19)	12% (32)¶	
Polich et al†	28% (39)		
Aminoff and Goodin[96]	61% (36)		
Patterson et al†	13% (15)	0% (8)**	
Neshige et al†	41% (27)		
Filipovic and Kostic[72]	70% (40)		14% (58)
Pokryszko-Dragan et al[76]	31% (13)		0% (13)
Bennys et al[80]	91% (30)		0% (10)
Total	56% (347)	11% (134)	8% (143)

*Percentage of patients in each diagnostic category who had P3 components with latencies more than 2 standard errors away from the normal age latency as determined separately by each group (see Table 29-2). Numbers in parentheses indicate number of patients studied in each category.

†Cited in Goodin.[36]

‡Diagnostic categories given in Table 29-4.

§The authors state that these patients suffered primarily from depression.

‖Thirty-four depressed patients and 20 schizophrenics.

¶Seventeen depressed patients and 15 schizophrenics.

**All patients were depressed.

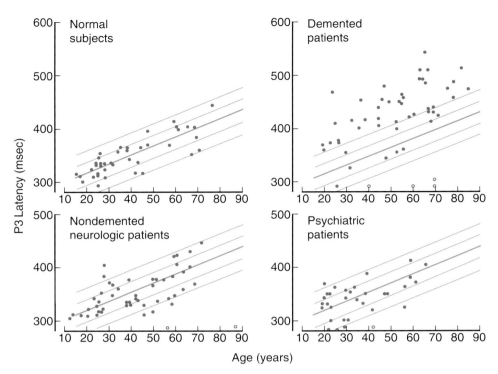

FIGURE 29-11 ■ The relationship between P3 latency and age in three patient groups (see Table 29-4) and in normal subjects. Open circles represent persons in whom no P3 response could be identified. Superimposed on each plot is the regression line for the normal subjects, as well as lighter lines representing 1 and 2 standard errors away from this regression line. Only 3 (3.5 percent) of the combined psychiatric and nondemented patients have P3 latencies that are more than 2 standard errors above the regression line, whereas 43 (74 percent) of the 58 demented patients have P3 latencies that are this prolonged. Subjects with no identifiable P3 response were considered normal. (Modified from Squires KC, Chippendale TJ, Wrege KS et al: Electrophysiological assessment of mental function in aging and dementia. p. 125. In Poon LW [ed]: Aging in the 1980s. American Psychological Association, Washington, DC, 1980, with permission.)

may be applicable to only a subset of depressed patients, as three recent studies have reported the P300 latency to be prolonged significantly in patients with major depressive disorders.[86–88] Moreover, there have also been conflicting data regarding the sensitivity and specificity of the test in a clinical setting. Thus, the false-positive rate generally is reported to be low (see Table 29-3). By contrast, the false-negative rate (reflecting the sensitivity of the test) has been more widely variable (see Table 29-3) and has led to some controversy regarding the clinical utility of measuring P3 latency.[89–91] This increased variability may be due, in part, to variations in task complexity used to elicit the P3 response. Consequently, when using ERPs in a clinical setting, it is important to employ the simplest paradigm to elicit the P3 response and thereby minimize normal intersubject variability. Another complicating factor is that the changes in P3 amplitude and latency are less marked in patients with early SDAT or "mild cognitive impairment" (MCI)

compared with the changes seen in patients with more advanced disease.[73,76,78,80,83] In such a circumstance, the sensitivity of the test would be expected to be less if the sample cohort included a greater proportion of only SDAT cases. Nevertheless, although this is the general finding in most reports, one group reported that the sensitivity and specificity of using P3 latency to distinguish MCI from controls were 75 percent and 80 percent, respectively. The important question, however, is whether those MCI patients with an abnormal P3 at baseline are more likely to progress to full-blown SDAT than are those who have a normal baseline P3. The answer to this question is not known, although in one study, it was reported that one of the two patients who progressed to SDAT over the course of the subsequent year had a markedly prolonged P3 latency at baseline,[74] and a longitudinal study by the same group showed a nonsignificant trend toward showing longer P3 latencies in MCI patients who convert to SDAT compared to

TABLE 29-4 ■ Event-Related Potentials in Dementia

Diagnosis	Number	P3 Latency (SE)*
DEMENTED PATIENTS		
Alzheimer type	13	2.79[†]
Uncertain cause	12	3.17
Toxic-metabolic	11	4.09[†]
Vascular disease	8	4.98[‡]
Hydrocephalus	7	2.84
Brain tumor	4	4.20
Multiple sclerosis	2	8.19
Herpes simplex encephalitis	1	−0.29
All	58	3.61
PSYCHIATRIC PATIENTS		
Depression	12	−0.22
Paranoid schizophrenia	11	−0.30[†]
Manic-depression	6	0.16
Acute schizophrenia	4	−0.23
All	33	−0.18
NONDEMENTED NEUROLOGIC PATIENTS		
Brain tumor	8	−0.52
Vascular disease	7	−0.41
Multiple sclerosis	6	−0.42
Parkinsonism	5	0.50[†]
Hydrocephalus	5	0.87
Trauma	3	0.41
Miscellaneous	17	0.20[†]
All	51	−0.30

*Average P3 latency expressed in units of standard error away from the normal age–latency regression line (see Fig. 29-11).

[†]One patient had no identifiable P3 response and is not included in the average.

[‡]Two patients had no identifiable P3 response and are not included in the average.

Modified from Squires KC, Chippendale TJ, Wrege KS et al: Electrophysiological assessment of mental function in aging and dementia. p. 125. In Poon LW (ed): Aging in the 1980s. American Psychological Association, Washington, DC, 1980, with permission.

MCI patients who are stable.[78] Clearly, this requires further investigation. A reduced sensitivity might also result from the inclusion of patients with distinctive forms of dementia other than SDAT in the demented cohort. For example, in one recent report, patients with frontotemporal dementia were found (as in MCI) to have P3 latencies intermediate between normal controls and patients with SDAT.[92] More important than the possibility that this might help to explain the variable sensitivity, however, is the possibility that this differential effect of frontotemporal dementia and SDAT on P3 could be exploited to help clinicians to distinguish one disorder from the other.

ERPs may also be useful in other clinical contexts. There has been considerable controversy regarding whether a distinction can be made between the dementia syndrome that results from diseases that predominantly affect the neocortex (e.g., Alzheimer disease) and the dementia that results from diseases in which the major pathologic changes are in subcortical structures (e.g., Huntington and Parkinson diseases).[93,94] By recording ERPs in a group of patients with clinically definite Huntington, Alzheimer, or Parkinson disease, however, Goodin and Aminoff were able to demonstrate clear electrophysiologic differences not only between the cortical and the subcortical dementias but also within the subcortical group.[95,96] Thus, only the N2 and P3 latencies were prolonged in Alzheimer disease. In both Huntington disease and Parkinson disease, there was, in addition, a delay in N1 latency, whereas only patients with Huntington disease had a delay in P2 latency. These differences were specific for the dementia because they were not seen in a group of nondemented patients with Parkinson disease of equivalent severity as judged by disease duration and by stage of the disease on the Hoehn and Yahr scale.[95] Other authors have also looked at the electrophysiologic changes in Parkinson, Huntington, and Alzheimer diseases (see Aminoff and Goodin[96] for a review), although no attempt has been made to compare the findings between the different groups. Nonetheless, the reported changes generally have paralleled those outlined earlier for each of the diagnostic groups considered separately. These findings provide direct evidence that different subtypes of dementia exist, and that electrophysiologic techniques may in the future prove useful both for diagnostic purposes and for selecting homogeneous patient populations for clinical trials. In addition, one recent study has suggested that the recording of ERPs in patients with Parkinson disease may be predictive of which patients will experience difficulties with their activities of daily living (ADLs).[97] Thus, of the 30 patients in this study, 8 had prolonged P3 latencies; and, in this latter group, either P3 amplitude or latency was correlated significantly with several ADL and neuropsychologic measures.[97] This is, however, only a single small cohort and, as a result, these observations require confirmation.

Multiple sclerosis (MS) is also a predominantly subcortical disease, although approximately 20 percent of MS plaques are known to involve the gray matter.[98] Moreover, cognitive dysfunction, often independent of any physical disability, is being recognized increasingly as a frequent accompaniment of MS.[99–104] The neuropsychologic pattern of cognitive abnormality in MS is quite reminiscent of that seen in the other subcortical dementias discussed above, with a disproportionate involvement of memory and information-processing compared with verbal performance, which is relatively spared.[99–104] Several groups have reported abnormalities of the ERP in MS and, as in other subcortical dementias, patients are reported to have abnormalities in both the early N1 and P2 components as well as in the later N2 and P3 components of the response.[105–112] However, unlike the other subcortical dementias, MS is associated with demyelination in the primary afferent pathways which, independently of any cognitive disturbance, is known to prolong the peak latencies of the different scalp-recorded evoked potential components (see Chapters 22 to 27). Consequently, interpretation of a prolonged ERP peak latency in an MS patient is ambiguous because any such observation could be caused by demyelination in either a subcortical location or an afferent pathway leading to the brain. In the former circumstance, the ERP change would be expected to reflect the cognitive deficit. In the latter circumstance, by contrast, the correlation between ERP change and cognitive dysfunction, presumably, would be minimal. Aminoff and Goodin explored these possibilities and found not only that the absolute peak latencies of all of the ERP components (N1, P2, N2, and P3) were delayed in MS patients, but also that the N1–N2 and N1–N3 interpeak latencies were both delayed and correlated with the patients' level of cognitive function.[111] This observation suggests that the changes in the later ERP components are not simply caused by alterations in the primary afferent pathways but are the consequence of central demyelination.

ERPs have also been studied in patients infected with human immunodeficiency virus (HIV), of whom some were asymptomatic from their infection and others were demented and met other diagnostic criteria for acquired immunodeficiency syndrome (AIDS).[113] As in other subcortical dementias, patients with the AIDS–dementia complex have a prolongation of the early components of the ERP, particularly the N1 component, in addition to the prolongation of later N2 and P3 components that occurs in other dementing disorders (see Table 29-4). Importantly, Bungener and colleagues have confirmed these general findings.[114] In addition, almost one-third of the asymptomatic patients infected by HIV have ERP changes similar to those with overt dementia, which suggests that these patients may be at particular risk for cognitive difficulties developing in the future.[115] Thus, it may be that the recording of ERPs will permit early recognition of HIV encephalopathy and thereby help to identify patients with a poor prognosis or in need of more aggressive management.

The recording of ERPs can be used to study sequentially the same individual, and thereby provide an objective measure of alteration in cognitive function with time (Fig. 29-12). Unlike SRPs, which may remain abnormal despite the restoration of function in the sensory system being tested, ERPs seem to fluctuate in parallel with the

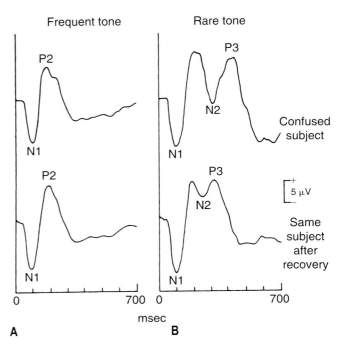

FIGURE 29-12 ■ Long-latency evoked potentials recorded from the vertex in a 60-year-old man admitted to the hospital in a hyponatremic coma. **A**, Responses to the frequent tone. **B**, Responses to the rare tone. The waveforms in the top row were obtained while the patient was still mentally slow. The waveforms in the bottom row were obtained when he was fully recovered, 2 weeks later. The stimulus-related N1 and P2 components are unchanged in amplitude or latency between recordings. The latency of the event-related components has shortened considerably in the recording made after full recovery. (Modified from Goodin DS, Starr A, Chippendale T et al: Sequential changes in the P3 component of the auditory evoked potential in confusional states and dementing illnesses. Neurology, 33:1215, 1983, with permission.)

clinical state.[51,115–120] For example, in one early report, P3 latency was shortened in uremic patients after dialysis.[115] In another, the authors were able to demonstrate that there was a sustained benefit on P3 latency in uremic patients receiving continuous ambulatory peritoneal dialysis compared with only a transient benefit in similar patients receiving standard (intermittent) hemodialysis.[116] Also, P3 latency has been used to assess the effectiveness of medications such as those for Parkinson disease and SDAT.[117–120] Thus, several studies have documented improvements in P3 latency following donepezil treatment in SDAT patients.[121–123] These results suggest that the recording of ERPs may be quite useful in assessing the effectiveness of specific therapies in individual patients with cognitive dysfunction or in evaluating the relative effectiveness of different therapeutic strategies in groups of cognitively impaired patients.

Other Disease States

The ERP has also been used to study disease states other than dementia, although at present the clinical role of the P3 response in these settings has not been defined clearly. For instance, several authors have reported a reduction in the amplitude of the P3 response in schizophrenia,[36,121–123] and some have reported prolongation in latency as well.[36,122,124] In addition, some studies have also demonstrated amplitude asymmetries of the P3 response with a relative attenuation of the response in the left temporal region in schizophrenic patients.[125,126] In general, however, these studies have been directed at theoretical issues (e.g., the nature of the cognitive defects in schizophrenia) rather than at clinical problems. Moreover, as discussed previously, amplitude is such a variable measure, even in the normal population, that although significant group differences may be demonstrated, the group to which an individual belongs (i.e., normal or schizophrenic) cannot be determined reliably on this basis.

Similarly, the P3 response has been studied in both acute alcohol intoxication and chronic alcohol abuse.[36] The general finding is that the P3 amplitude is reduced in both settings, although a few authors also report latency differences.[36] These studies have been largely of theoretical, rather than clinical, interest. There are also reports that subjects with a family history of alcoholism (and therefore at increased risk for becoming alcoholics) had large amplitude decrements in recorded ERPs, unlike subjects without such a history.[36] Such findings suggest that both the P3 response and susceptibility to alcoholism are under genetic control.[36] Moreover, it may be possible in the future to use these studies to identify individuals at particular risk for the development of alcoholism and thereby allow for early intervention.

DIFFICULTY IN ERP INTERPRETATION

During the recording and interpretation of ERPs, several difficulties may be encountered. First, it is difficult to interpret the absence of a P3 response, which may merely reflect the subject's inattention to the task. Moreover, the P3 response is occasionally absent in alert, attentive, and cooperative nondemented subjects (see Fig. 29-11). Consequently, the absence of a response cannot be interpreted as abnormal. This limitation does not, however, detract from the utility of the test in demented patients because most of them (93 percent from Table 29-4) have an identifiable P3 response. Moreover, the sensitivity figure of 74 percent (quoted previously) included the absence of a response as a normal variant (see Fig. 29-11).

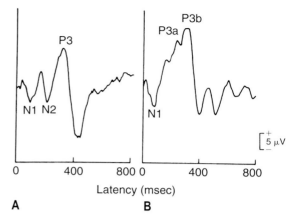

FIGURE 29-13 ■ Long-latency evoked potentials recorded from the vertex in response to the rare stimulus in two young subjects of similar age. One subject (**A**) had the typical complex described previously (see Fig. 29-1). In the other subject (**B**) the P3 was not a single peak but had two subcomponents, P3a and P3b.

The second difficulty that may be encountered is how to interpret a P3 peak when it consists of two subcomponents, P3a and P3b (Fig. 29-13). Typically, the P3a subcomponent is seen in the averaged response to the rare tones even when subjects are inattentive to the stimulus. It is reasonable to measure these two components separately, especially given the occasional reports that only one or the other of them may be abnormal in certain patient populations. As a practical matter, however, the P3a and P3b subcomponents are often fused into a single component (see Fig. 29-1). Nonetheless, it is possible that treating P3a and P3b as a single peak and taking a single latency measurement for the entire complex (see Fig. 29-13) may reduce the sensitivity of the test. Even so, such a procedure generally results in both small standard errors (see Table 29-2) and high sensitivities (see Table 29-3).

The third difficulty relates to intertrial variability of the P3 response in the same subject. Normally, the response is quite reproducible, although occasionally, especially when the P3 latency is considerably prolonged, its latency may be more variable from trial to trial (Fig. 29-14). Even in this latter circumstance, however, the variability rarely exceeds 5 percent of the mean P3 latency, and in general P3 latencies measured from individual trials fall on the same side of the limit of 2 standard errors. Rarely, the intertrial variability will just span this boundary, and conclusions about normality or abnormality cannot be made reliably. In such circumstances, repeating the test often resolves any ambiguity.

Finally, because of the dramatic changes that occur in the P3 response with maturation, separate normal data for the pediatric age group are required if this test is to be used in children.[36–39]

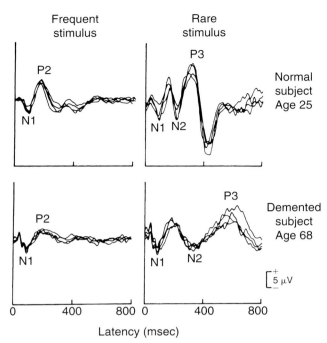

FIGURE 29-14 ■ Long-latency evoked potentials recorded from the vertex on several occasions in two subjects. The waveforms in the top traces are from a young normal subject; the variability in P3 latency is quite small (313 ± 7 msec). The waveforms in the bottom traces are from a 68-year-old demented subject; the P3 response is markedly delayed and the variability in P3 latency is considerably greater (589 ± 21 msec). However, when the latency variability (as measured in terms of standard deviation) is expressed as a percentage of the mean P3 latency, it is comparable in the two subjects (less than 5 percent).

CONCLUDING COMMENTS

ERPs have now been applied quite extensively in clinical settings, especially in circumstances where an individual either has, or is at risk to have, cognitive dysfunction. They are, for the most part, affected differentially by disorders such as dementia and depression or in different forms of dementing illness. They can shed light on clinical controversies, such as whether a distinction between cortical and subcortical dementias is possible. They may also be useful in identifying individuals with certain illnesses (e.g., HIV infection, MS, Parkinson disease) who are at risk for cognitive dysfunction and who, perhaps, are in need of special treatment. Clearly, there are areas of continuing controversy, such as the best recording design for optimizing the sensitivity and specificity of the test or the actual value of the ERP information in different clinical settings. Nonetheless, the recording of ERPs in clinical contexts has proven useful, and it seems likely that these potentials will continue to be used in the evaluation of patients who have or are at risk for

having dementing disorders, both as an aid in the diagnosis and management of patients and as a guide to their prognosis.

REFERENCES

1. Halliday AM: Evoked Potentials in Clinical Testing. 2nd Ed. Churchill Livingstone, Edinburgh, 1993
2. Picton TW: The P300 wave of the human event-related potential. J Clin Neurophysiol, 9:456, 1992
3. Polich J, Kok A: Cognitive and biological determinants of P300: an integrative review. Biol Psychol, 41:103, 1995
4. Muller-Gass A, Campbell K: Event-related measures of the inhibition of information processing: I. Selective attention in the waking state. Int J Psychophysiol, 46:177, 2002
5. Goodin DS, Aminoff MJ, Chequer RS et al: Response compatibility and the relationship between event-related potentials and the timing of a motor response. J Neurophysiol, 76:3705, 1996
6. Verleger R: On the utility of P3 latency as an index of mental chronometry. Psychophysiol, 34:131, 1997
7. Aminoff MJ, Goodin DS: The decision to make a movement: neurophysiological insights. Can J Neurol Sci, 24:181, 1997
8. Donchin E, Coles MGH: Context updating and the P300. Behav Brain Sci, 21:152, 1998
9. Goodin DS, Aminoff MJ: Event-related potentials in the study of sensory discrimination and motor response in simple and choice reaction tasks. J Clin Neurophysiol, 15:34, 1998
10. Leuthold H, Sommer W: Postperceptual effects and P300 latency. Psychophysiology, 35:34, 1998
11. Leppert DL, Goodin DS, Aminoff MJ: Stimulus recognition and its relationship to the cerebral event-related potential. Neurology, 61:1533, 2003
12. Verleger R, Jaskowski P, Wascher E: Evidence for an integrative role of P3b in linking reaction to perception. J Psychophysiol, 19:165, 2005
13. Polich J: Updating P300: an integrative theory of P3a and P3b. Clin Neurophysiol, 118:2128, 2007
14. Barcelo F, Perianez JA: Updating sensory versus task representations during task-switching: insights from cognitive brain potentials in humans. Neuropsychologia, 47:1160, 2009
15. Knight RT, Scabini D: Anatomic basis of event-related potentials and their relationship to novelty detection in humans. J Clin Neurophysiol, 15:3, 1998
16. Comerchero MD, Polich J: P3a and P3b from typical auditory and visual stimuli: typicality, task, and topography. Clin Neurophysiol, 110:24, 1999
17. Fjell AM, Wahlhovd KB: On the topography of P3a and P3b across the adult lifespan: a factor-analytic study using orthogonal procrustes rotation. Brain Topogr, 15:153, 2003
18. Federmeier KD, Van Petten C, Schwartz TJ et al: Sounds, words, sentences: age-related changes across levels of language processing. Psychol Aging, 18:858, 2003

19. Vidal F, Hasbroucq T, Grapperon J et al: Is the "error negativity" specific to errors? Biol Psychol, 51:109, 2000

20. Falkenstein M, Hoormann J, Hohnsbein J: Changes of error-related ERPs with age. Exp Brain Res, 138:258, 2001

21. Campbell K, Colrain IM: Event-related measures of the inhibition of information processing: II. The sleep onset period. Int J Psychophysiol, 46:197, 2002

22. Polich J: P300 clinical utility and control of variability. J Clin Neurophysiol, 15:14, 1998

23. Fallgatter AJ, Esienack SS, Neuhauser B et al: Stability of late event-related potentials: topographical descriptors of motor control compared with the P300 amplitude. Brain Topogr, 12:255, 2000

24. Lew HL, Gray M, Poole JH: Temporal stability of auditory event-related potentials in healthy individuals and patients with traumatic brain injury. J Clin Neurophysiol, 24:392, 2007

25. Yamaguchi S, Knight RT: Effects of temporal-parietal lesions on the somatosensory P3 to lower limb stimulation. Electroencephalogr Clin Neurophysiol, 84:139, 1992

26. Verleger R, Heide W, Butt C et al: Reduction of P3b in patients with temporo-parietal lesions. Brain Res Cogn Brain Res, 2:103, 1994

27. Kirino E, Belger A, Goldman-Rakic P et al: Prefrontal activation evoked by infrequent target and novel stimuli in a visual target detection task: an event-related functional magnetic resonance imaging study. J Neurosci, 20:6612, 2000

28. Kiehl KA, Laurens KR, Duty TL et al: Neural sources involved in auditory target detection and novelty processing: an event-related fMRI study. Psychophysiology, 38:133, 2001

29. Dien J, Spencer KM, Donchin E: Localization of the event-related potential novelty response as defined by principal components analysis. Brain Res Cogn Brain Res, 17:637, 2003

30. Folgelson N, Shah M, Scabini D et al: Prefrontal cortex is critical for contextual processing: evidence from brain lesions. Brain, 132:3002, 2009

31. Polich J, Comerchero MD: P3a from visual stimuli: typicality, task, and topography. Brain Topogr, 15:141, 2003

32. Stadler W, Klimesch W, Pouthas V et al: Differential effects of the stimulus sequence on CNV and P300. Brain Res, 1123:157, 2006

33. Bonala B, Boutros NN, Jansen BH: Target probability affects the likelihood that a P300 will be generated in response to a target stimulus, but not its amplitude. Psychophysiology, 45:93, 2008

34. Goodin DS, Aminoff MJ, Chequer RS: The effect of different high-pass filters on the long latency event-related potentials in normal human subjects and individuals infected with human immunodeficiency virus. J Clin Neurophysiol, 9:97, 1992

35. Goodin D, Desmedt J, Maurer K et al: IFCN recommended standards for long-latency auditory event-related potentials. Report of an IFCN committee. Electroencephalogr Clin Neurophysiol, 91:18, 1994

36. Goodin DS: Event-related potentials. p. 609. In Aminoff MJ (ed): Electrodiagnosis in Clinical Neurology. 5th Ed. Elsevier Churchill Livingstone, Philadelphia, 2005

37. Stige S, Fjell AM, Smith L et al: The development of visual P3a and P3b. Dev Neuropsychol, 32:563, 2007

38. Brinkman MJ, Stauder JE: The development of passive auditory novelty processing. Int J Psychophysiol, 70:33, 2008

39. Fuchigami Y, Okubo O, Fujita Y et al: Event-related potentials in response to 3-D auditory stimuli. Brain Dev, 31:577, 2009

40. Enoki H, Sanada S, Yoshinaga H et al: The effects of age on the N200 component of the auditory event-related potentials. Brain Res Cog Brain Res, 1:161, 1993

41. Iragui VJ, Kutas M, Mitchiner MR et al: Effects of aging on event-related brain potentials and reaction times in an auditory oddball task. Psychophysiology, 30:10, 1993

42. Polich J: Meta-analysis of P300 normative aging studies. Psychophysiology, 33:334, 1996

43. Anderer P, Semlitsch HV, Saletu B: Multichannel auditory event-related brain potentials: effects of normal aging on the scalp distribution of N1, P2, N2, and P300 latencies and amplitudes. Electroencephalogr Clin Neurophysiol, 99:458, 1996

44. Alain C, Woods DL: Age-related changes in processing auditory stimuli during visual attention: evidence for deficits in inhibitory control and sensory memory. Psychol Aging, 14:507, 1999

45. Walhovd KB, Fjell AM: Two- and three-stimuli auditory oddball ERP tasks and neuropsychological measures in aging. Neuroreport, 12:3149, 2001

46. Daffner KR, Ryan KK, Williams DM et al: Age-related differences in novelty and target processing among cognitively high performing adults. Neurobiol Aging, 26:1283, 2005

47. Golob EJ, Irimajiri R, Starr A: Auditory cortical activity in amnestic mild cognitive impairment: relationship to subtype and conversion to dementia. Brain, 130:740, 2007

48. Schiff S, Valenti P, Andrea P et al: The effect of aging on auditory components of event-related brain potentials. Clin Neurophysiol, 119:1795, 2008

49. Pontifex MB, Hillman CH, Polich J: Age, physical fitness, and attention: P3a and P3b. Psychophysiology, 46:379, 2009

50. Fjell AM, Walhovd KB: Age-sensitivity of P3 in high-functioning adults. Neurobiol Aging, 26:1297, 2005

51. Steffensen SC, Ohran AJ, Shipp DN et al: Gender-selective effects of the P300 and N400 components of the visual evoked potential. Vision Res, 48:917, 2008

52. Duarte JL, Alvarenge K de F, Banhara MR et al: P300-long-latency auditory evoked potential in normal hearing subjects: simultaneous recording value in Fz and Cz. Braz J Otorhinolaryngol, 75:231, 2009

53. Criado JR, Polich J: Neuropsychology and neuropharmacology of P3a and P3b. Int J Psychophysiol, 60:172, 2006

54. Galderisi S, Mucci A, Volpe U et al: Evidence-based medicine and electrophysiology in schizophrenia. Clin EEG Neurosci, 40:62, 2009

55. Ford JM, White PM, Csernansky JG et al: ERPs in schizophrenia: effects of antipsychotic medication. Biol Psychiatry, 36:153, 1994

56. Reeves RR, Struve FA, Patricks G et al: The effects of donepezil on the P300 auditory and visual cognitive evoked potentials of patients with Alzheimer's disease. Am J Geriatr Psychiatry, 7:349, 1999

57. Thomas A, Iacono D, Bonanni L et al: Donepezil, rivastigmine, and vitamin E in Alzheimer disease: a combined P300 event-related potential/neuropsychologic evaluation over 6 months. Clin Neuropharmacol, 24:31, 2001

58. Katada E, Sato K, Sawaki A et al: Long-term effects of donepezil on P300 auditory event-related potentials in patients with Alzheimer's disease. J Geriatr Psychiatry Neurol, 16:39, 2003

59. Hansenne M: The p300 cognitive event-related potential. I. Theoretical and psychobiologic perspectives. Neurophysiol Clin, 30:191, 2000

60. Meador KJ, Nichols ME, Franke P et al: Evidence for a central cholinergic effect of high-dose thiamine. Ann Neurol, 34:724, 1993

61. Easton CJ, Bauer LO: Beneficial effects of thiamine on recognition memory and P300 in abstinent cocaine-dependent patients. Psychiatry Res, 70:165, 1997

62. Meador KJ, Loring DW, Huh K et al: Comparative cognitive effects of anticonvulsants. Neurology, 40:391, 1990

63. Chen YJ, Kang WM, So WC: Comparison of antiepileptic drugs on cognitive function in newly diagnosed epileptic children: a psychometric and neurophysiological study. Epilepsia, 37:81, 1996

64. Panagopoulos GR, Thomaides T, Tigaris G et al: Auditory event-related potentials in patients with epilepsy on sodium valproate monotherapy. Acta Neurol Scand, 96:62, 1997

65. Enoki H, Sanada S, Oka E et al: Effects of high-dose antiepileptic drugs on event-related potentials in epileptic children. Epilepsy Res, 25:59, 1996

66. Lee HJ, Kim L, Suh KY: Cognitive deterioration and changes of P300 during total sleep deprivation. Psychiatry Clin Neurosci, 57:490, 2003

67. Dustman RE, Emmerson RY, Ruhling RO et al: Age and fitness effects on EEG, ERPs, visual sensitivity, and cognition. Neurobiol Aging, 11:193, 1990

68. Magnie MN, Bermon S, Martin F et al: P300, N400, aerobic fitness, and maximal aerobic exercise. Psychophysiology, 37:369, 2000

69. Pontifex MB, Hillman CH, Polich J: Age, physical fitness, and attention: P3a and P3b. Psychophysiology, 46:379, 2009

70. Geisler MW, Polich J: P300 and time-of-day: circadian rhythms, food intake, and body temperature. Biol Psychol, 31:117, 1990

71. Polich J, Herbst KL: P300 as a clinical assay: rationale, evaluation, and findings. Int J Psychophysiol, 38:3, 2000

72. Filipovic SR, Kostic VS: Utility of auditory P300 in detection of presenile dementia. J Neurol Sci, 13:150, 1995

73. Frodl T, Hampel H, Juckel G et al: Value of event-related P300 subcomponents in the clinical diagnosis of mild cognitive impairment and Alzheimer's disease. Psychophysiology, 39:175, 2002

74. Golob EJ, Johnson JK, Starr A: Auditory event-related potentials during target detection are abnormal in mild cognitive impairment. Clin Neurophysiol, 113:151, 2002

75. Braverman ER, Blum K: P300 (latency) event-related potential: an accurate predictor of memory impairment. Clin Electroencephalogr, 34:124, 2003

76. Pokryszko-Dragan A, Slotwinski K, Podemski R: Modality-specific changes in P300 parameters in patients with dementia of the Alzheimer type. Med Sci Monit, 9:CR130, 2003

77. Braverman ER, Chen TJ, Schoolfield J et al: Delayed P300 latency correlates with abnormal Test of Variables of Attention (TOVA) in adults and predicts early cognitive decline in a clinical setting. Adv Ther, 23:582, 2006

78. Golob EJ, Irimajiri R, Starr A: Auditory cortical activity in amnestic mild cognitive impairment: relationship to subtype and conversion to dementia. Brain, 130:740, 2007

79. Taylor JR, Olichney JM: From amnesia to dementia: ERP studies of memory and language. Clin EEG Neurosci, 38:8, 2007

80. Bennys K, Portet F, Touchon J et al: Diagnostic value of event-related evoked potentials N200 and P300 subcomponents in early diagnosis of Alzheimer's disease and mild cognitive impairment. J Clin Neurophysiol, 24:405, 2007

81. Juckel G, Clotz F, Kawohl W et al: Diagnostic usefulness of cognitive auditory event-related p300 subcomponents in patients with Alzheimer's disease? J Clin Neurophysiol, 25:147, 2008

82. Papaliagkas V, Kimiskidis V, Tsolaki M et al: Usefulness of event-related potentials in the assessment of mild cognitive impairment. BMC Neurosci, 9:107, 2008

83. van Deursen JA, Vuurman EF, Smits LL et al: Response speed, contingent negative variation and P300 in Alzheimer's disease and MCI. Brain Cogn, 69:592, 2009

84. Golob EJ, Ringman JM, Irimajiri R et al: Cortical event-related potentials in preclinical familial Alzheimer disease. Neurology, 73:1649, 2009

85. Lai CL, Lin RT, Liou LM et al: The role of event-related potentials in cognitive decline in Alzheimer's disease. Clin Neurophysiol, 121:194, 2010

86. Himani A, Tandon OP, Bhatia MS: A study of P300-event related evoked potential in the patients of major depression. Ind J Physiol Pharmacol, 43:367, 1999

87. Karaaslan F, Gonul AS, Oguz A et al: P300 changes in major depressive disorders with and without psychotic features. J Affect Disord, 73:283, 2003

88. Kemp AH, Pe Benito L, Quintana DS et al: Impact of depression heterogeneity on attention: an auditory oddball event related potential study. J Affect Disord, 123:202, 2010

89. Celesia GG: Clinical utility of long latency "cognitive" event-related potentials (P3): editorial comment. Electroencephalogr Clin Neurophysiol, 76:1, 1990

90. Goodin DS: Clinical utility of long latency "cognitive" event-related potentials (P3): the pros. Electroencephalogr Clin Neurophysiol, 76:2, 1990

91. Pfefferbaum A, Ford JM, Kraemer HC: Clinical utility of long latency "cognitive" event-related potentials (P3): the cons. Electroencephalogr Clin Neurophysiol, 76:6, 1990

92. Jimenez-Escrig A, Fernandez-Lorente J, Herrero A: Event-related evoked potential P300 in frontotemporal dementia. Dement Geriatr Cogn Disord, 13:27, 2002

93. Farlow MR, Cummings J: A modern hypothesis: the distinct pathologies of dementia associated with Parkinson's disease versus Alzheimer's disease. Dement Geriatr Cogn Disord, 25:301, 2008

94. Jellinger KA: The pathology of "vascular dementia": a critical update. J Alzheimers Dis, 14:107, 2008

95. Goodin DS: Electrophysiological correlates of dementia in Parkinson's disease. p. 199. In Huber SJ, Cummings JL (eds): Neurobehavior of Parkinson's Disease. Oxford University Press, New York, 1992

96. Aminoff MJ, Goodin DS: Electrophysiological evaluation of dementia. Handb Clin Neurol, 89:63, 2008

97. Maeshima S, Itakura T, Komai N et al: Relationships between event-related potentials (P300) and activities of daily living in Parkinson's disease. Brain Inj, 16:1, 2002

98. Bo L, Vedeler CA, Nyland HI et al: Subpial demyelination in the cerebral cortex of multiple sclerosis patients. J Neuropathol Exp Neurol, 62:723, 2003

99. Rao SM, Leo GJ, Bernardin L et al: Cognitive dysfunction in multiple sclerosis. I: Frequency, patterns, and prediction. Neurology, 41:685, 1991

100. Rao SM, Leo GJ, Ellington L et al: Cognitive dysfunction in multiple sclerosis II: Impact on employment and social functioning. Neurology, 41:692, 1991

101. Kujala P, Portin R, Ruutianen J: Memory deficits and early cognitive deterioration in MS. Acta Neurol Scand, 93:329, 1996

102. Pelosi L, Geesken JM, Holly M et al: Working memory impairment in early multiple sclerosis: evidence from an event-related potential study of patients with clinically isolated myelopathy. Brain, 120:2039, 1997

103. Paul RH, Beatty WW, Schneider R et al: Impairments of attention in individuals with multiple sclerosis. Mult Scler, 4:433, 1998

104. Demaree HA, DeLuca J, Guadino EA et al: Speed of information processing in multiple sclerosis: implications for rehabilitation. J Neurol Neurosurg Psychiatry, 67:661, 1999

105. Honig LS, Eugene-Ramsay R, Sheremata WA: Event-related potential P300 in multiple sclerosis. Arch Neurol, 49:44, 1992

106. Giesser BS, Schroeder MM, LaRocca NG et al: Endogenous event-related potentials as indices of dementia in multiple sclerosis patients. Electroencephalogr Clin Neurophysiol, 82:320, 1992

107. Polich J, Romine JS, Sipe JC et al: P300 in multiple sclerosis: a preliminary report. Int J Psychophysiol, 12:155, 1992

108. Triantafyllou NI, Voumvourakis K, Zalonis I et al: Cognition in relapsing-remitting multiple sclerosis: a multi-channel event-related potential (P300) study. Acta Neurol Scand, 85:10, 1992

109. Gil R, Zai L, Neau JP et al: Event-related auditory evoked potentials and multiple sclerosis. Electroencephalogr Clin Neurophysiol, 88:182, 1993

110. Slater JD, Wu FY, Honig LS et al: Neural network analysis of the P300 event-related potential in multiple sclerosis. Electroencephalogr Clin Neurophysiol, 90:114, 1994

111. Aminoff JC, Goodin DS: Long-latency cerebral event-related potentials in multiple sclerosis. J Clin Neurophysiol, 18:372, 2001

112. Piras MR, Magnano I, Canu ED et al: Longitudinal study of cognitive dysfunction in multiple sclerosis: neuropsychological, neuroradiological, and neurophysiological findings. J Neurol Neurosurg Psychiatry, 74:878, 2003

113. Goodin DS, Aminoff MJ, Chernoff DN et al: Long latency event-related potentials in patients infected with human immunodeficiency virus. Ann Neurol, 27:414, 1990

114. Bungener C, Le Houezc JL, Pierson A et al: Cognitive and emotional deficits in early stages of HIV infection. Prog Neuropsychopharmacol Biol Psychiatry, 20:1303, 1996

115. Gallai V, Alberti A, Buoncristiani U et al: Changes in auditory P3 event-related potentials in uremic patients undergoing haemodialysis. Electromyogr Clin Neurophysiol, 34:397, 1994

116. Buoncristiani U, Alberti A, Gubbiotti G et al: Better preservation of cognitive faculty in continuous ambulatory peritoneal dialysis. Perit Dial Int, 13:Suppl 2, S202, 1993

117. Prabhakar S, Syal P, Srivastava T: P300 in newly diagnosed non-dementing Parkinson's disease: effect of dopaminergic drugs. Neurol India, 48:239, 2000

118. Katada E, Sato K, Sawaki A et al: Long-term effects of donepezil on P300 auditory event-related potentials in patients with Alzheimer's disease. J Geriatr Psychiatry Neurol, 16:39, 2003

119. Onofrj M, Thomas A, Iacono D et al: The effects of a cholinesterase inhibitor are prominent in patients with fluctuating cognition: a part 3 study of the main mechanism of cholinesterase inhibitors in dementia. Clin Neuropharmacol, 26:239, 2003

120. Werber EA, Gandelman-Marton R, Klein C et al: The clinical use of P300 event related potentials for the evaluation of cholinesterase inhibitors treatment in demented patients. J Neural Transm, 110:659, 2003

121. Souza VB, Muir WJ, Walker MT et al: Auditory P300 event-related potentials and neuropsychological performance in schizophrenia and bipolar affective disorder. Biol Psychiatry, 37:300, 1995

122. Heidrich A, Strik WK: Auditory P300 topography and neuropsychological test performance: evidence for left hemispheric dysfunction in schizophrenia. Biol Psychiatry, 41:327, 1997

123. Martin-Loeches M, Molina V, Munoz F et al: P300 amplitude as a possible correlate of frontal degeneration in schizophrenia. Schizophr Res, 49:121, 2001

124. O'Donnell BF, Faux SF, McCarley RW et al: Increased rate of latency prolongation with age in schizophrenia: electrophysiological evidence for a neurodegenerative process. Arch Gen Psychiatry, 52:544, 1995

125. Porjesz B, Begleiter H: Genetic basis of event-related potentials and their relationship to alcoholism and alcohol use. J Clin Neurophysiol, 15:44, 1998

126. Hill SY, Steinhauer S, Park J et al: Event-related potential characteristics in children of alcoholics from high density families. Alcohol Clin Exp Res, 14:6, 1990

Intraoperative Monitoring by Evoked Potential Techniques

RONALD G. EMERSON and DAVID C. ADAMS

Over the past three decades, the field of intraoperative neurophysiologic monitoring has evolved and matured, and monitoring during procedures such as resection of acoustic nerve tumors and correction of spinal deformities is now considered the standard of care. Intraoperative monitoring can diminish the risk of neurologic injury during surgery in three ways. Nearly real-time functional surveillance of neural structures may enable detection of injury at a time when it can be reversed or minimized. For example, during surgery for correction of spinal deformities, monitoring by somatosensory evoked potential (SEP) and motor evoked potential (MEP) recordings can detect deteriorating long-tract function early enough to avert permanent spinal cord damage. Intraoperative neurophysiologic techniques can also be used to identify neural structures that are difficult to locate visually. SEPs, for example, are used commonly to identify the rolandic fissure during resective cerebral surgery. Finally, monitoring occasionally provides insights into the pathophysiology of intraoperative neurologic injury that may lead to improvements in surgical practice, anesthetic management, and neurophysiologic technique.[1]

The development of effective intraoperative neurophysiologic monitoring strategies has resulted from the combined efforts of neurophysiologists, anesthesiologists, and surgeons. For the neurophysiologist, transposition of neurophysiologic recording techniques from the traditional diagnostic laboratory setting to the operating room has entailed the modification of standard recording techniques

as well as the development of new ones. It has also been necessary to develop interpretative strategies appropriate for the operating room. For the anesthesiologist, this has meant adaptation of anesthetic techniques to facilitate neurophysiologic monitoring. For the surgeon, optimal utilization of intraoperative monitoring has required learning the appropriate questions to ask the neurophysiologist and what to do with the answers.

Careful examination of early reports of failures of evoked potential (EP) monitoring to detect neurologic injury reveals that some of these failures did not reflect limitations inherent to EP monitoring per se, but rather were the consequence of errors such as the failure to monitor for a sufficient time, failure to monitor the correct type of EP, and failure to recognize artifact.[2-4] The occurrence of these types of failures reflects the learning curve that is an inevitable part of the development of a new family of technical procedures. The field of intraoperative monitoring continues to evolve, and in some cases there are significant differences in the techniques used at various centers. The current literature contains an unending stream of papers describing innovative, imaginative, and often effective approaches to various aspects of intraoperative monitoring.[5] This chapter is not intended to serve as either an exhaustive reference or an instruction manual. Rather, it is intended to provide an introduction to the major clinical areas in which intraoperative monitoring is used currently and to illustrate how standard diagnostic laboratory techniques may be extended for use in the operating room.

LONG-TRACT MONITORING

One important application of intraoperative monitoring is the surveillance of long-tract function during procedures that place motor and sensory tracts at risk. These include certain orthopedic spinal procedures, invasive neuroradiologic procedures, spinal cord and brainstem surgery, and surgery involving the abdominal aorta.[5–14] Historically, the "wake-up" test was used to verify the functional integrity of the spinal cord during certain spinal procedures.[15] However, the wake-up test provides only a single, nonquantitative indication of spinal cord function, and it exposes the patient to additional risks including dislodgment of instrumentation, laminar fractures, pulmonary embolism, and accidental extubation. When the wake-up test is performed, its typical role is now confirmatory, rather than one of primary surveillance.

Because SEPs and MEPs are mediated by anatomically segregated pathways, independent intraoperative injury can occur to either pathway.[16–19] During surgery for intramedullary lesions, SEPs may be lost due to posterior column disturbance at the time of the initial myelotomy when there has been no injury to motor tracts, precluding further SEP monitoring.[20] The vascular anatomy of the spinal cord, with anterior and lateral portions being dependent on the anterior spinal artery and the posterior columns supplied independently and more robustly by the posterior spinal arteries, provides a further basis for independent injury. The anterior spinal artery has large watershed regions along its length, making the corticospinal tracts particularly vulnerable to ischemia resulting from hypotension and potentially producing loss of motor function without altering SEPs.[16] During scoliosis surgery, distraction or derotation may cause occlusion or spasm of the artery of Adamkiewicz, the major radicular branch supplying the lower portion of the anterior spinal artery. This can disrupt the blood supply to the corticospinal tracts, with preservation of posterior column perfusion leaving SEPs intact. For similar reasons, MEP monitoring is employed during thoracic abdominal aneurysm repair at some centers where it can have important input into real-time management decisions. These decisions include discontinuation of partial bypass, the selection of segmental arteries for reimplantation, and changes to blood pressure, cardiac output, and bypass flow rate.[21–26] Independent loss of MEPs and SEPs may be observed during provocative testing with intra-arterial lidocaine injection before endovascular embolization of spinal cord vascular malformations; the modality lost following injection of anterior or posterior circulation may be unpredictable because of abnormal angioarchitecture.[27]

In general, SEP and MEP monitoring are complementary, and optimal monitoring of long-tract function often entails concurrent recording of both SEPs and MEPs. Despite their dependence on distinct anatomic pathways, each modality provides good surveillance of spinal cord integrity in many cases. Experimental spinal cord injury caused by ischemia, compression, and blunt trauma produces graded changes of both MEPs and SEPs.[28–31] Operative injury, particularly injury caused by spinal cord compression, generally produces changes in both MEPs and SEPs.[32,33] Importantly, it is possible that either measure may be compromised by electrical interference or other factors that can make its interpretation difficult or ambiguous; for this reason, concurrent MEP and SEP recording can provide an added level of security. Additionally, concomitant monitoring of both upper and lower extremities can provide a basis for distinction of systemic or anesthetic effects from local surgical injury.[14,21,34]

SEP Monitoring

Although the techniques used for intraoperative SEP recording are similar to those used in the diagnostic laboratory, important differences exist. Among these are the effects of certain anesthetic agents that can attenuate the cortical components of SEPs, anesthetic agents that may augment intraoperative cortical recordings, and the use of paralytic drugs that can actually facilitate the recording of subcortical SEP components.

The montages used to record SEPs, both in the diagnostic laboratory and in the operating room, exploit the restricted scalp topographies of the primary cortical SEP components and the widespread distribution of the far-field subcortical components. For the median nerve SEP, the primary cortical N20 response is confined to the centroparietal portion of the scalp opposite the stimulated arm, whereas the subcortical P14 and N18 responses are widely distributed. Accordingly, a bipolar "scalp-to-scalp" recording between symmetric centroparietal scalp electrodes on either side of the head detects the N20 response in isolation. By contrast, a referential "scalp-to-noncephalic" recording, which uses a scalp electrode ipsilateral to the stimulated median nerve, detects only subcortical far-field potentials (Fig. 30-1). The topography of posterior tibial nerve SEPs is somewhat more complex, and varies considerably among individuals. The primary cortical P37 response may be largest at the vertex or over the scalp *ipsilateral* to the stimulated leg. For this reason, it is necessary to use at least two channels to record P37 reliably in all patients (e.g., CPz–CP contralateral as well as CP ipsilateral–CP contralateral),[35]

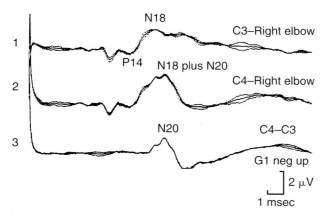

FIGURE 30-1 ■ Left median nerve somatosensory evoked potential demonstrating selective recording of subcortical (P14, N18; trace 1) and cortical (N20; trace 3) potentials. Trace 3 was obtained by digitally subtracting trace 1 from trace 2, equivalent to recording using a C4–C3 bipolar derivation.

or to determine the optimal derivation for recording P37 by mapping the response prior to monitoring.[36] (Electrode locations CP ipsilateral and CP contralateral refer to standard CP3 and CP4 locations, respectively ipsilateral and contralateral to the stimulated limb.) The subcortical P31 and N34 components are detected in isolation by using a referential Fpz electrode to a noncephalic derivation.

In the diagnostic laboratory, N20 and P37 cortical responses are typically easy to record, even in awake patients. The relatively short interelectrode distances minimize movement- and muscle-related artifacts. However, in the operating room, cortical SEP components can be difficult to record reliably because they are attenuated by most inhaled general anesthetic agents. This can cause cortical SEP components to be unstable and change in both amplitude and latency with variations in anesthetic drug concentration. These effects are greatest in infants and young children[37] and are generally more prominent

for lower-extremity SEP recordings. Both halogenated inhalational agents (e.g., halothane, isoflurane, sevoflurane, and desflurane) and nitrous oxide reduce cortical SEP amplitudes and prolong SEP latencies.[38–41] It appears that the combination of halogenated anesthetics with nitrous oxide has more profound effects on SEP latency and amplitude than equipotent doses of these anesthetic agents used alone.[41,42] Likewise, because sevoflurane, desflurane, and nitrous oxide are insoluble relative to halothane and isoflurane, anesthetic effects on the SEP may vary rapidly as delivered concentrations are changed intraoperatively. Most other agents (e.g., propofol, dexmedetomidine, opioids, benzodiazepines, and barbiturates) have similar but considerably less prominent effects.[38,41,43]

In the diagnostic laboratory, subcortical far-field potentials are often difficult to record, largely due to the susceptibility of noncephalic referential recordings to contamination by movement- and muscle-related artifacts. In the operating room, muscle-related noise can be eliminated, and the recording of subcortical signals correspondingly facilitated through the use of neuromuscular blocking agents (Fig. 30-2).[14] Subcortical SEP components are much less affected by anesthetic agents, and for this reason can be particularly useful indicators for intraoperative monitoring (Fig. 30-3).[43]

Subcortical signal can be occasionally difficult to record, particularly in patients with pre-existing neurologic deficits. Further, in cases where concurrent MEP or electromyographic (EMG) monitoring limits or precludes the use of neuromuscular blockade, it is particularly important to be able to monitor cortical responses. In these cases, agents that have less effect on cortical SEPs (e.g., propofol or dexmedetomidine) are desirable, and those that most attenuate the cortical SEPs (e.g., halogenated inhalational agents) should be limited.[43,44] Communication with the anesthesiologist is essential

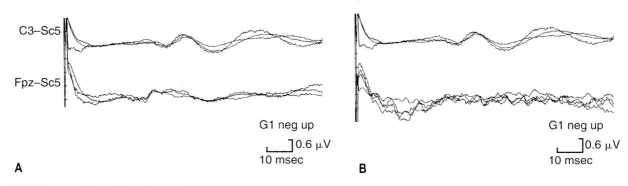

FIGURE 30-2 ■ Posterior tibial nerve somatosensory evoked potential recorded in a patient receiving nitrous oxide/fentanyl anesthesia with (**A**) and without (**B**) a paralytic agent. Neuromuscular blockade produced by a vecuronium infusion facilitated recording of a good-quality subcortical response (Fpz–Sc5). Sc5 designates an electrode position over the fifth cervical vertebra.

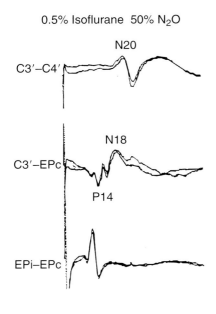

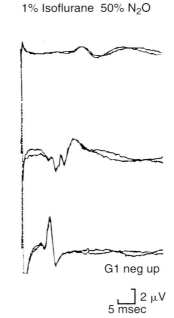

FIGURE 30-3 ■ Median nerve somatosensory evoked potential. Isoflurane suppresses the N20 cortical potential but not the subcortical N18 potential. C3′ and C4′ refer to electrode positions midway between C3 and P3, and C4 and P4, respectively. EPi and EPc refer to electrode positions over Erb's point ipsilateral and contralateral, respectively, to the stimulated median nerve.

because small variations in the doses of anesthetic drugs, particularly halogenated inhalational agents and nitrous oxide, may produce large variations in SEP amplitude that can mimic the effects of surgical injury. Cortical SEP amplitudes may exhibit similar sensitivity to fluctuations in blood pressure (Fig. 30-4). Additionally, etomidate, a gamma-aminobutyric acid (GABA)$_A$ receptor agonist, and ketamine, an antagonist of N-methyl-D-aspartate (NMDA) receptors—intravenous anesthetic agents that have been shown to increase the amplitude of cortical SEP components—can be used to augment cortical SEPs intraoperatively.[45-47] Figure 30-5 presents an example of SEP monitoring using subcortical and cortical SEPs and the use of etomidate to enhance the cortical signals.

Surgical injury to the spinal cord typically produces loss of EP amplitude and degradation of signal morphology; latency prolongations are a less prominent and consistent finding.[7,48] Interpretive strategies must therefore be different from those used in standard laboratory SEP testing, which are based primarily on response latencies.[35] Moreover, for intraoperative monitoring, a patient's EPs are compared primarily with that patient's baseline values rather than normative controls.

Two somewhat different approaches have been used to interpret intraoperative SEP recordings. One is to adopt predefined limits beyond which the risk of neurologic insult is considered to be substantial and to inform the surgeon when those limits have been reached. Many centers, somewhat arbitrarily, use a 50 percent decrement in amplitude or a 10 percent increase in latency for these limits. An alternative approach is to inform the surgeon of changes, even if small, in SEP amplitude, latency, and morphology that are determined by the neurophysiologist to have exceeded the baseline variability in that patient's recordings. The authors favor the

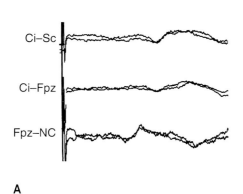

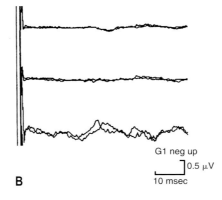

FIGURE 30-4 ■ Median nerve somatosensory evoked potential. An example of mild hypotension attenuating the cortical response but not substantially affecting the subcortical response. NC represents a noncephalic reference. Blood pressure was 120/70 mm Hg in **A**, and 90/50 mm Hg in **B**.

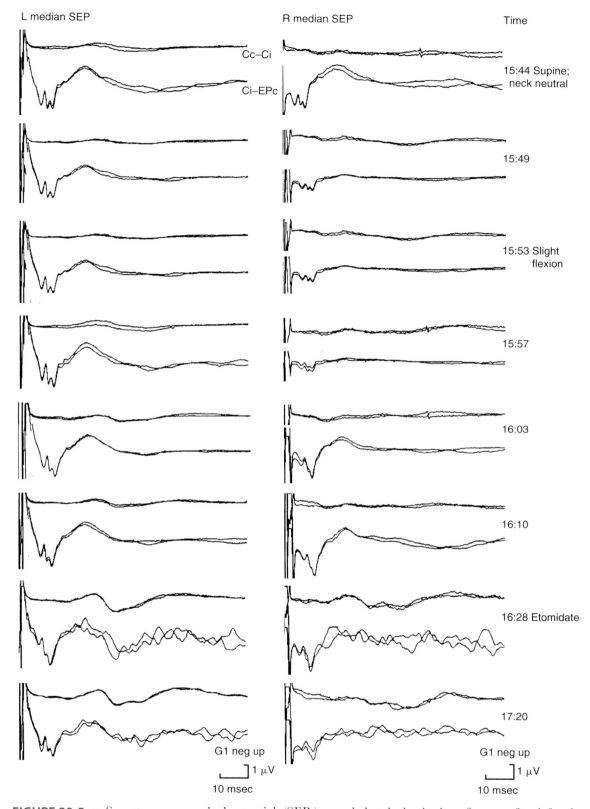

FIGURE 30-5 ▪ Somatosensory evoked potentials (SEPs) recorded at the beginning of surgery for cleft palate repair in a 3-year-old patient with achondroplasia. Initially, intact subcortical SEPs were recorded while the child was lying supine and receiving halothane anesthesia by mask. As expected for a young child receiving a halogenated anesthetic agent, the N20 cortical SEPs were of low voltage. With slight flexion of the neck during myringotomy, loss of N18 on the right was noted. The response returned when the head was returned to the neutral position. Surgery was deferred, and etomidate was used to facilitate monitoring of N20 for the remainder of the procedure. The patient awoke without neurologic deficits.

latter approach because it better enables the surgeon to identify the cause of SEP changes and to use that information to decide whether to take a "wait-and-see" approach or to act immediately.[49]

The implication of SEP deterioration is very much dependent on the surgery being performed. The loss of SEP amplitude during correction of spinal deformities is ominous and carries with it a high risk of serious neurologic injury in the absence of corrective measures.[7,50] By contrast, the loss of SEP amplitude during intramedullary surgery is often predictive of immediate postoperative neurologic deficits but is less often predictive of the eventual neurologic outcome.[51,52] Surgical manipulation of the spinal cord can cause transient conduction block without permanent axonal injury.[51] Further, while the stability of SEPs during intramedullary surgery can provide useful reassurance to the surgeon that neurologic injury has not occurred, the loss of SEPs tends to be abrupt and not serve as a warning of impending injury.[52]

MEP Monitoring

The integrity of descending motor pathways can be monitored intraoperatively by recording the signals from spinal cord or muscle that are evoked by transcranial stimulation. Transcranial stimulation may directly fire pyramidal neurons or may activate cortical interneurons, which then fire pyramidal cells indirectly. Intervening synapses prevent retrograde firing of sensory tracts. Direct pyramidal stimulation produces the earlier, more stable components of the MEP known as D waves, whereas indirect pyramidal activation via interneurons results in the longer-latency, less stable I waves (Fig. 30-6).[53] D waves are relatively resistant to attenuation by anesthetic drugs, including volatile anesthetics, while I waves are highly susceptible.[54,55] In general, the temporal summation of a series of descending volleys, either D wave followed by subsequent I wave or a series of closely spaced D waves, is required to activate spinal motor neurons.[5,56,57]

While motor pathways may be activated by both electrical and magnetic stimulation, transcranial magnetic MEPs are attenuated substantially by most commonly used anesthetics,[58–61] and are not sufficiently reliable for intraoperative monitoring. Instead, intraoperative MEP monitoring relies on transcranial electrical stimulation. Transcranial electrical MEPs are elicited using anodal stimulation. For lower-extremity stimulation, the anode may be placed at Cz, with the cathode at C1 or C2, C3 or C4, or Fz, or utilizing linked electrodes around the cranial base.[62,63] Alternatively, a single pair of electrodes may be used at C1 and C2 or C3 and C4,

reversing electrode polarity to produce greatest-amplitude compound muscle action potentials (CMAPs) contralateral to the anode.[64] Lower stimulation intensity generally is required to elicit MEPs from the upper extremities than from the lower; greater intensities are also likely to produce deeper effective stimulation, activating the corticospinal tracts at the level of the internal capsule.[63] MEPs may be elicited using either special purpose capacitive-coupled constant-voltage stimulators, or standard constant-current SEP-type stimulators. The former provide more rapid delivery of charges: 1 coulomb/sec compared to 0.1 coulomb/sec. Both types of stimulator provide satisfactory stimulation for MEP monitoring, although the capacitive-coupled constant-voltage type has been found to require lower total charge delivery.[65]

The effectiveness of transcranial electrical stimulation is enhanced considerably by using a series of rapidly delivered pulses rather than a single pulse.[66–69] This likely results from temporal summation at both cortical and spinal levels.[5,64,66–68,70] In one study, prominent increases in CMAP amplitude and decreases in latency occurred as the interpulse interval decreased from 10 msec to 1 msec (Fig. 30-7). In another study, simultaneous recordings from epidural space and muscle demonstrated only D waves and no muscle response to a single pulse, or to two transcranial pulses 2 msec apart. However, there were D waves, multiple I waves, and a CMAP to trains of three or four pulses.[67,70] In patients with no pre-existing motor deficits undergoing various neurosurgical procedures under total intravenous anesthesia without neuromuscular blockade, the lowest motor thresholds were achieved with a train of five monophasic constant-current 0.5-msec pulses with an interstimulus interval of 4 msec.[69] Dual train stimulation, in which the test stimulus train is preceded by a conditioning train that heightens motor neuron excitability, can be used to enhance MEPs further. Journee described a trimodal facilitation curve with optimal response at intertrain intervals of approximately 10 and 20 msec, and again at greater than approximately 150 msec. Proper selection of intertrain interval appears to be critical; intertrain intervals of 30 to 150 msec produced attenuation, rather than facilitation, of the response to the second stimulus train (Fig. 30-8).[71]

MEPs may be monitored by recording neural activity in the epidural space, subdural space, or peripheral nerve, or CMAPs from target muscles.[5,8,72] During 160 surgeries for intramedullary lesions, Kothbauer and associates reported success in recording epidural MEPS in about two-thirds of cases.[73] With adequate stimulation (i.e., 2 to 3 times threshold), epidural D waves to transcranial stimulation are robust and relatively stable.[74] Unchanged epidural MEPs were reported to be associated universally

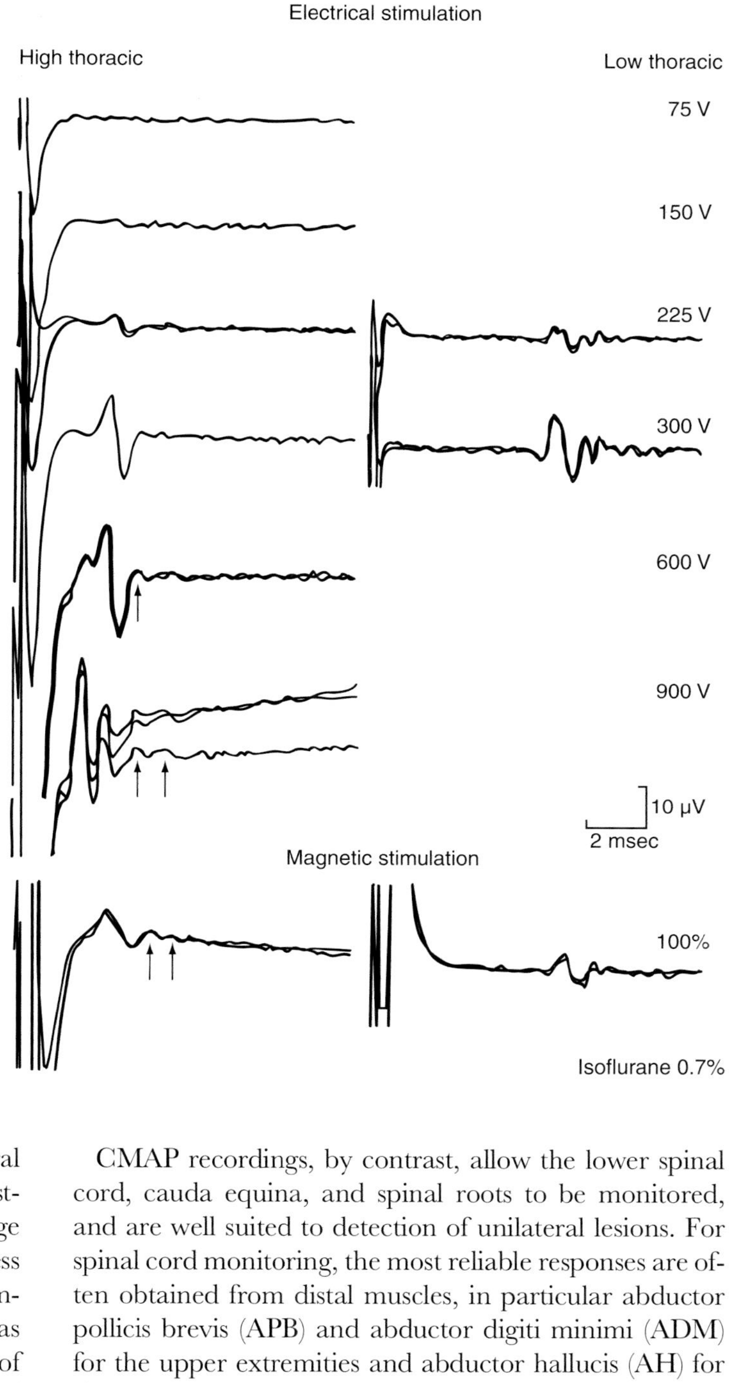

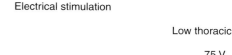

Electrical stimulation

High thoracic   Low thoracic

75 V

150 V

225 V

300 V

600 V

900 V

] 10 μV

2 msec

Magnetic stimulation

100%

Isoflurane 0.7%

FIGURE 30-6 ▪ Corticospinal volleys produced by electrical and magnetic transcranial stimulation, recorded epidurally in a 14-year-old girl. Although in this case the magnetic stimulation produced a D wave, it is smaller than that produced by electrical stimulation. Arrows denote I waves. (From Burke D, Hicks RG, Gandevia SC et al: Direct comparison of corticospinal volleys in human subjects to transcranial magnetic and electrical stimulation. J Physiol, 470:383, 1993, with permission.)

with preserved function, whereas reduction of epidural MEPs over 50 percent generally was associated with postoperative deficit.[73] Epidural recording has the advantage of reduced sensitivity to anesthetic agents,[54] which depress spinal motor neurons as well as cortical activity. It is compatible with the use of volatile anesthetics[54,55,74] as well as complete neuromuscular blockade. The amplitude of epidural D waves, however, is greatest rostrally, and diminishes substantially below T8.[21] Further, D-wave monitoring cannot detect spinal motor neuron ischemia. Epidural recordings therefore are not well suited to detecting lesions affecting lower spinal cord, cauda equina, or spinal roots, and cases in which detection of unilateral lesions is an important consideration.[21] During scoliosis surgery, spurious decreases, as well as increases in D-wave amplitude, have been reported, likely resulting from change in position of spinal cord relative to the epidural recording electrode during correction.[75]

CMAP recordings, by contrast, allow the lower spinal cord, cauda equina, and spinal roots to be monitored, and are well suited to detection of unilateral lesions. For spinal cord monitoring, the most reliable responses are often obtained from distal muscles, in particular abductor pollicis brevis (APB) and abductor digiti minimi (ADM) for the upper extremities and abductor hallucis (AH) for the lower extremities, perhaps reflecting their higher density of corticospinal tract innervation. For this reason, assuming that these muscles are functionally intact at baseline, they generally should be included in MEP monitoring of spinal cord function.[76] CMAP recordings are sensitive to commonly used inhalational anesthetics,[77–79] and total intravenous anesthetic techniques are preferred in some centers.[34,80,81] Anesthetic techniques that include a continuous infusion of propofol, a GABA$_A$ receptor agonist, or dexmedetomidine, a selective central alpha$_2$ receptor agonist, combined with an opioid (e.g., fentanyl,

Double pulses 300 V

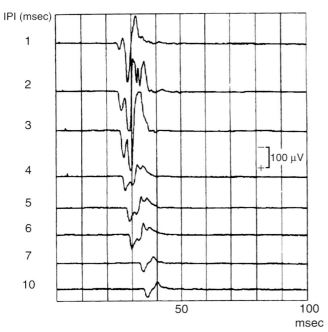

FIGURE 30-7 ■ Motor evoked potentials (MEPs) recorded from the abductor digiti minimi following transcranial stimulation using pulse pairs with varying interpulse intervals (IPIs). The largest and earliest MEPs were recorded at IPIs of less than 2 msec. (From Jones SJ, Harrison R, Koh KF et al: Motor evoked potential monitoring during spinal surgery: response of distal limb muscles to transcranial cortical stimulation with pulse trains. Electroencephalogr Clin Neurophysiol, 100:375, 1996, with permission.)

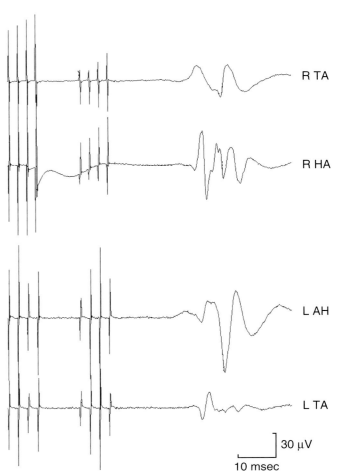

FIGURE 30-8 ■ Motor evoked potentials (MEPs) recorded using dual-train stimulation in a 2-year-old undergoing posterior spinal fusion under propofol, opioid, and ketamine anesthesia. Each stimulus train consisted of four 364-volt pulses; the interpulse interval was 2 msec and the intertrain interval was 20 msec. No MEPs were elicited by the first train in the pair, but the second train reliably elicited responses in abductor hallucis (AH) and tibialis anterior (TA) bilaterally.

sufentanil, or remifentanil) and occasionally supplemented by low-dose ketamine, are compatible with CMAP recording.[34,44] However, by employing high-output (500 V) multipulse stimulators, CMAP MEP monitoring can often be compatible with the use of either nitrous oxide or isoflurane anesthesia, or both.[82–85] Partial neuromuscular blockade, produced by an infusion of nondepolarizing muscle relaxant, may be used to reduce movements that would interfere with surgery and EMG activity that compromises SEP monitoring, yet still permit reliable monitoring of CMAP MEPs.[86] Figure 30-9 illustrates concurrent SEP and MEP recordings during surgery for correction of a spinal deformity in which there was unilateral loss of both SEPs and MEPs, with subsequent partial recovery of the SEP. Postoperative examination revealed a corresponding monoparesis.

Examination of adverse events in over 15,000 published and unpublished instances of patients monitored by transcranial electrical MEPs reveals a favorable safety profile. There is no apparent association of transcranial electrical MEPs with adverse cognitive, affective, or endocrine effects. The most common adverse events were bite injuries (29 patients) to lips or tongue, and a single mandibular fracture. Additional associated adverse events included cardiac arrhythmias (5 patients), seizures (5 patients), scalp burns (2 patients), and intraoperative awareness (1 patient).[87] The occurrence of bite-related injury has prompted the suggestion that soft bite-blocks, such as rolled gauze, be used. The rare arrhythmias and seizures may have been coincidental, although the authors have encountered one (additional) case of bradycardia that was associated reproducibly with transcranial electrical stimulation. This occurred in a 65-year-old patient with history of cardiac disease; bradycardia resolved promptly upon cessation of stimulation, and there were no sequelae.

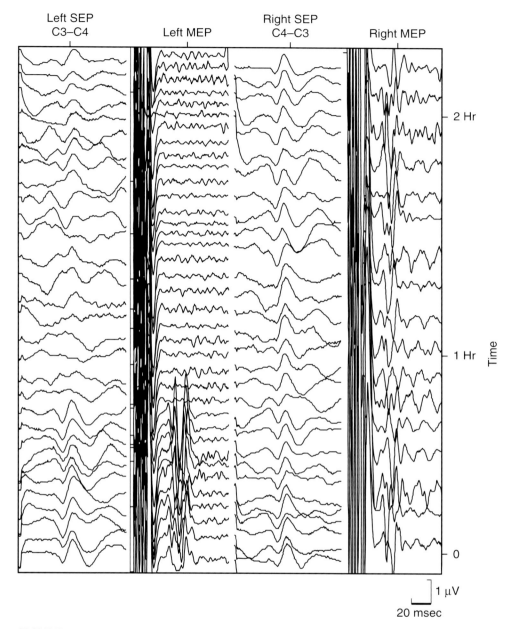

FIGURE 30-9 ■ Concurrent somatosensory evoked potentials (SEPs) and motor evoked potentials (MEPs) recorded during surgery for correction of kyphoscoliosis. During screw placement, there was loss of left SEPs and MEPs, with preservation of right-sided responses. A wake-up test confirmed a left-leg monoparesis. The left SEP demonstrated partial recovery, but the MEP remained absent. Postoperatively, the monoparesis persisted. MEPs illustrated are unaveraged responses of the abductor hallucis to a train of five stimuli, with an inter-stimulus interval of 285 msec. Calibration is the same for all recordings.

INTERPRETIVE CRITERIA

Unlike SEP recording, in which all stimuli produce identical responses, there is considerable within-patient, trial-to-trial variability of CMAPs elicited by both transcranial and direct spinal stimulation (Fig. 30-10).[64] This complicates the establishment of clear criteria for abnormality. Various criteria have been proposed, ranging from amplitude reduction to 50 percent or 20 percent of baseline, to complete loss of MEPs in consecutive trials.[19,23,88-90] Criteria based on MEP waveform morphology[91] and stimulus threshold intensity have also been suggested.[64,76]

As with SEP monitoring,[49] an alternative approach is to inform the surgeon of changes in MEP response (amplitude, latency, and morphology) that exceed the

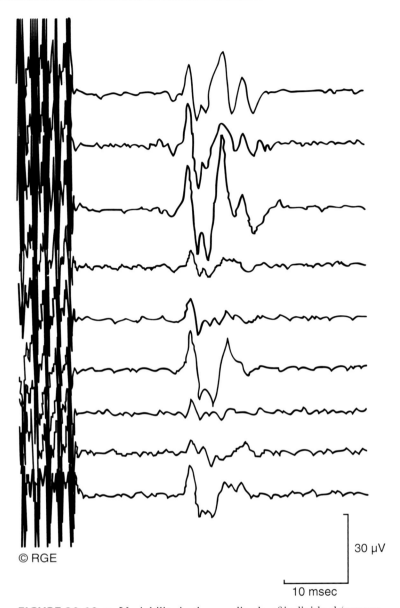

© RGE

30 μV

10 msec

FIGURE 30-10 ■ Variability in the amplitude of individual (unaveraged) motor evoked potential responses, recorded from the right tibialis anterior muscle in a patient receiving intravenous (propofol and narcotic) anesthesia, stimulated with trains of five pulses at 2-msec interpulse intervals.

baseline variability in the patient's recordings, realizing that the reproducibility of MEPs may be influenced by various factors, including anesthetic technique and stimulation protocol. Although this approach is somewhat subjective because the criteria employed are quantified less easily, we currently favor its use. It avoids application of arbitrary and simplistic criteria, and also enables the surgeon to best identify causes of MEP changes. For monitoring of thoracolumbar cord function, correlation with MEPs recorded from thenar muscles is useful for identifying confounding systemic effects.[23]

CRANIAL NERVE AND SPINAL ROOT MONITORING

Intraoperative electrophysiologic monitoring provides a means of identifying cranial nerves and spinal roots and allows continuous monitoring of their functional integrity. The facial nerve commonly is monitored during acoustic neuroma and other cerebellopontine angle surgery, where it is at risk for being injured or inadvertently severed. Particularly with large tumors, cranial nerve VII may be difficult to identify visually if it is spread apart by or enmeshed in the tumor or tumor capsule. Several early studies have confirmed the efficacy of facial nerve monitoring for reducing morbidity following acoustic neuroma surgery.[92,93] In a comparison of 91 consecutive monitored cases with 91 control subjects matched for age, tumor size, and year of surgery at the Mayo Clinic, 45 percent of the monitored but only 27 percent of the unmonitored patients were free from deficit. Two percent of the monitored and 6 percent of the unmonitored patients had no facial nerve function.[92-94]

Additionally, cranial nerves III, IV, and VI may be monitored during surgery involving the cavernous sinus.[95] Lower cranial nerves are monitored during skull base surgery, including resection of clivus tumors and tumors of the jugular foramen.[96] Spinal roots are monitored during procedures such as tumor resection, spinal cord untethering, and placement of pedicle screws, all of which carry the risk of injury.[97-100]

Triggered EMG

When cranial nerves or spinal roots are difficult to identify visually because of abnormalities such as scarring or anatomic distortion, they can be identified electrophysiologically by electrically stimulating the tissue in question and recording CMAPs over appropriate muscles. In contrast to transcutaneous stimulation, where constant-current stimulators generally are used, constant-voltage stimulators are often preferred for stimulation within the surgical site. Constant-current stimulators are favored in the standard laboratory setting because they deliver relatively constant depolarizing current to the nerve despite variations in electrode impedance. In the operative field, however, current shunting by ambient fluid, rather than contact impedance, is the major concern. Constant-current stimulators can deliver widely varying currents to a nerve, depending on whether the field is dry or covered by cerebrospinal fluid; a more uniform current actually is delivered to the nerve by a constant-voltage stimulator.[49,101]

Either surface or intramuscular electrodes are suitable for recording CMAPs following electrical nerve stimulation. If needed, partial neuromuscular blockade may be used to suppress movement, but typically is avoided altogether. CMAPs recorded from direct nerve stimulation are compatible with the use of either inhalational or intravenous anesthetic techniques. Stimulation is performed with a hand-held monopolar probe controlled by the surgeon. Initial "searching" for nerve roots is performed at relatively high stimulus intensities. The stimulus intensity is then decreased so that the target root is stimulated selectively to confirm its identity and establish its stimulation threshold. The stimulation threshold is about 0.03 to 0.1 mA for healthy bare cranial nerves and slightly higher for roots. Throughout dissection, the nerves are probed repeatedly. When the immediate objective is to confirm that the area to be resected or cauterized does not contain nerve, high stimulation intensities (about three times threshold) are used. To confirm the identity of the nerve, that nerve's threshold intensity is used. It is important to note that, besides lack of proximity to the nerve, failure to stimulate can reflect nerve injury causing conduction block or previous transection of the nerve proximal to the site of stimulation. The ease with which a nerve is stimulated may be predictive of postoperative function.

The proximity of muscles on the face can result in "crosstalk" between recording electrodes. Electrodes in muscles innervated by cranial nerve VII, for example, may also record signals generated by the masseter or temporalis muscles, which are innervated by cranial nerve V. Onset latencies of the CMAP can help to distinguish these responses. When stimulated intracranially, cranial nerve VII has a latency of about 6 msec, whereas cranial nerve V (motor) has a latency of about 3 msec. Stimulation of cranial nerve VI activates the lateral rectus muscle. This activity can be picked up in the "orbicularis oculi channel," but at a latency of about 2 msec (Fig. 30-11).[101]

Triggered EMG thresholds can also be used to assess pedicle screw placement during transpedicular lumbosacral fixation. Inadvertent penetration of the pedicle cortex during screw placement can result in postoperative radiculopathy. To test the integrity of a pedicle screw hole, the wall of the hole is stimulated prior to screw placement (Fig. 30-12), and the stimulation threshold for appropriate lower-extremity muscles is measured (Fig. 30-13). If the pedicle remains intact, the bone provides insulation, which raises the stimulation threshold of the adjacent root. If the cortex has been perforated, a low-impedance path is created between the probe and the nerve root, which reduces the stimulation threshold. Pedicle screws may also be stimulated after they have been inserted. Pedicle wall breakthrough has been associated with stimulation thresholds below 6 to 11 mA.[102-104] In a small series of 102 screws placed in 18 patients, stimulation results prompted redirection of 8 screws and detected 12 other instances of unsuspected cortical perforation.[103] Pre-existing radiculopathy can be an important source of false-negatives on pedicle screw testing, as chronically compressed nerve roots can have elevated stimulation thresholds in the 10 to 20 mA range, thus simulating the presence of intact pedicle wall.[105]

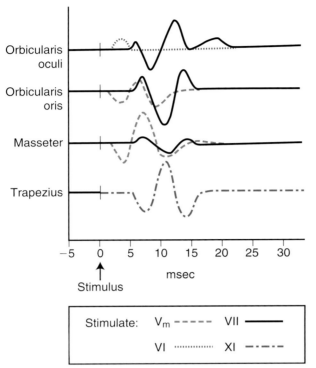

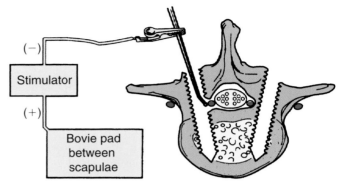

FIGURE 30-12 ■ Diagram illustrating testing of the integrity of a pedicle screw hole in a lumbar vertebra before placement of the screw. (From Calancie B, Madsen P, Lebwohl N: Stimulus-evoked EMG monitoring during transpedicular lumbosacral instrumentation. Spine, 19:2780, 1994, with permission.)

FIGURE 30-11 ■ Schematic diagram depicting compound muscle action potentials recorded from the orbicularis oculi, orbicularis oris, masseter, and trapezius. Although the proximity of recording sites causes crosstalk between recording sites, latency differences aid in distinguishing between responses to stimulation of cranial nerves V (motor), VI, VII, and XI. (From Yingling CD, Gardi JN: Intraoperative monitoring of facial and cochlear nerves during acoustic neuroma surgery. Otolaryngol Clin North Am, 25:413, 1992, with permission.)

extremity muscles, while probing the screw track with an electrode delivering high-frequency pulse-trains, has been suggested as a method for detection of medial thoracic pedicle wall breach.[106]

Neurotonic Discharges

Surgical stimulation of nerve can elicit two forms of "neurotonic" EMG activity. In contrast to CMAPs, neurotonic discharges are best recorded with intramuscular electrodes,[107,108] either standard EMG needles, electroencephalographic (EEG) scalp needles, or fine wires inserted through hypodermic needles. Furthermore, although controlled partial neuromuscular blockade generally does not interfere with monitoring of electrically elicited CMAPs, it may interfere with recording of mechanically elicited EMG activity.[101] For that reason, when neurotonic discharges are monitored it is best to avoid the use of neuromuscular blocking agents and instead rely on other techniques such as higher anesthetic concentrations to achieve relaxation.

Malposition of thoracic pedicle screws poses potentially greater risk to the patient than lumbosacral screws, as the spinal cord can be injured directly by medial breach of a thoracic screw. Triggered EMG testing for thoracic pedicle screw placement using abdominal or intercostal muscles has been proposed, but has proven difficult. Monitoring the stimulation threshold of lower-

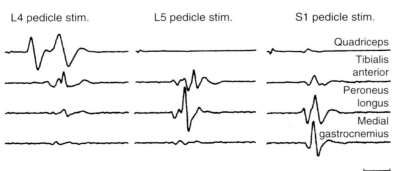

FIGURE 30-13 ■ Compound muscle action potentials recorded following stimulation of L4, L5, and S1 pedicle screws at stimulus intensities 1 to 2 mA above the response threshold. (From Calancie B, Madsen P, Lebwohl N: Stimulus evoked EMG monitoring during transpedicular lumbosacral instrumentation. Spine, 19:2780, 1994, with permission.)

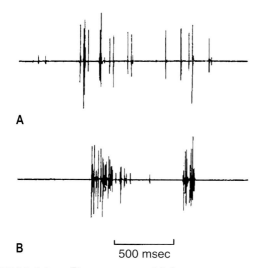

A

B

FIGURE 30-14 ◼ Electromyographic burst response recorded at the time of acoustic neuroma surgery (**A**) during blunt dissection and (**B**) following a rapid squirt with Ringer's solution. The tracings are from a "free-running" display, and the discharges occurred at the time of the stimulus. (From Prass RL, Lüders H: Acoustic [loudspeaker] facial electromyographic monitoring. Part 1. Evoked electromyographic activity during acoustic neuroma resection. Neurosurgery, 19:392, 1986, with permission.)

Mechanical stimulation resulting from, for example, direct manipulation of nerve by dissecting instruments or irrigation produces an EMG pattern consisting of relatively synchronous brief (less than 1 second) bursts of motor unit action potentials that occur coincident with the mechanical stimulus and tend to fatigue with repeated stimulation (Fig. 30-14). This pattern does not reflect injury. Easily elicited bursts to mechanical stimuli indicate functional integrity of the nerve distal to the stimulated site, and loss of this response to mechanical stimulation may signal that nerve injury has occurred.[109] However, it is possible to sever the nerve and produce only minimal EMG response. Furthermore, injured nerves may not be sensitive to mechanical stimulation. Therefore, mechanically elicited discharges alone should not be relied on for nerve identification but should be supplemented by frequent electrical stimulation. The presence of a response following surgical manipulation confirms continuity of the nerve. During pedicle screw placement, mechanically elicited neurotonic discharges warn of perforation of the cortical wall. These discharges are typically brief, even in cases of postoperative radiculopathy.[102]

Tonic "train" discharges signal nerve damage. These discharges are prolonged and asynchronous, and last up to several seconds or minutes. Their onset may be delayed for seconds to minutes after the insult (Fig. 30-15). They may be produced by ischemia, heating, or prolonged mechanical deformation. Two forms of tonic discharges are described and can be differentiated by their sound when monitored through a loudspeaker: 50 to 100 Hz "bomber" discharges[109] and 1 to 50 Hz "popcorn" discharges.[109] The presence of tonic discharges during surgery for acoustic neuroma has been associated with an inability to stimulate the nerve electrically following tumor removal and with postoperative deficit.[107] Based on experience with cranial nerve VII monitoring, Prass and co-workers described a modification of the surgical technique for minimizing lateral to medial traction on the facial nerve, a manipulation often associated with train EMG discharges.[110]

ACOUSTIC NERVE AND BRAINSTEM AUDITORY PATHWAY MONITORING

Brainstem auditory evoked potentials (BAEPs) reflect the integrity of cochlea, auditory nerve, and brainstem auditory pathways. The clinically important components of the BAEP are wave I, generated by the auditory nerve close to the cochlea; wave III, generated in the lower pons; and wave V, generated in the lower midbrain. Most commonly, BAEPs are monitored during surgery in the cerebellopontine angle with the goal of preserving auditory nerve function. They may also be recorded to assess brainstem function.

Intraoperatively, BAEPs are recorded in a manner similar to that used in the diagnostic laboratory. The bulky earphone used in the laboratory is replaced by a small insertable earphone or by a molded earplug connected by a thin tube to a remotely located transducer. Commonly, a faster stimulation rate is used for monitoring than in the diagnostic laboratory—typically about 30 Hz compared with 10 Hz. This faster stimulation rate results in a small reduction in signal voltage but allows more rapid signal acquisition. Stable, robust BAEPs are recorded readily in the presence of general anesthetic agents, although clinically used concentrations of halogenated inhalational agents can produce small increases in the latency of wave V.[111] Furthermore, a decrease in body core temperature produces an increase in wave V latencies of approximately 0.2 msec/°C, an effect that may be enhanced by local cooling at the surgical site.[101]

The utility of BAEPs in safeguarding acoustic nerve function was demonstrated first by Radke and colleagues, who compared the outcomes following 70 microvascular decompressions for trigeminal neuralgia or hemifacial spasm that were monitored with BAEPs with the outcomes of 152 similar procedures performed at the same institution prior to the introduction of monitoring. The incidence of profound hearing loss was 6.6 percent in

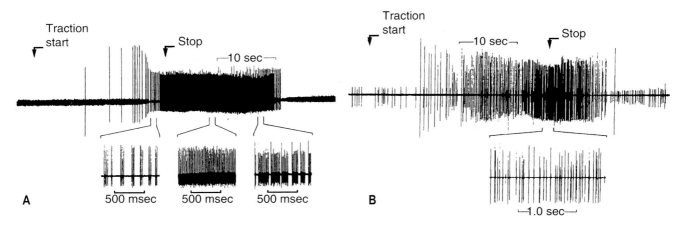

FIGURE 30-15 ▪ Examples of (**A**) "bomber" and (**B**) "popcorn" types of train discharges recorded during lateral-to-medial facial nerve traction. (From Prass RL, Lüders H: Acoustic [loudspeaker] facial electromyographic monitoring. Part 1. Evoked electromyographic activity during acoustic neuroma resection. Neurosurgery, 19:392, 1986, with permission.)

the unmonitored group compared to 0 percent in the monitored group.[112] The value of BAEP monitoring for hearing preservation during acoustic neuroma resection is well documented.[101,113–115] In a comparison of 90 consecutive patients undergoing acoustic neuroma resection with BAEP monitoring to 90 historical control subjects matched for preoperative hearing and tumor size, Harper and co-workers demonstrated hearing preservation in 79 percent of the monitored group, in contrast to 42 percent of the unmonitored group for tumors less than 1.1 cm.[113] Their data support the use of BAEP monitoring in patients with tumors up to 2 cm in diameter, but not in patients with larger tumors, for whom preservation of hearing is unlikely.

During surgical manipulation threatening the auditory nerve, a loss of wave V amplitude of 50 percent or more or an increase in wave V latency by 0.5 msec generally is recognized as a potentially important alteration, particularly when it occurs suddenly.[113,116] Correlation of alterations of the monitored signals with surgical manipulation permits identification of offending maneuvers (Fig. 30-16). Manipulations identified as most likely to cause deterioration of responses include coagulation near the auditory nerve, drilling of the internal auditory canal, pulling of the tumor nerve bundle, and direct manipulation of the auditory nerve.[117,118] BAEP monitoring is capable of providing feedback to the surgeon at approximately 1- to 2-minute intervals. By performing the most dangerous maneuvers in incremental steps rather than continuously, it is possible to use BAEP feedback to guide the resection. Often, simply pausing will cause the deteriorated signals to recover.[119]

A number of techniques have been introduced to facilitate more rapid feedback, including recording directly from the cochlear nerve[117,120] or from near the brainstem.[121,122] The improved signal-to-noise ratios achieved by these techniques mean that fewer samples need to be averaged to resolve signals and allow changes to be detected after seconds rather than minutes. Monitoring cochlear nerve action potentials, Colletti and associates identified resection of tumor from within the lateral end of the auditory meatus, where the cochlear nerve and the auditory artery and tumor are tightly confined, as posing the greatest risk of both change in the monitored signal and subsequent hearing loss. The use of a recording electrode probe to identify the acoustic nerve was also found helpful in cases in which it was obscured by tumor.[117]

BAEP monitoring also provides a means of assessing brainstem integrity, although it allows surveillance of only a limited portion of the brainstem between the lower pons and the lower midbrain. In patients with large tumors of the cerebellopontine angle, Angelo and Moller observed that BAEPs measured following stimulation of the ear opposite the lesions were sensitive to surgical manipulation of the brainstem. A consistent relationship between prolongation of wave V latency and surgical manipulation of the brainstem was observed. Wave V latency was related more closely to surgical manipulation than was either wave V amplitude or hemodynamic parameters.[123]

During suboccipital decompression for Chiari I malformation in children, BAEPs routinely demonstrate small decreases in the I–V interpeak latency. This improvement occurs almost entirely after bony decompression and before the dura is incised. Since the morbidity of posterior fossa decompression with duraplasty generally is associated with the dura having been opened, a safer and equally effective procedure might be limited to bony decompression alone (Fig. 30-17).[124]

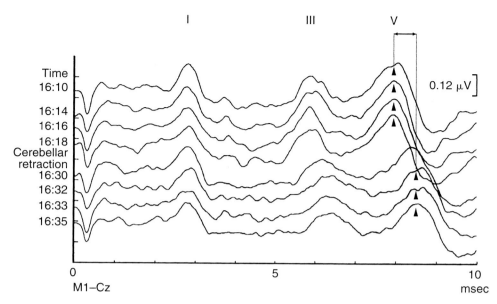

FIGURE 30-16 ▪ Increase in the I–III interpeak latency, together with a corresponding increase in wave V latency, in the brainstem auditory evoked potential after cerebellar retraction.

CORTICAL MONITORING BY SEPs

Detecting Cerebral Ischemia

Intraoperative SEP recording has been used as a warning of impending ischemic injury during cerebral vascular surgery. The generators of the primary cortical N20 component of the median SEP lie within the territory of the middle cerebral artery and, accordingly, are at risk during carotid cross-clamping. For this reason, median SEPs have been used to monitor cortical function during carotid endarterectomy. Loss of amplitude of N20, without alteration in subcortical (N18 and earlier) components, is the principal SEP abnormality observed during carotid cross-clamping. During 994 endarterectomies, Haupt and Horsch observed reversible changes of N20 in approximately 10 percent of cases and irreversible changes in 0.7 percent. All patients with irreversible changes had corresponding postoperative deficits. The incidence of SEP abnormalities during carotid cross-clamping correlated with the degree of contralateral carotid stenosis, and the most common cause of reversible N20 amplitude change was stenosis of the contralateral carotid artery.[125] SEPs have also been used to monitor cortical integrity during aneurysm surgery.[125,126] It is essential that the SEP monitored be appropriate for the territory at risk. For example, median nerve SEPs are appropriate for monitoring during surgery for internal carotid and middle cerebral artery aneurysms, but not anterior cerebral artery aneurysms. A study comparing SEP and EEG monitoring during carotid endarterectomy suggested that the two techniques have similar sensitivity and specificity.[127] Nonetheless, in comparison to SEP methods, EEG monitoring has the inherent advantages of being less complicated, providing continuous real-time feedback, and surveying the function of more widespread regions of cerebral cortex.

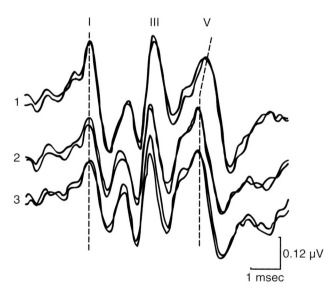

FIGURE 30-17 ▪ Brainstem auditory evoked potentials during suboccipital decompression with duraplasty for Chiari 1 malformation. 1, Baseline prone. 2, After bony decompression and division of atlanto-occipital membrane. 3, After duraplasty at closure. (From Anderson RC, Emerson RG, Dowling KC et al: Improvement in brainstem auditory evoked potentials after suboccipital decompression in patients with Chiari I malformation. J Neurosurg, 98:459, 2003, with permission.)

Functional Localization

It can be difficult to identify visually the central sulcus with certainty at surgery; however, the central sulcus is easily identified functionally by using SEPs recorded from a cortical electrode array following median nerve stimulation. The initial component of the N20 primary cortical response is that generated by activation of cortical area 3b on the posterior bank of the central fissure. Activation of this area produces a "horizontal dipole," which is recorded as a negativity postcentrally and simultaneously as a positivity precentrally (Fig. 30-18). Following N20, the P2 potential, probably reflecting concurrent activation of areas 1, 2, 3a, and 4, also phase reverses across the rolandic fissure. The large area of cortex contributing to the P2 potential, including area 4 on the crown of the anterior bank of the central fissure, probably explains the more gradual phase reversal observed with P2.[128,129] Use of the median SEP for localization of the rolandic fissure requires demonstration of these phase reversals. If the surgical exposure does not permit demonstration of these phase reversals in cortical recordings, comparison of cortical SEP waveforms with those recorded simultaneously from scalp electrodes may be helpful.[129]

Electrical stimulation can also be used to identify precentral cortex. The cortex is stimulated with sustained 60-Hz trains and target muscles are observed for movement. Stimulation intensities of up to 15 mA that do not produce sustained afterdischarges may be used. Electrical cortical stimulation may be problematic in young children, whose motor cortices are difficult to stimulate electrically.[128–130] An important limitation of this technique is incidence of intraoperative seizures: as high as 20 percent.[131] An alternative, recently introduced technique entails stimulating the cortex with brief-pulse, high-frequency trains and recording of MEPs over muscles of interest. In contrast to the 60-Hz method, seizures are much less likely, occurring in 0 of 70 patients in one series.[132]

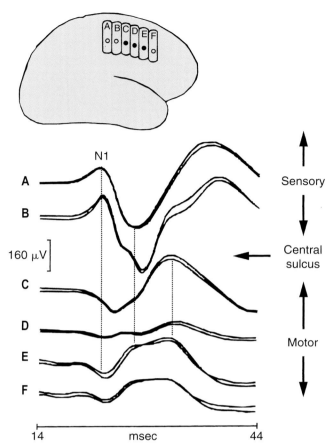

FIGURE 30-18 ■ Cortical recordings illustrating phase reversal of the primary cortical response (labeled N1) across the central fissure following median nerve stimulation (From Lüders H, Lesser RP, Hahn J et al: Cortical somatosensory evoked potentials in response to hand stimulation. J Neurosurg, 58:885, 1983, with permission.)

REFERENCES

1. Sloan TB: Advancing the multidisciplinary approach to spinal cord injury risk reduction in thoracoabdominal aortic aneurysm repair. Anesthesiology, 108:555, 2008

2. Ginsburg HH, Shetter AG, Raudzens PA: Postoperative paraplegia with preserved intraoperative somatosensory evoked potentials. Case report. J Neurosurg, 63:296, 1985

3. Lesser RP, Raudzens P, Lueders H et al: Postoperative neurological deficits may occur despite unchanged intraoperative somatosensory evoked potentials. Ann Neurol, 19:22, 1986

4. Molaie M: False negative intraoperative somatosensory evoked potentials with simultaneous bilateral stimulation. Clin Electroencephalogr, 17:6, 1986

5. Deletis V, Sala F: Intraoperative neurophysiological monitoring of the spinal cord during spinal cord and spine surgery: a review focus on the corticospinal tracts. Clin Neurophysiol, 119:248, 2008

6. Drenger B, Parker SD, McPherson RW et al: Spinal cord stimulation evoked potentials during thoracoabdominal aortic aneurysm surgery. Anesthesiology, 76:689, 1992

7. Forbes HJ, Allen PW, Waller CS et al: Spinal cord monitoring in scoliosis surgery. J Bone Joint Surg, 73-B:487, 1991

8. Burke D, Hicks R, Stephen J et al: Assessment of corticospinal and somatosensory conduction simultaneously during scoliosis surgery. Electroencephalogr Clin Neurophysiol, 85:388, 1992

9. Noordeen MHH, Lee J, Gibbons CER et al: Spinal cord monitoring in operations for neuromuscular scoliosis. J Bone Joint Surg, 79-B:53, 1997

10. Stechison MT: Neurophysiologic monitoring during cranial base surgery. J Neurooncol, 20:313, 1994

11. Matsui Y, Goh K, Shiiya N et al: Clinical application of evoked spinal cord potentials elicited by direct stimulation of the cord during temporary occlusion of the thoracic aorta. J Thorac Cardiovasc Surg, 107:1519, 1994

12. Padberg AM, Russo MH, Lenke LG et al: Validity and reliability of spinal cord monitoring in neuromuscular spinal deformity surgery. J Spinal Deformities, 9:150, 1996

13. Malhotra NR, Shaffrey CI: Intraoperative electrophysiological monitoring in spine surgery. Spine, 35:2167, 2010

14. Mendiratta A, Emerson RG: Neurophysiologic intraoperative monitoring of scoliosis surgery. J Clin Neurophysiol, 26:62, 2009

15. Vauzelle C, Stagnara P, Jouvinroux P: Functional monitoring of spinal cord activity during spinal surgery. Clin Orthop, 93:173, 1973

16. Zornow MH, Grafe MR, Tybor C et al: Preservation of evoked potentials in a case of anterior spinal artery syndrome. Electroencephalogr Clin Neurophysiol, 77:137, 1990

17. Noel P, Deltenre P, Lamoureaux J et al: Neurophysiologic detection of a unilateral motor deficit occurring during the noncritical phase of scoliosis surgery. Spine, 19:2399, 1994

18. Stephen JP, Sullivan MR, Hicks RG et al: Cotrel-Dubousset instrumentation in children using simultaneous motor and somatosensory evoked potential monitoring. Spine, 21:2450, 1996

19. Pelosi L, Lamb J, Grevitt M et al: Combined monitoring of motor and somatosensory evoked potentials in orthopedic spinal surgery. Clin Neurophysiol, 113:1082, 2002

20. Steinbok P, Cochrane D, Poskitt K: Intramedullary spinal cord tumors in children. Neurosurg Clin N Am, 3:931, 1992

21. MacDonald D, Janusz MT: An approach to intraabdominal neurophysiologic monitoring of thoracoabdominal aneurysm surgery. J Clin Neurophysiol, 19:43, 2002

22. Dong JCJ, MacDonald D, Janusz MT: Intraoperative spinal cord monitoring during descending thoracic and thoracoabdominal aneurysm surgery. Ann Thorac Surg, 74:S1873, 2002

23. Jacobs MJHM, Meylaerts SA, de Hann P et al: Strategies to prevent neurologic deficit based on motor-evoked potentials in type I and II thoracoabdominal aortic aneurysm repair. J Vasc Surg, 29:48, 1999

24. Jacobs MJ, Elenbaas TW, Schurink GWH et al: Assessment of spinal cord integrity during thoracoabdominal aortic aneurysm repair. Ann Thorac Surg, 74:S1864, 2002

25. Sueda T, Okada K, Orihashi K et al: Cold blood spinal cord plegia for prediction of spinal cord ischemia during thoracoabdominal aneurysm repair. Ann Thorac Surg, 73:1155, 2002

26. Shine TS, Harrison BA, De Ruyter ML et al: Motor and somatosensory evoked potentials: their role in predicting spinal cord ischemia in patients undergoing thoracoabdominal aortic aneurysm repair with regional lumbar epidural cooling. Anesthesiology, 108:580, 2008

27. Sala F, Niimi Y, Berenstein A et al: Neuroprotective role of neurophysiological monitoring during endovascular procedures in the spinal cord. Ann N Y Acad Sci, 939:137, 2001

28. Shiau JS, Zappulla RA, Nieves J: The effect of graded spinal cord injury on the extrapyramidal and pyramidal motor evoked potentials of the rat. Neurosurgery, 30:76, 1992

29. Machida M, Weinstein SL, Imamura Y et al: Compound muscle action potentials and spinal evoked potentials in experimental spine maneuver. Spine, 14:687, 1989

30. Reuter DG, Tacker WA Jr, Badylak SF et al: Correlation of motor-evoked potential response to ischemic spinal cord damage. J Thorac Cardiovasc Surg, 104:262, 1992

31. Fehlings MG, Tator CH, Linden RD: The relationships among the severity of spinal cord injury, motor and somatosensory evoked potentials and spinal cord blood flow. Electroencephalogr Clin Neurophysiol, 74:241, 1989

32. Nagle K, Emerson RG, Adams DA et al: Intraoperative motor and somatosensory evoked potential monitoring: a review of 116 cases. Neurology, 47:999, 1996

33. Padberg A, Bridwell H: Spinal cord monitoring. Current state of the art. Orthop Clin North Am, 30:407, 1999

34. Sloan T, Heyer EJ: Anesthesia for intraoperative neurophysiologic monitoring of the spinal cord. J Clin Neurophysiol, 19:430, 2002

35. American Clinical Neurophysiology Society Guideline 11B: Recommended standards for intraoperative monitoring of somatosensory evoked potentials, 2009 cited 2011; Available from:http://www.acns.org/pdfs/Guideline%2011B.pdf

36. MacDonald DB, Stigsby B, Zayed ZA: A comparison between derivation optimization and Cz0–FPz for posterior tibial P37 somatosensory evoked potential intraoperative monitoring. Clin Neurophysiol, 115:1925, 2004

37. Harper CM, Nelson KR: Intraoperative electrophysiological monitoring in children. J Clin Neurophysiol, 9:342, 1992

38. Perlik SJ, VanEgeren R, Fisher MA: Somatosensory evoked potential surgical monitoring. Observation during combined isoflurane-nitrous oxide anesthesia. Spine, 17:273, 1992

39. Browning JL, Heizer ML, Baskin DS: Variations in corticomotor and somatosensory evoked potentials: effects of temperature, halothane anesthesia, and arterial partial pressure of CO_2. Anesth Analg, 74:643, 1992

40. Sebel PS, Bowles SM, Saini V et al: EEG bispectrum predicts movement during thiopental/isoflurane anesthesia. J Clin Monit, 11:83, 1995

41. Clapcich AJ, Emerson RG, Roye DP Jr, et al: The effects of propofol, small-dose isoflurane, and nitrous oxide on cortical somatosensory evoked potential and bispectral index monitoring in adolescents undergoing spinal fusion. Anesth Analg, 99:1334, 2004

42. Sloan T, Sloan H, Rogers J: Nitrous oxide and isoflurane are synergistic with respect to amplitude and latency effects on sensory evoked potentials. J Clin Monit Comput, 24:113, 2010

43. Sloan TB, Heyer EJ: Anesthesia for intraoperative neurophysiologic monitoring of the spinal cord. J Clin Neurophysiol, 19:430, 2002

44. Bala E, Sessler DI, Nair DR et al: Motor and somatosensory evoked potentials are well maintained in patients given dexmedetomidine during spine surgery. Anesthesiology, 109:417, 2008

45. Agarwal R, Roitman KJ, Stokes M: Improvement of intraoperative somatosensory evoked potentials by ketamine. Paediatr Anaesth, 8:263, 1998

46. Erb TO, Ryhult SE, Duitmann E et al: Improvement of motor-evoked potentials by ketamine and spatial facilitation during spinal surgery in a young child. Anesth Analg, 100:1634, 2005

47. Schubert A, Licina MG, Lineberry PJ: The effect of ketamine on human somatosensory evoked potentials and its modification by nitrous oxide. Anesthesiology, 72:33, 1990

48. O'Brien MF, Lenke LG, Bridwell KH et al: Evoked potentials monitoring of upper extremities during thoracic and lumbar spinal deformity surgery: a prospective study. J Spinal Disord, 7:277, 1994

49. Moller AR: Intraoperative neurophysiological monitoring. Am J Otol, 16:115, 1992

50. Fehlings MG, Brodke DS, Norvell DC et al: The evidence for intraoperative neurophysiological monitoring in spine surgery: does it make a difference? Spine, 35:S37, 2010

51. Whittle IR, Johnston IH, Besser M: Recording of spinal somatosensory evoked potentials for intraoperative spinal cord monitoring. J Neurosurg, 64:601, 1986

52. Kearse LA, Lopez-Bresnahan M, McPeek K et al: Loss of intraoperative somatosensory evoked potentials during intramedullary spinal cord injury predicts postoperative neurological deficits in motor function. J Clin Anesth, 5:392, 1993

53. Rothwell J, Burke D, Hicks R et al: Transcranial electrical stimulation of the motor cortex in man: further evidence for the site of activation. J Physiol, 481:243, 1994

54. Hicks R, Woodforth I, Crawford M et al: Some effects of isoflurane on motor evoked potentials. Br J Anaesth, 69:130, 1992

55. Hicks R, Burke D, Stephen J et al: Corticospinal volleys evoked by electrical stimulation of human motor cortex after withdrawal of volatile anesthetics. J Physiol, 456:393, 1992

56. Taniguchi M, Cedzich C, Schramm J: Modification of cortical stimulation for motor evoked potentials under general anesthesia: technical description. Neurosurg, 32:219, 1993

57. Day B, Rothwell J, Thompson P et al: Motor cortex stimulation in intact man. Brain, 110:1191, 1987

58. Ghaly RF, Stone JL, Levy WJ et al: The effect of neuroleptanalgesia (droperidol-fentanyl) on motor potentials evoked by transcranial magnetic stimulation in the monkey. J Neurosurg Anesthesiol, 3:117, 1991

59. Kalkman CJ, Drummond JC, Kennely NA et al: Intraoperative monitoring of tibialis anterior muscle motor evoked responses to transcranial electrical stimulation during partial neuromuscular blockade. Anesth Analg, 73:584, 1992

60. Kalkman CJ, Drummond JC, Ribberink AA et al: Effects of propofol, etomidate, midazolam, and fentanyl on motor evoked responses to transcranial electrical or magnetic stimulation in humans. Anesthesiology, 76:502, 1992

61. Gugino L, Aglio L, Segal M: Use of transcranial magnetic stimulation for monitoring spinal cord motor pathways. Semin Spinal Surg, 9:315, 1997

62. Ubags L, Kalkman C, Been H et al: The use of a circumferential cathode improves amplitude of intraoperative electrical transcranial myogenic motor evoked responses. Anesth Analg, 82:1011, 1996

63. Deletis V: Intraoperative neurophysiology and methodologies used to monitor the functional integrity of the motor system. p. 25. In Deletis V, Shils J (eds): Neurophysiology and Neurosurgery: A Modern Intraoperative Approach. Academic Press, Amsterdam, 2002

64. Calancie B, Harris W, Broton JG et al: "Threshold-level" multipulse transcranial electrical stimulation of motor cortex for intraoperative monitoring of spinal motor tracts: description of methods and comparison to somatosensory evoked potential monitoring. J Neurosurg, 88:457, 1998

65. Hausmann ON, Min K, Boos N et al: Transcranial electrical stimulation: significance of fast versus slow charge delivery for intra-operative monitoring. Clin Neurophysiol, 113:1523, 2002

66. Taylor B, Fennelly M, Taylor A et al: Temporal summation— the key to motor evoked potential spinal cord monitoring in humans. J Neurol Neurosurg Psychiatry, 56:104, 1993

67. Jones SJ, Harrison R, Koh KF et al: Motor evoked potential monitoring during spinal surgery: response of distal limb muscles to transcranial cortical stimulation with pulse trains. Electroencephalogr Clin Neurophysiol, 100:375, 1996

68. Pechstein U, Cornelia C, Nadstawek J et al: Transcranial high-frequency repetitive electrical stimulation for recording myogenic motor evoked potentials with the patient under general anesthesia. Neurosurgery, 39:335, 1996

69. Szelenyi A, Kothbauer KF, Deletis V: Transcranial electric stimulation for intraoperative motor evoked potential monitoring: stimulation parameters and electrode montages. Clin Neurophysiol, 118:1586, 2007

70. Rodi Z, Delitis V, Morota N et al: Motor evoked potentials during brain surgery. Pflugers Arch Eur J Physiol, 431 (Suppl 2):R291, 1996

71. Journee H, Polak H, de Kleuver M: Conditioning stimulation techniques for enhancement of transcranially elicited evoked motor responses. Neurophysiol Clin, 37:423, 2007

72. Sala F, Palandri G, Basso E et al: Motor evoked potential monitoring improves outcome after surgery for intramedullary spinal cord tumors: a historical control study. Neurosurgery, 58:1129, 2006

73. Kothbauer K, Deletis V, Epstein F: Intraoperative spinal cord monitoring for intramedullary surgery: an essential adjunct. Pediatr Neurosurg, 26:247, 1997

74. Burke D, Hicks R: Surgical monitoring of motor pathways. J Clin Neurophysiol, 15:194, 1998

75. Ulkatan S, Neuwirth M, Bitan F et al: Monitoring of scoliosis surgery with epidurally recorded motor evoked potentials (D-wave) revealed false results. Clin Neurophysiol, 117:2093, 2006

76. Calancie B, Molano M: Alarm criteria for motor-evoked potentials. What's wrong with the "presence of absence" approach? Spine, 33:406, 2008

77. Kalkman CJ, Drummond JC, Ribberink AA: Low concentrations of isoflurane abolish motor evoked responses to transcranial electrical stimulation during nitrous oxide/opioid anesthesia in humans. Anesth Analg, 73:410, 1991

78. Zentner J, Albrecht T, Heuser D: Influence of halothane, enflurane, and isoflurane on motor evoked potentials. Neurosurgery, 31:298, 1992

79. Haghighi SS, Madsen R, Green KD et al: Suppression of motor evoked potentials by inhalation anesthetics. J Neurosurg Anesthesiol, 2:73, 1990

80. Pechstein U, Nadstawek J, Zentner J et al: Isoflurane plus nitrous oxide versus propofol for recording of motor evoked potentials after high frequency repetitive electrical stimulation. Electroencephalogr Clin Neurophysiol, 108:175, 1998

81. Scheufler KM, Zentner J: Total intravenous anesthesia for intraoperative monitoring of the motor pathways: an integral view combining clinical and experimental data. J Neurosurg, 96:571, 2002

82. Ubags L, Kalkman C, Been H: Influence of isoflurane on myogenic motor evoked potentials to single and multiple transcranial stimuli during nitrous oxide/opioid anesthesia. Neurosurgery, 43:90, 1998

83. Pelosi L, Stevenson M, Hobbs GJ et al: Intraoperative motor evoked potentials to transcranial electrical stimulation during two anesthetic regimens. Clin Neurophysiol, 112:1076, 2001

84. van Dongen EP, ter Beek HT, Schepens MA et al: The influence of nitrous oxide to supplement fentanyl/low-dose propofol anesthesia on transcranial myogenic motor-evoked potentials during thoracic aortic surgery. J Cardiothorac Vasc Anesth, 13:30, 1999

85. van Dongen EP, ter Beek HT, Schepens MA et al: Effect of nitrous oxide on myogenic motor potentials evoked by a six pulse train of transcranial electrical stimuli: a possible monitor for aortic surgery. Br J Anaesth, 82:323, 1999

86. Adams DC, Emerson RG, Heyer EJ et al: Monitoring of intraoperative motor evoked potentials under conditions of controlled neuromuscular blockade. Anesth Analg, 77:913, 1993

87. MacDonald D: Safety of intraoperative transcranial electrical stimulation motor evoked potential monitoring. J Clin Neurophysiol, 19:416, 2002

88. Lips J, de Hann P, de Jager SW et al: The role of transcranial motor evoked potentials in predicting neurologic and histopathologic outcome after experimental spinal cord ischemia. Anesthesiology, 97:183, 2002

89. de Haan P, Kalkman CJ, de Mol BA et al: Efficacy of transcranial motor-evoked myogenic potentials to detect spinal cord ischemia during operations for thoracoabdominal aneurysms. J Thorac Cardiovasc Surg, 113:87, 1997

90. Langeloo D, Journee H, de Kleuver M et al: Criteria for transcranial electrical motor evoked potential monitoring during spinal deformity surgery. A review and discussion of the literature. Neurophysiol Clin, 37:431, 2007

91. Quinones-Hinojosa A, Lyon R, Zada G et al: Changes in transcranial motor evoked potentials during intramedullary spinal cord tumour resection correlate with postoperative motor function. Neurosurgery, 56:982, 2005

92. Leonetti JP, Brackmann DE, Prass RL: Improved preservation of facial nerve function in the infratemporal approach to the skull base. Otolaryngol Head Neck Surg, 101:74, 1989

93. Harner SG, Daube JR, Beatty CW et al: Intraoperative monitoring of the facial nerve. Laryngoscope, 98:209, 1988

94. Niparko JK, Kileny PR, Kemink JL et al: Neurophysiologic intraoperative monitoring: II. Facial nerve function. Am J Otol, 10:55, 1989

95. Sekhar LN, Moller AR: Operative management of tumors involving the cavernous sinus. J Neurosurg, 64:879, 1986

96. Moller AR: Evoked Potentials in Intraoperative Monitoring. Williams & Wilkins, Baltimore, 1988

97. Herdmann J, Deletis V, Edmonds HL et al: Spinal cord and nerve root monitoring in spine surgery and related procedures. Spine, 21:879, 1996

98. Hormes JT, Chappuis JL: Monitoring of lumbosacral nerve roots during spinal instrumentation. Spine, 18:2059, 1993

99. Kothbauer K, Schmid UD, Seiler RW et al: Intraoperative motor and sensory monitoring of the cauda equina. Neurosurgery, 34:702, 1994

100. Epstein NE, Danto J, Nardi D: Evaluation of intraoperative somatosensory evoked potential monitoring during 100 cervical operations. Spine, 18:737, 1993

101. Yingling CD, Gardi JN: Intraoperative monitoring of facial and cochlear nerves during acoustic neuroma surgery. Otolaryngol Clin North Am, 25:413, 1992

102. Clements DH, Morledge DE, Martin WH et al: Evoked and spontaneous electromyography to evaluate lumbosacral pedicle screw placement. Spine, 21:600, 1996

103. Calancie B, Madsen P, Lebwohl N: Stimulus-evoked EMG monitoring during transpedicular lumbosacral instrumentation. Spine, 19:2780, 1994

104. Maguire J, Wallace S, Madiga R et al: Evaluation of intrapedicular screw position using intraoperative evoked electromyography. Spine, 20:1068, 1995

105. Holland N, Lukacyk T, Kostuik J: Higher electrical stimulus intensities are required to activate chronically compressed nerve roots: implications for intraoperative testing during transpedicular instrumentation. Spine, 23:224, 1998

106. Donohue M, Murtagh-Schaffer C, Basta J et al: Pulse-train stimulation for detecting medial malposition of thoracic pedicle screws. Spine, 33:E378, 2008

107. Daube JR, Harper CM: Surgical monitoring of cranial and peripheral nerves. p. 115. In Desmedt JE (ed): Neuromonitoring in Surgery. Elsevier, Amsterdam, 1989

108. Skinner S, Transfeldt E, Savik K: Surface electrodes are not sufficient to detect neurotonic discharges: observations in a

porcine model and clinical review of deltoid electrographic monitoring using multiple electrodes. J Clin Monit Comput, 22:131, 2008

109. Prass RL, Luders H: Acoustic (loudspeaker) facial electromyographic monitoring: Part 1. Evoked electromyographic activity during acoustic neuroma resection. Neurosurgery, 19:392, 1986

110. Prass RL, Kinney S, Hardy R et al: Acoustic (loudspeaker) facial EMG monitoring: II. Use of evoked EMG activity during acoustic neuroma resection. Otolaryngol Head Neck Surg, 97:541, 1987

111. Lloyd-Thomas AR, Cole PV, Prior PF: Quantitative EEG and brainstem auditory potentials: comparison of isoflurane with halothane using cerebral function analysing monitor. Br J Anaesth, 65:306, 1990

112. Radke RA, Erwin CW, Wilkins RH: Intraoperative brainstem auditory evoked potentials: significant decrease in postoperative morbidity. Neurology, 39:187, 1989

113. Harper CM, Harner SG, Slavit DH et al: Effect of BAEP monitoring on hearing preservation during acoustic neuroma resection. Neurology, 42:1551, 1992

114. Morioka T, Tobimatsu S, Fujii K et al: Direct spinal versus peripheral nerve stimulation as monitoring techniques in epidurally recorded spinal cord potentials. Acta Neurochir (Wien), 108:122, 1991

115. Kemink JL, LaRouere MJ, Kileny PR et al: Hearing preservation following suboccipital removal of acoustic neuromas. Laryngoscope, 100:597, 1990

116. Cheek JC: Posterior fossa intraoperative monitoring. J Clin Neurophysiol, 10:412, 1993

117. Colletti V, Fiorino FG: Vulnerability of hearing function during acoustic neuroma surgery. Acta Otolaryngol, 114:264, 1994

118. Matthies C, Samii M: Management of vestibular schwannomas (acoustic neuromas): the value of neurophysiology for intraoperative monitoring of auditory function in 200 cases. Neurosurgery, 40:459, 1997

119. Post KD, Eisenberg MB, Catalano PJ: Hearing preservation in vestibular schwannoma surgery: what factors influence outcome. J Neurosurg, 83:191, 1995

120. Roberson J, Senne A, Brackmann D et al: Direct cochlear nerve action potentials as an aid to hearing preservation in middle fossa acoustic neuroma resection. Am J Otol, 17:653, 1996

121. Matthies C, Samii M: Direct brainstem recording of auditory evoked potentials during vestibular schwannoma resection: nuclear BAEP recording. J Neurosurg, 86:1057, 1997

122. Moller AR, Jho HD, Janetta PJ: Preservation of hearing in operations on acoustic tumors: an alternative to recording brainstem auditory potentials. Neurosurgery, 34:688, 1994

123. Angelo R, Moller AR: Contralateral evoked brainstem auditory potentials as an indicator of intraoperative brainstem manipulation in cerebellopontine angle tumors. Neurol Res, 18:528, 1996

124. Anderson R, Dowling K, Feldstein N et al: Chiari I malformation: potential role of intraoperative electrophysiologic monitoring. J Clin Neurophysiol, 20:65, 2003

125. Haupt WF, Horsch S: Evoked potential monitoring in carotid surgery. A review of 994 cases. Neurology, 42:835, 1992

126. Schramm J, Koht A, Schmidt G et al: Surgical and electrophysiological observations during clipping of 134 aneurysms with evoked potential monitoring. Neurosurgery, 26:61, 1990

127. Lam AM, Manimen PH, Ferguson GG et al: Monitoring electrophysiologic function during carotid endarterectomy: a comparison of somatosensory evoked potentials and conventional electroencephalogram. Anesthesiology, 75:15, 1991

128. Lueders H, Lesser RP, Hahn J et al: Cortical somatosensory evoked potentials in response to hand stimulation. J Neurosurg, 58:885, 1983

129. Lueders H, Dinner DS, Lesser RP et al: Evoked potentials in cortical localization. J Clin Neurophysiol, 3:75, 1986

130. Ojemann G: Temporal lobectomy tailored to electrocorticography and functional mapping. p. 137. In Spencer SS, Spencer DD (eds): Surgery for Epilepsy. Blackwell Scientific, Oxford, 1991

131. Sartorius C, Wright G: Intraoperative brain mapping in a community setting. Surg Neurol, 47:380, 1997

132. Kombos T, Seuss O, Funk T et al: Intra-operative mapping of the motor cortex during surgery in and around the motor cortex. Acta Neurochir (Wien), 142:263, 2000

Bladder, Bowel, and Sexual Dysfunction

Electrophysiologic Evaluation of Sacral Function

SIMON PODNAR and DAVID B. VODUŠEK

Electrodiagnostic methods are well established in the evaluation of the sacral nervous system, which has a critical role in the control of bladder, bowel, and sexual functions. The application of electrodiagnostic techniques in this context closely followed their introduction into clinical neurology, the first technique being needle electromyography (EMG).[1] Electrodiagnostic methods have been proposed for both research and diagnostic applications in patients with suspected neurogenic sacral dysfunction.[2] The emphasis of this chapter is on established tests that are of diagnostic value in the assessment of individual patients. These include EMG, bulbocavernosus reflex studies, and pudendal somatosensory evoked potentials (SEPs). Other tests that are not of clinical diagnostic value are also presented briefly. Detailed descriptions of these investigational sacral electrodiagnostic tests are provided elsewhere.[2]

ESTABLISHED ELECTRODIAGNOSTIC TESTS

Electromyography

KINESIOLOGIC EMG

The aim of kinesiologic EMG is to assess the time course and intensity of activity of individual muscles during various maneuvers. Such recordings reveal the behavior of pelvic floor and sphincter muscles during bladder or rectal filling and emptying (cystometry and anal manometry studies, respectively). It usually is referred to simply as EMG, which causes confusion with needle EMG performed for the diagnosis of motor unit (MU) pathology.

There is no commonly accepted standardized technique. Bioelectrical activity typically is sampled from a

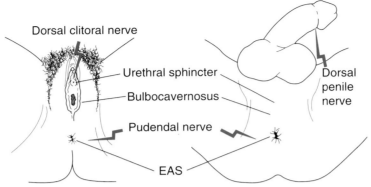

FIGURE 31-1 ■ Needle electrode insertions into the pelvic floor and sphincter muscles and positions for electrical stimulation of peripheral nerves in the female and male perineum. Insertion into the subcutaneous external anal sphincter (EAS) muscle is at about 1 cm from the anal orifice, to a depth of 3 to 6 mm. For the bulbocavernosus muscle, the needle is inserted 2 to 3 cm in front of the anal orifice, about 1 cm from the midline in men, and in women through the skin lateral to the labia majora. The urethral sphincter is reached from the perineum, about 4 cm in front of the anus toward the fingertip palpating the apex of the prostate in men, and in women 0.5 cm lateral to the urethral orifice. The puborectalis (part of levator ani) is inserted at a depth of 5 cm at the anal orifice, at an angle of about 30 degrees to the anal canal axis. The pubococcygeus (part of levator ani) muscle can be located by transrectal or transvaginal palpation and reached transcutaneously from the perineum or transvaginally. The dorsal penile nerves are stimulated in the midline with the cathode proximal, and the dorsal clitoral nerves are stimulated with the cathode applied to the dorsal clitoris and the anode lateral to it. The pudendal nerves are stimulated posterolateral to the anal orifice by applying firm compression against the medial aspect of the ischial bones.

single muscle detection site. Figure 31-1 shows the most useful sphincter and pelvic floor muscle insertion sites. Various types of surface or intramuscular (needle or wire) electrodes can record the kinesiologic EMG signal; the former have problems with artifacts and contamination from other muscles, whereas the latter have problems with representation of the large pelvic floor muscles. The quality of the EMG recorded from the external urethral sphincter (EUS) muscle is improved by a catheter-mounted surface electrode device that applies mild suction.[3] Although either standard EMG equipment or EMG facilities contained within urodynamic systems can be used, the better visual and audio control provided by standard EMG equipment facilitates optimal electrode placement and improves recordings.[4] Generally, the EMG signal is described only qualitatively, but quantitative techniques are also available and increase the validity of the findings.[5]

The normal sphincter EMG shows continuous activity of "low-threshold" MUs,[6] which persists even when subjects are asleep. Such activity can also be recorded in

many, but not all, sites of the levator ani[7] and the deeper external anal sphincter (EAS) muscle.[6] This continuous EAS activity is reduced in a subgroup of patients with idiopathic anal incontinence.[6] EMG activity may be increased voluntarily or reflexly (e.g., by talking, deep breathing, or coughing) when "high-threshold" MUs are recruited. Strong voluntary activation of sphincter and pelvic floor muscles can be sustained only for less than 1 minute. In health, all sphincter and pelvic floor EMG activity disappears on voiding and defecation. However, in central nervous system (CNS) disorders, detrusor contraction and straining may be associated with increased sphincter EMG activity ("detrusor–sphincter dyssynergia"[8] and "paradoxical puborectalis contraction,"[9,10] respectively). Neurogenic, uncoordinated sphincter behavior is sometimes difficult to differentiate from voluntary contractions that may occur in poorly compliant patients and in patients with dysfunctional voiding.[11,12]

Little is known about the normal activity patterns of different pelvic floor (i.e., parts of the levator ani) and sphincter muscles (i.e., sphincter urethrae, urethrovaginal sphincter, and the EAS). The assumption that they all act as one muscle may be incorrect because no relation is found between the ability to activate pelvic floor and the sphincter urethrae muscles.[13] Coordinated behavior is often lost in disease states.[9] A consistent contraction sequence of the superficial and deep pelvic floor muscles is found in continent but not in incontinent women.[14] Apart from polygraph urodynamic recordings to assess detrusor–sphincter coordination, the diagnostic usefulness of kinesiologic EMG has not been established. Needle electrodes are more useful than perineal patch electrodes to demonstrate MU quiescence during voiding.[15] In selected patients with neurogenic detrusor overactivity, EMG of the EUS muscle can also be used to demonstrate the onset of detrusor contractions.[16]

Needle EMG

Although abnormalities on needle EMG may be caused both by muscle disease and by changes in muscle innervation, sacral myopathies are of no clinical importance. Thus, the aim of needle EMG of the sacral myotomes is to differentiate abnormally from normally innervated striated muscle.

For needle EMG, an advanced EMG system with quantitative template-based analysis of motor unit potentials (MUPs) is ideal. The commonly used amplifier filter setting for needle EMG is 5 Hz to 10 kHz; this needs to be identical to that set when reference values for MUP parameters were compiled.

Because of easy access, bulk of the muscle, and the relative ease of its examination, the EAS is the most practical muscle for needle EMG of the lower sacral myotomes.[17] Examination of the subcutaneous EAS muscle is usually sufficient for most diagnostic purposes.[18] To reach this muscle, the needle is inserted about 1 cm from the anal orifice to a depth of 3 to 6 mm (see Fig. 31-1).[17] The left and right EAS muscles should be examined separately by systematic needle insertions into at least four muscle sites.

As with evaluation of other skeletal muscles, needle EMG of the sphincter and pelvic floor muscles is divided into observation of insertion activity, evaluation of any spontaneous activity, (quantitative) assessment of MUPs, and (qualitative) assessment of the interference pattern.[19] In addition, counting of the number of continuously firing MUs during relaxation[6] and observation of MU recruitment on reflex and voluntary activation are recommended.[19]

Insertion Activity and Spontaneous Activity

As in other skeletal muscles, needle movement in sphincter muscles elicits a short burst of insertion activity (gain: 50 μV/division; sweep speed: 10 msec/division).

Approximately 10 to 20 days after an axonal lesion, insertion activity becomes more prominent and prolonged, and abnormal spontaneous activity (i.e., fibrillation potentials and positive sharp waves) appears (Fig. 31-2). The absence of insertion activity with appropriate placement of the needle electrode[17] usually signifies an end-point state after complete muscle denervation.[18,20,21]

In partially denervated muscle, some MUPs remain and mingle with spontaneous denervation activity. Because the MUPs in sphincter muscles are short and mostly biphasic or triphasic[21,22] (as are fibrillation potentials), it takes considerable experience to differentiate one from the other. In this situation, examination of the bulbocavernosus muscle is particularly useful because, in contrast to sphincter muscles, it lacks ongoing activity of low-threshold MUs during relaxation (see Fig. 31-2). Needle insertion into the bulbocavernosus muscle is shown in Figure 31-1.

In long-standing, partially denervated muscles, simple or complex repetitive discharges may also be provoked by needle movement or muscle contraction, or may occur spontaneously (e.g., rhythmically). This activity is sometimes found in the urethral sphincters of patients without any other evidence of neuromuscular disease and, in that situation, is regarded as a nonspecific sign without predictive value for the outcome of surgery.[23]

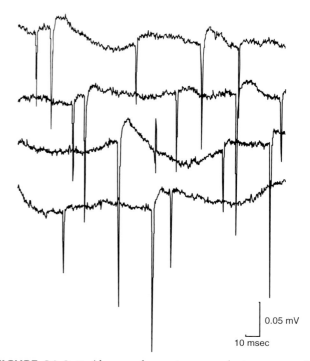

0.05 mV

10 msec

FIGURE 31-2 ■ Abnormal spontaneous electromyographic (EMG) activity recorded during relaxation by a concentric EMG needle in the right bulbocavernosus muscle of a 32-year-old man, 4 weeks after traumatic fracture of the pubic bones and rupture of the urethra.

However, profuse repetitive discharges (called decelerating bursts and complex repetitive discharges), which have been described in the urethral sphincter muscles of some young women with voiding dysfunction (Fig. 31-3), may be diagnostic of idiopathic urinary retention[11,24,25] (Fowler syndrome). The spontaneous discharges are thought to cause involuntary muscle contraction and secondary detrusor dysfunction.

In partially denervated sphincter muscle, a loss of MUs occurs and can be quantified by MUP count during relaxation. The sensitivity of this approach for the diagnosis of neuropathic lesions in the EAS muscle is low; however, MU count during relaxation was reduced in most patients with idiopathic fecal incontinence.[6] In limb muscles, qualitative assessment of the interference pattern (i.e., reduction in the number of activated MUs and increase in their firing rate) usually is performed for estimating MU loss. This is more difficult in the sphincter and pelvic floor muscles because concomitant assessment of the power of muscle contraction cannot be made.

MUP Analysis

With axonal reinnervation after complete denervation, short, low-amplitude, biphasic and triphasic nascent MUPs initially appear; these soon become polyphasic, serrated, and of prolonged duration. In small sphincter muscles with inefficient reinnervation after denervation, such a picture may persist, and on quantitative analysis, MUP area and duration may have values below the lower confidence limits ("pseudomyopathic" MUPs).[18]

By contrast, changes caused by collateral reinnervation after partial axon-loss lesions are reflected in prolongation of the MUP waveform, which may have small, late

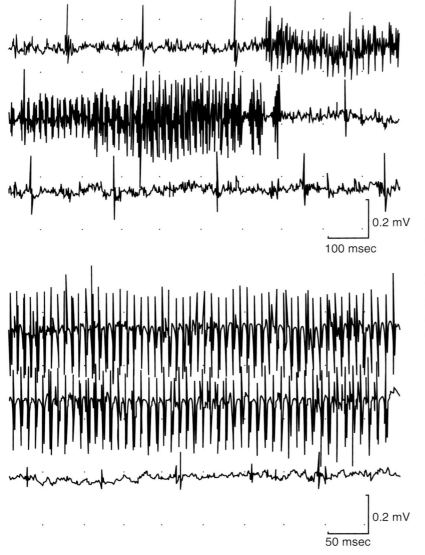

FIGURE 31-3 ■ Profuse pathologic spontaneous activity (complex repetitive discharges) in the urethral sphincter muscle of a 26-year-old, otherwise healthy woman with a 5-year history of difficult bladder emptying. Activity was provoked by movement of the concentric needle electrode or by voluntary muscle contraction. Note the different sweep speeds of the two traces.

components ("satellites"), as shown in Figure 31-4. These have been defined as late spikes firing concomitantly with the main component of the MUP and starting at least 3 msec after the end of it.[26] In newly formed axon sprouts and endplates, transmission is insecure, which may be reflected in MUPs as instability (i.e., jitter and blocking of individual components).[27] Over time, in the absence of further denervation, the reinnervating axonal sprouts increase in diameter so that activation of all parts of the reinnervated MU becomes nearly synchronous; this increases the amplitude and reduces the duration of the MUPs (see Fig. 31-4). This phenomenon may be different in sphincter muscles affected by degenerative disorders such as multisystem atrophy, where long-duration MUPs seem to remain a prominent feature (Fig. 31-5).[28,29]

Three quantitative analysis techniques are available for the systematic examination of individual MUPs, all of which have a similar sensitivity for detecting neuropathic changes.[21] Reference data for mean values and outliers for the EAS muscle have been published for each of these techniques.[21,22,30] The first technique follows an algorithm similar to that used many years ago by Buchthal, but the MUPs are analyzed on the screen. This modified manual-MUP technique is time-consuming (2 to 3 minutes per muscle site); demanding on the operator (reproducible MUPs have to be identified, the one with the smoothest baseline selected, and the duration cursors set); and

MUPs from the left EAS muscle

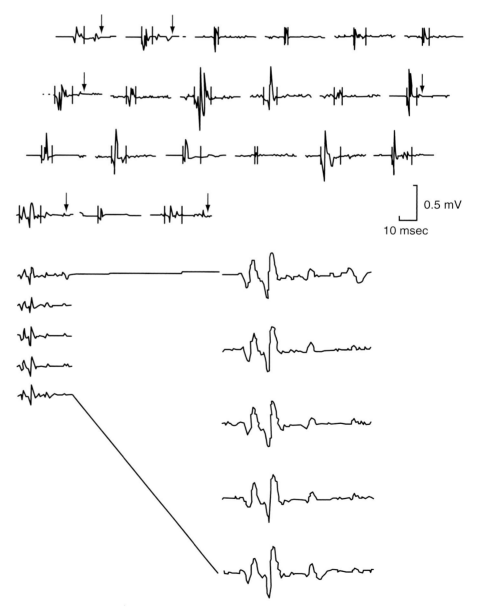

FIGURE 31-4 ▪ Electrodiagnostic findings in a 75-year-old woman with symmetric dopa-unresponsive parkinsonism and urinary and fecal incontinence, referred for sphincter electromyography because of suspected multisystem atrophy. On quantitative analysis of motor unit potentials (MUPs), late MUP components (satellites) were noted in 6 of 21 sampled MUPs, but they were excluded from automatic MUP duration measurements, which resulted in normal findings (duration: mean = 7.0 msec, Z value = 0.4, number of outliers = 1). However, after confirming the consistent simultaneous appearance of late components with the main MUP spike (presented for MUP 19), the position of the second duration markers was changed manually to include them in the MUP duration measurement (arrows), which resulted in a prolonged MUP duration (duration: mean = 10.1 msec, Z value = 3.4, number of outliers = 4). All other evaluated MUP parameters remained within normal limits.

0.5 mV

10 msec

MUPs from the left EAS muscle

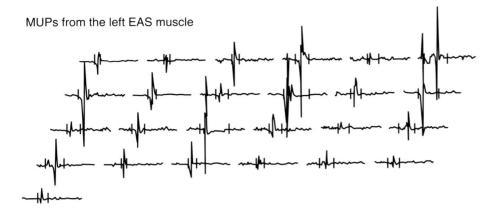

MUPs from the right EAS muscle

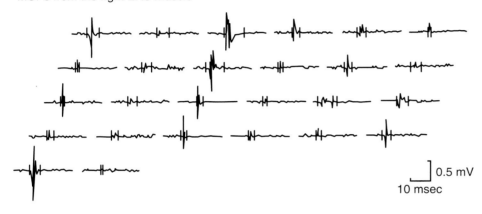

] 0.5 mV

10 msec

T/A analysis of the left EAS muscle

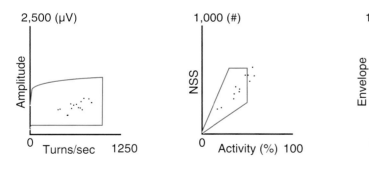

FIGURE 31-5 ■ Motor unit potentials (MUPs) and turns/amplitude (T/A) analysis of the interference pattern from the external anal sphincter (EAS) muscles of a 31-year-old man with a 14-month history of left-sided sciatica, atrophy of the left calf, and fasciculations in both calves. He denied any sacral (urinary, bowel, or sexual) dysfunction or sensory symptoms. Severe atrophy of the left calf, occasional fasciculations in both calves, nonelicitable bulbocavernosus reflex, and normal perineal sensation were found on clinical examination. Note the pronounced neuropathic MUP changes in the left and normal findings in the right EAS muscle. T/A analysis of the interference pattern in the left EAS muscle was normal (dots outside of the second and the third cloud indicate only very strong muscle contraction). Quantitative sphincter electromyography thus demonstrated an asymmetric cauda equina lesion clinically suspected because of fasciculations in both calves and nonelicitable bulbocavernosus reflex.

inevitably open to bias (especially in the determination of MUP duration).[21] The second technique uses a trigger and delay unit, which is set on a steadily firing MUP during a constant level of EMG activity. The MUP is averaged until the baseline becomes smooth (usually about 1 minute). This single-MUP analysis is also time-consuming, provides fewer MUPs than the other two techniques, and is again prone to personal bias.[21] In the template-operated techniques available only on advanced EMG systems (e.g., multi-MUP analysis), the operator

indicates when the computer takes the previous (last) 5 to 10 seconds of the signal. MUPs are extracted automatically from that signal and sorted into several classes, each representing the average of consecutive discharges of MUPs (see Fig. 31-5). MUPs with an unsteady baseline (i.e., unclear beginning or end) or MUPs distorted by averaging need to be recognized and deleted.[31] Multi-MUP analysis is the fastest and easiest to use of these three quantitative MUP analysis techniques.

In sphincter muscles, two MUP populations with different characteristics exist: (1) smaller, continuously firing, low-threshold MUPs; and (2) larger, recruited, high-threshold MUPs. To increase the accuracy of analysis it was proposed that MUPs should be sampled at an activity level permitting 3 to 5 MUPs to be evaluated by a template-operated multi-MUP technique.[21] In contrast to the manual-MUP technique (biased toward low-threshold MUPs) and single MUP (biased toward high-amplitude MUPs), the multi-MUP technique samples all consistently firing MUPs during sphincter muscle relaxation and at slight activation.[21]

In the small sphincter muscle, collecting ten different MUPs is held to be a minimal requirement for using single-MUP analysis. Using the manual-MUP and multi-MUP techniques, sampling of 20 MUPs (the standard number in limb muscles) from each EAS presents no problem in healthy controls[21,22] and in most patients.[18,20,21]

MUP Parameters

A number of MUP parameters are used in the quantitative EMG diagnosis of neuromuscular disease. Traditionally, amplitude and duration are measured and the number of phases is counted. In the EAS muscle, however, only the MUP area, duration, and number of turns are needed for optimal diagnostic power (sensitivity and specificity).[32] Criteria for the diagnosis of neuropathic conditions have also been validated.[33]

The MUP area reflects the sum of the total bioelectrical activity generated by the MU. It is the most sensitive MUP parameter for detecting neuropathic disorders in the EAS muscles.[32,34]

The MUP duration is the interval between the first consistent deflection of the MUP waveform and the point when it finally returns to the baseline. The difficulty with duration measurement is in the exact definition of the beginning and end of the MUP. Using manual positioning of duration cursors depends on amplifier gain; at a higher gain, MUPs seem longer.[26] Because of difficulty with automatic measurement, it has also been suggested that late (satellite) potentials should be excluded from the measurement.[26] However, in the sphincter muscles of patients with suspected multisystem atrophy, the diagnostic power of MUP analysis depends critically on the inclusion of late potentials when MUP duration is measured.[29]

The number-of-turns parameter is similar to the traditional MUP parameter of number of phases. A turn is defined as a change in direction of the MUP trace that is larger than a specified amount (e.g., 100 μV). The number of turns is an MUP parameter that is particularly sensitive to reinnervation changes in small muscles such as the EAS.[21,32,34]

With computer analysis, other MUP parameters are available. Thus, by advanced EMG systems, MUP duration of the negative peak can be measured,[22,34] and thickness (thickness = area/amplitude[35]) and size index (size index = $2 \times log$ [amplitude] + area/amplitude[36]) can be calculated automatically. It has been suggested that the combination of MUP thickness and number of turns might be even more accurate[37] than the previously suggested combination of MUP area, duration, and number of turns.[32]

Interference Pattern Analysis

At high levels of activation of sphincter and pelvic floor muscle, a dense interference pattern can be seen and can be assessed quantitatively using a number of automatic quantitative techniques, the turn/amplitude analysis being the most popular.[38–40] On applying turns/amplitude analysis in sacral electrodiagnosis, subjects contract muscles voluntarily or reflexly by coughing. The examiner selects 0.5-second time intervals of the crisp EMG signal to be analyzed using several interference pattern parameters measured automatically by the EMG system. Although interference pattern sampling using turns/amplitude analysis is even faster than MUP analysis using the multi-MUP technique, its sensitivity for detecting neuropathic EAS muscles is only about half that of MUP analysis techniques.[21] By contrast, turns/amplitude, but not MUP analysis, may detect evidence of denervation and subsequent reinnervation in postpartum women with mild anal incontinence.[41] Qualitative assessment of the interference pattern has been recommended in sphincter and pelvic floor muscles to assess MU loss.[42]

Summary

Template-based multi-MUP analysis is sensitive (equal to traditional MUP analysis techniques), fast (5 to 10 minutes per muscle), easy to apply, and less prone to personal bias.[21] In the EAS muscle, its use is supported by common normative data, which are unaffected by age,[22] gender,[22] number and characteristics of vaginal deliveries,[31] or mild chronic constipation.[43] All these factors make multi-MUP analysis the technique of choice for quantitative analysis of reinnervation of the EAS.

In practice, needle EMG examination can be extended in the same diagnostic session from the lumbar and upper sacral myotomes to the lower sacral myotomes, which commonly require study after a cauda equina lesion. A concentric needle electrode can also be employed at the same diagnostic session for recording evoked direct (M-wave) and reflex muscle responses (bulbocavernosus reflex).

Sacral Reflexes

Sacral reflexes are the electrophysiologically recordable responses of the pelvic floor and sphincter muscles to stimulation of sensory fibers in the uro-ano-genital region. Clinically, two reflexes commonly are elicited in the lower sacral segments: (1) the penilo- or clitoro-cavernosus (i.e., bulbocavernosus) reflex; and (2) the anal reflex.[44] The bulbocavernosus reflex is elicited by squeezing the glans penis and observing or palpating the resulting pelvic floor contraction. The anal reflex is evoked by perianal pinprick and is detected by observation of the anal wink. In both, the afferent and efferent limbs of the reflex arcs are in the pudendal nerves and cauda equina, and integration occurs centrally in the spinal cord at levels S2 to S4 (conus medullaris).

Electrophysiologic measurement of the sacral reflexes is quantitative, more sensitive, and more reproducible than are clinical methods, which may also produce false-positive results.[45] Changes in the threshold, amplitude, and latency of the bulbocavernosus reflex occur not only because of changes in conduction along peripheral and central neural pathways but also as a consequence of changes in transmission within the interneurons of the CNS. With a constant stimulus, they depend on the physiologic state of the pelvic viscera (e.g., bladder[46]) and are affected by pathologic conditions such as suprasacral spinal cord lesions.[47] Thus, electrophysiologic testing of sacral reflexes reveals not only the integrity of the sacral spinal reflex arc but also the excitation level of motor neurons in the sacral spinal cord.[46]

To elicit sacral reflexes, electrical,[48–55] mechanical,[52,53,56] or magnetic[57] stimulation can be used. Whereas the latter two modalities have only been applied to the penis,[54–56] clitoris, and the suprapubic area,[52] electrical stimuli can be applied to various sites: to the dorsal penile or clitoral nerve; perianally (see Fig. 31-1); and, using a catheter-mounted ring electrode, to the bladder neck/proximal urethra.[58] In clinical practice, electrical stimulation of the penis or clitoris is used most commonly (Fig. 31-6).

For electrical stimulation, placement of surface electrodes on the dorsum of the penis/clitoris and application of 10 single, 0.2-msec supramaximal stimuli at time intervals of 2 seconds (0.5 Hz) has been recommended.[2] In addition to single-pulse electrical stimulation, two identical electrical pulses separated by a 3-msec interval can be used (i.e., double-pulse electrical stimulation).[54,55] Double-pulse electrical stimulation is more efficient in eliciting sacral reflexes.[54] For mechanical stimulation, either a standard commercially available reflex hammer or a customized electromechanical hammer can be employed. Using a reflex hammer, the stimulus is applied to a wooden spatula placed on the glans penis or clitoris.[54,55] Such stimulation is painless and is particularly suitable for testing children.[56]

For reflex recordings, concentric needle or surface electrodes are placed into or over the bulbocavernosus or the EAS muscle. The use of filters (10 Hz to 10 kHz), a sweep speed of 10 msec/division, and a gain of 50 to 1000 μV/division are recommended. Traditionally, the onset latency of the sacral reflex has been the only measured parameter.[2] Onset latency provides information on the fastest nerve fibers in the sacral reflex arc. Latency of mechanically elicited bulbocavernosus reflex is comparable to that elicited by single and double electrical pulses.[54] However, using electrical stimulation, sensory threshold (lowest perceived stimulus intensity) and reflex threshold (minimum stimulus intensity eliciting sacral reflex) can also be measured. They evaluate lower sacral sensory pathways and excitation level of the sacral reflex pathway, respectively. Although, for men, confidence intervals for these two new parameters have been established,[54] their clinical utility has not yet been determined.

The sacral reflex evoked by dorsal penile or clitoral nerve stimulation consists of two components. The first, with a mean latency of 29.9 ± 5.7 msec in one study in men,[54] is stable, does not habituate, and is thought to be an oligosynaptic reflex.[49] In adults, values of 40, 36, and 36 m/sec have been suggested as the upper limit of normal for the shortest latency obtained on eliciting a series of reflex responses using single, double, and mechanical stimulation, respectively.[54] The second component, which is not always demonstrable as a discrete response, has a similar latency to the sacral reflexes evoked by stimulation perianally (anal reflex) or from the proximal urethra, and it is a polysynaptic reflex.[49] In normal subjects it is usually the first component that has a lower threshold. However, in some patients the first component of the bulbocavernosus reflex cannot be obtained with single electrical stimuli but, on strong stimulation, the second component appears and can be misinterpreted as a delayed early response. The situation may be clarified by using double electrical or mechanical stimuli that facilitate the reflex and reveal the first component.

Two unilateral arcs for the bulbocavernosus reflex have been demonstrated.[51] Thus, by recording of the bulbocavernosus reflex from the left and right bulbocavernosus or the EAS muscles, separate testing of both bulbocavernosus reflex arcs can be performed. This is important because in patients with unilateral disease

Electrical stimulation

Left   Right

FIGURE 31-6 ■ Bulbocavernosus reflex obtained on electrical and mechanical stimulation in a 60-year-old man 50 months after fracture of the L1 vertebra. Immediately after the trauma he noted transient difficulty in bladder emptying but no bowel or sexual dysfunction. Perianal sensation and the bulbocavernosus reflex were normal. Using a concentric needle recording electrode and electrical and mechanical stimulation, no bulbocavernosus reflex was recorded in the right bulbocavernosus muscle, whereas a normal latency response was recorded in the left.

Mechanical stimulation

] 0.5 mV

20 msec

(e.g., sacral plexopathy or pudendal neuropathy) or asymmetric lesions (e.g., cauda equina syndrome; see Fig. 31-6), a healthy bulbocavernosus reflex arc may obscure a pathologic one.

Sacral reflex responses on stimulation of the dorsal penile and clitoral nerve are of value in evaluating patients with cauda equina and other lower motor neuron lesions, although a response of normal latency does not exclude the possibility of a partial axonal lesion in its reflex arc. In men with chronic cauda equina lesions, the penilo-cavernosus reflex has a sensitivity of 81 to 83 percent (with different stimulation techniques), and higher specificity, predictive values, and likelihood ratios than clinical testing.[59] The value of sacral reflex testing is less clear in women. An abnormally short reflex latency of the bulbocavernosus reflex suggests an abnormally low position of the conus medullaris.[50]

Sacral reflex testing should be part of the diagnostic battery, of which needle EMG exploration of the sphincter and pelvic floor muscles is the most important part. Sensitivity of the combination of penilo-cavernosus reflex (using different stimulation techniques) and quantitative EMG was 94 to 96 percent in one study of men with chronic cauda equina or conus medullaris lesions.[60] The results, however, should always be interpreted in the clinical context.

Pudendal Somatosensory Evoked Potentials

The pudendal SEP is recorded easily following electrical[56,61-64] or mechanical[56] stimulation of the dorsal penile or clitoral nerves (see Fig. 31-1). The first positive peak, at 41 ± 2.3 msec in one study[61] (called P1 or P40), usually is defined clearly in healthy subjects after computer averaging of 100 responses on electrical stimulation that is 2 to 4 times stronger than the sensory threshold (Fig. 31-7). The response is, as a rule, of highest amplitude (0.5 to 12 μV) at the central recording site (Cz′–Fz of the international 10–20 system of electrode placement[62]) and is highly reproducible. Later negative (at about 55 msec) and subsequent positive waves show intersubject variability and have little clinical relevance.

Recording of pudendal SEPs sometimes is indicated in patients with a normal bulbocavernosus reflex who complain of abnormal sensation in the lower sacral segments, pointing to the possibility of a central (i.e., spinal cord) lesion above the sacral segments. It has been shown in such patients, however, that the tibial SEPs are more

often abnormal than is the pudendal SEP, as in multiple sclerosis.[64,65] Only rarely is the pudendal SEP abnormal and the tibial SEPs normal, suggesting a localized conus medullaris lesion.[64] Furthermore, in the investigation of urogenital symptoms, the pudendal SEP is reported to be of no greater value than a clinical examination focusing on signs of spinal cord disease in the lower limbs.[63] Abnormal pudendal SEPs seem to predict a poor surgical outcome after resection of a tight filum terminale.[66]

The method is valid and robust, but seems to be of minor clinical value. There may, however, be circumstances in which it is reassuring to be able to record a normal pudendal SEP (e.g., when a patient complains of loss of bladder, genital, or perianal sensation).

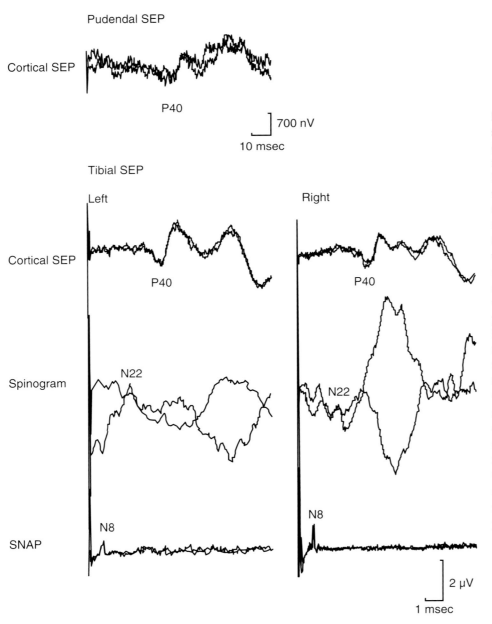

FIGURE 31-7 ■ Pudendal and tibial somatosensory evoked potentials (SEPs) recorded in a 28-year-old man 13 months after spinal fracture. Immediately after trauma the patient was unable to void or defecate, and some sacral dysfunction persisted. On clinical examination the anal sphincter tone and contraction were weakened and the bulbocavernosus reflex was not elicitable. Sensations of touch, vibration, and joint position were preserved in all areas, but pinprick and temperature were not felt bilaterally in all sacral dermatomes (S1–S5). On dorsal penile nerve stimulation, a pudendal SEP with a normal peak latency of the first positive wave (47 msec) was recorded, and normal tibial SEPs were recorded on tibial nerve stimulation at the ankles. The clinical picture, corroborated by electrodiagnostic findings, was consistent with a lesion of the anterior conus medullaris. SNAP represents the sensory nerve action potential.

Cerebral SEPs elicited by penile/clitoral stimulation have been reported as possibly valuable for intraoperative monitoring in patients in whom the cauda equina or conus medullaris is at risk during surgery.[67]

OTHER ELECTRODIAGNOSTIC TESTS

The Sacral Motor System

SINGLE-FIBER EMG

The aim of single-fiber EMG (SF-EMG) testing is similar to that of needle EMG: to differentiate normal from abnormal striated muscle. SF-EMG is most suitable for recording "instability" of MUPs (specifically, the jitter or variability in time interval between consecutive firings of muscle fibers, as discussed in Chapter 17. The jitter may be increased by recent reinnervation as well as by diseases affecting neuromuscular transmission. The SF-EMG parameter that reflects MU morphology is the fiber density, which is defined as the mean number of muscle fibers belonging to an individual MU per detection site (recorded from 20 intramuscular detection sites).[27]

SF-EMG has been applied in research into sacral nervous system physiology and into pelvic organ dysfunction. The normal fiber density for the EAS is below 2.0,[68] increases with age, and is affected by gender (greater in women).[68] Quantified needle EMG provides the same information on reinnervation in muscle as fiber density on SF-EMG,[69] but it also reveals the presence of spontaneous denervation activity. After severe partial denervation, areas of fibrosis in muscle are "silent" on EMG exploration, and the results of the examination are based only on the MUP activity in surviving muscle. Such muscle is easier to examine with conventional EMG, which records from a larger volume of tissue than a single-fiber electrode.

SURFACE EMG WITH NONINVASIVE ELECTRODE ARRAYS

Recently, surface EMG recording using noninvasive electrode arrays and multichannel EMG amplifiers was introduced to the sphincter and pelvic floor muscles (e.g., the EAS and puborectalis). Using this approach, investigators can localize muscle innervation zones and asymmetry in muscle innervation,[70] and analyze discharge patterns of MUPs and propagation velocities along the muscle fibers—some characteristics of MUPs.[71] Although comparisons with normal have been made of the findings in pathologic conditions,[72] the clinical value of these methods in diagnosing neurogenic sacral disorders has not been demonstrated.

MOTOR NERVE CONDUCTION STUDIES

Recording of the compound muscle action potential (CMAP) elicited by electrical stimulation of a motor nerve is hindered with regard to the lower sacral segments by access to stimulation sites and by difficulty in recording a reproducible supramaximal response. As a consequence, the only electrophysiologic parameter that can be measured in the pelvic floor is the pudendal nerve terminal motor latency (PNTML), which measures conduction in the fastest-conducting motor nerve fibers.

PNTML can be elicited by bipolar perianal stimulation (see Fig. 31-1) and recorded with a concentric needle electrode from the bulbocavernosus, EAS, or urethral sphincter muscles. Using this perianal technique, the PNTML is approximately 5 msec.[48] More often, a motor response is evoked by a bipolar stimulating electrode fixed onto a distal gloved index finger inserted into the rectum, and by the recording electrode pair placed 8 cm proximally on the base of the index finger (the "St. Mark's electrode").[73,74] It is assumed that, using this approach, the pudendal nerve is stimulated close to the ischial spine, and that the response recorded is of the EAS muscle. In women, intravaginal stimulation and recording from the bulbocavernosus muscles has also been undertaken, with similar distal latencies.[75] However, the latency of such a response is typically only around 2 msec, which seems unusually short compared with the perineal technique and with conduction in the much thicker motor fibers of peripheral nerves in the limbs. It seems unlikely that the PNTML using the St. Mark's electrode really evaluates conduction along the last 8 cm of the pudendal nerve. Stimulation of the terminal pudendal branches or pelvic floor muscles near their motor points seems more likely, and this is supported by the much longer PNTML (3.7 ± 0.9 msec) obtained with a monopolar intrarectal stimulation electrode.[73]

Prolongation of the PNTML as measured by the St. Mark's electrode has been found in several sacral disorders[74,76] and has also been claimed to predict the outcome of therapeutic interventions by some investigators[77] but not by others.[68,78-81] This prolongation was taken as a sign of damage to the pudendal nerves, leading to the term pudendal neuropathy, which is used particularly by proctologists. A prolongation of PNTML has been equated mistakenly with pelvic floor denervation, but studies have failed to demonstrate any correlation between a prolonged PNTML and morphologic (EAS thickness[79]) or functional signs of denervation.[80] The clinical significance of such prolongations in latency is unclear in the absence of relevant morphologic studies. The authors have found the PNTML unhelpful for diagnostic purposes in individual patients with pelvic floor disorders. In patients with fecal incontinence, conventional needle EMG[81] is more useful than the PNTML. Eliciting a CMAP in pelvic floor muscles using perianal stimulation may be helpful in excluding a complete peripheral (axonal) lesion.

CONDUCTION STUDIES WITH ROOT STIMULATION

The sacral roots can be stimulated electrically or magnetically at their exit from the lower spinal canal.[82,83] Typical mean latencies vary from 5 to 9 msec, depending on the stimulation site.[83] Lumbosacral stimulation often evokes a large stimulus artifact that can be decreased by positioning the ground electrode between the stimulating and recording electrodes.[84] Selective stimulation of individual sacral roots is possible by appropriate positioning of surface stimulating electrodes.[85] However, nonselective stimulation is applied more commonly and results in activation of all muscles innervated by lumbosacral segments; responses from the large gluteal muscles may contaminate surface recordings from the sphincter muscle, and needle detection is necessary.[86]

Recording the motor evoked potential (MEP) with lumbosacral magnetic stimulation has been less successful than with electrical stimulation.[87] It also often evokes a large stimulus artifact that can be decreased by positioning the ground electrode between the recording electrodes and the stimulating coil.[88] Demonstration of a perineal MEP on stimulation over the lumbosacral spine and recording with a concentric needle electrode occasionally may be helpful, but an absent response has to be evaluated with caution.

ASSESSMENT OF CENTRAL MOTOR PATHWAYS

Magnetic or electrical stimulation can be used to stimulate the brain, the response being recorded from the pelvic floor and sphincter muscles. The aim of these techniques is to assess conduction, not only in peripheral but also in central motor pathways. In contrast to magnetic stimulation, cerebral electrical stimulation is painful and nowadays is used only on anesthetized patients during intraoperative monitoring.[89]

In response to magnetic stimulation over the motor cortex of healthy subjects, MEPs in a variety of sphincter[83,84] and pelvic floor muscles[83] have been reported. As with measurements from limb muscles, only latencies are used in evaluating the response. When no facilitatory maneuver is used, mean latencies are 19 to 21 msec, but slight voluntary contraction of the sphincter and pelvic floor muscles shortens latencies by up to 3 msec.

By subtracting the latency of the MEPs obtained by stimulation over the scalp and at the L1 level, a central conduction time of 15 to 16 msec without and 13 to 14 msec with facilitation is obtained for pelvic floor and sphincter muscles.[82,83,90]

Although a substantially prolonged central conduction time usually is obtained in patients with multiple sclerosis[90,91] and myelopathy,[90] the diagnostic contribution of the technique is minor because these patients also have clinically evident spinal cord disease. However, MEPs may be useful in patients with unclear localization of spinal lesions.[90] In patients with peripheral (e.g., cauda equina) lesions, a concomitant spinal cord lesion may be obscured clinically but revealed neurophysiologically by prolongation of the central motor conduction time calculated using both lumbar magnetic stimulation and the F-wave latency measurement; patients without an additional spinal cord lesion only have central prolongation obtained by lumbar magnetic stimulation.[92] A well-formed sphincter MEP with a normal latency occasionally may be helpful in a patient with a possibly nonorganic disorder or in a medicolegal case.

The Sacral Sensory System

ELECTRONEUROGRAPHY OF DORSAL PENILE NERVES

In healthy men, a low-amplitude (10-μV) sensory nerve action potential (SNAP) is recorded by placing a pair of stimulating electrodes across the penile glans and placing a pair of recording electrodes across the base of the penis. The sensory conduction velocity of the dorsal penile nerve is 27 to 33 m/sec.[93] Measuring the conduction distance is difficult because penis length is readily changeable. The antidromic method of stimulating the pudendal nerve transrectally by the St. Mark's electrode and recording SNAPs from the penis seems more reproducible.[94] Nerve conduction studies of the dorsal penile nerve have been proposed as a means of assessing sensory function in the lower sacral segments. Theoretically, a normal-amplitude SNAP of the dorsal penile nerves in an insensitive penis distinguishes a sensory lesion proximal to the dorsal spinal ganglion (e.g., cauda equina, central pathways) from a lesion distal to the ganglion (e.g., sacral plexus, pudendal nerves). The test is not often used.

ELECTRICAL RESPONSES OF DORSAL SENSORY ROOTS

Using surface electrodes at the level of the lower thoracic and upper lumbar vertebrae, particularly in slim men, a low-amplitude (less than 1 μV) monophasic negative potential with a mean peak latency of about 12.5 msec can be recorded on stimulation of the dorsal penile nerves.[61] With epidural electrodes, sacral root potentials have been recorded in 59 percent, and postsynaptic cord potentials in 41 percent, of men.[95]

Intraoperatively, with the sacral roots exposed, SNAPs can be recorded more readily on stimulation of the dorsal penile and clitoral nerves. This has been helpful in preserving roots important for perineal sensation in spastic children undergoing dorsal rhizotomy, perhaps thereby decreasing the incidence of postoperative voiding dysfunction.[96] No use for such recordings has been established outside of the operating room.

CEREBRAL SEPs ON STIMULATION OF PELVIC VISCERA

Cerebral SEPs on stimulation of pelvic viscera are claimed to be more relevant to neurogenic sacral dysfunction than the pudendal SEP because the A-delta sensory afferents from pelvic viscera accompany the autonomic fibers in the pelvic nerves and also participate in visceral reflexes. To obviate depolarization of somatic afferents for such measurements, bipolar electrical stimulation applied by catheters and other special devices is required. These cerebral SEPs have been shown to have a maximum amplitude over the midline (Cz'–Fz). They are of low amplitude (1 μV or less) and of variable configuration, which makes their identification difficult, even in control subjects. On stimulation of the bladder,[58] urethra,[58] and sigmoid colon,[97] the typical latency of the most prominent negative potential (N1) is about 100 msec, whereas, with stimulation of the anal canal, the response has a slightly longer latency. On electrical and mechanical stimulation of the rectum, the cerebral SEP is similar in shape and latency to the pudendal SEP.[98] No clinical utility of such recordings has been established. Instead of recording the cortical response, the sympathetic skin response (SSR) can be recorded from the hand after bladder/urethral stimulation.[99] A preserved palmar SSR then demonstrates continuity of the sensory pathways from the bladder neck/posterior urethra to the cervical spinal cord level.[99]

ASSESSMENT OF SACRAL SENSATION

Although not strictly a neurophysiologic test, measurement of electrical thresholds adds clinically unobtainable information on sensory function of the lower urinary tract.[100] Electrical currents are applied to the bladder, urethra, or genital skin using catheter-mounted or surface electrodes. High-frequency stimulation (greater than 20 Hz), with a stimulus duration of 0.5 or 1 msec, is used because it is perceived more easily in the lower urinary tract. Measurement of sensory thresholds with such stimulation is reproducible, and normative data have been published.[100] To date it has been used in only a few conditions (e.g., painful bladder syndrome[101]). In addition, palmar SSR and perineal surface EMG recordings can be used for more objectively demonstrating sensations during cystometry. The activity of both appears and increases in parallel with the first sensation of bladder filling, and with the first desire to void, respectively.[5] Further studies using these methods are needed to establish their clinical utility.

Autonomic Nervous System Tests

The electrodiagnostic techniques just discussed assess only the somatic nervous system, whereas the autonomic nervous system is more relevant for sacral organ function. Although focal involvement of the sacral nervous system (trauma or compression) usually involves both somatic and autonomic fibers, in some circumstances the autonomic system is affected in isolation (e.g., after excision of mesorectal carcinoma[102] and prostatectomy[103]). Furthermore, some systemic disorders affect predominantly the autonomic nervous system.[104]

SYMPATHETIC SKIN RESPONSE

The SSR is a reflex subserved by myelinated sensory fibers (afferent limb), a complex central integrative mechanism, and sympathetic postganglionic nonmyelinated C fibers (efferent limb). The responses, which can be recorded from the perineum or penis, rapidly habituate and are critically dependent on a number of endogenous and exogenous factors, including skin temperature. The stimulus used in clinical practice is generally an electrical pulse delivered to a peripheral nerve in the limbs, but the genital organs can also be stimulated.

The SSR can be recorded on the penis following stimulation of the median nerve at the wrist in all control subjects; the response is variable in shape and has latencies of approximately 2 seconds.[105] Similarly, the SSR can be recorded from the genital region in women.[106] Only an absent SSR is considered abnormal. The SSR can also be recorded on bladder/urethral stimulation,[99] which in addition to central sympathetic pathways also tests thin afferent fibers from the pelvic viscera. The SSR is reportedly useful in the assessment of neuropathies involving unmyelinated nerve fibers,[107] and in patients with spinal cord injury, it may serve also as an indicator of bladder neck competence.[108] In men it may serve as a predictor of preserved psychogenic erections.[109]

DARTOS REFLEX

In men, another approach to test lumbosacral sympathetic function is by neurophysiologic measurement of the dartos reflex obtained by cutaneous stimulation of the thigh. The dartos muscle is a sympathetically innervated dermal layer within the scrotum, distinct from the somatically innervated cremasteric muscle. A reliable and reproducible dartos reflex (i.e., scrotal skin contraction) with a latency of about 5 seconds has been demonstrated in healthy men.[110]

SMOOTH MUSCLE EMG

Information on parasympathetic bladder innervation can, to some extent, be obtained by cystometry, although this cannot demonstrate directly the neuropathic etiology of the dysfunction. Electrodiagnostic tests of sacral parasympathetic nerve function (e.g., corpus cavernosum EMG,[111] clitoral EMG,[112] and detrusor EMG) would, in principle, constitute the most definitive indicator of neurogenic sacral organ involvement. Further studies to validate these tests would be necessary to clarify their place in research and clinical practice. At present, clinical application of these tests is premature.[113]

CLINICAL APPLICATION OF ELECTRODIAGNOSTIC TESTS

Electrodiagnostic tests are an extension of the clinical neurologic examination and are helpful in evaluating patients in whom a nervous system lesion is suspected.

However, they are not useful for screening purposes. They provide data on the physiologic integrity of various structures; document a clinically diagnosed nervous system lesion; assist in the precise localization of the lesion; aid in determination of the type, duration, and progression of the lesion; and help to define lesion severity (Table 31-1). In selected patients with sacral disorders, these data should be relevant for prognostication and may affect decisions regarding therapeutic (including surgical) intervention.

Electrodiagnostic tests, however, also have limitations. They are uncomfortable; localization is difficult in patients with multifocal lesions or with proximal peripheral sacral lesions (paravertebral muscles are absent in the lower sacral segments); and optimal timing of the investigation is limited (sensitivity is highest 3 weeks to several months after onset of focal peripheral sacral lesions). Test results do not correlate directly with bladder, anorectal, or sexual dysfunction.

An international consensus statement proposed that sacral electrodiagnostic studies are most useful in patients with suspected focal peripheral sacral lesions (e.g., conus medullaris, cauda equina, sacral plexus, and pudendal nerve lesions); in patients with multisystem atrophy; and in women with urinary retention.[2] Neurogenic sacral dysfunction can, of course, also be caused by a variety of other neurologic disorders, but the value of sacral electrodiagnostic studies in the evaluation of those patients is minor. In patients with brain disease, imaging studies are the most useful investigative approach. In spinal cord disease, EMG during cystometry may be performed to demonstrate detrusor–sphincter dyssynergia,

---

TABLE 31-1 ■ Information Provided by Sacral Electrodiagnostic Tests that is not Provided by Other Functional Tests

Information		Method	Finding
Integrity preserved	Lower motor neuron	EMG	No denervation activity
			Continuous MUP firing during relaxation
	Lower and upper motor neuron	EMG	Dense interference pattern on voluntary activation
	Sacral reflex arc	EMG	Dense interference pattern on reflex activation (touch)
		Sacral reflex response	Brisk bulbocavernosus reflex of normal latency
	Sensory pathways	Pudendal SEP	Normal shape and latency of responses
Localization of lesions	Root vs. plexus or nerve	EMG	Paravertebral denervation activity in neighboring myotomes
		SNAP	Normal (penile) SNAP with impaired (penile) skin sensation
Severity of lesions	Complete vs. partial	EMG	Profuse denervation activity, absent MUPs
	Severe vs. moderate	Sacral reflex response	Bulbocavernosus reflex not elicitable
Timing of lesions	Acute or subacute vs. chronic	EMG	Profuse denervation activity
			No MUP changes of chronic reinnervation
Progression of lesions	Progressive vs. nonprogressive	EMG	Denervation activity
			Subacute MUP changes
Type of lesion	Conduction block vs. axonotmesis	EMG	Absent or sparse denervation activity
	Axonotmesis vs. neurotmesis	EMG	Appearance of nascent MUPs after complete muscle denervation

EMG, concentric-needle electromyography; MUP, motor unit potential; SEP, somatosensory evoked potential; SNAP, sensory nerve action potential.

although videocystourethrography is the investigation of choice.[4] As an addition to the clinical examination and imaging studies, SEPs elicited by tibial nerve stimulation are probably more useful than are pudendal SEPs for demonstration of abnormal spinal cord conduction.[64] Similarly, in patients with sacral dysfunction caused by generalized peripheral neuropathies, nerve conduction studies performed in the lower limbs are a more sensitive adjunct to clinical examination than are sacral electrodiagnostic studies.[114]

In a personal series of 194 consecutive patients referred for electrodiagnostic evaluation, quantitative needle EMG of the EAS muscles supported a diagnosis of a cauda equina or conus medullaris lesion in 36 patients, a lesion of the EAS muscle in 6, a pudendal nerve lesion in 2, and a sacral plexus lesion in 1 patient. Furthermore, neuropathic findings in the EAS were compatible with a diagnosis of multisystem atrophy in 11, and most probably were caused by severe polyneuropathy in 2 patients. In another 11 patients, the etiology of the pathologic findings could not be established at the time of electrodiagnostic testing.[115]

Assessment of Patients Before Testing

Detailed clinical evaluation is necessary before electrodiagnostic testing. An inability to empty the bladder and saddle sensory loss in particular are predictive of a peripheral sacral nerve lesion amenable to electrodiagnostic studies.[115] In other patients, isolated urinary, bowel, or sexual dysfunction is more often than not non-neurogenic. In contrast, a neurogenic etiology for sacral dysfunction is likely in patients with a combination of sacral dysfunctions. Patients should be asked about conditions that predispose to neurogenic sacral dysfunction (e.g., extrapyramidal disorders). Neurogenic sacral dysfunction is common in patients after lower spinal and pelvic fractures.

To document and quantify the patient's complaints and to obtain additional data, functional investigations (e.g., urodynamics,[108,116,117] anorectal manometry,[80] cineradiography,[10] and colonic transit studies[118]) may be considered. The physiologic investigations used in the evaluation of pelvic organ disorders test function, whereas electrodiagnostic studies only reflect the neurologic lesion. As a consequence, electrodiagnostic tests are complementary and not an alternative to these other tests. Similarly, electrophysiologic tests are complementary to imaging studies such as ultrasound,[79,119] computerized tomography (CT), and magnetic resonance imaging (MRI[117]) of the anorectum and the lower urinary and genital tracts. Imaging studies reveal morphologic abnormalities (e.g., anal sphincter

tears, abnormal position of the bladder neck, or pelvic vascular stenosis) that are possibly causing or contributing to sacral dysfunction.[79,80] In addition, imaging studies may show structural changes in the brain, spinal canal,[108,116] or the pelvis relevant to sacral neurogenic dysfunction.

Cauda Equina and Conus Medullaris Lesions

Lesions of the cauda equina or conus medullaris commonly cause pelvic floor dysfunction. These mainly have been a consequence of neural compression within the spinal canal caused by intervertebral disc herniation, spinal fractures, epidural hematomas, and intraspinal tumors; or a result of spinal surgery, mainly on lumbar discs.[120,121] Electrodiagnostic tests are also useful in the assessment of neurogenic lesions in children with spinal dysraphism.[117]

After detailed clinical examination of the lumbosacral segments (with particular emphasis on perianal sensation), neurophysiologic testing assesses the severity of the lesion and may clarify the diagnosis. In the authors' series, 10 percent of patients with cauda equina lesions reported normal perianal sensation.[122] Electrodiagnostic tests that need to be considered are bilateral needle EMG of the EAS muscle (see Fig. 31-4) and the bulbocavernosus muscle in subacute situations (see Fig. 31-2); and electrophysiologic evaluation of the bulbocavernosus reflex[60] (see Fig. 31-6) when this is absent or equivocal clinically.[123] Detection of spontaneous denervation activity by needle EMG is common from approximately 3 weeks to several months after injury, and the bulbocavernosus muscle is particularly helpful in this respect. Later, MUP analysis becomes more important for demonstrating reinnervation. The bulbocavernosus reflex is useful for assessing the integrity of the sacral reflex arc in subjects with cauda equina or conus medullaris lesions.[123] Most of these lesions cause partial denervation; a traumatic lesion to the lumbosacral spine or pelvis is probably the only acquired condition in which complete denervation of the perineal muscles can be observed.[18,20,21]

Sacral Plexus and Pudendal Nerve Lesions

Vaginal delivery has been shown to cause pelvic floor and sphincter muscle lesions, mostly neurogenic.[124] After uncomplicated deliveries, these changes are minimal in the EAS muscle.[31] It is assumed commonly that these lesions are relevant in the pathogenesis of stress incontinence and pelvic organ prolapse in women. Electrodiagnostic testing in these patients, however, is recommended only when a proximal peripheral sacral neurogenic lesion is a possibility (see later discussion on urinary incontinence).[2]

Other lesions of the sacral plexus and pudendal nerves are less common than are cauda equina or conus medullaris lesions. They can be caused by pelvic fractures, hip surgery, complicated deliveries,[125] malignant infiltration, and local radiotherapy,[126] and by use of orthopedic traction tables.[127] They are usually unilateral. There are no validated techniques for distinguishing cauda equina lesions from more distal lesions.

Parkinsonism

Multisystem atrophy is a progressive neurodegenerative disease of unknown etiology that is often mistaken for Parkinson disease in its early stages. Prolonged duration[8,28,128,129] and increased polyphasicity of MUPs,[69] as well as a diminished number of continuously active low-threshold MUs and interference pattern abnormalities[130] in the sphincter and the bulbocavernosus muscles, have been described as markers for degeneration of Onuf's nucleus, which occurs in patients with this disorder. Changes consistent with chronic reinnervation can also be demonstrated as an increase in fiber density on SF-EMG.[69] Sphincter EMG may not be sensitive in the early phase of the disease[8,131] and is not specific after 5 years of parkinsonism.[128] Among 30 patients with a pathologic diagnosis of multisystem atrophy, 24 had abnormal, 5 had a borderline, and only 1 had a normal sphincter EMG.[132] Some studies have failed to demonstrate the effectiveness of MUP analysis in sphincter muscles,[133,134] probably because of the exclusion of late components from MUP duration (see Fig. 31-5).[29] The changes of chronic reinnervation may also be found in progressive supranuclear palsy,[135,136] and in Machado–Joseph disease,[137] in which neuronal loss in Onuf's nucleus has also been demonstrated histologically.[137,138]

Unilateral needle EMG, including observation of denervation activity[139] and quantitative MUP analysis,[8,28,69,128,129] is indicated in patients with suspected multisystem atrophy,[19] particularly in its early stages when the diagnosis is unclear.[128] If the test is normal, but suspicion of the diagnosis persists, it might be of value to repeat the test later.[8] EMG performed during urodynamics can also be valuable for documenting detrusor–sphincter dyssynergia in patients with Parkinson disease and multisystem atrophy.[8,139]

Urinary Retention in Women

Isolated urinary retention in young women traditionally was considered to be either psychogenic or the first symptom of multiple sclerosis; however, needle EMG of the urethral sphincter muscle has demonstrated that many such patients have profuse, complex repetitive discharges and decelerating burst activity (see Fig. 31-3).[11,24,25] The presence of such activity in the needle EMG of the EUS of young women with nonobstructive urinary retention (Fowler syndrome) is the only predictor of the long-term success of therapeutic sacral neuromodulation.[140] The cause of this activity is unknown, but an association with polycystic ovaries has been described[141] and in some women it may be the expression of an occult generalized dysautonomia.[142] Typically, women with this syndrome are premenopausal, with a maximum incidence under the age of 30 years.[25] The spontaneous activity persists during attempted micturition and may obstruct flow,[11] leading to secondary detrusor instability or failure to contract.[25]

Because needle EMG of the urinary sphincter detects changes related to denervation and reinnervation, as well as this peculiar abnormal spontaneous activity, it has been proposed that needle EMG of the urinary sphincter muscle should always be undertaken in women with unexplained urinary retention.[2]

Miscellaneous Disorders

Neurophysiologic studies have been undertaken in a variety of other clinical contexts but their utility is less clear. Only a brief summary therefore is provided here concerning these applications.

EMG performed as a part of urodynamic studies may be useful in patients with CNS disease and a pelvic floor disorder. Electrodiagnostic tests of central conduction (MEP, SEP) do not correlate with urodynamic abnormalities[116] and probably will contribute to the neurologic diagnosis only in selected patients. In one study, pudendal SEPs were found to provide relevant information in the initial diagnostic evaluation of patients with multiple sclerosis and were also suggested as a screening test for cystometric evaluation in this population.[143] Needle EMG is not indicated in the evaluation of central lesions unless sacral spinal cord involvement is suspected.

URINARY INCONTINENCE

EMG has been used to examine the extent of nerve damage following childbirth[144–146] and in the assessment of stress incontinence in women. Needle EMG and muscle biopsy of the urethral sphincter showed more severe neuropathic changes in women with stress incontinence than in controls.[147] There is a general consensus that changes occur in the urethral sphincter after vaginal delivery; however, the incidence of more extensive involvement of pelvic floor muscles as a consequence of pudendal nerve and sacral plexus injury is controversial. Sacral plexus lesions certainly occur as a consequence of childbirth,[125] but the prevalence and relevance of minor injuries is not known. Partial reinnervation changes have been found in the EAS and pubococcygeus muscles in women with stress incontinence and genital prolapse using SF-EMG (fiber density), as have changes in interference pattern consistent with MU loss and failure of central activation using turns/amplitude analysis.[39] In addition, age-related neurogenic changes have been found. Needle EMG examination of the pubococcygeus muscle revealed a significant increase in MUP duration following vaginal delivery; this was most marked in women with urinary incontinence 8 weeks after delivery, a prolonged second stage, and heavier babies.[148] However, a study using less biased automated MUP and interference pattern analysis techniques[31] questioned the widely held notion that significant damage to the innervation of the EAS occurs even during uncomplicated deliveries.[148] Although vaginal delivery was related to minor EMG abnormalities, there was no indication that this correlated with loss of sphincter function. (Parous women with stress incontinence had less "neuropathic" MUP changes than continent women.) EMG performed as a part of the urodynamic evaluation may show loss of coordination between the two sides of the pubococcygeus muscle in patients with stress incontinence.[149]

In individual patients without clinical evidence of a neurologic lesion, sacral electrodiagnostic testing is unlikely to be either helpful or necessary.[2] EMG of the EAS muscle may be contributory in patients with urinary incontinence associated with other evidence of sacral dysfunction by history (e.g., bowel or sexual disturbances) or examination. Concentric needle EMG of the EAS revealed neurogenic changes in a similar proportion of women with urinary and fecal incontinence or fecal incontinence alone.[150]

ANAL INCONTINENCE

Needle EMG of the EAS may be useful in patients with anal incontinence[151] following anal ultrasound examination to exclude structural lesions of the sphincter mechanism.[152] Clinical and electrophysiologic signs of more generalized (as in multisystem atrophy) or proximal (e.g., cauda equina or conus medullaris) involvement of the lower sacral myotomes should be sought. In a subgroup of patients in whom no cause of anal incontinence can be established (i.e., idiopathic anal incontinence), the only electrophysiologic abnormality found is a diminished number (absence) of continuously firing low-threshold MUs during relaxation.[6] In patients with fecal incontinence and an increased fiber density on SF-EMG, lower anal squeeze pressures and diminished rectal sensation

have been demonstrated.[80] Evidence of denervation and subsequent reinnervation has been found on amplitude/turn analysis of the interference pattern, but not on MUP analysis, in a group of postpartum women with mild anal incontinence.[41]

There is no consensus regarding the utility of electrophysiologic testing in neurologically normal patients with isolated anal incontinence.

CHRONIC CONSTIPATION

Constipation occurs for a variety of reasons; its prevalence depends on the diagnostic criteria applied. Radiographic methods can demonstrate prolonged colonic transit (using radio-opaque markers) and abnormal pelvic floor movement during defecation (cinedefecography), which are the main mechanisms of constipation.[10,118] EMG may demonstrate continuous puborectalis muscle contraction characteristic of a subtype of obstructed defecation ("nonrelaxing puborectalis syndrome").[9,10]

Chronic constipation with repetitive straining has been proposed to be the main cause of advancing pudendal neuropathy in patients with urinary and anal incontinence; SF-EMG (fiber density[74,153]) and semiquantitative[154] or quantitative MUP changes on conventional EMG of the EAS muscles of severely constipated subjects have been reported by some[74,153] but not all investigators.[154] In one study using advanced MUP and interference pattern analysis, no abnormalities were demonstrated in the EAS muscles of patients with mild chronic constipation.[43] The finding is important for the interpretation of EMG findings in patients with other conditions, a significant proportion of whom also suffer from chronic constipation.

SEXUAL DYSFUNCTION

Neurophysiologic techniques have been applied extensively in research into erectile dysfunction, substantiating the hypothesis that a proportion of such patients have nervous system involvement.[103,104,114] Sensory conduction studies of the dorsal penile nerves were used to support the view that sensory penile neuropathy is an important cause of erectile dysfunction.[93] Testing of the bulbocavernosus reflex to electrical stimulation of the dorsal penile nerves has also been proposed, but its sensitivity and specificity are poor. In diabetics with suspected neurogenic erectile dysfunction, motor and sensory nerve conduction studies in the limbs are more sensitive in revealing peripheral neuropathy than bulbocavernosus reflex latencies.[114] Pudendal SEP recordings have also been employed in men with neurogenic erectile dysfunction and in women with sexual dysfunction because of spinal cord lesions, multiple sclerosis,[155] or diabetes.[114] However, pudendal SEPs were of no greater value than clinical examination in detecting spinal cord disease.[65] Autonomic function tests may be worthwhile. The SSR recorded at the penis is reported to be especially sensitive because it assesses local sympathetic pathways and is sometimes the only evidence for an autonomic deficit.[105] The penile smooth muscle is an obvious target for electrophysiologic recordings in patients with erectile dysfunction, but EMG of this muscle is of uncertain utility.[111,113] Quantitative sensory testing of thermal[103,104] and vibratory[103,104,155] thresholds was reported to be most sensitive for the detection of neuropathy in patients with erectile dysfunction. Although electrodiagnostic tests may be contributory in establishing a neurologic diagnosis in selected patients with erectile dysfunction, abnormal test results do not correlate with dysfunction.

Sacral electrodiagnostic studies may be useful for characterization of spinal cord lesions. A normal bulbocavernosus reflex indicates preservation of the parasympathetic sacral center (and reflex erections in men and lubrication in women[156]); a normal SSR indicates preservation of the sympathetic lumbosacral center (and psychogenic erections), and in men with a lesion level below T12 also preserved ejaculation.[156] A normal pudendal SEP correlates with preserved sacral sensation (and the ability to maintain an erection).[109]

The consensus is that neurophysiologic testing (EMG and bulbocavernosus reflex) is helpful only in selected patients who are suspected of having a neurogenic condition on the basis of the clinical neurologic examination.[157]

APPLICATION OF ELECTRODIAGNOSTIC TESTS IN INVASIVE TREATMENTS OF SACRAL DYSFUNCTION

Surgery

Several studies have demonstrated the utility of neurophysiologic studies in the assessment of surgical candidates with neurogenic sacral disorders. Abnormal tibial SEPs recorded in the lumbosacral region predicted patients with chronic high spinal cord injury in whom sphincterotomy failed to improve bladder emptying,[158] probably due to an additional peripheral lesion resulting in detrusor failure. An abnormal pudendal SEP similarly predicted a poor surgical outcome after resection of a tight filum terminale.[66] Cerebral SEPs elicited by penile/clitoral stimulation may be useful for intraoperative monitoring of patients in whom the cauda equina or conus medullaris is at risk during surgery.[67] In patients with tethered cord syndrome, an electrophysiologic approach, using both threshold-based and continuous EMG monitoring, provides a means to identify and untether autonomous placodes,[159] and safely section the filum terminale,[160] possibly resulting in decreased retethering rates. Other studies have also reported the utility of sacral neurophysiologic methods in intraoperative mapping of neural structures.[96]

Intraoperative MEP monitoring of the EUS and EAS is a feasible method, best achieved by cortical stimulation directed from C4 to C3 or C2 to C1 points.[161,162]

Neuromodulation

In recent years, chronic sacral or pudendal nerve stimulation (i.e., neuromodulation) has become increasingly important in the management of patients with neurogenic sacral disorders involving the control of the bladder or anal sphincters. In spite of wide clinical application, the mechanism of neuromodulation remains unexplained. In patients with neurogenic incontinence who underwent sacral nerve stimulation, the poor response in patients with complete spinal cord injury suggested that neuromodulation involves suprasacral (probably spino-bulbo-spinal) pathways.[163] Symptom benefit in patients with fecal incontinence is associated with a reversible reduction in cortico-anal excitability following neuromodulation by sacral nerve stimulation.[164] Pudendal SEP latency, which is decreased significantly by sacral neuromodulation, may serve as a prognostic factor for clinical outcome.[165] As mentioned earlier, decelerating burst and complex repetitive discharge activity in the EMG of the EUS of young women with nonobstructive urinary retention (Fowler syndrome) is the only predictor of long-term success of therapeutic sacral neuromodulation.[140] Neurophysiologic guidance is mandatory for placement of the lead for chronic pudendal nerve stimulation.[166] Recently, a technique was described for percutaneous S3 spinal nerve stimulation, which enables noninvasive screening of candidates for chronic neurostimulation before the invasive peripheral nerve evaluation test.[85] Adding neurophysiologic monitoring to the biologic monitoring was associated with a reduction in the percentage of patients denied implantation for sacral neuromodulation (from 50 to 20 percent).[167]

Botulinum Toxin Injections

Treatment of detrusor–sphincter dyssynergia in patients with suprasacral nervous lesions may involve transperineal injection of botulinum toxin into the EUS.

For exact muscle localization, combined fluoroscopic and EMG guidance is safe, accurate, easy to perform, and effective.[168]

CONCLUDING COMMENTS

Several electrodiagnostic tests have been proposed for evaluation of the sacral nervous system in patients with bladder, bowel, and sexual dysfunction. All tests discussed in this chapter are of research interest. EMG is of definite utility in the diagnostic evaluation of selected groups of patients with pelvic floor dysfunction, those with traumatic lesions, and those with atypical parkinsonism. In addition, bulbocavernosus reflex and pudendal SEP studies are useful in the evaluation of selected patients with suspected peripheral or central neurogenic sacral lesions. Probably the only patients in whom sacral dysfunction in itself should be considered an indication for EMG (of the urethral sphincter) are women with unexplained urinary retention.

REFERENCES

1. Beck A: Elektromyographische Untersuchungen am Sphincter Ani. Pflugers Arch, 224:278, 1930
2. Vodušek DB, Amarenco G, Podnar S: Clinical neurophysiological tests. p. 523. In Abrams P, Cardozo L, Khoury S (eds): Incontinence. Health Publication, Plymouth (UK), 2009
3. Stafford RE, Sapsford R, Ashton-Miller J et al: A novel transurethral surface electrode to record male striated urethral sphincter electromyographic activity. J Urol, 183:378, 2010
4. De EJ, Patel CY, Tharian B et al: Diagnostic discordance of electromyography (EMG) versus voiding cystourethrogram (VCUG) for detrusor-external sphincter dyssynergy (DESD). Neurourol Urodyn, 24:616, 2005
5. Reitz A, Schmid DM, Curt A et al: Electrophysiological assessment of sensations arising from the bladder: are there objective criteria for subjective perceptions? J Urol, 169:190, 2003
6. Podnar S, Mrkaic M, Vodušek DB: Standardization of anal sphincter electromyography: quantification of continuous activity during relaxation. Neurourol Urodyn, 21:540, 2002
7. Deindl FM, Vodušek DB, Hesse U et al: Activity patterns of pubococcygeal muscles in nulliparous continent women. Br J Urol, 72:46, 1993
8. Stocchi F, Carbone A, Inghilleri M et al: Urodynamic and neurophysiological evaluation in Parkinson's disease and multiple system atrophy. J Neurol Neurosurg Psychiatry, 62:507, 1997
9. Mathers SE, Kempster PA, Swash M et al: Constipation and paradoxical puborectalis contraction in anismus and Parkinson's disease: a dystonic phenomenon? J Neurol Neurosurg Psychiatry, 51:1503, 1988
10. Jorge JM, Wexner SD, Ger GC et al: Cinedefecography and electromyography in the diagnosis of nonrelaxing puborectalis syndrome. Dis Colon Rectum, 36:668, 1993
11. Deindl FM, Vodušek DB, Bischoff C et al: Dysfunctional voiding in women: which muscles are responsible? Br J Urol, 82:814, 1998
12. Groutz A, Blaivas JG, Pies C et al: Learned voiding dysfunction (non-neurogenic, neurogenic bladder) among adults. Neurourol Urodyn, 20:259, 2001
13. Kenton K, Brubaker L: Relationship between levator ani contraction and motor unit activation in the urethral sphincter. Am J Obstet Gynecol, 187:403, 2002
14. Devreese A, Staes F, Janssens L et al: Incontinent women have altered pelvic floor muscle contraction patterns. J Urol, 178:558, 2007
15. Mahajan ST, Fitzgerald MP, Kenton K et al: Concentric needle electrodes are superior to perineal surface-patch electrodes for electromyographic documentation of urethral sphincter relaxation during voiding. BJU Int, 97:117, 2006
16. Hansen J, Borau A, Rodriguez A et al: Urethral sphincter EMG as event detector for neurogenic detrusor overactivity. IEEE Trans Biomed Eng, 54:1212, 2007
17. Podnar S, Rodi Z, Lukanovic A et al: Standardization of anal sphincter EMG: technique of needle examination. Muscle Nerve, 22:400, 1999
18. Podnar S: Electromyography of the anal sphincter: which muscle to examine? Muscle Nerve, 28:377, 2003
19. Podnar S, Vodušek DB: Protocol for clinical neurophysiologic examination of the pelvic floor. Neurourol Urodyn, 20:669, 2001
20. Podnar S, Oblak C, Vodušek DB: Sexual function in men with cauda equina lesions: a clinical and electromyographic study. J Neurol Neurosurg Psychiatry, 73:715, 2002
21. Podnar S, Vodušek DB, Stalberg E: Comparison of quantitative techniques in anal sphincter electromyography. Muscle Nerve, 25:83, 2002
22. Podnar S, Vodušek DB, Stalberg E: Standardization of anal sphincter electromyography: normative data. Clin Neurophysiol, 111:2200, 2000
23. FitzGerald MP, Blazek B, Brubaker L: Complex repetitive discharges during urethral sphincter EMG: clinical correlates. Neurourol Urodyn, 19:577, 2000
24. Fowler CJ, Kirby RS: Electromyography of urethral sphincter in women with urinary retention. Lancet, 1:1455, 1986
25. Swinn MJ, Wiseman OJ, Lowe E et al: The cause and natural history of isolated urinary retention in young women. J Urol, 167:151, 2002
26. Stalberg E, Andreassen S, Falck B et al: Quantitative analysis of individual motor unit potentials: a proposition for standardized terminology and criteria for measurement. J Clin Neurophysiol, 3:313, 1986
27. Stalberg E, Trontelj JV: Single Fiber Electromyography: Studies in Healthy and Diseased Muscle. Raven, New York, 1994
28. Palace J, Chandiramani VA, Fowler CJ: Value of sphincter electromyography in the diagnosis of multiple system atrophy. Muscle Nerve, 20:1396, 1997

29. Podnar S, Fowler CJ: Sphincter electromyography in diagnosis of multiple system atrophy: technical issues. Muscle Nerve, 29:151, 2004

30. Del Rey AP, Entrena BF: Reference values of motor unit potentials (MUPs) of the external anal sphincter muscle. Clin Neurophysiol, 113:1832, 2002

31. Podnar S, Lukanoviè A, Vodušek DB: Anal sphincter electromyography after vaginal delivery: neuropathic insufficiency or normal wear and tear? Neurourol Urodyn, 19:249, 2000

32. Podnar S, Mrkaic M: Predictive power of motor unit potential parameters in anal sphincter electromyography. Muscle Nerve, 26:389, 2002

33. Podnar S: Criteria for neuropathic abnormality in quantitative anal sphincter electromyography. Muscle Nerve, 30:596, 2004

34. Podnar S, Vodušek DB: Standardization of anal sphincter electromyography: utility of motor unit potential parameters. Muscle Nerve, 24:946, 2001

35. Nandedkar SD, Barkhaus PE, Sanders DB et al: Analysis of amplitude and area of concentric needle EMG motor unit action potentials. Electroencephalogr Clin Neurophysiol, 69:561, 1988

36. Sonoo M, Stalberg E: The ability of MUP parameters to discriminate between normal and neurogenic MUPs in concentric EMG: analysis of the MUP "thickness" and the proposal of "size index". Electroencephalogr Clin Neurophysiol, 89:291, 1993

37. Pino LJ, Stashuk DW, Podnar S: Bayesian characterization of external anal sphincter muscles using quantitative electromyography. Clin Neurophysiol, 119:2266, 2008

38. Nandedkar SD, Sanders DB, Stalberg EV: Automatic analysis of the electromyographic interference pattern. Part II: Findings in control subjects and in some neuromuscular diseases. Muscle Nerve, 9:491, 1986

39. Weidner AC, Barber MD, Visco AG et al: Pelvic muscle electromyography of levator ani and external anal sphincter in nulliparous women and women with pelvic floor dysfunction. Am J Obstet Gynecol, 183:1390, 2000

40. Gregory WT, Clark AL, Simmons K et al: Determining the shape of the turns-amplitude cloud during anal sphincter quantitative EMG. Int Urogynecol J Pelvic Floor Dysfunct, 19:971, 2008

41. Gregory WT, Lou JS, Simmons K et al: Quantitative anal sphincter electromyography in primiparous women with anal incontinence. Am J Obstet Gynecol, 198:550.e1, 2008

42. Podnar S: Electrodiagnosis of the anorectum: a review of techniques and clinical applications. Tech Coloproctol, 7:71, 2003

43. Podnar S, Vodušek DB: Standardization of anal sphincter electromyography: effect of chronic constipation. Muscle Nerve, 23:1748, 2000

44. Podnar S: Nomenclature of the electrophysiologically tested sacral reflexes. Neurourol Urodyn, 25:95, 2006

45. Wester C, FitzGerald MP, Brubaker L et al: Validation of the clinical bulbocavernosus reflex. Neurourol Urodyn, 22:589, 2003

46. Kaiho Y, Namima T, Uchi K et al: Electromyographic study of the striated urethral sphincter by using the bulbocavernosus reflex: study on change of sacral reflex activity caused by bladder filling. Nippon Hinyokika Gakkai Zasshi, 91:715, 2000

47. Sethi RK, Bauer SB, Dyro FM et al: Modulation of the bulbocavernosus reflex during voiding: loss of inhibition in upper motor neuron lesions. Muscle Nerve, 12:892, 1989

48. Vodušek DB, Janko M, Lokar J: Direct and reflex responses in perineal muscles on electrical stimulation. J Neurol Neurosurg Psychiatry, 46:67, 1983

49. Vodušek DB, Janko M: The bulbocavernosus reflex. A single motor neuron study. Brain, 113:813, 1990

50. Hanson P, Rigaux P, Gilliard C et al: Sacral reflex latencies in tethered cord syndrome. Am J Phys Med Rehabil, 72:39, 1993

51. Amarenco G, Kerdraon J: Clinical value of ipsi- and contralateral sacral reflex latency measurement: a normative data study in man. Neurourol Urodyn, 19:565, 2000

52. Amarenco G, Bayle B, Ismael SS et al: Bulbocavernosus muscle responses after suprapubic stimulation: analysis and measurement of suprapubic bulbocavernosus reflex latency. Neurourol Urodyn, 21:210, 2002

53. Amarenco G, Ismael SS, Bayle B et al: Dissociation between electrical and mechanical bulbocavernosus reflexes. Neurourol Urodyn, 22:676, 2003

54. Podnar S: Neurophysiologic studies of the penilo-cavernosus reflex: normative data. Neurourol Urodyn, 26:864, 2007

55. Podnar S: The penilo-cavernosus reflex: comparison of different stimulation techniques. Neurourol Urodyn, 27:244, 2007

56. Podnar S, Vodušek DB, Trsinar B et al: A method of uroneurophysiological investigation in children. Electroencephalogr Clin Neurophysiol, 104:389, 1997

57. Loening-Baucke V, Read NW, Yamada T et al: Evaluation of the motor and sensory components of the pudendal nerve. Electroencephalogr Clin Neurophysiol, 93:35, 1994

58. Hansen MV, Ertekin C, Larsson LE: Cerebral evoked potentials after stimulation of the posterior urethra in man. Electroencephalogr Clin Neurophysiol, 77:52, 1990

59. Podnar S: Predictive value of the penilo-cavernosus reflex. Neurourol Urodyn, 28:390, 2009

60. Podnar S: Sphincter electromyography and the penilo-cavernosus reflex: are both necessary? Neurourol Urodyn, 27:813, 2008

61. Vodušek DB: Pudendal SEP and bulbocavernosus reflex in women. Electroencephalogr Clin Neurophysiol, 77:134, 1990

62. Guerit J, Opsomer R: Bit-mapped imaging of somatosensory evoked potentials after stimulation of the posterior tibial nerves and dorsal nerve of the penis/clitoris. Electroencephalogr Clin Neurophysiol, 80:228, 1991

63. Delodovici ML, Fowler CJ: Clinical value of the pudendal somatosensory evoked potential. Electroencephalogr Clin Neurophysiol, 96:509, 1995

64. Rodi Z, Vodušek DB, Denislic M: Clinical uroneurophysiological investigation in multiple sclerosis. Eur J Neurol, 3:574, 1996

65. Betts CD, Jones SJ, Fowler CG et al: Erectile dysfunction in multiple sclerosis. Associated neurological and neurophysiological deficits, and treatment of the condition. Brain, 117:1303, 1994

66. Selcuki M, Coskun K: Management of tight filum terminale syndrome with special emphasis on normal level conus medullaris (NLCM). Surg Neurol, 50:318, 1998

67. Vodušek DB, Deletis V, Abbott R et al: Prevention of iatrogenic micturition disorders through intraoperative monitoring. Neurourol Urodyn, 9:444, 1990

68. Jameson JS, Chia YW, Kamm MA et al: Effect of age, sex and parity on anorectal function. Br J Surg, 81:1689, 1994

69. Rodi Z, Denislic M, Vodušek DB: External anal sphincter electromyography in the differential diagnosis of parkinsonism. J Neurol Neurosurg Psychiatry, 60:460, 1996

70. Enck P, Franz H, Davico E et al: Repeatability of innervation zone identification in the external anal sphincter muscle. Neurourol Urodyn, 29:449, 2010

71. Merletti R, Holobar A, Farina D: Analysis of motor units with high-density surface electromyography. J Electromyogr Kinesiol, 18:879, 2008

72. Cescon C, Bottin A, Fernandez Fraga XL et al: Detection of individual motor units of the puborectalis muscle by non-invasive EMG electrode arrays. J Electromyogr Kinesiol, 18:382, 2008

73. Lefaucheur J, Yiou R, Thomas C: Pudendal nerve terminal motor latency: age effects and technical considerations. Clin Neurophysiol, 112:472, 2001

74. Snooks SJ, Barnes PR, Swash M et al: Damage to the innervation of the pelvic floor musculature in chronic constipation. Gastroenterology, 89:977, 1985

75. Cavalcanti GA, Manzano GM, Giuliano LM et al: Pudendal nerve latency time in normal women via intravaginal stimulation. Int Braz J Urol, 32:705, 2006

76. Bakas P, Liapis A, Karandreas A et al: Pudendal nerve terminal motor latency in women with genuine stress incontinence and prolapse. Gynecol Obstet Invest, 51:187, 2001

77. Gilliland R, Altomare DF, Moreira H Jr, et al: Pudendal neuropathy is predictive of failure following anterior overlapping sphincteroplasty. Dis Colon Rectum, 41:1516, 1998

78. Chen AS, Luchtefeld MA, Senagore AJ et al: Pudendal nerve latency. Does it predict outcome of anal sphincter repair? Dis Colon Rectum, 41:1005, 1998

79. Voyvodic F, Schloithe AC, Wattchow DA et al: Delayed pudendal nerve conduction and endosonographic appearance of the anal sphincter complex. Dis Colon Rectum, 43:1689, 2000

80. Osterberg A, Graf W, Edebol Eeg-Olofsson K et al: Results of neurophysiologic evaluation in fecal incontinence. Dis Colon Rectum, 43:1256, 2000

81. Thomas C, Lefaucheur JP, Galula G et al: Respective value of pudendal nerve terminal motor latency and anal sphincter electromyography in neurogenic fecal incontinence. Neurophysiol Clin, 32:85, 2002

82. Opsomer RJ, Caramia MD, Zarola F et al: Neurophysiological evaluation of central-peripheral sensory and motor pudendal fibres. Electroencephalogr Clin Neurophysiol, 74:260, 1989

83. Brostrom S: Motor evoked potentials from the pelvic floor. Neurourol Urodyn, 22:620, 2003

84. Lefaucheur JP: Intrarectal ground electrode improves the reliability of motor evoked potentials recorded in the anal sphincter. Muscle Nerve, 32:110, 2005

85. Pelliccioni G, Scarpino O: External anal sphincter responses after S3 spinal root surface electrical stimulation. Neurourol Urodyn, 25:788, 2006

86. Brostrom S, Jennum P, Lose G: Motor evoked potentials from the striated urethral sphincter: a comparison of concentric needle and surface electrodes. Neurourol Urodyn, 22:123, 2003

87. Morren GL, Walter S, Lindehammar H et al: Latency of compound muscle action potentials of the anal sphincter after magnetic sacral stimulation. Muscle Nerve, 24:1232, 2001

88. Jost WH, Schimrigk K: A new method to determine pudendal nerve motor latency and central motor conduction time to the external anal sphincter. Electroencephalogr Clin Neurophysiol, 93:237, 1994

89. Inoue S, Kawaguchi M, Takashi S et al: Intraoperative monitoring of myogenic motor-evoked potentials from the external anal sphincter muscle to transcranial electrical stimulation. Spine, 27:E454, 2002

90. Schmid DM, Curt A, Hauri D et al: Motor evoked potentials (MEP) and evoked pressure curves (EPC) from the urethral compressive musculature (UCM) by functional magnetic stimulation in healthy volunteers and patients with neurogenic incontinence. Neurourol Urodyn, 24:117, 2005

91. Brostrom S, Frederiksen JL, Jennum P et al: Motor evoked potentials from the pelvic floor in patients with multiple sclerosis. J Neurol Neurosurg Psychiatry, 74:498, 2003

92. Di Lazzaro V, Pilato F, Oliviero A et al: Role of motor evoked potentials in diagnosis of cauda equina and lumbosacral cord lesions. Neurology, 63:2266, 2004

93. Bradley WE, Lin JT, Johnson B: Measurement of the conduction velocity of the dorsal nerve of the penis. J Urol, 131:1127, 1984

94. Amarenco G, Kerdraon J: Pudendal nerve terminal sensitive latency: technique and normal values. J Urol, 161:103, 1999

95. Ertekin C, Mungan B: Sacral spinal cord and root potentials evoked by the stimulation of the dorsal nerve of penis and cord conduction delay for the bulbocavernosus reflex. Neurourol Urodyn, 12:9, 1993

96. Huang JC, Deletis V, Vodušek DB et al: Preservation of pudendal afferents in sacral rhizotomies. Neurosurgery, 41:411, 1997

97. Loening-Baucke V, Read NW, Yamada T: Further evaluation of the afferent nervous pathways from the rectum. Am J Physiol, 262:G927, 1992

98. Chan YK, Herkes GK, Badcock C et al: Alterations in cerebral potentials evoked by rectal distension in irritable bowel syndrome. Am J Gastroenterol, 96:2413, 2001

99. Schmid DM, Reitz A, Curt A et al: Urethral evoked sympathetic skin responses and viscerosensory evoked potentials as diagnostic tools to evaluate urogenital autonomic afferent innervation in spinal cord injured patients. J Urol, 171:1156, 2004

100. Wyndaele JJ, Van Eetvelde B, Callens D: Comparison in young healthy volunteers of 3 different parameters of constant current stimulation used to determine sensory thresholds in the lower urinary tract. J Urol, 156:1415, 1996

101. Fitzgerald MP, Koch D, Senka J: Visceral and cutaneous sensory testing in patients with painful bladder syndrome. Neurourol Urodyn, 24:627, 2005

102. Pietrangeli A, Bove L, Innocenti P et al: Neurophysiological evaluation of sexual dysfunction in patients operated for colorectal cancer. Clin Auton Res, 8:353, 1998

103. Lefaucheur JP, Yiou R, Salomon L et al: Assessment of penile small nerve fiber damage after transurethral resection of the prostate by measurement of penile thermal sensation. J Urol, 164:1416, 2000

104. Lefaucheur JP, Yiou R, Colombel M et al: Relationship between penile thermal sensory threshold measurement and electrophysiologic tests to assess neurogenic impotence. Urology, 57:306, 2001

105. Daffertshofer M, Linden D, Syren M et al: Assessment of local sympathetic function in patients with erectile dysfunction. Int J Impot Res, 6:213, 1994

106. Secil Y, Ozdedeli K, Altay B et al: Sympathetic skin response recorded from the genital region in normal and diabetic women. Neurophysiol Clin, 35:11, 2005

107. Ertekin C, Ertekin N, Mutlu S et al: Skin potentials (SP) recorded from the extremities and genital regions in normal and impotent subjects. Acta Neurol Scand, 76:28, 1987

108. Rodic B, Curt A, Dietz V et al: Bladder neck incompetence in patients with spinal cord injury: significance of sympathetic skin response. J Urol, 163:1223, 2000

109. Schmid DM, Curt A, Hauri D et al: Clinical value of combined electrophysiological and urodynamic recordings to assess sexual disorders in spinal cord injured men. Neurourol Urodyn, 22:314, 2003

110. Yilmaz U, Yang CC, Berger RE: Dartos reflex: a sympathetically mediated scrotal reflex. Muscle Nerve, 33:363, 2006

111. Colakoglu Z, Kutluay E, Ertekin C: The nature of spontaneous cavernosal activity. BJU Int, 83:449, 1999

112. Yilmaz U, Soylu A, Ozcan C et al: Clitoral electromyography. J Urol, 167:616, 2002

113. Vardi Y, Gruenwald I, Sprecher E: The role of corpus cavernosum electromyography. Curr Opin Urol, 10:635, 2000

114. Vodušek DB, Ravnik-Oblak M, Oblak C: Pudendal versus limb nerve electrophysiological abnormalities in diabetics with erectile dysfunction. Int J Impot Res, 5:37, 1993

115. Podnar S: Which patients need referral for anal sphincter electromyography? Muscle Nerve, 33:278, 2006

116. Kalita J, Shah S, Kapoor R et al: Bladder dysfunction in acute transverse myelitis: magnetic resonance imaging and neurophysiological and urodynamic correlations. J Neurol Neurosurg Psychiatry, 73:154, 2002

117. Torre M, Planche D, Louis-Borrione C et al: Value of electrophysiological assessment after surgical treatment of spinal dysraphism. J Urol, 168:1759, 2002

118. Snape WJ Jr: Role of colonic motility in guiding therapy in patients with constipation. Dig Dis, 15(Suppl 1):104, 1997

119. Osterberg A, Edebol Eeg-Olofsson K, Graf W: Results of surgical treatment for faecal incontinence. Br J Surg, 87:1546, 2000

120. Podnar S: Cauda equina lesions as a complication of spinal surgery. Eur Spine J, 19:451, 2010

121. Podnar S: Epidemiology of cauda equina and conus medullaris lesions. Muscle Nerve, 35:529, 2007

122. Podnar S: Saddle sensation is preserved in a few patients with cauda equina or conus medullaris lesions. Eur J Neurol, 14:48, 2007

123. Podnar S: Clinical and neurophysiologic testing of the penilo-cavernosus reflex. Neurourol Urodyn, 27:399, 2008

124. Mallet VT, Hosker GL, Smith ARB et al: Pelvic floor damage and childbirth: a neurophysiologic follow-up study. Neurourol Urodyn, 12:357, 1993

125. Feasby TE, Burton SR, Hahn AF: Obstetrical lumbosacral plexus injury. Muscle Nerve, 15:937, 1992

126. Vock P, Mattle H, Studer M et al: Lumbosacral plexus lesions: correlation of clinical signs and computed tomography. J Neurol Neurosurg Psychiatry, 51:72, 1988

127. Amarenco G, Ismael SS, Bayle B et al: Electrophysiological analysis of pudendal neuropathy following traction. Muscle Nerve, 24:116, 2001

128. Libelius R, Johansson F: Quantitative electromyography of the external anal sphincter in Parkinson's disease and multiple system atrophy. Muscle Nerve, 23:1250, 2000

129. Tison F, Arne P, Sourgen C et al: The value of external anal sphincter electromyography for the diagnosis of multiple system atrophy. Mov Disord, 15:1148, 2000

130. Gilad R, Giladi N, Korczyn AD et al: Quantitative anal sphincter EMG in multisystem atrophy and 100 controls. J Neurol Neurosurg Psychiatry, 71:596, 2001

131. Yamamoto T, Sakakibara R, Uchiyama T et al: When is Onuf's nucleus involved in multiple system atrophy? A sphincter electromyography study. J Neurol Neurosurg Psychiatry, 76:1645, 2005

132. Paviour DC, Williams D, Fowler CJ et al: Is sphincter electromyography a helpful investigation in the diagnosis of multiple system atrophy? A retrospective study with pathological diagnosis. Mov Disord, 20:1425, 2005

133. Schwarz J, Kornhuber M, Bischoff C et al: Electromyography of the external anal sphincter in patients with Parkinson's disease and multiple system atrophy: frequency of abnormal spontaneous activity and polyphasic motor unit potentials. Muscle Nerve, 20:1167, 1997

134. Giladi N, Simon ES, Korczyn AD et al: Anal sphincter EMG does not distinguish between multiple system atrophy and Parkinson's disease. Muscle Nerve, 23:731, 2000

135. Valldeoriola F, Valls-Sole J, Tolosa ES et al: Striated anal sphincter denervation in patients with progressive supranuclear palsy. Mov Disord, 10:550, 1995

136. Winge K, Jennum P, Lokkegaard A et al: Anal sphincter EMG in the diagnosis of parkinsonian syndromes. Acta Neurol Scand, 121:198, 2009

137. Shimizu H, Yamada M, Toyoshima Y et al: Involvement of Onuf's nucleus in Machado–Joseph disease: a morphometric and immunohistochemical study. Acta Neuropathol (Berl), 120:439, 2010

138. Scaravilli T, Pramstaller PP, Salerno A et al: Neuronal loss in Onuf's nucleus in three patients with progressive supranuclear palsy. Ann Neurol, 48:97, 2000

139. Sakakibara R, Hattori T, Uchiyama T et al: Urinary dysfunction and orthostatic hypotension in multiple system atrophy: which is the more common and earlier manifestation? J Neurol Neurosurg Psychiatry, 68:25, 2000

140. De Ridder D, Ost D, Bruyninckx F: The presence of Fowler's syndrome predicts successful long-term outcome of sacral nerve stimulation in women with urinary retention. Eur Urol, 51:229, 2007

141. Fowler CJ, Christmas TJ, Chapple CR et al: Abnormal electromyographic activity of the urethral sphincter, voiding dysfunction, and polycystic ovaries: a new syndrome? Br Med J, 297:1436, 1988

142. Amarenco G, Raibaut P, Ismael SS et al: Evidence of occult dysautonomia in Fowler's syndrome: alteration of cardiovascular autonomic function tests in female patients presenting with urinary retention. BJU Int, 97:288, 2006

143. Sau G, Siracusano S, Aiello I et al: The usefulness of the somatosensory evoked potentials of the pudendal nerve in diagnosis of probable multiple sclerosis. Spinal Cord, 37:258, 1999

144. South MM, Stinnett SS, Sanders DB et al: Levator ani denervation and reinnervation 6 months after childbirth. Am J Obstet Gynecol, 200:519.e1, 2009

145. Weidner AC, Jamison MG, Branham V et al: Neuropathic injury to the levator ani occurs in 1 in 4 primiparous women. Am J Obstet Gynecol, 195:1851, 2006

146. Weidner AC, South MM, Sanders DB et al: Change in urethral sphincter neuromuscular function during pregnancy persists after delivery. Am J Obstet Gynecol, 201:529.e1, 2009

147. Hale DS, Benson JT, Brubaker L et al: Histologic analysis of needle biopsy of urethral sphincter from women with normal and stress incontinence with comparison of electromyographic findings. Am J Obstet Gynecol, 180:342, 1999

148. Allen RE, Hosker GL, Smith AR et al: Pelvic floor damage and childbirth: a neurophysiological study. Br J Obstet Gynaecol, 97:770, 1990

149. Deindl FM, Vodušek DB, Hesse U et al: Pelvic floor activity patterns: comparison of nulliparous continent and parous urinary stress incontinent women. A kinesiological EMG study. Br J Urol, 73:413, 1994

150. Lacima G, Pera M, Valls-Solé J et al: Electrophysiologic studies and clinical findings in females with combined fecal and urinary incontinence: a prospective study. Dis Colon Rectum, 49:353, 2006

151. Aanestad O, Flink R: Interference pattern in perineal muscles. A quantitative electromyographic study in patients with faecal incontinence. Eur J Surg, 160:111, 1994

152. Enck P, von Giesen HJ, Schafer A et al: Comparison of anal sonography with conventional needle electromyography in the evaluation of anal sphincter defects. Am J Gastroenterol, 91:2539, 1996

153. Fink RL, Roberts LJ, Scott M: The role of manometry, electromyography and radiology in the assessment of intractable constipation. Aust N Z J Surg, 62:959, 1992

154. Vaccaro CA, Cheong DM, Wexner SD et al: Pudendal neuropathy in evacuatory disorders. Dis Colon Rectum, 38:166, 1995

155. Yang CC, Bowen JR, Kraft GH: Cortical evoked potentials of the dorsal nerve of the clitoris and female sexual dysfunction in multiple sclerosis. J Urol, 164:2010, 2000

156. Tas I, Yagiz On A, Altay B et al: Electrophysiological assessment of sexual dysfunction in spinal cord injured patients. Spinal Cord, 45:298, 2007

157. Lundberg PO, Brackett NL, Denys P et al: Neurological disorders: erectile and ejaculatory dysfunction. p. 593. In Jardin A, Wagner G, Khoury S et al, (eds): Erectile Dysfunction. Health Publication, Plymouth (UK), 2000

158. Light JK, Beric A, Wise PG: Predictive criteria for failed sphincterotomy in spinal cord injury patients. J Urol, 138:1201, 1987

159. Pouratian N, Elias WJ, Jane JA et al: Electrophysiologically guided untethering of secondary tethered spinal cord syndrome. Neurosurg Focus, 29:E3, 2010

160. Quinones-Hinojosa A, Gadkary CA, Gulati M et al: Neurophysiological monitoring for safe surgical tethered cord syndrome release in adults. Surg Neurol, 62:127, 2004

161. Haghighi SS, Agrawal S: Cortical localization of external urethral sphincter activation by transcranial electrical stimulation. Electromyogr Clin Neurophysiol, 46:343, 2006

162. Haghighi SS, Zhang R: Activation of the external anal and urethral sphincter muscles by repetitive transcranial cortical stimulation during spine surgery. J Clin Monit Comput, 18:1, 2004

163. Schurch B, Reilly I, Reitz A et al: Electrophysiological recordings during the peripheral nerve evaluation (PNE) test in complete spinal cord injury patients. World J Urol, 20:319, 2003

164. Sheldon R, Kiff ES, Clarke A et al: Sacral nerve stimulation reduces corticoanal excitability in patients with faecal incontinence. Br J Surg, 92:1423, 2005

165. Malaguti S, Spinelli M, Giardiello G et al: Neurophysiological evidence may predict the outcome of sacral neuromodulation. J Urol, 170:2323, 2003

166. Spinelli M, Malaguti S, Giardiello G et al: A new minimally invasive procedure for pudendal nerve stimulation to treat neurogenic bladder: description of the method and preliminary data. Neurourol Urodyn, 24:305, 2005

167. Benson JT: Sacral nerve stimulation results may be improved by electrodiagnostic techniques. Int Urogynecol J Pelvic Floor Dysfunct, 11:352, 2000

168. Tsai SJ, Ying TH, Huang YH et al: Transperineal injection of botulinum toxin A for treatment of detrusor sphincter dyssynergia: localization with combined fluoroscopic and electromyographic guidance. Arch Phys Med Rehabil, 90:832, 2009

Tests of Vestibular Function

Vestibular Laboratory Testing

JOSEPH M. FURMAN and FLORIS L. WUYTS

The purpose of vestibular laboratory testing is to assess the peripheral and central vestibular system in patients with suspected labyrinthine dysfunction. Such information can be used to help establish a diagnosis and develop a treatment plan. Vestibular laboratory testing sometimes provides lateralizing information (i.e., information regarding whether the lesion is on the left or the right). It also can help to assess the status of central nervous system (CNS) compensation for a unilateral peripheral vestibular loss.

The majority of the involved laboratory techniques focus on the assessment of the horizontal vestibulo-ocular reflex (VOR). Newer technologies such as vestibular evoked myogenic potentials, galvanic vestibular stimulation, and off-axis rotation (unilateral centrifugation) may allow a more thorough assessment of the vestibular system. This chapter focuses on how and why the VOR is assessed in the vestibular laboratory. Additionally, computerized dynamic posturography and newer technologies are discussed that assess other aspects of vestibular function. The clinical application of vestibular laboratory testing is also considered in selected disorders. Figure 32-1 provides an overview of those portions of

the vestibular labyrinth that are assessed by the various tests discussed in this chapter.

INDICATIONS FOR VESTIBULAR TESTING

Table 32-1 lists the uses of vestibular laboratory testing. A specialist with a high level of suspicion that a vestibular disorder is present typically requests evaluation in the laboratory. Such testing can aid in determining whether a vestibular system abnormality is present, whether the problem can be localized to the central or peripheral vestibular system, whether the problem can be lateralized to the left or right side, and whether a peripheral abnormality can be localized to the semicircular canals or otolith organs. Vestibular testing provides quantitative information useful for documenting the presence of an abnormality only suspected by bedside evaluation. Moreover, vestibular laboratory testing can provide information that may be useful in deciding about treatment with balance rehabilitation. Occasionally, by repeating some of the tests, vestibular laboratory testing is helpful in the long-term management of patients.

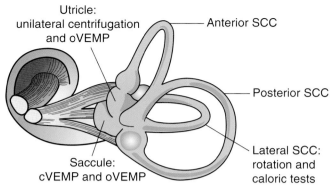

FIGURE 32-1 ■ Diagram of the vestibular labyrinth showing the three semicircular canals (SCCs; i.e., the anterior, posterior, and lateral or horizontal SCCs) and the two otolith organs (the utricle and the saccule). The lateral SCC can be assessed using rotational and caloric tests. The utricle can be assessed using unilateral centrifugation. The saccule can be assessed using vestibular evoked myogenic potentials. oVEMPs, ocular vestibular evoked myogenic potentials; cVEMPs, cervical vestibular evoked myogenic potentials.

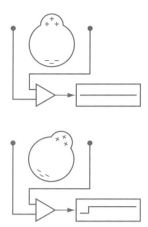

FIGURE 32-2 ■ The corneo-retinal dipole potential has a magnitude of approximately 1 μV, with the cornea being positive with respect to the retina. The filled circles represent the electrodes. A rightward deviation of the eye makes the right electrode more positive, resulting, by convention, in an upward deflection on the recording.

TECHNIQUES FOR RECORDING EYE MOVEMENTS

Electro-Oculography

Electro-oculography (EOG), also called electronystagmography (ENG), is based on the corneo-retinal dipole potential of the eyeball (Fig. 32-2). This potential is thought to result from the metabolic activity of the retina. When the eye rotates in the orbit, the dipole also rotates. Silver–silver chloride electrodes placed near the orbit can be used to record this dipole and, thus, eye position. The combined movement of both eyes can be recorded with one pair of electrodes placed bitemporally. The movement of each eye can be recorded separately (Fig. 32-3) by placing electrodes to the left and right of each eye. A reference electrode typically is placed on the forehead. The electrodes should not be placed too

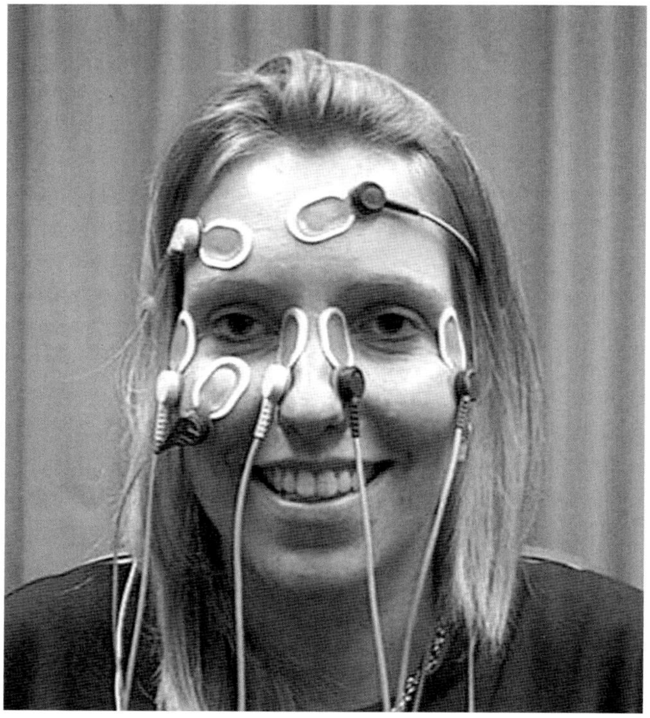

TABLE 32-1 ■ Uses of Vestibular Laboratory Testing
Aids in diagnosis
Localization: central versus peripheral localization
Lateralization
Semicircular canal vs. otolith organ
Documentation of an abnormality suspected by bedside evaluation
Aids in devising a treatment plan
Aids in long-term management

From Baloh RW, Halmagyi GM (eds): Disorders of the Vestibular System. Oxford University Press, New York, 1996, with permission.

FIGURE 32-3 ■ Placement of electrodes for horizontal and vertical electro-oculographic eye-movement recording. For horizontal recordings, each eye is recorded separately. The two horizontal signals can be summed by the recording equipment to enhance the signal-to-noise ratio. The forehead electrode serves as a common ground electrode. The vertical electrodes typically are used for vertical eye-movement detection and artifact identification.

close to the lateral canthi because this sometimes causes frequent blinking and thereby increases artifacts.

Before the application of the electrodes, the skin is cleansed and prepared thoroughly so as to reduce its impedance to less than 25k ohms. Electrode impedance should not vary from one electrode to another by more than 10k ohms. The electrical signal from the electrodes is amplified using direct-current (DC) rather than alternating-current (AC) coupling because this type of recording provides a more reliable measurement of eye position, especially during visual fixation. For vertical eye-movement recording, electrodes are placed above and below one eye. The signal from vertically placed electrodes is useful, but eyelid movement, muscular activity near the eyebrow, and eye blinks cause artifacts that interfere with the reliability of the recording. Frequent eye blinks can also interfere with horizontal recordings and render the horizontal EOG recording uninterpretable (Fig. 32-4).

The corneo-retinal dipole potential fluctuates during laboratory assessment, especially with changes in ambient luminance (Fig. 32-5). Thus, before the test begins,

the patient is kept in a semidarkened room for at least 5 minutes so that the eyes can adapt to the near-darkness. Even with this precaution, the variability in the corneo-retinal dipole potential makes it imperative that calibrations of the EOG signal are performed repeatedly throughout the assessment. Calibration of the EOG signal is performed by asking the patient to look at visual targets placed at 10 degrees to the left and right of center. Most ENG systems use computer-based analysis techniques. Laboratories should adhere to a standardized method of stimulus presentation (e.g., as proposed in the American National Standards Institute [ANSI] protocols). Additionally, the interpretation of eye-movement data should never rely solely on a computer output; rather, an experienced individual should inspect the eye-movement recordings independently.

Video-Oculography

Video-oculography (VOG) is replacing EOG as the eye-movement recording system of choice. The main component of a VOG system, also sometimes called

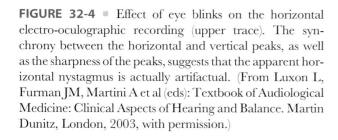

FIGURE 32-4 ▪ Effect of eye blinks on the horizontal electro-oculographic recording (upper trace). The synchrony between the horizontal and vertical peaks, as well as the sharpness of the peaks, suggests that the apparent horizontal nystagmus is actually artifactual. (From Luxon L, Furman JM, Martini A et al (eds): Textbook of Audiological Medicine: Clinical Aspects of Hearing and Balance. Martin Dunitz, London, 2003, with permission.)

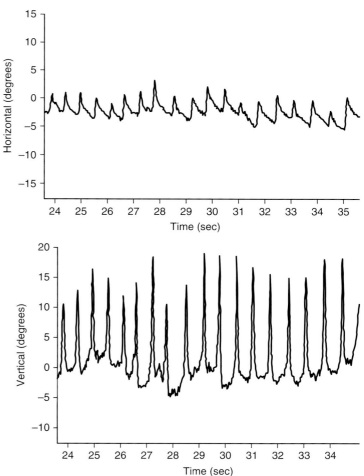

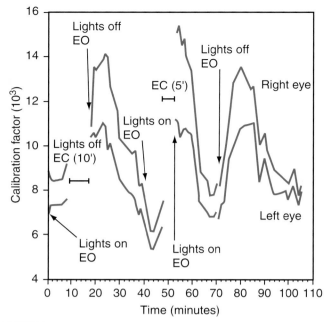

FIGURE 32-5 ▪ Corneo-retinal potential (CRP) variation during 105 minutes of recording in one subject. EO, eyes open; EC, eyes closed. A change in ambient luminance produces a change in the corneo-retinal dipole potential of up to 100 percent. Note that the eyes did not change their CRP equally. (From Luxon L, Furman JM, Martini A et al (eds): Textbook of Audiological Medicine: Clinical Aspects of Hearing and Balance. Martin Dunitz, London, 2003, by permission.)

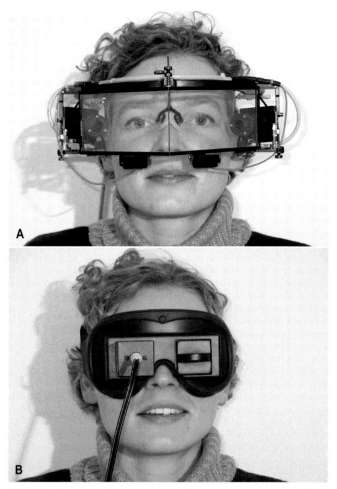

FIGURE 32-6 ▪ Photographs of a patient wearing video-oculography goggles. **A**, See-through system. **B**, Non-see-through system.

video-ENG or VNG, is a small video camera that sends images to a personal computer for image processing. A representative VOG system is illustrated in Figure 32-6. Two-dimensional VOG systems extract horizontal and vertical eye movements from the video images using the pupil; three-dimensional VOG systems additionally extract torsional eye position using iris landmarks. Most VOG systems use infrared light and thus can function in complete darkness. VOG systems may be monocular or binocular. Most commercial VOG systems have a standard frame rate of 50 or 60 Hz, which may limit the accuracy of VOG for some ocular motor testing (e.g., assessment of saccades). Some manufacturers offer a higher frame-rate system, but these are considerably more expensive. Two-dimensional VOG, because of its reliable vertical as well as horizontal eye-movement detection, has an advantage over conventional EOG. With VOG, it is essential that the goggles are attached firmly to the patient's head because any relative movement of the goggles with respect to the head will result in an artifactual change in eye position during the

recording. Table 32-2 compares the properties of EOG (or ENG), two-dimensional VOG, and three-dimensional VOG systems.

Scleral Search Coil

The scleral search coil method is based on the recording of small electric currents induced by a magnetic field in a coil of very narrow-gauge wire embedded in a pliable donut-shaped plastic ring that is placed on the eye (Fig. 32-7).[1] The scleral search coil method has emerged as the "gold standard" for the accurate recording of eye movements; however, it is an invasive technique that may cause discomfort for the patient. Also, recording time is limited to approximately 30 minutes. The scleral search coil technique generally is confined to research purposes.

TABLE 32-2 ■ Comparison Between Electronystagmography and Video-Oculography

Characteristics	Electronystagmography	Two-Dimensional Video-Oculography	Three-Dimensional Video-Oculography
Recording device	Paste-on electrodes (AgCl–Ag)	Video camera	Video camera
Principle	Corneo-retinal dipole potential	Image processing	Image processing
Contrast enhancement of pupil	Pupil and iris structure analysis	Cross-correlation or neural network	
Horizontal eye movement	Reliable	Very reliable	Very reliable
Vertical eye movement	Unreliable	Very reliable	Very reliable
Torsional eye movement	Not possible	Not possible	Reliable
Approximate accuracy	1–2 degrees	1–2 degrees	1 degree
Head movement resistance	High	If properly secured	If properly secured
Sampling rate	> 150 Hz	25–60 Hz	25–60 Hz
Iris structure dependence	None	No	Yes
Amplifier drift	Yes	No	No
Calibration	Repeatedly	Once	Once
Sensitive to			
Blink artifacts	Yes	Yes	Yes
Changes in room lighting	Yes	No	No
Myogenic activity	Yes	No	No
Vestibular stimuli possible	Yes	Yes	Yes
Functions in total darkness	Yes	Yes	Yes
Patient tolerance	About 1 hour	About ½ hour	About ½ hour

From Luxon L, Furman JM, Martini A et al (eds): Textbook of Audiological Medicine: Clinical Aspects of Hearing and Balance. Martin Dunitz, London, 2003, with permission.

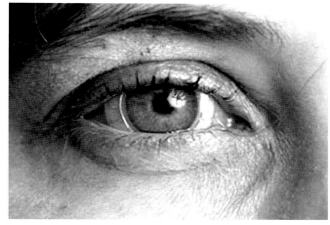

FIGURE 32-7 ■ A scleral coil placed on the right eye. Note the fine wire running from the coil across the bridge of the nose.

Choice of Eye-Movement Recording Technique

EOG has, for many decades, been the standard eye-movement measurement technique. It is a safe, convenient, and efficient means of recording eye position in persons of all ages. The primary limitation of EOG is its inability to provide consistently reliable vertical eye-movement recording. Also, eye blinks produce problematic artifacts, and fluctuations in the corneo-retinal dipole potential can reduce the accuracy of the technique. VOG will replace EOG eventually as the method of choice for recording eye movements during vestibular laboratory testing. It has the advantage of allowing both horizontal and vertical eye-movement recording. As with EOG, eye blink artifacts can be problematic during VOG recordings. Also, relative movement between the VOG goggles and head can produce artifacts.

Definition of Nystagmus

By convention, the eye position that is displayed on a computer screen or chart recorder represents rightward eye movement by an upward deflection and leftward eye movement by a downward deflection. Torsional eye movements should be described from the patient's viewpoint (i.e., movement of the upper pole of the eye toward the right ear should be displayed as an upward deflection). A slow eye movement followed by a fast movement in the opposite direction is called jerk nystagmus; by convention, this is named after its fast component. Nystagmus is analyzed by computing the slow component velocity (SCV) because the slow movement reflects that portion of the nystagmus generated by the VOR, whereas the fast component is merely a saccadic reset movement (Fig. 32-8).

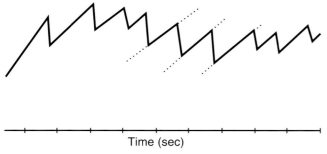

FIGURE 32-8 ■ Nystagmus analysis. Note the slow and quick components of nystagmus illustrated from an electronystagmography (ENG) recording. The three oblique dashed lines indicate the slope of the slow components (i.e., the slow-component velocities). Computerized ENG has automatic algorithms for nystagmus analysis.

VESTIBULAR LABORATORY TESTING

Reducing Visual Fixation

When testing requires the absence of visual input, two different methods can be used: (1) eyes opened in darkness or (2) eyes closed in a semi-darkened room. The former method is recommended by ANSI because it produces more reliable and reproducible results. Also, closing the eye induces the Bell phenomenon, which may interfere with nystagmus production. Testing with eyes opened in darkness may lead to excessive eye blinking; this sometimes produces artifacts that should not be confused with eye movement (see Fig. 32-4). Regardless of the mechanism used to remove visual input, patients should be kept alert because drowsiness reduces the consistency of the VOR. Alerting is often accomplished by asking patients to perform simple mental tasks.

Ocular Motor Screening Battery

The purpose of the ocular motor screening battery is to uncover eye-movement abnormalities that may interfere with the interpretation of the positional, caloric, or rotational tests. Furthermore, the ocular motor screening battery can provide some information concerning CNS abnormalities and, in particular, can provide information regarding CNS function that relates to balance. The ocular motor screening battery consists of several tests, including an assessment of spontaneous nystagmus, gaze-evoked nystagmus, saccadic eye movements, pursuit eye movements, and optokinetic nystagmus.

The term *spontaneous nystagmus* sometimes denotes a nystagmus that occurs during visual fixation; at other times it denotes nystagmus that occurs only with loss of visual fixation. The term *spontaneous vestibular nystagmus* should be used to describe nystagmus that is of significantly greater magnitude when visual fixation is lost (Fig. 32-9) and is thus likely to be of vestibular origin. Spontaneous nystagmus should be used for nystagmus seen with visual fixation. Thus, the search for spontaneous vestibular nystagmus should be performed with the patient in darkness. To maintain alertness, the patient should be asked to perform simple mental tasks such as counting backward by threes. To confirm the presence and direction of a spontaneous nystagmus, the patient is asked to look left and right while in darkness. The nystagmus should change its magnitude according to Alexander's law (i.e., it should increase when the patient looks in the direction of the fast component). Normal individuals may have spontaneous nystagmus, but the SCV of this nystagmus should not exceed about 4 deg/sec. Also, a clinically significant spontaneous nystagmus should be observed consistently during testing; a few isolated beats of nystagmus should not be considered abnormal. Spontaneous vestibular nystagmus is typically

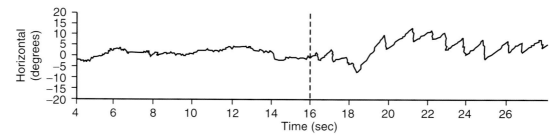

FIGURE 32-9 ■ Example of spontaneous vestibular nystagmus seen only with loss of fixation. Note that the right side of the figure illustrates left-beating nystagmus recorded with the patient's eyes open in the dark. At timing marker 16 seconds, the patient was asked to close the eyes. Before then, the patient was looking at a fixation target.

horizontal-torsional. As a result, both EOG and two-dimensional VOG will record only the horizontal component of this nystagmus. Spontaneous nystagmus may be either pendular (i.e., having no clearly defined fast and slow components) or jerk (i.e., with clearly defined fast and slow components). Pendular nystagmus may be congenital or acquired. Spontaneous jerk nystagmus most commonly occurs as the result of an acute vestibular lesion. In this case, the spontaneous vestibular nystagmus usually beats away from the impaired labyrinth. For example, an acute right-sided peripheral vestibular lesion usually will be associated with a left-beating spontaneous vestibular nystagmus. Vertical nystagmus seen during ocular motor screening suggests a central abnormality. Different facilities have different criteria to define the limits of normality during ocular motor screening, as is discussed later.

To search for gaze-evoked nystagmus, the patient should be asked to look at visual targets directly in front of him or her and at 30 degrees left and right and 15 degrees up and down. The most common type of gaze-evoked nystagmus is bidirectional, as illustrated in Figure 32-10. Gaze-evoked nystagmus is considered a result of an abnormal "ocular motor integrator." Gaze-evoked nystagmus typically is seen with both leftward and rightward gaze and may be seen with upgaze as well. By definition, the fast component of gaze-evoked nystagmus is always in the direction of gaze. Because of Alexander's law, a spontaneous vestibular nystagmus may be evident only with gaze deviation. For example, a patient with a right-sided peripheral vestibular lesion may demonstrate a left-beating nystagmus only with gaze to the left.

Saccadic eye movements (i.e., rapid eye movements) are tested by asking the patient to look at small visual targets that move abruptly to the left or right at random times, in random directions, and for random distances. Saccadic eye movement typically is recorded monocularly from each eye to uncover abnormalities in voluntary gaze, limitations of gaze, and dysconjugacies. Eye position is used to evaluate the latency, accuracy, and velocity of saccades. Normal values for peak velocity and latency of saccades differ in different laboratories (Table 32-3), as is discussed later. The presence of abnormal saccadic eye movements usually suggests a CNS abnormality, assuming that vision is normal.

To assess smooth pursuit, the patient should be asked to follow a visual target moving slowly horizontally. The total excursion of the visual target should be restricted to 30 degrees. Figure 32-11 illustrates asymmetric smooth pursuit while a patient follows a target moving horizontally in a sinusoidal pattern. This type of abnormality suggests a CNS problem. Table 32-3 provides normal values for smooth pursuit gain.

Optokinetic nystagmus is elicited by asking the patient to look at a large visual moving stimulus such as full-field vertical stripes. When the stripes are moved at a constant velocity, the patient should experience circular vection (i.e., an illusory sense of motion of self rather than of the surrounding world). Both clockwise and counterclockwise optokinetic stimuli should be presented. Eye position during optokinetic nystagmus is analyzed by computing the magnitude of the SCV and relating this magnitude to the stimulus velocity. The amount of left–right asymmetry of optokinetic nystagmus should also be computed. Optokinetic nystagmus provides information that is largely redundant because of that provided by ocular pursuit testing. Table 32-3 provides normative data for optokinetic nystagmus.

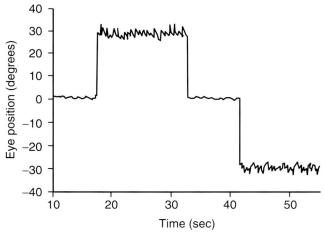

FIGURE 32-10 ■ Gaze-evoked nystagmus. There is right-beating nystagmus on rightward gaze and left-beating nystagmus on leftward gaze, with an absence of nystagmus when looking straight ahead. (From Luxon L, Furman JM, Martini A et al (eds): Textbook of Audiological Medicine: Clinical Aspects of Hearing and Balance. Martin Dunitz, London, 2003, with permission.)

Positional and Positioning Testing

Positional testing is performed by placing the patient in one of the head lateral positions including the supine, supine-head right, supine-head left, right lateral, and left lateral positions (Fig. 32-12). The nystagmus elicited during positional testing may be direction-fixed or direction-changing. If direction-changing, the nystagmus may be either ageotropic (i.e., beating away from the earth) or geotropic (i.e., beating toward the earth).

Table 32-3 ■ Normative Data					
Test Items	**Normative Limits***	**Reference No.**	**Test Items**	**Normative Limits***	**Reference No.**
Spontaneous nystagmus is	> 4 deg/sec	3, 4	0.05 Hz, 50 deg/sec	0.24–0.85	13
abnormal if slow component	> 5 deg/sec	5, 6	0.05 Hz, 60 deg/sec	0.38–0.98	19
velocity is	> 6 deg/sec	7, 8	Phase		
	> 7 deg/sec	2, 9, 10	0.05 Hz, 60 deg/sec	6–14 deg	20
	> 6 beats/10 sec	5	0.05 Hz, 60 deg/sec	2–20 deg	21
Ocular motor testing			0.05 Hz, 50 deg/sec	−1–18 deg	13
Saccades			0.05 Hz, 50 deg/sec	−1.9–24 deg	22
Lower limit of peak velocity for	210 deg/sec	6, 11	0.05 Hz, 60 deg/sec	0.8–20.2	19
20-deg saccade	252 deg/sec	12	Directional preponderance		
	283 deg/sec	13	0.05 Hz, 60 deg/sec	> 15 %	19
Latency for 20-deg saccade	104–365 msec	14	0.05 Hz, 50 deg/sec	> 24 %	13
	128–255 msec	13	Velocity step testing at 90 deg/sec		
Smooth pursuit gain at 0.3 Hz	> 0.80	3, 4, 15	Gain	0.33–0.72	23
Optokinetic nystagmus asymmetry	< 13 %	13	Time constant	11–26 sec	23
	< 16 %	3	Directional preponderance	> 22 %	23
Positional testing	< 6 deg/sec	7	Velocity step testing at 100 deg/sec		
Caloric testing			Gain	0.27–0.99	3
Reduced vestibular response	> 25 %	7	Time constant	5–19.4 sec	3
	> 20 %	5	Cervical vestibular evoked myogenic		
	> 19 %	13	potentials		
	> 15 %	16	Interaural ratio	< 36%	24
	> 22 %	3, 17		< 32%	25
	> 20 %	9		< 35%	26
	> 20 %	18		< 52%	27
	> 25 %	19	Threshold	69–92 dB nHL	24
General reduced vestibular	> 22 %			68–108 dB nHL	28
response limit				65–89 dB nHL	25
Directional preponderance	> 23 %	7		58–93 dB nHL	26
	> 23 %	5	Latency		
	> 16 %	13	p13	< 18.4 msec	24
	> 18 %	16		< 15.4 msec	28
	> 28 %	3, 17		< 17.8 msec	25
	> 26 %	9		< 17.9 msec	26
	> 27 %	18		< 18.2 msec	27
	> 32 %	19	n23	< 28.1 msec	24
General directional preponderance limit	> 26 %	Meta-analysis		< 23.1 msec	28
Rotational chair test				< 26.8 msec	25
Sinusoidal testing				< 28.1 msec	26
Gain				< 25.4 msec	27
0.05 Hz, 60 deg/sec	0.20–0.80	20			
0.05 Hz, 60 deg/sec	0.13–0.77	21			

*Mean ± 2 standard deviations.

An example of positional nystagmus is shown in Figure 32-12. Persistent positional nystagmus is considered a nonspecific, nonlocalizing abnormality that can be caused by a central or peripheral vestibular abnormality. However, persistent ageotropic horizontal positional nystagmus, especially one of high magnitude, may suggest horizontal semicircular canal cupulolithiasis. Paroxysmal rather than persistent geotropic positional nystagmus seen in the ear-down positions (i.e., paroxysmal left-beating in the head left and left lateral positions

and paroxysmal right-beating in the head right and right lateral positions) suggests horizontal semicircular canal canalithiasis.

Positioning nystagmus refers to paroxysmal nystagmus that occurs after the patient is moved rapidly into an ear-down position using the Dix–Hallpike maneuver, which is illustrated in Figure 32-13. The most common form of positioning nystagmus is that associated with benign paroxysmal positional vertigo (BPPV) as a result of movement of free-floating debris in the

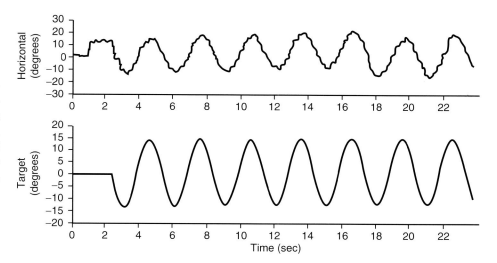

FIGURE 32-11 ▪ Example of asymmetric smooth pursuit eye movements. The lower trace illustrates the position of a small LED target. The upper trace illustrates horizontal eye position and indicates difficulty with pursuit of the target, more so when it is moving to the right.

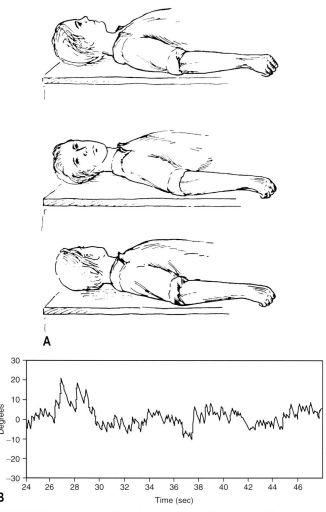

FIGURE 32-12 ▪ **A**, Positional testing illustrating (from top): the supine, head-right and head-left positions. **B**, Electronystagmographic recording of a persistent right-beating positional nystagmus. (**A** From Baloh RW: Dizziness, Hearing Loss, and Tinnitus: The Essentials of Neurotology. FA Davis, Philadelphia, 1984, by permission.)

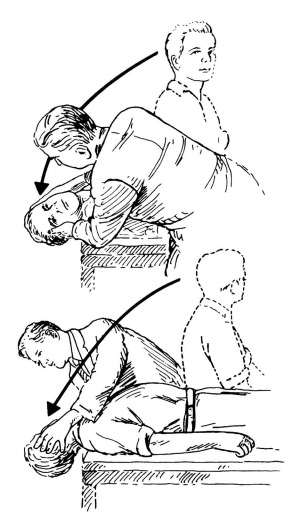

FIGURE 32-13 ▪ The Dix–Hallpike maneuver shown for the right (upper panel) and left (lower panel) ear. (From Baloh RW: Dizziness, Hearing Loss, and Tinnitus: The Essentials of Neurotology. FA Davis, Philadelphia, 1984, with permission.)

posterior semicircular canal. The nystagmus is predominantly torsional with a small upbeating component. Thus, only with three-dimensional VOG is this type of nystagmus recorded adequately; when using EOG or two-dimensional VOG, reliable information is not obtained.

Caloric Testing

Despite its numerous disadvantages, the caloric test remains the most established test that can provide lateralizing information about a peripheral vestibular lesion. In particular, caloric testing has low sensitivity and specificity, and assesses only the function of the horizontal semicircular canal. The patient is placed supine with the head tilted up by 30 degrees. In this way, the horizontal semicircular canal is oriented in a vertical plane. After careful inspection of the external auditory canals to exclude a perforated tympanic membrane or other adverse conditions (e.g., impacted cerumen), the external auditory canal is warmed or cooled with water or air sequentially for 30 to 40 seconds. A thermal gradient across the horizontal semicircular canal thus develops and produces a convection current within the endolymph (Fig. 32-14). The warm stimulus induces utriculopetal endolymph flow, which corresponds to

an excitation of the horizontal semicircular canal and results in a nystagmus that beats toward the stimulated ear. The cool stimulus induces utriclofugal endolymph flow, which corresponds to an inhibition of the horizontal semicircular canal and results in nystagmus that beats away from the stimulated ear. Although thermal convection accounts for the majority of the caloric response, direct thermal stimulation of the vestibular labyrinth and neural elements appears to account for some of the response. During caloric testing, patients may feel vertiginous. It is very important that patients be informed about this physiologically normal response in an effort to minimize anxiety.

The order in which the four caloric irrigations are performed is not standardized, but the Dutch Vestibular Society suggests that they be delivered in the following order: warm right, warm left, cold right, and finally cold left.[2] The patient should be kept alert using mental tasks. When water is used, a typical stimulus consists of a 30- to 40-second irrigation with water of 30 degrees C and 44 degrees C using a flow rate of 350 ± 30 ml per minute. Following each irrigation, at least 5 minutes are needed to allow temperature stabilization of the labyrinth. To analyze the eye movement induced by caloric stimulation, a computer calculates the maximum slow component velocity during the eye movement response for each stimulus. This usually is accomplished by computing the average slow component velocity during about 5 to 10 seconds around the time of the peak eye velocity response (Figs. 32-15 and 32-16). If the magnitude of the response to one of the four caloric responses is not in agreement with the responses to the other three, this irrigation should be repeated. Reduced vestibular response (RVR), also sometimes known as labyrinthine asymmetry, and directional preponderance (DP) are calculated using Jongkees' formula:

$$RVR = \frac{(\text{right-cold} + \text{right-warm}) - (\text{left-cold} + \text{left-warm})}{(\text{left-cold} + \text{right-cold} + \text{left-warm} + \text{right-warm})}$$

$$DP = \frac{(\text{left-cold} + \text{right-warm}) - (\text{right-cold} + \text{left-warm})}{(\text{left-cold} + \text{right-cold} + \text{left-warm} + \text{right-warm})}$$

Table 32-3 provides a list of normal limits for RVR and DP from several laboratories. The authors prefer values of 25 percent or greater for RVR and 30 percent or greater for DP.

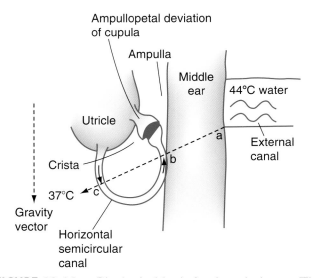

FIGURE 32-14 ■ Biophysical basis for the caloric test. The thermal gradient (along the a–b–c line) across the semicircular canal produces a convection current, deflecting the cupula. For illustrative purposes, the cupular deflection is exaggerated because it deflects only 1.5 to 2.6 μm for cold (10°C) water irrigation. (From Baloh RW, Honrubia V: Clinical Neurophysiology of the Vestibular System. 2nd Ed. FA Davis, Philadelphia, 1990, with permission.)

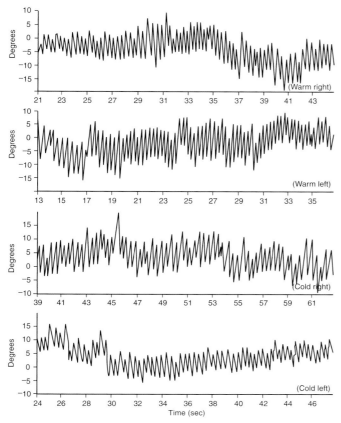

FIGURE 32-15 ▪ Caloric responses in a normal individual. Unprocessed eye-movement response.

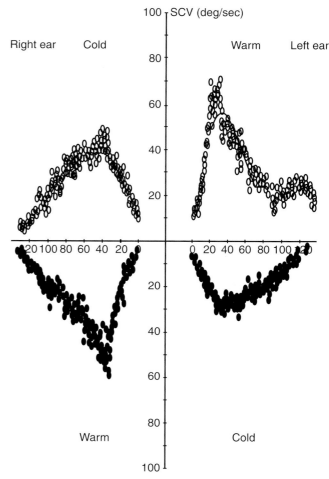

FIGURE 32-16 ▪ Caloric responses in a normal individual (same subject as in Fig. 32-5). Slow component velocity (SCV) shown for each of four irrigations in a "butterfly plot." Note that the time axis runs from the center in both directions and that responses above the horizontal axis denote left-beating nystagmus and responses below the horizontal axis denote right-beating nystagmus.

A unilateral RVR (Figs. 32-17 and 32-18) indicates a unilateral peripheral vestibular ailment. However, abnormalities on caloric testing can result from an abnormality in the vestibular labyrinth itself, in the vestibular nerve, or in the vestibular nucleus in the brainstem. When there is no consistent response from an ear with caloric testing, ice water irrigation should be performed, if possible. A patient's response to ice water irrigation should be recorded with the patient both supine and prone to assure that the nystagmus reverses direction and is thus a result of labyrinthine stimulation rather than a spontaneous nystagmus activated by stimulation of the external auditory canal. Bilaterally reduced responses to caloric testing suggest bilateral vestibular loss. However, patients with absent caloric responses, including patients with absent responses to ice water caloric irrigation, often have preserved rotational responses, especially at higher rotational frequencies. Thus, a diagnosis of bilateral vestibular loss should not be based solely on caloric testing but rather should be corroborated by a finding of reduced gain on rotational testing. A directional preponderance on caloric testing (Figs. 32-19 and 32-20) is a nonspecific abnormality.

Rotational Testing

Rotational testing, which employs the natural stimulus to the labyrinth, is performed in darkness while patients perform mental arithmetic to maintain alertness (Fig. 32-21). Patients are seated in a chair that rotates under computer control. Rotational testing can be categorized according to the vestibular subsystem that it tests; this is determined by the orientation of the axis of rotation with respect to gravity and by the orientation of the patient with respect to the axis of rotation. The most common type of rotational testing uses earth-vertical axis rotation with the patient seated upright. This type of rotation stimulates primarily the horizontal semicircular canals. Earth-vertical axis rotational testing typically is performed using both sinusoidal and constant-velocity

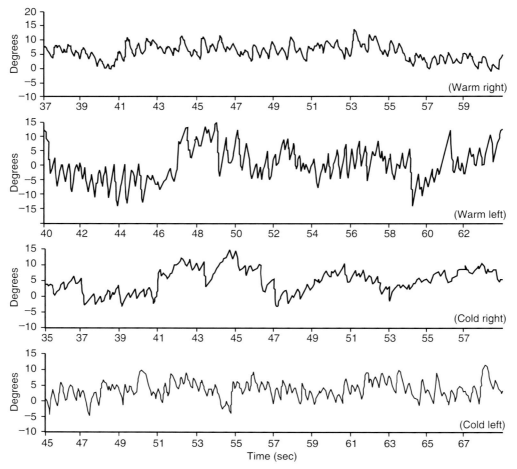

FIGURE 32-17 ■ Example of caloric responses in a patient with a right unilateral reduced vestibular response. Horizontal nystagmus recorded with warm and cold stimulation of the right and left ears. Note the obvious reduction in the magnitude of the response to stimulation of the right ear.

motion, though sinusoidal motion is the most commonly used rotational stimulus. In this test the patient is rotated alternately to the left and right following a sinusoidal pattern. Typical sinusoidal frequencies range from 0.02 Hz to 1.0 Hz with a maximal velocity of 50 to 60 deg/sec. VOR magnitude typically increases with higher rotational frequencies. Thus, at low frequency (e.g., at 0.02 Hz and below) VOR responses may be nearly absent despite normal responses at higher frequencies (e.g., above 0.1 Hz).

Although the VOR works best at frequencies above 0.1 Hz, physical constraints and cost dictate that most earth-vertical axis rotational testing is performed at frequencies of less than 0.1 Hz. Constant-velocity rotation typically is performed using a 60 deg/sec or 90 deg/sec movement in darkness until nystagmus becomes negligible. This decay of the rotational response occurs because the semicircular canals are sensitive to acceleration, which is nil during constant-velocity rotation, except at its onset. Shortly after the nystagmus ceases, the rotation

is stopped abruptly. This results in a deceleration exceeding 100 deg/sec per second and induces a post-rotatory nystagmus that usually decreases exponentially over time. Rotational testing is typically well tolerated.

The relationship between a sinusoidal earth-vertical axis rotational stimulus and the eye-movement response can be described by three parameters: (1) VOR gain (peak eye velocity divided by peak stimulus velocity); (2) VOR phase (the timing relationship between the stimulus and the response); and (3) VOR symmetry, which corresponds to directional preponderance for caloric testing and is a measure of the amount of right-beating versus left-beating nystagmus. When the VOR gain is too small (i.e., below about 0.1), the phase and asymmetry measures should be interpreted cautiously or disregarded entirely because they become unreliable. The exponential rate of decay of nystagmus produced by constant velocity earth-vertical axis rotation is called the VOR time constant and can be related mathematically to the phase of the response to sinusoidal rotation.

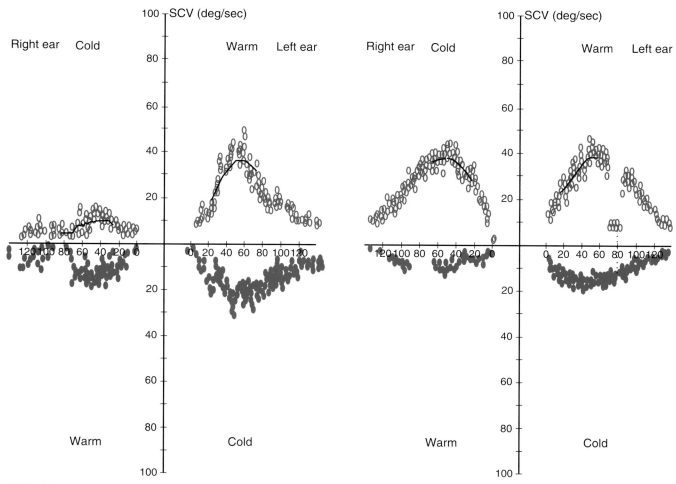

FIGURE 32-18 ■ "Butterfly" plot of the slow component velocity (SCV) response shown in Figure 32-17. Note the marked reduction of responsiveness of the right ear.

FIGURE 32-19 ■ "Butterfly" plots of the responses shown in Figure 32-20. Note the preponderance of the right-cold and left-warm responses as compared to the right-warm and left-cold responses, indicating a left directional preponderance. SCV, slow component velocity.

A small decrease in gain on rotational testing is seen with a significant unilateral reduced vestibular response or a mild bilateral vestibular loss. A large decrease in gain on rotational testing suggests bilateral peripheral vestibular loss. Rarely, VOR gain is increased; this may indicate an impairment of cerebellar function. Increased phase lead and shortened time constant are nonspecific and nonlocalizing VOR abnormalities but often are associated with a unilateral or bilateral peripheral vestibular loss. In patients with unilateral vestibular loss, an asymmetry (i.e., a directional preponderance) on rotational testing suggests incomplete central compensation for the unilaterally reduced vestibular response (Fig. 32-22). Also, a directional preponderance on rotational testing can be seen in patients without evidence for a peripheral vestibular ailment. Such patients include some individuals with migraine-related dizziness and some with anxiety.

There are several other types of rotational testing in addition to earth-vertical axis rotation. Visual–vestibular interaction testing combines rotation with visual stimuli including small fixation targets that rotate with the patient or earth-fixed full-field stripes. In this way, vision can be used either to reduce or to augment the VOR. Visual–vestibular interaction testing is most helpful when evaluating central vestibular abnormalities. Testing usually consists of rotation at a single sinusoidal frequency (e.g., 0.05 Hz) under three conditions: (1) in darkness; (2) with a chair-fixed fixation target; and (3) with earth-fixed full-field stripes. Analysis of the response is similar to that for rotation in darkness and is designed to yield gain and phase. An inability to suppress the VOR during visual–vestibular interaction testing suggests poor vision, poor attention, or a central abnormality and often corresponds with impaired ocular pursuit.

Head-only rotational testing, which has not yet been accepted widely, assesses the VOR at frequencies of 1 Hz and above, where the VOR is the most efficient.[29]

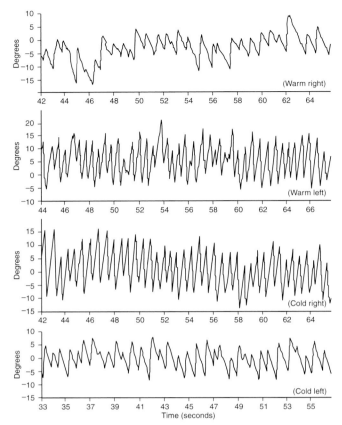

FIGURE 32-20 ■ Example of a directional preponderance in the response to caloric stimulation. Horizontal nystagmus recorded with warm and cold irrigation of the right and left ears. Note the preponderance of left-beating nystagmus as compared with right-beating nystagmus. This is the unprocessed eye-movement response for which the "butterfly" plot is shown in Figure 32-19.

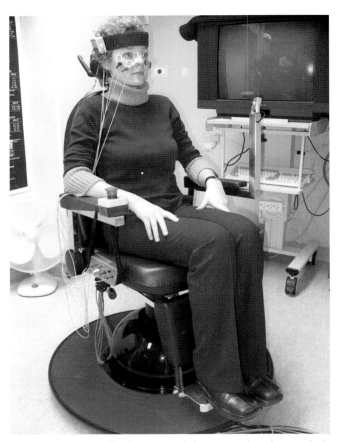

FIGURE 32-21 ■ Patient seated in a rotational test chair. Note the electro-oculography electrodes for recording eye movement and the angular rate sensor on the head.

This type of testing requires the patient's cooperation. Numerous technical issues have limited the number of laboratories that use this technique.

Unilateral Centrifugation

In this test, subjects are rotated about an earth-vertical axis at a velocity that is relatively high (e.g., 300 to 400 deg/sec). After rotating at constant velocity for several seconds, the subject is translated gradually 4 cm to the right and then to the left along an interaural axis, to a position at which one utricle and then the other becomes aligned with the axis of rotation. At these points, one utricle is exposed to the combination of gravity and a centrifugal acceleration of 0.4 g, corresponding to an apparent roll-tilt of 21.7 degrees. The other utricle is exposed only to gravity. In Figure 32-23, the subject is being rotated with the axis of rotation passing through the

left ear. Note that the long earrings indicate the forces. Because the earring on the right ear is deflected considerably, whereas the one on the left ear is nearly vertical, it is the right utricle that is being stimulated. This stimulus induces ocular counter-rolling (i.e., ocular torsion), which is measured using three-dimensional VOG (Fig. 32-24). This test dates from the early 1990s, as described by Wetzig and co-workers[30] and was developed further by others.[31] The amount of ocular counter-rolling is a linear function of the apparent gravito-inertial tilt of the head during the lateral translation.[32] Using this method, utricular sensitivity and the preponderance of the right or left utricle can be assessed separately. This method is much more powerful than the simple lateroflexion test because it allows localization of the side of utricular dysfunction.[33,34]

Cervical Vestibular Evoked Myogenic Potentials

The vestibulocollic reflex can be used to assess saccular function via a cervical vestibular evoked myogenic potential (cVEMP). The stimulus is a loud sound that

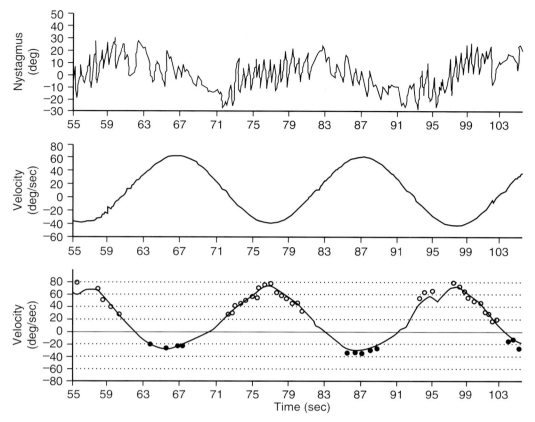

FIGURE 32-22 ■ Example of directional preponderance seen with earth-vertical axis rotational testing. The middle trace illustrates the rotational velocity of the patient in a rotational test chair with a frequency of 0.05 Hz and a peak amplitude of 50 deg/sec. The upper trace illustrates the horizontal nystagmus induced by the rotational stimulus. The lower trace illustrates the slow component velocity of the nystagmus. Note the preponderance of left-beating nystagmus in the upper trace and the concomitant asymmetric slow component velocity shown in the lower trace with a preponderance of rightward slow component velocity.

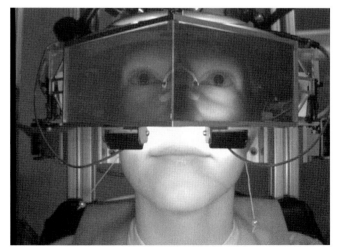

FIGURE 32-23 ■ Patient undergoing unilateral centrifugation. The patient is being rotated at 400 degrees/second with the axis of rotation passing through the left ear. The long earrings indicate the gravito-inertial force. Note that the earring on the right ear is deflected considerably, whereas the earring on the left ear is nearly vertical.

stimulates the saccule. Through the inferior vestibular nerve, the response travels to the vestibular nuclei in the brainstem, from where it projects via the vestibulospinal tract to the motor neurons of the sternocleidomastoid muscle. There, the response modulates the tonically contracted muscle (Fig. 32-25) by means of an inhibitory pulse. Although initially discovered in the 1960s by Bickford and co-workers,[35] it is only since the work of Colebatch and associates[36] that the clinical significance of the cVEMP has been demonstrated. These authors showed that the first two peaks, i.e., p13 and n23, of a cVEMP have a vestibular origin because they are abolished after a vestibular nerve section, and that they do not have a cochlear origin because the response is preserved in subjects with severe hearing loss.[36]

The cVEMP is an ipsilateral reflex, faster than the startle reflex; unlike the startle reflex, it is not fatigable. The ipsilateral inhibitory aspect of the cVEMP may imply

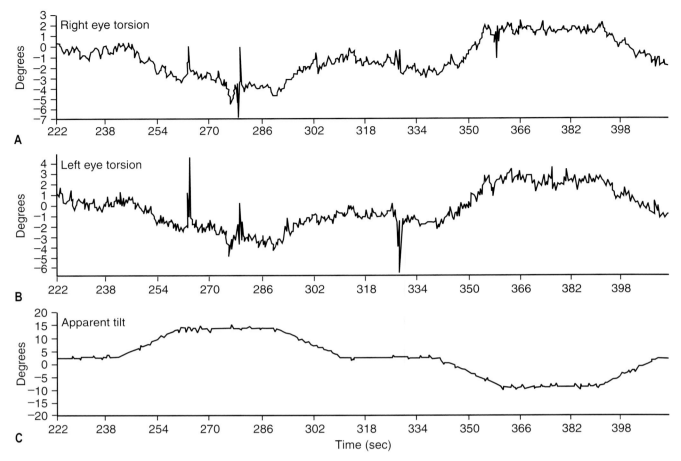

FIGURE 32-24 ■ Ocular torsion during unilateral centrifugation in a normal person. Note that there is conjugate ocular torsion induced by stimulation of the otolith organs. **A**, Right eye torsion. **B**, Left eye torsion. **C**, Apparent tilt measured by an inclinometer placed at the center of the head.

that the reflex redirects the head in the direction of the loud noise.

The equipment necessary to record cVEMPs is standard for evoked potential studies. Surface electrodes typically are placed as follows: the active electrode on the belly of the ipsilateral sternocleidomastoid muscle, the reference electrode on the sternum, and the common ground electrode on the forehead. The cVEMP has a typical biphasic waveform and a latency in the order of 10 to 30 msec (Fig. 32-26). Loud stimuli are necessary to elicit the response. Recording a cVEMP requires approximately 30 seconds per trace because the repetition rate is 5 to 10 Hz; about 250 stimuli are sufficient to record a response. As with other evoked potentials, it is advisable to repeat each recording at least once. Initially, 100-μs clicks at 100 dB HL were used, but more recently, short tone bursts of 500 Hz (100 dB HL, rise/fall-time 1 msec, plateau 2 msec) are used. Tapping the head is also used but is less popular. In that case, the vestibular system on each side is triggered simultaneously.

The amplitude of the cVEMP, measured from the maximum of the p13 peak to the maximum of the n23 peak, is proportional to the contraction state of the sternocleidomastoid muscle; a small contraction produces only a slight cVEMP response. Different methods are used to contract the sternocleidomastoid muscle appropriately. Ideally, the electromyogram of the contracted sternocleidomastoid is monitored throughout the examination, and the rectified mean voltage is used for normalization.[24] The seated subject, for example, is asked to turn the head and push against the hand of the examiner (or against a solid obstacle) in the direction contralateral to the stimulated ear. Alternatively, the subject can be tested supine on a bed while attempting to lift the head and orient it contralaterally to the side of the stimulated ear. This method is relatively demanding for the sternocleidomastoid muscles and can be difficult for older patients.

The cVEMPs have been obtained from patients with vestibular neuritis,[37] Ménière's disease,[38,39] superior

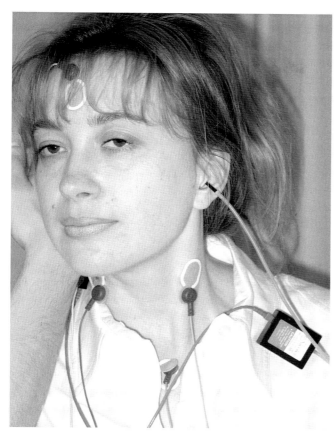

FIGURE 32-25 ▪ A patient undergoing the recording of a cervical vestibular evoked myogenic potential. Note that the auditory stimulus is delivered to the left ear while a surface recording electrode is placed over the contracted left sterno-cleidomastoid muscle.

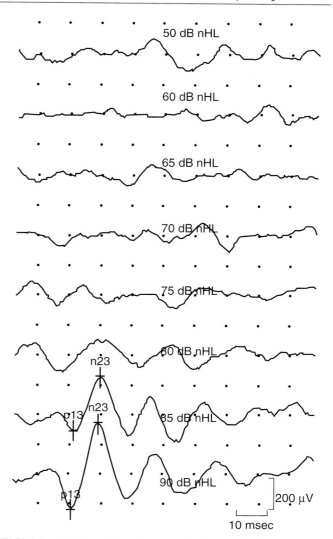

FIGURE 32-26 ▪ Cervical vestibular evoked myogenic potential. From top, the intensities of the auditory stimulus are 50, 60, 65, 70, 75, 80, 85, and 90 dB nHL. Note that only the highest intensities of 85 and 90 dB nHL give rise to a reliable response. The stimulus consisted of 500-Hz tone bursts lasting for 4 msec.

canal dehiscence,[40,41] and vestibular schwannoma.[42] They have become a common component of the battery of tests used to assess vestibular function because they test a portion of the vestibular system not tested otherwise, i.e., the sacculus and inferior vestibular nerves. Normative values for cVEMP parameters are given in Table 32-3. Whereas the caloric test assesses the horizontal semicircular canal, the vestibulo-ocular reflex, and the superior vestibular nerve, the cVEMP tests the integrity of the saccule, the vestibulocollic reflex, and the inferior vestibular nerve.

Computerized Dynamic Posturography

Computerized dynamic posturography has become an established vestibular laboratory test. The most commonly used device, which is commercially available under the trade name EquiTest, is illustrated in Figure 32-27. In this type of testing, patients are asked to stand quietly on a computer-monitored platform that is surrounded by a

visual scene. The most useful portion of computerized dynamic posturography, when assessing a patient with a possible vestibular abnormality, is the sensory organization test. This test is designed to alter vision and somatic sensation in such a way that patients are forced to rely on various combinations of sensory inputs to maintain upright balance. Figure 32-28 illustrates the physiologic basis for the sensory organization test portion of computerized dynamic posturography.

The basic principle underlying computerized dynamic posturography is a technique called sway referencing, in which the platform on which the patient is standing or the visual surroundings are rotated in unison with the patient's spontaneous sway. In this way, the sensory

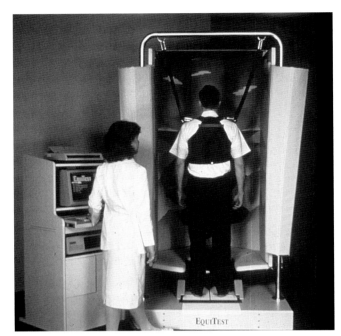

FIGURE 32-27 ■ Computerized dynamic posturography (EquiTest System, NeuroCom International). The patient stands on a force platform enclosed by a visual surround. A safety harness is used to prevent injury should the patient lose balance. The system is used for the sensory organization test, which is illustrated separately. (With permission from Neuro-Com International Inc., Clackamas, OR.)

inputs from vision or somatic sensation can be distorted selectively. The six sensory conditions are designed to provide patients with various combinations of sensory inputs important for balance. The surface on which the patient stands is monitored by a computer that processes the postural sway data. Figure 32-29 illustrates the analysis of postural sway during computerized dynamic posturography for a patient with bilateral vestibular loss. Note that the patient was unable to stand during sensory conditions 5 and 6 but was able to stand normally during the first four sensory conditions. In conditions 5 and 6, the patient is deprived of reliable visual and somatosensory information and thus is forced to rely on vestibular information to maintain upright postural sway. This vestibular pattern can be seen in patients with bilateral vestibular loss and in patients with unilateral loss who have not compensated for their peripheral vestibular abnormality.

Advantages of computerized dynamic posturography include the following: (1) it evaluates balance while standing, and in this way is a functional measure that depends upon vestibulospinal function; (2) it provides information that is different from that provided by vestibulo-ocular tests such as caloric and rotational testing; and (3) it is easily administered and repeatable. The disadvantages of computerized dynamic posturography include the requirement that patients cooperate fully.

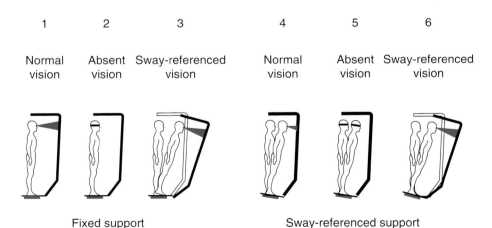

1	2	3	4	5	6
Normal vision	Absent vision	Sway-referenced vision	Normal vision	Absent vision	Sway-referenced vision

Fixed support   Sway-referenced support

FIGURE 32-28 ■ The sensory organization portion of computerized dynamic posturography includes six paradigms: (1) eyes open, platform stable; (2) eyes closed, platform stable; (3) eyes open with visual surroundings moving and platform stable; (4) eyes open, platform moving; (5) eyes closed, platform moving; and (6) both visual surround and platform moving. The movements of the visual surroundings, the platform, or both are designed to parallel movements of the patient's center of mass, so-called sway referencing, thereby providing a distorted visual or proprioceptive input. The fifth and sixth conditions, wherein the patient's eyes are closed or the patient is viewing moving visual surroundings while the floor moves, force the patient to rely on the vestibulospinal system to maintain balance. (With permission from NeuroCom International Inc., Clackamas, OR.)

EQUILIBRIUM SCORE

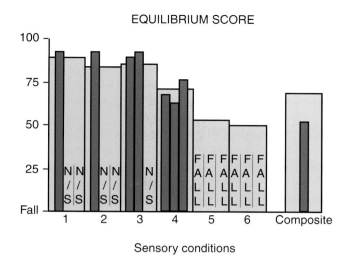

FIGURE 32-29 ▪ Computer analysis of postural sway provided by EquiTest for a patient who was able to stand during the first four sensory conditions but unable to stand during the fifth and sixth conditions. Light shading represents normal limits and dark columns represent patient trials. N/S, no score; FALL indicates a fall, so that the score for that trial was 0. This patient has a vestibular pattern on posturography, suggesting an ongoing vestibulospinal abnormality. (From Furman JM, Cass SP: Vestibular Disorders: A Case Study Approach. 2nd Ed. Oxford University Press, New York, 2003.)

Additionally, abnormalities are often nonspecific and nonlocalizing, and do not provide information regarding the activity of specific labyrinthine sensors or the laterality or etiology of any disturbance. Despite these disadvantages, computerized dynamic posturography is an appropriate test for patients whose symptoms of "dizziness" are accompanied by complaints of imbalance while standing or walking.

Test Batteries

Vestibular laboratory testing may involve several different types of assessment tools. The standard tests have just been discussed and three emerging technologies are described below. Table 32-4 provides an itemization of what is considered appropriate to include in a basic battery of tests performed to evaluate a patient with a suspected peripheral or central vestibular abnormality. The parameters of interest for these tests are shown in Table 32-5. Computerized dynamic posturography is appropriate for an evaluation of patients with imbalance thought to be related to vestibular dysfunction. Three other tests, ocular vestibular evoked myogenic potentials, galvanic vestibular stimulation, and gaze stability testing/dynamic visual acuity, cannot yet be recommended

TABLE 32-4 ▪ Vestibular Test Batteries
SUSPECTED PERIPHERAL VESTIBULAR ABNORMALITY
Ocular motor screening battery
Search for vestibular nystagmus
Positional testing
Caloric testing
Rotational testing
Computerized dynamic posturography
Cervical vestibular evoked myogenic potentials
SUSPECTED CENTRAL VESTIBULAR ABNORMALITY
Ocular motor screening battery
Search for vestibular nystagmus
Positional testing
Rotational testing: visual–vestibular interaction

Adapted from Baloh RW, Halmagyi GM (eds): Disorders of the Vestibular System. Oxford University Press, New York, 1996, with permission.

TABLE 32-5 ▪ Main Parameters of Interest in the Standard Vestibular Test Protocol	
Protocol Item	**Parameters of Interest**
Ocular motor screening battery	
Spontaneous nystagmus detection	Nystagmus direction, and SCV
Gaze-evoked nystagmus	Nystagmus at different positions of gaze
Saccades	Velocity, latency, accuracy, binocular asymmetry
Optokinetic nystagmus	Gain, left/right asymmetry
Smooth pursuit	Gain, left/right asymmetry, morphology
Position tests	
Positional testing	Nystagmus direction and SCV, fixation suppression
Positioning testing	Nystagmus direction, latency, fatigability
Caloric test	Reduced vestibular response, directional preponderance, total responsiveness
Rotatory chair test	Gain, phase, time constant, directional preponderance (asymmetry)
Computerized dynamic posturography	EquiTest scores
Cervical vestibular evoked myogenic potentials	Asymmetry, threshold, latency

SCV, slow component velocity.
Adapted from Luxon L, Furman JM, Martini A et al (eds): Textbook of Audiological Medicine: Clinical Aspects of Hearing and Balance. Martin Dunitz/Taylor & Francis, London, 2003, with permission.

as part of a routine vestibular test battery. Their value as adjuncts to more established tests is discussed in a later section.

Normative Laboratory Values

There is considerable variation among the results of different studies of normative vestibular function. This variability probably is based on differences of equipment, technique, and analysis methods. The published results from several facilities are shown in Table 32-3. Each laboratory should decide on a set of normal limits that are applied consistently.

VESTIBULAR TEST ABNORMALITIES IN CLINICAL DISORDERS

Benign Paroxysmal Positional Vertigo

A definitive diagnosis of BPPV can be established by confirming a positive Dix–Hallpike maneuver with characteristic torsional-vertical nystagmus. Unless a laboratory is equipped with three-dimensional VOG, vestibular laboratory testing cannot confirm the diagnosis of BPPV. However, because about 25 percent of such patients have a unilateral RVR on caloric testing, vestibular laboratory testing can be useful in the assessment of patients with BPPV. Other patients with BPPV may have a spontaneous nystagmus, a persistent positional nystagmus, or a directional preponderance.[43,44] These abnormalities would suggest a more widespread vestibular abnormality other than simply posterior semicircular canal canalithiasis.

Ménière Disease

The most common vestibular laboratory abnormality seen in Ménière disease is a unilateral reduced vestibular response on caloric testing[45,46]; however, some patients with Ménière disease have normal testing, especially if they are early in the course of their disorder and have not had a recent attack of vertigo.[46] Patients with a recent attack of Ménière disease may manifest a spontaneous nystagmus, a positional nystagmus, or a directional preponderance, indicating active vestibular disease. Patients with bilateral Ménière disease may show a reduction in the total slow component velocity across the four irrigations and a reduced gain on rotational testing. Recently, cVEMPs have been shown to be reduced in Ménière disease.[47] Overall, vestibular laboratory testing is not especially useful for establishing a diagnosis of Ménière disease because the diagnosis depends primarily upon a history of episodic vertigo with associated unilateral hearing loss and tinnitus and audiometric evidence of a low-frequency sensorineural hearing loss. However, vestibular laboratory testing can provide information that may be useful for management.

Migraine-Related Vestibulopathy

Recently, migraine-related vestibulopathy has become recognized as a common cause of "dizziness."[48,49] Many patients with migraine headache have vestibular abnormalities, even if they do not suffer from migraine-related dizziness. There is a great deal of variability among migraineurs regarding vestibular test results. Nonetheless, documenting an abnormality such as a unilateral reduced vestibular response, which is seen in about 25 percent of patients with migraine-related vestibulopathy, or a directional preponderance on rotational testing can be useful in the assessment of these patients.

Cerebellopontine Angle Tumors

Patients with cerebellopontine angle tumors, including acoustic neuromas, usually have a unilaterally reduced vestibular response on caloric testing on the side of the lesion.[50,51] However, these patients usually have minimal, if any, vestibular-related symptoms, probably because of the gradual onset of their peripheral vestibular loss, which allows compensation to occur. With large cerebellopontine angle tumors, especially those associated with compression of the cerebellum, patients usually have abnormalities on ocular motor testing, including abnormal ocular pursuit, optokinetic nystagmus, and, in some instances, Brun nystagmus.[52] Although vestibular testing is not required for establishing the diagnosis of an eighth nerve tumor, knowledge of remaining vestibular function may be useful in planning management. Specifically, following surgical treatment, the amount of postoperative vertigo can be predicted by the extent of preoperative vestibular loss.

Ototoxic Drug Exposure

Patients who have received ototoxic drugs (e.g., aminoglycoside antibiotics and certain chemotherapeutic agents such as cisplatin) may suffer from bilateral vestibular loss. Unfortunately, during the course of treatment with these vestibulotoxic medications, there may be no warning that a patient is losing vestibular function. Bilateral caloric reduction and reduced gain on rotational testing, both of which indicate bilateral vestibular loss, are the most common abnormalities seen following ototoxic drug exposure.[53] Occasionally, patients suffering from ototoxic drug exposure demonstrate an asymmetric caloric response or a directional preponderance on rotational testing. Overall, laboratory testing of patients who have received ototoxic medications provides extremely useful information regarding the severity of vestibular damage.

EMERGING TECHNOLOGIES

Ocular Vestibular Evoked Myogenic Potentials

Ocular VEMPs (oVEMPs) have emerged recently as a method for measuring utricular function, under the condition that bone-conducted vibration is used, preferably with a "minishaker" (Fig. 32-30). Extraocular electromyography (EMG) responses are recorded with surface electrodes placed over the inferior oblique muscles. Ocular VEMPs are a crossed response, so the left eye response represents the excitability of the right utricular macula, and in particular the striolar zone. Currently, the method for recording oVEMPs is still under debate, as is its interpretation.[54] Within the next few years, the usefulness and reliability of oVEMPs undoubtedly will be established further.

Galvanic Vestibular Stimulation

Galvanic vestibular stimulation has been studied since the time of Barany but has not become a routine vestibular laboratory test. It is performed by applying small electrical currents to the vestibular labyrinth using electrodes while recording either eye movements[55] or postural sway.[56–58] Typical electrode arrangements are

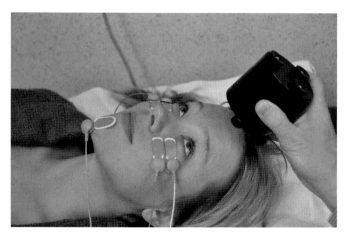

FIGURE 32-30 ■ A patient undergoing the recording of an ocular vestibular evoked myogenic potential. Note that the stimulus is a bone-conducted vibration to the forehead while surface recording electrodes capture extraocular electromyographic activity of the inferior oblique muscles. It is essential that the patient is looking up during the test.

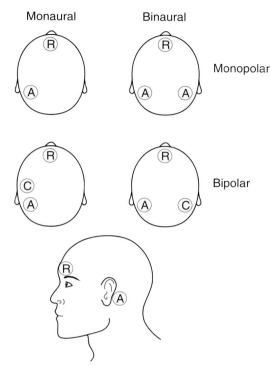

FIGURE 32-31 ■ Electrode configurations for galvanic vestibular stimulation. Illustrated are monaural and binaural configurations for both monopolar and bipolar stimulation. Electrodes are designated as reference (R), anode (A), and cathode (C).

illustrated in Figure 32-31. By placing an electrode on each mastoid (one positive and one negative), medial-lateral sway (Fig. 32-32) and horizontal/torsional eye movement can be produced by stimulating both labyrinths in opposite directions simultaneously. An alternate electrode configuration allows the method to assess each labyrinth separately, which can now be accomplished only with caloric testing. This attribute is also an advantage of VEMPs and unilateral centrifugation, discussed earlier in this chapter.

It is unknown exactly which portions of the vestibular labyrinth are responsible for the eye movements and postural sway induced by galvanic vestibular stimulation. The technique is believed to excite the synapse between vestibular hair cells and the eighth nerve afferents. Thus, it can provide information regarding "neural" rather than "sensory" function. Patients with hair-cell damage (e.g., from ototoxic drug exposure) who have preserved eighth nerve afferent function may have normal or even increased responses to galvanic vestibular stimulation despite absent responses to caloric and rotational testing.

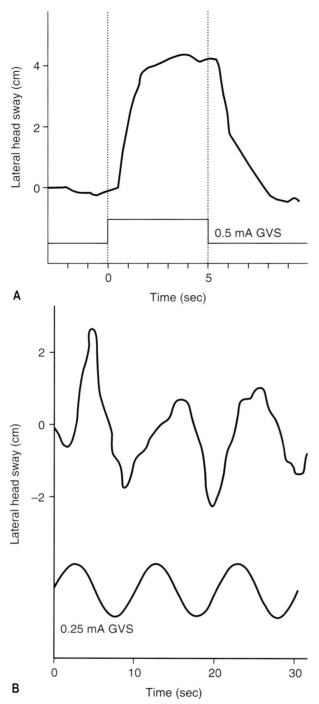

A

B

FIGURE 32-32 ■ Postural responses to galvanic vestibular stimulation (GVS). **A**, Head movement response (shown above) to a 5-second pulse of binaural bipolar 0.5 mA galvanic stimulation (shown below). **B**, Head movement response (shown above) to a sinusoidal galvanic stimulation of 0.25 mA at 0.1 Hz (shown below).

Technical challenges of the method include the fact that the eye movement produced is primarily torsional and of small magnitude, which renders accurate measurement difficult. Also, the postural sway induced by

galvanic vestibular stimulation is of low amplitude, variable, and complex biomechanically. Unresolved issues concerning galvanic vestibular stimulation include the following: (1) the influence of the orientation of the head on the torso; (2) the electrical waveform that is most useful (i.e., whether constant current or sinusoidal currents should be used); and (3) when the delivery of a constant current should begin with respect to a patient's spontaneous sway. Despite these challenges, three-dimensional VOG and lower-cost motion-analysis systems increase the possibility that galvanic vestibular stimulation may become clinically useful.

Gaze Stability Testing/Dynamic Visual Acuity

Gaze stability testing and dynamic visual acuity represent two recently introduced functional tests of vestibulo-ocular function.[59,60] They both rely on patients' voluntary head movement and subjective responses to visual stimuli rather than on recording of eye movements. In both tests, the patient looks at a computer monitor while turning the head left and right or up and down (Fig. 32-33). A computer monitors head velocity and displays an optotype (e.g., the letter "E") in a random orientation on the computer monitor when the head achieves a requisite velocity. The ability of the patient to indicate accurately the orientation of the optotype depends on the VOR and vision. The influence of vision is largely eliminated by basing the size of the optotype on the patient's visual acuity when the head is still. In dynamic visual acuity (DVA) testing, the optotype is presented when the

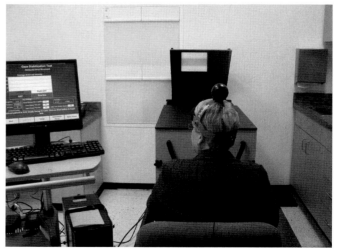

FIGURE 32-33 ■ Device used for gaze stability testing and dynamic visual acuity testing. Note the velocity sensor on the patient's head, the separate monitor for the technician, and the precise distance between the patient and the display.

head is moving faster than a predetermined velocity (e.g., 80 deg/sec). The size of the optotype is varied by the computer to determine the smallest optotype whose orientation can be recognized reliably. The reported result is the difference between baseline visual acuity and visual acuity while the head is moving at a preselected velocity. In gaze stability testing (GST), the size of the optotype is held constant (e.g., two logMAR units above baseline visual acuity) while the patient is asked to move the head faster and faster. The optotype is displayed when the head velocity exceeds a certain threshold, which varies in a controlled way as the test proceeds. The reported result is the fastest head velocity at which the patient can identify the orientation of the optotype reliably.

The basis for both DVA testing and the GST is the ability of the patient to hold a visual target accurately on the fovea with minimal visual motion. To accomplish this, the eyes must move in precisely the opposite direction to the head, an ability that depends on the VOR. Theoretically, the GST is more representative of actual VOR function because the head naturally moves at various velocities while visual targets retain their size. However, the DVA test may be more reliable because the optotype is presented when the head achieves a set velocity. Studies of patients with vestibular disorders suggest that both tests reflect abnormalities of the VOR.[59,60] The usefulness of DVA testing and the GST remains to be determined. However, the studies published to date suggest that both tests may become valuable additions to quantitative vestibular laboratory testing primarily because these tests assess the functional status of the VOR.

CONCLUDING COMMENTS

Patients with complaints suggestive of vestibular dysfunction, such as of "dizziness", vertigo, disequilibrium, or unsteadiness, are commonly encountered by clinicians, especially primary care physicians, neurologists, and otolaryngologists. The etiology of such symptoms must be identified so that they can be managed effectively. A clinical history and competent physical examination are important in the evaluation of such patients, but vestibular function tests provide useful additional information. They may confirm the clinical diagnosis or suggest the diagnosis when it is clinically uncertain. They help to localize and lateralize the underlying disorder, and the quantitative information obtained in the vestibular laboratory allows the course of a disorder or its response to treatment to be monitored. The emergence of new methods for evaluating utricular function, the

introduction of new approaches for testing vestibulo-ocular function, and the development of means for galvanic vestibular stimulation will add to the repertoire of techniques that are available for studying derangements of vestibular function in the laboratory for clinical purposes.

REFERENCES

1. Robinson DA: A method of measuring eye movement using a scleral search coil in a magnetic field. IEEE Trans Biomed Elect, 10:137, 1963
2. Committee on Hearing, Bioacoustics, and Biomechanics Commission on Behavioral and Social Sciences and Education, National Research Council: Evaluation of tests for vestibular function. Aviat Space Environ Med, 63:A1, 1992
3. Baloh RW, Honrubia V: Clinical Neurophysiology of the Vestibular System. Oxford University Press, New York, 2001
4. Jacobson GP, Newman CW, Kartush JM: Handbook of Balance Function Testing. Mosby–Year Book, St. Louis, 1993
5. Proctor L, Glackin R, Shimizu H et al: Reference values for serial vestibular testing. Ann Otol Rhinol Laryngol, 95:83, 1986
6. Shepard NT, Telian SA: Practical Management of the Balance Disorder Patient. Singular, London, 1996
7. Barber HO, Stockwell CW: Manual of Electronystagmography. Mosby, St. Louis, 1980
8. Mulch G, Lewitzki W: Spontaneous and positional nystagmus in healthy persons demonstrated only by electronystagmography: physiological spontaneous nystagmus or "functional scar"? Arch Otorhinolaryngol, 215:135, 1977
9. Coats AC: Directional preponderance and spontaneous nystagmus as observed in the electronystagmographic examination. Ann Otol Rhinol Laryngol, 75:1135, 1966
10. Fischer AJ, Huygen PL, Folgering HT et al: Vestibular hyperreactivity and hyperventilation after whiplash injury. J Neurol Sci, 132:35, 1995
11. Baloh RW, Konrad HR, Sills AW et al: The saccade velocity test. Neurology, 25:1071, 1975
12. Henriksson NG, Pyykko I, Schalen L et al: Velocity patterns of rapid eye movements. Acta Otolaryngol, 89:504, 1980
13. Van der Stappen A, Wuyts FL, Van de Heyning P: Computerized electronystagmography: normative data revisited. Acta Otolaryngol, 120:724, 2000
14. Abel LA, Troost BT, Dell'Osso LF: The effects of age on normal saccadic characteristics and their variability. Vision Res, 23:33, 1983
15. Leigh RJ, Zee DS: The Neurology of Eye Movements. Oxford University Press, New York, 1999
16. Jongkees LBW, Philipszoon AJ: Electronystagmography. Acta Otolaryngol, 42:Suppl 189,1, 1964
17. Sills AW, Baloh RW, Honrubia V: Caloric testing 2. Results in normal subjects. Ann Otol Rhinol Laryngol Suppl, 86:7, 1977

18. Boniver R, Demanez JP, Lennes G: Epreuves rotatoires et caloriques chez le sujet normal. p. 195. In Proceedings of the Neurootological and Equilibriometric Society. Vol. 1, Medicine und Pharmacie, Frankfurt, 1975

19. Peterka RJ, Black FO, Schoenhoff MB: Age-related changes in human vestibulo-ocular reflexes: sinusoidal rotation and caloric tests. J Vestib Res, 1:49, 1990

20. Baloh RW, Sakala SM, Yee RD et al: Quantitative vestibular testing. Otolaryngol Head Neck Surg, 92:145, 1984

21. Hess K, Baloh RW, Honrubia V et al: Rotational testing in patients with bilateral peripheral vestibular disease. Laryngoscope, 95:85, 1985

22. Wall C, Black FO, Hunt AE: Effects of age, sex and stimulus parameters upon vestibulo-ocular responses to sinusoidal rotation. Acta Otolaryngol, 98:270, 1984

23. Theunissen EJ, Huygen PL, Folgering HT: Vestibular hyperreactivity and hyperventilation. Clin Otolaryngol, 11:161, 1986

24. Vanspauwen R, Wuyts FL, Van de Heyning PH: Vestibular evoked myogenic potentials: test-retest reliability and normative values obtained with a feedback method for the sternocleidomastoid muscle contraction. J Vestib Res, 19:127, 2009

25. Maes L, Vinck BM, DeVel E et al: The vestibular evoked myogenic potential: a test-retest reliability study. Clin Neurophysiol, 120:594, 2009

26. Tal D, Hershkovitz D, Kaminski G et al: Vestibular evoked myogenic potential threshold and seasickness susceptibility. J Vestib Res, 16:273, 2006

27. Isaradisaikul S, Strong DA, Moushey JM et al: Reliability of vestibular evoked myogenic potentials in healthy subjects. Otol Neurotol, 29:542, 2008

28. Wang SJ, Yeh TH, Chang CH et al: Consistent latencies of vestibular evoked myogenic potentials. Ear Hear, 29:923, 2008

29. Furman JF, Durrant JD: Head-only rotational testing: influence of volition and vision. J Vestib Res, 5:323, 1995

30. Wetzig J, Reiser M, Martin E et al: Unilateral centrifugation of the otoliths as a new method to determine bilateral asymmetries of the otolith apparatus in man. Acta Astronaut, 21:519, 1990

31. Clarke AH, Engelhorn A: Unilateral testing of utricular function. Exp Brain Res, 121:457, 1998

32. Wuyts FL, Hoppenbrouwers M, Pauwels G et al: Utricular sensitivity and preponderance assessed by the unilateral centrifugation test. J Vestib Res, 13:227, 2004

33. Clarke AH: Perspectives for the comprehensive examination of semicircular canal and otolith function. Biol Sci Space, 15:393, 2001

34. Buytaert KI, Nooij SAE, Neyt X et al: A new model for utricular function testing using a sinusoidal translation profile during unilateral centrifugation. Audiol Neurootol, 15:343, 2010

35. Bickford RG, Jacobson JL, Cody DT: Nature of average evoked potentials to sound and other stimuli in man. Ann N Y Acad Sci, 112:204, 1964

36. Colebatch JG, Halmagyi GM, Skuse NF: Myogenic potentials generated by a click-evoked vestibulocollic reflex. J Neurol Neurosurg Psychiatry, 57:190, 1994

37. Murofushi T, Halmagyi GM, Yavor RA et al: Absent vestibular evoked myogenic potentials in vestibular neurolabyrinthitis. An indicator of inferior vestibular nerve involvement? Arch Otolaryngol Head Neck Surg, 122:845, 1996

38. de Waele C, Huy PT, Diard JP et al: Saccular dysfunction in Menière's disease. Am J Otol, 20:223, 1999

39. Young YH, Huang TW, Cheng PW: Assessing the stage of Menière's disease using vestibular evoked myogenic potentials. Arch Otolaryngol Head Neck Surg, 129:815, 2003

40. Brantberg K, Bergenius J, Tribukait A: Vestibular-evoked myogenic potentials in patients with dehiscence of the superior semicircular canal. Acta Otolaryngol, 119:633, 1999

41. Streubel SO, Cremer PD, Carey JP et al: Vestibular-evoked myogenic potentials in the diagnosis of superior canal dehiscence syndrome. Acta Otolaryngol Suppl, 545:41, 2001

42. Patko T, Vidal PP, Vibert N et al: Vestibular evoked myogenic potentials in patients suffering from a unilateral acoustic neuroma: a study of 170 patients. Clin Neurophysiol, 114:1344, 2003

43. Baloh RW, Honrubia V, Jacobson K: Benign positional vertigo: clinical and oculographic features in 240 cases. Neurology, 37:371, 1987

44. McClure J, Lycett P, Rounthwaite J: Vestibular dysfunction associated with benign paroxysmal vertigo. Laryngoscope, 87:1434, 1977

45. Hulshof JH, Baarsma EA: Vestibular investigations in Menière's disease. Acta Otolaryngol, 92:75, 1981

46. Hulshof JH, Baarsma EA: Follow-up vestibular examination in Menière's disease. Acta Otolaryngol, 92:397, 1981

47. Rauch SD, Zhou G, Kujawa SG et al: Vestibular evoked myogenic potentials show altered tuning in patients with Menière's disease. Otol Neurotol, 25:333, 2004

48. Neuhauser H, Leopold M, von Brevern M et al: The interrelations of migraine, vertigo, and migrainous vertigo. Neurology, 56:436, 2001

49. Furman JM, Marcus DA, Balaban CD: Migrainous vertigo: development of a pathogenetic model and structured diagnostic interview. Curr Opin Neurol, 16:5, 2003

50. Tos M, Thomsen J: Epidemiology of acoustic neuromas. J Laryngol Otol, 98:685, 1984

51. Baloh RW, Konrad HR, Dirks D et al: Cerebellar-pontine angle tumors. Results of quantitative vestibulo-ocular testing. Arch Neurol, 33:507, 1976

52. Nedzelski JM: Cerebellopontine angle tumors: bilateral flocculus compression as cause of associated oculomotor abnormalities. Laryngoscope, 93:1251, 1983

53. Hess K: Vestibulotoxic drugs and other causes of acquired bilateral peripheral vestibulopathy. p. 360. In Baloh RW, Halmagyi GM (eds): Disorders of the Vestibular System. Oxford University Press, New York, 1996

54. Welgampola MS, Carey JP: Waiting for the evidence: VEMP testing and the ability to differentiate utricular

versus saccular function. Otolaryngol Head Neck Surg, 143:281, 2010

55. Severac Cauquil A, Faldon M, Popov K et al: Short-latency eye movements evoked by near-threshold galvanic vestibular stimulation. Exp Brain Res, 148:414, 2003

56. Benson AJ, Jobson PH: Body sway induced by a low frequency alternating current. Int J Equilib Res, 3:55, 1973

57. Hlavacka F, Njiokiktjien C: Postural responses evoked by sinusoidal galvanic stimulation of the labyrinth. Influence of head position. Acta Otolaryngol, 99:107, 1985

58. Tokita T, Ito Y, Takagi K: Modulation by head and trunk positions of the vestibulo-spinal reflexes evoked by galvanic stimulation of the labyrinth. Observations by labyrinthine evoked EMG. Acta Otolaryngol, 107:327, 1989

59. Ward BK, Mohammad MT, Whitney SL et al: The reliability, stability, and concurrent validity of a test of gaze stabilization. J Vestib Res, 20:363, 2010

60. Herdman SJ, Schubert MC, Das VE et al: Recovery of dynamic visual acuity in unilateral vestibular hypofunction. Arch Otolaryngol Head Neck Surg, 129:819, 2003

Electrophysiologic Evaluation in Special Situations

Polysomnographic Evaluation of Sleep Disorders

VIVIEN C. ABAD and CHRISTIAN GUILLEMINAULT

The term *polysomnography* (PSG) describes the overnight monitoring during sleep of multiple biologic variables and the evaluation of their relationships within a specific state of alertness. It uses the 10–20 international electrode placement system for electroencephalography (EEG) in addition to monitoring respiratory parameters (airflow, snoring, effort, oxygen saturation, with or without carbon dioxide [CO_2] monitoring), cardiac monitoring, electromyographic recording, and video recording. Clinical PSG allows a broad investigation of biologic functions during different states of alertness. PSG can facilitate the investigation of the impact of sleep stages on the control of vital organs and on the autonomic nervous system. It can illustrate the impact of circadian rhythms on diverse biologic functions. Additionally, PSG can help evaluate the efficacy of treatment for various sleep disorders.

HISTORY OF POLYSOMNOGRAPHY

Hans Berger recorded the first continuous overnight EEG tracing in 1929 and demonstrated patterns that correlated with sleep and wakefulness.[1] Loomis and colleagues devised a classification system for EEG during sleep in the late 1930s.[2] In their classic paper in 1953, Aserinsky and Kleitman reported the cyclic occurrence during sleep of rapid eye movements associated with a specific EEG pattern of low-voltage, fast EEG activity.[3] Dement and Kleitman in 1957 reported on the cyclic nature of two different states of alertness, using the terms *rapid eye movement* (REM) and *non–rapid eye movement* (non-REM).[4] The term *REM sleep* still has a number of synonymous names. Among the most common are desynchronized sleep; D (for desynchronized and dreaming) states, commonly used in animal research; active sleep, used mainly during the neonatal period; and paradoxical sleep.

Non-REM sleep was defined better following the initial efforts of Loomis and his team.[2] An international conference of sleep researchers in 1968 led to the publication of the Rechtschaffen and Kales manual, which, until recently, was the most commonly utilized standardized scoring of PSG.[5] This manual gives specific instructions on how to score sleep states and stages, and defines four sleep stages of non-REM sleep (also called synchronized sleep; slow-wave sleep; and, in infants, quiet sleep). These criteria utilize scoring by epochs (i.e., 30-second recording) and the "majority of epoch" rule. This rule applies when more than one stage occurs in an epoch, so that the stage that constitutes greater than 50 percent of the epoch is the stage with which the epoch is scored. These definitions are valid for children over 2 years of age and for young or middle-aged adults, but are not as accurate for the elderly.

A second consensus conference produced a second manual for scoring sleep in premature and newborn infants that generally was used until the 50th to 52nd postgestational week of age (i.e., until an infant born at term is 10 to 12 weeks old).[6] This atlas, edited by Anders and colleagues, recognizes the postnatal maturation processes that occur in the brain and the difficulties of subdividing quiet (non-REM) sleep into stages. Only four states are defined: wakefulness and quiet, active, and indeterminate sleep. The last of these indicates that, even in full-term newborns, EEG and other criteria may be insufficient to separate quiet from active sleep.

In 2007, the American Academy of Sleep Medicine (AASM) introduced the AASM Manual for the Scoring of Sleep and Associated Events,[7] which has replaced the Rechtschaffen and Kales scoring system.[5] The major changes set forth by AASM included primarily changes in EEG derivations, reduction in number of sleep stages (Rechtschaffen and Kales: wake, stages 1,2,3,4 non-REM sleep and stage REM sleep) by merging stages 3 and 4 and the elimination of movement time (AASM: N1, N2, N3, and stage R), the simplification of many context rules, and recommendations on sampling rates and filter settings for polysomnographic reporting and user interfaces for computer-assisted analysis.

SLEEP OVERVIEW

Human existence represents a continuum of three states of being: (1) wakefulness; (2) non-REM sleep; and (3) REM sleep. Wakefulness is associated with an alert state; eye movements with eyes open; erect, sitting, or recumbent posture; normal responsiveness to stimuli; and normal mobility. Sleep, by contrast, is associated with reversible unconsciousness, a closed-eye position with or without eye movements, recumbent posture, mild to moderate reduction in responsiveness to stimuli, and reduced or absent mobility.

Sleep Onset and Behavioral Correlates

Sleep onset is associated with perceptual disengagement from visual and auditory stimuli, discriminant response to meaningful versus nonmeaningful stimuli, impairment of memory, occurrence of hypnic myoclonia, and "automatic behavior."[8] Guilleminault and colleagues presented light flashes and instructed EEG-monitored subjects to press a microswitch taped to their hands.[9] When the EEG patterns were consistent with stage 1 or stage 2 sleep, responses were absent 85 percent of the time, and subjects later reported that they did not see the light flash.[9] Others reported that subjects exhibited longer reaction times in response to auditory tones presented close to the onset of stage 1 sleep, and responses were absent during unequivocal sleep.[9] Soft calling of one's name during light sleep may evoke an arousal, whereas a nonmeaningful stimulus may not. It has been hypothesized that sleep may close the gate between short-term memory and long-term memory stores. An experiment in which word pairs were presented at 1-minute intervals to volunteers demonstrated that when subjects were awakened 30 seconds after sleep onset, they could recall words presented 4 to 10 minutes (defined as long-term memory) and 0 to 3 minutes (defined as short-term memory) before EEG-defined sleep onset.[10] By contrast, if they were awakened 10 minutes after sleep onset, they could recall words presented at 4 to 10 minutes but not words presented at 0 to 3 minutes before sleep onset.[10] This experiment suggested that sleep inactivates the transfer of storage from short-term to long-term memory or that the encoding of the material presented before sleep onset was not of sufficient strength to allow recall.[8,10] General or local muscle contraction (hypnic myoclonus), often associated with visual imagery, may be noted at sleep onset. "Automatic behavior" (e.g., subjects continuing to tap a switch for a few seconds after sleep onset) has also been reported.[9]

EEG at sleep onset demonstrates a change from rhythmic alpha (8- to 13-Hz) activity to a relatively low-voltage mixed-frequency pattern. This change usually occurs seconds to minutes after the electro-oculogram (EOG) shows slow, often asynchronous, eye movements. The electromyogram (EMG) demonstrates gradual diminution in level.

Temporal Organization of Normal Sleep

Nocturnal sleep is associated with a regular pattern. A normal adult first enters non-REM sleep and then goes into REM sleep after about 80 or 90 minutes. Thereafter, non-REM and REM sleep alternate throughout the night with a periodicity of about 100 minutes. The combination of one non-REM sleep segment and one REM sleep segment is a sleep cycle.

SLEEP STAGES

Under the criteria of Rechtschaffen and Kales, non-REM sleep consists of four stages (1 to 4). Stage 1 sleep is associated with slow eye movements; EMG levels below those of relaxed wakefulness; and low-voltage, mixed-frequency EEG in the 2- to 7-Hz frequencies (Fig. 33-1). During the latter part of stage 1, vertex sharp waves may appear associated with high-amplitude 2- to 7-Hz activity. Scoring of stage 1 sleep requires an absolute absence of clearly defined K-complexes and sleep spindles. Stage 2 sleep is defined by the presence of K-complexes or sleep spindles and by the presence of sleep-delta activity for less than 20 percent of the epoch (Fig. 33-2). K-complexes are seen maximally over the vertex regions and represent EEG waveforms consisting of a well-defined negative sharp wave immediately followed by a positive component, with the entire complex exceeding 0.5 seconds in duration. Waves of 12- to 14-Hz activity may or may not be part of the complex. Stages 3 and 4 comprise slow-wave sleep. Stage 3 is scored when at least 20 percent but not more than 50 percent of the epoch consists of slow delta waves (i.e., 2 Hz or less, with amplitude greater than 75 μV measured from peak to peak) (Fig. 33-3). Stage 4 is scored when at least 50 percent of the epoch consists of such delta waves. Sleep spindles may or may not be present in stage 3 or 4.

The 2007 AASM scoring manual designates three stages of non-REM sleep (N1, N2, N3) and one stage of REM sleep (R). N1 is equivalent to stage 1 non-REM sleep, N2 to stage 2 non-REM sleep, N3 to stages 3 and 4 non-REM sleep, and R to stage REM sleep.

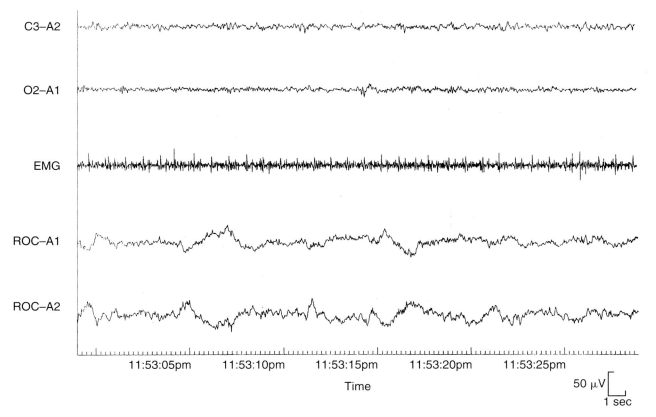

FIGURE 33-1 ▪ Stage 1 sleep. Note the low-voltage, mixed-frequency electroencephalogram, presence of muscle tone, and slow rolling eye movements.

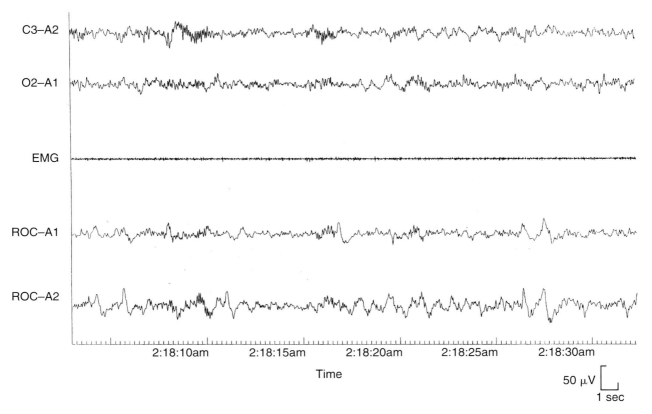

FIGURE 33-2 ■ Stage 2 sleep showing the presence of sleep spindles. K-complexes (not clearly shown) are also classically present.

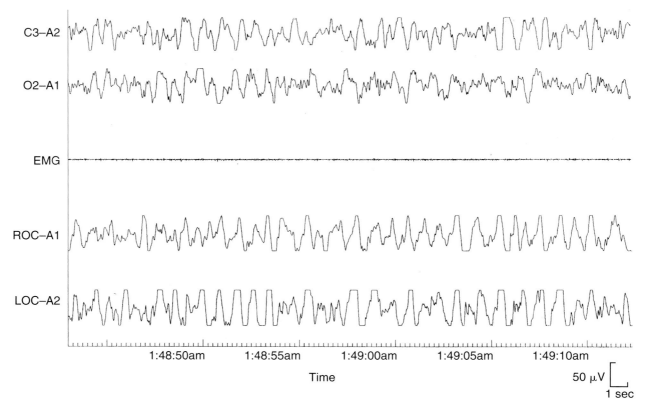

FIGURE 33-3 ■ Stage 3 (N3) sleep. High-amplitude, low-frequency delta activity is present in the electroencephalogram (EEG). The eye movement channels (frontally placed) are reflective of the EEG.

EEG during REM sleep demonstrates the concomitant appearance of low-voltage, mixed-frequency EEG activity and episodic rapid eye movements. During REM sleep, "sawtooth" (i.e., 2- to 3-Hz, sharply contoured, triangular) waves can be noted in the vertex and frontal regions in conjunction with bursts of REM (Fig. 33-4). Alpha activity can also be seen, but its frequency is 1 to 2 Hz slower than during wakefulness. There is an absolute absence of sleep spindles and K-complexes during REM sleep. REM sleep can be divided into tonic REM sleep and phasic REM sleep. During tonic REM sleep, the EEG is desynchronized; there is hypotonia or atonia of major muscle groups and depression of monosynaptic and polysynaptic reflexes. Tonic EMG activity is low in amplitude. Phasic REM sleep is associated with rapid eye movements; irregularities in blood pressure, heart rate, and respiration; spontaneous muscle activity; and tongue movements.

FIRST SLEEP CYCLE

In a normal young adult, the first sleep cycle begins with stage 1 sleep, which generally lasts for only a few (1 to 7) minutes. Stage 1 non-REM sleep is interrupted easily, and oscillations from wakefulness to stage 1 are often observed during the sleep-onset period. Stage 2 non-REM sleep follows this short stage 1 transition from wakefulness and continues for 10 to 25 minutes. Progressive, gradual appearance of high-voltage slow-wave activity signals the evolution toward stage 3 non-REM sleep. This stage usually lasts only a few minutes and represents a transition to stage 4 non-REM sleep as more and more high-voltage activity is seen. Stage 4 non-REM sleep lasts for 20 to 40 minutes during the first cycle. If body movements occur, there is a transient switch to lighter sleep (i.e., stage 1 or stage 2).

Often, a brief switch from stage 4 to stage 2 non-REM sleep occurs several minutes before the subject goes into REM sleep. The passage from non-REM to REM sleep is not abrupt; the EMG may decline long before the switch to REM sleep occurs. Although the EEG pattern characteristic of REM sleep will become more and more prominent, REM sleep cannot be declared before identification of the first rapid eye movement. One must go back from this first eye movement to pinpoint the onset of the first REM period using EEG and EMG criteria. This first REM sleep period is short, lasting between 2 and 6 minutes. It may be suppressed easily if any discomfort occurs (which may be related to the recording apparatus). REM sleep often ends with a short body movement, and a new cycle begins.[5]

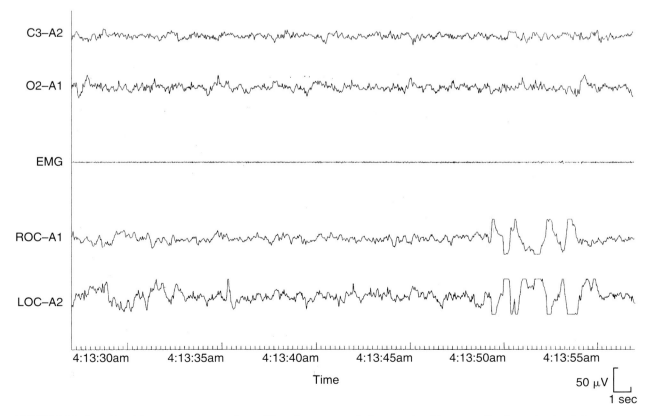

FIGURE 33-4 ■ Rapid eye movement sleep. The electroencephalogram is of low amplitude and mixed frequency, and muscle atonia and rapid eye movements are present.

LATER SLEEP CYCLES

Non-REM and REM sleep continue to alternate throughout the night in a cyclic fashion. As the night progresses, each sleep cycle differs slightly from the previous one. The average length of the second and later sleep cycles is about 100 to 120 minutes. The last sleep cycle is usually the longest.

DISTRIBUTION OF SLEEP STAGES THROUGHOUT THE NIGHT

The distribution of sleep stages varies slightly during the night from sleep cycle to sleep cycle, with stage 3 and stage 4 non-REM sleep occurring mainly during the first two sleep cycles and the REM sleep period growing progressively longer in the last two sleep cycles. Stage 3 and stage 4 non-REM sleep, also known as slow-wave sleep or N3 sleep, is most prominent during the first third of the night. The preferential distribution of slow-wave sleep toward the beginning of nocturnal sleep is related to the length of prior wakefulness, the time at which sleep onset occurs, and the time course of sleep per se. Factor "S" (for slow-wave activity) may be manipulated by conditions such as sleep deprivation, sleep satiety, and time of sleep; it is the object of theoretical investigations and mathematic modeling. The preferential distribution of REM sleep toward the latter portion of the night in young adults is hypothesized to be linked to a circadian oscillator, which can be investigated by monitoring the 24-hour core body temperature. In an adult, non-REM sleep takes up approximately 80 percent of the total sleep time, with stage 1 occupying 5 percent; stage 2, 50 to 55 percent; stages 3 and 4, 20 percent; and REM sleep, 20 to 22 percent.

EFFECT OF AGE

Sleep patterns vary with age (Fig. 33-5). In the neonate, active (REM) sleep usually consumes 50 percent of the total sleep time. Before puberty, this percentage rapidly declines and then stabilizes at around 20 percent until old age. Stages 3 and 4 of non-REM sleep are usually of maximal duration in childhood and decline progressively in adulthood, with fairly low levels attained around 50 to 55 years of age. Although several studies of sleep changes during aging have been performed, normative data are still relatively few, and a number of areas must still be explored.

Development of Sleep in Infancy

It has been established clearly that the basic rest–activity cycle originates during fetal life. REM sleep has been recognized in infants near 28 weeks gestational age (GA), but non-REM sleep is very difficult to identify before

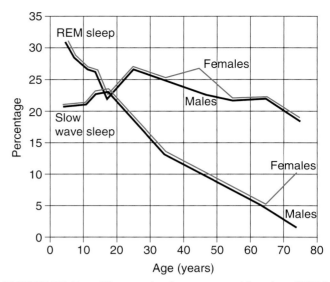

FIGURE 33-5 ■ Changes in sleep states with aging. REM, rapid eye movement.

34 to 35 weeks GA. It is only near the 36th week GA that observable variables such as body movement, eye movements, and changes in heart rate and respiratory patterns allow the scoring of both sleep states without much difficulty. Between the 40th week GA and the 3rd month of postnatal life in a full-term infant, a tighter association between physiologic and behavioral variables allows even easier definition of sleep and its states. During that period, the polyphasic sleeping–waking pattern, which seems to be associated with the 4-hour feeding cycle, changes to a diurnal pattern. Thus, a full-term infant has, at birth, a rhythm that is generally longer than 24 hours. A full-term newborn spends 70 to 80 percent of life asleep.

At birth, the lack of concordance between EEG, eye movements, and chin EMG results in the classifications of quiet, active, and indeterminate sleep. During active (REM) sleep, fast eye movements can be seen, often behind closed eyelids, but at times are associated with brief eye openings. Smiles, facial grimaces, frowns, blinking, and bursts of sucking are observed.[6] Gross body writhing admixed with limb twitching is noted. Vocalizations consisting of brief grunts, whimpers, or cries are heard.[6] The heart rate and respiratory rate are characterized by abrupt, short-lived irregularities. One breath may be missing, prolonged, or shortened. The EMG is variable but often low. The EEG during active sleep demonstrates any of the following patterns: a low-voltage (14- to 35-μV) irregular pattern admixed with slower activity (1 to 5 Hz), a mixed pattern with high- and low-voltage polyrhythmic waves intermingled without periodicity, or a high-voltage slow (HVS) pattern with continuous rhythmic medium to high voltage (50- to 150- μV) slow (0.5- to 4-Hz) waves.[6]

During quiet sleep, the newborn has eyes closed and no fast eye movements are noted. There are no body movements except for occasional startles and mouth movements. Respiration is quiet and very regular, as is the heart rate. EMG activity is variable, but usually tonus is maintained. The EEG demonstrates one of the following patterns: *tracé alternant* pattern of bursts of high-voltage slow waves (0.5 to 3 Hz) with superimposed rapid low-voltage waves and with sharp waves of 2 to 4 Hz interspersed between the slow waves; a low-voltage irregular pattern; or a mixed pattern.

It is usual to require that, during a given "epoch" (usually 30 to 60 seconds of a recording), three variables (i.e., EEG, EMG, and EOG) be concordant for the state in order for it to be scored. If concordance is lacking, indeterminate sleep is the recommended label.[7] Identification of various non-REM and REM features of sleep becomes easier with increasing age of the subject. By 3 months of age, non-REM and REM sleep can be recognized. At this age, non-REM sleep can be subdivided into two stages: 1 and 2; and 3 and 4 (or delta) sleep. Theta activity (4- to 7-Hz) is prominent during stage 1 or 2, but sleep spindles can be recognized by their synchronous or asynchronous occurrence over both hemispheres. When 20 percent or more of an epoch contains delta waves, stage 3 or stage 4 (delta) sleep is scored. By 3 months of age, stage 3 or stage 4 sleep has become prominent at the beginning of the night; the prominence of REM sleep during the second half of the night is noted clearly after 6 months of age. The classic stages 1 to 4 of non-REM sleep can be dissociated completely from one another by 6 months of age.

Sleep states can be recognized more easily with increasing age. Total sleep time takes up about 70 percent of the 24-hour period at birth. Between the ages of 6 and 10 weeks, a circadian rhythm emerges, the timing of which suggests interaction between environmental and maturational influences. At about 3 months of age, a rhythm has been established, with sleep occurring predominantly in the nocturnal period. Once this longest sleep period has been established, the longest period of wakefulness is established in the late afternoon or early evening, just before the nocturnal period. With maturation, wakefulness progressively increases, and by 6 months of age the infant remains awake for about 50 percent of the 24-hour period. The increase in wakefulness at this age occurs mainly through a decrease in the proportion of REM sleep from one-third to one-quarter of the sleep time. As children age, the proportion of time spent in REM sleep declines. By the age of 5 years, REM sleep is reduced further to between 20 and 22 percent of the total sleep time, whereas the time spent in stage 4 non-REM sleep increases from 14 to 18 percent between the ages of 2 and 5 years. So begins the pattern of sleep and wakefulness that will continue more or less throughout life. The distribution of sleep and wakefulness in the morning hours and early afternoon is still variable. At this age, the maturational processes have been such that sleep scoring can be based on classic EEG, EMG, and EOG criteria.

Recognition of these stages in infants is important. A lack of concordance for scoring states or a disturbance in maturation that impairs the scoring of stages at the appropriate time indicates that a pathologic process has interacted or is interacting with development of the sleep–wake cycle. During the first year of life, the nocturnal organization of sleep that will continue throughout life is established.

In summary, the basic sleep–wake organization of adults is present in infants by 3 months of age. Some changes do occur thereafter, but they are much less profound than those occurring during the first 3 months. All of the sleep stages observed in the adult can be identified and scored by 6 months of age, and it appears that the initial organization of wakefulness follows the organization of sleep.

The AASM pediatric taskforce indicated that Anders infant sleep criteria remain suitable for scoring sleep–wake states in infants of 46 to 48 weeks conceptional age, until sleep spindles are observed.[7] With the Anders criteria, the newborn infant has four states: quiet sleep, active sleep, indeterminate sleep, and wakefulness.[6] The 2007 AASM scoring rules for wakefulness and sleep are applicable to children older than 2 months post-term. Arousals are also defined. Caution is advised in adopting the new scoring criteria in children, since significant differences have been demonstrated between the two scoring systems: N1 (AASM) percentage is significantly higher than stage 1 (Rechtschaffen and Kales) while N2 and R percentages are significantly lower than stage 2 and REM (Rechtschaffen and Kales). Additionally, there is relatively low concordance for scoring stage shifts per hour between the two systems.

Sleep in Older Children

In prepubertal and pubertal children, slow-wave sleep (stage 3 and stage 4 non-REM sleep) undergoes further changes. The slow-wave sleep seen in the first sleep cycle in this age group appears resistant to arousal compared with that found in any other age group. For example, in one study, no sign of arousal with 123-dB tone stimuli presented during stage 3 or stage 4 non-REM sleep could be found in a group of 10-year-olds.[9] This finding is interesting because most parasomnias during childhood (particularly sleepwalking and night terrors) occur during the first slow-wave cycle. In specific experiments, children of this age were moved into an upright position during slow-wave sleep without being awakened fully. In most cases, sleepwalking episodes were triggered. These experiments indicate that deambulation (automatic walking) may be induced in normal children. The children will go back to sleep immediately if helped back to bed and will have complete amnesia for the event the following morning (Guilleminault, unpublished data). A decrease in slow-wave sleep of nearly 40 percent during the pubertal years has been reported. It has been hypothesized that the age-related decline in slow-wave sleep may run parallel to a loss of cortical synaptic density. The AASM 2007 manual has suggested grouping stages 3 and 4 together as N3 sleep, even in children. However, objections have been raised, as reduction in stage 4 percentage may affect hormonal secretion significantly, while N3 percentage may appear normal or minimally reduced. Growth hormone secretion is much more linked to stage 4 sleep in prepubertal children.

Sleep in the Elderly

In a meta-analysis of sleep parameters by age, Ohayon and colleagues showed that, in healthy adults, total sleep time, sleep efficiency, REM latency, percentage of slow-wave sleep, and percentage of REM sleep all decline with age, whereas sleep latency, wake after sleep onset, and percentages of stages 1 and 2 non-REM sleep increase.[11] However, after age 60 years, only sleep efficiency continues to decrease significantly.[11] The major change in sleep in the elderly is the decreased percentage of slow-wave sleep and increased stage 1 sleep, which is more pronounced in men. The amplitude of slow-wave sleep declines with age, but in parallel to EEG waves of other frequencies. The Visual Scoring Task Force and the Geriatric Task Force of the AASM voted to retain the 75-μV criterion for all ages and recommended that the frontal derivation be utilized for scoring slow-wave sleep. N3 sleep is scored when 20 percent or more of an epoch consists of 0.5- to 2-Hz frequencies with peak-to-peak amplitude exceeding 75 μV in the frontal derivation.[12]

SLEEP AND ITS PATHOLOGY

Disturbances of sleep lead to three different complaints:

1. "Tiredness," "fatigue," and "sleepiness" at times when the subject would like to be awake and alert
2. Difficulty in falling asleep or in maintaining sleep; or complaints of unrefreshing sleep, associated with fear of a decrease in performance during wakefulness because of lack of sleep

3. Complaints by spouses or roommates that their own sleep is disturbed by the abnormal behavior presented by the index case during sleep.

These three very different complaints have led to the creation of three major subcategories of pathology: excessive daytime sleepiness, insomnias, and parasomnias.

Epidemiologic studies in many Westernized countries have revealed that sleep disorders are a dominant health problem. Investigations performed in Italy, Finland, Israel, and several metropolitan areas of the United States have found that excessive daytime sleepiness affects between 3.7 and 4.2 percent of the general population. By comparison, Parkinson disease has an overall incidence of 1 percent among the population older than 50 years of age, and the prevalence of epilepsy is calculated at 0.5 percent.

The incidence of complaints of insomnia varies with age and gender, with prevalence ranging from 10 to 28 percent.[13,14] Chronic hypnotic usage has varied between 10 and 16 percent in Western civilizations.[13,14] In general, surveys have found that chronic and frequent usage of hypnotics increases with age, and that the most common consumer is a widowed, divorced, or separated woman older than 50 years. However, in surveys in the San Francisco Bay area and in San Diego, 58 percent of those aged 6 to 14 years and 56 percent of those aged 15 to 19 years reported a sleep problem at the time of the survey; few sought medical attention. Such data indicate that many subjects with sleep problems go unrecognized.

The epidemiology of parasomnias has not been studied adequately in the general population. Arousal disorders such as sleepwalking, confusional arousals, and sleep terrors occur primarily during childhood and rarely persist during adulthood. The prevalence of sleep terrors in childhood ranges from 1.0 to 6.5 percent, whereas the prevalence in adults is not known. Sleepwalking has a prevalence in adults ranging from 0.5 to 3 percent and is not gender related.[13]

DIAGNOSTIC TESTS

Different approaches have been used to investigate sleep and its pathologies. Subjective ratings, validated scales, and questionnaires such as the Stanford Sleepiness Scale and Epworth Sleepiness Scale have often been used to determine levels of sleepiness. Sleep disorders can be evaluated utilizing polygraphic monitoring of sleep and wakefulness. Currently, the most commonly utilized tests include the following:

1. Nocturnal or 24-hour polygraphic monitoring, i.e., PSG
2. Portable monitoring

3. The multiple sleep latency test (MSLT)
4. The maintenance of wakefulness test (MWT)
5. Psychomotor vigilance testing
6. Videopolysomnography
7. Pupillography
8. Actigraphy.

Polysomnography

The term *polysomnography* denotes the nocturnal or 24-hour monitoring of sleep and wakefulness and their impact on biologic functions. PSG generally is performed under conditions conducive to natural sleep, with the patient monitored remotely from a separate room. The ideal setting for the patient is a private, quiet room that can be darkened as necessary. Numerous variables are recorded during sleep including EEG (sleep staging), EOG, submental EMG, nasal or oral airflow, respiratory effort, oximetry, electrocardiogram (ECG), tibialis anterior EMG, and position monitoring. Depending upon the clinical diagnosis and protocol implemented, other measurable factors such as transcutaneous carbon dioxide (CO_2) or end-tidal gas analysis, extremity muscle activity, motor activity/movement, extended video-EEG, penile tumescence, esophageal pressure, gastroesophageal reflux, continuous blood pressure, and snoring activity may be added.[7,15] To determine the type of study required, it is important to know the reason that the PSG is being undertaken.

INDICATIONS

PSG is indicated routinely in the following circumstances[15–17]:

1. Diagnosis of sleep-related breathing disorders (a full-night PSG is recommended).
2. Titration of positive airway pressure in patients with sleep-related breathing disorders (a full night of PSG is recommended). PSG with titration is indicated for patients with respiratory disturbance index (RDI) of greater than 15 or patients with RDI greater than or equal to 5 who are excessively sleepy. A cardiorespiratory PSG (without EEG leads) should not be utilized for titration. A split-night study (initial diagnostic followed by titration of continuous positive airway pressure, or CPAP, during PSG on the same night) is an alternative to the full-night diagnostic followed by a full night of titration under the following four criteria:
   a. An apnea-hypopnea index of at least 40 is documented during a minimum of 2 hours of diagnostic PSG.
   b. An apnea-hypopnea index of 20 to 40 (based on clinical judgment) is documented during a minimum of 2 hours of diagnostic PSG.
   c. At least 3 hours of CPAP titration is carried out and PSG documents that CPAP eliminates or nearly eliminates the respiratory events during REM and non-REM sleep, including during supine REM sleep.
   d. A second full night of PSG for CPAP titration is performed if the diagnosis of sleep-related breathing is confirmed but criteria (b) and (c) are not met.
3. Preoperative evaluation for obstructive sleep apnea (OSA) in all patients prior to undergoing surgery of the upper airway for snoring or sleep apnea.
4. Assessment of treatment results of oral appliance therapy.
5. Assessment of treatment results after sleep apnea surgery in patients with moderate to severe OSA.
6. Evaluation of patients with sleep apnea whose symptoms recur after initial good response to either surgical or dental treatment.
7. Assessment of treatment results in patients on CPAP therapy who have either gained or lost substantial weight to determine the need for continued therapy or for the assessment of adequacy of CPAP pressures in symptomatic patients.
8. Evaluation of patients with systolic or diastolic heart failure with nocturnal symptoms of sleep-related breathing disorders (snoring, disturbed sleep, nocturnal dyspnea) who remain symptomatic despite optimal medical management of congestive heart failure. Additionally, as guidelines, the AASM recommends that patients with coronary artery disease be evaluated for sleep apnea and a sleep study be performed if OSA is suspected. Patients referred for evaluation of significant tachyarrhythmias or bradyarrhythmias should be questioned about symptoms of sleep apnea. A sleep study is indicated if questioning results in a reasonable suspicion that OSA or central sleep apnea (CSA) is present.
9. Evaluation of patients with neuromuscular disorders and sleep-related symptoms.
10. Evaluation of patients with suspected narcolepsy. (A whole night of attended PSG is followed the next day by a multiple sleep latency test.)
11. Evaluation of periodic limb movement disorder.
12. Evaluation of insomnia when the diagnosis is uncertain, when behavioral or pharmacologic treatment fails, or when precipitous arousals occur with violent or injurious behavior.

PSG with video and extended bilateral EEG montage is indicated in evaluating the following: sleep-related epilepsy and potentially injurious sleep-related behaviors; unusual or atypical parasomnias; situations with forensic considerations, and presumed parasomnia or sleep-related epilepsy that is unresponsive to therapy.[15] PSG is not useful in differentiating insomnia associated with dementia from other forms of insomnia, including insomnia with depression, or for establishing the diagnosis of insomnia associated with fibromyalgia or chronic fatigue syndrome. It is not indicated for the routine evaluation of transient or chronic insomnia. PSG is not indicated routinely for the diagnosis or treatment of restless legs syndrome except when the diagnosis is uncertain.[15]

OTHER CONSIDERATIONS

In choosing a protocol, various factors must be considered. First, subjects must be able to sleep despite the equipment used. As a result, several nights of recording may be needed to determine the overall problem and its severity. Lighter equipment should be used on certain nights to provide information on sleep and sleep-structure changes; on other nights, more invasive equipment (with poorer sleep) may be used to evaluate the "end-organ" changes during the different sleep states. Second, a general diagnostic protocol may not uncover the cause of a sleep disturbance but may indicate the disturbance and its frequency. Clinical information then refocuses the emphasis of the test so that subsequent nocturnal investigations can affirm the etiologic diagnosis

Third, clinical PSG implies monitoring during the total longest sleeping period, which for most people takes place during the night. Daytime nap testing periods are unacceptable because of the circadian distribution of REM and slow-wave sleep, with REM sleep peaking between 3 and 6 A.M. and slow-wave sleep peaking between 11 P.M. and 2 A.M. Care must be taken to avoid prior sleep deprivation and the use of any pharmacologic agent to induce sleep. Sleep deprivation has an impact on the arousal threshold. Moreover, several investigations performed after one night of sleep deprivation have shown significant changes in respiratory control. Pharmacologic agents affect the control of sleep states and stages.

AASM (2007) SCORING RULES

Controversies have arisen since the establishment of the AASM 2007 rules. Comparison of AASM scoring to Rechtschaffen and Kales scoring in adults has shown significant differences in time in minutes and percentage of total sleep time, such that stage 1 increased compared to N1, stage 2 decreased significantly compared to N2, and wake after sleep onset increased significantly, while stage R changes were age-dependent. Such significant differences in results utilizing the two scoring systems imply that previously collected age-dependent normative values for these parameters using Rechtschaffen and Kales methodology cannot be applied and underscores the need to gather new normative data utilizing AASM criteria from large and representative control groups. In children, comparison of the two scoring systems has also shown significant differences: N1 was significantly greater than stage 1, whereas N2 and R were significantly less than stage 2 and REM sleep. Additionally, there was a relatively low concordance between the two systems for scoring the number of stage shifts per hour, and minutes and percentages of N1/stage 1 and N2/stage 2. The most important controversy involves grouping stages 3 and 4 under the label "N3," particularly in children As mentioned above, association with specific physiologic activities, such as secretion of growth hormone in children, is linked to delta sleep and such linkage is described much better by separating stage 3 from stage 4 non-REM sleep. There is also controversy over the description of sleep-disordered breathing in children. In nonoverweight children with mild hypopneas but important daytime complaints, N3 may be within the expected range, but tabulation of stage 3 and stage 4 separately showed a disappearance of stage 4 in these cases with hyperinflation of stage 3 non-REM sleep. A final commentary is on the absence of a more robust definition of arousals in the 2007 AASM scoring manual, which has been linked to low inter-rater reliability correlation for N2 staging. Understanding arousals may give us a better understanding of the organization of sleep and how it is affected by various disorders.

By contrast, the Cyclic Alternating Pattern (CAP) atlas, which is utilized more in Europe than in North America, places greater emphasis on arousals. CAP is a normal physiologic EEG pattern that is observed commonly during non-REM sleep; periodic recurrence of phasic morphologic patterns are compounded by the alternation of activation phases (Phase A) followed by inhibition phases (Phase B). Three main Phase A EEG patterns are: A1 subtype, with predominantly synchronized EEG activity; A2 subtype, with synchronized and desynchronized EEG activity; and A3 subtype, consisting of primarily desynchronized EEG activity. The Phase A1 subtype is involved in the buildup and maintenance of deep non-REM sleep and may have a protective role in maintaining sleep continuity. Phases A2 and A3 are implicated in maintaining subject arousability. There is a significantly greater opportunity to see Phases A2 and A3 during stage 3 non-REM sleep and Phase A1 during stage 4 non-REM sleep. As Phases A2 and A3 involve scoring of an arousal not necessarily scored with AASM or the Rechtschaffen and Kales criteria, scoring stages 3 and 4 separately may still have advantages compared to combining them under N3.

Sleep Recording

Regardless of the subject's age, the 10–20 electrode placement system recommended by the International Federation of Clinical Neurophysiology is used for polysomnographic recording during sleep. The 2007 AASM scoring manual recommends at least 6 hours of overnight recording for routine PSG and lists technical and digital specifications, including desirable and minimal sampling rates for various parameters and rules for PSG display and manipulation.[7] Differential alternating-current (AC) amplifiers are utilized to record EEG, EOG, EMG, and ECG. Airflow and effort of breathing can be recorded using either AC or direct-current (DC) amplifiers. Oximetry and esophageal pressure monitoring utilize DC channels. EEG and EOG electrodes should have impedance less than 5,000 ohms.

Minimum parameters to be recorded include specified EEG derivations, EOG derivations, chin EMG, leg EMG derivations, airflow parameters, effort parameters, oxygen saturation, and body position. The recommended derivations are right frontal (F4), right central (C4), and right occipital (O2) electrodes referenced to the contralateral mastoid electrode (M1), with backup electrodes at the left frontal (F1), left central (C3), and left occipital (O1) sites referenced to the contralateral mastoid (M2). There is a small electropotential difference between the front and back of the eyeball, with the cornea positive relative to the retina. The EOG records the movement of the corneoretinal potential difference that occurs in the eye. The EOG derivations are: E1–M2 (E1 is placed 1 cm below the left outer canthus); E2–M2 (E2 is placed 1 cm above the right outer canthus). The eye electrodes allow monitoring of the slow, rolling eye movements commonly associated with sleep onset and the rapid eye movements of REM sleep. If needed, additional electrodes can be added infraorbitally or supraorbitally for either the right or left eye to allow detection of vertical eye movements. EMG from the chin is recorded from three electrodes (one in the midline 1 cm above the inferior edge of the mandible; another located 1 cm below the inferior edge of the mandible and 2 cm to the right; and a third electrode located 1 cm below the inferior edge of the mandible and 2 cm to the left).

PSG in children utilizes the same derivations for EEG, EOG, and chin EMG. However, in children and infants with small head size, the distance between the chin EMG electrodes is often reduced from 2 cm to 1 cm and the distance from the eyes in the EOG electrodes is often reduced from 1 cm to 0.5 cm.

The chin EMG electrodes are important for sleep staging, especially REM sleep. Bilateral leg EMG recordings are standard and are utilized to diagnose periodic limb movements of sleep (PLMS). Upper-extremity EMG electrodes are added if REM sleep behavior disorder, parasomnias, or nocturnal seizures are suspected. Snoring is recorded with a microphone. Airflow through the nose is recorded through a nasal pressure monitor and a thermistor monitors oral breathing. The thermistor measures changes in electrical conductance in response to temperature changes in the probe induced by inspiration or expiration. Several scientific bodies over the last 10 years have emphasized that usage of nasal thermistor or oronasal thermocouple should be forbidden when investigating abnormal breathing during sleep as they do not allow the appropriate scoring of hypopneas. However, when the nasal pressure sensor is not working, the AASM (2007) manual allows the use of an oronasal thermal sensor to score hypopneas.

Respiratory effort is monitored either through an esophageal pressure sensor or through calibrated or uncalibrated inductance plethysmography (RIP). The AASM recommends low-frequency filter settings of 0.1 and high-frequency settings of 15 for RIP. At times, a low-frequency setting of 0.05 to 0.01 Hz can allow visualization of possible flattening in the thorax belt, which can occur along with a flattening of the observed signal from a pressure transducer. In a RIP effort belt, the sensing element is a zigzagging wire that runs the entire length of the belt. Since the sensing element covers the entire circumference, all changes in breathing are detected, regardless of the patient's position. The chest and abdominal signals can be summed mathematically or represented individually. Paradoxical breathing leads to a significant decrease of the summed signal. RIP effort sensors are better than Piezo sensors. However, poor signals in RIP effort can occur if the belts are applied either too tightly (leading to cross-sectional change of the chest or abdomen) or too loosely (leading to belt movement and overlapping). To obtain good RIP signals, the belts should be placed near the nipple line (midchest) and just above the umbilicus. An alternative sensor for effort is diaphragmatic/intercostal EMG. Integration of this EMG signal can give even better semiquantitative information on increased inspiratory effort. Monitoring of expiratory muscle EMGs can be useful in recognizing the presence of mild sleep-disordered breathing and neuro-muscular disorders, and during nasal CPAP calibration as an indicator of the persistence of an abnormal active expiration.

Capnography is the continuous recording of the partial pressure of CO_2 in inspiratory and expiratory gas. A capnometer provides numeric PCO_2 values during inhalation and exhalation. A capnogram continuously depicts PCO_2 as a function of either time or volume. Carbon dioxide monitoring can be performed through either end-tidal capnography ($PEtCO_2$) or transcutaneous CO_2 monitoring. Mainstream or side-stream sampling of the gas is utilized with $EtCO_2$. Side-stream sampling is utilized in most sleep laboratories because the mainstream sensor may not be well tolerated during sleep. Transcutaneous CO_2 monitoring ($tcPCO_2$) is an alternative and is accomplished with pH electrodes placed on the skin (usually the chest). The skin is warmed to 42 to 44°F to increase perfusion; CO_2 diffuses through the skin and is measured. The system has to be calibrated for each use and about 30 minutes of placement on the skin are required before stable measurements can be obtained. The sensor must be moved during the night to prevent skin burns. Capnography is useful in detecting pediatric OSA, alveolar hypoventilation, Cheyne–Stokes respiration, and central sleep apnea.

Body position is recorded continuously by an accelerometer but should be correlated with video or technologist notes (if no video recording is available) during calibration to verify that the position stated is confirmed. Single-lead ECG recording and oximetry are standard. Commercially available oximeters give accurate measurements down to 60 to 50 percent oxygen saturation. It is important to know the sensitivity of the equipment; today, good oximeters use 2 heart beats to provide 1 point on the oximetry curve. In infants, transcutaneous oxygen tension and CO_2 tension are measured with electrodes. It is as simple to derive from the finger oximetry signal a finger plethysmography curve that will show similar data and also identify artifactual pulse oximetry values, which commonly occur in association with body movements and artifactually lower oximetry values. By convention, a downward movement of the finger-plethysmography curve indicates sympathetic activation that may or may not be associated with an EEG arousal. Sympathetic activations are seen commonly with events disturbing sleep such as PLMS or sleep-disordered breathing (SDB) events. The potential negative impact on the cardiovascular system of these repetitive autonomic activations is unknown and is being studied.

Sleep Staging Rules

Sleep stages are scored in 30-second sequential epochs based on EEG, EOG, and EMG findings. If two or more stages are seen in one epoch, the epoch is assigned the stage comprising the greatest portion of the epoch. The reader is referred to the AASM criteria for details of scoring sleep in adults and children.[7] Sleep in infants is variable and the following guidelines for sleep stage scoring are recommended.[6] If there are no recognizable sleep spindles, K-complexes, or high-amplitude 0.5- to 2-Hz slow-wave activity, all epochs of non-REM sleep are scored as stage N. Stage N2 is scored for non-REM epochs that contain sleep spindles or K-complexes. If the remaining non-REM epochs have 20 percent or more of slow-wave sleep, they are scored as stage N. Stage N3 is scored for non-REM epochs with more than 20 percent slow-wave sleep. If the remaining non-REM epochs have no K-complexes or sleep spindles, they are scored as stage N. If non-REM sleep has some epochs containing sleep spindles or K-complexes and other epochs contain sufficient slow-wave activity, it is scored as either N1, N2, or N3. Arousals are scored during N1, N2, or N3, or R if there is an abrupt shift in EEG frequency, including alpha, theta, and/or other frequencies exceeding 16 Hz that last at least 3 seconds, preceded by at least 10 seconds of stable sleep.[6] Arousal during stage R needs concurrent increase in chin EMG tone lasting at least 1 second.

Respiratory Rules

The AASM-specified sensor for detecting absence of airflow (apnea) is an oronasal thermal sensor, with a nasal pressure transducer designated as an alternate sensor, if the thermistor is malfunctioning. Determination of an apnea is more accurate when both oral thermistor and the nasal cannula pressure transducer waveforms are associated. The sensor for detecting absence of airflow (apnea) is an oronasal sensor, while the sensor for detection of airflow for identification of a hypopnea is a nasal air pressure transducer with or without square root transformation of the signal. If the nasal pressure sensor fails, then the oronasal thermal sensor should be used for scoring hypopneas. The sensor for detection of respiratory effort is either esophageal manometry or RIP. Piezoelectric sensors and strain gauges are qualitative monitors and are not recommended by the AASM. The sensor for detection of blood oxygen is pulse oximetry with a maximum acceptable signal averaging time of 3 seconds. This is because longer averaging times dampen the signal and lead to underestimation of oxygen saturation. Acceptable methods for assessing alveolar hypoventilation are either transcutaneous PCO_2 or end-tidal PCO_2 monitoring.

For adults, the AASM scoring manual classifies respiratory events based upon various parameters which include event duration, amplitude of the breath, associated desaturation, and/or arousal. An apnea refers to a reduction of 90 percent or more in flow. A hypopnea consists of at least a 30 percent reduction in flow associated with a 4 percent desaturation or a reduction in flow of at least 50 percent associated with a 3 percent desaturation. Apneas and hypopneas are classified as either obstructive, central, or mixed, depending upon the presence of effort in the thoracic or abdominal sensors. Respiratory event-related arousals (RERA) consist of a sequence of breaths lasting at least 10 seconds associated with increasing respiratory effort or flattening of the nasal pressure waveform associated with an arousal; the event does not meet criteria for either apnea or hypopnea. Apneas, hypopneas, and RERA should last at least 10 seconds. Cheyne–Stokes respiration refers to a crescendo–decrescendo pattern of breathing that lasts at least 10 minutes or recurs in at least 5 cycles per hour of sleep. Hypoventilation in adults refers to an increase of more than 10 mm Hg in $PaCO_2$ during sleep, in comparison to an awake, supine value.

Criteria for respiratory events during sleep for infants and children can be used for children younger than 18 years, but the individual physician can choose to score children aged 13 years or more using adult criteria. Definitions of apneas, hypopneas, and RERAs differ from the adult criteria. For mixed and obstructive apneas, the event duration in children is at least two missed breaths. Central apneas in children are either (1) 20 seconds or more or (2) two or more missed breaths in duration, associated with either arousal or awakening or a desaturation of 3 percent or more. A hypopnea is scored when there is a reduction of 50 percent or more in nasal pressure amplitude lasting at least the duration of two missed breaths and is associated with an arousal, awakening, or more than 3 percent desaturation. A RERA in children consists of flattening and an amplitude drop of less than 50 percent of the nasal waveform or an esophageal pressure (Pes) crescendo of inspiratory effort lasting at least the duration of two missed breaths and is associated with noisy breathing, snoring, and elevation in end-tidal PCO_2 or transcutaneous PCO_2, or visual evidence of increased respiratory effort. Classifying hypopneas into obstructive, central, or mixed types requires the use of either esophageal manometry or calibrated RIP sensors. Sleep-related hypoventilation is diagnosed when 25 percent or more of the total sleep time is spent with either end-tidal or transcutaneous PCO_2 exceeding 50 mmHg. Periodic breathing is scored if there are more than three episodes of central apnea lasting more than 3 seconds, separated by no more than 20 seconds of normal breathing.

There are controversies concerning these rules, mainly regarding the definition of hypopnea. Limitations of the current definitions have led several groups to present different scoring systems, more particularly in Europe, but also in North America. The dissension is particularly important when scoring sleep-disordered breathing events in children.

Cardiac Event Scoring Rules

These rules provide definitions for various arrhythmias noted during the sleep period. (The ECG sensor is lead II.[7]) Unlike definitions during the wake period, sinus tachycardia during sleep refers to sustained heart rate exceeding 90 beats per minute, while sinus bradycardia during sleep refers to sustained heart rate of less than 40 beats per minute.

Movement Rules

These clarify definitions for scoring significant leg movement events and series of periodic leg movements (PLM).[7] Electrode placement on the anterior tibialis, amplitude of the baseline deflection, impedance, and sensitivity settings are specified in the AASM scoring manual.

Periodic Leg Movements

A significant leg movement is characterized by an increase equal to or greater than 8 µV in EMG voltage over resting EMG with a duration of between 0.5 and 10 seconds. A PLM series consists of at least four consecutive significant leg movements with an interonset interval of 5 to 90 seconds.

Bruxism

Bruxism is a stereotyped disorder during sleep characterized by either tooth grinding or clenching. Jaw contractions can either be tonic, sustained jaw clenching, or phasic repetitive muscle contractions termed rhythmic masticatory muscle activity (RMMA). Bruxism is scored under the following circumstances: (1) if there are brief elevations of chin EMG that are 0.25 to 2 seconds in duration and if at least three elevations occur in a regular sequence; or (2) if sustained chin EMG duration exceeds 2 seconds.

REM Sleep Behavior Disorder

This disorder is characterized by either or both of the following: sustained muscle activity (tonic activity) in REM sleep in the chin EMG or excessive transient muscle activity during REM sleep in the chin or limb EMG (in a 30-second epoch of REM sleep divided into 10 sequential 3-second mini-epochs, at least 5 of the mini-epochs contain a burst of transient muscle activity). Amplitude is at least four times the amplitude in the background and phasic bursts are 0.1 to 5.0 seconds in duration.

Rhythmic Movement Disorder

This refers to a cluster of rhythmic movements (four or more individual movements of 0.5- to 2-Hz frequency with amplitude twice that of the background EMG activity). Time-synchronized video PSG in addition to polysomnographic criteria is needed for the diagnosis. Bipolar surface electrodes should be placed to record from the large muscle groups involved.

Optional Movements to Score

1. Alternating leg muscle activation (ALMA) series consists of four or more ALMAs (discrete and alternating bursts of leg muscle activity with a frequency of 0.5 Hz to 3.0 Hz).
2. Hypnagogic foot tremor (HFT) consists of a train of four or more bursts with a frequency of 0.3 to 4 Hz.
3. Excessive fragmentary myoclonus (EFM) consists of five or more EMG potentials per minute with maximum EMG burst duration of 150 msec. At least 20 minutes of non-REM sleep with EFM must be recorded.

Portable Monitoring

There are three categories of portable monitoring devices: (1) type 2, comprehensive portable PSG with a minimum of seven channels (EEG, EOG, chin EMG, ECG, airflow, respiratory effort, and oxygen saturation); (2) type 3, modified portable sleep apnea testing that includes a minimum of four channels (at least two channels of respiratory movement or airflow and respiratory movement plus ECG and oxygen saturation); and (3) type 4, continuous single or dual biparameter recording. (Type 1 is the polysomnogram with all regular channels.) A high rate of data loss in the unattended setting has been reported with type 2 devices.[17]

The AASM's Portable Monitoring (PM) Taskforce[18] issued updated clinical guidelines in 2007 for the use of portable monitoring in the diagnosis of OSA in adults. The taskforce limited their review to type 3 devices. The taskforce guidelines specifically recommend that these studies be performed only in conjunction with a comprehensive sleep evaluation by a board-certified or board-eligible sleep specialist. It is important to understand the indications, limitations, and contraindications for these various tests, as advised by the 2007[18] and 2003 taskforces.[17]

Multiple Sleep Latency Test

The MSLT (Fig. 33-6) is the gold standard for objective measurement of sleepiness by quantifying the time required for falling asleep. The AASM's 2005 practice parameters detail the indications and protocol for the MSLT.[19,20] The MSLT is used as part of the clinical evaluation of patients with suspected narcolepsy or idiopathic hypersomnia. The MSLT is not routinely indicated in the initial evaluation and workup of OSA or in the assessment of change following treatment with CPAP. The MSLT is not routinely indicated for evaluation of sleepiness in medical and neurologic disorders (other than narcolepsy), insomnia, or circadian rhythm disorders. Standardized MSLT protocols must be followed strictly.[19]

The patient completes a 1-week sleep log prior to the MSLT so that the sleep–wake schedule can be assessed. This is important in that cumulative sleep deprivation could affect the MSLT results. Stimulants, stimulant-like medications, and REM-suppressing medications ideally should be stopped 2 weeks before the MSLT. The timing of the patient's other medications (e.g., antihypertensives, insulin, etc.) should be reviewed by the sleep clinician before MSLT testing in order to minimize any undesired stimulating or sedating properties of the medications. A urine drug screen is performed on the day of the MSLT to detect the presence of drugs that could affect sleep. The MSLT must be performed immediately following PSG recorded during the individual's major sleep period. The PSG is done in order to detect nocturnal sleep disorders that might artifactually produce short daytime sleep latencies. The test should not be performed after a split night recording. The total sleep time (TST) on the preceding night should be 6 hours or more. This point is crucial because abnormal nocturnal sleep negates the usefulness of the MSLT as a diagnostic tool (e.g., in narcolepsy).

The MSLT consists of five nap opportunities performed at 2-hour intervals. The initial nap opportunity begins 1.5 to 3 hours after termination of the nocturnal recording.

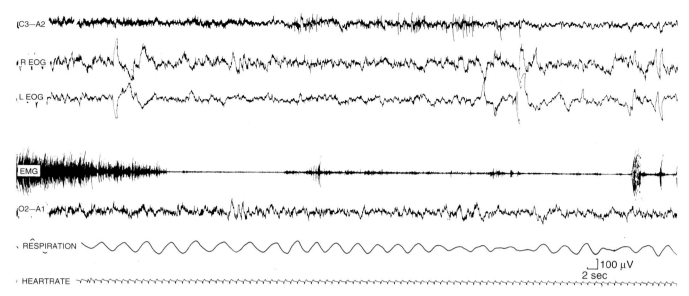

FIGURE 33-6 ■ Example of a sleep-onset period of rapid eye movement (REM) in a narcoleptic. Note the abrupt disappearance of muscle tone (channel 4 from the top); appearance of rapid eye movements of REM sleep (channels 2 and 3, left part of the figure); and low-amplitude, mixed-frequency electroencephalogram (channels 1 and 5). This REM sleep period does not differ from one seen in a normal subject. Its early appearance at sleep onset is the abnormal feature.

A shorter four-nap test may be performed but this test is not reliable for the diagnosis of narcolepsy unless at least two sleep-onset REM periods have occurred. Standardization of test conditions is critical for obtaining valid results. Sleep rooms should be dark and quiet during testing. Room temperature should be set based on the patient's comfort level. Smoking should be stopped at least 30 minutes prior to each nap opportunity. Vigorous physical activity should be avoided during the day and any stimulating activities by the patient should end at least 15 minutes prior to each nap opportunity. The patient must abstain from any caffeinated beverages and avoid unusual exposures to bright sunlight. A light breakfast is recommended at least 1 hour prior to the first trial, and a light lunch is recommended immediately after the termination of the second noon trial. The conventional recording montage for the MSLT includes central EEG (C3–A2, C4–A1) and occipital (O1–A2, O2–A1) derivations, left and right eye EOGs, mental/submental EMG, and ECG. Prior to each nap opportunity, patients should be asked if they need to go to the bathroom or need other adjustments for comfort. With each nap opportunity the subject is instructed to lie quietly, in a comfortable position, with eyes closed, and try to fall asleep. The same instructions should be given prior to every test. Immediately after these instructions, bedroom lights are turned off, signaling the start of the test. Between naps, the patient should be out of bed and prevented from sleeping. This generally requires continuous observation by a laboratory staff member.

Sleep-onset latency refers to the interval in minutes from lights out to the first epoch of any stage of sleep, including stage 1 sleep. Sleep onset is defined as the first epoch exceeding 15 seconds of cumulative sleep in a 30-second epoch. The absence of sleep on a nap opportunity is recorded as a sleep latency of 20 minutes. This latency is included in the calculation of mean sleep latency (MSL). In order to assess for the occurrence of REM sleep, the clinical MSLT continues for 15 minutes from after the first epoch of sleep. The duration of 15 minutes is determined by "clock time," and is not determined by a sleep time of 15 minutes. REM latency is taken as the time of the first epoch of sleep to the beginning of the first epoch of REM sleep, regardless of the intervening stages of sleep or wakefulness. A nap session is terminated after 20 minutes if sleep does not occur. Events that represent deviation from standard protocol or conditions should be documented by the sleep technologist for review by the interpreting sleep clinician. The MSLT report should include the start and end times of each nap or nap opportunity, latency from lights out to the first epoch of sleep, mean sleep latency (arithmetic mean of all naps or nap opportunities), and number of sleep-onset REM periods (defined as greater than 15 seconds of REM sleep in a 30-second epoch).

The International Classification of Sleep Disorders categorizes sleepiness as mild (10 to 15 minutes sleep-onset latency), moderate (5 to 10 minutes), and severe (less than 5 minutes).[21] Various physiologic factors affect mean sleep latency.[20] Sleep deprivation, hypnotic ingestion, barbiturate disruption, or sleep fragmentation decreases mean sleep latency.[20] Stimulant ingestion increases mean sleep latency.[20] Age also influences mean sleep latency; young adults have the shortest MSL while prepubescent children have the longest latencies.[20] Anxiety and stress can prolong sleep latency, whereas depression may shorten sleep latency in some patients.[20] Moscovitch and associates reported that 85 percent of narcoleptic subjects have mean sleep latency scores of 5 minutes or less.[22]

Although the MSLT is utilized primarily to evaluate complaints of sleepiness, it can also help to distinguish physical tiredness or fatigue from true sleepiness, because the former can show prolonged sleep latencies.[23] In addition to the mean sleep latency, the number of sleep-onset REM periods, defined as REM sleep occurring within 15 minutes of sleep onset, is determined. The presence of two or more of such periods during an MSLT has been noted in 80 percent of narcoleptic subjects and in 6.6 percent of non-narcoleptic subjects.[23] However, some subjects with typical narcolepsy-cataplexy show no sleep-onset REM periods at first testing; in some cases, the test must be performed for four successive days to demonstrate the presence of two or more sleep-onset REM periods in these subjects.[9] Sleep-onset REM periods have been reported in non-narcoleptic adolescents who were phase-delayed and who were tested at a time when their circadian system had a high probability of initiating REM sleep.[24] In addition, they have been described in 17 percent of normal young adults who were probably chronically sleep-deprived.[25]

Maintenance of Wakefulness Test

The MWT measures the ability to stay awake under soporific conditions for a defined period of time.[19] A valid MWT can be obtained only after the patient has experienced an adequate quantity and quality of nocturnal sleep during the night prior to the MWT and the patient reports feeling normally awake and alert on the day of the test. The findings on the test are correlated with the clinical history. The MWT 40-minute protocol is recommended when objective data are needed to assess an individual's ability to remain awake. Performance of PSG the night before is optional. The MWT 40 can be used to assess an individual's ability to remain awake when inability to remain awake constitutes a public or personal safety issue, and to assess the response to treatment in patients with excessive sleepiness.

The recommended 40-minute MWT protocol is published elsewhere.[19] The test should be performed by an experienced technologist. In brief, the MWT consists of four trials performed at 2-hour intervals, with the first trial beginning about 1.5 to 3 hours after the patient's usual wake-up time. The first trial usually starts at 0900 or 1000 hours. The clinician decides on whether to use sleep logs prior to the MWT or to perform a PSG prior to MWT (i.e., PSG on the night preceding the MWT is not mandatory). The room should be insulated maximally from external light. The light source should be positioned slightly behind the subject's head such that it is just out of the field of vision, and should deliver an illuminance of 0.10 to 0.13 lux at the corneal level. (A 7.5-W night light can be used, placed 1 foot off the floor and 3 feet laterally removed from the subject's head.) Room temperature should be based on the patient's comfort level. The subject should be seated in bed, with the back and head supported by a bed rest (bolster pillow), such that the neck is not flexed or extended uncomfortably. The use of tobacco, caffeine, and any medications by the patient before and during MWT should be decided by the sleep clinician before MWT. Drug screening may be indicated to ensure that sleepiness–wakefulness on the MWT is not influenced by substances other than medically prescribed drugs. A light breakfast is recommended at least 1 hour prior to the first trial, and a light lunch is recommended immediately after the termination of the second noon trial. The conventional recording montage for the MWT includes central EEG (C3–A2, C4–A1) and occipital (O1–A2, O2–A1) derivations, left and right eye EOGs, mental/submental EMG, and ECG. Prior to each trial, patients should be asked if they need to go to the bathroom or need other adjustments for comfort. The subject is instructed to lie still and remain awake for as long as possible, looking directly ahead, and not directly at the light.

Sleep onset is defined as the first epoch exceeding 15 seconds of cumulative sleep in a 30-second epoch. Trials are ended after 40 minutes if no sleep occurs, or after unequivocal sleep, defined as three consecutive epochs of stage 1 sleep, or one epoch of any other stage of sleep. A record is made of start and stop times for each trial, sleep latency, total sleep time, stages of sleep achieved for each trial, and the mean sleep latency (the arithmetic mean of the four trials).

The MWT is most useful in assessing the effects of sleep disorders or of medications upon the ability to remain awake. Compared to the MSLT, the MWT may be more sensitive in detecting treatment effects and in detecting the effects of the manipulation of the previous night's sleep quality and quantity on daytime alertness. The MWT has been utilized in clinical practice to help determine efficacy of therapy and for the determination of work status in individuals whose occupations carry a high risk of injury should the patient fall asleep (e.g., truck drivers, pilots). The average sleep latency for normal individuals for the 40-minute MWT is 35.2 minutes.[26] Narcoleptic patients have a mean sleep latency of 10 minutes.

Pupillometry

Electronic pupillometry documents pupillary size and changes in diameter. Wakefulness is associated with a large, stable pupil, whereas a constricted, unstable pupil suggests sleepiness. There are no reference standards for this method. A study comparing narcoleptics with normal controls showed greater pupillary instability in narcoleptics with no difference in pupillary diameter.[27]

Vigilance Performance Tests

The psychomotor vigilance task (PVT), a computer-based test, is a chronometric measure of an individual's reaction to specified small changes in a labile environment. Subjects are instructed to respond to a digital signal on a computer terminal by pressing a key. Errors of omission and commission are recorded. The primary outcome measures of PVT performance, lapses, are defined as reaction times exceeding 500 msec or failure to react.[28] The PVT lapses are believed to represent perceptual, processing, or executive failures in the central nervous system (CNS). Lapses constitute highly sensitive measures of the effects of sleep deprivation, or sleep restriction, on attention and vigilance.[29–31] Impairment in executive functioning is reflected in another measure, the PVT count of false responses (responding when no stimulus is presented).[32] PVT has been utilized as an objective indicator of cognitive impairment in conditions of chronic sleep restriction,[29,33,34] partial sleep loss, sleepiness,[35] and napping.[36] Primary insomniacs responded faster on simple vigilance tasks and slower on complex vigilance tasks than controls.[37] Sleep therapy effectively restored normal performance, suggesting that performance decline with increasing neurocognitive tasks may be an early measure of neurocognitive sequelae of insomnia.[37] The PVT results also correlated with objective measures of sleepiness in studies of OSA patients and sleep-deprived patients.[29,38] In patients with OSA, vigilance and sustained attention are impaired, as shown by PVT results.[39] The decline in PVT performance is worse in older female subjects,[40] subjects with higher body mass index,[40] more sleep loss (total sleep deprivation, chronic partial sleep restriction, and sleep fragmentation),[21] and

higher apnea-hypopnea index.[39] PVT performance may also be a good marker of fatigue.[41]

Sleep deprivation leads to lapses in attention and to slowed responses during driving. Driving simulation tests measure the effects of sleep deprivation and alertness through the use of repetitive tasks and evaluation of declining performance. For instance, Steer Clear is a driving simulator that tests the ability to avoid obstacles on a monotonous drive, without steering or tracking. Using Steer Clear, Findley and co-workers reported that narcoleptic patients and patients with sleep apnea hit more obstacles than did control subjects.[42] Patients who performed poorly on this test manifested decreased vigilance, and these patients actually had a significantly higher number of vehicular accidents. The divided-attention driving task simulator utilizes tracking and visual search in its performance evaluation. The subject must observe visual cues in the periphery and steer. Using this simulator, George and colleagues reported that, as a group, patients with untreated sleep apnea or narcolepsy performed worse than did the control group, although some patients performed as well or better than some controls.[43] These findings indicate that vigilance is not always impaired in sleepy patients.

Videoelectroencephalography-Polysomnography

Videoelectroencephalography-polysomnography (VEEG-PSG) combines simultaneous PSG and video-EEG to evaluate nocturnal events in patients with sleep disorders such as epilepsy, rhythmic movement disorder, non-REM arousal disorders, REM sleep behavior disorder, and psychiatric disorders (e.g., panic attacks or dissociative disorders). This technique provides the capability to record, study, and correlate behavior with neurophysiologic and cardiorespiratory parameters and to detect ictal and interictal epileptiform abnormalities. The AASM Standards of Practice Committee stated that PSG, including video-EEG with an extended bilateral montage, is indicated in the diagnosis of paroxysmal arousals or other sleep disruptions that are thought to be seizure-related when the initial evaluation and results of a standard EEG are inconclusive.[15]

Actigraphy

Actigraphy utilizes small, portable devices that record movement over extended periods of time. A minimum recording of three consecutive 24-hour periods is required. The indications for actigraphy were updated in the AASM 2007 practice parameters.[44] Actigraphy is a valid tool to assist in determining sleep patterns in normal, healthy adult populations, normal infants and children, and patients suspected of certain sleep disorders. It is indicated in the evaluation of patients with advanced sleep-phase syndrome (ASPS), delayed sleep-phase syndrome (DSPS), and shift work disorder. Some evidence suggests its usefulness in evaluating other circadian rhythm disorders, such as jet-lag disorder and non–24-hour sleep–wake syndrome (including that associated with blindness). It can also characterize the circadian rhythms and sleep patterns and disturbances of patients with insomnia and hypersomnia. When PSG is not available, actigraphy can be utilized to estimate total sleep time in patients with OSA.

EXAMPLES OF POLYGRAPHIC PROTOCOLS

Polygraphic Monitoring of Patients with Suspected Sleep Apnea Syndromes

The sensors and derivations follow AASM 2007 Scoring Guidelines.[7] Prior to starting the recording, physiologic calibrations are performed and artifacts should be corrected. After satisfactory calibration, the patient is told to assume a comfortable sleeping position and attempt to fall asleep. Monitoring and recording during the night with appropriate documentation are performed. When the study is ended, the equipment is calibrated, and the patient completes the morning questionnaire. Although the procedure described here is utilized commonly, specialized protocols may be helpful for evaluating specific conditions.

Upper airway resistance and respiratory efforts can be evaluated indirectly with measurement of esophageal pressure changes by using a calibrated esophageal balloon or Milliard catheter. To obtain direct measurement of upper airway resistance, an oronasal mask, a heated pneumotachometer, and a transducer have to be used to determine flow.

Measuring endoesophageal pressure by inserting either an endoesophageal balloon (Anode Rubber Plating Company, Houston, TX) or a catheter-tip pressure transducer (Bio-Tech BT6F, Bio-Tech Instruments, Pasadena, CA) on an infant feeding tube also conclusively determines the type of apnea. A series of increasingly negative endoesophageal pressures, following from and terminated by an interval during which the pressure variation with respiratory effort is consistent with waking values, may indicate the presence of airway obstruction indirectly. When esophageal pressure measurements are not available,

pulse transit time has been utilized. Pulse transit time, defined as the time taken for pulse pressure to travel from the aortic valve to the periphery, is correlated inversely with blood pressure. It is measured as the time between the R wave on the ECG and the arrival of the pulse wave at the finger as detected by photoplethysmography.

Cardiac and Hemodynamic Studies and the Sleep–Wake Cycle

PSG may also allow monitoring of risk factors or medical problems that are linked or worsened by sleep and sleep states. Cardiovascular variables can be monitored with invasive and noninvasive techniques. With Swan–Ganz catheters, right ventricular, pulmonary arterial, and wedge pressures can be measured without great difficulty. Systemic arterial lines permit the monitoring of systemic pressures with any of the standard pressure transducers (e.g., model MP-15, Micron Instrument, Los Angeles, CA) coupled to optically isolated polygraph preamplifiers (Model 8805c pressure amplifiers, Hewlett-Packard, Waltham, MA). These studies have been helpful in monitoring the circadian appearance of some types of angina pectoris, particularly Prinzmetal angina. With accurate noninvasive blood pressure recorders, long-term studies of blood pressure in normal and hypertensive subjects using Doppler or Finapres (Ohmeda, Inc., Englewood, CO) systems are possible. Noninvasive electrical impedance systems have been validated to measure heart rate, stroke volume, and cardiac output (BioMed Diagnostics, San Jose, CA). These systems are particularly useful when the number of ventricular arrhythmias is limited. Impedance cardiography (BioZ system, Cardiodynamics, San Diego, CA) utilizes baseline and dynamic impedance to calculate various hemodynamic parameters.[45] Autonomic testing can also be conducted and correlated with PSG recordings. Batteries of tests, such as those proposed by Valensi,[46] can be utilized to determine parasympathetic and sympathetic integrity. A recent study in children with OSA demonstrated increased basal sympathetic activity during wakefulness and an impaired reaction to several physiologic stimuli, which was dependent on disease severity.[47]

Studies indicate a direct relationship between sleep stages and arterial pressure changes. The lowest systolic and diastolic values are always noted in stage 3 and 4 non-REM sleep. During REM sleep, there is a variability in systemic arterial pressure that does not correlate with changes in heart rate or arterial tone. Systemic arterial pressure during REM sleep may increase abruptly with bursts of random eye movements.

There have been lengthy speculations on the diurnal variation in heart rate observed in normal volunteers and patients with heart disease. Although the overall trend is for ventricular arrhythmias to decrease during sleep, some patients may demonstrate an increase in ventricular irritability consistently during sleep.

Studies of Gastrointestinal Secretions

Gastroesophageal reflux during sleep has a dual component: the retrograde flow of gastric contents through the gastroesophageal junction and impaired esophageal acid clearing. For most patients with gastroesophageal reflux, ambulatory pH monitoring is performed. The pH probe is positioned 5 cm above the lower esophageal sphincter. Dual pH probes can record from the proximal and distal esophagus. The pH can also be monitored by wireless telemetry. Patients suspected of having sleep-related reflux and pulmonary aspiration may benefit from PSG recording during overnight pH monitoring.[48] This may also

help demonstrate whether reflux itself is triggered by arousal responses due to disturbed sleep. To evaluate sphincter pressure and determine the presence of abnormal reflux, gastrointestinal secretions from normal volunteers and patients have been studied in relation to the REM–non-REM cycle (Fig. 33-7). The most commonly performed sphincter and reflux studies involve the gastroesophageal or gastroduodenal junctions. Reflux is defined as a decline in pH of the distal esophagus below a level of 4.0, and clearance is characterized by a return of esophageal pH to this level. A recent study utilized overnight PSG with manometry, multichannel impedance/pH recordings, and synchronization devices to determine upper esophageal sphincter and gastroesophageal junction pressure change during OSA and characterize the gastroesophageal and esophagopharyngeal reflux events during sleep.[49] The study confirmed that the intraesophageal pressure decreased during apneic events.[49] However, this decrease was counterbalanced by an increase in upper esophageal sphincter and gastroesophageal junction pressures during apnea, with

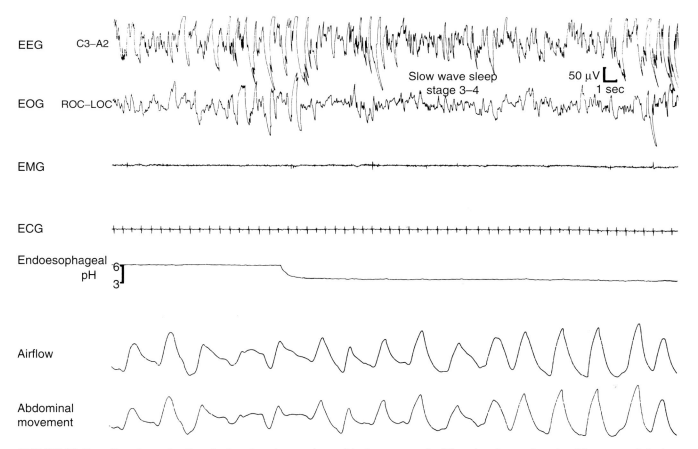

FIGURE 33-7 ■ Esophageal reflux during sleep in a patient with dysautonomia. Note the abrupt drop in pH measured during sleep with an esophageal pH electrode (channel 5 from the top). This figure also illustrates very clear stage 4 sleep with high-amplitude slow waves (delta sleep). The submental electromyogram is low (channel 3), not uncommon in stage 3 and stage 4 sleep.

changes of a magnitude that precluded both gastroesophageal and esophagopharyngeal reflux. The pressure changes with inspiration at the gastroesophageal junction likely resulted from contraction of the diaphragmatic crura, rather than from a change in the tone of the smooth muscle lower esophageal sphincter. As a consequence, no gastroesophageal or esophagopharyngeal reflux events were seen during apnea. The prevalence of these events in patients with OSA was similar to that in both healthy subjects and patients with gastroesophageal reflux disease. According to these findings, OSA does not seem to induce either gastroesophageal or esophagopharyngeal reflux events.

These findings differ from results in a prior study which showed that patients with OSA had significantly more gastroesophageal reflux events (number of reflux events over 8 hours and percentage of time spent at pH less than 4) than did normal controls, and 53.4 percent of these events were related temporally to apneas or hypopneas.[50] The latter study only recorded pH from the distal esophagus. Treatment of gastroesophageal reflux may improve OSA. Using omeprazole for 30 days to treat reflux resulted in a 31 percent decline of the mean apnea index and a 25 percent decrease in the respiratory disturbance index in 10 men aged 20 to 64 years.[51]

Sleep-related gastroesophageal reflux has been implicated in sudden infant death syndrome, repetitive bronchopneumonia, and asthma attacks in children, and in the sudden appearance of sleep-related laryngospasm in adults. The Tuttle test (continuous monitoring of esophageal pH over a 24-hour period during nocturnal sleep), performed with monitoring of the heart and respiration, is helpful in determining the frequency or duration of reflux episodes during sleep and their impact on cardiorespiratory variables. A pH probe is placed in the esophagus 5 cm above the esophagogastric junction (cardia). Reflux is documented if the pH drops below 4.0. In children, the mean duration of reflux episodes during sleep positively correlated with the presence of respiratory symptoms.[52]

Studies of Organic Causes of Impotence

The polysomnogram is useful for investigating organic causes of impotence and may help to determine the underlying cause. Studies are usually based on two nights of recording physiologic erections related to REM sleep. Penile rigidity is the single most important polysomnographic measure in assessing erectile dysfunction.[53,54] Rigidity (penile buckling pressure) refers to the minimum force capable of buckling the penile shaft. At the peak of the erection, the buckling pressure is determined and the penis is examined directly. Buckling pressure, which must be measured on a different night from the basic penile tumescence monitoring (Fig. 33-8), can identify an early deficiency when there is some degree of erection but objective signs of impaired function. A system continuously measuring circumference and pressure is commonly used. Axial rigidity of 750 to 1200 grams is seen in normal males. Rigidities of 500 to 749 grams are potentially functional, while rigidities less than 500 grams are abnormal and are rarely sufficient for penetration.[54] An average minimum rigidity of 500 to 650 grams force is needed to achieve vaginal penetration. A general rule is that a rigid, normal-magnitude erection during REM sleep with sustained full tumescence for 5 to 10 minutes represents documentation of adequate erectile capacity and maintenance; therefore, erectile dysfunction under these conditions suggests psychogenic or behavioral etiologies. Exceptions to this rule include pelvic steal syndrome, sensory nerve deficit, acute androgen deficiency, and anatomic problems preventing normal intercourse.[54]

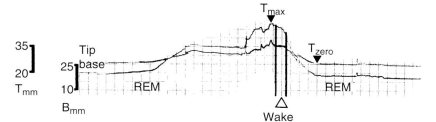

FIGURE 33-8 ■ Measurement of nocturnal penile tumescence during rapid eye movement (REM) sleep to investigate organic impotence in a young insulin-dependent diabetic. Along with the standard polygraphic sleep variables, penile tumescence is measured by using strain gauges placed at the tip and base of the penis. The maximum dilatation (T_{max}) is measured. The patient is awakened, and a picture taken. Detumescence and return to a flaccid penis (T_{zero}) is recorded.

Continuously measured systemic blood pressure may also yield clues about the cause of the problem. Evaluating systemic arterial pressure at the penile dorsal midline with a Doppler system may give valuable information on the presence or absence of localized atheromatous plaque, particularly in patients with diabetes or vascular disorders. In conjunction with evaluation of penile tumescence, samples of blood are obtained at frequent intervals for studying prolactin and testosterone release and their relationship to the sleep–wake and REM–non-REM cycle.

Evaluation of Suspected Sleep-Related Seizures

Many epileptics have seizures that occur mostly or exclusively at night (i.e., "sleep-related epilepsy"). A patient with suspected sleep-related seizures needs detailed clinical evaluation. A comprehensive clinical history must be obtained, and the patient should have a neurologic examination and a routine 2-hour EEG, including wakefulness and sleep, following a night of sleep deprivation. When the initial clinical evaluation and the results of a standard EEG are inconclusive, PSG with additional EEG derivations in an extended bilateral montage and synchronized video recording is recommended.

However, the optimal number and location of electrodes and channels have not been standardized. When the number of EEG channels is limited, the montage selected depends upon the suspected seizure focus. If the history does not localize the seizure focus clinically, published guidelines should be followed; these recommend that at least six channels of EEG be utilized in patients with suspected seizures.[55] The montage should include the following electrode placements: Fp1, Fp2, C3, C4, O1, O2, T3 (now T7), and T4 (now T8).[55]

Foldvary and co-workers conducted a study of blinded EEG analysis of seizures and arousals during video-PSG. Detection of temporal lobe seizure was better using 7 and 18 EEG channels (sensitivity of 82 percent and 86 percent, respectively) than 4 channels (sensitivity of 67 percent).[56] The number of EEG channels did not affect the accuracy of frontal lobe seizure detection.[56] In addition, the training of the readers affected the sensitivity rates when EEG channels were increased.[56] EEG-trained readers increased their accuracy of identifying seizures from 71 percent using 4 channels of EEG at 10 mm/sec to 90 percent on viewing 18 channels at 30 mm/sec. Increasing the number of EEG channels did not improve the accuracy of the sleep medicine–trained readers.[56]

Video recordings are essential in the differentiation of seizures and other nocturnal events. PSG technologists should be trained to recognize behaviors that are likely to be epileptic in nature, to test patients during and after nocturnal events to establish the degree of unresponsiveness and recollection of ictal content, and to determine the presence of lateralizing signs. Technologists should be capable of managing patients during generalized motor seizures and be able to recognize potentially injurious situations such as prolonged seizures or aspiration. In addition, they must be able to cope with postictal violence or aggression.

Long-Term Evaluation of Sleep Disorders

Clinical PSG has its limitations. To evaluate sleep and its pathology in the home environment or outside the sleep laboratory, nonattended monitoring has been implemented. Such monitoring does not replace clinical PSG but is used in conjunction with it to document the patient's complaint and its impact better. Actigraphy is one of the simplest approaches. It may give important information about rest and activity during the 24-hour period and is very helpful in investigating complaints of insomnia or dyschronosis.

Systems that evaluate heart rate, snoring, oxygen saturation, body position, and respiratory variables are helpful in screening for OSA and snoring. Some are pocket-sized and are able to record for 12 hours without an external power source. Others have more channels, transmit over a wireless ethernet link, or record on a palm-sized enclosure. Although these ambulatory devices have many channels and leads, and some can replicate full polysomnograms, they may be prone to gathering more artifactual data.

CLINICAL DISORDERS OF SLEEP IDENTIFIED BY POLYSOMNOGRAPHY

The AASM diagnostic and coding manual classifies sleep disorders into four main categories: (1) dyssomnias; (2) parasomnias; (3) sleep disorders associated with mental, neurologic, or other medical disorders; and (4) proposed sleep disorders.[21] The following is a brief summary of the principal sleep disorders that can be identified with clinical PSG.

Breathing Disorders during Sleep and Sleep Apnea Syndrome

In the United States, adult OSA has a reported prevalence of 4 percent in men and 2 percent in women between the ages of 30 and 60 years,[57] but the actual prevalence may be higher.[58] About 70 to 80 percent of patients with sleep apnea are estimated to be undiagnosed.[59,60] Several books and many review articles have been devoted to this syndrome.[61–64] Symptoms include excessive daytime sleepiness (EDS) or insomnia; fatigue; multiple awakenings at night and nocturia; dryness of the mouth or sore throat on awakening; morning headaches; mood changes with either depression or anxiety; sexual dysfunction with decreased libido and impotence; cognitive deficits with memory and intellectual impairment; decreased vigilance; nocturnal symptoms of restless sleep; loud snoring; frequent episodes of obstructed breathing during the night with gasping or choking; and, occasionally, confusion or disorientation. Children with sleep-disordered breathing have a threefold increase in neurocognitive and behavioral abnormalities. Chervin and co-workers estimated that 5 to 39 percent of attention deficit hyperactivity disorders in children could be attributed to abnormalities in breathing during sleep.[65] Untreated, moderate to severe sleep apnea results in higher accident rates, increased all-cause mortality,[66] and increased heart failure, myocardial infarction, and stroke risk, metabolic dysfunction, and cognitive dysfunction.[67–70] OSA is an independent risk factor for coronary artery disease.[71] The risk of nocturnal (between midnight and 6 A.M.) sudden cardiac death increases with OSA severity, whereas cardiovascular events mostly occur between 6 A.M. and midnight in subjects from the general population.[72] Sleep apnea prevalence is six times higher in patients whose myocardial infarction occurred between midnight and 6 A.M. than in the remaining hours of the day, suggesting that sleep apnea increases the risk of infarction during the night.[73] CPAP treatment reduces the risk for fatal and nonfatal cardiovascular events.[74] OSA is an independent risk factor for hypertension, and hypertension is often associated with sleep apnea.[70–72] The Cochrane Collaboration review found that CPAP therapy reduced mean 24-hour systolic pressure (-7.24 mmHg) and mean diastolic pressure (-3.07 mmHg).[75] Cor pulmonale develops in the most severe forms. Of 500 patients reviewed at the Stanford Sleep Disorders Clinic, two-thirds were at least 10 percent above their ideal weight, although only 7 percent were morbidly obese.[9]

The diagnosis of upper-airway sleep apnea syndrome is based on a nocturnal PSG recording of at least one night's duration. Central, mixed, and obstructive apneas (Figs. 33-9, 33-10, and 33-11) recorded on the polygraphic tracing can be identified, with simultaneous oxygen desaturation and associated cardiac and hemodynamic changes. Over the duration of a sleep period, repetitive obstructive apneic episodes lead to clear hemodynamic changes. In some individuals, systemic arterial blood pressure can increase to dangerously high values (up to 300/220 mmHg). Pulmonary arterial and wedge pressures also increase significantly. Abnormalities in pulmonary wedge pressures during sleep may approach pressures producing pulmonary edema in some patients.[9] Hemodynamic changes are less pronounced if the apnea is intermittent and not repetitive; nocturnal monitoring can be used to ascertain the type of apneic event and thereby select appropriate treatment. Cardiac arrhythmias occur with repetitive, mixed, and obstructive apneas during sleep. They most commonly involve sinus arrest but can also include other types of arrhythmias, including a serious increase in premature ventricular contractions.

OSA syndrome is more common in men than in premenopausal women. When it occurs before menopause in women, the OSA syndrome is usually secondary to micrognathia, other anatomic facial risk factors, or coexisting disease, such as acromegaly or hypothyroidism. Other predisposing factors in patients with sleep apnea include a small oropharynx, macroglossia, enlarged uvula, low-lying soft palate, and enlarged lymphoid tissue. In children, enlarged tonsils and adenoids may play a major role in the appearance of the syndrome. Crowding of the oropharynx, together with absent oropharyngeal muscle contraction during sleep to counteract the increasingly negative pressure of diaphragmatic inspiratory movements, leads to upper-airway collapse. Initially, local abnormalities (type II malocclusion) may induce heavy snoring at night without complete obstruction of the airway. However, factors such as aging, weight increase, oropharyngeal fatty infiltration, upper mandibular overjet, infection, repetitive alcohol intake, sleep fragmentation, and smoking slowly decrease the diameter of the airway until the full-blown syndrome develops. Both progressive hypoxia and sleep fragmentation seriously inhibit the responsiveness of the neuronal network controlling the airway and respiratory-related muscles. The severe repetitive oxygen desaturation, the strong autonomic nervous system changes induced by the repetitive Müller maneuver (an inverse Valsalva maneuver) during sleep, and the resulting cardiovascular abnormalities can be responsible for death during sleep.

The severity of the sleep apnea, presence of coexisting conditions, preferences of patient and physician, and efficacy of the various options determine the treatment regimen. Nonsurgical options include weight loss (10 to 20 percent of body weight in obese individuals); behavioral modification (i.e., avoidance of alcohol, nicotine, sedatives, and sleep deprivation); and positional therapy (i.e., avoidance of supine posture). Modafinil or armodafinil may be utilized as an adjunctive measure for persistent symptomatic sleepiness despite optimal therapy with either surgery or use of mechanical devices (oromandibular appliance or CPAP). The mainstay of therapy for moderate and severe OSA is CPAP. For such patients who are unable or unwilling to tolerate CPAP, surgical options[61,76–79] are available

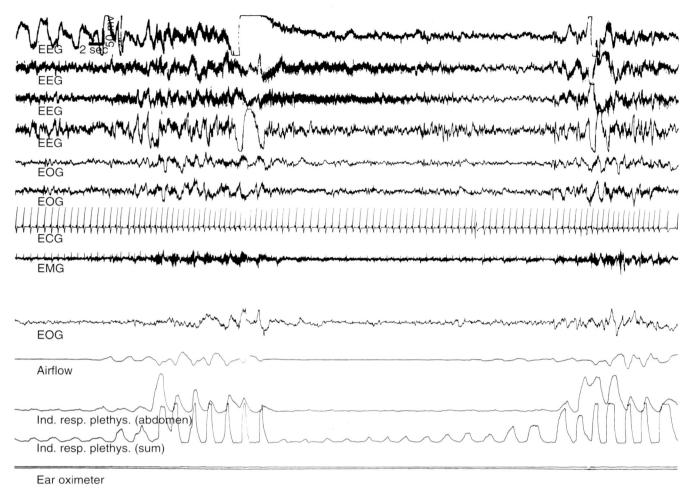

FIGURE 33-9 ■ Example of obstructive sleep apnea in an obese patient. Note the interruption of airflow (channel 10 from the top) with persistence of respiratory efforts (channel 12 from the top). These efforts are monitored with inductive respiratory plethysmography (Ind. resp. plethys.). Abdominal movements (channel 11) are minimal, but efforts increase with a progressive decrease in oxygen saturation (channel 13). On channel 13, the top line indicates the 95 percent SaO_2 level and the bottom line is the patient's SaO_2 measurement by pulse oximetry. The decrease seen here is equal to 10 percent (right side). An increase in systolic and diastolic blood pressure can be seen with arousal and hyperventilation (channel 14).

to relieve site-specific obstruction. Tracheostomy has been shown to be an effective single intervention for OSA but should be considered only when other options do not exist, have failed, or are refused, or when this operation is deemed clinically urgent.[76]

Narcolepsy

Gélineau coined the term *narcolepsy* in 1880 to describe a 38-year-old man with a history of frequent sleep attacks, cataplexy, and sleep paralysis.[80] Despite its long history, narcolepsy is still not well recognized; a 10-year lag between symptom onset and diagnosis is not unusual.[81]

In patients with prepubertal onset of narcolepsy, Guilleminault and Pelayo reported that children with cataplexy had been misdiagnosed previously with seizures, while older children who had been referred for sleepiness or abnormal behavior had been labeled with attention deficit or school performance complaints.[82]

The narcoleptic symptom pentad consists of disturbed nocturnal sleep, excessive daytime sleepiness, cataplexy, hypnagogic hallucinations, and sleep paralysis.[83-85] At night, nearly 50 percent of narcoleptic patients report disturbed sleep with frequent awakenings and prolonged wakefulness, interspersed with frightening dreams. Indeed, REM sleep behavior disorder, sleepwalking, sleep

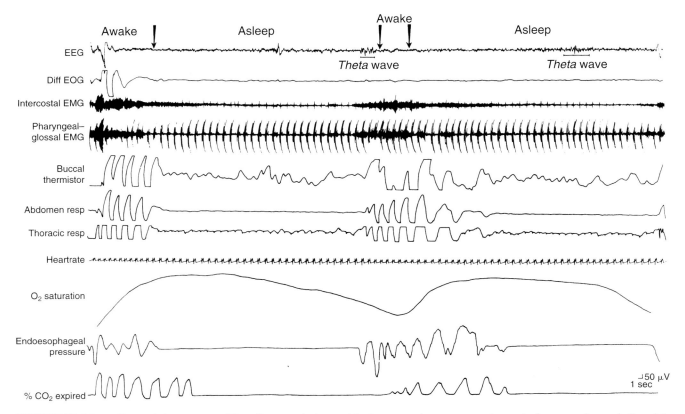

FIGURE 33-10 ■ Central sleep apnea. Note (from top) channel 1, the arousal response at the end of apnea; channels 3 and 4, the disappearance of muscle tone; channel 5, artifact resulting from mouth movements without airflow; channel 9, the drop in oxygen saturation; and channel 10, the absence of esophageal pressure changes.

terrors, and PLMS have a higher prevalence in narcoleptic patients. For many narcoleptics, excessive sleepiness is the first symptom and the most troublesome. Patients can fall asleep readily under monotonous and sedentary conditions. Subjects experience an overwhelming desire to sleep, usually several times daily. These may occur even while performing demanding physical or mental activities. Drowsiness is frequent and interspersed with short micro sleep events characterized by "blanking out" that last a few seconds to minutes. Automatic behavior may result when these occur in salvo. Patients may try to resist drowsiness, but the number of micro sleep events greatly increases. Occasionally, these episodes can last for an hour, if the patient is recumbent. Reduced alertness and vigilance may contribute to the increased frequency of industrial, home, and automobile accidents reported.[86–88] In addition to feeling sleepy, patients report blurred vision, a burning sensation in the eyes, poor memory, impaired thinking, and a "heavy" feeling in the head. As drowsiness worsens, hypnagogic hallucinations or vivid dreamlike states surge. These experiences may be visual, auditory, tactile, or olfactory and can be very complex. Others report floating sensations (levitation) or extracorporeal sensations ("I am above my bed outside my body"). Similar

events can occur on awakening (hypnopompic hallucinations). These hallucinations can be so realistic and vivid that patients act on them upon awakening. The unpleasant effect of hypnagogic hallucinations can be intensified if the patient also experiences sleep paralysis. In 40 to 80 percent of narcoleptic patients, sleep paralysis occurs during the transition between sleep and wakefulness and can be terrifying. Patients are unable to move, open their eyes, speak, or even breathe deeply, but are intensely aware of their weakness and can recollect these events.

Cataplexy is a classic symptom that occurs in 60 to 70 percent of narcolepsy patients. Cataplexy starts within 3 months to 5 years of onset of excessive somnolence.[84] It involves an episodic inhibition of voluntary movements secondary to a sudden drop in muscle tone triggered by emotional factors, such as laughter or surprise, and less frequently by anger or frustration. Episodes usually last a few seconds to 2 minutes, but sometimes up to 30 minutes. Such attacks may occur several times a day or less than once a month. The severity and extent of attacks vary from a state of absolute powerlessness involving the entire musculature to no more than a fleeting sensation of weakness throughout the body. The respiratory and eye muscles usually are

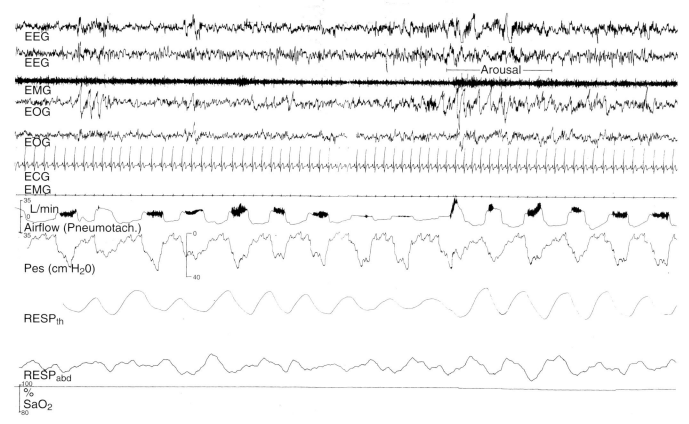

FIGURE 33-11 ■ Example of monitoring of breathing with a pneumotachograph and a facemask, which allows quantification of flow (channel 8). Note on channel 8 the snores associated with each breath. Near the center of the figure, flow abruptly decreases for two breaths. This decrease is associated with a more negative esophageal pressure (channel 9). An arousal is triggered, as indicated by the electroencephalographic channels (1, 2), with an increase in chin electromyogram (channel 3). Following arousal, there is a decrease in the esophageal pressure (Pes) nadir (channel 9), but the subject begins snoring again and the inspiratory esophageal pressure nadir becomes more negative. Oxygen saturation (channel 12) is hardly affected by the two obstructed breaths, but an arousal has been triggered.

spared. Fortunately, falls and injury are rare, as the patient usually has time to stand against a wall or sit while the attack occurs. Consciousness is preserved, although prolonged episodes may lead directly into REM sleep. Cataplexy may be elicited by emotion, stress, or fatigue.[83] Positive emotions, such as laughter, amusement, elation, and repartee, seem to be the most common precipitants, but attacks can also be induced by exercise, frustration, or anger, or by sexual intercourse.[83] Figure 33-12 shows the electrophysiologic features of a cataplectic attack in a patient with narcolepsy. Cataplexy is associated with inhibition of the monosynaptic H and muscle stretch reflexes; during an attack, noting the absence of patellar reflexes may help with the diagnosis.

Status cataplecticus is rare; it is characterized by cataplexy that lasts for hours or days and usually confines the subject to bed. It can be triggered by withdrawal from anticataplectic drugs, such as clomipramine,[89] or by taking prazosin. Functional magnetic resonance imaging

(MRI) studies suggest involvement of the striatal dopaminergic system.[90,91] Single-photon emission computed tomography (SPECT) imaging during status cataplecticus resembles normal REM sleep (with high cingular, orbitofrontal, and putamen activity) but without the other imaging characteristics of REM sleep (no hyperactivation of the pons, amygdala, or occipital cortex), leading to the hypothesis that cataplexy is an intermediate stage between REM sleep and wakefulness.[91]

The prevalence of narcolepsy with cataplexy is estimated at 25 to 50 per 100,000.[92] Among various ethnic groups, 0.03 to 0.16 percent of the general population are affected, with equal predominance among men and women.[83,85]

Symptom onset is usually after age 5 but children with secondary narcolepsy from Niemann–Pick disease type C, diencephalic tumors, or unspecified neurologic causes can present before age 5.[93] Narcolepsy occurs sporadically in most cases, but genetic predisposition and environmental factors are important for the development of

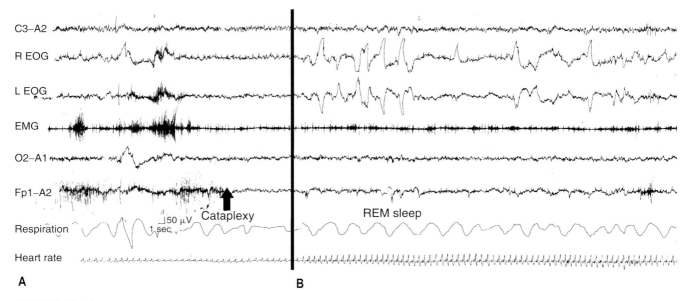

FIGURE 33-12 ▪ **A**, Example of a cataplectic attack in a narcoleptic patient. Abrupt drops in muscle tone accompany the intermittent burst of electromyographic activity (channel 4 from the top). The patient is awake and trying to overcome the mild attack. **B**, Rapid eye movement (REM) sleep in the same patient. Note the bursts of rapid eye movements on channels 2 and 3 from the top. Twitches are present, however, and it is difficult to dissociate cataplexy from REM sleep. The electroencephalographic frequency is 2 Hz slower during REM sleep.

narcolepsy and up to 5 percent of cases may occur in families. First-degree relatives of narcolepsy patients have a 1 to 2 percent risk of development of narcolepsy, which is 10 to 40 times higher than in the general population. Across various ethnic groups, HLA DQB1*0602 is the most specific genetic marker for narcolepsy and it is found in 95 percent of patients with narcolepsy and cataplexy. Low cerebrospinal fluid levels of hypocretin-1 are highly associated with narcolepsy with cataplexy (89.5 percent), particularly in patients with cataplexy who are HLA DQB1*0602-positive (95.7 percent).[94-96] Cerebrospinal fluid hypocretin levels less than 110 pg have a high positive predictive value (94 percent) for narcolepsy with cataplexy.[85,97] Most patients with narcolepsy with cataplexy have hypocretin ligand deficiency resulting from postnatal cell death of approximately 70,000 hypocretin neurons.[97] Involvement of autoimmune mechanisms has been suggested.[97]

The clinical diagnosis of narcolepsy with cataplexy is based on a history of excessive daytime sleepiness occurring almost daily for at least 3 months and a definite history of cataplexy.[21] The diagnosis should be confirmed by overnight PSG followed by MSLT. Overnight polysomnographic findings include sleep latency of less than 10 minutes and the presence of sleep-onset REM periods. The MSLT demonstrates a mean latency of less than 8 minutes (usually less than 5 minutes) and at least two sleep-onset REM periods. Sleep duration prior to the MSLT must be at least 6 hours.

For the correct interpretation of the MSLT, the patient must be free of drugs that influence sleep for at least 15 days or for at least 5 times the half-life of the drug and its longest-acting metabolite; the sleep–wake schedule must have been standardized for at least 7 days before the PSG and documented by sleep log or actigraphy, and nocturnal PSG the night before to exclude other sleep disorders that could mimic narcolepsy with cataplexy. Narcolepsy without cataplexy is diagnosed by excessive daytime sleepiness occurring almost daily for at least 3 months. Cataplexy episodes are either doubtful or atypical. The diagnosis must be confirmed by nocturnal PSG followed by MSLT the next day. If doubt exists, measurement of cerebrospinal fluid hypocretin will resolve the problem. If cataplexy is absent and HLA DQB1*0602 is negative, the chance of having narcolepsy is less than 1 percent, independent of MSLT results.

Idiopathic Hypersomnia

The prevalence of idiopathic hypersomnia currently is estimated at 50 per million.[98] Patients report daytime sleepiness that is not overwhelming; taking long naps (exceeding 1 hour and up to 4 hours) which are not refreshing; difficulty in awakening to usual stimuli; and sleep drunkenness (automatic behavior, confusion, disorientation, and repeated return to sleep).[98-102] Symptoms usually start within the first two decades (mean 16.6 ± 9.4 years[101]) but diagnosis may be delayed until the mid-30s.[98,100] Excessive daytime sleepiness may occur first following a bout of transient insomnia, overexertion, viral illness, general anesthesia, or an abrupt change in the sleep–wake schedule. Two separate groups are recognized: idiopathic hypersomnia with or without long sleep time.[21] Characteristic differences between the two groups have been described.[100] Patients with idiopathic hypersomnia with long sleep time sleep for longer than 10 hours. In contrast, those without a long sleep time have either a normal sleep duration or slightly longer sleep period but less than 10 hours. Hypersomniacs have more frequent slow-wave sleep episodes at the end of the night and more sleep cycles than controls.[100] MSLT demonstrates a mean sleep latency of less than 8 minutes and fewer than two sleep-onset REM periods.[21]

Idiopathic hypersomnia is suspected clinically when the only complaint is constant daytime sleepiness. The absence of auxiliary symptoms (e.g., snoring at night, chronic pulmonary or chest wall diseases, nocturnal sleep disturbances, clear neurologic disorders, depression, and drug intake) is an important negative finding, but polysomnographic evaluation and MSLT currently determine the diagnosis.[102]

Disorders of Initiating and Maintaining Sleep (DIMS)

DIMS AND PSYCHIATRIC DISORDERS

DIMS may be associated with psychiatric disorders, and insomnia is often described as one of the symptoms of the psychiatric syndrome. Generalized anxiety disorders, panic disorders, phobic disorders, hypochondriasis, obsessive-compulsive disorders, and personality disorders can lead to difficulty in falling asleep and frequent awakenings, sometimes with anxiety-provoking dreams. Anxiety or anxiety derivatives (e.g., hypochondriacal concerns) are thought to be responsible for the long sleep latency and the frequent awakenings noted on objective polygraphic monitoring in these subjects. The PSG in anxiety disorders shows increased sleep latency, decreased REM sleep, and reduced sleep efficiency. Patients with panic disorders report difficulty in initiating and maintaining sleep, nonrestorative sleep, and, often, sleep panic attacks. These attacks are non-REM sleep phenomena from which the patient arouses abruptly with shortness of breath, sweating, palpitations, and intense fear. Patients with post-traumatic stress disorder (PTSD) experience difficulty in falling asleep or staying asleep. Such patients have abnormalities in REM sleep including increased REM sleep density, greater sleep fragmentation during REM sleep, and increased transitions from REM sleep to stage 1 or wakefulness.[103]

Insomnia may herald the onset of a first episode of mania or depression. Two types of DIMS can accompany the major affective disorders. The manic phase of bipolar illness may be associated with sleep-onset insomnia and shortened sleep period together with sleep-maintenance problems. Polysomnographic findings during manic episodes show disrupted sleep continuity, short REM latency, and increased REM density,[104] whereas unipolar depression may be associated with early morning awakening and short REM sleep latency. In unipolar depression, the sleep disturbance consists of repeated awakenings in the night, premature (or early morning) awakenings, significantly reduced total sleep time with reduced stage 3 and 4 non-REM sleep, and a short REM sleep latency.[105] In bipolar depression, REM sleep latencies are short, and total sleep time increases whereas stage 3 and stage 4 non-REM sleep decrease. The short REM sleep latency after sleep onset, increased first REM period duration, and increased REM density are important biologic markers of depression.[106]

PSYCHOPHYSIOLOGIC DIMS

Insomnia or difficulty in sleeping is common in the general population, especially in women and non-Caucasians.[106] Psychophysiologic problems are a common cause of DIMS in patients surveyed in American sleep clinics. Psychophysiologic insomnia refers to maladaptive sleep-preventing behaviors, which perpetuate the sleep disturbance. Based on duration of symptoms, psychophysiologic insomnia has been subdivided into two groups: (1) transient and situational; and (2) persistent.

Transient and situational DIMS involves brief periods of disturbed sleep, often induced by an acute emotional arousal or conflict. Transient DIMS does not usually last longer than 3 weeks after the traumatic event. This particular problem is probably the one that should be treated by hypnotics. Individuals with a low threshold for emotional arousal appear to be most vulnerable.

Persistent DIMS[105–109] is defined as a sleep-onset and intermediary sleep-maintenance insomnia that develops as a result of mutually reinforcing factors of chronic, somatized tension and negative conditioning to sleep.[105–109] These two elements interact with cumulative results. Patients, however, are not usually aware of the factors maintaining their sleeplessness. They consider themselves light sleepers and often have multiple somatic complaints (e.g., tension headaches, palpitations, and low back pain). In the few studies in which persistent DIMS has been monitored systematically, resting muscle activity has been high.

Polysomnographic monitoring demonstrates increased sleep latency with reduced sleep efficiency and an increased number of awakenings despite the absence of any causative medical or mental disorders.[21]

Most of these patients are tense and anxious, but many deny that these factors are responsible for their distress. They worry about their inability to fall asleep, a lack of "good" sleep, and overtiredness the next day. A vicious cycle develops: the more they strive to sleep, the less they can. The continuous effort, which involves somatic participation (e.g., muscle contractions), results in bombardment of the CNS arousal structures. Stress of any type exacerbates persistent DIMS.

DIMs and Drug and Alcohol Use

The second most common cause of DIMS is drug and alcohol use.[9] It is linked to a tolerance to or withdrawal from a CNS depressant after sustained use. During withdrawal, sleep medications seriously disrupt sleep architecture such that PSG monitoring demonstrates an increase in stages 1 and 2 non-REM sleep, decreases in stages 3 and 4 non-REM sleep, increases in REM sleep, and decreases in sleep "efficiency" (i.e., sleep stage and sleep pattern are maintained with the intrusion of light sleep or a short EEG arousal pattern). Sleep stage transitions are frequent, and sleep spindles are reduced in association with an increase in pseudospindles at 14 to 18 Hz.

Patients often experience an abrupt rebound of severe insomnia when they stop taking a hypnotic agent, thus reinforcing their "need" for pharmacologic treatment. They may also experience residual daytime side-effects (e.g., sluggishness, poor coordination, atonia, slurred speech, locomotor problems, muscle aches, sleepiness, and afternoon restlessness) and attribute these symptoms to lack of sleep rather than to drug intake. An important neurotic psychopathology may have existed before the drug intake. Depression, at times with suicidal ideation, is common, with patients using their stock of drugs in a suicide attempt. These patients need careful supervision during treatment. It may be necessary to hospitalize them, but the authors have been able to achieve drug withdrawal in these patients on an outpatient basis in 95 percent of cases.

If rapid drug reduction or abrupt withdrawal occurs, sleep is disrupted very severely, with major decreases in total sleep time and the development of REM sleep rebounds with many phasic events such as twitches, eye movements, and irregular respiratory pauses. Severe dream-anxiety attacks occur during this extended period of REM sleep. A typical withdrawal syndrome with nausea, tension, aches, restlessness, and nervousness occurs during the daytime. The circadian rhythm of many

biologic variables is disrupted profoundly, with a dissociation between sleep–wake cycles and day–night rhythm. To avoid these problems, drug withdrawal should be gradual, with elimination of one therapeutic unit per week.[108–110] A therapeutic unit varies with the drug considered (e.g., 5 mg with diazepam and 25 mg with doxepin or imipramine). The schedule must be adapted to the patient's response and severity of withdrawal symptoms. Polygraphic monitoring during sleep has demonstrated that, after complete withdrawal and re-entrainment with the day–night cycle, total sleep time and sleep organization improve spontaneously compared with sleep before withdrawal, although some disruptions may persist. A thorough evaluation of a subject's underlying psychopathology and a supportive psychotherapy program during the withdrawal period help to ensure successful withdrawal. Withdrawal from all chronic CNS stimulant drugs, including caffeine, should be dealt with in a similar fashion. A stepped care approach in hypnotic withdrawal together with cognitive behavioral therapy may be an alternative strategy.[108–110]

Parasomnias

Parasomnias are characterized by undesirable physical phenomena or behaviors that occur predominantly during sleep, associated with prominent skeletal muscle activity and autonomic nervous system changes. It has been proposed that most, if not all, of them are related to disorders of arousal rather than epilepsy despite features such as abrupt sleep onset, confusion, disorientation during the episode, retrograde amnesia following the event, and occasional bodily injury incurred during the seizure-like attack.[9] Since that time, several systematic studies have been performed on these "disorders of arousal" or "non-REM sleep dyssomnia." Parasomnias are composed of disorders of arousal and partial arousal, sleep–wake transition, and REM sleep. Disorders of arousal (e.g., sleep terrors, sleepwalking, and confusional arousals) are the most common form of parasomnias.

Parasomniac events often occur during the first half of the night, in many cases during the first sleep cycle. As noted by several authors, most events are seen during stages 3 and 4 non-REM (slow-wave) sleep.[9,111,112] The abnormal nocturnal behavior is preceded by generalized, symmetric, hypersynchronous delta activity. This pattern persists after the sleepwalking event or night terror has started, while the patient is arising from bed. With VEEG-PSG, ambulation is documented. Polysomnographic recordings in sleepwalkers demonstrate two abnormalities during the first sleep cycle: frequent, brief, nonbehavioral EEG-defined arousals before the somnambulistic episode; and abnormally low delta (0.75 to 2.0 Hz) EEG power on EEG spectral analysis, correlating with the occurrence of high-voltage hypersynchronous delta waves lasting 10 to 15 seconds just before the movement.[9] This is followed by stage 1 non-REM sleep without evidence of complete awakening. Usage of the CAP atlas has shown that the succession of high-amplitude slow-wave bursts followed by return to a baseline background EEG is characteristic of a CAP sequence. Further investigations by several different authors have shown that an abnormal CAP rate during non-REM sleep is seen in sleepwalking and sleep terrors in children and adults, indicating instability of non-REM sleep in these subjects. The abnormality of sleep concerns Phase B of the CAP cycle. Normally, subjects attempt to reach a stable non-REM sleep stage: either a stable sleep-spindle stage or a delta stage, supported by hypersynchronization either in the thalamus (sleep spindle) or in the cortex (delta). Successful passage from one stable stage to another is associated with a short-lived period of instability (stage 1 or stage 3 of non-REM sleep). However, an underlying cause disturbing sleep will lead to persistence of unstable non-REM sleep, which will be manifested when using the CAP scoring system by an increase in CAP rate.

In sleep-transition disorders (e.g., rhythmic movement disorder), VEEG-PSG demonstrates rhythmic movements during any stage of sleep or in wakefulness with no associated seizure activity. In the case of sleep starts, VEEG-PSG during the event demonstrates either brief, high-amplitude muscle potentials during the transition from wakefulness to sleep or arousals from light sleep.

Another parasomnia, *REM behavior disorder* (RBD), spans various age groups and has an acute and chronic form. Acute RBD usually is associated with medication toxicity, drug abuse, or drug or alcohol withdrawal. Medications implicated in RBD are fluoxetine, mirtazapine, venlafaxine, selegiline, tricyclic antidepressants, and biperiden. Chronic RBD is more prevalent in elderly men. Major diagnostic features include harmful or potentially harmful sleep behaviors that disrupt sleep continuity and dream enactment during REM sleep.[113–118] About 32 percent of patients report self-injury ranging from falling out of bed to striking or bumping into the furniture or walls, and 64 percent of spouses report being assaulted during sleep.[113] Treatment of RBD consists of medications such as clonazepam or melatonin; prevention of harm by environmental safety precautions is also important.[114]

RBD may be associated with synucleinopathy in up to 65 percent of patients (e.g., Parkinson disease, dementia with Lewy bodies, and multiple system atrophy). Other comorbid conditions may include narcolepsy, agrypnia excitata, sleepwalking, and sleep terrors. REM behavior disorder is hypothesized to be caused by primary dysfunction of the pedunculopontine nucleus or other key brainstem structures associated with basal ganglia pathology; or, alternatively, by abnormal afferent signals in the basal ganglia leading to dysfunction in the midbrain extrapyramidal area and pedunculopontine nucleus.

In patients with RBD, the polysomnogram during REM sleep demonstrates excessive augmentation of chin EMG or excessive chin or limb phasic EMG twitching.[21,114–116] EMG activity is more prominent in distal rather than proximal muscles. Simultaneous recording of the mentalis, flexor digitorum superficialis, and extensor digitorum brevis muscles provides the highest rates of REM sleep phasic EMG activity.[117] VEEG-PSG of patients with RBD requires monitoring of all four limbs because the arms and legs may move independently. During REM sleep, patients may show excessive limb or body jerking, or both; complex movements; or vigorous or violent movements. However, no epileptic activity is associated with the disorder.

Subclinical RBD refers to a subset of patients with REM without atonia who may remain asymptomatic, progress to clinical RBD, develop clinical RBD with progression to Parkinson disease, or progress directly to Parkinson disease without clinical RBD. Patients with subclinical RBD have high EMG tone during at least 15 to 20 percent of REM sleep.

Disorders of the Sleep–Wake Schedule

Disorders of the sleep–wake schedule are often related to the schedule changes imposed by industrial development that do not conform to the sleep–wake periods and day–night cycles on which society normally bases its work–rest cycle. Some problems are transient, such as jet lag, a syndrome related to rapid time-zone change.[119,120] Sleepiness, fatigue, and disrupted sleep result when an attempt is made to follow the day–night cycle of a new time zone while the body's circadian rhythms are still based on the old one. It takes a mean of 8 days to reset biologic variables, even if the sleep complaint has since abated.

Shift work, equivalent to rapid, multiple time-zone changes, is a major problem of industrial medicine. *Shift work disorder* results when the patient's internal circadian clock is misaligned with the desired sleep–wake schedule. Between 25.8 and 37.8 million Americans are shift workers on a regular or rotating basis.[120] Shift work disorder results in reduced alertness and increased accident rates, reduced productivity, increased absenteeism, and impairment of quality of life. Health risks with shift work disorder include an increased rate of breast cancer, duodenal ulcers, and cardiovascular morbidity and mortality.[120] The development of shift work disorder depends on the frequency of shift rotations, scheduling differences, shift duration, family and social responsibilities, and differences in sleep and circadian physiology. Analysis of 2-week sleep–wake diaries focusing on activities prior to bedtime, regularity and timing of bedtimes, and duration of sleep, together with actigraphy, confirms the pattern of sleep disturbance and circadian disruption. PSG is not performed routinely, but is helpful to exclude other sleep disorders. It shows increased sleep latency, numerous arousals during sleep, early awakening, and reduced sleep efficiency of below 85 percent.

Repetitive shift work and many other medical and social conditions can lead to a specific syndrome: the *delayed sleep-phase syndrome*. This biologic rhythm disorder induces a complaint of insomnia. Although sleep onset and awakening are stable, they come later than desired. Subjects may go to bed early without falling asleep for several hours; when morning comes, they have difficulty in waking up and achieve peak alertness only late in the day. A sleep log and actigraphy (for a minimum of 7 days) are useful tools to evaluate this disorder. Treatment involves phase advancement of the circadian clock through chronotherapy, carefully timed "morning" light administration, or "evening" melatonin administration. These subjects can be helped easily through chronotherapy (i.e., delaying their bedtime by a maximum of 3 hours every day during the therapeutic period and rotating their sleep–wake cycle in a clockwise fashion until they are back to a sleep–wake cycle in phase with the night–day cycle). Reinforcing external cues (e.g., fixed time for meals, exercise, and bedtime) once the resetting is performed is important for successful chronotherapy. *Advanced sleep-phase syndrome* has a reported prevalence of 1 percent in middle-aged adults. Affected individuals have uniformly earlier sleep and wake times than desired; body temperature cycles are uniformly advanced (measured in constant routine conditions to avoid masking) compared with those in younger men. PSG monitoring during a 24- to 36-hour period demonstrates an advance in the timing of the habitual sleep period.

Sleep-Related Epilepsy

Between 7.5 and 45 percent of epileptic patients have seizures occurring either exclusively or predominantly during sleep.[121] Clinical presentations of nocturnal seizures may be difficult to distinguish from parasomnias. Seizures are more frequent during non-REM sleep but can also occur during REM sleep. The events are stereotyped and repetitive, and disrupt the sleep of the patient and often the bed partner. Epilepsies that predominantly occur during sleep include nocturnal temporal lobe epilepsy, benign epilepsy of childhood with centrotemporal spikes, nocturnal paroxysmal dystonia, supplementary sensorimotor seizures, autosomal-dominant nocturnal frontal lobe epilepsy, epilepsy with continuous spike-wave activity during sleep, juvenile myoclonic epilepsy, and generalized tonic-clonic seizures on awakening.[121]

Polysomnographic studies have shown reduced total and REM sleep time on the nights when seizures occurred.[122–124] In patients with temporal lobe epilepsy, wake time after sleep onset increased, N3 sleep and REM sleep decreased, and REM sleep latency was prolonged during ictal nights when compared to seizure-free nights.[125] The more common sleep-related epilepsy syndromes and associated VEEG-PSG findings are discussed in this section.

BENIGN FOCAL EPILEPSY OF CHILDHOOD

Benign childhood epilepsy with centrotemporal spikes, or *rolandic epilepsy*, has a peak incidence between 7 and 10 years of age.[120,126–129] Seizures typically occur during non-REM sleep, and VEEG-PSG may document oropharyngeal disturbances (guttural sounds and excessive salivation) associated with hemiconvulsions or tonic–clonic seizures followed by postictal paresis. The interictal EEG shows stereotypic high-voltage centrotemporal sharp waves, which may be unilateral or bilateral, superimposed on normal background activity.

Early-onset *benign childhood occipital seizures*, also called benign childhood epilepsy with occipital paroxysms, usually presents between the ages of 1 and 12 years, with a peak at age 5 years.[126] Seizures commonly occur during non-REM sleep but may also occur in wakefulness. VEEG-PSG can document ictal behavioral changes of irritability; pallor; vomiting; coughing; speech disturbances; oropharyngolaryngeal movements; altered consciousness; and hemiclonic, complex partial, or generalized tonic–clonic convulsions. EEG channels demonstrate occipital paroxysms or bilateral generalized discharges. Interictal EEG findings include high-amplitude, rhythmic, posterior temporal or occipital sharp waves or spikes during eye closure, attenuated by eye opening.

AUTOSOMAL-DOMINANT NOCTURNAL FRONTAL LOBE EPILEPSY

Pedley and Guilleminault described "episodic nocturnal wanderings," characterized by paroxysmal attacks in sleep of ambulation and bizarre behavior, as summarized elsewhere.[9] Interictal frontal epileptiform activity was noted, and PSG revealed minor seizures in sleep with dystonic, autonomic, and affective features; patients responded to anticonvulsants (e.g., carbamazepine and phenytoin).[9] In 1981, Lugaresi and Cirignotta described motor attacks characterized by complex behavior with dystonic-dyskinetic or ballistic movements occurring during non-REM sleep associated with tonic spasms and occasional vocalizations or laughter.[9] They called this syndrome hypnogenic paroxysmal dystonia, which was later renamed nocturnal paroxysmal dystonia. A third category, paroxysmal arousals, consists of brief, sudden awakenings associated with stereotyped dystonic-dyskinetic movements, at times accompanied by frightened behavior and screaming. These three presentations encompass the spectrum of nocturnal frontal lobe epilepsy.[130,131] An autosomal-dominant form has been linked to chromosome 20q13.2 and 15q24 mutations in the coding of the neuronal nicotinic and acetylcholine receptor subunits.[132,133] In a series of 38 affected individuals from 30 unrelated Italian families, Oldani and colleagues reported that mean age of onset was 11.8 years, with frequent, nocturnal seizures occurring 1 to 20 times per week and persisting into adulthood in almost 94 percent of subjects.[133,134] VEEG-PSG documented sudden awakenings with dystonic/dyskinetic movements (42.1 percent), complex behaviors (13.2 percent), and sleep-related violent behavior (5.3 percent) accompanied by ictal epileptiform abnormalities over the frontal areas (31.6 percent) and ictal rhythmic slowing anteriorly (47.4 percent).[133,134] Stereotyped motor attacks lasted 5 to 30 seconds, with sudden head and trunk elevation, fearful facial expression, dystonic or clonic movements of the arms, and occasional vocalization lasting 1 minute or longer. Seizures occurred during stage 2 and slow-wave sleep, but sleep architecture remained normal.

FRONTAL LOBE EPILEPSIES

Seizures arising from the frontal lobe occur commonly or almost exclusively during sleep in more than half of affected patients.[133–135] The different syndromes include seizures arising from the supplementary sensorimotor, orbitofrontal, anterior frontopolar, and dorsolateral frontal areas. Manifestations include version, complex motor automatisms with kicking and thrashing movements, sexual automatisms, laughter, vocalizations, and the common development of complex partial status epilepticus. The EEG demonstrates lateralized or localized discharges in one-third of patients; nonlateralized slowing, rhythmic activity, or repetitive spiking in another one-third; and no EEG accompaniments in the remaining one-third.[135–137] Sleep organization is normal.[136]

TEMPORAL LOBE EPILEPSY

Mesial and lateral (neocortical) syndromes are well recognized, as discussed in earlier chapters. Sleep in patients with temporal lobe epilepsy is altered. Decreased sleep efficiency and increased awakenings have been found in both treated and untreated patients, in addition to increased non-REM stage 4 sleep in untreated patients.[9] There is an increase in wakefulness after sleep onset and shifting of sleep stages with an increase in stages 1 and 2 non-REM sleep, as detailed elsewhere.[9]

ELECTRICAL STATUS EPILEPTICUS IN SLEEP

This disorder encompasses patients with continuous spike-wave activity during slow-wave sleep or with Landau–Kleffner syndrome. A subset initially presents with benign childhood epilepsy with centrotemporal spikes. Tassinari first described this syndrome in six children in 1971 and called it encephalopathy with electrical status epilepticus during sleep.[138] It is an age-related disorder of unknown etiology associated with regression of expressive language and cognition, motor impairment, epilepsy, and status epilepticus during sleep. Seizures present between 2 months and 12 years of age and can be either generalized motor seizures or focal motor status epilepticus arising from sleep. The EEG during wakefulness shows diffuse 2- to 3-Hz spike-wave complexes with or without clinical manifestations. The criterion for this disorder is that epileptiform activity occupies at least 86 percent of sleep recordings. During REM sleep, epileptiform activity becomes fragmented, less frequent, and less continuous. No specific treatment has been advocated. Sodium valproate, benzodiazepines, and adrenocorticotropic hormone (ACTH) control the seizures and status epilepticus during sleep, although often temporarily. Subpial transection has been proposed in some instances of nonregressive acquired aphasia.

Restless Legs Syndrome and Periodic Leg Movement Disorder

Restless legs syndrome, a sensorimotor disorder, is a clinical diagnosis that is based primarily upon fulfillment of specific clinical criteria.[139] More than 80 percent of patients with restless legs syndrome manifest periodic leg movements during sleep and polysomnographic monitoring demonstrates limb movements at sleep onset.[21] Polysomnographic reports typically detail periodic leg movements during sleep, a periodic limb movement index (PLMI), and a periodic limb movement arousal index (PLMAI).[139] Periodic limb movement disorder (PLMD), by contrast, is a clinical diagnosis based on a sleep complaint (either insomnia or daytime sleepiness) that is associated with increased periodic leg movements during sleep and is made only after other sleep disorders that could produce similar symptoms have been excluded.[139] The 2004 AASM review paper clarifies the distinctions between these terms.[139]

Since the first reports of the relationship between periodic leg movements (nocturnal myoclonus) and disturbed nocturnal sleep, several studies have confirmed the relationship and linked it to a complaint of insomnia or daytime tiredness and fatigue.[9] The myoclonic jerks are generally bilateral, but they can involve only one leg without an apparent pattern. The myoclonus is usually independent of generalized body movements during sleep and is not observed during wakefulness. The contraction consists of an extension of the big toe and sometimes partial flexing of the ankle, knee, and, occasionally, hip. Patients rarely complain of sore legs in the morning. Bed partners report rhythmic leg-kicking. Periodic limb movements are seen most commonly without other associated medical or neurologic problems. They are often associated with restless legs syndrome, which can be familial (autosomal-dominant) or associated with a number of general medical conditions. The myoclonic jerks are followed by a K-complex, a lightening of sleep stages, and a partial EEG arousal or awakening (Fig. 33-13). EMG monitoring of the tibialis anterior muscle shows repetitive myoclonic contractions lasting from 0.5 to

10 seconds. The interval between jerks is typically 20 to 40 seconds, with a maximum variation of 5 to 90 seconds. The contractions can occur throughout nocturnal sleep but most often happen during one part of it. A recent study reported that patients with periodic leg movements during sleep exhibit a circadian rhythm that is maximal in the late evening or early night, similar to patients with restless legs syndrome.[140] Periodic leg movements during sleep are also seen with OSA, upper airway resistance syndrome, and RBD.

CONCLUDING COMMENTS

Sleep is a complex process that oscillates between several states of being: wakefulness, non-REM sleep, and REM sleep. Age-related changes, sleep deprivation, circadian rhythm abnormalities, medications, and the presence of primary sleep disorders can affect sleep architecture. Autonomic functions vary with the different states of alertness and circadian time. Any understanding of the physiology of sleep and the various sleep disorders is enhanced greatly by the capacity to investigate these through PSG and related tests. Specific risk factors underlying various sleep disorders that are sleep-state–related autonomic events can be unmasked through electrophysiologic monitoring. PSG and related procedures permit a better understanding of patients' problems and risks, and hence can facilitate better treatment.

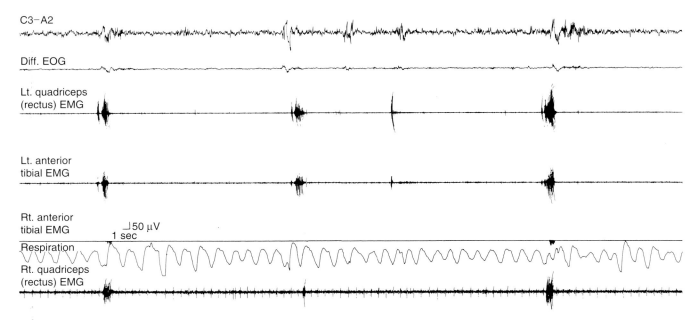

FIGURE 33-13 ▪ Example of periodic leg movements. Note the periodicity of the electromyographic discharge and the associated electroencephalographic arousal during stage 2 non-REM sleep.

REFERENCES

1. Berger H: Über das Elektroenkephalogramm des Menschen. Arch Psychiatr Nervenkr, 87:527, 1929 [in German]

2. Loomis AL, Harvey EN, Hobart G: Cerebral states during sleep as studied by human brain potentials. J Exp Psychol, 21:127, 1937

3. Aserinsky E, Kleitman N: Regularly occurring periods of eye motility and concomitant phenomena during sleep. Science, 118:273, 1953

4. Dement W, Kleitman N: Cyclic variations in EEG during sleep and their relation to eye movements, body motility, and dreaming. Electroencephalogr Clin Neurophysiol, 9:673, 1957

5. Rechtschaffen A, Kales AD: A Manual of Standardized Terminology, Techniques and Scoring System for Sleep Stages of Human Subjects. Brain Information Service, UCLA, Los Angeles, 1968

6. Anders T, Emde R, Parmelee A (eds): A Manual of Standardized Terminology, Techniques and Criteria for the Scoring of States of Sleep and Wakefulness in Newborn Infants. Brain Information Service, UCLA, Los Angeles, 1971

7. American Academy of Sleep Medicine: AASM Manual for the Scoring of Sleep and Associated Events: Rules, Terminology and Technical Specification. American Academy of Sleep Medicine, Darien, IL, 2007

8. Carskadon M, Dement W: Normal human sleep: an overview. p. 15. In Kryger M, Roth T, Dement W (eds): Principles and Practice of Sleep Medicine. 3rd Ed. WB Saunders, Philadelphia, 2000

9. Guilleminault C, Abad VC: Polysomnographic evaluation of sleep disorders. p. 701. In Aminoff MJ (ed): Electrodiagnosis in Clinical Neurology. 5th Ed. Elsevier Churchill Livingstone, Philadelphia, 2005

10. Wyatt J, Bootzin R, Anthony J et al: Does sleep onset produce retrograde amnesia? Sleep Res, 21:113, 1992

11. Ohayon MM, Carskadon MA, Guilleminault C et al: Meta-analysis of quantitative sleep parameters from childhood to old age in healthy individuals: developing normative sleep values across the human lifespan. Sleep, 27:1255, 2004

12. Silber M, Anconi-Israel S, Bonnet M et al: The visual scoring of sleep in adults. J Clin Sleep Med, 3:121, 2007

13. Ohayon M, Guilleminault C: Epidemiology of sleep disorders. p. 285. In Chokroverty S (ed): Sleep Disorders Medicine. 3rd Ed. Butterworth–Heinemann, Woburn, MA, 2009

14. Partinen M, Hublin C: Epidemiology of sleep disorders. p. 626. In Kryger M, Roth T, Dement W (eds): Principles and Practice of Sleep Medicine. 4th Ed. WB Saunders, Philadelphia, 2005

15. Kushida CA, Littner MR, Morgenthaler T et al: Practice parameters for the indications for polysomnography and related procedures: an update for 2005. Sleep, 28:499, 2005

16. Standards of Practice Committee of the American Academy of Sleep Medicine: Practice parameters for using polysomnography to evaluate insomnia: an update for 2002. Sleep, 26:754, 2003

17. Chesson AL, Berry RB, Pack A: Practice parameters for the use of portable monitoring devices in the investigation of suspected obstructive sleep apnea in adults. Sleep, 26: 907, 2003

18. Collop NA, Anderson WM, Boehlecke B et al: Clinical guidelines for the use of unattended portable monitors in the diagnosis of obstructive sleep apnea in adult patients. J Clin Sleep Med, 3:737, 2007

19. Littner MR, Kushida C, Wise M et al: Practice parameters for clinical use of the multiple sleep latency test and the maintenance of wakefulness test. Sleep, 28:113, 2005

20. Arand D, Bonnet M, Hurwitz T et al: The clinical use of the MSLT and MWT. Sleep, 28:123, 2005

21. American Academy of Sleep Medicine: International Classification of Sleep Disorders, Revised: Diagnostic and Coding Manual. American Academy of Sleep Medicine, Rochester, MN, 2000

22. Moscovitch A, Partinen M, Patterson-Rhoads N et al: Cataplexy in differentiation of excessive daytime somnolence. Sleep Res, 20:303, 1991

23. Aldrich M, Chervin R, Malow B: Value of the multiple sleep latency test for the diagnosis of narcolepsy. Sleep, 20:520, 1997

24. Carskadon M, Wolfson A, Acebo C et al: Adolescent sleep patterns, circadian timing and sleepiness at a transition to early school days. Sleep, 21:871, 1998

25. Bishop C, Rosenthal L, Helmus T et al: The frequency of multiple sleep onset REM periods among subjects with no excessive daytime sleepiness. Sleep, 19:727, 1996

26. Doghramji K, Mitler M, Sangal RB et al: A normative study of the maintenance of wakefulness test (MWT). Electroencephalogr Clin Neurophysiol, 103:554, 1997

27. Newman J, Broughton R: Pupillometric assessment of excessive daytime sleepiness in narcolepsy-cataplexy. Sleep, 14:121, 1991

28. Lim J, Dinges DF: Sleep deprivation and vigilant attention. Ann N Y Acad Sci, 1129:305, 2008

29. Dinges DF, Pack F, Williams K et al: Cumulative sleepiness, mood disturbance and psychomotor vigilance performance decrements during a week of sleep restricted to 4–5 hours per night. Sleep, 20:267, 1997

30. Doran SM, Van Dongen HP, Dinges DF: Sustained attention performance during sleep deprivation: evidence of state instability. Arch Ital Biol, 139:253, 2001

31. Banks S, Dinges DF: Behavioral and physiological consequences of sleep restriction. J Clin Sleep Med, 3:519, 2007

32. Dinges DF: Probing the limits of functional capability: the effects of sleep loss on short-duration tasks. p. 177. In Broughton RJ, Ogilvie R (eds): Sleep, Arousal and Performance: Problems and Promises. Birkhauser, Boston, 1992

33. Belenky G, Wesensten NJ, Thorne DR et al: Patterns of performance degradation and restoration during sleep restriction and subsequent recovery: a sleep dose–response study. J Sleep Res, 12:1, 2003

34. Van Dongen HP, Maislin G, Mullington JM: The cumulative cost of additional wakefulness: dose–response effects on neurobehavioral functions and sleep physiology from

chronic sleep restriction and total sleep deprivation. Sleep, 26:117, 2003

35. Philip P, Sagaspe P, Moore N et al: Fatigue, sleep restriction and driving performance. Accid Anal Prev, 37:473, 2005

36. Dinges DF: Adult napping and its effects on ability to function. p. 118. In Stampi C (ed): Why We Nap. Birkhauser, Boston, 1992

37. Altena E, Van Der Werf YD, Strijers RL et al: Sleep loss affects vigilance: effects of chronic insomnia and sleep therapy. J Sleep Res, 17:335, 2008

38. Kribbs NB, Pack AI, Kline LR et al: Effects of one night without nasal CPAP treatment on sleep and sleepiness in patients with obstructive sleep apnea. Am Rev Respir Dis, 147:1162, 1993

39. Kim H, Dinges DF, Young T: Sleep-disordered breathing and psychomotor vigilance in a community-based sample. Sleep, 30:1309, 2007

40. Blatter K, Graw P, Munch M et al: Gender and age differences in psychomotor vigilance performance under differential sleep pressure conditions. Behav Brain Res, 168:312, 2006

41. Lee IS, Bardwell WA, Ancoli-Israel S et al: Number of lapses during the psychomotor vigilance task as an objective measure of fatigue. J Clin Sleep Med, 6:163, 2010

42. Findley L, Unverzagt M, Guchu R et al: Vigilance and automobile accidents in patients with sleep apnea or narcolepsy. Chest, 108:619, 1995

43. George C, Boudreau A, Smiley A: Comparison of simulated driving performance in narcolepsy and sleep apnea patients. Sleep, 19:711, 1996

44. Morgenthaler T, Alessi C, Friedman L et al: Practice parameters for the use of actigraphy in the assessment of sleep and sleep disorders: an update for 2007. Sleep, 30:519, 2007

45. Soll BA, Yeo KK, Davis JW et al: The effect of posture on Cheyne–Stokes respirations and hemodynamics in patients with heart failure. Sleep, 32:1499, 2009

46. Valensi P, Sachs RN, Harfouche B et al: Predictive value of cardiac autonomic neuropathy in diabetic patients with or without silent myocardial ischemia. Diabetes Care, 24:339, 2001

47. Montesano M, Miano S, Paolino MC et al: Autonomic cardiovascular tests in children with obstructive sleep apnea syndrome. Sleep, 33:1349, 2010

48. Orr W, Chen CL: Gastrointestinal monitoring techniques. p. 1454. In Kryger MH, Roth T, Dement WC (eds): Principles and Practice of Sleep Medicine. Elsevier Saunders, Philadelphia, 2005

49. Kuribayashi S, Massey BT, Hafeezullah M et al: Upper esophageal sphincter and gastroesophageal junction pressure changes act to prevent gastroesophageal and esophagopharyngeal reflux during apneic episodes in patients with obstructive sleep apnea. Chest, 137:769, 2010

50. Ing AJ, Ngu MC, Breslin AG: Obstructive sleep apnea and gastroesophageal reflux. Am J Med, 6:120S, 2000

51. Senior BA, Khan M, Schwimmer C et al: Gastroesophageal reflux and obstructive sleep apnea. Laryngoscope, 111:2144, 2001

52. Halpern LM, Jolley SG, Tunell WP et al: The mean duration of gastroesophageal reflux during sleep as an indicator of respiratory symptoms from gastroesophageal reflux in children. J Pediatr Surg, 26:686, 1991

53. Ware JC, Hirshkowitz M: Assessment of sleep-related erections. p. 1394. In Kryger MH, Roth T, Dement WC (eds): Principles and Practice of Sleep Medicine. Elsevier Saunders, Philadelphia, 2005

54. Hirshkowitz M: Monitoring penile erections during sleep. p. 673. In Lee-Chiong T, Sateia M, Carskadon M (eds): Sleep Medicine. Hanley & Belfus, Philadelphia, 2002

55. American Electroencephalographic Society: Guidelines for polygraphic assessment of sleep-related disorders (polysomnography). J Clin Neurophysiol, 11:111, 1994

56. Foldvary N, Caruso AC, Mascha E et al: Identifying montages that best detect electrographic seizure activity during polysomnography. Sleep, 23:221, 2000

57. Young T, Palta M, Dempsey J et al: The occurrence of sleep disordered breathing among middle-aged adults. N Engl J Med, 328:1230, 1993

58. Punjabi NM: The epidemiology of adult obstructive sleep apnea. Proc Am Thorac Soc, 5:136, 2008

59. Young T, Evans L, Finn L et al: Estimation of the clinically diagnosed proportion of sleep apnea syndrome in middle-aged men and women. Sleep, 20:705, 1997

60. Kapur V, Strohl KP, Redline S et al: Underdiagnosis of sleep apnea syndrome in US communities. Sleep Breath, 6:49, 2002

61. Pack A (ed): Sleep Apnea. Pathogenesis, Diagnosis, and Treatment. Marcel Dekker, New York, 2002

62. Guilleminault C, Dement WC (eds): Sleep Apnea Syndromes. Alan R Liss, New York, 1978

63. Yaggi HK, Strohl KP: Adult obstructive sleep apnea/hypopnea syndrome: definitions, risk factors, and pathogenesis. Clin Chest Med, 31:179, 2010

64. Abad VC, Guilleminault C: Treatment options for obstructive sleep apnea. Curr Treat Options Neurol, 11:358, 2009

65. Chervin RD, Archbold KH, Dillon JE et al: Inattention, hyperactivity, and symptoms of sleep-disordered breathing. Pediatrics, 109:449, 2002

66. Marshall NS, Wong KK, Liu PY et al: Sleep apnea as an independent risk factor for all-cause mortality: the Busselton Health Study. Sleep, 31:1079, 2008

67. Kato M, Adachi T, Koshino Y et al: Obstructive sleep apnea and cardiovascular disease. Circ J, 73:1363, 2009

68. Dart RA, Gregoire JR, Gutterman DD et al: The association of hypertension and secondary cardiovascular disease with sleep-disordered breathing. Chest, 123:24, 2003

69. Pepperell JC, Davies RJ, Stradling JR: Systemic hypertension and obstructive sleep apnoea. Sleep Med Rev, 6:157, 2002

70. Lattimore JD, Celermajer DS, Wilcox I: Obstructive sleep apnea and cardiovascular disease. J Am Coll Cardiol, 41:1429, 2003

71. Shahar E, Whitney CW, Redline S et al: Sleep-disordered breathing and cardiovascular disease: cross-sectional results

of the Sleep Heart Health Study. Am J Respir Crit Care Med, 163:19, 2001

72. Gami AS, Howard DE, Olson EJ et al: Day-night pattern of sudden death in obstructive sleep apnea. N Engl J Med, 352:1206, 2005

73. Kuniyoshi FH, Garcia-Touchard A, Gami AS et al: Day-night variation of acute myocardial infarction in obstructive sleep apnea. J Am Coll Cardiol, 52:343, 2008

74. Marin JM, Carrizo SJ, Vicente E et al: Long-term cardiovascular outcomes in men with obstructive sleep apnoea-hypopnoea with or without treatment with continuous positive airway pressure: an observational study. Lancet, 365:1046, 2005

75. Giles T, Lasserson T, Smith B et al: Continuous positive airways pressure for obstructive sleep apnoea in adults. Cochrane Database Syst Rev, 3:CD001106, 2006

76. Aurora RN, Casey KR, Kristo D et al: Practice parameters for the surgical modifications of the upper airway for obstructive sleep apnea in adults. Sleep, 33:1408, 2010

77. Caples SM, Rowley JA, Prinsell JR et al: Surgical modifications of the upper airway for obstructive sleep apnea in adults: a systematic review and meta-analysis. Sleep, 33:1396, 2010

78. Powell N, Riley R: Surgical management for obstructive sleep-disordered breathing. p. 1250. In Kryger M, Roth T, Dement W (eds): Principles and Practice of Sleep Medicine. 5th Ed. Elsevier Saunders, St. Louis, MO, 2011

79. Won CH, Li KK, Guilleminault C: Surgical treatment of obstructive sleep apnea: upper airway and maxillomandibular surgery. Proc Am Thorac Soc, 5:193, 2008

80. Schenck CH, Bassetti CL, Arnulf I et al: English translations of the first clinical reports on narcolepsy and cataplexy by Westphal and Gélineau in the late 19th century, with commentary. J Clin Sleep Med, 3:301, 2007

81. Morrish E, King MA, Smith IE et al: Factors associated with a delay in the diagnosis of narcolepsy. Sleep Med, 5:37, 2004

82. Guilleminault C, Pelayo R: Narcolepsy in prepubertal children. Ann Neurol, 43:135, 1998

83. Guilleminault C, Abad VC: Narcolepsy. p. 379. In Chokroverty S (ed): Sleep Disorders Medicine. Basic Science, Technical Considerations and Clinical Aspects. 3rd Ed. Elsevier Saunders, Philadelphia, 2009

84. Aran A, Einen M, Lin L et al: Clinical and therapeutic aspects of childhood narcolepsy-cataplexy: a retrospective study of 51 children. Sleep, 33:1457, 2010

85. Nishino S: Clinical and neurobiological aspects of narcolepsy. Sleep Med, 8:373, 2007

86. Philip P, Sagaspe P, Lagarde E et al: Sleep disorders and accidental risk in a large group of regular registered highway drivers. Sleep Med, 11:973, 2010

87. Findley L, Unverzagt M, Guchu R et al: Vigilance and automobile accidents in patients with sleep apnoea or narcolepsy. Chest, 108:619, 1995

88. Kotterba S, Mueller N, Leidag M et al: Comparison of driving simulator performance and neuropsychological testing in narcolepsy. Clin Neurol Neurosurg, 106:275, 2004

89. Martínez-Rodríguez J, Iranzo A, Santamaría JR: Status cataplecticus induced by abrupt withdrawal of clomipramine. Neurologia, 17:113, 2002

90. Eisensehr I, Linke R, Tatsch K et al: Alteration of the striatal dopaminergic system in human narcolepsy. Neurology, 60:1817, 2003

91. Chabas D, Habert MO, Maksud P et al: Functional imaging of cataplexy during status cataplecticus. Sleep, 30:153, 2007

92. Longstreth WT Jr, Koepsell TD, Ton TG et al: The epidemiology of narcolepsy. Sleep, 30:13, 2007

93. Challamel MJ, Mazzola ME, Nevsimalova S et al: Narcolepsy in children. Sleep, 17:Suppl S17, 1994

94. Mignot E, Lammers GJ, Ripley B et al: The role for cerebrospinal fluid hypocretin measurement in the diagnosis of narcolepsy and other hypersomnias. Arch Neurol, 59:1553, 2002

95. Krahn LE, Pankratz VS, Oliver L et al: Hypocretin (orexin) levels in cerebrospinal fluid of patients with narcolepsy: relationship to cataplexy and HLA DQB1*0602 status. Sleep, 25:733, 2002

96. Kanbayashi T, Inoue Y, Chiba S et al: CSF hypocretin-1 (orexin-A) concentrations in narcolepsy with and without cataplexy and idiopathic hypersomnia. J Sleep Res, 11:91, 2002

97. Ritchie C, Okuro M, Kanbayashi T et al: Hypocretin ligand deficiency in narcolepsy: recent basic and clinical insights. Curr Neurol Neurosci Rep, 10:180, 2010

98. Bassetti C, Dauvilliers Y: Idiopathic hypersomnia. p. 969. In Kryger M, Roth T, Dement W (eds): Principles and Practice of Sleep Medicine. 5th Ed. Elsevier Saunders, St. Louis, MO, 2011

99. Ali M, Auger RR, Slocumb NL et al: Idiopathic hypersomnia: clinical features and response to treatment. J Clin Sleep Med, 5:562, 2009

100. Vernet C, Arnulf I: Idiopathic hypersomnia with and without long sleep time: a controlled series of 75 patients. Sleep, 32:753, 2009

101. Anderson KN, Pilsworth S, Sharples LD et al: Idiopathic hypersomnia: a study of 77 cases. Sleep, 30:1274, 2007

102. Guilleminault C, Brooks S: Idiopathic hypersomnia: a neurological dilemma. Sleep Med Rev, 5:347, 2001

103. Ramsawh H, Stein M, Mellman TA: Anxiety disorders. p. 1474. In Kryger M, Roth T, Dement W (eds): Principles and Practice of Sleep Medicine. 5th Ed. Elsevier Saunders, St. Louis, MO, 2011

104. Hudson JI, Lipinski JF, Keck PE Jr et al: Polysomnographic characteristics of young manic patients. Comparison with unipolar depressed patients and normal control subjects. Arch Gen Psychiatry, 49:378, 1992

105. Morin C, Hauri P, Espie C et al: Nonpharmacologic treatment of chronic insomnia. An American Academy of Sleep Medicine review. Sleep, 22:1134, 1999

106. Bixler E, Vzontzas A, Lin H et al: Insomnia in central Pennsylvania. J Psychosom Res, 53:589, 2002

107. Petit L, Azad N, Byszewski A et al: Nonpharmacological management of primary and secondary insomnia among older people: review of assessment tools and treatments. Age Ageing, 32:19, 2003

108. Morgenthaler T, Kramer M, Alessi C et al: Practice parameters for the psychological and behavioral treatment of insomnia: an update. An American Academy of Sleep Medicine report. Sleep, 29:1415, 2006

109. Schutte-Rodin S, Broch L, Buysse D et al: Clinical guideline for the evaluation and management of chronic insomnia in adults. J Clin Sleep Med, 4:487, 2008

110. Belanger L, Bellville G, Morin C: Management of hypnotic discontinuation in chronic insomnia. Sleep Med Clin, 4:583, 2009

111. Guilleminault C, Palombini L, Pelayo R et al: Sleepwalking and sleep terrors in prepubertal children: what triggers them? Pediatrics, 111:e17, 2003

112. Guilleminault C, Poyares D, Abat F et al: Sleep and wakefulness in somnambulism. A spectral analysis study. J Psychosom Res, 51:411, 2001

113. Olson E, Boeve B, Silbert M: Rapid eye movement sleep behaviour disorder: demographic, clinical and laboratory findings in 93 cases. Brain, 123:331, 2000

114. Abad VC, Guilleminault C: Review of rapid eye movement behavior sleep disorders. Curr Neurol Neurosci Rep, 4:157, 2004

115. Boeve BF: REM sleep behavior disorder: updated review of the core features, the REM sleep behavior disorder–neurodegenerative disease association, evolving concepts, controversies, and future directions. Ann N Y Acad Sci, 1184:15, 2010

116. Schenck C, Mahowald M: REM sleep behavior disorder: clinical, developmental, and neuroscience perspectives 16 years after its formal identification in sleep. Sleep, 25:120, 2002

117. Frauscher B, Iranzo A, Högl B et al: Quantification of electromyographic activity during REM sleep in multiple muscles in REM sleep behavior disorder. Sleep, 31:724, 2008

118. Aurora RN, Zak RS, Maganti RK et al: Best practice guide for the treatment of REM sleep behavior disorder (RBD). J Clin Sleep Med, 6:85, 2010

119. Cvengros J, Wyatt J: Circadian rhythm disorders. Sleep Med Clin, 4:495, 2009

120. Drake C, Wright K: Shift work, shift-work disorder, and jet lag. p. 784. In Kryger M, Roth T, Dement W (eds): Principles and Practice of Sleep Medicine. 5th Ed. Elsevier Saunders, St Louis, MO, 2011

121. Zucconi M: Sleep-related epilepsy. Handbk Clin Neurol, 99:1109, 2011

122. Baldy-Moulinier M: Sleep architecture and childhood absence epilepsy. Epilepsy Res Suppl, 6:195, 1992

123. Bazil CW: Epilepsy and sleep disturbance. Epilepsy Behav, 4:Suppl 2, S39, 2003

124. Kotagal P: The relationship between sleep and epilepsy. Semin Pediatr Neurol, 8:241, 2001

125. de Almeida CA, Lins OG et al: Sleep disorders in temporal lobe epilepsy. Arq Neuropsiquiatr, 61:979, 2003

126. Foldvary-Schaefer N: Salient video-PSGs of unexpected seizures during sleep. In PSG 2003: Advanced Polysomnographic Interpretation Course. APSS annual meeting, Chicago, 2003

127. Eeg-Olofsson O: Rolandic epilepsy. p. 257. In Bazil CW, Malow BA, Sammaritano MR (eds): Sleep and Epilepsy: The Clinical Spectrum. Elsevier, Amsterdam, 2002

128. Lundberg S, Eeg-Olofsson O: Rolandic epilepsy: a challenge in terminology and classification. Eur J Paediatr Neurol, 7:239, 2003

129. Gelisse P, Corda D, Raybaud C et al: Abnormal neuroimaging in patients with benign epilepsy with centrotemporal spikes. Epilepsia, 44:372, 2003

130. Provini F, Plazzi G, Tinuper P et al: Nocturnal frontal lobe epilepsy. A clinical and polygraphic overview of 100 consecutive cases. Brain, 122:1017, 1999

131. Provini F, Plazzi G, Montagna P et al: The wide clinical spectrum of nocturnal frontal lobe epilepsy. Sleep Med Rev, 4:375, 2000

132. Phillips HA, Scheffer IE, Berkovic SF et al: Localization of a gene for autosomal dominant nocturnal frontal lobe epilepsy to chromosome 20q 13.2. Nat Genet, 10:117, 1995

133. Oldani A, Zucconi M, Asselta R et al: Autosomal dominant nocturnal frontal lobe epilepsy. A video-polysomnographic and genetic appraisal of 40 patients and delineation of the epilepsy syndrome. Brain, 121:205, 1998

134. Oldani A, Zucconi M, Ferini-Strambi L et al: Autosomal dominant nocturnal frontal lobe epilepsy: electroclinical picture. Epilepsia, 37:964, 1996

135. Jobst BC, Siegel AM, Thadani VM et al: Intractable seizures of frontal lobe origin: clinical characteristics, localizing signs, and results of surgery. Epilepsia, 41:1139, 2000

136. Crespel A, Baldy-Moulinier M, Coubes P: The relationship between sleep and epilepsy in frontal and temporal lobe epilepsies: practical and physiopathologic considerations. Epilepsia, 39:1150, 1998

137. Laskowitz DT, Sperling MR, French JA et al: The syndrome of frontal lobe epilepsy. Neurology, 45:780, 1995

138. Tassinari CA, Rubboli G, Volpi L et al: Encephalopathy with electrical status epilepticus during slow sleep or ESES syndrome including the acquired aphasia. Clin Neurophysiol, 111:Suppl 2, S94, 2000

139. Restless Legs Syndrome Task Force of the Standards of Practice Committee of the American Academy of Sleep Medicine: An update on the dopaminergic treatment of restless legs syndrome and periodic limb movement disorder. Sleep, 27:560, 2004

140. Duffy JF, Lowe AS, Silva EJ et al: Periodic limb movements in sleep exhibit a circadian rhythm that is maximal in the late evening/early night. Sleep Med, 12:83, 2011

Electrophysiologic Evaluation of Patients in the Intensive Care Unit

G. BRYAN YOUNG and CHARLES F. BOLTON

Despite challenges, electrophysiologic studies can be performed readily in the intensive care unit (ICU) in a sensitive, reliable, and quantifiable manner.[1-4] They assess nervous system functions that are clinically inaccessible. For example, most cases of septic encephalopathy or critical illness polyneuropathy cannot be confirmed without electrophysiologic studies.[5,6] Treatable conditions such as nonconvulsive status epilepticus and myasthenia gravis may be disclosed. The prognosis of anoxic-ischemic encephalopathy or neuromuscular conditions causing difficulty in weaning from the ventilator is determined more readily. Various tests provide objective methods of monitoring the course of disease and the effects of therapy. Newer techniques, notably those testing the control of respiration, will enhance the value of neuroelectrophysiology in the future and offer new avenues of research. These studies can be applied in adult,[7] pediatric,[8] neonatal, and neurologic-neurosurgical ICUs.[3]

ROLE OF ELECTROPHYSIOLOGIC TESTS

Diagnosis

Electroencephalography (EEG) assists in the diagnosis of certain specific conditions such as nonconvulsive status epilepticus, herpes simplex encephalitis, and barbiturate intoxication. A normal EEG with reactivity to passive eye opening in an apparently obtunded patient raises the possibility of psychogenic unresponsiveness or locked-in syndrome from a brainstem lesion or neuromuscular paralysis. More often, disease categories can be classified only broadly. The EEG patterns can differentiate cortical gray matter involvement (mild slowing and spikes) from white matter (delta activity) and combined cortical and subcortical nuclear involvement (periodic discharges, as in some cases of anoxic encephalopathy). Typical triphasic waves or frontally predominant, generalized rhythmic delta activity on a slowed background is strongly suggestive of a metabolic encephalopathy but not specific to one disease process.

Electrophysiologic studies of the limbs and respiratory structures are indicated when a neuromuscular cause of respiratory insufficiency is suspected or when focal or generalized limb weakness and reduced deep tendon reflexes are present. Even in the absence of these signs, if the patient has established sepsis for more than 3 weeks, the tests should be performed. Localization within the peripheral nervous system is usually possible. Polyneuropathies, mononeuropathies, neuromuscular transmission defects, and myopathies usually can be distinguished, and neuropathies can be subclassified into axonal and demyelinating varieties. Specific patterns in certain disorders allow for more precise diagnoses. When electrophysiologic features are combined with clinical information and (in selected cases) neuroimaging, serum creatine kinase determination, and muscle biopsy, the differential diagnosis can be narrowed further.

Assessment of Disease Course and Effects of Therapy

Continuous EEG (CEEG) monitoring is of great value in the ongoing management of patients with unstable but potentially reversible conditions such as status epilepticus. In conditions associated with decreased perfusion (e.g., stroke, vasospasm, and microvascular compression from mass effect), the EEG reveals frequency and amplitude changes caused by ischemia before irreversible tissue damage occurs.[9] The benefit of therapeutic maneuvers such as induced hypertension in cases of vasospasm can be monitored. In routine management, CEEG can be used for monitoring the depth of sedation with, for example, midazolam or other sedative drugs. This application of CEEG is especially useful for paralyzed patients. Because excessive sedation prolongs length of stay in the ICU, CEEG may be useful for ensuring optimal utilization of resources.

Electrophysiologic studies of the limbs and respiration should be performed early and then repeated. Such studies often establish the diagnosis and indicate the course of the disorder, thereby allowing a prognostic estimate of recovery and expected length of stay in the ICU.

Prognosis

With central nervous system (CNS) disorders, the neurologic or electrophysiologic determination of prognosis is valid only for conditions that are capable of causing neuronal death. (Some systemic disorders, such as sepsis, multiple organ failure, or intoxication, may compromise CNS function in a reversible manner.) Determination of the prognosis of comatose patients with intact brainstem function requires months of clinical evaluation.[10] Electrophysiologic tests can, in some circumstances, establish a reliable prognosis at an early stage. In anoxic-ischemic encephalopathy, a "flat" or diffusely suppressed EEG is strongly suggestive of a prognosis no better than a permanent vegetative state. Invariant or deteriorating patterns, provided that no confounding elements such as sedatives and sepsis are present, are also strongly supportive of a poor prognosis.[11,12] Somatosensory evoked potentials (SEPs) are objective and quantified. The early components from activation of the primary somatosensory cortex, especially the N20 response to median nerve stimulation, are very robust. If peripheral nerve and spinal cord components (as well as subcortical waves) are present, but the cortical component is absent, either severe cortical damage or disconnection from subcortical sites is likely.

Research

The ICU provides opportunities for clinical research that have been neglected by clinical neurophysiologists. Valuable contributions in patient care guidelines should result from research in the ICU. Much future effort will be spent in the execution of controlled studies that examine the usefulness of various electrophysiologic investigations or monitoring systems in different conditions and with varying severity of illness. Guidelines should be formulated through an evidence-based approach. In clinical research, the classification of electroclinical phenomena should use strategies with high intrarater and interrater reliability.

INITIAL CLINICAL EVALUATION

A careful clinical evaluation is essential to allow the clinician to pose suitable questions to be addressed by electrophysiologic testing. The clinical neurophysiologist must be aware of the key issues to plan appropriate investigations.

Clinical assessment of ICU patients is often difficult. Commonly, a history cannot be obtained because the patient has impaired consciousness or an endotracheal tube is in place. Relatives are often absent, and charts are voluminous. Sedating and paralyzing drugs and numerous lines and catheters further hamper clinical assessment. Nonetheless, as much clinical information as possible should be obtained. Relatives can be contacted by telephone; residents and bedside nurses can provide helpful information. Details of the admitting illness and past history (including drugs and previous illnesses) should be noted. In addition, details of current therapy, including procedures such as insertion of Swan–Ganz or aortic catheters, drugs (especially sedatives, antibiotics, aminophylline, vasopressor agents, corticosteroids, and neuromuscular blocking agents), and surgical procedures of the head, neck, chest, or abdomen are often relevant. One should look for evidence of sepsis and multiorgan failure and for episodes of significant hypotension or hypoxemia. Laboratory data, including neuroimaging, are then reviewed.

The physical examination is often limited. The patient should be observed for spontaneous movement and patterns of respiration before assessment of reactivity to increasing stimulation, beginning with auditory, then tactile, and then noxious stimuli to the limbs and face. Examination of most of the cranial nerves, tendon reflexes, and plantar responses is usually feasible unless the patient has received a neuromuscular blocking agent. Flaccidity, reduced tendon reflexes, and absent plantar responses may result from conditions varying as widely as acute encephalopathy; acute myelopathy with spinal shock; polyneuropathy; defects in neuromuscular transmission; and, occasionally, a myopathy.

In association with drug overdose, sustained pressure on various parts of the body by hard objects may induce local necrosis of skin, subcutaneous tissue, and occasionally the underlying muscle, and may also be associated with severe compressive focal neuropathy. The examiner should look for characteristic erythematous blisters of the skin at the site of compression and suspect injury to an underlying nerve if the latter lies nearby. Electrophysiologic techniques help to identify these mononeuropathies.

Rapid, shallow respirations and a rising $PaCO_2$ are supportive of neuromuscular respiratory insufficiency and should prompt electrophysiologic studies, including electromyography (EMG) of the diaphragm, which can localize and classify the problem and gauge its severity.

ELECTROPHYSIOLOGIC TECHNIQUES

For many disorders, electrophysiologic tests enhance the clinical assessment in a sensitive and quantifiable manner. This extension of the clinical examination is particularly valuable when the aforementioned confounding factors compromise assessment. Electrophysiologic testing is a component in the care of the patient. Clinical interpretation is incorporated with other information to formulate a diagnostic and prognostic evaluation or to monitor the effects of treatment.

The choice of electrophysiologic test to be performed in the ICU depends on the nature of the clinical problem. For example, sedation monitoring requires an EEG of four or fewer channels. For seizures, long-term monitoring for at least 48 hours is optimal.[13] Quantitative CEEG monitoring can be useful in detecting ischemia at a reversible stage when due to vasospasm from subarachnoid hemorrhage.[14] The EEG can help to narrow the differential diagnoses, for example, by differentiating seizures from metabolic encephalopathies. "Trending" or recording serial EEGs or evoked responses may clarify the prognosis in certain circumstances. Thus, although a standard EEG may have a role in assessing comatose victims of cardiac arrest, there is more prognostic promise in trending the automated or raw EEG over 48 hours or more to determine whether there is variability (invariant EEGs carry a worse prognosis), improvement, or worsening.[15] It is also important to consider which patients should be monitored. Some groups—such as those with recent convulsive seizures and with acute structural brain lesions—are at especially high risk for seizures.[16]

In patients with suspected neuromuscular diseases, the clinical picture guides the electrophysiologic approach and—when results are equivocal, as in some cases of critical illness neuromyopathy—percutaneous muscle biopsy may be important in supplementing the electrophysiologic tests.

Specific Tests

The following electrophysiologic tests have proven or potential usefulness in the study of nervous system disorders of patients in the ICU.

STANDARD EEG, CEEG, AND QUANTITATIVE EEG (QEEG)

Standard EEG consists of 20- to 30-minute single or serial recordings; CEEG and QEEG are discussed in Chapters 6 and 8 respectively. Digital EEG has paved the way for bedside monitoring, quantification of EEG signals, automated detection strategies, and the instantaneous transmission of EEG data from the bedside to the office of the electroencephalographer. The authors have developed an EEG classification system (Table 34-1) for comatose patients that is relatively unambiguous, is easy to apply, and shows excellent interobserver reliability.[17] Polysomnography has been underexplored in ICU patients, but holds promise in the approach to delirium and in assisting in prognostic determination after stroke, trauma, and other conditions.[18,19]

TABLE 34-1 ■ Electroencephalographic Classification of Coma

Category	Subcategory
I. Delta/theta >50% of the record (not theta coma)	A. Reactivity B. No reactivity
II. Triphasic waves	
III. Burst-suppression	A. With epileptiform activity B. Without epileptiform activity
IV. Alpha/theta/spindle coma (unreactive)	
V. Epileptiform activity (not in burst-suppression pattern)	A. Generalized B. Focal or multifocal
VI. Suppression	A. <20 μV but >10 μV B. ≤10 μV

GUIDELINES

1. Burst-suppression pattern should have generalized flattening at standard sensitivity for ≥1 second at least every 20 seconds
2. Suppression: for this category, voltage criteria should be met for the entire record; there should be no reactivity
3. When more than one category applies, the worst (most advanced) is selected

Modified from Young GB, McLachlan RS, Kreeft JH et al: An electroencephalographic classification system for coma. Can J Neurol Sci, 24:320, 1997, with permission.

EMG AND NERVE CONDUCTION TESTS

All the tests routinely performed in the EMG laboratory can be done in the ICU (Table 34-2). The choice of tests and sequence of testing will vary according to the circumstances. In the limbs, standard motor and sensory nerve conduction studies, needle EMG, and repetitive nerve stimulation are of great value. Phrenic nerve conduction studies and needle EMG of the diaphragm are performed if there is any possibility of a nervous system cause for respiratory insufficiency. The other respiratory electrophysiologic tests probably will prove valuable in the future. Preliminary studies indicate that stimulated single-fiber EMG and direct muscle stimulation may also be useful. Motor unit number estimates and muscle force and sound have yet to be tried, but are of great theoretical interest.

EVOKED POTENTIALS

SEPs are especially useful, inasmuch as they assess somatosensory pathways from the entry point of the sensory nerve to the cerebral cortex. Brainstem auditory evoked potential and blink reflex testing assess intrinsic brainstem circuitry and the integrity of extra-axial components of the relevant cranial nerves (see Chapters 19, 24 and 25). Preliminary work has shown that later potentials (event-related or cognitive-evoked responses, discussed in Chapter 29) hold promise for detecting cognitive processing in patients who are not capable of showing behavioral responses.[20] Such patients may have favorable outcomes, but this awaits further study.

TRANSCRANIAL AND TRANSCERVICAL MAGNETIC STIMULATION

Motor evoked potentials are discussed in Chapter 28. Such techniques may help in assessing cerebral motor control, spinal cord dysfunction, and respiratory function,[21] but their role in the ICU is still uncertain.

TABLE 34-2 ■ Electrophysiologic Tests of Neuromuscular Function Used in the Intensive Care Unit

Conditions	Site of Dysfunction	Electrophysiologic Test
Neurologic respiratory insufficiency	Brain, spinal cord, peripheral nerves, neuromuscular junction, or diaphragm	Transcranial and cervical magnetic stimulation Phrenic nerve somatosensory evoked potentials Phrenic nerve conduction Repetitive phrenic nerve stimulation Needle EMG of the diaphragm Automated interference pattern analysis of the diaphragm Power spectral analysis of the diaphragm
Polyneuropathies	Peripheral nerves	Motor and sensory nerve conduction, needle EMG
Neuromuscular transmission defects	Neuromuscular junction	Repetitive nerve stimulation Stimulated single-fiber EMG
Myopathies	Skeletal muscle	Motor and sensory nerve conduction, needle EMG Direct muscle stimulation Measurement of duration of compound muscle action potential
Other tests		Measurement of muscle force and sound

EMG, electromyography.

Technical and Patient-Related Considerations

When performing needle EMGs, it should be kept in mind that underlying nerve, muscle, and bone may be near the skin surface. The needle electrode should be advanced through the skin very carefully while constantly monitoring for the presence of insertion activity to ensure that the electrode is in muscle. This caution is particularly relevant to needle EMG of the diaphragm in young children, in whom the underlying muscle, including the diaphragm itself, is quite near the skin surface.

The relief of discomfort in conscious patients is worthy of comment. (Unconscious patients usually do not require analgesia or sedation for diagnostic tests.) Patients with Guillain–Barré syndrome find nerve conduction studies and EMG testing especially uncomfortable. Appropriate analgesia is therefore necessary for EMG procedures. Sedative drugs (especially midazolam) have profound effects on EEG recordings and should be used only when absolutely necessary.

Electrical interference is common in the ICU, and 60-Hz notch filters are therefore useful for both EMG and EEG machines. Adjacent machines or poorly grounded plugs may cause interference. The EMG machine must have adequately shielded cables. If other electrical devices are causing interference, these devices should be unplugged if safe to do so without harming the patient. Even then, 60-Hz artifact may be difficult to eliminate entirely.

Artifact from intravenous accurate control (IVAC) machines, movement artifact with ventilation, perspiration artifact, and current induction from proximity to other cables are common; static charge from drip chambers, fluid moving in ventilator tubing, and persons moving near or touching, moving, or percussing the patient are additional, commonly encountered sources of environmental and biologic artifact.[21] With long-term EEG monitoring, problems with electrode impedance, especially ground and reference electrodes, may render the recording unreliable. The collodion technique of securing EEG electrodes is recommended. Wrapping the head in a bandage and taping the electrode wires together helps to preserve contacts and prevents traction and excessive movement artifact. Subdermal wire electrodes allow for artifact-free recording for days.[22] The application of noncephalic leads or simultaneous video recording may help in detecting movement artifact. In applying EMG electrodes, it may be necessary, particularly in young children, to splint the limb to avoid excessive movement that may loosen the contact.

Electrical safety in the ICU is of special concern. Two-wire ungrounded devices that are not essential to patient survival should be unplugged with the agreement of the attending staff. If needed, these instruments must be grounded properly and plugged into an isolation transformer. The EEG or EMG machine must be plugged into a three-wire grounded outlet located in the same circuit branch that is used to power the other instruments connected to the patient. Extension cords must not be used. The reference or common line from the patient must be isolated electrically from the power line ground or include an appropriate type of current-limiting device. No additional ground electrode should be used. Switching the machine on and calibrating the EEG machine before the patient is connected, and disconnecting the patient before switching off the instrument, are recommended. Electrical interference should be investigated promptly because this may indicate current leakage through the patient.

When indwelling catheters or pacemaker electrodes are already connected to the patient, special precautions must be taken to ensure that these connections are isolated properly or current-limited. Application of an electrical stimulus near an intravascular line that terminates close to the heart is of theoretical concern in regard to the induction of arrhythmias or asystole. However, one of the authors (CFB) often stimulates at these sites in adults and children and has never had such a complication. This has been borne out in the study by Schoeck and colleagues.[23] Such stimuli should, however, be avoided in patients with temporary transvenous pacemakers.

CENTRAL NERVOUS SYSTEM DISORDERS

The role of the EEG in the evaluations of different neurologic disorders is considered in detail in Chapters 3 and 4. Attention here is confined to disorders encountered in the ICU.

Seizures

Overt convulsive seizures, either generalized or focal, can be seen and managed clinically. However, the EEG allows the physician to look for nonconvulsive seizures, which may be clinically inapparent (Fig. 34-1). Some evidence indicates that varieties of nonconvulsive status epilepticus other than absence status epilepticus can damage the brain, but this is controversial.[24,25] Prompt treatment of such patients should improve outcome and will shorten ICU and hospital stays. Continuous EEG monitoring is the optimal method of gauging the effects of antiepileptic drug therapy for status epilepticus. Problems of undertreatment or overtreatment can be minimized.

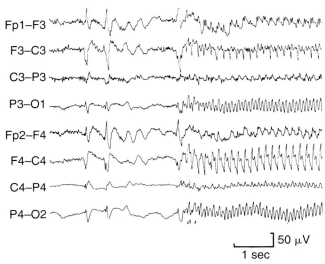

FIGURE 34-1 ■ A generalized nonconvulsive seizure is captured in a 73-year-old woman in coma 2 days after cardiac arrest. Isolated generalized spike-wave complexes are succeeded by a seizure that consists of rhythmic waves posteriorly and rapid, bisynchronous, sequential spike-wave complexes more anteriorly.

Impairment of consciousness may be attributed mistakenly to the cumulative effects of sedative drugs, intercurrent systemic (especially inflammatory) illness, or organ failure when, in fact, it is caused by nonconvulsive status epilepticus. The occurrence of nonconvulsive status is suggested by several clinical circumstances[26,27]:

1. An apparently prolonged "postictal state" following generalized convulsive seizures or a prolonged reduction of alertness after an operative procedure or neurologic insult
2. Acute onset of impaired consciousness or a fluctuating disturbance of consciousness with episodes of normal mentation
3. Impaired mentation or consciousness with myoclonus of the facial muscles or nystagmoid eye movements
4. Episodic blank staring, aphasia, automatisms (e.g., lip smacking, fumbling with fingers), or perseverative activity
5. Aphasia without an acute structural lesion
6. Other acute behavioral disturbances or impaired consciousness without obvious or adequate cause.

In such circumstances, an EEG should be obtained. If seizures or abundant epileptiform activity, such as periodic lateralized epileptiform discharges (PLEDs) or generalized epileptiform activity, is seen, more intensive monitoring with CEEG or serial recordings is indicated.[28,29]

Continuous EEG is valuable in the management of status epilepticus, especially for the diagnosis of nonconvulsive seizures and for monitoring the success of antiepileptic drug regimens.[30] In refractory status epilepticus, operationally defined as status epilepticus that continues for 60 to 90 minutes or more from the onset of therapy, full anesthesia usually is required to arrest the seizures. Agents include intravenous barbiturate anesthetic agents (e.g., thiopental and pentobarbital), inhalational agents (e.g., isoflurane), and intravenous nonbarbiturate anesthetics (e.g., midazolam, propofol, and etomidate). These drugs usually produce a burst-suppression pattern on the EEG to achieve control of seizures. In the authors' experience, generalized suppression for 2 to 30 seconds is effective. Greater periods of suppression, at least with barbiturate anesthetics, are associated with profound depression of the vasomotor center and hypotension. Monitoring allows optimal administration of the necessary agent and therefore avoidance of underdosing as well as excessive administration, which can be followed by complications or protracted recovery.

Continuous EEG can be helpful in estimating the prognosis in various conditions: normalization of the EEG is associated with a good outcome, whereas burst-suppression (provided that it is not caused by drugs), recurring ictal discharges, and (to a lesser extent) PLEDs are less favorable.[31] The cause of the seizures undoubtedly contributes to the prognosis. The duration of status epilepticus is also an independent determinant of mortality, thus emphasizing the importance of detection and prompt control of such seizures in the ICU.[27]

The most common cause of myoclonic status epilepticus in coma is the postanoxic state after cardiac arrest. The EEG findings are variable. One of the most common patterns is generalized burst-suppression, often with epileptiform potentials occurring within the bursts. Myoclonus often accompanies the EEG bursts, but the temporal relationship may be inconsistent. Other patterns include periodic complexes against a suppressed background; again, the relationship of the myoclonus to the complexes is variable. Some EEGs show no cortical spiking or complexes; in these situations the myoclonus probably arises entirely from a subcortical structure such as the brainstem reticular formation. Thus, EEG monitoring allows insight into the site of seizure origin in the brain and is of great assistance in classification. The syndromic classification and clinical background are of great importance in guiding further management.

Trauma

Trauma may affect the brain by a number of mechanisms such as intraparenchymal or extraparenchymal hemorrhage, ischemia, axonal shear injury, and a variety of metabolic derangements. These conditions may occur in any combination, and a rich variety of EEG abnormalities thus may be encountered. Their prognostic significance rests not only on their severity but also on the reversibility of the responsible pathogenetic mechanisms.

The following EEG patterns have been described: slowing in the theta range; delta activity, including continuous focal arrhythmic, diffuse rhythmic or arrhythmic, or intermittent rhythmic patterns; faster frequencies; epileptiform activity, including focal spikes or seizures, either clinical or electrographic; synchronous periodic slow-wave bursts; triphasic waves; focal suppression; other asymmetries; and alpha, theta, or spindle coma patterns.

The timing of the EEG in head injury is important with respect to the types of abnormalities and their associated etiologic, prognostic, and management implications.

Localized abnormalities at any stage should raise the possibility of structural lesions. Changes in amplitude, especially localized attenuation of activity, should be considered to reflect an intracranial hematoma until proved otherwise, provided that local scalp swelling is excluded. Focal slowing sometimes is associated with such lesions but can occur as a transient phenomenon. Electrographic seizures usually reflect severe brain injury, are of reliable lateralizing value, and should prompt urgent brain imaging and treatment.

When the recording shows continuous rhythmic activity (including sleep phenomena), the presence of variability in frequencies and amplitude is more favorable for outcome than are recordings showing no such variability.[32] Any reactivity is associated with a better prognosis than is no reactivity.[32]

Sometimes trauma affects the brain indirectly. Fat embolism to the brain and lungs is a complication of fractures of long bones. The patient may be asymptomatic for 12 to 36 hours after the injury and then become obtunded in association with pulmonary symptoms and tachycardia. The EEG shows replacement of normal rhythms with diffuse polymorphic delta and theta activity accentuated over the frontal regions. Trauma to the neck may cause delayed occlusion of the carotid or vertebral arteries and clinical and EEG features of strokes in these territories.

Serial EEGs or continuous monitoring may be useful in determining prognosis and in detecting potentially treatable conditions such as seizure activity, brain herniation, hydrocephalus, and intracerebral or subdural hematomas. The latter should be suspected if the EEG shows increasing slow-wave activity, focal suppression, or chronically persisting focal abnormalities along with intermittent rhythmic delta activity. These EEG findings and their timing need to be considered along with the integrity of brainstem function and clinical responsiveness when formulating a prognosis for a particular patient.

With regard to traumatic brain injury, the conduction time of the median-derived SEP through the brain (central conduction time) determined at a single time-point in the first few days after injury does not predict the outcome accurately in individual cases. However, bilaterally absent, cortically generated N20 waveforms in the early stages after a head injury nearly always predict death or a persistent vegetative state, whereas normal cortical SEPs are associated with recovery of conscious awareness and lack of severe motor deficits in adult patients.[33–35] Intermediate grades of SEP abnormality, in which the N20 responses are present but delayed or reduced in amplitude, have less precise or useful predictive value.[35]

Anoxic-Ischemic Encephalopathy

Anoxic-ischemic encephalopathy shares many features with metabolic encephalopathies but also has distinct clinical and electrophysiologic features. Unlike most other metabolic disorders, it is often associated with neuronal death.

Anoxic-ischemic encephalopathy because of cardiac arrest is the third leading cause of coma in ICU patients, following trauma and drug overdose.[36] Among comatose survivors of cardiopulmonary resuscitation, only about 1 in 4 survives to discharge; only 1 in 5 is able to return home; and fewer than 1 in 10 returns to former status, employability, and independence.[36] It is desirable to have reliable, early predictors of both favorable and unfavorable outcomes for resource allocation, management, and counseling of family members. Clinical, EEG, SEP, and biochemical studies have correlated outcomes in patients after cardiac arrest, but few have examined combined variables prospectively in the same patients while ensuring that patients survived for at least several days, to prevent premature "self-fulfilling prophecies."[37–39] SEP results serve as a reliable predictor of poor outcome; bilateral abolition of N20 indicates with close to 100 percent specificity that the patient will not recover.[40] However, preservation of the N20 response does not guarantee awakening; more than 40 percent of such patients do not recover conscious awareness.[41] Long-latency SEPs might reliably provide early identification of patients with favorable outcome because they provide a better evaluation of cortical integrity than short-latency responses.[42] In a preliminary study, patients whose N70 response was preserved consistently recovered awareness, with about half making a good recovery and the other half remaining disabled but still interactive and aware.[43] Further studies on the role of long-latency responses, including cognitive event-related potentials, clearly are needed.

EEG can play a useful role in prognosis, especially when the N20 response of the median-derived SEP is preserved. Patients with diffuse but variable and reactive theta and delta patterns (not theta-pattern coma, in which there is little or no variability or reactivity) recover awareness.[43] Similarly, those with more "malignant" EEG patterns, especially with generalized suppression of less than 20 μV or a burst-suppression pattern containing generalized epileptiform activity, do not recover awareness and either die in coma or remain in a vegetative state.

Metabolic Disorders

Anesthesia and metabolic encephalopathies share a number of features: EEG patterns show similarities, the graded EEG response to increasing anesthetic administration is similar to the evolutionary changes seen with increasing severity of metabolic or toxic derangement, and with some exceptions the changes are reversible.

In such a model the anesthetic dose, like the severity of metabolic encephalopathy, shows an inverse relationship with EEG frequency and a direct relationship with amplitude. Such slowing accompanies decreased unitary activity of cerebral cortical neurons.[44] This linearity breaks down at high doses, with the appearance of a burst-suppression pattern or epileptiform activity. The following sequential EEG changes are common to increasing levels of anesthesia and to most metabolic encephalopathies of increasing severity:

1. Desynchronization of background activity, followed by the appearance of increasing amounts of theta activity
2. Increase in the rhythmicity and voltage of delta activity, initially mixed with faster frequencies
3. Simplified delta activity (without faster frequencies)
4. Burst-suppression pattern, with the duration of suppression becoming longer with deeper levels
5. Suppression leading to an isoelectric EEG.

This progression applies to sedative drug intoxication and to most metabolic encephalopathies, including hepatic and renal failure, septic encephalopathy, carbon dioxide narcosis, and adrenal failure.[44] This analogy has limitations, however, and is not perfect. First, with certain clinical conditions capable of causing neuronal death (e.g., anoxic-ischemic encephalopathy), the EEG changes are not reversible and may progress, if severe enough, to permanent suppression. Second, in some diseases, specific features are superimposed on the patterns of sinusoidal waves or suppression, such as triphasic waves in hepatic encephalopathy, renal failure, and septic encephalopathy, and spikes in anoxia and penicillin-induced encephalopathy. Third, the number of metabolic encephalopathies that progress to a burst-suppression or suppression pattern is limited. Examples of the latter include anoxic-ischemic encephalopathy, septic encephalopathy, drug-induced coma (especially from barbiturates and benzodiazepines), hypothermia, and extreme hypoglycemic encephalopathy. Most others do not progress to this degree of abnormality unless the encephalopathy is associated with raised intracranial pressure and resultant global ischemia, as in the cerebral edema accompanying acute hepatic encephalopathy or Reye syndrome.[44]

Age has a bearing on EEG phenomena in coma. Triphasic waves are not found in children, whereas 14- and 6-Hz positive spikes have been described in comatose children with Reye syndrome or hepatic encephalopathy.[44]

Table 34-3 lists a number of metabolic conditions, along with special caveats that depart from the anesthetic model, and the degree of reversibility of a suppression or burst-suppression pattern. Examples include drug intoxication, hepatic failure, Reye syndrome, uremia, dialysis encephalopathy, septic encephalopathy, porphyria, hypothyroidism, Wernicke encephalopathy, Addison disease, hypercalcemia, hypocalcemia, hypoglycemia, and hypothermia.[44]

Infections

Bacterial and tuberculous meningitis usually produce irregular, widespread delta activity as the predominant EEG abnormality. Background activity usually is preserved better than in encephalitis. The improvement in frequencies parallels clinical resolution. In patients with a good prognosis, the EEG shows rapid normalization within 6 to 9 days. Prolongation of EEG abnormalities beyond 2 weeks suggests a complication such as infarction from vasculitis, hydrocephalus, or subdural hygromas (the latter in young children).

Encephalitis also usually produces delta activity as the predominant EEG abnormality. Multifocal epileptiform activity commonly occurs and is a reflection of cortical gray matter disease. In herpes simplex encephalitis, the temporal regions are the site of maximal slowing; between the 2nd and 14th days of illness these may contain PLEDs with a repetition rate of 0.5 to 2 per second. This feature is important in suggesting herpes simplex

TABLE 34-3 ■ Metabolic Encephalopathies Related to the Anesthetic Model

Etiology	Additional Features	Reversibility and Implication of Burst-Suppression or Suppression
Anoxia	Epileptiform activity	Usually not reversible
	Alpha/theta coma*	Usually unfavorable
	Generalized periodicity	Usually unfavorable[‡]
Drug intoxication	Some may produce epileptiform activity; a mixture of beta plus theta/delta suggests barbiturate or benzodiazepine overdose	Completely reversible for all patterns
Hepatic failure	Triphasic waves[†]	Not reversible (older literature)
		? Potentially reversible if liver function improves or with detoxification
Reye syndrome	14- and 6-Hz positive spikes in 50% (controversial significance)	Probably not reversible (dependent on damage from brain swelling and/or hypoglycemia)
Uremic encephalopathy	Triphasic waves[†] or epileptiform activity in some; photic sensitivity	Probably reversible
Septic encephalopathy	Triphasic waves[†] in some	Potentially reversible if the patient survives multiple organ failure
Dialysis encephalopathy	Epileptiform activity (generalized spike-wave abnormality)	Not reversible in advanced cases
Porphyria	Focal features (e.g., spikes, suppression) occasionally seen; usually transient	Largely reversible; EEG may be slow to improve
Hypothyroidism	Low amplitude	Should resolve, except in cretinism
Wernicke encephalopathy	May show sharp and slow-wave complexes, periods of suppression in advanced cases	EEG may improve; many patients have severe amnesia and ataxia
Addison disease	Majority are normal; others show diffuse slowing	Resolves, especially with corticosteroids
Hypercalcemia	May have triphasic waves or FIRDA	Rare, resolves
Hypocalcemia	Bursts of generalized spikes	Interictal suppression reversible
Hypoglycemia	May show epileptiform activity, periodic complexes	Partly reversible
Hypothermia	No change until <30°C	Completely reversible
	Burst-suppression at 20°C to 22°C	Completely reversible
	Suppression at <18°C	Completely reversible

*Alpha or theta coma patterns have been described in anoxic-ischemic encephalopathy, brainstem lesions, and drug intoxication, especially with barbiturates. In intoxication, the prognosis is favorable. In anoxic-ischemic encephalopathy or brainstem lesions, these patterns usually but not invariably are associated with a poor prognosis for recovery of full conscious awareness. The alpha-theta coma pattern is unstable and usually changes to a more definitive prognostic pattern in 5 to 6 days from coma onset.

[†]Triphasic waves were thought originally to be specific for hepatic encephalopathy but can occur in a variety of metabolic encephalopathies, septic encephalopathies, and neurodegenerative conditions. In the context of an acute alteration in alertness, however, they are highly suggestive of metabolic encephalopathy. Hepatic or renal failure and septic encephalopathy are the most common underlying causes in this situation.

[‡]A burst-suppression pattern after cardiac arrest is associated with 96 percent mortality rate; recordings should be done more than 24 hours after arrest and repeated to help establish the prognosis.

EEG, electroencephalogram; FIRDA, frontal irregular rhythmic delta activity.

From Young GB, Leung LS, Campbell V et al: The electroencephalogram in metabolic/toxic coma. Am J EEG Technol, 32:243, 1992, with permission.

encephalitis, which is treatable with the antiviral agent acyclovir. Multifocal delta activity may accompany acute disseminated encephalomyelitis, a postinfectious, immunologically mediated syndrome characterized by perivenous demyelination.

Septic encephalopathy, in which the brain appears to be affected in an indirect, reversible fashion (at least in the early, acute stage), behaves like most metabolic encephalopathies in that it closely follows the "anesthetic model" (Figs. 34-2 and 34-3). Cerebrospinal fluid analysis and imaging studies are usually unremarkable.

Structural Lesions

Single structural lesions in the supratentorial compartment produce coma mainly by compression of deeper structures such as the diencephalon or midbrain tegmentum. The EEG manifestations may be diffuse by the time the patient is in coma, but a supratentorial lesion should be suspected if significant and consistent asymmetry in voltage is noted between the two hemispheres or if intermittent rhythmic delta activity is exclusively frontal.[44] Another mechanism by which supratentorial lesions produce coma is by causing seizures. Epileptiform activity on EEG may suggest that an earlier seizure was missed clinically and that the comatose patient is in a postictal state. Alternatively, electrographic seizure activity may indicate a nonconvulsive seizure or status epilepticus.

Lesions limited to the brainstem often do not produce much EEG slowing; however, sleep potentials sometimes are found. Often the EEG shows an alpha pattern that may be more marked posteriorly. Care should be taken to ensure that the patient is in coma and not in a locked-in state, as discussed in Chapter 3.

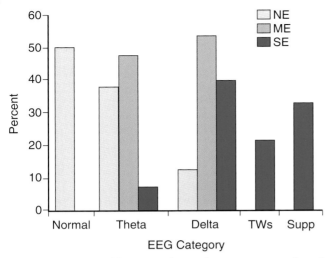

FIGURE 34-2 ▪ A histogram shows the percentages of septic patients with various electroencephalographic (EEG) abnormalities. Encephalopathic patients have EEG abnormalities that correspond to the severity of the encephalopathy. Theta, EEG dominated by frequencies in theta range; Delta, EEG dominated by delta frequencies; TWs, presence of triphasic waves; Supp, generalized suppression or burst-suppression pattern; NE, nonencephalopathic; ME, mildly encephalopathic; SE, severely encephalopathic. (From Young GB, Bolton CF, Archibald YM et al: The electroencephalogram in sepsis-associated encephalopathy. J Clin Neurophysiol, 9:145, 1992, with permission.)

Cerebrovascular Diseases

Cerebrovascular disorders typically cause focal structural brain lesions. Sometimes, however, the lesions are not single. In subarachnoid hemorrhage, for example, multifocal vasospasm may cause multifocal delta or epileptiform activity. Watershed ischemia also shows bilateral abnormalities but with maximal localization over the posterior temporal-occipital-parietal regions. The background is slow and often accompanied by periodic epileptiform activity.[45] Thrombosis of the superior sagittal sinus and draining veins would be expected to produce a somewhat similar picture of bilateral arrhythmic delta and epileptiform activity, but this activity may not consistently be maximal posteriorly in the head.

Metabolic consequences of cerebrovascular diseases (e.g., inappropriate antidiuretic hormone secretion and hyponatremia) may alter the EEG diffusely, as may hydrocephalus with coma.

PERIPHERAL NERVOUS SYSTEM DISORDERS

A variety of electrophysiologic tests may be applied to the peripheral nervous system, including tests of respiratory function (see Table 34-2). This section indicates the role of such studies, notably in the common ICU problem of difficulty in weaning from the ventilator, and then discusses specific causes of generalized limb and respiratory muscle weakness according to its time of onset in relation to admission to the ICU. Mononeuropathies, also important ICU complications, are then discussed.

Respiratory Studies

Most patients in the ICU are maintained on ventilators, and in many the reason is neurologic.[46,47] The ventilator alters abnormal patterns of CNS dysfunction, such as Cheyne–Stokes respiration, which may be of localizing value. Decreased tidal volume, increased respiratory rate, and increased CO_2 with paradoxical chest and abdominal wall movements, which suggest neuromuscular respiratory insufficiency, may be absent or, if present, are nonspecific. Decreased vital capacity and maximum inspiratory pressure, which also suggest a neuromuscular cause, may be caused by decreased central drive or by a disorder of the phrenic nerves, neuromuscular junctions, or diaphragm muscle. Electrophysiologic tests have now been developed that can test specifically the site of dysfunction in the peripheral and central nervous systems (see Table 34-2, Fig. 34-4). In addition to the various nerve conduction studies, needle EMG of the diaphragm is an important test, evaluating disorders of both the central and peripheral nervous systems affecting respiration. An ultrasound-guided technique is valuable in patients who are obese or edematous, or who have other structural changes that make the technique difficult.[48] Pneumothorax is a rare complication, occurring in two patients of the authors who were on a ventilator and had chronic obstructive lung disease.[48] Application of these respiratory electrophysiologic tests will be described in conjunction with discussion of the peripheral nervous system.

DIFFICULTY IN WEANING FROM THE VENTILATOR

Difficulty in weaning a patient from ventilation is the most common reason for a neuromuscular electrophysiologic consultation in the ICU. After diseases of the lungs and heart have been excluded, clinical examination alone suggests a neurologic cause in 40 percent of cases.[49] Maher and co-workers performed electrophysiologic studies of the limbs, phrenic nerve conduction studies, and needle EMG of the diaphragm and showed that 38 of 40 such patients had a neuromuscular cause[50] (Fig. 34-5). Spitzer and associates made similar observations.[51] In most cases the cause was critical illness

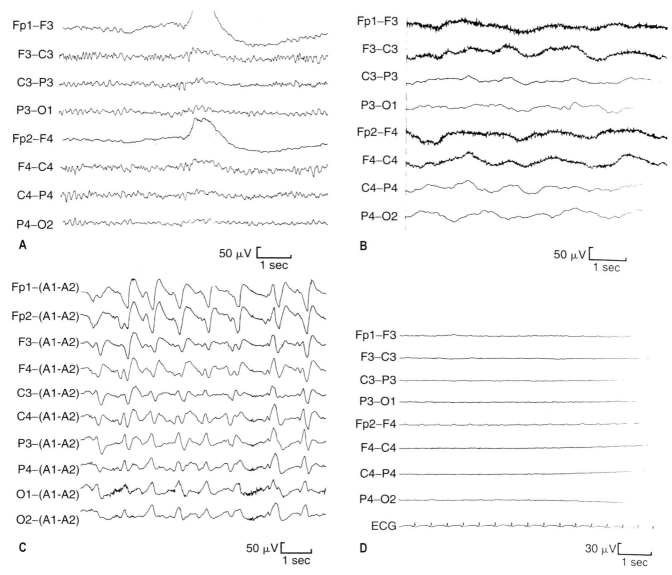

FIGURE 34-3 ▪ **A**, Electroencephalogram (EEG) of a mildly encephalopathic patient, showing excessive theta. **B**, EEG dominated by excessive delta in a comatose septic patient. **C**, Abundant triphasic waves in a 73-year-old comatose patient with septic encephalopathy. **D**, Nearly complete generalized suppression of the EEG in a 75-year-old comatose patient 1 day after cardiac arrest.

polyneuropathy, but there were varying combinations of this disorder with impaired central drive, unilateral phrenic nerve damage, neuromuscular transmission defects, and primary myopathies. The information was valuable in determining long-term prognosis. It will be important in future studies to apply the more recently developed techniques (see Table 34-2), which may clarify further the nature and incidence of lack of central drive and conditions primarily affecting the diaphragm (e.g., neuromuscular transmission defects and the phenomenon of diaphragmatic fatigue). A shift of the mean electrical frequency in the diaphragm from a higher to a lower frequency, as demonstrated by power spectral

analysis, suggests diaphragmatic fatigue. Automated interference pattern analysis may provide specific information about the nature of primary myopathies affecting the diaphragm.

Acute Weakness Developing Before ICU Admission

Patients may have rapidly developing paralysis that includes the respiratory muscles, making endotracheal intubation and mechanical ventilation necessary. The course may be so rapid that time is insufficient for an

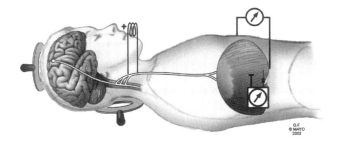

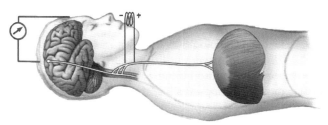

FIGURE 34-4 ▪ Electrophysiologic studies of respiration. The motor pathways (upper figure) are tested by magnetic stimulation of the motor cortex or cervical spinal cord with recording from the opposite hemidiaphragm, or by stimulation of the phrenic nerve in the neck by an electrical stimulus and recording from the ipsilateral hemidiaphragm, or by recording from the diaphragm with a needle electrode. Sensory pathways (lower figure) are tested by the somatosensory evoked potential technique. The phrenic nerve is stimulated by an electrical stimulus in the neck and the evoked potential recorded from the opposite sensory cortex, i.e., between CP3 and F2. (From Bolton CF, Chen R, Wijdicks EFM et al: Neurology of Breathing. Butterworth–Heinemann, Philadelphia, 2004, with permission.)

accurate diagnosis.[52] Thus, investigations must proceed after admission to the ICU. In this acutely developing situation, clinical signs may be confusing. The differential diagnosis should be approached systematically (Fig. 34-6).

SPINAL CORD COMPRESSION

In acute disorders of the high cervical spinal cord (e.g., compression caused by neoplasm or infection) or acute transverse myelitis, the traditional signs of localized spinal cord disease may be absent. Hyporeflexia induced by spinal shock is present, and the sensory level may be difficult to determine. Thus, magnetic resonance imaging (MRI) of the spinal cord on an emergency basis is often necessary.

On electrophysiologic assessment, motor conduction studies show decreased amplitudes of compound muscle action potentials caused by anterior horn cell disease if at least 5 days have elapsed since the injury. If sensory conduction is normal despite clinical sensory loss, the lesion

lies proximal to the dorsal root ganglion and is usually a myelopathy. Needle EMG abnormalities will appear after a 10- to 20-day interval, depending on the distance between the site of injury along the nerve and the muscle. The pattern of affected muscles assists in localizing the segmental level, in determining whether the pathology is unilateral or bilateral, and in providing a guide to the number of segments involved, although because of the considerable segmental overlap (particularly in paraspinal muscle innervation) the results may not be precise. In SEP studies, scalp recordings reveal delayed or absent potentials. Normal peripheral nerve and T12 responses localize the lesion to above the T12 level; absent or delayed T12 responses suggest that the lesion is in the region of the cauda equina or lumbosacral plexus if peripheral nerve responses are normal. Unless the spinal cord lesion clearly involves the posterior-column somatosensory pathways, SEP results may be normal in the presence of a spinal cord lesion of considerable size.

Transcutaneous magnetic stimulation of the brain and spinal cord, phrenic nerve conduction studies, and needle EMG of the diaphragm will aid further in localizing the lesion.

MOTOR NEURON DISEASE

Motor neuron disease may present initially as severe respiratory insufficiency.[53] The clinical signs of combined upper and lower motor neuron deficits, hyporeflexia or hyperreflexia, muscle wasting and fasciculations, and atrophy and fasciculations of the tongue may not be clearly

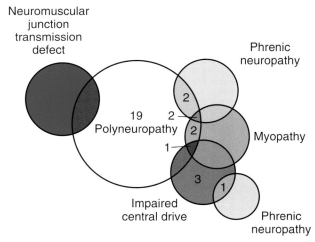

FIGURE 34-5 ▪ Types of neuromuscular disorders among 40 patients who failed to wean from ventilation. Thirty-eight (95 percent) had a neuromuscular disorder, and 15 (38 percent) had a combination of disorders. (From Maher J, Rutledge F, Remtulla H et al: Neurophysiological assessment of failure to wean from a ventilator. Can J Neurol Sci, 20:S28, 1995, with permission.)

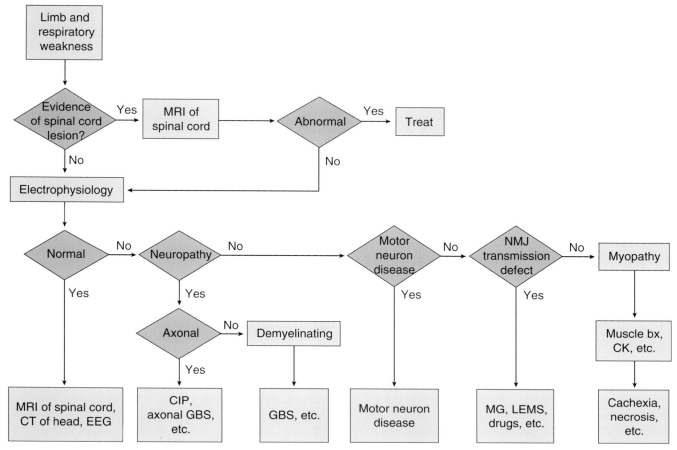

FIGURE 34-6 ■ Algorithm to guide the approach to the investigation of intensive care unit patients who have weakness of limb and respiratory muscles. Note: Positive serology or stool culture for *Campylobacter jejuni* may be the earliest warning of the axonal form of Guillain–Barré syndrome (GBS). MRI, magnetic resonance imaging; NMJ, neuromuscular junction; bx, biopsy; CK, serum creatine kinase; CT, computed tomography; EEG, electroencephalogram; CIP, critical illness polyneuropathy; MG, myasthenia gravis; LEMS, Lambert–Eaton myasthenic syndrome. (From Bolton CF, Young GB: The neurological consultation and neurological syndromes in the intensive care unit. Baillieres Clin Neurol, 5:447, 1996, with permission.)

present. Electrophysiologic studies, including phrenic nerve conduction studies and needle EMG of the chest wall and diaphragm, as well as comprehensive needle EMG of limb muscles, often will suggest the diagnosis.[50,54] Even then, it may be necessary to proceed with MRI. Disorders simulating motor neuron disease (e.g., motor neuropathy with multifocal conduction block) should be excluded.

Acute Polyneuropathy

Polyneuropathy is suggested by the presence of muscle weakness, hyporeflexia, and distal sensory loss, and by the absence of upper motor neuron signs or bladder dysfunction, but these signs may not always be clearly present. For example, bladder dysfunction and extensor plantar responses are occasionally seen in Guillain–Barré syndrome. Electrophysiologic studies are thus of great value in establishing the diagnosis.

Acute Inflammatory Demyelinating Polyneuropathy (Guillain–Barré Syndrome)

The electrophysiologic features are those of demyelination of peripheral nerves. In the initial stages, nerve conduction velocities may be only mildly depressed, but prolonged or absent F waves, evidence of conduction block, and absence of abnormal spontaneous activity in muscle with a reduced number of rapidly firing motor unit potentials all suggest this diagnosis. Thus, even within hours of onset, the findings are often strongly suggestive of Guillain–Barré syndrome. Phrenic nerve conduction studies and needle EMG of the diaphragm are particularly valuable in establishing the nature and severity of the involvement of these sites, even when performed within the first 3 days of onset.[55] Serial electrophysiologic studies to monitor the course of treatment are valuable. Intravenous immunoglobulin and plasmapheresis may both be effective. Corticosteroids are not.[56]

This applies to axonal forms, as well. However, symptomatic improvement may precede electrophysiologic improvement. Several variants of Guillain–Barré syndrome are now recognized that are primarily axonal rather than demyelinating. All are likely to have *Campylobacter jejuni* infection as the factor precipitating the immune-mediated polyneuropathy. These variants are discussed in the following sections, except for the Miller Fisher variant of ophthalmoplegia, ataxia, and areflexia, which rarely requires admission to the ICU. Positive serology or stool culture for *C. jejuni* may be the earliest evidence of these axonal forms.

Acute Motor and Sensory Axonal Neuropathy

This acute axonal form of Guillain–Barré syndrome usually is manifested as a rapidly developing paralysis that reaches completion within a matter of hours and requires early admission to the ICU and full ventilatory assistance. Although its severity varies, all muscles of the body, including the cranial musculature and even the eye muscles and pupils, may be totally paralyzed. Thus, clinically, the syndrome of brain death may be simulated, but the EEG is relatively normal. All peripheral nerves, including cranial nerves, may be unresponsive to electrical stimulation, even when the stimuli are of high voltage and long duration. Often, sensory as well as muscle compound action potentials are reduced or absent. Needle EMG initially will show no abnormal spontaneous activity and an absence of motor unit potentials. Denervation potentials appear after 10 to 20 days. Recovery is often quite prolonged and incomplete.

Acute Motor Axonal Neuropathy

This acute paralytic syndrome of children and young adults consists of a symmetric, ascending weakness that progresses over days and is associated with normal sensation, with often preserved tendon reflexes, and with an increased cerebrospinal fluid protein concentration.[57] The electrophysiologic features are consistent with pure motor dysfunction, a primary dysfunction of anterior horn cells or proximal motor axons. Compound muscle action potential amplitudes are reduced, but motor latencies are normal. Sensory conduction is normal. Needle EMG reveals varying degrees of denervation of affected muscle. Significant respiratory paralysis may be present, but good recovery eventually occurs. This neuropathy is a variant of Guillain–Barré syndrome and may be related to *C. jejuni* enteritis and anti-GM antibodies.[57]

Other polyneuropathies such as acute porphyria should also be considered and excluded when necessary. If Lyme disease or human immunodeficiency virus infection is suspected even remotely, appropriate antibody tests should be performed.

Chronic Polyneuropathies

Chronic polyneuropathies occasionally evolve as a rapidly developing respiratory insufficiency. Although rare, such insufficiency may occur in chronic inflammatory demyelinating polyneuropathy and diabetic polyneuropathy. In addition to the more typical clinical and electrophysiologic signs of these polyneuropathies, it is worthwhile performing phrenic nerve conduction studies and needle EMG of the diaphragm to show that the respiratory insufficiency is caused by the neuropathy.

Neuromuscular Transmission Defects

Defects in neuromuscular transmission are rare but present particular challenges in diagnosis. Both myasthenia gravis and Lambert–Eaton myasthenic syndrome may be manifested initially as respiratory insufficiency.[58] The diagnosis of myasthenia gravis rests on the presence of variability in the weakness of eye and facial muscles, a positive Tensilon test, and the findings on single-fiber EMG. Phrenic nerve conduction and needle EMG studies of the diaphragm may reveal partial denervation of the diaphragm. These patients improve with immunosuppressive therapy. The respiratory muscles strengthen, and successful weaning from the ventilator is achieved.[58]

Lambert–Eaton myasthenic syndrome may also be manifested initially as an acute, severe respiratory failure requiring management on a ventilator in the ICU.[59] Clinical signs may be equivocal. The pattern of reduced compound muscle action potentials; normal sensory nerve action potentials; no abnormal spontaneous activity; and small, short-duration motor units on needle EMG suggests this diagnosis, which is confirmed by repetitive stimulation studies at slow and fast rates. Phrenic nerve conduction, including repetitive stimulation,[60] and needle EMG of the diaphragm shows abnormalities including denervation. Improvement occurs with immunosuppression and facilitates weaning from the ventilator.[59]

Other types of presynaptic neuromuscular transmission defects (e.g., hypocalcemia, hypermagnesemia, and wound botulism) may also be identified electrophysiologically. In organophosphate poisoning, a repetitive muscle action potential discharge after a single electrical shock to a peripheral nerve is diagnostic. The effective maneuver in diagnosing tick bite paralysis is to search carefully for the tick and remove it.

MYOPATHIES

Myopathies do not usually present a difficult diagnostic problem. The respiratory muscles occasionally are involved, and if so, may necessitate intubation and admission to the ICU, but the diagnosis is usually evident or has been established previously in chronic cases. Comprehensive electrophysiologic testing, including transcranial magnetic stimulation, will identify impaired central drive (Fig. 34-7) or a primary myopathy (Fig. 34-8) as the cause of the respiratory insufficiency.[61] In more acute

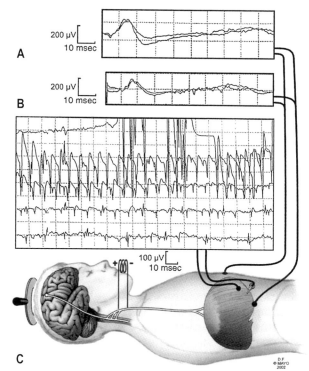

FIGURE 34-8 ▪ A patient with myotonic dystrophy. The diaphragmatic compound muscle action potential on (**A**) direct phrenic nerve electrical stimulation and (**B**) cortical magnetic stimulation was low in amplitude. **C**, Needle electromyography of the diaphragm revealed myotonic discharge and positive sharp waves, indicating a primary myopathy. (From Bolton CF, Chen R, Wijdicks EFM et al: Neurology of Breathing. Butterworth–Heinemann, Philadelphia, 2004, with permission.)

myopathies (e.g., necrotizing myopathy with myoglobinuria), the diagnosis is clearly evident from the very high serum levels of creatine kinase; myoglobinuria may also occur and muscle necrosis may be evident on muscle biopsy.

Acute Weakness Developing After ICU Admission

In large medical and surgical ICUs, the authors estimate that at least 50 percent of patients have significant involvement of the nervous system. Neuromuscular problems are much more common than is generally recognized. Sepsis and multiple organ failure now occur in 20 to 50 percent of patients in a medical ICU, and 70 percent of such patients have critical illness polyneuropathy.[62,63] Neuromuscular blocking agents and corticosteroids may cause further distinctive neuromuscular syndromes.[54] Because of difficulties in clinically evaluating such patients, identification of neuromuscular

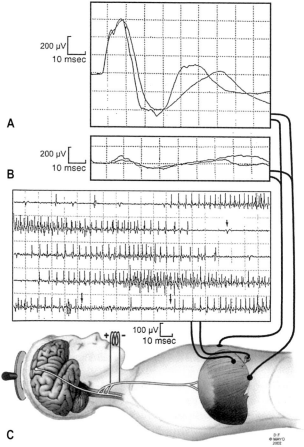

FIGURE 34-7 ▪ A patient with myotonic dystrophy. **A**, The diaphragmatic compound muscle action potential on direct electrical stimulation was normal but (**B**) was markedly reduced on cortical magnetic stimulation. **C**, Needle electromyography of the diaphragm showed that only a few motor unit potentials fired with each inspiration. The findings indicated impaired central respiratory drive. The short arrow indicates electrocardiogram artifact; the two long arrows bracket a low-amplitude myotonic discharge. (From Bolton CF, Chen R, Wijdicks EFM et al: Neurology of Breathing. Butterworth–Heinemann, Philadelphia, 2004, with permission.)

problems can be established only through electrophysiologic tests, at times supplemented by muscle and, rarely, nerve biopsy. These investigations aid in managing conditions such as difficulty in weaning from the ventilator and limb weakness during recovery. The subject has been reviewed elsewhere.[54,64-66]

MYELOPATHY

Myelopathies seen in the ICU are traumatic; compressive, caused by neoplasm, hemorrhage, or infection in the epidural space; and vascular, such as spinal cord infarction secondary to surgical procedures on the aorta. However, in almost all instances, the myelopathy will have occurred from the aforementioned circumstances before admission to the ICU and will have been managed as described earlier. If not, MRI is of great diagnostic value.

ACUTE POLYNEUROPATHY

Critical Illness Polyneuropathy

Since its initial description, critical illness polyneuropathy has come to be recognized as a common polyneuropathy, occurring in 50 to 70 percent of patients who are critically ill or injured.[67,68] Such patients have a syndrome now termed the systemic inflammatory response syndrome.[66] This syndrome occurs in response to both infection and several forms of trauma, including major surgery and burns. The neuropathy has been reviewed elsewhere.[64,66,69]

The relationship of critical illness polyneuropathy and critical illness myopathy has been established. In a systematic review, Stevens et al evaluated 21 studies involving 1,421 critically ill patients.[70] Among these patients, 46 percent had critical illness neuromuscular abnormalities and these were linked to hyperglycemia, the systemic inflammatory response syndrome, sepsis, renal replacement therapy, and catecholamine administration, all markers of severe sepsis and multiple organ failure.

After the development of systemic inflammatory response syndrome in the critical care unit, the earliest nervous system manifestation is septic encephalopathy. If the syndrome responds to antibiotics, surgical drainage of an infected focus, and supportive measures, the encephalopathy usually improves rapidly, but at this time difficulty in weaning from the ventilator may be noted. The most common neuromuscular cause for such weaning difficulty, after cardiac and pulmonary causes have been excluded, is critical illness polyneuropathy.

However, clinical signs of polyneuropathy, including depressed tendon reflexes, are present in only half of these patients. Hence, electrophysiologic studies are necessary to establish the diagnosis. A more severe polyneuropathy can, however, be suspected when, on deep painful stimulation of the distal extremities, limb movements seem weak despite strong grimacing of facial musculature.

In the critical care unit, central respiratory drive may be assessed by temporarily decreasing ventilatory support to 5 to 8 cm H_2O of pressure support or continuous positive airway pressure (to overcome airway/ventilator resistance) for a maximum of 15 minutes. Mechanical ventilation is restored if evidence of respiratory distress is present, arterial oxygen saturation declines to less than 90 percent (based on a pulse oximeter reading), or a significant rise in heart rate or blood pressure is noted. It is advantageous to decrease ventilatory support at the time of needle EMG of the diaphragm. The presence and type of any disorder of central drive then can be assessed more accurately.

The earliest electrophysiologic sign of the neuropathy is a reduction in amplitude of compound muscle action potentials with a minor change in latency. The duration of the compound muscle action potential is not prolonged, as it is in critical illness myopathy. This pattern is typical of axonal damage and occurs within 1 week.[71] Fibrillation potentials and positive sharp waves may not appear in muscle until 3 weeks. Motor unit potentials, if they can be activated voluntarily by the patient (which may not be possible because of sedation or septic encephalopathy), will often appear normal or somewhat low in amplitude and polyphasic in configuration and suggest an associated primary myopathy. Hence, it is important to demonstrate depression in amplitude of sensory nerve action potentials before a firm electrophysiologic diagnosis of polyneuropathy is made. Using several methods of testing peripheral nerve excitability in patients with critical illness polyneuropathy, it was observed that nerve membranes were depolarized by two possible mechanisms: raised extracellular potassium or hypoperfusion.[72]

Repetitive nerve stimulation studies should also be performed to seek a defect in neuromuscular transmission. Such a defect does not occur in sepsis but will be present if neuromuscular blocking agents have been used. The effects of these agents may persist beyond several hours to a number of days if the patient is in renal or liver failure.[73] Phrenic nerve conduction studies and needle EMG of the chest wall and diaphragm are important in establishing that the difficulty in weaning from the ventilator is, in fact, caused by critical illness polyneuropathy.[74]

Knowledge of the presence of critical illness polyneuropathy aids management on the ventilator and indicates that prolonged care in the ICU may be necessary. If the polyneuropathy is mild, recovery occurs within a matter of weeks; if severe, it may take months. In especially severe cases, recovery may not occur.[75] Despite improvement, clinical and electrophysiologic signs of critical illness polyneuropathy of varying severity may persist for 5 years or longer.[76,77] In unusually severe cases, recovery may not occur, and the patient remains quadriplegic.[63] In patients who are recovering, physiotherapy and appropriate rehabilitation measures should be instituted. In a prospective study by Leijten and co-workers, critical illness polyneuropathy was associated with increased mortality and rehabilitation problems.[75] Other than management of the systemic inflammatory response syndrome, no specific treatment of the neuropathy is known. Wijdicks and Fulgham failed to observe any improvement after treatment with high-dose intravenous immunoglobulin.[78] A few instances of critical illness polyneuropathy in children have been observed.[79-81] Intensive insulin therapy in critically ill patients reduces the mortality and morbidity, including a 44 percent reduction in the incidence of critical illness polyneuropathy.[82] This supports the earlier conjecture by Witt and associates that elevated blood glucose levels might play a direct role in the genesis of critical illness polyneuropathy.[63]

The morphologic features of critical illness polyneuropathy have been revealed through biopsy of peripheral nerve and muscle and comprehensive autopsy study of both the central and peripheral nervous systems. There is primary distal axonal degeneration of peripheral motor and sensory fibers. Muscle shows scattered atrophic fibers in acute denervation and grouped atrophy in chronic denervation. Occasional necrotic muscle fibers are present and suggest an associated primary myopathy.

NEUROMUSCULAR BLOCKING AGENTS

Neuromuscular blocking agents are used in the ICU to facilitate mechanical ventilation. Phrenic nerve conduction studies, repetitive phrenic nerve stimulation, needle EMG of the diaphragm, and automated interference pattern analysis of the diaphragm are valuable in investigating patients with muscle weakness and difficulty in weaning from the ventilator in the ICU (see Tables 34-2 and 34-4). Power spectral analysis of the diaphragm may also prove useful in such circumstances.

A pure axonal motor neuropathy or critical illness myopathy may develop in patients who have been in the ICU for several days, or longer, and have received competitive neuromuscular blocking agents such as

TABLE 34-4 ■ Normal Values of Various Respiratory Electrophysiologic Studies

Pathway		Mean ± SD	Normal Values
MOTOR CENTRAL RESPIRATORY PATHWAY			
Transcortical magnetic stimulation (n = 35) (response recorded from the diaphragm)			
Latency	(msec)	13.5 ± 1.4	<16.3
Amplitude	(μV)	263 ± 144	>100
Threshold	(%)	49.1 ± 7.5	<65
Cervical magnetic stimulation (n = 35) (response recorded from the diaphragm)			
Latency	(msec)	8.3 ± 1.2	<10.7
Amplitude	(μV)	281 ± 128	>100
Threshold	(%)	31.4 ± 9.0	<50
Central motor conduction time	(msec)	5.3 ± 1.1	<7.5
SENSORY PERIPHERAL RESPIRATORY PATHWAY			
Phrenic nerve somatosensory evoked potentials (n = 3)			
P1 latency	(msec)	12 ± 0.8	
N1 latency	(msec)	17 ± 1.3	
Amplitude	(μV)	0.3 ± 0.6	
MOTOR PERIPHERAL RESPIRATORY PATHWAY			
Phrenic nerve conduction (n = 25)			
Latency	(msec)	6.5 ± 0.8	<8.1
Amplitude	(μV)	669 ± 159	>300
Area	(μV. msec)	7.3 ± 2.1	>4.0
Duration	(msec)	19.4 ± 2.7	<25
3-Hz repetitive phrenic nerve stimulation (n = 6)			
Amplitude	(%)	12.1 ± 8.3	
Area	(%)	−2.2 ± 4.3	
Duration	(%)	−8.7 ± 9.6	<10.8

From Zifko U, Chen R: The respiratory system. Baillieres Clin Neurol, 5:477, 1996, with permission.

pancuronium bromide or the shorter-acting vecuronium to ease mechanical ventilation.[83,84] These agents, possibly in combination with corticosteroids, generally will have been used for longer than 48 hours, occasionally for days or weeks. When they are discontinued, difficulty in weaning from the ventilator and limb paralysis are noted. The serum creatine kinase concentration is mildly or moderately elevated. Electrophysiologic testing sometimes reveals a defect in neuromuscular transmission at slower rates of stimulation, as expected with a postsynaptic defect. Nerve conduction and needle EMG studies provide evidence of severe, primary axonal degeneration of predominantly motor fibers. Phrenic nerve conduction studies and needle EMG of the diaphragm may indicate involvement of the phrenic nerves. Muscle biopsy shows varying degrees of denervation atrophy, muscle necrosis, or a myosin-deficient myopathy.

Although the mechanism for the pure axonal motor neuropathy is unknown, it is likely a variant of critical illness polyneuropathy, and sepsis appears to be an important underlying factor in most, if not all, cases.[54] Thus, if the various systemic complications can be treated successfully, the neuromuscular disorder improves spontaneously and good recovery may occur, sometimes quite rapidly. The authors[63] and others[67,68,85] have failed to implicate neuromuscular blocking agents as a cause of critical illness polyneuropathy; however, these agents probably have an additional toxic effect on nerve and muscle, and their use should be avoided if possible.

Competitive neuromuscular blocking agents may also cause a transient neuromuscular blockade. They are metabolized or cleared by the liver and kidney; with failure of these organs, the effect of these agents may be prolonged for a number of days after their withdrawal.[73] Repetitive nerve stimulation studies will identify the defect in neuromuscular transmission. However, by the time of testing, critical illness polyneuropathy or myopathy will also have developed in many of these patients; electrophysiologic studies should disclose the disorder or combination of disorders.

CRITICAL ILLNESS MYOPATHY

An acute myopathy may affect a variety of critically ill patients. This myopathy has many names, including critical care myopathy, acute necrotizing myopathy of intensive care, thick filament myopathy, acute quadriplegic myopathy, critical illness myopathy, acute corticosteroid myopathy, acute hydrocortisone myopathy, acute myopathy in severe asthma, and acute corticosteroid and pancuronium-associated myopathy. The term *critical illness myopathy* is now considered the most appropriate description for this syndrome. It includes at least three different types of muscle abnormalities: thick filament myopathy, cachectic myopathy, and acute necrotizing myopathy.

There has been much debate as to the incidence of critical illness myopathy, which may occur independently of or in association with critical illness polyneuropathy. A relationship between the early onset and severity of critical illness polyneuropathy and myopathy and the severity of critical illness and sepsis has been described.[86] Critical illness myopathy develops in at least one-third of ICU patients treated for status asthmaticus,[87] in 7 percent of patients after orthoptic liver transplantation,[88] and in an unknown percentage of adults and children with other critical illnesses.[89]

The major feature is flaccid weakness, which tends to be diffuse, involving all limb muscles and the neck flexors and often involving the facial muscles and diaphragm. Thus, most patients are also difficult to wean from mechanical ventilation. Ophthalmoplegia may be present.[90] Tendon reflexes are often, but not always, depressed. Myalgias are uncommon. Although the myopathy occurs acutely, the time of onset is usually difficult to determine because of commonly associated encephalopathy, administration of neuromuscular blocking agents, sedation, or other neuromuscular disease.

The clinical distinction between an axonal motor neuropathy and myopathy in critically ill patients is often impossible. Therefore, electrophysiologic studies are mandatory to separate these disorders. The typical features of critical illness myopathy on nerve conduction studies are low-amplitude compound muscle action potentials.

The duration of the compound muscle action potential in critical illness myopathy is often prolonged. There is little change in latency. The size and shape of the compound muscle action potential is quite similar with both proximal and distal nerve stimulation, implying dysfunction of the muscle membrane. Studies by Allen and co-workers[91] confirm earlier reports[92] that the excitation threshold is increased and that the prolonged duration of the compound muscle action potential results from decreased membrane conduction velocity. This may relate to dysfunction of sodium channels. In critical illness myopathy this abnormality is present in all muscles tested. Normal values for duration of the compound muscle action potential for key muscles in upper and lower limbs have been reported by Goodman and associates.[93]

Sensory nerve action potentials should be preserved; however, interpretation of sensory nerve conduction studies is often limited because of tissue edema. Reliable examination of volitionally activated motor unit potentials on needle EMG is also difficult with severe muscle weakness or impaired central drive to limb muscles. Hence, the needle EMG findings may be limited to interpretation of spontaneous activity. Abnormal spontaneous activity may be less prominent than with denervation from polyneuropathy, but its presence cannot be used to distinguish critical illness myopathy from polyneuropathy. Electrical inexcitability of the muscle membrane can be demonstrated by direct needle muscle stimulation in patients with severe myopathy who have markedly reduced or absent compound muscle action potentials. Direct muscle stimulation therefore may be helpful in the differentiation of critical illness myopathy and neuropathy.[92]

Determination of serum creatine kinase levels may be helpful in differential diagnosis; significantly elevated levels suggest a necrotizing myopathy. In these cases, myoglobinuria may be present. Serum levels become elevated between the 2nd and 16th days after corticosteroid exposure. Normal serum levels of creatine kinase, obtained 3 or more weeks after probable onset of weakness, do not exclude critical illness myopathy. Definite diagnosis is often possible only by light-microscopic examination of muscle tissue. Pathologic findings depend on the type of myopathy.

Phrenic nerve conduction studies and needle EMG of diaphragm and chest wall muscles are valuable in assessing patients with suspected critical illness myopathy. Phrenic nerve conduction studies typically show normal latencies, but the amplitude of distal compound muscle action potentials may be reduced. Needle EMG may reveal positive sharp waves and fibrillation potentials in respiratory muscles. Motor unit potentials, as in other myopathies, may be difficult to interpret in the diaphragm because they normally have a "myopathic" appearance. Follow-up phrenic nerve conduction studies may show a return toward normal as the patient recovers.

Lacomis and associates proposed criteria emphasizing the electrodiagnostic features for a diagnosis of probable critical illness myopathy and requiring histopathologic identification of myosin loss for a definite diagnosis.[89] The proposed major diagnostic features are as follows:

1. Sensory action potentials with amplitude exceeding 80 percent of the lower limit of normal (LLN) in two or more nerves
2. Needle EMG showing short-duration, low-amplitude motor unit potentials with early or normal full recruitment, with or without fibrillation potentials

3. Absence of a decremental response on repetitive nerve stimulation
4. Muscle histopathologic findings of myopathy with myosin loss.

Supportive features are:

1. Compound muscle action potentials with amplitude exceeding 80 percent of the LLN in two or more nerves without conduction block
2. Elevated serum creatine kinase levels (best assessed in the first week of illness)
3. Demonstration of muscle inexcitability. By definition, patients are or were critically ill, and weakness should have started after the onset of critical illness.

Added to these criteria, possibly as the most important diagnositic feature, should be the characteristic increase in the duration of the compound muscle action potential (discussed earlier).

These criteria are for research protocols. Whether a clinician should routinely pursue a muscle biopsy in order to distinguish critical illness myopathy from other myopathies or from critical illness polyneuropathy is questionable. A muscle biopsy should be considered if another myopathic process (e.g., an inflammatory myopathy) is suspected or if the histologic findings are likely to affect management. For example, a firm diagnosis of critical illness myopathy may lead to avoidance of intravenous corticosteroids or neuromuscular blocking agents. As indicated in Table 34-5,[94] the

---

TABLE 34-5 ■ Neuromuscular Conditions in the Critical Care Unit Associated with the Systemic Inflammatory Response Syndrome

Condition	Incidence	Clinical Features	Electrophysiologic Findings	Creatine Kinase	Muscle Biopsy
POLYNEUROPATHY					
Critical illness	Common	Flaccid limbs and respiratory weakness	Axonal degeneration of motor and sensory fibers	Nearly normal	Denervation atrophy
Motor neuropathy	Common with neuromuscular blocking agents and sepsis	Flaccid limbs and respiratory weakness	Axonal degeneration of motor fibers	Nearly normal	Denervation atrophy
NEUROMUSCULAR TRANSMISSION DEFECT					
Transient neuromuscular blockade	Common with neuromuscular blocking agents	Flaccid limbs and respiratory weakness	Abnormal repetitive nerve stimulation studies	Normal	Normal
CRITICAL ILLNESS MYOPATHY					
Thick-filament myopathy	Common with steroids, neuromuscular blocking agents, and sepsis	Flaccid limbs and respiratory weakness	Abnormal spontaneous activity in muscle	Elevated	Central loss of thick filaments
Disuse (cachectic) myopathy	Common (?)	Muscle wasting	Normal	Normal	Normal or type 2 fiber atrophy
Necrotizing myopathy of intensive care	Rare	Flaccid weakness and myoglobinuria	Abnormal spontaneous activity in muscle	Markedly elevated	Necrotic fibers

From Bolton CF, Young GB, Zochodne DW: Neurological changes during severe sepsis. p. 180. In Dobb GJ, Bion J, Burchardi H et al (eds): Current Topics in Intensive Care. WB Saunders, Philadelphia, 1994, with permission.

types of critical illness myopathy (i.e., myosin-deficiency myopathy, acute necrotizing myopathy, and cachectic myopathy) can be distinguished by clinical, electrophysiologic, and, if necessary, histologic features. This is important for prognosis. The necrotizing myopathy, if severe, may have a poor prognosis for recovery of muscle strength, whereas the prognosis is much better for cachectic myopathy and myosin-deficiency myopathy.[95]

Thick-Filament Myopathy

This distinctive syndrome occurs in children or adults in the setting of sudden, severe asthma[96–100] or in the setting of the ICU after organ transplantation.[101] Endotracheal intubation and placement on a ventilator are necessary. High-dose corticosteroids to treat the asthma and neuromuscular blocking agents to ease mechanical ventilation are administered, often for a number of days. On attempted weaning from the ventilator, the patient is found to have severe neuromuscular respiratory insufficiency and limb weakness. Ophthalmoplegia may be present.[90] Serum creatine kinase concentrations are normal or mildly increased. Repetitive nerve stimulation studies are usually normal. Sensory and motor conduction studies are normal, except for low-amplitude compound muscle action potentials. On needle EMG, motor unit potentials tend to be low in amplitude, of short duration, and polyphasic, thus indicating a primary myopathy. Direct electrical stimulation of the muscle membrane may reveal it to be inexcitable.[102] Muscle biopsy shows a loss of structure centrally in muscle fibers. Under the electron microscope, this loss of structure has been related to destruction of the thick myosin filaments.[97] Corticosteroids may activate an adenosine triphosphate–ubiquitin proteolytic system, which seemed to be the mechanism of myosin degradation in the muscle biopsies of two patients.[99] Another possible mechanism for proteolysis was shown in five patients by Showalter and Engel.[103] Calpain expression, which alters calcium homeostasis, was markedly enhanced. It is of interest that all the patients of Showalter and Engel were critically ill, and one had not received either corticosteroids or neuromuscular blocking agents. Thus, the systemic inflammatory response syndrome appears to be the common etiologic factor.

Recovery occurs rapidly. The clinical and electrophysiologic features are usually so distinctive that muscle biopsy is often not necessary.

Although the subject is still controversial, the authors believe that neuromuscular blocking agents should be used to ease mechanical ventilation in asthmatics only when the indications are clear; their use should be in as low a dosage and for as short a time as possible.

Cachectic Myopathy

Cachectic myopathy, disuse atrophy, and catabolic myopathy are often cited as complications of critical illness. However, even though these disorders cause muscle weakness and wasting, all are ill-defined in clinical terms. Motor and sensory nerve conduction studies, needle EMG, and serum creatine kinase concentrations are all normal. Muscle biopsy may be normal or show type 2 muscle fiber atrophy as a nonspecific finding. An exception is the report by Gutmann and co-workers of two critically ill patients who had severe muscle weakness and unusually severe atrophy of type 2 muscle fibers with regenerative changes on muscle biopsy.[104]

Acute Necrotizing Myopathy of Intensive Care

Rare but better-defined is acute necrotizing myopathy of intensive care.[105,106] It may be precipitated by a variety of infective, chemical, and other insults, basically involving the differential diagnosis of acute myoglobinuria.[54] Electrophysiologic studies are consistent with a severe myopathy, and muscle biopsy shows widespread necrosis of muscle fibers. Rapid and spontaneous recovery is expected in mild cases, but in more severe cases the prognosis may be poor.[106]

Mild increases in serum creatine kinase concentrations and scattered necrosis of muscle fibers on muscle biopsy occur in some critically ill patients and is suggestive of primary involvement of muscle as well as denervation atrophy. This finding may be caused by a reduction in bioenergetic reserves as measured by ^{31}P nuclear magnetic resonance spectroscopy because two such patients had very low ratios of phosphocreatine/inorganic phosphate, which would not be expected from denervation of muscle alone.[54] These abnormalities returned toward normal as the patients recovered. Nonetheless, biopsies performed in 11 of these patients (because of uncertainty about the nature of their neuromuscular conditions) were all notable for denervation atrophy, presumably secondary to a critical illness polyneuropathy.[107] The authors also believe that the syndrome of acute quadriplegic myopathy,[97,99,101] which has been attributed to the use of neuromuscular blocking agents and steroids, has sepsis as the main underlying factor.

Critical Illness Polyneuropathy and Myopathy

Considering the widespread effects of sepsis and multiple organ failure, both muscle and nerve are likely to be affected. Needle EMG in some patients reveals motor unit potentials that are small and polyphasic, suggesting associated myopathy. Morphologic studies of muscle reveal varying degrees of scattered necrosis in addition to denervation. Moreover, serum creatine kinase levels may be elevated more than would be expected from sepsis alone. Studies have indicated that, in patients with a neuromuscular cause for failure to wean from mechanical ventilation, there is evidence of myopathy in addition to neuropathy.[50,51] The compound muscle action potential amplitude in the early stages in sepsis, in addition to being reduced in amplitude, is prolonged in duration without change in latency, suggesting primary, energy-deficient involvement of the muscle fiber membrane.[54] Nuclear magnetic resonance spectroscopy of muscle in two patients with critical illness polyneuropathy revealed a marked reduction in bioenergetic reserves, more marked than in other patients who were not septic and had denervation of muscle alone.[54]

Other studies have further established the concept of sepsis affecting both nerve and muscle. In prospective studies of critically ill patients,[85,108] electrophysiologic studies indicated an axonal polyneuropathy; but muscle biopsy, in addition to showing signs of denervation, also showed signs of a primary myopathy. De Letter and associates showed that scores of the severity of critical illness and the presence of systemic inflammatory response syndrome both were able to predict the later development of a combined critical illness polyneuropathy and myopathy.[86]

In a study by Sander and co-workers, eight patients with "quadriplegic areflexic ICU illness" had clinical, electrophysiologic, and light microscopic findings of an axonal polyneuropathy. Peripheral nerve morphology was reported as normal, however, and electron microscopy of muscle revealed a thick filament-loss myopathy.[109] This unusual result may be explained by failure to perform teased-fiber preparations and semi-thin sections to observe early changes of peripheral nerve morphology. Furthermore, as observed by Latronico and colleagues, electrophysiologic signs of neuropathy may be present despite normal peripheral nerve morphology,[85] suggesting that functional derangement precedes structural change. In rats, denervation of muscle accompanied by corticosteroid administration induces a thick filament-loss myopathy.[110]

Thus, it appears that a significant number of patients will show combined critical illness polyneuropathy and myopathy. In this instance, it would be appropriate to apply the term "critical illness polyneuromyopathy," as originally suggested by Op de Coul and associates in 1991.[111]

In some ICUs, patients are now taken off sedation at regular intervals.[112] At that time, muscle strength can be assessed. If there is significant weakness that does not improve in follow-up, electrophysiologic studies

and a muscle biopsy are performed. This protocol allows for early physical therapy and rehabilitation and the determination of long-term prognosis.[113,114] Early mobilization also shortens length of stay in the ICU.[113]

Electrophysiologic studies are important in identifying these entities and determining prognosis. In one prospective study of 6 patients with myopathy followed for 1 year, 1 died and 5 recovered completely; of 3 with combined neuropathy and myopathy, 1 died, 1 recovered, and 1 remained tetraplegic; of 4 with neuropathy, 1 recovered, 2 had persisting muscle weakness, and 1 remained tetraplegic.[115] In general, myopathy has a better prognosis than neuropathy.

MONONEUROPATHIES

Lumbosacral or brachial plexopathies may be secondary to direct trauma, usually from motor vehicle accidents or surgery. Insertion of catheters into the iliac arteries or aorta may dislodge thrombi; the resulting embolization impairs the vascular supply to nerves and, in this manner, induces focal ischemic plexopathy. Direct surgical trauma to vessels may also induce vascular insufficiency.

Motorcycle accidents commonly injure the brachial plexus. Proximal lesions are suggested by Horner syndrome, winging of the scapula, and diaphragmatic paralysis. Electrophysiologic studies, ideally performed after 3 weeks, will help to localize the lesion further. Myelography, CT myelography, or MRI may provide more positive evidence of root avulsion, which would preclude attempts at operative nerve repair.

Fractures of the pelvis may cause varying patterns of damage to the lumbosacral plexus. Observations of focal weakness on reflex or voluntarily induced movement and abnormalities of the tendon reflexes may provide an initial clue to the presence of such damage. Thus, weakness of hip adduction and flexion and of knee extension and an absent patellar reflex suggest damage to the L2–4 roots of the lumbosacral plexus.

Electrophysiologic studies should demonstrate abnormalities on motor and sensory conduction studies and, in particular, on needle EMG that localize the lesion to the brachial or lumbosacral plexus. There are several types of mononeuropathies. If the patient's primary reason for admission to the ICU was the postoperative state, the initial surgery may have induced a mononeuropathy when operating room equipment or perhaps the surgery itself directly damaged peripheral nerves. A variety of limb nerves may be damaged by trauma. For example, weakness of extension of the wrist and digits and an absent triceps reflex suggest radial nerve damage in the spiral groove of the humerus by fracture or direct compression. Phrenic nerves, either bilaterally or unilaterally, may be damaged at the time of surgery by direct trauma or by the application of cold, as with hypothermia associated with cardiac operations.

More distal nerves may be damaged by impairment of nutrient blood supply through distal embolization. Thus, after cardiac or vascular surgery, patients may manifest varying combinations of involvement of the femoral or sciatic nerves. Electrophysiologic studies show a relatively pure axonal degeneration of motor and sensory fibers.

Patients who are receiving anticoagulants run the risk of hemorrhage, and a sudden rise in tissue pressure produces a "compartment syndrome," the severe compression resulting in ischemia to nerve as well as muscle. The compartments most commonly involved are the iliopsoas and the gluteal, which produce acute femoral or sciatic neuropathies, respectively; or a lumbosacral plexopathy may occur with bleeding in the retroperitoneal space. An immediate CT scan should be ordered, which will show the hemorrhage. Surgical decompression may successfully decompress the nerve. The situation is so acute that electrophysiologic studies are of little value.

REFERENCES

1. Bolton CF: Electrophysiological studies of critically ill patients. Muscle Nerve, 10:129, 1987

2. Young GB, Bolton CF, Archibald YM et al: The electroencephalogram in sepsis-associated encephalopathy. J Clin Neurophysiol, 9:145, 1992

3. Chiappa KH, Hoch DB: Electrophysiologic monitoring. p. 147. In Ropper AH (ed): Neurological and Neurosurgical Intensive Care. 2nd Ed. Butterworth–Heinemann, Boston, 1993

4. Bolton CF, Young GB (eds): Electrophysiological studies in the critical care unit. Can J Neurol Sci, 25:Suppl 1, S1, 1998

5. Young GB, Bolton CF, Austin TW et al: The encephalopathy associated with septic illness. Clin Invest Med, 13:297, 1990

6. Witt NJ, Zochodne DW, Bolton CF et al: Peripheral nerve function in sepsis and multiple organ failure. Chest, 99:176, 1991

7. Bolton CF: Electromyography in the critical care unit. p. 675. In Brown WF, Bolton CF (eds): Clinical Electromyography. 2nd Ed. Butterworth–Heinemann, Boston, 1993

8. Bolton CF: Electromyography in the critical care unit. p. 445. In Jones HR, Bolton CF, Harper CM (eds): Pediatric Electromyography. Lippincott–Raven, Philadelphia, 1996

9. Jordan KG: Continuous EEG and evoked potential monitoring in the neuroscience intensive care unit. J Clin Neurophysiol, 10:445, 1993

10. Multi-Society Task Force on PVS: Medical aspects of the persistent vegetative state (second of two parts). N Engl J Med, 330:1572, 1996

11. Tsubokawa T, Yamamoto T, Katayama Y: Prediction of outcome of prolonged coma caused by brain damage. Brain Inj, 4:329, 1990

12. Young GB, Blume WT, Campbell VM et al: Alpha, theta and alpha-theta coma: a clinical outcome study using serial recordings. Electroencephalogr Clin Neurophysiol, 91:93, 1994

13. Claassen J, Meyer SA, Kowalski RG et al: Detection of electrographic seizures with continuous EEG monitoring in critically ill patients. Neurology, 62:1743, 2004

14. Claassen J, Mayer SA, Hirsch LJ: Continuous EEG monitoring in patients with subarachnoid hemorrhage. J Clin Neurophysiol, 22:92, 2005

15. Hebb MO, McArthur DL, Alger J et al: Impaired percent alpha variability on continuous electroencephalography is associated with thalamic injury and predicts poor long-term outcome after human traumatic brain injury. J Neurotrauma, 24:579, 2007

16. Young GB, Doig GS: Continuous EEG monitoring in comatose intensive care unit patients: epileptiform activity in etiologically distinct groups. Neurocrit Care, 2:5, 2005

17. Young GB, McLachlan RS, Kreeft JH et al: An electroencephalographic classification system for coma. Can J Neurol Sci, 24:320, 1997

18. Figueroa-Ramos MI, Arroyo-Novoa CM, Lee KA et al: Sleep and delirium in ICU patients: a review of mechanisms and manifestations. Intensive Care Med, 35:781, 2009

19. Chéliout-Heraut F, Rubinsztajn R, Ioos C et al: Prognostic value of evoked potentials and sleep recordings in the prolonged comatose state of children. Preliminary data. Neurophysiol Clin, 3:283, 2001

20. Connolly JF, D'Arcy RCN: Innovations in neuropsychological assessment using event-related brain potentials. Int J Psychophysiol, 37:31, 2000

21. Young GB, Campbell VC: EEG monitoring in the intensive care unit: pitfalls and caveats. J Clin Neurophysiol, 16:40, 1999

22. Young B, Ives J, Chapman M et al: A comparison of subdermal wire electrodes with collodion-applied disk electrodes in long-term EEG recordings in ICU. Clin Neurophysiol, 117:1376, 2006

23. Schoeck AP, Mellion ML, Gilchrist JM et al: Safety of nerve conduction studies in patients with implanted cardiac devices. Muscle Nerve, 35:521, 2007

24. Facco E, Munari M, Baratto F et al: Multimodality evoked potentials (auditory, somatosensory and motor) in coma. Neurophysiol Clin, 23:237, 1993

25. Young GB, Jordan KG, Aminoff MJ et al: Controversies in neurology. Do nonconvulsive seizures damage the brain? Arch Neurol, 55:117, 1998

26. Shorvon S: Status Epilepticus: Its Clinical Features and Treatment in Children and Adults. Cambridge University Press, Cambridge, 1994

27. Young GB, Jordan KG, Doig GS: An assessment of nonconvulsive seizures in the intensive care unit using continuous

EEG monitoring: an investigation of variables associated with mortality. Neurology, 47:83, 1996

28. Grand'maison F, Reiher J, Leduc CP: Retrospective inventory of EEG abnormalities in partial status epilepticus. Electroencephalogr Clin Neurophysiol, 79:264, 1991

29. Reiher J, Grand'Maison F, Leduc CP: Partial status epilepticus: short-term prediction of seizure outcome from on-line EEG analysis. Electroencephalogr Clin Neurophysiol, 82:17, 1992

30. Young GB, Wijdicks EFM: Seizures and status epilepticus. p. 495. In Young GB, Ropper AH, Bolton CF (eds): Coma and Impaired Consciousness: A Clinical Perspective. McGraw–Hill, New York, 1998

31. Jaitly R, Sgro JA, Towne AR et al: Prognostic value of EEG monitoring after status epilepticus: a prospective audit study. J Clin Neurophysiol, 14:326, 1997

32. Rath SA, Klein HJ: Current applications of the EEG in the comatose patient. Am J EEG Technol, 31:65, 1991

33. Houlden DA, Li C, Schwartz ML et al: Median nerve somatosensory evoked potentials and the Glasgow Coma Scale as predictors of outcome in comatose patients with head injuries. Neurosurgery, 27:701, 1990

34. Chiappa KH, Hill RA: Evaluation and prognostication in coma. Electroencephalogr Clin Neurophysiol, 106:149, 1998

35. Wang JT, Young GB, Connolly JF: Prognostic value of evoked responses and event-related brain potentials in coma. Can J Neurol Sci, 31:438, 2004

36. Bassetti C, Bromio F, Mathis J et al: Early prognosis in coma after cardiac arrest: a prospective clinical, electrophysiological and biochemical study of 60 patients. J Neurol Neurosurg Psychiatry, 61:610, 1996

37. Pohlmann-Eden B, Dingethal K, Bender H-J et al: How reliable is the predictive value of SEP (somatosensory evoked potentials) patterns in severe brain damage with special regard to the bilateral loss of cortical responses? Intensive Care Med, 23:301, 1997

38. Rothstein TL, Thomas EM, Sumi SM: Predicting outcome in hypoxic-ischemic coma. A prospective clinical and electrophysiological study. Electroencephalogr Clin Neurophysiol, 79:101, 1991

39. Zandbergen EG, de Haan RJ, Stoutenbeek CP et al: Systematic review of early prediction of poor outcome in anoxic-ischaemic coma. Lancet, 352:1796, 1998

40. Rothstein TL: The role of evoked potentials in anoxic-ischemic coma and severe brain trauma. J Clin Neurophysiol, 17:486, 2000

41. Logi F, Fischer C, Murri L et al: The prognostic value of evoked responses from primary somatosensory and auditory cortex in comatose patients. Clin Neurophysiol, 114:1615, 2003

42. Madl C, Grimm G, Kramer L et al: Early prediction of individual outcome after cardiopulmonary resuscitation. Lancet, 341:855, 1993

43. Young B, Doig G, Ragazzoni A: Anoxic-ischemic encephalopathy: clinical and electrophysiological associations with outcome. Neurocrit Care, 2:159, 2005

44. Young GB, Leung LS, Campbell V et al: The electroencephalogram in metabolic/toxic coma. Am J EEG Technol, 32:243, 1992

45. Niedermeyer E: Cerebrovascular disorders and the EEG. p. 275. In Niedermeyer E, Lopes da Silva F (eds): Electroencephalography: Basic Principles, Clinical Applications and Related Fields. 2nd Ed. Urban & Schwarzenberg, Baltimore, 1987

46. Bolton CF, Chen R, Wijdicks EFM et al: Neurology of Breathing. Butterworth–Heinemann, Philadelphia, 2004

47. Zifko U, Chen R: The respiratory system. Baillieres Clin Neurol, 5:477, 1996

48. Boon AJ, Alsharif KI, Harper CM: Ultrasound-guided EMG of the diaphragm: technique description and case report. Muscle Nerve, 38:1623, 2008

49. Lemaire F: Difficulty weaning. Intensive Care Med, 19: Suppl 2, S69, 1993

50. Maher J, Rutledge F, Remtulla H et al: Neurophysiological assessment of failure to wean from a ventilator. Can J Neurol Sci, 20:S28, 1995

51. Spitzer AR, Giancarlo T, Maher L et al: Neuromuscular causes of prolonged ventilator dependency. Muscle Nerve, 15:682, 1992

52. Bolton CF, Young GB: The neurological consultation and neurological syndromes in the intensive care unit. Baillieres Clin Neurol, 5:447, 1996

53. Chen R, Grand'Maison F, Strong MJ et al: Motor neuron disease presenting as acute respiratory failure. A clinical and pathological study. J Neurol Neurosurg Psychiatry, 60:455, 1996

54. Bolton CF, Young GB, Zochodne DW: Neurological changes during severe sepsis. p. 180. In Dobb GJ, Bion J, Burchardi H et al (eds): Current Topics in Intensive Care. WB Saunders, Philadelphia, 1994

55. Zifko U, Chen R, Remtulla H et al: Respiratory electrophysiologic studies in Guillain–Barré syndrome. J Neurol Neurosurg Psychiatry, 60:191, 1996

56. Vucic S, Kiernan MC, Cornblath DR: Guillain–Barré syndrome: an update. J Clin Neurosci, 16:733, 2009

57. McKhann GM, Cornblath DR, Ho T et al: Clinical and electrophysiological aspects of acute paralytic disease of children and young adults in northern China. Lancet, 338:593, 1991

58. Maher J, Grand'Maison F, Nicolle MW et al: Diagnostic difficulties in myasthenia gravis. Muscle Nerve, 21:577, 1998

59. Nicolle MW, Stewart DJ, Remtulla H et al: Lambert–Eaton syndrome presenting with severe respiratory failure. Muscle Nerve, 19:1328, 1996

60. Zifko U, Nicolle MW, Remtulla H et al: Repetitive phrenic nerve stimulation study in normal subjects. J Clin Neurophysiol, 14:235, 1997

61. Zifko UA, Hahn AF, George CF et al: Central and peripheral respiratory electrophysiological studies in myotonic dystrophy. Brain, 119:1911, 1996

62. Tran DD, Groeneveld ABJ, Nauta JJP et al: Age, chronic disease, sepsis, organ system failure and mortality in a medical intensive care unit. Crit Care Med, 18:474, 1990

63. Witt NJ, Zochodne DW, Bolton CF et al: Peripheral nerve function in sepsis and multiple organ failure. Chest, 99:176, 1991

64. Leijten FSS, de Weerd AW: Critical illness polyneuropathy. A review of the literature, definition and pathophysiology. Clin Neurol Neurosurg, 96:10, 1994

65. Hund EF: Neuromuscular complications in the ICU: the spectrum of critical illness-related conditions causing muscular weakness and weaning failure. J Neurol Sci, 136:10, 1996

66. Bolton CF: Sepsis and the systemic inflammatory response syndrome: neuromuscular manifestations. Crit Care Med, 24:1408, 1996

67. Leijten FSS, De Weerd AW, Poortvliet DC et al: Critical illness polyneuropathy in multiple organ dysfunction syndrome and weaning from the ventilator. Intensive Care Med, 22:856, 1996

68. Berek K, Margreiter J, Willeit J et al: Polyneuropathies in critically ill patients: a prospective evaluation. Intensive Care Med, 22:849, 1996

69. Leijten FSS: Critical Illness Polyneuropathy. A Longitudinal Study. Doctoral thesis. Rijksuniversiteit te Leiden, The Netherlands, 1996

70. Stevens RD, Dowdy DW, Michaels RK et al: Neuromuscular dysfunction in critical illness: a systematic review. Intensive Care Med, 33:1876, 2007

71. Tennila A, Salmi T, Pettila V et al: Early signs of critical illness polyneuropathy in ICU patients with systemic inflammatory response syndrome or sepsis. Intensive Care Med, 26:1360, 2000

72. Z'Graggen WJ, Lim CS, Howeard RS et al: Nerve excitability changes in critical illness polyneuropathy. Brain, 129:2461, 2006

73. Segredo V, Caldwell JE, Matthay MA et al: Persistent paralysis in critically ill patients after the long-term administration of vecuronium. N Engl J Med, 327:524, 1992

74. Bolton CF: Clinical neurophysiology of the respiratory system. Muscle Nerve, 16:809, 1993

75. Leijten FSS, Harinck-de-Weerd JE, Poortvliet DCJ et al: The role of polyneuropathy in motor convalescence after prolonged mechanical ventilation. JAMA, 274:1221, 1995

76. Zifko UA: Long-term outcome of critical illness polyneuropathy. Muscle Nerve Suppl, 9:S49, 2000

77. Fletcher S, Kennedy DD, Ghosh IR et al: Persistent neuromuscular and neurophysiologic abnormalities in long-term survivors of prolonged critical illness. Crit Care Med, 31:1012, 2003

78. Wijdicks EFM, Fulgham JR: Failure of high dose intravenous immunoglobulin to alter the clinical course of critical illness polyneuropathy. Muscle Nerve, 17:1494, 1994

79. Sheth RD, Pryse-Phillips WEM: Post-ventilatory quadriplegia: critical illness polyneuropathy in childhood. Neurology, 44:A169, 1994

80. Dimachkie M, Austin SG, Slopis JM et al: Critical illness polyneuropathy in childhood. J Child Neurol, 9:207, 1994

81. Bolton CF: EMG in the paediatric critical care unit. p. 459. In Jones HR, Bolton CF, Harper M (eds): Pediatric Electromyography. Raven, New York, 1996

82. van den Berghe G, Wouters P, Weekers F et al: Intensive insulin therapy in the critically ill patients. N Engl J Med, 345:1359, 2001

83. Barohn RJ, Jackson CE, Rogers SJ et al: Prolonged paralysis due to nondepolarizing neuromuscular blocking agents and corticosteroids. Muscle Nerve, 17:647, 1994

84. Giostra E, Magistris MR, Pizzolato G et al: Neuromuscular disorder in intensive care unit patients treated with pancuronium bromide. Chest, 106:210, 1994

85. Latronico N, Fenzi F, Recupero D et al: Critical illness myopathy and neuropathy. Lancet, 347:1579, 1996

86. de Letter MA, Schmitz PI, Visser LH et al: Risk factors for the development of polyneuropathy and myopathy in critically ill patients. Crit Care Med, 29:2281, 2001

87. Douglas JA, Tuxen DV, Horne M et al: Myopathy in severe asthma. Am Rev Respir Dis, 146:517, 1992

88. Campellone JV, Lacomis D, Kramer DJ et al: Acute myopathy after liver transplantation. Neurology, 50:46, 1998

89. Lacomis D, Zochodne DW, Bird SJ: Critical illness myopathy. Muscle Nerve, 23:1785, 2000

90. Sitwell LD, Weinshenker BG, Monpetit V et al: Complete ophthalmoplegia as a complication of acute corticosteroid- and pancuronium-associated myopathy. Neurology, 41:921, 1991

91. Allen DC, Arunachalum R, Mills KR: Critical illness myopathy: further evidence for muscle fiber inexcitability: studies of an acquired channelopathy. Muscle Nerve, 37:14, 2008

92. Rich MM, Bird SJ, Raps EC et al: Direct muscle stimulation in acute quadriplegic myopathy. Muscle Nerve, 20:665, 1997

93. Goodman BP, Harper CM, Boon AJ: Prolonged compound muscle action potential in critical illness myopathy. Muscle Nerve, 30:1040, 2009

94. Bolton CF: Sepsis and the systemic inflammatory response syndrome: neuromuscular manifestations. Crit Care Med, 24:1408, 1996

95. Bolton CF: Critical illness polyneuropathy and myopathy. Crit Care Med, 29:2388, 2001

96. Lacomis D, Smith TW, Chad DA: Acute myopathy and neuropathy in status asthmaticus: case report and literature review. Muscle Nerve, 16:84, 1993

97. Danon MJ, Carpenter S: Myopathy and thick filament (myosin) loss following prolonged paralysis with vecuronium during steroid treatment. Muscle Nerve, 14:1131, 1991

98. Douglass JA, Tuxen DV, Horne M et al: Myopathy in severe asthma. Am Rev Respir Dis, 146:517, 1991

99. Hirano M, Ott BR, Raps EC et al: Acute quadriplegic myopathy: a complication of treatment with steroids, nondepolarizing blocking agents, or both. Neurology, 42:2082, 1992

100. Minetti C, Hirano M, Morreale G et al: Ubiquitin expression in acute steroid myopathy with loss of myosin thick filaments. Muscle Nerve, 19:94, 1996

101. Lacomis D, Giuliani MJ, Van Cott A et al: Acute myopathy of intensive care: clinical, electromyographic, and pathological aspects. Ann Neurol, 40:645, 1996

102. Rich MM, Teener JW, Raps EC et al: Muscle is electrically inexcitable in acute quadriplegic myopathy. Neurology, 46:731, 1996

103. Showalter CJ, Engel AG: Acute quadriplegic myopathy: analysis of myosin isoforms and evidence for calpain-mediated proteolysis. Muscle Nerve, 20:316, 1997

104. Gutmann L, Blumenthal D, Gutmann L et al: Acute type II myofiber atrophy in critical illness. Neurology, 46:819, 1996

105. Zochodne DW, Ramsay DA, Saly V et al: Acute necrotizing myopathy of intensive care. Electrophysiological studies. Muscle Nerve, 17:285, 1994

106. Ramsay DA, Zochodne DW, Robertson DM et al: A syndrome of acute severe muscle necrosis in intensive care unit patients. J Neuropathol Exp Neurol, 52:387, 1993

107. Pringle CE, Bolton CF, Ramsay DA et al: Muscle biopsy in critical illness. Electrophysiological and morphological correlations. Can J Neurol Sci, 2:297, 1992

108. De Jonghe B, Sharshar T, Lefaucheur JP et al: Paresis acquired in the intensive care unit: a prospective multicenter study. JAMA, 288:2859, 2002

109. Sander HW, Golden M, Danon MJ: Quadriplegic areflexic ICU illness: selective thick filament loss and normal nerve histology. Muscle Nerve, 26:499, 2002

110. Massa R, Carpenter S, Holland P et al: Loss and renewal of thick myofilaments in glucocorticoid-treated rat soleus after denervation and reinnervation. Muscle Nerve, 15:1290, 1992

111. Op de Coul AAW, Werheul GAM, Leyten ACM et al: Critical illness polyneuromyopathy after artificial respiration. Clin Neurol Neurosurg, 93:27, 1991

112. Kress JP, Pohlman AS, O'Connor ME et al: Daily interruption of sedation infusions in critically ill patients undergoing mechanical ventilation. N Eng J Med, 342:1471, 2000

113. De Jonghe B, Cook D, Sharshar T et al: Acquired neuromuscular disorders in critically ill patients: a systematic review. Intensive Care Med, 24:1242, 1998

114. O'Connor ED, Walsham J: Should we mobilize critically ill patients? A review. Crit Care Resusc, 11:290, 2009

115. Guarneri B, Bertolini G, Latronico N: Long-term outcome in patients with critical illness myopathy or neuropathy: the Italian multicentre CRIMYNE study. J Neurol Neurosurg Psychiatry, 79:838, 2008

Electrophysiologic Evaluation of Brain Death: A Critical Appraisal

THOMAS P. BLECK

Traditionally, death was defined in medicine as the permanent cessation of heartbeat and respiration. When the loss of these functions is not reversed promptly by resuscitative measures, profound and irreversible pathologic alterations occur in the brain within minutes under normothermic conditions. The increasing effectiveness of resuscitative techniques and life-support systems has restored and artificially maintained cardiovascular and respiratory functions in countless individuals. However, the extreme vulnerability of the brain to anoxia, which exceeds that of other systems of the body, remains the major factor limiting a favorable outcome of resuscitation. In patients who have suffered a sufficiently prolonged arrest, restoring and maintaining pulmonary, cardiac, and other functions does not lead to recovery of conscious behaviors and higher mental faculties that represent the very essence of human life. Because preservation of other organs is inconsequential in the face of complete and permanent abolition of brain function, these states of *coma dépassé*[1] (a state beyond coma) or *brain death*[1] have been equated with death of the person by medical, legal, and religious authorities. It has been recognized that the use of extraordinary measures to support bodily functions in individuals with dead brains demands an unreasonable expenditure of human and financial resources, unnecessarily prolongs the sorrow and grief of relatives and friends, and is contrary to the individual's right to die with dignity. The rapid progress of organ transplantation surgery provides further impetus to redefining death of the individual as death of the brain because the success of such surgery depends on the use of viable organs removed from a patient with permanently abolished brain function before the circulation fails.

This chapter has been updated by the present author from the chapter of the same name that appeared in earlier editions of this book, authored by Professor Gian-Emilio Chatrian, who has now retired.

DEFINITION AND NEUROPATHOLOGY OF BRAIN DEATH

Two opposing concepts of death by neurologic criteria exist. In the United States, death by neurologic criteria is defined as "irreversible loss of function of the brain, including the brainstem,"[2] whereas in the United Kingdom it is characterized as an "irreversible cessation of brainstem function."[3] That irreversible cessation of brain function involves the whole brain is demonstrated irrefutably by electrophysiologic, i.e., electroencephalographic (EEG) and evoked potential tests, brain blood-flow studies, and pathologic findings. However, the opposing views of brain death expressed by British and American students of this condition are not irreconcilable; no fundamental contradiction appears to exist between the concept that brain death is characterized by the irreversible loss of function of the whole brain, including the brainstem, and the belief that permanent abolition of brainstem function "is the physiologic kernel of brain death, the anatomic substratum of its cardinal signs (apnoeic coma with absent brainstem function) and the main determinant of its invariable cardiac prognosis: asystole within hours or days."[4] This last observation has been challenged by Shewmon,[5] although not without debate.[6]

As the concept of brain death evolved, so did knowledge of the neuropathologic changes characterizing this condition. Early work suggested that marked edema, extensive softening, necrosis (particularly in the gray matter), and severe neuronal alterations without inflammatory reaction or vascular thrombosis characterized the brains of individuals who had been in *coma dépassé* and artificially ventilated.[1,2] However, subsequent research revealed a greater diversity of findings in individuals with brain death maintained on a respirator for variable periods. Most commonly, swelling and softening as well as transtentorial herniation, hemorrhage, infarction, and necrosis were found in the cerebrum, cerebellum, and brainstem of individuals with brain death. These alterations varied considerably in extent, severity, and distribution.[7] In addition, the brains of some patients who died within about 24 hours after the onset of coma and apnea displayed minimal or no pathologic abnormalities, thus indicating that some time must elapse after the onset of coma and apnea for the changes of the "respirator brain" to develop.[7]

Brain death defined as irreversible loss of function of the whole brain must be distinguished from:

1. *Cortical death*, characterized by acute failure of forebrain with variable preservation of brainstem function
2. *Primary brainstem death*, defined as acute loss of brainstem function with substantial preservation of cortical function.

CLINICAL DIAGNOSIS OF BRAIN DEATH IN ADULTS

Acceptance of the notion of brain death, and identification of this condition with death of the individual, required operational criteria for diagnosing this state in persons with artificially sustained cardiac and respiratory functions. The definition of these standards was intended to help physicians identify the circumstances under which continuation of extraordinary supportive measures was both unnecessary and inadvisable, as well as to protect patients against premature termination of these efforts. Following earlier formulations, guidelines for determining brain death in adults were published by the American Academy of Neurology.[2]

Prerequisites for Applying the Criteria of Brain Death

Certain conditions must be satisfied before the diagnosis of brain death is considered,[2] including:

1. Demonstration by clinical and neuroimaging studies that an acute central nervous system (CNS) catastrophe has occurred that is compatible with brain death. Brain death from primary neurologic disease is often the result of severe head injury, aneurysmal subarachnoid hemorrhage, orintracerebral hemorrhage. In intensive care units (ICUs), hypoxic-ischemic encephalopathy after prolonged cardiac resuscitation or asphyxia, large ischemic strokes associated with brain swelling and herniation, and massive brain edema in patients with fulminant hepatic failure are the most common causes of brain death.
2. Exclusion of conditions that may reversibly produce or may contribute to cause clinical manifestations mimicking brain death, including:
   a. *Hypothermia.* Prerequisite core temperature must be equal to or greater than 36 °C or 96.8 °F
   b. *Drug intoxication or poisoning,* including the effects of sedatives, aminoglycoside antibiotics, tricyclic antidepressants, anticholinergics, antiepileptic drugs, and chemotherapeutic agents or neuromuscular blocking drugs causing total paralysis
   c. *Profound hypotension.* Prerequisite systemic blood pressure must be equal to or greater than 100 mm Hg
   d. *Severe metabolic (electrolyte and acid-base) derangements and endocrine crises.*

Clinical Observations that Establish Brain Death

Provided all prerequisites are satisfied, the following clinical findings establish the diagnosis of brain death[2]:

1. Unresponsiveness, defined as the absence of motor responses of the limbs and lack of facial grimacing to noxious stimuli such as pressure on the supraorbital ridge, the nail bed, or the temporomandibular joint.
2. Absent brainstem reflexes, including pupillary, oculocephalic, oculovestibular, corneal, jaw, pharyngeal, and tracheal reflexes.
3. Apnea demonstrated by a strictly standardized test that entails interrupting artificial ventilation long enough to allow the $PaCO_2$ to rise to levels producing maximal stimulation of the brainstem respiratory center while providing adequate oxygenation. This level usually is specified as 60 mm Hg in North America and 50 mm Hg in the United Kingdom. However, since the pH, not the $PaCO_2$, is the major determinant of respiratory drive, the observer should ensure that the arterial pH declines to 7.3 or lower during the apnea test.

Some potentially misleading clinical observations that do not invalidate the diagnosis of brain death are detailed in the guidelines of the American Academy of Neurology.[2]

Induced hypothermia for the treatment of patients in coma after cardiac arrest does not alter these criteria, but they can be applied only after the patient's core temperature has been returned to normothermia. During the period of induced hypothermia, the usual prognostic significance of the clinical and electrophysiologic variables used to predict death or survival should not be used, with the possible exception of the median nerve somatosensory evoked response.[8]

CONFIRMATORY TESTS IN ADULTS

The guidelines of the American Academy of Neurology affirm that brain death is a clinical diagnosis.[2] However, the guidelines recognize that in some circumstances specific components of the clinical examination cannot be tested or evaluated reliably. These conditions include severe facial trauma; pre-existing pupillary abnormalities; instability of the cervical spine; petrous bone fracture; and toxic blood levels of sedative drugs, aminoglycosides, tricyclic antidepressants, anticholinergics, antiepileptic drugs, chemotherapeutic agents, or neuromuscular blocking drugs. When these conditions exist, laboratory tests are desirable but are not required. Prolonged clinical observation, sometimes over a period of days, may be necessary to establish by clinical means that irreversible loss of brain function has occurred. This approach appears to be justified only when the instrumentation and human skills required for ancillary studies are not available.

In the author's opinion, when the diagnosis of brain death is in doubt, no effort should be spared to decrease the chance of error, expedite the diagnosis, and provide objective proof of irreversible extinction of brain function by using appropriate confirmatory procedures. At present, these methods primarily include: (1) electrophysiologic methods; and (2) tests of cerebral blood flow. In most of the United States, the choice of the confirmatory test is left to the discretion of the physician, consideration being given to the laws of the individual states and to institutional directives. Some jurisdictions require specific tests by law, requiring that they be performed even when the history and clinical examination are conclusive. Because confounding conditions (e.g., the administration of high doses of sedative drugs, sometimes combined with neuromuscular junction blocking agents) are increasingly common in ICUs, the contribution of laboratory tests to the determination of brain death has acquired special significance.[9] This chapter examines the role of electrophysiologic testing in the confirmation of suspected brain death.

The Electroencephalogram

ELECTROCEREBRAL INACTIVITY: DEFINITION

In a substantial proportion of patients with clinically diagnosed brain death (as many as 80 percent in a report by Grigg and associates[10]), EEG recording shows a pattern of "electrocerebral inactivity" (ECI) defined as "absence over all regions of the head of identifiable electrical activity of cerebral origin, whether spontaneous or induced by physiological stimuli and pharmacological agents,"[11] and electrical activity of cerebral origin is identified when it exceeds an assumed instrumental noise of 2 μV (Fig. 35-1). The use of nonphysiologic terms to describe ECI, such as "electrocerebral silence" (ECS), "isoelectric," "flat," and "null" EEG, is discouraged.

Early cortical and depth recordings in patients who satisfied all prerequisites and clinical criteria of brain death demonstrated that ECI in scalp EEGs was associated with absence of electrocerebral activity at all cortical and subcortical sites explored, indicating global loss of brain function.[12,13]

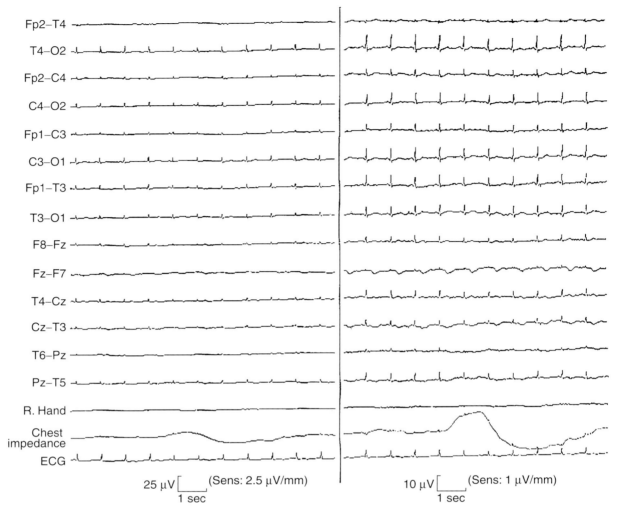

FIGURE 35-1 ▪ Electrocerebral inactivity in a 23-year-old hypertensive woman 2 days after intracerebral hemorrhage. This patient was unresponsive to noxious and other stimuli and had absent brainstem reflexes, fixed dilated pupils, and apnea. Three hours after this recording, respiratory support was discontinued and she was pronounced dead.

As defined, ECI excludes the following:

1. Records displaying a "burst-suppression" pattern that consists of "bursts of theta and/or delta waves, at times intermixed with faster waves, and intervening periods of low amplitude" that commonly are found in conditions such as severe hypoxic-ischemic encephalopathies, acute intoxication with CNS depressants, deep hypothermia, late-stage status epilepticus, and general anesthesia. In patients who are drug-intoxicated, the EEG activity may be reduced to isolated waves separated by apparently quiescent intervals lasting several minutes, but may subsequently recover (Fig. 35-2).
2. Low-voltage, slow EEGs primarily consisting of delta and theta activity generally unreactive to stimuli such as are demonstrated in deeply comatose or brain-dead patients with widespread brain damage.
3. Low-voltage waking EEGs that are "characterized by activity of amplitude not greater than 20 μV/mm over all head regions." Using high instrumental sensitivities, these EEGs are shown to be composed of beta, theta, and (to a lesser degree) delta waves, with or without alpha activity over the posterior areas.[12] These recordings "are susceptible to change under the influence of certain physiological stimuli, sleep, pharmacological agents and pathological processes."
4. EEGs showing no detectable electrocerebral activity, but recorded only over limited areas of the scalp.

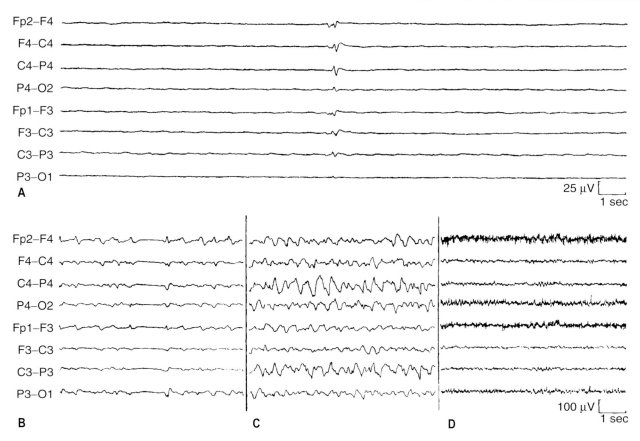

FIGURE 35-2 ■ Electroencephalogram (EEG) of a 30-year-old woman with secobarbital overdose. **A,** On the second day of hospitalization she was unresponsive to all stimuli and had apnea, no brainstem reflexes, constricted unreactive pupils, and a blood barbiturate level of 36 mg/100 ml. Her EEG showed pseudoperiodic sharp-and-slow waves more prominent on the right than left hemisphere, with intervening periods of "suppression" lasting up to 22 seconds. **B,** On the following day she was clinically unchanged, and demonstrated bilateral asymmetric sharp waves repeating at 1 to 2 Hz. **C,** Four days after admission, she withdrew to noxious stimuli and her pupils reacted to light stimulation. High-voltage 2- to 3-Hz waves occurred bilaterally in her EEG. **D,** Eight days later she was alert, followed commands, and had an EEG displaying a 9- to 10-Hz posterior rhythm attenuated by eye opening. The patient recovered without neurologic sequelae.

DEMONSTRATION OF ELECTROCEREBRAL INACTIVITY

Demonstrating ECI in patients with suspected brain death requires rigorous recording technique. The EEG examination should begin with a brief recording using a montage and the instrumental settings utilized in ordinary EEG recording. If this preliminary sampling produces either no evidence or questionable evidence of activity of cerebral origin, the technique should be modified promptly to demonstrate ECI according to stringent standards. These technical requirements (summarized in Table 35-1) are in substantial harmony with the guidelines of the American Clinical Neurophysiology Society.[14]

Artifacts (electrical potentials generated by extracerebral sources) commonly contaminate EEG records designed to demonstrate ECI. These spurious electrical events include potentials generated by instruments close to or connected with the patient, such as electrocardiographic (ECG)

monitors, pacemakers, warming blankets, and dialysis units, as well as biopotentials of cardiac, muscular, and respiratory origin. These have been described and illustrated in detail elsewhere.[15]

The most common and disturbing of all biologic artifacts is the ECG (see Fig. 35-1). ECG potentials are especially prominent in ear-reference montages. They occasionally resemble sharp-and-slow-wave complexes or triphasic waves.[15] Premature ventricular depolarizations or ventricular tachycardia may produce potentials that appear on the scalp as sharp transients and theta or delta rhythms, respectively. In addition, rhythms of mostly alpha frequency occasionally result from head vibration caused by the systolic pulse wave (ballistocardiogram). Disconnecting existing ECG monitors, repositioning the patient's head, and selecting montages less prone to ECG pickup may reduce, but generally do not eliminate, the ECG artifact.

TABLE 35-1 ■ Suggested Requirements for Demonstrating Electrocerebral Inactivity in the Adult

1. Following an initial study using all electrodes of the 10–20 system, the recording should utilize a minimum of 8 scalp electrodes, 2 earlobe reference electrodes, and 2 electrodes for electrocardiographic (ECG) monitoring. Additional electrodes may be required, including 2 electrodes on the dorsum of the right hand to monitor artifacts from the surroundings, and special transducers for monitoring respiration and related artifacts.[14]

2. A minimum of 8 channels of EEG recording should be obtained, and additional recording channels should be used to monitor the ECG and other variables simultaneously as required.

3. Interelectrode impedance should be below 10,000 but above 1,000 ohms.

4. The integrity of the entire recording system should be checked.[14]

5. Instrumental sensitivities should be no less than 2 μV/mm for at least 30 minutes of recording time, and calibrations should use appropriate voltages.[14]

6. Low-frequency cut-off should be no higher than 1 Hz, and high-frequency cut-off should be no lower than 50 Hz. The use of a 60- (50-)Hz notch filter is acceptable to reduce interference but is no substitute for good preparation of the patient. Excessive electromyographic activity should be eliminated by administering a neuromuscular blocking agent, except when contraindicated.[16]

7. Recordings taken with analog instruments and online data display and offline data review of digitally recorded EEGs should include bipolar (anteroposterior and transverse) and referential montages. Bipolar montages should consist primarily of derivations with interelectrode distances of at least 10 cm.[14]

8. EEG reactivity to noxious, auditory, and visual stimuli should be tested repeatedly but cautiously.

9. The recording should be performed by a qualified technologist experienced in EEG recordings in the ICU and working under the direction of a qualified electroencephalographer. The latter should be responsible for providing timely interpretation of the test.

10. Whenever electrocerebral inactivity is doubtful, the whole test should be repeated after an interval (e.g., 6 hours).[14]

11. Special precautions should be taken against electrical hazard, transmission of infection, and harmful effects of patient manipulations, especially head lifting and strong stimulation.

12. The minimal duration of actual, interpretable recording should be at least 30 minutes.

13. Following resuscitation from circulatory arrest, at least 8 hours should elapse between the onset of coma and the EEG examination.

Thus, having attempted these and other maneuvers, the technologist can generally do little but acknowledge the presence of this artifact and try to prove its origin by monitoring an ECG lead simultaneously with the scalp activity (see Fig. 35-1).

Electromyographic (EMG) potentials may obscure possible electrocerebral activity unless nondepolarizing neuromuscular blocking agents such as vecuronium or cisatracurium are given. However, caution is suggested by a report of cardiac arrest and death following administration of the depolarizing agent succinylcholine to reduce myogenic artifacts, as this agent rarely may produce severe hyperkalemia.[16]

Respiration-related artifacts may pose special problems. Delivery of a bolus of gas to the patient through flexible tubes may cause vibration of the head, resulting in rhythmic activity of alpha or other frequencies. Other head movements associated with respiration may generate large transients resembling periodic paroxysmal discharges. Monitoring respiration with appropriate transducers helps to determine the origin of these artifacts. On occasion it may even be necessary to stop the respirator briefly to assess questionable activity. However, if this disconnection test must be carried out over minutes, adequate oxygenation must be provided to avoid additional anoxic damage.

Identifying beyond doubt and eliminating or reducing and monitoring all sources of artifact are time-consuming tasks that often seriously challenge the competence, ingenuity, and determination of the EEG technologist. Preparing with special prudence the patient with suspected brain death for EEG monitoring, and sometimes interrupting the EEG examination to allow the performance of essential therapeutic maneuvers, often cause additional delays. Thus, the production of at least 30 minutes of interpretable recording satisfying current technical requirements may take as long as 2 hours and sometimes longer.

DETERMINATION THAT ELECTROCEREBRAL INACTIVITY IS IRREVERSIBLE

The EEG pattern of ECI indicates loss of cerebral function but does not imply that this loss is permanent. This pattern must be regarded as potentially reversible in the presence of those same conditions that also transiently cause clinical manifestations mimicking brain death (e.g., intoxication with CNS depressants, hypothermia, profound hypotension, and severe metabolic and endocrine disorders). When these potentially confounding conditions are excluded, ECI is highly likely to be irreversible and confirms the diagnosis of brain death.

CNS Depressant Drugs

Most reports of ECI persisting for 24 hours or longer in patients intoxicated with CNS depressants described EEGs that probably were not electrocerebrally inactive by current standards. The EEGs of these patients more commonly demonstrate prolonged periods of markedly diminished EEG activity rather than ECI (see Fig. 35-2, *A*). Major reversible decrease in EEG activity also characterizes patients treated in the ICU with high doses of barbiturates, sometimes combined with neuromuscular blocking agents and hypothermia.

Hypothermia

ECI occurs at a mean core temperature of 24 °C[17]; however, this pattern does not occur at the body temperatures that usually are encountered in the ICU. EEG activity recovers in hypothermic individuals with viable brains who are warmed to normal temperature.[18] Profound reversible depression, but not ECI as currently defined, has been reported in a patient with hyperthermia (rectal temperature of 42.5 °C).[19]

Profound Hypotension

EEG activity may be abolished by cardiovascular shock with consequent low cerebral perfusion pressure and may be restored when blood pressure is raised above shock levels. However, because patients are treated routinely in ICUs with intravenous volume expansion and vasopressors, hypotension generally does not play a major role in causing ECI.

Severe Metabolic and Endocrine Disorders

Severe metabolic and endocrine disorders (e.g., profound abnormalities of serum electrolytes, acid–base balance, and blood gases) and illnesses caused by severe dysfunction of the liver, kidney, and pancreas may also contribute to the generation of ECI.

PERSISTENCE OF ELECTROENCEPHALOGRAPHIC ACTIVITY

A substantial proportion of individuals who satisfy all preconditions and clinical criteria of brain death still demonstrate persistent electrocerebral activity in their EEGs several hours to several days after death of their brains has been diagnosed clinically. Grigg and associates observed this activity in 12 of 56 patients examined 2 to 168 hours after the diagnosis of brain death was established clinically,[10] and characterized it as follows:

1. Low-voltage theta or beta activity that occurred in 9 patients (16 percent) whose brains demonstrated hypoxic alterations involving diffusely the cerebral cortex, basal ganglia, brainstem, and cerebellum (Fig. 35-3)
2. Theta and delta waves intermixed with 10- to 12-Hz spindle-like potentials that were found in 2 individuals with extensive ischemic necrosis of the entire brainstem and cerebellum, with relative sparing of the cerebrum
3. Monotonous, unreactive, anterior-predominant activity of alpha frequency that was recorded in 1 patient in whom no autopsy was performed.

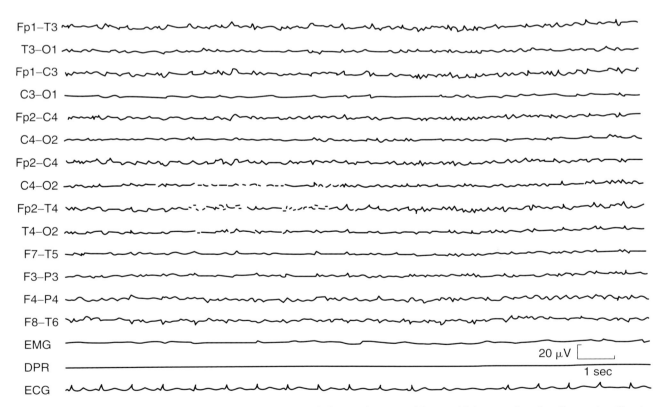

FIGURE 35-3 ■ This electroencephalogram was recorded on a 35-year-old man 32 hours after the diagnosis of brain death was made. Low-voltage 5- to 7-Hz activity was intermixed with some beta potentials and scattered delta waves. DPR, "dummy patient" resistor. (From Grigg MM, Kelly MA, Celesia GG et al: Electroencephalographic activity after brain death. Arch Neurol, 44:948, 1987, with permission.)

The presence of persistent electrocerebral activity and the pathologic alterations associated with this EEG finding indicate that relatively preserved areas of brain tissue in otherwise nonfunctional brains may still be capable of generating EEG potentials in individuals who are clinically brain dead.[11] In harmony with this contention, pathologic studies have shown that residual EEG activity is most common among individuals whose brain shows only patchy swelling, edema, infarction, and necrosis, whereas more extensive necrosis, swollen brain, and cerebral herniations are especially common among patients with ECI. Individuals with EEGs classified as equivocal demonstrate pathologic changes intermediate between these two groups.[20,21] The slow activity intermixed with spindle-like potentials sometimes found in the EEG of patients with extensive necrosis of the brainstem and cerebellum appears to be characteristic of "acute failure of brainstem function."

In five of six brain-dead individuals with preserved EEG activity studied by Grigg and colleagues,[10] radioisotope scintigraphy demonstrated absent cerebral perfusion. This finding adds substance to the belief that persistent electrocerebral activity in patients with clinically established brain death does not portend lasting survival and any form of residual sentience.[11] However, how much residual EEG activity is compatible with irreversible loss of brain function has not been determined. Thus, hesitant interpretations are justifiably common when electrocerebral activity is detected in patients with suspected brain death.

COMPUTER ANALYSIS OF THE ELECTROENCEPHALOGRAM

Attempts have been made to use computer techniques to analyze the EEGs of patients with suspected brain death in the hope of facilitating and increasing the objectivity and reliability of their interpretation. The earliest and most ambitious of these undertakings was the design by Bickford and co-workers of a central computer facility capable of analyzing EEGs transmitted via telephone to the center from any of a number of hospitals and automatically generating estimates of "brain output" as well as verbal interpretations.[22] Limitations and fallacies of this method were recognized,[23] and telephone transmission of EEGs to determine ECI was discouraged.[14] However, continuous monitoring and quantification of electrocerebral activity from limited areas of the scalp, pioneered by Prior and Maynard,[24] can signal the onset of brain death and suggest the need for a more complete EEG or other study.[25]

SUITABILITY OF THE ELECTROENCEPHALOGRAM AS A CONFIRMATORY TEST OF BRAIN DEATH IN ADULTS

The EEG has long enjoyed the status of a test of choice for the confirmation of clinically diagnosed brain death. Factors that account for this pre-eminent role included the noninvasive and safe nature of the test, its feasibility at the bedside in the ICU, its well-established technique and modest cost, the strong statistical association of ECI with brain death, and the high reproducibility of this pattern in successive recordings in the absence of the reversible conditions already alluded to in this chapter. However, the EEG suffers from major limitations and poses technical and interpretive problems that substantially diminish its utility as a confirmatory test of irreversible loss of brain function.[4] These difficulties include the following:

1. The EEG tests cortical but not brainstem function.
2. EEG recording of patients suspected of having dead brains is not available around the clock in many hospitals in the United States.
3. EEGs obtained in the ICU according to stringent technical standards, including high sensitivities (see Table 35-1), are difficult and time-consuming tests.
4. Some EEGs obtained in these circumstances contain irreducible artifacts that hamper their interpretation.
5. ECI can be caused by reversible conditions that hamper the clinical examination (i.e., in those same circumstances in which laboratory confirmation is most needed).
6. EEG activity persists in a substantial proportion of clinically brain-dead patients even in the face of absent measurable brain perfusion.
7. ECI does not differentiate between (whole) brain death and "cortical death" with substantially preserved brainstem function.
8. Recordings obtained to confirm clinically suspected brain death must be interpreted by physicians with special training in clinical neurophysiology and experience with recordings in the ICU.
9. Inter- and intra-interpreter disagreements occur even among qualified interpreters.[7,15,26]

The author believes that, because of these shortcomings, limitations, and pitfalls, relying on the EEG as the confirmatory test of choice is not justified. This view is not accepted universally. In several countries in Europe, Central and South America, and Asia, the demonstration of an EEG showing ECI is mandated by law for the certification of brain death. In France, two EEGs showing ECI at least 4 hours apart or an angiogram showing absence of intracranial circulation similarly is required.[27] Existing guidelines of the American Academy of Neurology suggest confirmatory tests only in those circumstances in which the diagnosis of brain death is suspected but cannot be established fully by the clinical examination.[28] In Canada, the EEG is not recommended as a confirmatory test.[29] Confirmation of brain death by EEG as well as other laboratory tests is neither required nor recommended in the United Kingdom.

Evoked Potentials

Computer-averaged evoked potentials (EPs) elicited by somatosensory, auditory, and visual stimuli offer an alternative to or may complement the EEG in the confirmation of clinically suspected brain death.

SOMATOSENSORY EVOKED POTENTIALS
Recording Methodology, Components, and Postulated Origin

In normal subjects, short-latency somatosensory evoked potentials (SEPs) to electrical stimulation of the median nerve at the wrist consist of a sequence of waves that are generated by the ascending volley at progressively higher levels of the somatosensory pathway from the sensory periphery to the cerebral cortex. Because appropriate

technique is critically important for the recording of SEPs, the following minimal montage was recommended by the American Clinical Neurophysiology Society[30]:

Channel 1: CPc–CPi (contralateral to ipsilateral centroparietal)
Channel 2: CPi–EPc (ipsilateral centroparietal to contralateral Erb's point)
Channel 3: C5S–EPc or AN (C5 spine to contralateral Erb's point or anterior neck)
Channel 4: EPi–EPc (ipsilateral to contralateral Erb's point).

SEP components most relevant to the assessment of brain death are designated N9, N13, P14, N18, and N20 (Fig. 35-4). Reviews published elsewhere[31,32] and Chapters 26 and 27 in the present volume analyze the features, topography, and putative generators of individual response components. Although the specific identity of these generators is still controversial, the following broad notions provide a framework for interpreting SEPs in brain-dead patients. The N9 potential recorded at Erb's point (see Fig. 35-4, *A*, channel 4) is generated by the brachial plexus afferent volley ("brachial plexus" or "peripheral" potential). The N13 peak detected over the fifth cervical spinous process (C5S; see Fig. 35-4, *A*, channel 3) reflects postsynaptic activity in central gray matter of the cervical cord ("spinal" or "cervical" potential). The P14 component (Fig. 35-4, channel 2) is widely distributed

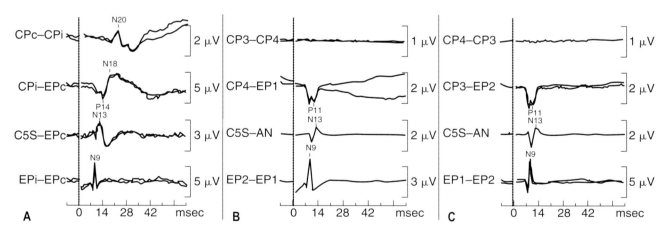

FIGURE 35-4 ■ Short-latency somatosensory-evoked potentials to electrical median nerve stimulation. **A**, Normal subject. CPc and CPi, centroparietal electrodes contralateral and ipsilateral to the limb stimulated, halfway between standard central and parietal electrodes. EPc and EPi, contralateral and ipsilateral Erb's point. C5S, C5 spine. AN, anterior surface of the neck just above the thyroid cartilage. Main response components are: N9 (brachial plexus), N13 (cervical cord), P14 and N18 (brainstem), and N20 (cortical) potentials. **B** and **C**, A 41-year-old woman showing unresponsiveness to all stimuli, absent brainstem reflexes, and apnea 5 days after an episode of ventricular fibrillation, perhaps caused by benzodiazepine overdose. Electrical stimulation of the right (*B*) and left (*C*) median nerves elicited N9, P11, and N13 potentials, but neither brainstem (P14 and N18) nor cortical (N20) responses. EP1 and EP2, left and right Erb's point; C5S, C5 spine; AN, anterior neck; CP3 and CP4, left and right centroparietal electrodes.

over the scalp with a frontal maximum, and is demonstrated by scalp–noncephalic reference derivations (e.g., CPi–EPc or Fz–EPc) but not by scalp-to-scalp recordings. The designation "P14" is used commonly in the literature to describe the "P13–P14 complex." This complex consists of two potentials, P13 and P14, which cannot always be differentiated clearly. Observations in normal subjects and individuals with cervicomedullary or high cervical cord lesions indicate that P13 and P14 are distinct potentials with different generators; P13 is generated in high segments of the cervical cord, whereas P14 arises in the low brainstem close to the cervicomedullary junction. Because of its widespread acceptance, the designation P14 is used in this review to describe the P13–P14 complex, but any reference to P14 as a "brainstem" potential should be interpreted as applying solely to the P14 component of the P13–P14 complex. An earlier, variably identifiable P11 potential preceding P13 is believed to reflect the ascending volley in the fibers of the dorsal column at the cervical level. The long-lasting N18 potential has a wide distribution on the scalp similar to that of the P14 and is demonstrated best by scalp–noncephalic reference derivation (CPi–EPc or Fz–EPc) (see Fig. 35-4, *A*, channel 2). This potential is believed to reflect postsynaptic activity in brainstem gray matter structures. As opposed to P14 and N18, the N20 is localized to the parietal region contralateral to the limb stimulated and represents the first response of the primary somatosensory cortex to the ascending volley ("cortical" potential) (see Fig. 35-4, *A*, channel 1).

Unlike the EEG, SEPs are not abolished by hypothermia and overdoses of CNS depressants,[33] which facilitates their use in the confirmation of the diagnosis of brain death.

Alterations in Brain-Dead Patients

In patients with clinically diagnosed brain death, SEPs typically show either obliteration of all SEP components excluding the brachial plexus (N9) or cervical cord (N13) potentials, or obliteration of the entire SEP including these early components.

Abolition of brainstem (P14 and N18) and cortical (N20) with preserved brachial plexus (N9) and/or cervical cord (N13) potentials to stimulation of each median nerve (see Fig. 35-4, *B* and *C*) is observed in the scalp–noncephalic recordings of a large proportion of patients with a clinical diagnosis of brain death[34–38] (93.8 percent in one series[39]). The possible relevance to brain death of abolished P14, N18, and N20 responses cannot be determined without first excluding pre-existing neurologic conditions that may cause severe dysfunction of brainstem somatosensory pathways (e.g., multiple sclerosis, degenerative diseases,

and Arnold–Chiari malformation) or an extensive primary brainstem lesion.[40] When none of these potentially confounding conditions exists, abolition of brainstem and cortical components of SEPs in the face of peripheral and spinal components suggests severe dysfunction of somatosensory pathways above the foramen magnum, in keeping with the diagnosis of brain death.

At variance with other authors, Wagner found that loss of P14 in scalp–noncephalic recordings (such as CPi–EPc) occurred in only 9.8 percent of brain-dead individuals, whereas a special midfrontal–nasopharyngeal derivation (Fz–Phz) demonstrated it in 100 percent.[41] According to Wagner, the positive potential that persists in scalp–noncephalic derivations in a proportion of brain-dead patients is a caudally generated P14 component spared by the brain-death process rather than a distinct P13 potential generated in high cervical cord segments. Whatever the interpretation of this finding, according to Wagner[41] the Fz–Phz derivation is uniquely suited to distinguish brain-dead patients (in whom P14 invariably would be abolished) from comatose individuals (in whom P14 unfailingly would be preserved). Setting aside some perplexities, the author believes that this special derivation may be a worthwhile addition to the standard recommended montage for the study of patients with suspected brain death.

Bilateral abolition of the cortical (N20) potential with preserved peripheral (N9) and spinal (N13) potentials occurs in most, if not all, brain-dead patients[34,37,38,41,42] (see Fig. 35-4), but it also occurs in a substantial proportion of individuals who are comatose rather than brain-dead (36 percent according to Wagner[41]). Because of its low specificity, the bilateral obliteration of N20 is of little assistance in confirming the diagnosis of brain death. This is in sharp contrast to the remarkable prognostic power of bilaterally abolished N20 in comatose patients with hypoxic-ischemic encephalopathies, which is unmatched by other neurophysiologic measures.[43–45] The unilateral loss of N20 has uncertain significance. Corroboration of the suspected diagnosis of brain death by SEPs requires the additional demonstration of extinguished brainstem P14 and N18 in the presence of preserved N9 and N13.

In a small proportion of patients with brain death (3.1 percent in the series by Facco and associates[39]), all SEPs after N9 are abolished. This is especially true in individuals whose condition is complicated by injury to the brachial plexus or cervical roots or cord. In the absence of demonstrable peripheral or spinal responses, one cannot determine whether the loss of subsequent response components reflects lack of input to or severe dysfunction of the brainstem somatosensory pathways and the receiving cortex. Thus, this finding cannot be regarded as confirmatory evidence of brain death.

In still other individuals who satisfy all clinical criteria of brain death (3.2 percent according to Facco and co-workers[39]), P14 and/or N18 are preserved, suggesting brainstem dysfunction less global than the clinical examination suggests.

BRAINSTEM AUDITORY EVOKED POTENTIALS

Recording Methodology, Components, and Postulated Origin

Short-latency auditory evoked potentials, commonly (and improperly) referred to as brainstem auditory evoked potentials (BAEPs), primarily consist of five successive waves named I through V. These generally are elicited by monaural clicks and are recorded in a vertex–ipsilateral earlobe derivation (Cz–Ai) (Fig. 35-5, bottom trace). Although multiple generators probably contribute to individual response components, the broad

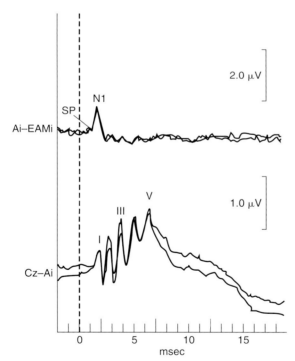

FIGURE 35-5 ■ Electrocochleogram (ECochG) (top traces) and brainstem auditory potentials (BAEPs) (bottom traces) in response to monaural clicks in an audiometrically normal subject. The ECochG was recorded with a noninvasive electrode in the external auditory meatus near the tympanic membrane.[45] Ai, earlobe ipsilateral to the stimulus. EAMi, ipsilateral external auditory meatus. Cz, vertex. SP, cochlear summating potential. N1, compound auditory nerve action potential simultaneous with but generally larger in amplitude than wave I. Waves III and V, main brainstem components of BAEPs. Appropriate instrumentation and technique make it possible to eliminate or markedly reduce the stimulus artifact.

localization (if not specific identity) of the main generators of individual response components helps to interpret the results of BAEP studies in brain-dead patients. Waves I and II are generated mostly by volleys of action potentials arising in the distal (closer to the cochlea) and proximal portions, respectively, of the auditory nerve. The subsequent waves III to V arise at successively higher levels along the brainstem auditory pathways, from the lower pons to the midbrain, as discussed in Chapters 24 and 25. Using special electrodes introduced into the external auditory meatus, it is also possible to record the electrocochleogram (ECochG), which demonstrates the compound auditory nerve action potential (N1; same as wave I of BAEPs), and the preceding summating potential (SP) of cochlear hair cells (see Fig. 35-5, top trace).[46] Much additional information on the features and putative generators of these potentials is offered in other reviews.[47,48]

Like SEPs, BAEPs are not abolished by toxic doses of barbiturates and other CNS depressants or by hypothermia, at least for temperatures as low as 20 °C.[49]

Alterations in Brain-Dead Patients

In patients with clinically suspected diagnosis of brain death, BAEP testing typically demonstrates either obliteration of all BAEPs including wave I or loss of all BAEPs excluding wave I (or waves I and II).

Obliteration of all BAEPs including wave I is demonstrated by a substantial majority of patients with clinically established brain death[36,37,39,42,50,51] (and occurred in 70.8 percent in one recent series[39]). Extinction of wave I indicates functional failure of the cochlea, the auditory nerve, or both. In individuals who have suffered cardiorespiratory arrest, obliteration of wave I likely is caused by cochlear ischemia secondary to arrest of the intracranial circulation. In patients who are brain-dead following head injury, loss of wave I often is related to fracture of the temporal bone with damage to the cochlea and auditory nerve, injury to the middle ear or tympanic membrane, and collection of blood in the external auditory canal. The detection of wave I may be hindered further by pre-existing deafness or profound hearing loss (e.g., as may be caused by treatment with ototoxic drugs) and by conductive deficits resulting from prolonged nasotracheal intubation and positive-pressure ventilation that interfere with eustachian tube function and may cause middle ear effusions. In the absence of wave I, it is impossible to determine whether the obliteration of all BAEPs is caused by lack of input to or severe dysfunction of brainstem auditory pathways. In these circumstances, BAEP testing provides no confirmatory evidence of brain death.

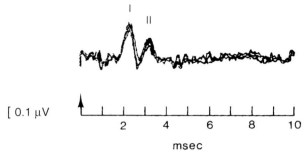

FIGURE 35-6 ■ Brainstem auditory evoked potentials demonstrating preservation of waves I and II in a clinically brain-dead individual. The patient died 2 hours after this recording. (Modified from Stockard JJ, Stockard JE, Sharbrough FW: Brainstem auditory evoked potentials in neurology: methodology, interpretation, and clinical application. p. 370. In Aminoff MJ (ed): Electrodiagnosis in Clinical Neurology. 2nd Ed. Churchill Livingstone, New York, 1980, with permission.)

In a minority of clinically brain-dead patients (24.6 percent in a recent study[39]), stimulation of each ear shows obliteration of all BAEPs except wave I (or waves I and II) (Fig. 35-6).[39,42,50] This finding indicates severe dysfunction of the auditory pathways in the brainstem such as occurs in brain death. Because confirmation of death of the brain by BAEPs depends on the demonstration of wave I, failure to detect this potential in ordinary testing should be scrutinized with special care. Malfunction of the stimulus circuit, the recording circuit, or both, should be tested and excluded. Additional recordings with electrodes in the external auditory meatus may improve the chances of detecting an elusive wave I, which is often small in voltage and delayed in latency in brain death.[50]

Loss of all BAEPs following wave I (or waves I and II) to stimulation of each ear typically distinguishes brain-dead individuals, in whom these potentials are abolished, from comatose patients, in whom they are preserved.[37,39,50] In keeping with this belief, serial recordings in patients with central herniation syndrome undergoing rostrocaudal deterioration show sequential, orderly loss of BAEPs generated at progressively lower levels of the brainstem. Obliteration of all BAEPs except wave I is not complete until all clinical criteria of brain death are met (Fig. 35-7).[50]

A small proportion of individuals who satisfy all clinical criteria of brain death (4.6 percent in one series[50]) demonstrate preservation of all BAEPs (I through V), suggesting that, in these individuals, brainstem dysfunction may be less global than the clinical examination indicates.

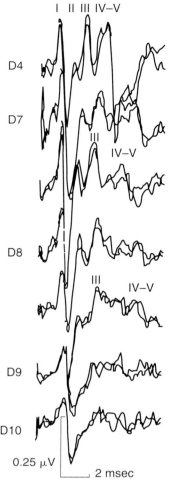

FIGURE 35-7 ■ Patient found unresponsive after an anoxic episode. The designations on the left (i.e., D4 to D10) refer to the days of hospitalization. On days 7 and 8, the top tracings were taken in the morning and the bottom tracings in the afternoon. On day 4 the patient was comatose but withdrew to noxious stimuli and had spontaneous respiration and preserved cephalic reflexes. One day earlier his electroencephalogram (EEG) showed widespread delta activity. On the 7th day, cephalic reflexes were no longer present, there were decerebrate responses to noxious stimuli, and low-voltage delta activity was detected in the EEG. On days 8 and 10, responses to noxious stimuli and spontaneous respiration were absent, and EEG showed electrocerebral inactivity. The patient expired 14 days after admission. Sequential loss of brainstem auditory evoked potentials of progressively shorter latency paralleled the craniocaudal deterioration of the patient's clinical status. Only wave I persisted on days 9 and 10, at which time the patient was brain-dead. (Modified from Starr A: Auditory brainstem responses in brain death. Brain, 99:543, 1976, with permission.)

VISUAL EVOKED POTENTIALS

It has long been known that potentials evoked by flashes in visual and related cortices (VEPs) are abolished in brain-dead patients[34,52,53] (Fig. 35-8). However, the

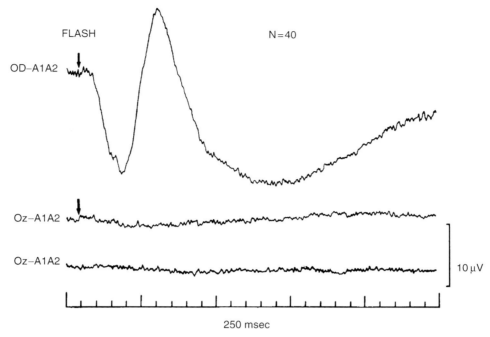

FLASH   N=40

OD–A1A2

Oz–A1A2

Oz–A1A2   10 µV

250 msec

FIGURE 35-8 ■ Preserved averaged electroretinogram (top trace) but abolished cerebral visual evoked potentials (middle trace) to light flashes in a 42-year-old clinically brain-dead patient. Bottom trace, control record without stimulus. OD, right infraorbital. Oz, midline occipital. A1A2, interconnected earlobes. (Modified from Wilkus RJ, Chatrian GE, Lettich E: The electroretinogram during terminal anoxia in humans. Electroencephalogr Clin Neurophysiol, 31:537, 1971, with permission.)

use of these potentials in the confirmation of suspected brain death is limited by their variability and vulnerability to sedative and anesthetic drugs and to hypothermia, among other factors. Loss of cerebral VEPs over the posterior head regions of brain-dead individuals is often associated with preservation of other stimulus-locked potentials over the anterior areas (see Fig. 35-8). The topography of these potentials with a maximum close to the eyes indicates that they are electroretinograms (ERGs). Their retinal origin can be demonstrated further by occluding either or both eyes during photic stimulation, recording simultaneously from scalp and periorbital electrodes, or both.[23] In the absence of those conditions that may reversibly cause an EEG pattern of ECI, abolished cerebral VEPs with preserved ERGs indicate severe cortical dysfunction in harmony with the diagnosis of brain death.

MOTOR EVOKED POTENTIALS

In patients with a clinical diagnosis of brain death, motor evoked potentials (MEPs)[54,55] are absent in response to transcranial magnetic (or electrical) stimulation of the motor cortex[56,57] but generally are preserved in response to cervical excitation.[56] However interesting, these motor responses have not won acceptance and are not suggested for the routine confirmation of brain death.

SUITABILITY OF EVOKED POTENTIALS FOR CONFIRMING BRAIN DEATH IN ADULTS

Unlike the EEG, evoked potentials are not abolished by CNS depressant drugs, deep hypothermia, profound hypotension, severe metabolic derangements, or endocrine crises, and they are capable of assessing brainstem function. However, short-latency SEPs, BAEPs, and VEPs do not contribute equally in confirming the diagnosis of brain death. SEPs are capable of assessing the functional integrity of the somatosensory pathways at multiple levels from sensory periphery to cerebral cortex and are inconclusive, because of the lack of wave N9 or N13, in only about 5 percent of brain-dead individuals. In contrast, BAEPs do not assess the functional state of the cerebral cortex and are unhelpful in 70 percent or more of brain-dead patients because of the absence of wave I. VEPs provide only limited insight into cortical function and are vulnerable to many influences.

Although SEPs are far more likely than BAEPs to provide confirmatory evidence of brain death, eliciting both SEPs and BAEPs helps to obviate some of the limitations inherent in single-modality testing. For example, BAEPs may provide evidence of loss of brainstem function in individuals in whom peripheral or spinal injury precludes the clinical assessment of somatosensory pathways.

Similarly, SEP testing may prove helpful when injury to the cochlea and the auditory nerve prevents the demonstration of BAEPs. When the confounding conditions alluded to earlier are excluded, the combined abolition of brainstem and cortical components of SEPs in the presence of peripheral or spinal potentials and the obliteration of brainstem components of BAEPs with preserved wave I confirm the suspected diagnosis of brain death in a high proportion of patients (93 percent in one series[40]). The addition of VEPs to SEPs, BAEPs, and the EEG is desirable to distinguish electrophysiologically between patients with (whole) brain death and individuals with cortical or primary brainstem death.

The author believes that, even when SEP testing gives evidence of severe dysfunction of the somatosensory pathways at multiple levels from periphery to cortex, the exploration of at least one additional pathway is needed to warrant the generalization that the loss of neural function likely involves the whole brain, and to provide the degree of reassuring redundancy demanded by the gravity of the diagnosis of brain death.

That multimodality evoked potentials have the capability of dependably confirming brain death in the adult does not imply that they are the method of choice for corroborating this diagnosis. Multimodality studies performed in the ICU according to rigorous standards are a difficult and time-consuming method that demands special technical expertise and interpretive skills often not available outside major medical centers. Four-vessel angiography remains the gold standard for confirming brain death, but it is invasive and is not free of risks. Thus, at present, the routine confirmation of irreversible loss of brain viability most commonly relies in the United States on other tests of cerebral blood flow, including radioisotope scintigraphy,[9,58] transcranial Doppler ultrasonography,[59] and single-photon emission computed tomography (SPECT).[60]

SELECTIVE FAILURE OF FOREBRAIN OR BRAINSTEM FUNCTION

Brain death as defined by the American Academy of Neurology is characterized by "irreversible loss of function of the brain, including the brainstem."[2] However, in some circumstances, acute functional failure selectively involves the forebrain, with substantially preserved brainstem function or, conversely, the brainstem with relative sparing of the forebrain. The term "death" used in the literature to designate these conditions is expedient but objectionable in several respects.

Acute Forebrain Failure (Cortical Death)

Some patients examined shortly after resuscitation from cardiorespiratory arrest demonstrate acute failure of the forebrain with variable sparing of brainstem function. This condition of "neocortical death,"[61] "cortical death,"[62] or "complete apallic syndrome"[63] is characterized by unresponsiveness to noxious and other stimuli, variable preservation of brainstem reflexes, and common preservation of spontaneous respiration. The EEG of cortically dead patients demonstrates ECI (Fig. 35-9), and cortical evoked potentials are abolished whereas brainstem and earlier response components are preserved.[63–65] Typically, flash VEPs are obliterated bilaterally but the ERGs are preserved (Fig. 35-10).[62–64,66] BAEPs, and ECochGs, when recorded, are often preserved (Fig. 35-11) but may be absent because of cochlear ischemia. Median nerve SEPs show bilateral abolition of the cortical N20 with preservation of brainstem (P14 and N18), spinal (N13), and peripheral (N9) components. Cortically dead patients generally do not survive, and their brains typically demonstrate widespread cortical necrosis with no or only minor changes in the thalamus and brainstem.

Acute Brainstem Failure (Primary Brainstem Death)

Acute infarction or hemorrhage sometimes transects the pons variably, involving the medulla and cerebellum but sparing the midbrain except for its lowermost portion. Individuals with this lesion typically demonstrate unresponsiveness to noxious stimuli, loss of brainstem reflexes, and apnea.[66–71] Because they are completely de-efferented, it is impossible to determine clinically whether they are aware of themselves and of the environment. Despite this uncertainty, their condition has been termed "rhombencephalic death," "brainstem death," and "primary brainstem death."

Unlike patients with (whole) brain death, individuals with brainstem death demonstrate preserved electrocerebral activity. Their EEGs may show a posterior alpha rhythm with or without intermixed theta and delta waves (Fig. 35-12) or may consist of low-voltage potentials primarily in the theta range.[67–72] Flash stimulation typically elicits cerebral responses over the posterior head regions, often visible even in unaveraged recordings and unresponsive to noxious stimuli. By contrast, SEPs generally show abolition of brainstem (P14, N18) and cortical (N20) components with preserved peripheral and spinal

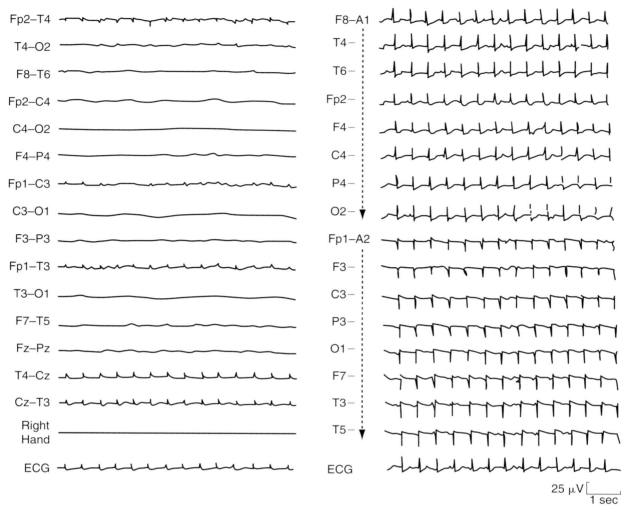

FIGURE 35-9 ■ Electroencephalogram demonstrating electrocerebral inactivity in a 45-year-old woman 3 days after an episode of ventricular fibrillation following coronary artery bypass graft. The patient was unresponsive to noxious stimuli and was artificially ventilated but exhibited intermittent spontaneous respiration and had intact brainstem reflexes. Right hand, dorsum of right hand. She died 6 days later and her brain demonstrated pseudolaminar necrosis of the whole cerebral cortex and necrosis of other forebrain structures, with substantial preservation of brainstem and spinal cord. (Modified from Wytrzes LM, Chatrian G-E, Shaw C-M et al: Acute failure of forebrain with sparing of brain-stem function: electroencephalographic, multimodal evoked potentials, and pathologic findings. Arch Neurol, 46:93, 1989, with permission.)

potentials (N9 and N13). BAEPs, often including wave I, are extinguished. Persistence of electrocerebral activity in patients with primary brainstem lesions is in harmony with the results of rostropontine transection in animals.[72] Figure 35-13 shows the extent of the lesion in one patient.

The EEGs of patients with primary brainstem death do not differ substantially from those of individuals with less extensive infarction or hemorrhage destroying the ventral pons bilaterally with no or variable extension into the pontine tegmentum. In these "locked-in" individuals,[73] VEPs

are usually present, but BAEP and SEP studies give variable results, presumably reflecting the extent and indirect effects of the lesion.[74]

EVALUATION OF BRAIN DEATH IN THE DEVELOPMENTAL PERIOD

Guidelines for establishing brain death in young patients, issued and widely disseminated in the United States by the Special Task Force for the Determination of Brain

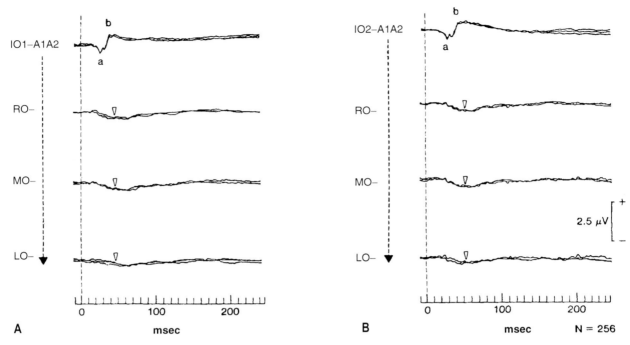

FIGURE 35-10 ■ Retinal, but no cerebral, responses to flash stimulation of (**A**) the left and (**B**) the right eye in the same patient as in Figure 35-9. Electroretinograms (ERGs) (waves a and b) were recorded between left and right infra-orbital electrodes (IO1 and IO2) and interconnected earlobe reference (A1A2). Slow downgoing potentials (open arrows) in recordings from right and left occipital electrodes (RO and LO) are ERGs detected by the A1A2 reference. (Modified from Wytrzes LM, Chatrian G-E, Shaw C-M et al: Acute failure of forebrain with sparing of brain-stem function: electroencephalographic, multimodal evoked potentials, and pathologic findings. Arch Neurol, 46:93, 1989, with permission.)

Death in Children, warned that it was not possible to establish cessation of cerebral and brainstem functions and determine its irreversibility following severe brain insults in newborns earlier than 7 days after term.[75] Clinical criteria of brain death applicable after this age did not differ from those recommended for adults. However, between the ages of 7 days and 1 year, the validity of these clinical standards depended on their persistence over specified periods and on their confirmation by EEG, cerebral radionuclide or contrast angiography, or both. No such constraints were advocated after the age of 1 year (Tables 35-2 and 35-3). These recommendations drew sharp criticism from some authors, who believed that the proposed standards were based on combined clinical criteria and laboratory tests, none of which had been validated.[76,77] Subsequent surveys of pediatric hospitals and neurosurgeons in the United States[78,79] revealed only scant adherence to the guidelines of the Special Task Force. In the United Kingdom, a Working Party of the British Paediatric Association believed that the concept itself of brain ("brainstem") death was "inappropriate" before 37 weeks' gestation, and that a confident diagnosis of this condition was "rarely possible" between

the ages of 37 weeks' gestation and 2 months.[80] For children older than 2 months, the assessment of brain death should be "approached in an unhurried manner" to ensure that all preconditions and clinical criteria are satisfied. The Working Party also denied the need to perform EEG, evoked potential, angiographic, radioisotope, and Doppler studies to confirm the diagnosis of brain death in a developing child. The present review of the literature reveals that the determination of brain death in children remains complex and controversial.

Clinical Criteria

It generally is agreed that attempting to determine by clinical observation and ancillary methods that brain function has ceased in newborns and young infants, and establishing that this functional failure is irreversible, are associated with unique problems. In a thoughtful introductory commentary to the report of the Special Task Force,[80] Volpe emphasized that "many of the critical functions to be assessed are either still in the process of developing or have only recently developed" and that

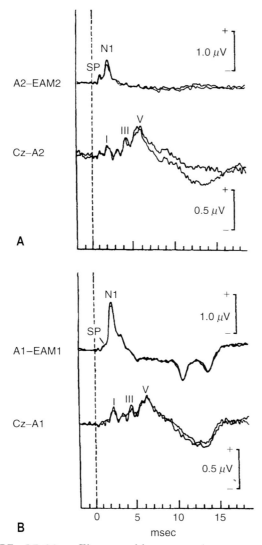

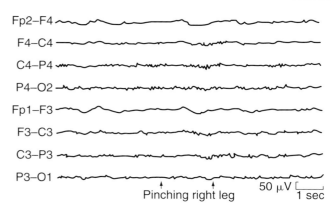

FIGURE 35-12 ◼ Eight hours after severe head injury, a 59-year-old man was unresponsive to noxious stimuli and visual threat, had rapid but deep and labored respiration, absent oculocephalic reflexes but preserved pupillary responses to light stimuli, and displayed bilateral extensor rigidity. His electroencephalogram demonstrated a posterior alpha rhythm at 8 to 10 Hz, best developed on the right hemisphere, and scattered 2- to 7-Hz potentials, most prominent on the left side. This pattern was unmodified by noxious stimuli. (Modified from Chatrian GE, White LE, Jr, Shaw CM: EEG pattern resembling wakefulness in unresponsive decerebrate state following traumatic brainstem infarct. Electroencephalogr Clin Neurophysiol, 16:285, 1964, with permission.)

FIGURE 35-11 ◼ Electrocochleograms (top traces) and brainstem auditory potentials (BAEPS) (bottom traces) in response to click stimulation of (**A**) the right and (**B**) the left ear. A2 and A1, right and left earlobes. EAM2 and EAM1, right and left external auditory meatuses. Cz, vertex. SP, cochlear summating potential. N1, compound auditory nerve action potential, simultaneous with wave I. Waves III and V, main brainstem components of BAEPs. The latency of N1 (and I) was prolonged on stimulation of the right but not of the left ear and all remaining latencies and interpeak intervals were normal. This is the same patient as in Figures 35–9 and 35–10. (Modified from Wytrzes LM, Chatrian GE, Shaw CM et al: Acute failure of forebrain with sparing of brain-stem function: electroencephalographic, multimodal evoked potentials, and pathologic findings. Arch Neurol, 46:93, 1989, with permission.)

"developing systems or recently acquired developmental functions are exquisitely vulnerable to injury by exogenous insults."[81] Rapid changes occur during the last 12 to 15 weeks of gestation in such functions as level of alertness; pupillary size and reaction to light; and the control of ventilation, eye movements, and bulbar reflexes. Some brainstem reflexes (e.g., pupillary and oculocephalic reflexes) are not fully developed before 32 weeks of gestation, and caloric stimulation is difficult to perform and assess in neonates.[82] Even the reliability of apnea tests in this age group has been questioned.[83]

In addition to developmental factors, other conditions may confound the clinical assessment of brain viability in the early developmental period. Among them, profound systemic hypotension, common among newborns and young infants suspected of having dead brains, may so reduce cerebral perfusion as to cause potentially reversible clinical manifestations of loss of brain function. In addition, neonates and infants suspected of having dead brains are often treated with high-dose intravenous pentobarbital to control intracranial pressure or have received high-dose intravenous phenobarbital loading because of proven or suspected seizures. Barbiturates have profound depressing effects on the CNS of severely brain-damaged neonates[83] and older children, and the inclusion in the treatment protocol of neuromuscular blocking agents and hypothermia further complicates the clinical assessment of these young patients.

A large proportion of newborns with suspected irreversible loss of brain function suffer from hypoxic-ischemic encephalopathies secondary to perinatal asphyxia of unclear duration and severity. In this age group, the extent and

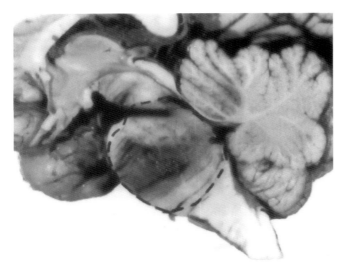

FIGURE 35-13 ■ Sagittal midline section of brain showing an infarct that transects the pons and lowermost portion of the midbrain (dashed line). The lesion was caused by pinching of the basilar artery in vertical midline fracture of the clivus. This is the same patient as in Figure 35-12. (Modified from Chatrian GE, White LE, Jr, Shaw CM: EEG pattern resembling wakefulness in unresponsive decerebrate state following traumatic brainstem infarct. Electroencephalogr Clin Neurophysiol, 16:285, 1964, with permission.)

gravity of the hypoxic-ischemic injury are assessed inadequately by clinical examination.[81] These factors, among others, limit the validity of the clinical criteria of deep coma, absent brainstem reflexes, and apnea as indicators of loss of brain function in neonates and young infants, and periods of observation longer than those in older patients are essential to establish their irreversibility.[82,83]

The Electroencephalogram

PECULIARITIES IN THE DEVELOPMENTAL PERIOD: TECHNICAL AND INTERPRETIVE REQUIREMENTS

The EEGs of neonates and small infants have peculiar features that differ sharply from those of older children as well as adults and that evolve particularly rapidly from prematurity to 2 months after term. Specifically, neonates, especially premature infants, display characteristically discontinuous electrocerebral activity consisting of bursts of EEG potentials separated by periods of voltage attenuation that decrease in duration with increasing age. This discontinuous pattern is associated with cyclic variations in the state of consciousness of the neonate.[84-87] Increasing duration of interburst intervals, widespread voltage attenuation, and, ultimately, ECI may develop under the influence of various conditions (e.g., hypoxia, hypotension, hypothermia, drug intoxication, and metabolic disorders).[85,86,88]

Because of the small head size of neonates and other developmental factors, obtaining EEGs on neonates ranging in age from prematurity to 4 to 8 weeks after term requires the use of fewer scalp electrodes than in older children and adults. In addition, neonatal recordings must include the monitoring of measures other than the EEG (typically, eye movements, mental EMG, respiration, and ECG) to identify sleep stages and demonstrate artifacts.[86,89,90] Actual recording time for these polygraphic studies should be at least 45 minutes,[90] but longer recordings are often indicated. Recording technique in children older than 4 to 8 weeks does not differ from that recommended for similarly unresponsive adults.[14]

Because the EEGs of neonates and infants are extremely sensitive to a variety of endogenous and exogenous factors, recordings demonstrating ECI in these patients are best repeated after an interval to ensure persistent lack of electrocerebral activity. A standard interval of 24 hours seems reasonable but is arbitrary.[82] Also, the peculiarities of the EEG in normal neonates and infants as well as neonates and infants presumed to be brain dead require that these tests be performed by qualified technologists and interpreted by clinical neurophysiologists with special expertise in this age group.

ASSESSMENT OF THE ELECTROENCEPHALOGRAM

Assessing the literature on the EEG as a confirmatory test of brain death in the developmental period is difficult because of paucity of data; common failure to report

Physical Examination	EEG	Cerebral Angiography
1. Coma and apnea 2. Absence of brainstem function 3. Lack of significant hypothermia or hypotension for age 4. Absence of spontaneous or reflex movements excluding spinal cord events such as reflex withdrawal or spinal myoclonus. The above findings should remain constant throughout the observation period	Electrocerebral inactivity over a 30-minute period according to guidelines of the American Clinical Neurophysiology Society. Drug concentrations should be insufficient to suppress EEG activity	Lack of visualization of intracranial arterial circulation in cerebral radionuclide angiography or lack of blood flow to brain in contrast angiography. Value of cerebral radionuclide angiography in infants under 2 months is under investigation

TABLE 35-2 ■ **Physical Examination and Laboratory Criteria for Determining Brain Death in Children***

*Summary of Report of Special Task Force on Brain Death in Children: Guidelines for the determination of brain death in children. Pediatrics, 80:298, 1987.
Note: The above guidelines have been questioned, as indicated in the text.

TABLE 35-3 ■ Types of Studies and Observation Periods for Determining Brain Death in Children*

Patient Age	Types of Studies and Observation Periods
7 days to 2 months	Two physical examinations and two EEGs demonstrating ECI at least 24 hours apart
2 months to 1 year	Two physical examinations and two EEGs showing ECI at least 24 hours apart; or a physical examination, an EEG demonstrating ECI, and a cerebral radionuclide angiogram demonstrating nonvisualization of cerebral arteries
Over 1 year	Assuming demonstration of irreversible cause of coma, two physical examinations 24 hours apart should fulfill the criteria of brain death when laboratory testing is not to be performed. The period of observation should be prolonged by at least 24 hours if the extent and irreversibility of brain damage are uncertain (especially in hypoxic-ischemic encephalopathy), or it may be reduced if the EEG demonstrates ECI or if cerebral radionuclide angiography does not visualize cerebral arteries

EEG, electroencephalogram; ECI, electrocerebral inactivity.
*Summary of Report of Special Task Force on Brain Death in Children: Guidelines for the determination of brain death in children. Pediatrics, 80:298, 1987.
Note: The above guidelines have been questioned, as indicated in the text.

results in newborns, infants, and older children separately; and the use of EEG and evoked potential techniques that are not described or are described incompletely, or are inadequate by current standards. Provided these limitations are recognized, the following observations on the EEG of neonates with presumed brain death deserve consideration:

1. A substantial proportion of neonates satisfying the clinical criteria of brain death demonstrate electrocerebral activity rather than ECI in their only or first EEG. In two different series, Ashwal found ECI in only 12 of 30 (40 percent) and 19 of 37 (51.4 percent) brain-dead neonates.[91,92] Persistent EEG activity in the remaining patients was characterized as "low voltage" or "suppression bursts."[92]

2. When present in a first EEG, ECI (Fig. 35-14) persists in subsequent recordings in neonates who remain clinically brain-dead.[92] Recovery of some electrocerebral activity after ECI lasting more than 24 hours may occur in patients receiving sedative drugs[93] but also, occasionally, in the absence of these medications.[89]

3. Newborns with ECI may demonstrate at least partially preserved brainstem function; Scher and associates reported this finding in as many as 15 of 18 patients (83.3 percent) who were not pharmacologically paralyzed.[93]

4. Very few newborns with clinical signs of brain death persisting for 24 hours or longer survive, whether their EEG shows ECI or preserved electrocerebral activity.[93] Whether their demise is caused by cardiac death or discontinuation of respiratory support is often unclear. However, some newborns with ECI survived, and a few were said to show ECI for as long as 2 years.[89]

5. Striking discrepancies have been reported in brain-dead neonates between the results of EEG and of cerebral blood-flow studies. In a paper by Ashwal, 8 of 12 newborns with ECI had no cerebral blood flow but so did 11 of 18 patients who demonstrated preserved EEG activity.[91]

However limited, these data suggest that the EEG is of questionable assistance, if any, in confirming brain death in neonates and should not be given major weight in deciding whether to continue respiratory support.

The demonstration of ECI more dependably corroborates the clinical diagnosis of brain death in patients older than 2 to 3 months. In a study by Alvarez and co-workers, even a single EEG demonstrating ECI in the absence of hypothermia, hypotension, and toxic or metabolic disorders was sufficient to confirm the permanent loss of brain viability after the age of 3 months.[94] However, some children in this study demonstrated variably preserved electrocerebral activity rather than ECI in the face of persistent clinical manifestations of extinguished brain function, sometimes associated with absent or critically reduced cerebral blood flow.

Evoked Potentials

Early evoked potential observations on neonates, infants, and small children with impaired responsiveness mostly consist of anecdotal reports describing the often reversible loss of BAEPs following hypoxic insults in neonates, infants, and even older children.[95-97] Most of these young patients did not fulfill all clinical criteria of brain death and survived, although some experienced neurologic sequelae. More recently, Ruíz-López and associates studied 51 children aged 7 days to 16 years with brain death of various, but predominantly traumatic, etiologies.[98] They found abolition of all BAEPs, including wave I, in the first test performed in 27 patients (53 percent); loss of all BAEPs, except wave I, to stimulation of each ear in 9 (17.6 percent); obliteration of BAEPs with preserved wave I to stimulation of one ear in 9 (17.6 percent); and preservation of (abnormal) BAEPs to stimulation of each ear in 6 children (11.8 percent). These authors interpreted their results as fulfilling criteria of brain death in 46 of 51 of their patients (90.2 percent). However, analysis of these data based on currently

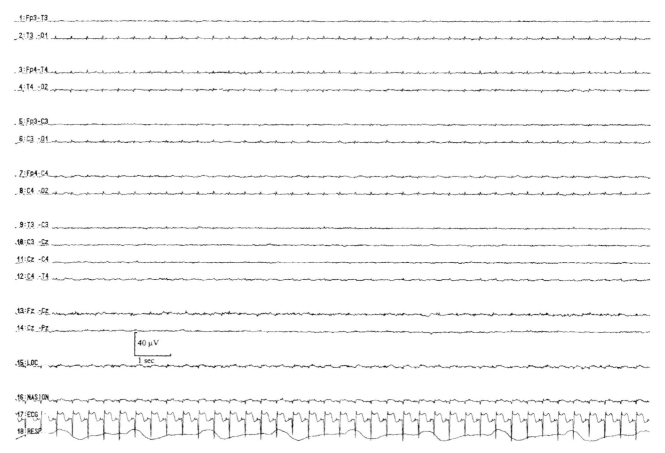

FIGURE 35-14 ■ Electrocerebral inactivity in a neonate with a conceptional age of 39 weeks who was clinically brain dead because of severe hypoxic-ischemic encephalopathy. (Modified from Clancy RR, Bergqvist AGC, Dlugos DJ: Neonatal electroencephalography. p. 160. In Ebersole TA, Pedley TA (eds): Current Practice of Clinical Electroencephalography. 3rd Ed. Lippincott, Williams & Wilkins, Philadelphia, 2003, with permission.)

accepted criteria detailed in this chapter indicates that BAEPs confirmed brain death in only 9 patients (17.6 percent) in whom stimulation of each ear demonstrated loss of all BAEPs after wave I. In this work, SEP testing was somewhat more successful in that obliteration of all response components in the face of preserved spinal N13 occurred in 10 of 16 patients (62.5 percent). Ruíz-García and colleagues performed BAEPs and SEPs in children ranging in age from 18 days to 17 years who suffered from brain death of various but predominantly infectious etiologies.[99] They reported that these combined tests provided conclusive evidence of brain death in 100 of 107 patients (93 percent) but did not specify their interpretive criteria. In neither of these last two studies were the results broken down according to age.

The present author believes that because of lack of adequate information, SEPs and BAEPs should not be relied upon at present to confirm irreversible loss of brain viability in neonates, infants, and small children.

REFERENCES

1. Adams RD, Jequier M: The brain death syndrome: hypoxemic panencephalopathy. Schweiz Med Wochenschr, 99:65, 1969
2. Wijdicks EF, Varelas PN, Gronseth GS et al: Evidence-based guideline update: determining brain death in adults: report of the Quality Standards Subcommittee of the American Academy of Neurology. Neurology, 74:1911, 2010
3. Working Group convened by the Royal College of Physicians and endorsed by the Conference of Medical Royal Colleges and their Faculties in the United Kingdom: Criteria for the diagnosis of brain stem death. J R Coll Physicians Lond, 29:381, 1995
4. Pallis C: ABC of brainstem death: the arguments about the EEG. Br Med J, 286:284, 1983
5. Shewmon DA: Chronic "brain death": meta-analysis and conceptual consequences. Neurology, 51:1538, 1998
6. Wijdicks EF, Bernat JL: Chronic "brain death": meta-analysis and conceptual consequences. Neurology, 53:1369, 1999
7. Walker AE: Cerebral Death. 3rd Ed. Urban & Schwarzenberg, Baltimore, 1985

8. Rossetti AO, Oddo M, Logroscino G et al: Prognostication after cardiac arrest and hypothermia: a prospective study. Ann Neurol, 67:301, 2010

9. Goodman KM: Brain death documentation: analysis and issues. Neurosurgery, 52:1242, 2003

10. Grigg MM, Kelly MA, Celesia GG et al: Electroencephalographic activity after brain death. Arch Neurol, 44:948, 1987

11. Noachtar S, Binnie C, Ebersole J et al: A glossary of terms most commonly used by clinical electroencephalographers, and proposal for the report form for the EEG findings. The International Federation of Clinical Neurophysiology. Electroencephalogr Clin Neurophysiol Suppl, 52:21, 1999

12. Waltregny A, Bonnal J, LeJeune G: Mort cérébrale et homotransplant: critères utilisés pour établir rapidement le diagnostic de coma dépassé. Rev Neurol, 122:406, 1970

13. Velasco M, Lopez-Portillo M, Olvera-Rabiela JE et al: EEG y registros profundos en casos de coma post traumático irreversible. Arch Invest Med, 2:1, 1971

14. American Clinical Neurophysiology Society: Guideline 3: Minimum technical standards for EEG recording in suspected cerebral death. J Clin Neurophysiol, 23:9, 2006

15. Bennett DR, Hughes JR, Korein J et al: Atlas of Electroencephalography in Coma and Cerebral Death. EEG at the Bedside or in the Intensive Care Unit. Raven, New York, 1976

16. Verma A, Bedlack RS, Radtke RA et al: Succinylcholine induced hyperkalemia and cardiac arrest: death related to an EEG study. J Clin Neurophysiol, 16:46, 1999

17. Guérit JM, Amantini A, Amodio P et al: Consensus on the use of neurophysiological tests in the intensive care unit (ICU): electroencephalogram (EEG), evoked potentials (EP), and electroneuromyography (ENMG). Neurophysiol Clin, 39:71, 2009

18. NINCDS Monograph No. 81–2286. The NINCDS Collaborative Study of Brain Death. Bethesda, MD, 1980

19. Cabral R, Prior PF, Scott DF et al: Reversible profound depression of cerebral electrical activity in hyperthermia. Electroencephalogr Clin Neurophysiol, 42:697, 1977

20. Moseley JI, Molinari GF, Walker AE: Respirator brain: report of a survey and review of current concepts. Arch Pathol Lab Med, 100:61, 1976

21. Hughes JR, Boshes B, Leestma J: Electro-clinical and pathological correlations in comatose patients. Clin Electroencephalogr, 7:13, 1976

22. Bickford RG, Sims JK, Billinger TW et al: Problems in EEG estimation of brain death and use of computer techniques for their solution. Trauma, 12:61, 1971

23. Chatrian GE: Electrophysiological evaluation of brain death: a critical appraisal. p. 525. In Aminoff MJ (ed): Electrodiagnosis in Clinical Neurology. Churchill Livingstone, New York, 1980

24. Prior PF, Maynard DE: Monitoring Cerebral Function. Long-term Monitoring of EEG and Evoked Potentials. Elsevier, Amsterdam, 1986

25. Dunham CM, Katradis A, Williams MD: The bispectral index, a useful adjunct for the timely diagnosis of brain death in the comatose trauma patient. Am J Surg, 198:846, 2009

26. Buchner H, Schuchardt V: Reliability of electroencephalogram in the diagnosis of brain death. Eur Neurol, 30:138, 1990

27. Sediri H, Bourriez JL, Derambure P: Place de l'EEG dans le diagnostic de mort encéphalique. Rev Neurol (Paris), 163:248, 2007

28. Wijdicks EF: The diagnosis of brain death. N Engl J Med, 344:1215, 2001

29. Young GB, Shemie SD, Doig CJ et al: Brief review: the role of ancillary tests in the neurological determination of death. Can J Anaesth, 53:620, 2006

30. American Clinical Neurophysiology Society: Guideline 9D: Guidelines on short-latency somatosensory evoked potentials. J Clin Neurophysiol, 23:1, 2006

31. Aminoff MJ, Eisen A: Somatosensory evoked potentials. p. 570. In Aminoff MJ (ed): Electrodiagnosis in Clinical Neurology. 5th Ed. Elsevier Churchill Livingstone, Philadelphia, 2005

32. Emerson RG, Pedley TA: Somatosensory evoked potentials. p. 892. In Ebersole JS, Pedley TA (eds): Current Practice of Clinical Electroencephalography. 3rd Ed. Lippincott Williams & Wilkins, Philadelphia, 2003

33. Rumpl E, Prugger M, Gerstenbrand F et al: Central somatosensory conduction time and acoustic brainstem transmission time in post-traumatic coma. J Clin Neurophysiol, 5:237, 1988

34. Trojaborg W, Jørgensen EO: Evoked cortical potentials in patients with "isoelectric" EEGs. Electroencephalogr Clin Neurophysiol, 35:301, 1973

35. Anziska BJ, Cracco RQ: Short-latency somatosensory evoked potentials in brain dead patients. Arch Neurol, 37:222, 1980

36. Goldie WD, Chiappa KH, Young RR et al: Brainstem auditory and short-latency somatosensory evoked responses in brain death. Neurology, 31:248, 1981

37. Mauguière F, Grand C, Fisher C et al: Aspects des potentiels évoqués auditifs et somesthésiques précoces dans les comas neurologiques et la mort cérébrale. Rev EEG Neurophysiol Clin, 12:280, 1982

38. Belsh JM, Chokroverty S: Short-latency somatosensory-evoked potentials in brain-death patients. Electroencephalogr Clin Neurophysiol, 68:75, 1987

39. Facco EE, Munari M, Gallo F et al: Role of short latency evoked potentials in the diagnosis of brain death. Clin Neurophysiol, 113:1855, 2002

40. Mauguière F, García-Larrea L, Murray NMF et al: Evoked potential diagnostic strategies: EPs in coma. p. 482. In Osselton JW (ed): Clinical Neurophysiology: EMG, Nerve Conduction, and Evoked Potentials. Butterworth–Heinemann, Oxford, 1995

41. Wagner W: Scalp, earlobe and nasopharyngeal recordings of the median nerve somatosensory evoked P14 potential in coma and brain death. Detailed latency and amplitude analysis in 181 patients. Brain, 119:1507, 1996

42. Machado C: Multimodality evoked potentials and electroretinography in a test battery for an early diagnosis of brain death. J Neurosurg Sci, 37:1225, 1993

43. Rothstein TL, Thomas EM, Sumi SM: Predicting outcome in hypoxic-ischemic coma. A prospective clinical and electrophysiologic study. Electroencephalogr Clin Neurophysiol, 79:101, 1991

44. Rothstein TL: The role of evoked potentials in anoxic-ischemic coma and severe brain trauma. J Clin Neurophysiol, 17:486, 2000

45. Zandbergen EGJ, de Haan RJ, Koelman JHTM et al: Prediction of poor outcome in anoxic-ischemic coma. J Clin Neurophysiol, 17:498, 2000

46. Chatrian GE, Wirch AL, Lettich E et al: Click-evoked human electrocochleogram. Noninvasive recording method, origin, and physiological significance. Am J EEG Technol, 22:151, 1982

47. Legatt AD: Brainstem auditory evoked potentials in neurology. p. 517. In Aminoff MJ (ed): Electrodiagnosis in Clinical Neurology. 5th Ed. Elsevier Churchill Livingstone, Philadelphia, 2005

48. Erwin CW, Husain AM: Brainstem auditory evoked potentials. p. 864. In: Ebersole JS, Pedley TA (eds): Current Practice of Clinical Electroencephalography. Lippincott Williams & Wilkins, Philadelphia, 2003

49. Markand ON, Lee BI, Warren C et al: Effects of hypothermia on BAEPs in humans. Ann Neurol, 22:507, 1987

50. Starr A: Auditory brain stem responses in brain death. Brain, 99:543, 1976

51. Facco E, Casartelli-Liviero M, Munari M et al: Short-latency evoked potentials: new criteria for brain death? J Neurol Neurosurg Psychiatry, 53:351, 1990

52. Arfel G: Stimulations visuelles et silence cérébral. Electroencephalogr Clin Neurophysiol, 23:172, 1967

53. Ganes T, Lundar T: EEG and evoked potentials in comatose patients with severe brain damage. Electroencephalogr Clin Neurophysiol, 69:6, 1988

54. Murray NMF: Motor evoked potentials. p. 600. In Aminoff MJ (ed): Electrodiagnosis in Clinical Neurology. 5th Ed. Elsevier Churchill Livingstone, Philadelphia, 2005

55. Rothwell JC, Hallett M, Berardelli A et al: Magnetic stimulation: motor evoked potentials. The International Federation of Clinical Neurophysiology. Electroencephalogr Clin Neurophysiol Suppl, 52:97, 1999

56. Firsching R, Wilhelms S, Cséscei G: Pyramidal tract function during onset of brain death. Electroencephalogr Clin Neurophysiol, 84:321, 1992

57. Ying Z, Schmid UD, Schmid J et al: Motor and somatosensory evoked potentials in coma: analysis and relation to clinical status and outcome. J Neurol Neurosurg Psychiatry, 55:470, 1992

58. Conrad GR, Sinha P: Scintigraphy as a confirmatory test of brain death. Semin Nucl Med, 33:312, 2003

59. Petty GW, Mohr JP, Pedley TA et al: The role of transcranial Doppler in confirming brain death: sensitivity, specificity, and suggestions for performance and interpretation. Neurology, 40:300, 1990

60. Bonetti MG, Ciritella P, Valle G et al: 99 mTc HM-PAO brain perfusion SPECT in brain death. Neuroradiology, 37:365, 1995

61. Brierly JB, Adams JH, Graham DI et al: Neocortical death after cardiac arrest: a clinical, neurophysiological, and neuropathological report of two cases. Lancet, 2:560, 1971

62. Wytrzes LM, Chatrian G-E, Shaw C-M et al: Acute failure of forebrain with sparing of brain stem function. Electroencephalographic, multimodality evoked potentials, and pathologic findings. Arch Neurol, 46:93, 1989

63. Biniek R, Ferbert A, Rimpl J et al: The complete apallic syndrome: a case report. Intensive Care Med, 15:212, 1989

64. Brunko E, Delecluse F, Herbaut AG et al: Unusual pattern of somatosensory and brainstem auditory evoked potentials after cardio-respiratory arrest. Electroencephalogr Clin Neurophysiol, 62:338, 1985

65. Rothstein TL, Austin E, Sumi SM: Evoked responses in neocortical death. Electroencephalogr Clin Neurophysiol, 56:S162, 1983

66. Chatrian GE, White LE Jr, Shaw CM: EEG patterns resembling wakefulness in unresponsive decerebrate state following traumatic brainstem infarct. Electroencephalogr Clin Neurophysiol, 16:285, 1964

67. Chase TN, Moretti L, Prensky AL: Clinical and electroencephalographic manifestations of vascular lesions of the pons. Neurology, 18:357, 1968

68. Ferbert A, Buchner H, Ringelstein EB et al: Isolated brainstem death. Case report with demonstration of preserved visual evoked potentials (VEPs). Electroencephalogr Clin Neurophysiol, 65:157, 1986

69. Ogata J, Imakita M, Yutani C et al: Primary brainstem death: a clinicopathological study. J Neurol Neurosurg Psychiatry, 51:646, 1988

70. Rodin E, Tahir S, Austin D et al: Brainstem death. Clin Electroencephalogr, 16:63, 1985

71. Zwarts MJ, Kornips FHM: Clinical brainstem death with preserved electroencephalographic activity and visual evoked response. Arch Neurol, 58:1010, 2001

72. Moruzzi G: The sleep-waking cycle. Ergebn Physiol, 64:1, 1972

73. Posner JB, Saper CB, Schiff ND et al: Plum and Posner's Diagnosis of Stupor and Coma. Oxford University Press, Oxford, 2007

74. Towle VL, Babikian V, Maselli R et al: A comparison of multimodality evoked potentials, computed tomography findings and clinical data in brainstem vascular infarcts. p. 383. In Morocutti C, Rizzo PA (eds): Evoked Potentials: Neurophysiological and Clinical Aspects. Elsevier, Amsterdam, 1985

75. Report of Special Task Force for the Determination of Brain Death in Children: Guidelines for the determination of brain death in children. Pediatrics, 80:298, 1987

76. Freeman JM, Ferry PC: New brain death guidelines in children: further confusion. Pediatrics, 81:301, 1988

77. Shewmon DA: Commentary on guidelines for the determination of brain death in children. Ann Neurol, 24:789, 1988

78. Meija RE, Pollack MM: Variability in brain death determination practices in children. JAMA, 274:550, 1995

79. Chang MY, McBride LA, Ferguson MA: Variability in brain death in declaration practices in pediatric head trauma patients. Pediatr Neurosurg, 39:7, 2003

80. Working Party Report on the Diagnosis of Brain Stem Death in Children. British Paediatric Association, London, 1991

81. Volpe JJ: Brain death determination in the newborn. Commentary. Pediatrics, 80:293, 1987

82. Ashwal S, Schneider S: Brain death in children: Part I. Pediatr Neurol, 3:5, 1987

83. Drake B, Ashwal S, Schneider S: Determination of cerebral death in the pediatric intensive care unit. Pediatrics, 78:107, 1986

84. Dreyfus-Brisac C, Larroche J-C: Discontinuous EEGs in prematures and full-term neonates. Electroencephalogr Clin Neurophysiol, 32:575, 1972

85. Stockard-Pope JE, Werner SS, Bickford RG et al: Atlas of Neonatal Electroencephalography. 2nd Ed. Raven, New York, 1992

86. Hahn JS, Tharp BR: Neonatal and pediatric electroencephalography. p. 123. In Aminoff MJ (ed): Electrodiagnosis in Clinical Neurology. 5th Ed. Elsevier Churchill Livingstone, Philadelphia, 2005

87. Clancy RR, Bergqvist C, Dlugos DJ: Neonatal electroencephalography. p. 160. In Ebersole JS, Pedley TA (eds): Current Practice of Clinical Electroencephalography. 3rd Ed. Lippincott Williams & Wilkins, Baltimore, 2003

88. Hrachovy RA, Mizrahi EM, Kellaway P: Electroencephalography of the newborn. p. 201. In Daly DD, Pedley TA (eds): Current Practice of Clinical Electroencephalography. 2nd Ed. Raven, New York, 1990

89. American Clinical Neurophysiology Society: Guideline 2: Minimum technical standards for pediatric electroencephalography. J Clin Neurophysiol, 23:92, 2006

90. De Weerd AW, Despland PA, Plouin P: Neonatal EEG. The International Federation of Clinical Neurophysiology. Electroencephalogr Clin Neurophysiol Suppl, 52:149, 1999

91. Ashwal S, Schneider S: Brain death in the newborn. Pediatrics, 84:429, 1989

92. Ashwal S: Brain death in the newborn. Current perspectives. Clin Perinatol, 24:859, 1997

93. Scher M, Barabas R, Barmada M: Clinical examination findings in neonates with the absence of electrocerebral activity: an acute or chronic encephalopathic state? J Perinatol, 16:455, 1996

94. Alvarez LA, Moshé SL, Belman AL et al: EEG and brain death determination in children. Neurology, 38:227, 1988

95. Taylor MJ, Houston BD, Lowry NJ: Recovery of auditory brainstem responses after a severe hypoxic ischemic insult. N Engl J Med, 309:1169, 1983

96. Dear PRF, Godfrey DJ: Neonatal auditory brainstem response cannot reliably diagnose brainstem death. Arch Dis Child, 60:17, 1985

97. Steinhart CM, Weiss IP: Use of brainstem auditory evoked potentials in pediatric brain death. Crit Care Med, 13:560, 1985

98. Ruíz-López MJ, Martínez de Azagra A, Serrano A et al: Brain death and evoked potentials in pediatric patients. Crit Care Med, 27:412, 1999

99. Ruíz-García M, González-Astiazarán A, Collado-Corona MA et al: Brain death in children: clinical, neurophysiological and radioisotopic angiography findings in 125 patients. Childs Nerv Syst, 16:40, 2000

Electrophysiologic Techniques in the Evaluation of Patients with Suspected Neurotoxic Disorders

MICHAEL J. AMINOFF and JAMES W. ALBERS

In recent years, both the general public and health-care professionals have become increasingly aware of the potential hazards of exposure to certain chemicals. At the same time, the introduction of more chemical agents into the work and social environments has led to an increased risk of exposure to potential neurotoxins. Similarly, many pharmacologic agents have adverse effects that include neurotoxicity. The neurologic consequences of toxin exposure vary, depending on the agents to which exposure has occurred, but either the central or peripheral nervous systems, or both, may be affected. Central disturbances are manifested most commonly as neurobehavioral changes, but sometimes more specific deficits affect cognition, motor or sensory function of the limbs, cerebellar function, or the autonomic nervous system.

The published literature concerning the consequences of exposure to neurotoxic agents is extensive, but many publications fail to permit valid conclusions to be reached concerning the risks or consequences of exposure to particular chemical agents. Clinical reports are often of anecdotal material, and interpretation is confounded by the multiplicity of factors that may have led to the occurrence of symptoms or neurologic signs. Formal studies in humans to evaluate the neurotoxicity of particular agents are often confounded, in turn, by inadequacies of study design, concomitant use of alcohol or psychoactive medication, exposure to multiple chemical agents, and the nonspecific nature of many of the complaints attributed to toxic exposure. Careful matching of subjects for age, sex, and educational and cultural background is important in epidemiologic studies but is often neglected.

In this setting, electrodiagnostic studies should have an important role in helping to:

1. Confirm the organic basis of symptoms
2. Define the nature of clinical disturbances and their anatomic sites of origin
3. Determine the severity of any dysfunction
4. Monitor progression of the disorder
5. Recognize early neurologic involvement after known exposure to a neurotoxic agent so that further exposure can be limited.

Electrophysiologic approaches have been especially helpful in evaluating the peripheral rather than the central nervous system. Both will be considered briefly in this chapter.

NEUROTOXIC DISORDERS OF THE CENTRAL NERVOUS SYSTEM

A number of medications are neurotoxic and lead to behavioral or other neurologic disturbances when taken either in excessive amounts or at recommended doses for therapeutic purposes.[1] Drugs taken for recreational purposes also have well-recognized neurotoxicity.[2] Concern has increased, however, about the potential neurotoxicity of chemicals encountered in other contexts such as the work environment. Many of the symptoms that are alleged to reflect a toxin-related neurobehavioral disorder are common in the general population, and their relationship to chemical exposure is therefore hard to ascertain. In consequence, claims for the occurrence of certain cognitive or neurobehavioral disorders as a result of toxin exposure are difficult to validate scientifically. Many published clinical and epidemiologic studies provide limited information about the degree of exposure; vary in the manner in which exposed individuals are identified; or involve exposure to a variety of different chemicals, which complicates interpretation of the findings.

Some published studies involve self-reports by one or more individuals of subjective neurologic complaints without adequate control populations. The nonspecific nature of such complaints and the failure to control other variables confound interpretation of these studies. Studies in animals are sometimes helpful in confirming a relationship between clinical disorders and toxin exposure, but animal models of neurobehavioral disorders are difficult to find. Again, when the occurrence of a neurobehavioral disorder in exposed workers is compared, for example, with the incidence of this same disorder in a suitable control group, the toxic basis for the disorder may not be evident. Reports of single or small series of subjects with symptoms attributed to toxin exposure are common, but their significance is uncertain, especially when the clinical disorder develops after an interval rather than in close temporal relationship to the exposure. Indeed, it may not be possible to accept a causal relationship between toxin exposure and the later development of a neurobehavioral disorder when several years elapse between exposure and the clinical disorder. It is especially difficult to recognize such an association when symptoms are nonspecific ones that could relate to a variety of different causes, rather than unusual ones

that are difficult to explain by other means. Some studies involve information derived from death certificates, but major methodologic concerns detract from such reports. For example, toxin exposure often is not indicated in the report and has to be inferred from the patient's occupation. Exposure to certain toxins may indeed occur in relation to various occupations, but the one occupation listed on a death certificate is typically the final or usual one and therefore may be misleading.

The importance of adequate control subjects cannot be overemphasized. For example, if intellectually less capable persons are hired to work in less desirable occupational settings, it will not be surprising if behavioral testing shows differences between them and normal college students. This concern is more than theoretical. For example, Errebo-Knudsen and Olsen, in their review of the so-called painters' syndrome, noted that approximately 28 percent of boys who later became painters were from the lowest IQ group and none was from the highest; 77 percent of those who became painters had IQs below the median of a group of 11,352 boys who were studied.[3] Careful examination of the methodologies of the Scandinavian studies that established the existence of a painters' encephalopathy in the 1970s reveals them to be so methodologically flawed that they are invalid.

Electrophysiologic studies have been used to evaluate patients with presumed dysfunction of the central nervous system as a result of neurotoxic exposure. In general, the findings have been of limited utility and uncertain clinical relevance.

Electroencephalography

The electroencephalogram (EEG) has been used widely to evaluate patients with neurobehavioral disturbances related to possible neurotoxic exposure. The marked variability of the EEG in normal subjects, however, has limited its utility. As indicated in Chapter 3, the EEG generally is evaluated subjectively, and such evaluation may lead to interpretive differences between different observers. Moreover, a number of variables (e.g., age, level of arousal, and certain medications) are known to affect the EEG, and these variables render comparison between individuals difficult, especially when only nonspecific abnormalities that have a high incidence in the general (unexposed) population are encountered.

In many patients with encephalopathies related to medication (including chemotherapy), recreational drugs, or chemical exposure in other contexts, the EEG shows nonspecific slowing. In some instances, paroxysmal epileptiform activity is also found, as with mercury or lead poisoning; exposure to chlorinated hydrocarbons (as in the manufacture of DDT); organophosphate poisoning; or patients receiving aminophylline, isoniazid, lithium, high-dose penicillin therapy, or neuroleptic drugs. The EEG changes with clozapine have been particularly well described and relate to serum levels.[4] Patients with a history of alcohol abuse may have focal epileptiform or slow-wave abnormalities, but the EEG is often normal; during acute intoxication, however, the EEG is slowed. The findings during acute alcohol-withdrawal states are varied; mild generalized slowing is often found, and photoparoxysmal responses and generalized epileptiform discharges may also be present. Stimulant drugs (e.g., amphetamines and cocaine) are associated with an increase in frequency of background rhythms.[5] Benzodiazepines and barbiturates lead to an increase in beta activity and then, with increasing doses, to some slowing of the EEG. The effects of antiepileptic drugs are considered in Chapter 3.

Attempts have been made to objectify EEG interpretation by using quantitative techniques, as discussed in Chapter 8. The use of such techniques to evaluate workers with possible exposure to neurotoxic agents generally has been unrewarding. This is because most studies have involved multiple comparisons of different aspects of the EEG, and false-positive results are therefore likely to occur on the basis of chance alone. Quantitative approaches require comparison of a test group to a reference sample and also require that the same approach be used to collect and analyze EEG data. The two groups must be matched for factors such as age, sex, social class, educational and occupational backgrounds, alcohol and substance abuse, medication use, and level of arousal and cognitive function. All too often, comparisons are made to groups that are not matched in this way, so any departure from normality is of uncertain relevance. Alterations in the level of arousal may lead to marked changes in the EEG that may be attributed mistakenly to toxin exposure if the true basis of the altered EEG is not recognized. Furthermore, other artifacts must be excluded before computerized analysis of the EEG if misinterpretation is to be avoided. Any computerized EEG analysis must also be interpreted cautiously because many thousands of separate statistical results may be generated by the analysis, and chance alone therefore may result in apparent deviations from normality in a number of instances. This problem, discussed further in Chapter 8, is pertinent when studies involving quantitative EEG are interpreted to determine the presence or nature of neurotoxic disorders. The sensitivity and specificity of EEG abnormalities are poor when the EEG is used to screen for the development of subclinical encephalopathies, and more studies are necessary to clarify the role, if any, of quantitative EEG analysis in this context.[6,7] Certainly, at the present time, it is hard to justify the use of quantitative EEG for medicolegal purposes to establish the presence of an encephalopathy that might have an occupational or toxic basis, and this accords with the position adopted by the American Academy of Neurology.[6] The EEG findings, whether analyzed subjectively or quantitatively, are not a reliable means of distinguishing between different types of encephalopathic disorder. Even when changes have been noted by individual observers, their relevance for clinical diagnosis or screening purposes is uncertain.

These various issues have limited the utility of the EEG and continue to confound its application as a means of monitoring for neurotoxic exposure. The EEG certainly may be abnormal when acute encephalopathy is caused by neurotoxicity, but in such circumstances additional ancillary investigations are usually unnecessary to confirm the presence of an organic disorder, and the EEG findings in themselves do not reveal the underlying cause of cerebral dysfunction. In patients referred for EEG evaluation after any acute encephalopathic process has resolved, the presence of a normal EEG is not helpful in excluding the possibility of a prior encephalopathic process.

Evoked Potential Studies

Evoked potential studies have been used for a number of years to evaluate the functional status of certain afferent systems. Because they provide quantitative data, they permit objective evaluation and facilitate comparisons between subjects or comparisons of the same subject at different times. As indicated in Chapters 22 to 27, a standardized protocol is used to record the response of the central nervous system following visual, auditory, or somatosensory stimuli. Depending on the sensory modality being tested, the latency, amplitude, and intercomponent latency of the response is determined and compared with values obtained in normal age- and sex-matched subjects. Alterations in the configuration or duration of a response are more difficult to quantify, and criteria for abnormality have not been agreed. Because the range of normal values is affected by numerous technical factors, a control population of normal subjects should be studied under the same conditions as individual subjects or any test populations are studied. Technical details are provided in earlier chapters. Evoked potential studies are important in determining the organic basis of complaints involving various afferent systems and in helping to indicate the likely site of the responsible pathology. In occasional instances, they may be helpful in detecting toxin-related changes at a subclinical stage so that further damage is avoided by preventing further exposure to the offending agent. For example, evoked potentials are particularly sensitive to the toxic effects of ethambutol on the visual system. In general, however, the findings are not specific to any individual disorder but provide information about the pathophysiologic basis of symptoms. Furthermore, certain evoked potentials (e.g., brainstem auditory evoked potentials) are generally resistant to changes related to metabolic or toxic disorders.

Endogenous Potentials

Endogenous potentials are considered in detail in Chapter 29. They are recorded over the vertex of the scalp in response to a stimulus to which the subject directs attention to distinguish it from other, more frequently occurring stimuli. Endogenous potentials depend on the setting in which the target stimulus is delivered rather than on the physical characteristics of that stimulus. In patients with cognitive changes, endogenous potentials may be delayed in comparison with age-matched control subjects. The size of the response is of little clinical consequence because it varies between subjects and depends on the level of attention of the subject. Endogenous potentials are recorded mainly to evaluate patients with suspected cognitive deficits and, in particular, to distinguish between dementia and depression. They have been used only on limited occasions to evaluate patients with neurobehavioral disturbances related to neurotoxic exposure, and their utility in this context is uncertain.

Evaluation of Central Neurotoxic Disorders

General comment was made earlier on the EEG findings in certain toxic encephalopathies. The use of electrophysiologic techniques to evaluate the central nervous system following exposure to selected chemical agents, particularly in an industrial or occupational setting, is discussed in this section. It is not intended to provide a comprehensive account, however, but only to exemplify the utility and limitations of these approaches.

N-HEXANE

n-Hexane is an organic solvent that has been used in paints, lacquers, and glues, and in the printing and rubber industries. Exposure to it has occurred in various occupational settings and following inhalation of certain glues for recreational purposes. Oxidative metabolism of n-hexane occurs in the liver, forming 2,5-hexanedione,

the purported neurotoxic component. The most conspicuous feature is a peripheral neuropathy, discussed on page 822, but evoked potential studies have also revealed central effects of exposure to it. Chang performed multimodality evoked potential studies in 22 patients with polyneuropathy, 5 with subclinical polyneuropathy, and 7 unaffected workers.[8] Pattern-evoked visual evoked potentials (VEPs) were prolonged in the patients with clinical or subclinical polyneuropathy when compared with normal control subjects, and the VEPs were somewhat attenuated in amplitude in the group with clinically evident neuropathy. Others have also noted reversible changes in the latency of VEPs.[9] Their occurrence supports an organic basis for the visual symptoms that may follow n-hexane exposure, but whether they relate to cerebral involvement or pathology of the optic nerve or macula is unclear. Brainstem auditory evoked potentials (BAEPs) showed a prolongation in the I–V interpeak latency that corresponded to the severity of the polyneuropathy, whereas somatosensory evoked potentials (SEPs) showed prolonged absolute latencies and central conduction time in patients with clinical or subclinical polyneuropathy.[8] The BAEP abnormalities support a central (brainstem) effect of the toxin exposure, but in the presence of peripheral pathology it is hard to determine the significance of the SEP findings reported by Chang.[8] SEP abnormalities have not always been found in patients with toxic polyneuropathy who were exposed to a variety of industrial toxins, including n-hexane. Nevertheless, evoked potential studies have revealed clearly that the neurologic disorder following n-hexane exposure may involve the central as well as the peripheral nervous system.

TOLUENE

Toluene is used widely for industrial purposes both as a solvent in paints and glues and to synthesize certain compounds (e.g., benzene). Exposure occurs especially among painters and linoleum layers and in the printing industry. Toluene inhalation for recreational purposes is also problematic.

Hormes and colleagues reported residual damage in 20 chronic solvent vapor abusers when evaluated at least 4 weeks after total abstinence from intoxicants.[10] Exposure had been primarily to toluene for 2 or more years. In 13 of the 20 patients, neurologic abnormalities included cognitive, pyramidal, cerebellar, and cranial nerve findings. The pattern of cognitive dysfunction suggested a subcortical dementia, with apathy, poor concentration, impaired memory, visuospatial dysfunction, and impaired complex cognition. The EEG was recorded in 7 neurologically impaired patients, and 3 had an excess of slow activity that was diffuse and continuous in one instance and intermittent in two. BAEPs were abnormal in 3 of 4 patients, with prolongation of the I–III interpeak latencies or abnormalities of waves III, IV, and V bilaterally. In one patient no other evidence of brainstem involvement was noted. In a subsequent study, Rosenberg and co-workers defined the BAEP findings in 11 chronic toluene abusers.[11] In 5, the BAEPs were abnormal, and analysis of the group showed a prolongation of the absolute latency of wave V and the I–V and III–V interpeak latencies when compared with control subjects. Two of the 5 patients with abnormal BAEPs had normal findings on neurologic examination and magnetic resonance imaging (MRI). These findings and other reports of BAEP abnormalities in toluene abusers[12] suggest a possible role for the BAEP in the early detection of central nervous system injury from toluene inhalation when clinical MRI findings are normal.

CARBON DISULFIDE

Carbon disulfide has been used as a soil fumigant in various industrial and manufacturing processes, as a constituent of certain insecticides and varnishes, and as a solvent for various chemicals. Acute exposure to high concentrations may lead to an encephalopathy with marked behavioral disturbances, whereas lower levels of exposure may lead to a mild encephalopathic disturbance that is revealed only by neurologic testing. The EEG has been used to evaluate exposed workers and reportedly has shown abnormalities more commonly in such workers than in healthy control subjects, but the findings are not consistent and their nonspecific nature suggests that the EEG has little practical utility as a screening technique. Thus, a study of 10 patients showed that none had abnormal EEGs,[13] another study revealed that the EEG findings were inconsistent but mostly normal,[14] and a third study showed frequency changes of dubious relevance.[15] Carbon disulfide may also lead to optic neuropathy as well as a clinical or subclinical polyneuropathy that is similar to that produced by *n*-hexane (see p. 822). Whether VEP studies have any role in monitoring for the development of optic neuropathy is uncertain.

CARBON MONOXIDE

Exposure to carbon monoxide may lead to cerebral hypoxia with neurologic sequelae. Such cases may result from industrial exposure, especially in miners or gas workers. The effect of acute exposure depends on the severity of intoxication, but cognitive or behavioral disturbances may occur, and focal neurologic deficits may also be evident. Generalized or lateralized EEG abnormalities have been described. After hyperbaric oxygen therapy, improvement of occipital alpha activity on quantitative EEG analysis (increased peak alpha frequency and relative alpha power) has suggested that monitoring of peak alpha frequency may be a useful indicator of therapeutic efficacy,[16] but this requires substantiation. Whether chronic low-level exposure to carbon monoxide leads to an encephalopathy is uncertain, and electrophysiologic techniques have not been helpful as a means of detecting such an encephalopathy at a subclinical stage.

ORGANOPHOSPHATES

Organophosphate compounds are used as pesticides and herbicides. Acute toxicity relates to anticholinesterase activity and is characterized by both central and peripheral manifestations. The central effects include behavioral disturbances, seizures, and eventually coma or death. Visual inspection of the EEG does not permit central neurotoxicity to be recognized in individual subjects. Quantitative analysis of the EEG recorded 1 year or more after exposure has revealed statistically significant group differences when compared with normal subjects, and similar changes are seen after acute exposure; however, their significance is uncertain. Cognitive processing may be delayed[17] and abnormalities of endogenous potentials have been described after chronic exposure to organophosphate pesticides,[18] but the significance of such findings is uncertain. Organophosphates may affect neuromuscular transmission (p. 827). Certain organophosphates also lead to the development of a delayed polyneuropathy about 2 to 3 weeks after acute exposure (see page 821).

METHYLMERCURY

A well-recognized syndrome follows poisoning with organic mercury compounds. Numbness and paresthesias occur initially, followed by constriction of the visual fields, blindness, hearing loss, pyramidal deficits, and dyskinesias. Electrophysiologic studies have shown VEP abnormalities in monkeys and dogs, which is in keeping with a central origin of the visual disturbance and with reports of pathologic changes in the visual cortex. The VEP changes may involve morphology, which is difficult to quantify, and amplitude, which is variable even in normal subjects. Median-derived SEPs show loss of the cortically generated N20 response that presumably relates to pathology in the somatosensory cortex. Thus, electrophysiologic findings indicate that neurologic disturbances have a central rather than peripheral origin in patients with methylmercury poisoning. Studies of preschool Inuit children suggest that VEPs can be used to assess the developmental neurotoxicity of methylmercury and other contaminants in fish-eating populations.[19] However, subtle changes, possibly due to low-level methylmercury exposure, are of uncertain clinical relevance and must be interpreted cautiously.[20]

STYRENE

Styrene is a colorless, volatile organic solvent that has been associated with behavioral effects, as well as with a possible peripheral neuropathy.[21,22] It has widespread application in the plastics industry, particularly in the polyester resin boat industry. Styrene is absorbed readily following inhalation.[23] Numerous studies published over the years have suggested that an encephalopathy may result from styrene exposure. A critical review of the literature by Rebert and Hall provided no indication of persisting neurologic damage following styrene exposure.[24] Much of the literature was flawed methodologically, and conclusions from it therefore were invalid.

Electrophysiologic studies have not been used widely in the evaluation of patients with suspected neurobehavioral disorders attributed to styrene exposure. Even when the EEG has been used, the changes have varied markedly between subjects and have not been consistent. Problems referred to earlier with regard to the EEG as a means of evaluating behavioral disorders are particularly apparent in the literature concerning the potential neurotoxicity of styrene. Matikainen and associates did undertake a quantitative evaluation of the EEG in patients from several plastics factories.[25] They attempted to minimize the effects of drowsiness by recording the EEG in the morning and discarding EEG epochs obtained during periods of obvious drowsiness, but it is not clear how drowsiness was assessed. Various quantitative abnormalities were identified but, as pointed out by Rebert and Hall,[24] these authors made some 798 comparisons, so by chance alone about 40 significant results would be expected with a significance criterion of 0.05. When several redundant parameters were eliminated and the channel count was restricted, the number of comparisons was reduced to 192, from which 10 significant findings would still be expected by chance alone. In fact, the number of significant comparisons was markedly less than expected by chance, and the biologic meaning of the finding is unclear because of the absence of an adequate control group. Neurometric discriminant analysis was used for classifying subjects in terms of EEG abnormalities, but the reference normative data were not an appropriate standard. Finally, even if abnormalities had been detected in this study of apparently healthy workers, there is no justification in concluding that the EEG changes reflect subclinical dysfunction related to neurotoxic exposure.

CHRONIC PAINTERS' ENCEPHALOPATHY

Gade and colleagues reanalyzed the psychologic test data in a group of subjects who were reported to have chronic painters' syndrome and compared the findings with those of matched controls.[26] They could not confirm previous impressions of significant intellectual impairment in the solvent-exposed subjects when the influence of age, education, and intelligence was taken into account. This study is of particular note because it was performed in the same department as the original studies that identified this syndrome. The use of electrophysiologic tests (often subjected to sophisticated quantitative analysis) to validate the existence of a syndrome that, on clinical grounds, is now questionable[26,27] seems difficult to justify. The relevance and validity of any electrophysiologic abnormalities detected are uncertain.

NEUROTOXIC DISORDERS OF THE PERIPHERAL NERVOUS SYSTEM

Patients with suspected neurotoxic disorders are often referred for neurophysiologic examination, which plays an important role in their evaluation. This role includes documenting the organic nature of a suspected disorder; classifying the abnormalities in a way that reduces the number of possible diagnoses in the differential diagnosis; and, occasionally, identifying the underlying pathophysiology. More recently, electrophysiologic studies have had application as screening instruments in clinical pharmaceutical and occupational or environmental studies. These applications include use as endpoint measures (as in a pharmaceutical trial) and to identify unsuspected adverse neurotoxicity. Because iatrogenic toxic neuropathies are common, this latter role is increasingly important.

Electrophysiologic tests have limitations, and their indiscriminate use in the evaluation of occupational or environmental disorders is inconsistent with their intended application. Few, if any, neurotoxic disorders are associated with electrophysiologic features that are so characteristic as to be diagnostic. In most instances, electrophysiologic abnormalities are nonspecific and of limited use in establishing the cause of neurologic impairment. Although toxic neuropathies are common, they probably are overdiagnosed, so that idiopathic neuropathies sometimes are attributed erroneously to toxic-metabolic causes. Toxic neuropathies are important to recognize, however, because improvement may occur once exposure is reduced or eliminated. With regard to cross-sectional group evaluations of persons with suspected neurotoxic disorders, electrophysiologic measures purporting to identify subclinical abnormalities must be interpreted cautiously because of numerous potential confounders that influence such data.

The role of electrophysiologic studies relates to their sensitivity in identifying abnormalities, sometimes in the absence of clinical symptoms or signs, and the ability to localize abnormalities to a specific level of the nervous system. The application and limitations of conventional electrophysiologic studies in the evaluation of suspected neurotoxic disorders are relatively well established, especially with regard to individual patient evaluations. Because the most common peripheral nervous system toxins produce neuropathy, this discussion will emphasize those disorders.

Clinical Examination

The electrodiagnostic examination is never performed in isolation but is designed in the context of the patient's complaints and clinical abnormalities. The nature of peripheral abnormalities simplifies the physician's task in terms of establishing the presence of neuropathy. Unfortunately, most neurotoxic disorders have no specific features to distinguish them from neurologic disorders arising from other causes. Importantly, the neuroanatomic diagnoses of neuropathy, myopathy, or defective neuromuscular transmission are established independently from an etiologic diagnosis. Most peripheral neurotoxic disorders are symmetric, however, and only rare exceptions to this rule exist. Occasionally, identification of some cardinal abnormality will be the first clue in identifying a specific toxic disorder, although recognition usually stems from a high level of suspicion. More commonly, a systematic neurologic examination focuses the subsequent electrodiagnostic and other laboratory evaluations. Clinical symptoms and signs are used to identify the presence of a peripheral disorder and to formulate a differential diagnosis. The differential diagnosis is used to select among the variety of clinical and laboratory tests available to confirm the presence of peripheral dysfunction and refine the diagnosis, as discussed in the following sections.

Electrodiagnostic Evaluation

Most electromyographers consider nerve conduction studies and needle electromyography (EMG) as extensions of the neurologic examination. These studies can be repeated at intervals to confirm previous findings and to document progression or improvement. The most important role of electrodiagnostic testing is to localize abnormality to specific levels of the peripheral nervous system. A secondary role includes identification of the most likely pathophysiology to produce a more manageable differential diagnosis that may include a toxic etiology after competing causes have been eliminated.

Standardized techniques should be used when performing nerve conduction studies to evaluate the nervous system, as discussed in Chapter 13. Normal values depend on numerous factors including technique, patient age and size, temperature, and even occupation. A major source of variability is limb temperature; cooling decreases the rate at which ionic channels open, thereby producing an increased response amplitude and decreased conduction velocity. To reduce the effect of temperature, standard practice requires monitoring of limb temperatures and warming to approximately 32° to 36°C, if necessary.

Sensory nerve action potentials and compound muscle action potentials are recorded in response to percutaneous electrical stimulation of peripheral nerves with surface electrodes. Measurement of response amplitude is very important because it reflects in part the number and size of functioning nerve or muscle fibers. Any disorder causing a substantial loss of axons or muscle fibers (e.g., a toxic neuropathy or myopathy) produces a response of reduced amplitude. Conventional recordings of nerve conduction velocity measure conduction in the fastest conducting fibers. Distal latency reflects conduction along the terminal portion of the nerve. In contrast, F-wave latency (see Chapter 18) reflects transmission time from the stimulation site to the spinal cord and then back along the entire nerve to the recording site. The long distance along the entire nerve accentuates minor conduction abnormalities. Blink reflex studies (see Chapter 19) record involuntary reflexes that occur in response to stimulation of the trigeminal nerve. These reflexes involve peripheral and brainstem connections, and they have occasional application in the evaluation of neurotoxic disorders.

Sensory conduction studies primarily evaluate the large myelinated sensory axons. One means of assessing smaller axons involves evaluation of the autonomic nervous system (see Chapter 21). Skin potential or sympathetic skin responses are mediated by small nerve fibers and represent a measure of autonomic function. They are recorded from the skin, between areas of high and low sweat gland density. They occur spontaneously or in response to a variety of stimuli, including electrical stimulation or startle. They have limited sensitivity and specificity, but intact responses argue against a significant abnormality of autonomic sudomotor function.

The method most commonly used to evaluate neuromuscular transmission is repetitive motor nerve stimulation (see Chapter 17). Impaired neuromuscular transmission is identified by a decrement in the amplitude of compound muscle action potentials with repeated percutaneous nerve stimulation. Low-rate stimulation of motor nerves challenges neuromuscular transmission by taking advantage of the normal decrease in the availability of acetylcholine immediately after discharge, before replenishment by mobilization. The primary role of these studies in neurotoxic disorders is to identify impaired neuromuscular transmission in acute organophosphorus poisoning, botulinum intoxication, and penicillamine-induced myasthenia gravis. Single-fiber EMG (see Chapter 17) is the most sensitive measure of neuromuscular transmission, but it has limited application in the evaluation of neurotoxic disorders.

The conventional needle examination (see Chapter 11) is a sensitive indicator of partial denervation or muscle fiber necrosis. It is an important component of the electrodiagnostic examination but has a secondary role in the evaluation of neurotoxic disorders when compared with nerve conduction studies. An exception is in the evaluation of toxic myopathy, although the abnormalities are nonspecific. Separation of a muscle fiber from its nerve supply, regardless of cause, results within weeks in the appearance of abnormal insertion activity characterized by positive waves and fibrillation potentials. These spontaneous discharges represent involuntary muscle fiber action potentials associated with denervation hypersensitivity caused by proliferation of acetylcholine receptors on the muscle fiber surface. They are recognized easily, are not confused easily with other EMG signals, and are not present in normal muscle.

Application of Electrodiagnostic Studies in Peripheral Neurotoxic Disorders

Electrodiagnostic examination is important in the following:

1. Identifying polyneuropathy, mononeuropathy multiplex, or polyradiculopathy
2. Recognizing selective involvement of sensory or motor fibers

3. Revealing substantial conduction slowing (suggesting a disturbance of myelin or membrane) or amplitude loss (axon degeneration)
4. Detecting impaired neuromuscular transmission
5. Indicating isolated muscle fiber involvement.

The findings do not address whether a specific toxin is responsible for the findings, but instead begin by localizing any abnormality to a focal, multifocal, or diffuse distribution. In the case of a diffuse polyneuropathy, the presence of predominant sensory or motor involvement is established, followed by determination of whether the abnormalities are characterized by substantial conduction slowing or simply by loss of response amplitude. Electrodiagnostic test results are used to classify peripheral disorders. This classification is easy to apply and reduces, to an extent not clinically possible, the number of disorders that must be considered in the differential diagnosis. Neurotoxic disorders may present with very different electrophysiologic features, however, depending on their severity and the time of testing in relation to the clinical course.

An important part of the classification system involves a determination of whether motor nerve conduction velocity is decreased to an extent greater than can be caused by axonal loss alone. This determination is often difficult, and existing criteria for conduction slowing are relatively insensitive.[28] Most criteria represent attempts to identify a surrogate electrophysiologic measure for segmental demyelination. Unfortunately, other pathologies (e.g., axonal inclusions, axonal stenosis, channelopathies, and selective loss of large myelinated motor fibers) produce substantial slowing. In the classification scheme, conduction slowing is used in a general sense to include any slowing unlikely to result from axon-loss lesions alone, regardless of cause. In this context, conduction velocities less than 80 percent of the lower limit of normal or distal and F-wave latencies exceeding 125 percent of the upper limit of normal usually fulfill this requirement. Before any problem can be attributed to a toxic neuropathy, hereditary disorders causing conduction slowing must be excluded. Partial conduction block and abnormally increased temporal dispersion are important features of acquired neuropathies. Their absence suggests uniform involvement of all fibers and supports a hereditary etiology.

Establishing the cause of any disorder is difficult, and many common diseases of the peripheral nervous system are of unknown etiology. Nevertheless, diagnosing a toxic neuropathy implies that the etiology has been established. Clinical medicine is based on the scientific method of hypothesis generation and testing, and most clinicians apply general scientific principles in the formulation of a differential diagnosis without giving thought to the process. Formal criteria exist, however, for establishing the cause of a problem. In the appropriate clinical setting, laboratory tests are useful in establishing an increased body burden of a potential neurotoxin or in identifying characteristic pathologic features of toxic exposure. However, in general, the electrodiagnostic examination represents the most important clinical measure in identifying a toxic neuropathy. Among the criteria useful in establishing a toxic etiology, electrodiagnostic studies have their most important role in establishing the presence of abnormality and in identifying competing explanations.

Certain pathophysiologic changes are relevant to the clinical electrodiagnosis of neuropathy. The most important changes include axonal degeneration, axonal atrophy, demyelination, and metabolic changes that alter nerve conduction. Examples follow with disorders separated into broad categories based on electrodiagnostic evidence of sensory or motor involvement combined with evidence of axonal loss or definite conduction slowing.

PREDOMINANTLY MOTOR AXONAL NEUROPATHIES

Predominantly motor neuropathies are uncommon, and identification of such disorders suggests a relatively limited differential diagnosis. Many neuropathies in this category have toxic causes, often involving medications.

Dapsone

Dapsone produces a neuropathy characterized by weakness and muscle wasting that often involves the arms more than the legs. It is one of several toxins associated with motor or predominantly motor involvement and is characterized by axonal loss without conduction slowing.[29] Mild sensory abnormalities may also be present. The neuropathy usually develops after prolonged (years-long) use. Dapsone is metabolized by acetylation in the liver, and neuropathy may be related to abnormal metabolism in slow acetylators. Dapsone motor neuropathy occasionally resembles multifocal motor neuropathy or mononeuropathy multiplex. Electrodiagnostic testing demonstrates normal sensory nerve conduction studies; motor responses may be asymmetric and characterized by borderline-low or reduced amplitudes in multiple locations but without conduction block. On needle EMG examination, fibrillation potentials and large-amplitude,

long-duration, polyphasic motor unit potentials are present in the upper and lower extremities in an asymmetric distribution involving the distal muscles of different peripheral nerve and root innervation. This asymmetry is not characteristic of most toxic neuropathies and may suggest a diagnosis of motor neuron disease. A slow but progressive improvement in motor function occurs after discontinuing dapsone use. Most patients recover in 1 to 3 years.

Nitrofurantoin

The primary toxicity of nitrofurantoin is neuropathy, but this sequela is rare.[30] Initial sensory involvement with paresthesias and sometimes pain is followed by the rapid onset of severe weakness, especially in elderly women with impaired renal function and presumably high nitrofurantoin blood levels. The neuropathy is a mixed sensorimotor polyneuropathy. The disorder may progress to respiratory failure and superficially resembles acute Guillain–Barré syndrome. When nitrofurantoin use is discontinued, most patients improve or recover, although recovery may be incomplete. In its most severe form, the neuropathy involves motor more than sensory fibers; it is characterized by a markedly reduced response amplitude but no conduction slowing, a finding that cannot be explained by isolated loss of myelinated nerve fibers.

Organophosphates

Organophosphates (see p. 817) produce a slowly reversible inactivation of acetylcholinesterase and accumulation of acetylcholine in cholinergic neurons.[31,32] Muscarinic overactivity results in miosis, increased secretions, profuse sweating, gastric hyperactivity, and bradycardia. Nicotinic overactivity results in fasciculations and weakness. If not fatal, the acute effects resolve, but some organophosphates produce a rapidly progressive neuropathy 2 to 4 weeks after acute exposure. Organophosphate-induced delayed neuropathy is manifested by dysesthesias and progressive weakness, especially distally. Reflexes are reduced at the ankles, but they may be normal or brisk elsewhere. Recovery is often incomplete, and spasticity later becomes a prominent feature. Clinically evident or subclinical neuropathy does not appear to result from exposures to organophosphate insecticides at levels that do not produce cholinergic toxicity.[33,34] During acute organophosphate intoxication, repetitive compound muscle action potentials occur after a single stimulus, presumably from recurrent postsynaptic depolarization by persistent acetylcholine.[35] Other electrodiagnostic findings are consistent with axonal degeneration of motor and, to a lesser extent, sensory fibers. Conduction velocity remains essentially normal, but amplitudes of compound muscle and sensory nerve action potentials are reduced and there is needle EMG evidence of severe denervation characterized by diffuse fibrillation potentials.

Vincristine

Vincristine usually produces an axonal sensorimotor neuropathy with sensory involvement exceeding motor involvement. However, a form of rapidly progressive weakness is associated with vincristine and can result in functional quadriplegia with little associated increase in sensory involvement. In some patients, the arms initially may be involved more than the legs, and the disorder resembles a pure motor neuropathy or neuronopathy. The electrodiagnostic findings then are those of an axonal neuropathy in which motor nerve abnormalities predominate, with evidence of severe neurogenic changes on needle EMG.

PREDOMINANTLY MOTOR NEUROPATHIES WITH CONDUCTION SLOWING

Amiodarone

Amiodarone is associated with a slowly progressive motor neuropathy with prominent conduction slowing, often in the range of 20 to 30 m/sec. Abnormal temporal dispersion and partial conduction block are not features of this neuropathy, and the conduction slowing is related to preferential loss of the largest myelinated fibers. The motor abnormalities are associated with low-amplitude sensory responses when the neuropathy is severe.

Arsenic

Acute arsenical neuropathy is one component of a systemic illness characterized by nausea, vomiting, diarrhea, pancytopenia with basophilic stippling, and abnormal liver function tests reflecting hepatic damage. Features of chronic toxicity include dermatitis (hyperkeratosis, pigmented dermatitis), cardiomyopathy, portal hypertension with esophageal varices, and splenomegaly.[36] Nerve conduction studies performed shortly after acute exposure may be suggestive of Guillain–Barré syndrome with reduced conduction velocity, increased temporal dispersion, partial conduction block, and low-amplitude or absent sensory responses.[37,38] Serial studies suggest a dying-back neuropathy with progressive axonal degeneration. The initial findings are probably secondary and appear before generalized axonal failure. Mees lines appear on the nails about 1 month after exposure. (See page 824 for additional findings of chronic arsenic intoxication.)

Disulfiram

Disulfiram (Antabuse) is metabolized to acetaldehyde when combined with alcohol, which forms the rationale for promoting alcohol abstinence. Disulfiram is associated with a progressive, predominantly motor neuropathy. The onset of weakness is sometimes abrupt and mimics Guillain–Barré syndrome. The electrodiagnostic findings may be indistinguishable from those of the axonal form of Guillain–Barré syndrome or may show substantial motor conduction slowing in association with axonal degeneration with paranodal and internodal swellings due to accumulation of neurofilaments, similar to the abnormalities attributed to *n*-hexane neuropathy (see below).[39,40]

n-Hexane

Excessive exposure to *n*-hexane produces a dying-back neuropathy characterized by distal weakness, stocking-glove sensory loss, and absent ankle reflexes.[41] In most reports, motor signs predominate, but this feature is not invariable. Clinical progression for several weeks after cessation of exposure is typical of many toxic neuropathies and is called "coasting." Nerve conduction studies reveal reduced sensory and motor response amplitudes and conduction velocities, sometimes to 35 or 40 percent of the lower limit of normal. The conduction slowing is often associated with partial conduction block and is typically sufficient to suggest acquired demyelination.[41–43] These findings are atypical of toxic neuropathy but are consistent with acute Guillain–Barré syndrome. Laboratory support for a diagnosis of Guillain–Barré syndrome also includes a slightly elevated cerebrospinal fluid protein concentration early in the course of illness. It is now established that the reduced conduction velocity and partial conduction block are explained by secondary myelin changes caused in part by axonal swelling in peripheral and central nerve fibers. Sural nerve biopsy demonstrates multifocal axonal distension with paranodal swelling and neurofilamentous masses. The axonal swellings consist of neurofilament aggregates, which may accumulate because of abnormalities in fast and slow axonal transport mechanisms. Improvement follows removal from exposure, although conduction slowing may persist in severely involved patients.

Tetrodotoxin and Saxitoxin

Neurotoxins that block sodium channels include tetrodotoxin derived from the puffer fish and saxitoxin derived from contaminated shellfish (red tide).[44] These natural toxins are of interest because they produce a neuropathy characterized by conduction slowing, a finding typically associated with demyelinating neuropathies. The sodium channel blockade produced by these neurotoxins decreases the local currents associated with action potential propagation, thereby slowing conduction velocity, an effect similar to that seen with reduced temperature. Amplitudes of compound muscle action potentials are reduced, but no abnormal temporal dispersion or partial conduction block is present.

SENSORY AXONAL NEUROPATHIES

Sensory involvement is common in mixed sensorimotor polyneuropathy, but exclusive and severe sensory involvement is unusual. Axonal sensory neuropathies or neuronopathies include those associated with pyridoxine, cisplatin, small-cell lung cancer, Sjögren's syndrome, the Miller Fisher variant of Guillain–Barré syndrome, and Friedreich ataxia. All present subacutely with unpleasant paresthesias and evidence of reduced vibration and joint position sensation, areflexia, and minimally decreased pain sensation; weakness is not observed. Electrodiagnostic findings include markedly reduced or absent sensory nerve action potentials with normal motor conduction studies. Sequential studies demonstrate a progressive decline in the amplitude of sensory nerve action potentials. There is no needle EMG evidence of denervation. It is difficult, if not impossible, to distinguish a sensory neuropathy from a neuronopathy, although a length-dependent process suggests the former.

Cisplatin

Cisplatin is an antineoplastic agent. Its major dose-limiting toxicity relates to the central and peripheral nervous systems, with preferential uptake in the posterior root ganglia producing a profound sensory neuropathy or neuronopathy. Toxicity is dose-related, but most patients completing a full course of cisplatin chemotherapy develop a clinically detectable sensory neuropathy.[45] Sensory symptoms and signs usually develop several weeks to months after administration. Absent reflexes are an early finding. Occasional patients report distal weakness, but this "weakness" probably reflects impaired proprioception, not true weakness. Cisplatin neuronopathy is indistinguishable from the paraneoplastic sensory neuronopathy associated with small-cell lung cancer and anti-Hu antibodies. Sequential studies of patients receiving cisplatin chemotherapy demonstrate a progressive reduction in the amplitude of sensory nerve action potentials with no clear abnormality in motor nerve conduction studies and no needle EMG evidence of denervation. Neuroprotective therapies have been sought to limit the neurotoxicity of cisplatin and related antineoplastic agents, and nerve conduction studies have been used to evaluate their efficacy.[45,46]

Pyridoxine

Pyridoxine is a vitamin (vitamin B_6) that occasionally is taken in "megadoses" by health faddists to treat a variety of nonspecific syndromes. It also is used to treat poisoning or exposure to several toxins, including the false morel *Gyromitra esculenta*. Like cisplatin, it has been associated with a profound sensory neuropathy.[47,48] Neurologic toxicity either is related to long-term cumulative exposure or occurs after short-term administration of large doses. With particularly large exposures, sensory loss may be virtually complete, including facial and mucous membrane areas, and produces ataxia and choreoathetoid movements. Such profound loss is consistent with a sensory neuronopathy. Apparent weakness may relate to impaired proprioception. Pyridoxine-induced sensory neuronopathy is indistinguishable from paraneoplastic sensory neuronopathy. Sequential electrophysiologic studies demonstrate progressive attenuation of sensory nerve action potentials with no clear abnormality in motor conduction and no needle EMG evidence of partial denervation.

Styrene

Workers with chronic styrene exposure may develop paresthesias in the fingers and toes without clear neurologic abnormalities, but electrodiagnostic evaluation reveals mild findings consistent with a sensory neuropathy. Mild sensory nerve conduction deficits were reported in 23 percent of workers exposed to less than 50 ppm styrene and in 71 percent of workers exposed to more than 100 ppm, but no conduction slowing was found in a small group of 5 men exposed to more than 100 ppm for less than 4 weeks.[22] These results of styrene-induced neurotoxicity have not been confirmed in animal models, and failure to identify a clear dose–response relationship in human subjects reduces the clinical significance of the reported work, although a possible peripheral neurotoxic effect cannot be excluded.

Thalidomide

Thalidomide is associated with a predominantly sensory, axonal, length-dependent neuropathy that presents typically with painful paresthesias or numbness. Electrodiagnostic studies may show reduced sensory nerve action potentials[49]; sural nerve biopsies may show evidence of Wallerian degeneration and loss of myelinated fibers.[50] Reports of proximal weakness being greater than distal weakness suggest anterior horn cell degeneration.

Thallium

Thallium intoxication is associated with a small-fiber neuropathy and alopecia. Clinical symptoms include a severe, painful, distal sensory neuropathy associated with evidence of dysautonomia including abdominal pain, constipation, and nausea.[51] Distal weakness may be present, but weakness is a minor complaint in comparison to the severe painful distal dysesthesias. Pin-pain sensation is the most markedly impaired, and muscle stretch reflexes may remain normal.

Sensorimotor Axonal Polyneuropathy

Distal axonopathy is the most common finding in a variety of toxic or metabolic disorders. Presumably, failure of axonal transport of some nutrient required for maintenance of the distal axon occurs in response to the metabolic abnormality. Axonal atrophy may precede axonal degeneration. Conduction velocity is proportional to axonal diameter and is reduced along the atrophic axon. Most toxic or metabolic neuropathies demonstrate axonal degeneration (dying back) of sensory and motor axons. Unfortunately, they are difficult to distinguish from each other electrodiagnostically. Sensory symptoms and signs initially predominate and include dysesthesias, paresthesias, distal sensory loss, and loss of Achilles' reflexes. Weakness and atrophy of the distal muscles develop, followed by more proximal involvement as a late finding. Amplitudes of sensory nerve action potentials are typically abnormal, even early in the course of disease. Compound muscle action potentials subsequently become attenuated, particularly in the legs. Conduction velocity, distal latency, and F-wave latency remain normal until the loss of large myelinated fibers is substantial. Distal latency may be abnormal with normal proximal conduction, a reflection of axonal atrophy. Fibrillation potentials and positive waves appear in distal extremity muscles before clinical evidence of weakness. Motor unit recruitment is reduced, and motor unit action potentials are increased in amplitude and duration.

Axonal sensorimotor neuropathies are the most common forms of toxic neuropathy. A description of all potential neurotoxicants producing this type of neuropathy is beyond the scope of this section. However, in addition to the chemicals described in the following sections, other substances that may produce a neuropathy characterized by sensory or sensorimotor involvement without conduction slowing include acrylamide, amitriptyline, carbon monoxide, ethambutol, ethylene oxide, elemental mercury, gold, hydralazine, isoniazid, lithium, metronidazole, nitrous oxide (myeloneuropathy), perhexiline, phenytoin, thallium, and zinc (myeloneuropathy).

Arsenic

Acute arsenical neuropathy was discussed on page 822. Once developed, chronic arsenical neuropathy is characterized by sensorimotor neuropathy of the axonal type.[37]

Colchicine

Colchicine is associated with mild axonal neuropathy among patients who are receiving it for gout prophylaxis. Associated weakness has been attributed to an underlying myopathy, and the combined abnormality has been referred to as a myopathy–neuropathy syndrome.[52,53]

Ethyl alcohol

Ethyl alcohol is associated with several neurologic disorders related to the direct neurotoxic effects of alcohol or its metabolites, to nutritional deficiency, to genetic factors, or to some combinations of these factors.[54] Clinically similar neuropathies occur in vitamin-deficient states, including thiamine and other B vitamins. However, a typical alcohol neuropathy may occur with normal nutrition, perhaps in association with impaired axonal transport.[55] The incidence of neuropathy in alcoholic patients is high, usually consisting of a nonspecific sensorimotor neuropathy, although some patients present with subacute-onset sensory neuropathy. Paresthesias and painful distal dysesthesias are early symptoms and are followed by distal sensory loss; distal weakness; and gait ataxia, often accompanied by dysautonomia. Tendon reflexes are absent or hypoactive. Nerve conduction studies and needle EMG are characteristic of an axonal neuropathy.

Vincristine

The major dose-limiting toxicity of vincristine, an antineoplastic alkaloid, is neuropathy, the onset and severity of which are dose-dependent. Initial symptoms appear within weeks of a single dose and include distal paresthesias, absent ankle reflexes, superficial sensory loss, and diminished vibration sensation.[56] Minimal distal weakness, particularly of toe extensor and hand intrinsic muscles, may be apparent. With increasing severity, dysautonomia characterized by constipation, abdominal pain, ileus, impotence, and orthostatic hypotension may become evident. Treatment with vincristine and other potentially neurotoxic medications at dosages considered "nontoxic" can produce significant worsening of a pre-existing neuropathy.[57] Electrophysiologic findings in mild neuropathy are consistent with a predominantly sensory axonal polyneuropathy. Amplitudes of sensory nerve action potentials and compound muscle action potentials are reduced, but conduction velocities are essentially normal or reduced only slightly, consistent with the loss of large myelinated fibers. An early finding is persistent H waves when ankle reflexes are absent. This paradox relates to early involvement of muscle spindles that interrupt the muscle stretch reflex arc. H-reflex studies depolarize large myelinated fibers directly, independent of muscle spindles. Partial denervation can be seen on needle EMG examination, particularly in distal limb muscles.

POLYRADICULONEUROPATHY WITH CONDUCTION SLOWING

Aerosolized Porcine Neural Tissue

Exposure to aerosolized porcine brain tissue among slaughterhouse workers has been associated recently with a sensory-predominant polyradiculoneuropathy, sometimes with additional features of a transverse myelitis, meningoencephalitis, or aseptic meningitis.[58] The polyradiculopathy is characterized by painful paresthesias, distal sensory loss and weakness, impaired tendon reflexes, and autonomic dysfunction developing at least 1 month after initial exposure. Cerebrospinal fluid protein concentrations are generally high. Electrophysiologic findings include a reduction in amplitude of sensory responses. The combination of normal motor conduction velocities without conduction block or abnormal temporal dispersion and prolonged F-wave, blink reflex, and motor latencies localizes abnormalities to the most proximal and distal nerve segments where the blood–nerve barrier is most permeable. Prominent MRI abnormalities have confirmed proximal involvement at nerve roots or ganglia, showing ganglia enlargement, T2 hyperintensity, or enhancement in posterior roots and enlarged (mostly anterior) roots in the cauda equina. Sural nerve biopsies reveal mild inflammatory demyelination, axonal degeneration, and perivascular foci of inflammation. No systemic disorder or infectious agent has been identified that could trigger a similar neurologic disease. However, sera from affected and many unaffected workers but not from community controls have a distinctive neural-reactive immunoglobulin (Ig)G that correlates with exposure risk. Among cases, 75 percent had sera showing an IgG specific to myelin basic protein. Although not typical of most neurotoxic conditions, the evidence suggests that this polyradiculoneuropathy has an autoimmune origin and likely is related to occupational exposure to multiple aerosolized porcine brain-tissue antigens. Similar immune-based mechanisms are associated with penicillamine-induced myasthenia gravis and Guillain–Barré syndrome attributed to some vaccinations.

MULTIFOCAL SENSORIMOTOR NEUROPATHY (MONONEUROPATHY MULTIPLEX)

Dapsone

As indicated on page 821, dapsone-associated neuropathy can mimic multiple entrapment neuropathies, although the paucity of sensory abnormality is atypical of a nerve entrapment syndrome. Electrodiagnostic evaluation demonstrates evidence of neurogenic atrophy with chronic denervation and reinnervation. Compound muscle action potentials are reduced in amplitude, but sensory studies are usually normal. Conduction slowing, when present, presumably relates to loss of the largest motor fibers.

L-Tryptophan

Few neurotoxicants produce a clinical picture of mononeuritis multiplex. In fact, it is difficult to propose how a systemic exposure could cause a multifocal, asymmetric mononeuropathy. Nevertheless, the eosinophilia–myalgia syndrome is a multifocal disorder of the peripheral nervous system associated with the ingestion of L-tryptophan. Eosinophilia, skin changes (peau d'orange), arthralgia, myalgia, fatigue, painful paresthesias, sensory loss, and weakness occur. Sensory loss may predominate and is typically asymmetric, but most patients have distal sensory loss and weakness. Reflexes are sometimes absent distally, but they may be preserved depending on the distribution of abnormality. Electrodiagnostic evaluation confirms multifocal involvement (axonal loss) of sensory more than motor fibers and suggests a mononeuropathy multiplex. Sensory responses for some nerves may be markedly abnormal with little accompanying motor response abnormality and no needle EMG evidence of denervation in appropriate muscles.

This sensory-motor dissociation is reminiscent of the abnormalities seen in lepromatous neuropathy, in which individual sensory nerves occasionally are involved in the subcutaneous tissue, whereas deeper motor branches are spared. Sural nerve biopsies demonstrate axonal degeneration with epineural and perivascular mononuclear inflammation.

A dose–response relationship exists, although the greatest neurologic impairment occasionally develops months after discontinuing L-tryptophan use. Epidemiologic investigations have linked the syndrome to L-tryptophan produced by using a strain of *Bacillus amyloliquefaciens* that possibly contained impurities consisting of a novel form of tryptophan that contributed to the toxicity.[59,60] Discontinuation of the process and decreased use of L-tryptophan have resulted in disappearance of the syndrome. The combined evidence suggests that an immune response to the novel amino acid contaminant resulted in an inflammatory vasculopathy, with mononeuritis multiplex being one component of a systemic response, as opposed to a direct neurotoxic effect.

Lead

In children, toxic exposure to lead produces encephalopathy; in adults, exposure produces peripheral abnormalities, although lead neuropathy is among the rarest of neurologic disorders. The neuropathy is described as involving the upper before the lower limbs, with preferential extensor involvement resulting in weakness of wrist and finger extensors that later extends to other muscles.[61] Associated systemic features include a microcytic, hypochromic anemia and basophilic stippling. The distribution may be asymmetric and involves motor more than sensory fibers. These peripheral findings are similar to those of porphyric neuropathy, with multifocal motor involvement suggestive of a neuronopathy with variable amounts of sensory loss. Like porphyria, lead toxicity demonstrates abnormal excretion of heme precursors, delta-aminolevulinic acid, and coproporphyrin, perhaps related to aminolevulinic acid dehydratase inhibition. Lead lines may be apparent on gums or on bone radiographs. Few patients have been studied with modern techniques. Existing studies describe mild slowing of motor and sensory velocity, but in severe cases there is evidence of severe axonal loss.[62,63] Needle EMG shows findings consistent with axonal involvement. Sural nerve biopsy has shown similar axonal loss. The multifocal, asymmetric involvement on EMG is consistent with mononeuropathy multiplex or a diffuse neuronopathy, although sensory studies could be interpreted as consistent with a sensory neuronopathy.

IMPAIRED NEUROMUSCULAR TRANSMISSION

Many drugs are known to exert effects at the neuromuscular junction, aggravating weakness among patients with myasthenia gravis or inducing myasthenic syndromes among "normal" individuals. Nevertheless, the neuromuscular junction is an uncommon target for neurotoxic medications compared with the peripheral nerves or muscles. Botulinum toxin, perhaps the most potent natural neurotoxin, does, however, directly assault the neuromuscular junction. Fortunately, electrophysiologic measures are sensitive indicators of defective neuromuscular transmission.

Botulinum Toxin

Botulinum toxin is a presynaptic neuromuscular junction poison that inhibits acetylcholine release. Food-borne and infantile botulism are the most common forms of botulinum toxicity.[64,65] Of the seven types of botulinum toxin, three (types A, B, and E) produce human disease.[64] Signs of botulinum poisoning include internal and external ophthalmoplegia with skeletal muscle weakness or paralysis involving bulbar, respiratory, and extremity muscles. The irreversible neuromuscular blockade produced by botulinum toxin results in a flaccid paralysis that typically appears about 12 to 72 hours after exposure.[65] Because involved muscle fibers are functionally denervated, recovery is prolonged. Electrophysiologic evaluation is important in identifying evidence of impaired neuromuscular transmission, localizing the impairment to the presynaptic neuromuscular junction, and establishing the magnitude of denervation. Cherington described the most consistent electrophysiologic abnormality as a low-amplitude motor response in a clinically affected muscle.[66] Less consistently, abnormal post-tetanic facilitation is identified in affected muscles. These abnormalities are similar to those of the Lambert–Eaton myasthenic syndrome, but they tend to be more variable in magnitude and distribution than the relatively severe and uniform involvement typically observed in that disorder. Single-fiber EMG shows markedly increased jitter and prominent muscle-fiber action potential blocking, which become less marked following activation.[66] Shortly after onset of weakness, conventional needle EMG shows only decreased recruitment, but serial examinations confirm the presence of severe denervation characterized by profuse fibrillation potentials.

Penicillamine

Penicillamine is associated with a disorder of neuromuscular transmission that is distinguishable from idiopathic myasthenia gravis only by the complete and permanent resolution of all symptoms, signs, and laboratory abnormalities after removal from additional penicillamine exposure. Although many medications interfere with neuromuscular transmission by a pharmacologic effect, penicillamine does so by means of an immunologic assault that involves the production of acetylcholine receptor antibodies. The resultant immune-mediated damage to the neuromuscular junction results in abnormal fatigability of skeletal muscle, involving primarily ocular, bulbar, and proximal limb muscles. Patients with penicillamine-induced myasthenia gravis display varying degrees of diplopia, ptosis, and generalized weakness. Electrophysiologic tests are valuable in documenting defective neuromuscular transmission in the form of a decremental response on repetitive motor nerve stimulation or increased jitter on single-fiber EMG, but the findings are identical to those in idiopathic myasthenia gravis.

Organophosphate Compounds

Gutmann and Besser reported that electrophysiologic studies performed during acute organophosphate intoxication demonstrated repetitive discharges to a single depolarizing stimulus, presumably related to recurrent depolarization of the postsynaptic endplate by persistent acetylcholine.[67] Others showed that increasing neuromuscular blockade was associated with a decline in motor response amplitudes among patients with organophosphate poisoning from attempted suicide.[68] The decremental response associated with acute organophosphate intoxication differs from the abnormalities observed in postsynaptic or presynaptic disorders such as myasthenia gravis or the myasthenic syndrome, showing a decremental response at high rates of stimulation (30 Hz and occasionally at 10 Hz) but not at lower rates of stimulation (3 Hz).[68] During the 24 to 96 hours after acute organophosphate poisoning, occasional patients develop an intermediate syndrome that is characterized by weakness of cranial, respiratory, and proximal limb muscles, a distribution resembling that of myasthenia gravis.[35] Electrodiagnostic studies performed in these patients reportedly have shown evidence of a presynaptic defect,[35] although repetitive motor nerve stimulation at low rates did not produce a decremental response. Many of the observations involving the results of repetitive motor nerve stimulation in organophosphate poisoning are difficult to reconcile with our current understanding of neuromuscular physiology.

MYOPATHY

The muscle fiber is the target of numerous myotoxicants, mainly in the form of medications, as is reviewed in detail elsewhere.[69]

Cholesterol-Lowering Medications

The cholesterol-lowering medications in general and the statin medications (HMG-CoA reductase inhibitors) in particular are among the medications associated most commonly with myopathy. Cholesterol-lowering agent myopathy is a syndrome characterized by muscle pain, weakness, elevated serum creatine kinase levels, and EMG evidence of muscle fiber necrosis confirmed by muscle biopsy.[70] The myopathy may be severe enough to produce fulminant disintegration of skeletal muscle cells, with resultant rhabdomyolysis, myoglobinuria, and acute renal failure. Most patients who develop a statin-induced myopathy have complicated medical problems or are receiving combined therapies with other cholesterol-lowering agents or medications that share common metabolic pathways.[69] The precise underlying mechanisms are unknown, but a relationship between mitochondrial dysfunction and muscle cell degeneration is speculated.

Electrophysiologic abnormalities associated with the disorder are those of any myopathy producing muscle fiber necrosis. The results of the EMG evaluation are important in confirming the presence of myopathy and in identifying the underlying pathophysiology, but they are nonspecific as to the cause of the myopathy. Muscle fiber necrosis of any cause produces a profound abnormality of spontaneous activity, with profuse fibrillation potentials and positive waves. Fibrillation potential and positive waves are most apparent in proximal muscles, reflecting the distribution of clinical involvement. Other features of myopathy (e.g., increased motor unit recruitment and abnormal motor unit potential configuration) may also be encountered but are not specific.

Colchicine

Colchicine is a potential cause of a myopathy–neuropathy syndrome.[71] Colchicine myopathy is associated with an elevated serum creatine kinase level. Rhabdomyolysis may occur with sufficient myoglobinuria to produce acute renal failure, typically in association with multiple risk factors in addition to colchicine.[72] The needle EMG examination in colchicine myopathy is reported to show proximal muscle abnormalities characterized by profuse fibrillation potentials and positive waves, complex repetitive discharges, and "myopathic" motor unit potentials.[73] In muscle biopsies, the presence of a vacuolar myopathy with acid phosphatase-positive vacuoles, myofibrillar disarray foci, and degenerating and regenerating muscle fibers, without evidence of inflammation, vasculitis, or connective tissue disease, has been documented.[74]

The mechanism by which colchicine produces myopathy is thought to involve membrane disruption and segmental necrosis of muscle fibers. The myopathy improves, sometimes dramatically, shortly after discontinuation of the colchicine.[75]

Nondepolarizing Neuromuscular Blockade and Corticosteroids

Critical illness myopathy is characterized by a rapidly evolving quadriparesis with normal sensation. It typically emerges in a critically ill patient in the setting of a systemic inflammatory response syndrome with sepsis; most (but not all) patients who develop critical illness myopathy have received nondepolarizing neuromuscular blocking agents during respiratory support and corticosteroids.[76,77] Serum creatine kinase levels may be elevated or normal.[78] Electrophysiologic studies show low-amplitude motor responses but normal sensory potentials, unless there is a coexisting critical illness neuropathy.[79] Normal neuromuscular transmission studies exclude the possibility of a prolonged neuromuscular blockade caused by nondepolarizing neuromuscular blocking agents. Needle EMG typically demonstrates a full interference pattern with minimal muscle contraction, often in the presence of complete paralysis (electromechanical dissociation). Some patients develop myonecrosis and show profuse fibrillation potentials,[80] whereas others show only loss of muscle excitability, perhaps because of muscle membrane depolarization or alteration in sodium channels.[78] Light microscopy may show few abnormalities, but electron microscopy evidence of myosin-deficient muscle fibers confirms the presence of a critical illness myopathy.[77] The biopsy results differ from the marked atrophy of type 2 muscle fibers associated with a chronic corticosteroid myopathy. The combined electrophysiologic and biopsy abnormalities suggest that critical illness myopathy results from several different pathophysiologic mechanisms.[78] The prognosis for recovery is excellent.[81] The combination of sepsis and concomitant use of high-dose corticosteroids, often with nondepolarizing neuromuscular blocking agents, suggests the myotoxic potential of these events.

CONCLUDING COMMENTS

Despite early optimism, electrophysiologic studies generally have been disappointing as a means of detecting early or subclinical encephalopathies resulting from exposure to neurotoxins. Routine EEG is generally too nonspecific for this purpose. Quantitative EEG analysis may be rewarding, but its utility in this context remains to be established. Evoked potential studies sometimes may be helpful in revealing involvement of central afferent pathways or in suggesting the basis of symptoms of uncertain origin.

By contrast, electrophysiologic evaluation is important in establishing the presence and etiology of peripheral neuropathy and permits toxic neuropathies to be identified. The patient's history and clinical findings provide important clues in establishing the diagnosis or in suggesting studies important in identifying the cause. Knowledge of potential exposure (e.g., occupational, social, or pharmacologic) may suggest the cause of a patient's neuropathy. Electrophysiologic classification of the neuropathy focuses the differential diagnosis and the subsequent evaluation and often suggests a specific diagnosis. Although many toxic neuropathies exhibit nonspecific axonal loss, several have distinguishing electrical features that help establish the diagnosis. Establishing a toxic etiology is difficult and depends on the temporal relationship between exposure and clinical disturbance and the use of available epidemiologic information.

REFERENCES

1. Mastaglia FL: Iatrogenic (drug-induced) disorders of the nervous system. p. 695. In Aminoff MJ (ed): Neurology and General Medicine. 4th Ed. Elsevier Churchill Livingstone, New York, 2008
2. Ricaurte GA, Langston JW, McCann UD: Neuropsychiatric complications of substance abuse. p. 735. In Aminoff MJ (ed): Neurology and General Medicine. 4th Ed. Elsevier Churchill Livingstone, New York, 2008
3. Errebo-Knudsen EO, Olsen F: Organic solvents and presenile dementia (the painters' syndrome). A critical review of the Danish literature. Sci Total Environ, 48:45, 1986
4. Freudenreich O, Weiner RD, McEvoy JP: Clozapine-induced electroencephalogram changes as a function of clozapine serum levels. Biol Psychiatry, 42:132, 1997
5. Herning RI, Guo X, Better WE et al: Neurophysiological signs of cocaine dependence: increased electroencephalogram beta during withdrawal. Biol Psychiatry, 41:1087, 1997
6. Nuwer M: Assessment of digital EEG, quantitative EEG, and EEG brain mapping: report of the American Academy of Neurology and the American Clinical Neurophysiology Society. Neurology, 49:277, 1997
7. Nuwer MR: Quantitative EEG analysis in clinical settings. Brain Topogr, 8:201, 1996
8. Chang Y-C: Neurotoxic effects of n-hexane on the human central nervous system: evoked potential abnormalities in n-hexane polyneuropathy. J Neurol Neurosurg Psychiatry, 50:269, 1987

9. Kutlu G, Gomceli YB, Sonmez T et al: Peripheral neuropathy and visual evoked potential changes in workers exposed to n-hexane. J Clin Neurosci, 16:1296, 2009

10. Hormes JT, Christopher MF, Rosenberg NL: Neurologic sequelae of chronic solvent vapor abuse. Neurology, 36:698, 1986

11. Rosenberg NL, Spitz MC, Filley CM et al: Central nervous system effects of chronic toluene abuse—clinical, brainstem evoked response and magnetic resonance imaging studies. Neurotoxicology, 10:489, 1988

12. Vrca A, Karacić V, Bozicević D et al: Brainstem auditory evoked potentials in individuals exposed to long-term low concentrations of toluene. Am J Ind Med, 30:62, 1996

13. Huang C-C, Chu C-C, Chen R-S et al: Chronic carbon disulfide encephalopathy. Eur Neurol, 36:364, 1996

14. Aaserud O, Hommeren OJ, Tvedt B et al: Carbon disulfide exposure and neurotoxic sequelae among viscose rayon workers. Am J Ind Med, 18:25, 1990

15. Sińczuk-Walczak H, Szymczak M: Rhythm patterns of basic brain bioelectric activity in workers chronically exposed to carbon disulfide. Int J Occup Med Environ Health, 10:429, 1997

16. Murata M, Suzuki M, Hasegawa Y et al: Improvement of occipital alpha activity by repetitive hyperbaric oxygen therapy in patients with carbon monoxide poisoning: a possible indicator for treatment efficacy. J Neurol Sci, 235:69, 2005

17. Dassanayake T, Weerasinghe V, Dangahadeniya U et al: Cognitive processing of visual stimuli in patients with organophosphate insecticide poisoning. Neurology, 68:2027, 2007

18. Dassanayake T, Weerasinghe V, Dangahadeniya U et al: Long-term event-related potential changes following organophosphorus insecticide poisoning. Clin Neurophysiol, 119:144, 2008

19. Saint-Amour D, Roy MS, Bastien C et al: Alterations of visual evoked potentials in preschool Inuit children exposed to methylmercury and polychlorinated biphenyls from a marine diet. Neurotoxicology, 27:567, 2006

20. Murata K, Grandjean P, Dakeishi M: Neurophysiological evidence of methylmercury neurotoxicity. Am J Ind Med, 50:765, 2007

21. Murata K, Araki S, Yokoyama K: Assessment of the peripheral, central, and autonomic nervous system function in styrene workers. Am J Ind Med, 20:775, 1991

22. Cherry N, Gautrin D: Neurotoxic effects of styrene: further evidence. Br J Ind Med, 47:29, 1990

23. O'Donoghue JL: Styrene. p. 1116. In Spencer PS, Schaumburg HH (eds): Experimental and Clinical Neurotoxicology. 2nd Ed. Oxford University Press, New York, 2000

24. Rebert CS, Hall TA: The neuroepidemiology of styrene: a critical review of representative literature. Crit Rev Toxicol, 24:S57, 1994

25. Matikainen E, Forsman-Gronholm L, Pfaffli P et al: Nervous system effects of occupational exposure to styrene: a clinical and neurophysiological study. Environ Res, 61:84, 1993

26. Gade A, Mortensen EL, Bruhn P: "Chronic painter's syndrome". A reanalysis of psychological test data in a group of diagnosed cases, based on comparisons with matched controls. Acta Neurol Scand, 77:293, 1988

27. Lees-Haley PR, Williams CW: Neurotoxicity of chronic low-dose exposure to organic solvents: a skeptical review. J Clin Psychol, 53:699, 1997

28. Bromberg MB: Comparison of electrodiagnostic criteria for primary demyelination in chronic polyneuropathy. Muscle Nerve, 14:968, 1991

29. Gutmann L: Dapsone. p. 464. In Spencer PS, Schaumburg HH (eds): Experimental and Clinical Neurotoxicology. Oxford University Press, New York, 2000

30. Jain KK: Drug-induced peripheral neuropathies. p. 209. In Jain KK (ed): Drug-Induced Neurological Disorders. Hogrefe & Huber, Seattle, 1996

31. Richardson RJ: Assessment of the neurotoxic potential of chlorpyrifos relative to other organophosphorus compounds: a critical review of the literature. J Toxicol Environ Health, 44:135, 1995

32. Lotti M: The pathogenesis of organophosphate polyneuropathy. Crit Rev Toxicol, 21:465, 1991

33. Lotti M: Low-level exposures to organophosphorus esters and peripheral nerve function. Muscle Nerve, 25:492, 2002

34. Albers JW, Garabrant DH, Mattsson JL et al: Dose-effect analyses of occupational chlorpyrifos exposure and peripheral nerve electrophysiology. Toxicol Sci, 97:196, 2007

35. Senanayake N, Karalliedde L: Neurotoxic effects of organophosphorus insecticides. N Engl J Med, 316:761, 1987

36. Hall AH: Chronic arsenic poisoning. Toxicol Lett, 128:69, 2002

37. Donofrio PD, Wilbourn AJ, Albers JW et al: Acute arsenic intoxication presenting as Guillain–Barré-like syndrome. Muscle Nerve, 10:114, 1987

38. Oh SJ: Electrophysiological profile in arsenic neuropathy. J Neurol Neurosurg Psychiatry, 54:1103, 1991

39. Bergouignan FX, Vital C, Henry P et al: Disulfiram neuropathy. J Neurol, 235:382, 1988

40. Filosto M, Tentorio M, Broglio L et al: Disulfiram neuropathy: two cases of distal axonopathy. Clin Toxicol, 46:314, 2008

41. Smith G, Albers JW: n-Hexane neuropathy due to rubber cement sniffing. Muscle Nerve, 20:1445, 1997

42. Yokoyama K, Feldman RG, Sax DS et al: Relation of distribution of conduction velocities to nerve biopsy findings in n-hexane poisoning. Muscle Nerve, 13:312, 1990

43. Pastore C, Izura V, Marhuenda D et al: Partial conduction blocks in n-hexane neuropathy. Muscle Nerve, 26:132, 2002

44. Long RR, Sargent JC, Hammer K: Paralytic shellfish poisoning: a case report and serial electrophysiologic observations. Neurology, 40:1310, 1990

45. Albers J, Chaudhry V, Cavaletti G et al: Interventions for preventing neuropathy caused by cisplatin and related compounds. Cochrane Database Syst Rev, CD005228, 2007

46. Cavaletti G, Bogliun G, Marzorati L et al: Early predictors of peripheral neurotoxicity in cisplatin and paclitaxel combination chemotherapy. Ann Oncol, 15:1439, 2004

47. Windebank AJ, Blexrud MD, Dyck PJ et al: The syndrome of acute sensory neuropathy: clinical features and electrophysiologic and pathologic changes. Neurology, 40:584, 1990

48. Berger AR, Schaumburg HH, Schroeder C et al: Dose response, coasting, and differential fiber vulnerability in human toxic neuropathy: a prospective study of pyridoxine neurotoxicity. Neurology, 42:1367, 1992

49. Molloy FM, Floeter MK, Syed NA et al: Thalidomide neuropathy in patients treated for metastatic prostate cancer. Muscle Nerve, 24:1050, 2001

50. Chaudhry V, Cornblath DR, Corse A et al: Thalidomide-induced neuropathy. Neurology, 59:1872, 2002

51. Kalantri A, Kurtz E: Electrodiagnosis in thallium toxicity: a case report. Muscle Nerve, 11:968A, 1988

52. Kuncl RW, Duncan G, Watson D et al: Colchicine myopathy and neuropathy. N Engl J Med, 316:1562, 1987

53. Palopoli JJ, Waxman J: Colchicine neuropathy or vitamin B_{12} deficiency neuropathy? N Engl J Med, 317:1290, 1987

54. Charness ME, Simon RP, Greenberg DA: Ethanol and the nervous system. N Engl J Med, 321:442, 1989

55. McLane JA: Decreased axonal transport in rat nerve following acute and chronic ethanol exposure. Alcohol, 4:385, 1987

56. DeAngelis LM, Gnecco C, Taylor L et al: Evolution of neuropathy and myopathy during intensive vincristine/corticosteroid chemotherapy for non-Hodgkin's lymphoma. Cancer, 67:2241, 1991

57. Chaudhry V, Chaudhry M, Crawford TO et al: Toxic neuropathy in patients with pre-existing neuropathy. Neurology, 60:337, 2003

58. Lachance DH, Lennon VA, Pittock SJ et al: An outbreak of neurological autoimmunity with polyradiculoneuropathy in workers exposed to aerosolized porcine neural tissue: a descriptive study. Lancet Neurol, 9:55, 2010

59. Mayeno AN, Belongia EA, Lin F et al: 3-(Phenylamino) alanine, a novel aniline-derived amino acid associated with the eosinophilia–myalgia syndrome: a link to the toxic oil syndrome? Mayo Clin Proc, 67:1134, 1992

60. Belongia EA, Hedberg CW, Gleich GJ et al: An investigation of the cause of the eosinophilia–myalgia syndrome associated with tryptophan use. N Engl J Med, 323:357, 1990

61. Thomson RM, Parry GJ: Neuropathies associated with excessive exposure to lead. Muscle Nerve, 33:732, 2006

62. Wu PB, Kingery WS, Date ES: An EMG case report of lead neuropathy 19 years after a gunshot injury. Muscle Nerve, 18:326, 1995

63. Ehle AL: Lead neuropathy and electrophysiological studies in low level lead exposure: a critical review. Neurotoxicology, 7:203, 1986

64. Goetz CG, Meisel E: Biological neurotoxins. Neurol Clin, 18:719, 2000

65. Arnon SS, Schechter R, Inglesby TV et al: Botulinum toxin as a biological weapon: medical and public health management. JAMA, 285:1059, 2001

66. Cherington M: Clinical spectrum of botulism. Muscle Nerve, 21:701, 1998

67. Gutmann L, Besser R: Organophosphate intoxication: pharmacologic, neurophysiologic, clinical, and therapeutic considerations. Semin Neurol, 10:46, 1990

68. Wadia RS, Chitra S, Amin RB et al: Electrophysiological studies in acute organophosphate poisoning. J Neurol Neurosurg Psychiatry, 50:1442, 1987

69. Wald JJ: The effects of toxins on muscle. Neurol Clin, 18:695, 2000

70. Argov Z: Drug-induced myopathies. Curr Opin Neurol, 13:541, 2000

71. Kuncl RW, Duncan G, Watson D et al: Colchicine myopathy and neuropathy. N Engl J Med, 316:1562, 1987

72. Melli G, Chaudhry V, Cornblath DR: Rhabdomyolysis: an evaluation of 475 hospitalized patients. Medicine, 84:377, 2005

73. Kuncl RW, Cornblath DR, Avila O et al: Electrodiagnosis of human colchicine myoneuropathy. Muscle Nerve, 12:360, 1989

74. Fernandez C, Figarella-Branger D, Alla P et al: Colchicine myopathy: a vacuolar myopathy with selective type I muscle fiber involvement. An immunohistochemical and electron microscopic study of two cases. Acta Neuropathol (Berl), 103:100, 2002

75. Tapal MF: Colchicine myopathy. Scand J Rheumatol, 25:105, 1996

76. al-Lozi MT, Pestronk A, Yee WC et al: Rapidly evolving myopathy with myosin-deficient muscle fibers. Ann Neurol, 35:273, 1994

77. Bolton CF: Sepsis and the systemic inflammatory response syndrome: neuromuscular manifestations. Crit Care Med, 24:1408, 1996

78. Ruff RL: Acute illness myopathy. Neurology, 46:600, 1996

79. Bird SJ, Rich MM: Critical illness myopathy and polyneuropathy. Curr Neurol Neurosci Rep, 2:527, 2002

80. Lacomis D, Petrella JT, Giuliani MJ: Causes of neuromuscular weakness in the intensive care unit: a study of 92 patients. Muscle Nerve, 21:610, 1998

81. Gutmann L, Blumenthal D, Schochet SS: Acute type II myofiber atrophy in critical illness. Neurology, 46:819, 1996

Index

Note: Page numbers followed by *f* indicate figures and *t* indicate tables.